seventeenth edition

Rypins' Basic Sciences Review

Rypins' Basic Sciences Review

seventeenth edition

Edited by

Edward D. Frohlich, MD, MACP, FACC
Alton Ochsner Distinguished Scientist
Vice President for Academic Affairs
Alton Ochsner Medical Foundation;
Staff Member, Ochsner Clinic; Professor of
Medicine and of Physiology, Louisiana State
University School of Medicine; Adjunct Professor
of Pharmacology and Clinical Professor of
Medicine, Tulane University School of Medicine
New Orleans, Louisiana

With the Collaboration of a Review Panel

Lippincott - Raven
PUBLISHERS
Philadelphia • New York

Acquisitions Editor: Richard Winters
Developmental Editor: Mary Beth Murphy
Senior Production Editor: Molly Connors
Production Service: Colophon, Inc.

Seventeenth Edition

Library of Congress Cataloging-in-Publication Data

Rypins' basic sciences review.—17th ed. / edited by Edward D. Frohlich ; with the collaboration of a review panel.
p. cm.
Includes bibliographical references and index.
ISBN 0-397-51488-3
1. Medical sciences—Handbooks, manuals, etc. 2. Medical sciences—Examinations, questions, etc. I. Rypins, Harold, 1892–1939. II. Frohlich, Edward D., 1931– .
[DNLM: 1. Medicine—examination questions. 2. Licensure, Medical—examination questions. W 18.2 R995 1997]
R834.5.R963 1997
610'.76—dc20
DNLM/DLC
for Library of Congress 96-34954
CIP

Care has been taken to confirm the accuracy of the information presented and to describe generally accepted practices. However, the authors, editors, and publisher are not responsible for errors or omissions or for any consequences from application of the information in this book and make no warranty, express or implied, with respect to the contents of the publication.

The authors, editors and publisher have exerted every effort to ensure that drug selection and dosage set forth in this text are in accordance with current recommendations and practice at the time of publication. However, in view of ongoing research, changes in government regulations, and the constant flow of information relating to drug therapy and drug reactions, the reader is urged to check the package insert for each drug for any change in indications and dosage and for added warnings and precautions. This is particularly important when the recommended agent is a new or infrequently employed drug.

Some drugs and medical devices presented in this publication have Food and Drug Administration (FDA) clearance for limited use in restricted research settings. It is the responsibility of the health care provider to ascertain the FDA status of each drug or device planned for use in their clinical practice.

9 8 7 6 5 4 3 2 1

To the deep-seated commitment of all physicians to continuing education. The source of this drive is the need for a better understanding of disease and disease mechanisms, the maintenance of wellness, and the need to practice medicine at the ''cutting edge.'' It is the patient, then, that is the source for the need for new knowledge; and it is the patient that is the inspiration for new thinking, research, and clinical investigation. Without this clinical inspiration medicine loses its art, its science, its status as a profession, and its exciting future. Hence, this textbook is dedicated to the students of medicine of today and tomorrow and their patients.

Editorial Review Panel

Pathology

Ivan Damjanov, MD, PhD
Professor and Chair
Department of Pathology
University of Kansas
Kansas City, Kansas

Peter J. Goldblatt, MD
Professor and Chair
Department of Pathology
Medical College of Ohio
Toledo, Ohio

Philip B. Conran, DVM, PhD
Professor
Department of Pathology
Medical College of Ohio
Toledo, Ohio

Pharmacology

Margaret A. Reilly, PhD
Adjunct Assistant Professor
Department of Pharmacology
New York Medical College
Valhalla, New York
Adjunct Assistant Professor of Pharmacology
Concordia College
Bronxville, New York
Instructor in Pharmacology
Phillips-Beth Israel School of Nursing
New York, New York

Behavioral Sciences

Ronald S. Krug, PhD
David Ross Boyd Professor and Interim Chairman
Department of Psychiatry and Behavioral Sciences
University of Oklahoma Health Sciences Center
Oklahoma City, Oklahoma

Preface

These are indeed very exciting times in medicine. Having made this statement, one's thoughts immediately reflect on the major changes that are occurring in our overall healthcare delivery system, utilization-review and shortened hospitalizations, issues concerning quality/assurance, ambulatory surgical procedures and medical clearances, and the impact of managed care on the practice of internal medicine and primary care. Each of these issues has had a considerable impact on the approach to the patient and in the practice of medicine.

But, even more mind-boggling than the foregoing changes, are the dramatic changes imposed on the practice of medicine by fundamental conceptual scientific innovations engendered by advances in basic science that no doubt will affect medical practice of the immediate future. Indeed, much of that which we have thought of as having a potential impact on the practice of medicine of the future has already been perceived. One need only take a cursory look at our weekly medical journals to realize that we are practicing "tomorrow's medicine today." And consider the goal (a few years ago) of actually describing the human genome, which is now near reality.

Reflect, then, for a moment on our current thinking about genetics, molecular biology, cellular immunology, and other areas that have impacted upon our current understanding of the underlying mechanisms of the pathophysiological concepts of disease. Moreover, paralleling these innovations have been remarkable advances in the so-called "high tech" and "gee-whiz" aspects of how we diagnose disease and treat patients. We can now think with much greater perspective about the dimensions of: more specific biological diagnoses concerned with molecular perturbations; gene therapy not only affecting genetic but oncological diseases; more specific pharmacotherapy involving highly specific receptor inhibition, alterations of intracellular signal transduction, manipulations of cellular protein synthesis; immunosuppressive therapy not only with respect to organ transplantations but also of autoimmune and other immune-related diseases; and therapeutic means for manipulating organ remodeling or the intravascular placement of stents. Each of these concepts has become inculcated into our everyday medical practice within the past decade. The reason why these changes have so rapidly promoted an upheaval in medical practice is continuing medical education, a constant awareness of the current medical literature, and a thirst for new knowledge.

In no area is this lesson more apparent than in the field of internal medicine. To assist the student and practitioner in that review process the publisher and I have initiated a new approach in the publication of RYPINS' BASIC AND CLINICAL SCIENCES REVIEWS. Thus, when I assumed responsibility to edit this long-standing board review series with the 13th edition of the textbook (first published in 1933), it was with a feeling of great excitement. I perceived that great changes would be coming to medicine, and I believed that this would be one ideal means of not only facing these changes head on, but also for me, personally, to cope and keep up with these changes. Over the subsequent editions, this confidence was reassured and rewarded. The presentation for the updating of medical information was tremendously enhanced by the substitution of new authors as the former authority "standbys" stepped down or retired from our faculty. Each of the authors who continues to be selected for maintaining the character of our textbook is an authority in his/her respective area having had considerable pedagogic and formal examination experience. One dramatic recent example of the changes in author replacement just came about with our forthcoming 17th edition. When I invited Doctor

Peter Goldblatt to participate in the authorship of the Pathology chapter of the textbook, his answer was "what goes around, comes around." You see, Doctor Goldblatt's father Doctor Harry Goldblatt, a major contributor to the history of hypertensive disease, was the first author of the Pathology chapter in 1931. What a satisfying experience for me, personally. Other less human changes in our format came with the establishment of two soft cover volumes, the current basic and clinical sciences review volumes, replacing the single volume text of earlier years. Then, a third supplementary volume concerned with questions and answers for the basic science volume appeared. Accompanying these more obvious changes were the constant updating of the knowledge base of each of the chapters; and this continues on into the present 17th edition.

And, now, we have introduced another major innovation in our presentation of the basic and clinical sciences reviews. This change is evidenced by the introduction of four new review volumes during 1996, drawn from four important chapters presented in the parent textbook: internal medicine, surgery, psychiatry and behavioral medicine, and behavioral sciences. Additional volumes, drawn from each of the other chapters of the parent textbook, will be published in subsequent years 1996, drawn from this new series, *Rypins' Intensive Reviews*, has been designed to be used separately from the parent textbook. Each will not only contain the material published in their respective chapters of the textbook, but will be considerably "fleshed out" in the discussions, tables, figures, and questions and answers. Thus, we hope that the new series will serve as an important supplement to the overall review process, and that it will also provide a study guide for those already in practice in preparing for specific specialty board certification and re-certification examinations.

Therefore, with continued confidence and excitement, I am pleased to present these innovations in review experience for your consideration. As in the past, I look forward to learning of your comments and suggestions. In doing so, we continue to look forward to our continued growth and acceptance of the RYPINS' review experience.

Edward D. Frohlich, M.D., M.A.C.P, F.A.C.C.
New Orleans, LA
June 1995

Preface to the First Edition

This book is an expression of the writer's conviction that the average American medical graduate of today is well prepared for the practice of his profession and that consequently there is little basis for the obvious dread with which he approaches the ordeal of the licensing examination. It is based on fifteen years' experience as Secretary of the New York State Board of Medical Examiners, during which period he has had intimate contact not only with medical schools and boards of medical examiners throughout the country, but also with large numbers of candidates for the licensing examination.

After a critical survey of many thousands of questions actually used throughout the whole United States, a selection of typical questions has been made, and these immediately follow the review presented in each of the nine major medical subjects. By placing these questions at the end of the chapters the thought processes of the student are stimulated and his best interests more fully served than in the older forms of questions and answers.

It is the proper function of the state to submit to examination all candidates for the right to practice medicine, and the state medical licensing examination can, and in some instances does, serve as a valuable check upon the work of the medical schools. There should be, however, closer co-operation between licensing boards and medical schools. Medical faculties should recognize more clearly the function and intention of the licensing boards, and licensing boards should be more clearly aware of the progress which is being made in medical schools. It is evident that the examining boards are slowly realizing that medical schools are in better position than themselves to test the student's academic or encyclopedic knowledge of such subjects as anatomy, chemistry, and bacteriology; that such testing may be safely left in the hands of medical faculties; and that examining boards should limit themselves to inquiring into the ability of the medical graduate to apply such knowledge clinically.

As for the graduate's attitude toward the state licensing examination, his fear arises from failure to understand the point of view of the state examiners as well as from an ability to muster in due proportion the vast amount of material presented to him during his medical course.

Careful study of licensing examinations throughout the United States indicates a general agreement among examiners regarding the material essential for the candidate. It is this ground, and only this ground, that the present volume aims to cover.

Every effort has been made to treat as concisely as possible those portions of the medical curriculum generally selected for use by the various examining boards. Repetition and overlapping have been avoided. Where a subject such as rabies, for example, has been covered in the chapter on Preventive Medicine, it is not repeated under the consideration of the Filtrable Viruses in Bacteriology. The arrangement of the material emphasizes the relations of the whole and its parts. It is taken for granted that the student has been adequately trained in the medical sciences and there is no attempt to teach him anything new. The object is, not to cram his mind, rather, to assist him in selecting and rearranging his material intelligently and practically.

Deliberate omission has been made of nearly all technical procedures, such as physical diagnosis, blood-counting and blood-chemistry, basal metabolism, x-ray, or surgical technic. Technical procedures cannot be taught in books and the ability to employ them properly should be assumed in the modern graduate. For similar reasons there is no separate section on materia medica or prescription-writing. References to the use of therapeutic agents are included in the consideration of the disease for which they are indicated.

To the authors in the various fields of medicine from whose books and articles he has freely drawn, the author desires to express his appreciative thanks. His gratitude to Miss E. Marion Pilpel, Miss Florence S. Muffson, and particularly to his wife, Senta Jonas Rypins, for invaluable secretarial assistance, he is most happy to acknowledge.

HAROLD RYPINS
Albany, N.Y.

Acknowledgments

In no other writing experience is one more dependent upon others than in a textbook, especially a textbook that provides a broad review for the student and fellow practitioner. In this spirit, I am truly indebted to all who have contributed to our past and current understanding of the fundamental and clinical aspects related to the practice of medicine. No one individual ever provides the singular ''breakthrough'' so frequently attributed as such by the news media. Knowledge develops and grows as a result of continuing and exciting contributions of research from all disciplines, academic institutions and nations. Clearly, outstanding investigators have been credited for major contributions, but those with true and understanding humility are quick to attribute the preceding input of knowledge by others to the growing body of knowledge. In this spirit, we acknowledge the long list of contributions to medicine over the generations. We also acknowledge that in no century has man so exceeded the sheer volume of these advances than in the current. Indeed, it has been said by many that the sum of new knowledge over the past 50 years most likely has exceeded all that which had been contributed in the prior years.

With this spirit of more universal acknowledgment I wish to recognize personally the interest, support and suggestions made by my colleagues in my own institution as well as elsewhere. I specifically refer to those people from my institution who were of particular help and listed at the outset of the internal medicine chapter and monograph. But, in addition to these colleagues, I want to express my deep appreciation to my institution and clinic for providing the opportunity and ambiance to maintain and continue these academic pursuits. As I have often said, the primary mission of a school of medicine is that of education and research; the care of patients, long a secondary mission to insure the conduct of the primary goal, has now also become a primary commitment in these more pragmatic times. In contrast, the primary mission of the major multispecialty clinics has been the care of patients, with education and research assuming secondary roles as these commitments become affordable in commitment. It is this distinction that sets the multispecialty clinic apart from other modes of medical practice.

Over-and-above a personal commitment and drive to assure publication of a textbook such as this, is the tremendous support and loyalty of a hard-working and dedicated office staff. To this end, I am tremendously grateful and indebted to Mrs. Lillian Buffa and Mrs. Caramia Fairchild. Their long hours of unselfish work in my behalf as well as to satisfy their own interest in participating in this major educational effort is appreciated no end; and I am personally deeply honored and thankful for their important roles in the publication of the Rypins' books.

Words of appreciation must be extended to the staff of Lippincott–Raven Publishers. It is over 25 years since I have become associated with this publishing house, one of the first to be established in our nation. Over these years I have become closely related with Mr. Richard Winters, not only with the Rypins' editions but also with other textbooks. His has been a labor of commitment, interest, and full support — not only because of his responsibility to his institution, but also to the excitement of the publication of new knowledge.

In recent years we discussed at length the merits of adding the monograph supplements to the parent textbook and, together, we worked out the details that have become the substance of our present ''joint venture.'' Moreover, together we are willing to make the necessary changes to assure the intellectual success of this series. To this end, we are delighted to include a new member in our team effort, Ms. Susan Kelly. She joined our cause to assure that the format of questions, the reference process of answers to those questions within the text itself, and the editorial process involved be natural and clear to readers.

I am grateful to many members of the Lippincott–Raven staff involved in the overall publication process.

Not the least, is my everlasting love and appreciation to my family. I am particularly indebted to my parents who, at a very early age, inculcated in me the love of education, the respect for study and hard work, and the honor for those who share these values. In this regard, it would have been impossible for me to accomplish any of my academic pursuits without the love, inspiration and continued support of my wife Sherry. Not only has she maintained the personal encouragement to initiate and continue with these labors of love, but she has sustained and supported our family and home life so that these activities could be encouraged. Hopefully, these pursuits have not detracted from the development and love of our children, Margie, Bruce, and Lara. I assume that this has not occurred; we are so very proud that each is also personally committed to education and research. How satisfying it is to realize that these ideals remain a familial characteristic.

Contents

seventeenth edition

Rypins' Basic Sciences Review

Rypins' Basic Sciences Review, 17th Edition,
edited by Edward D. Frohlich. Lippincott–Raven Publishers,
Philadelphia © 1997.

1

Medical Qualifying Examinations

Edward D. Frohlich, M.D., M.A.C.P.
Alton Ochsner Distinguished Scientist
Vice President for Academic Affairs
Alton Ochsner Medical Foundation;
Staff Member, Ochsner Clinic; Professor of
Medicine and of Physiology, Louisiana State
University School of Medicine; Adjunct Professor
of Pharmacology and Clinical Professor of
Medicine, Tulane University School of Medicine
New Orleans, Louisiana

The testing of professional competence before certifying for public responsibilities is an age-old practice. In China, for example, candidates for public service were required to submit to special examinations at least 3,000 years ago, and the tests were said to be not unlike those employed today. In the United States the practice developed slowly, first as a kind of contribution by the profession itself to public welfare; later as a responsibility of the state. In New York State the problem arose in the early 19th century as far as the practice of medicine is concerned. At that time, the Legislature found that attempts to control the practice of ''physic and surgery'' in unorganized fashion had been most unsatisfactory, since charlatans and quacks abounded, and passed ''an act to incorporate Medical Societies for the purpose of regulating the practice of Physic and Surgery in this state.'' This law provided for the establishment of a medical society in each county and gave to the practicing physicians themselves, thus legally organized, the power to grant licenses to qualified applicants and to regulate the practice of medicine in their counties.

Methods of testing varied. In general, tests were clinical and practical, limited to questions or discussions concerning the diagnosis and the treatment of diseases, for the candidates were chiefly those who had received their training as apprentices to practicing physicians. Not until nearly midcentury did the number of physicians who had their education and training in medical schools predominate. Soon thereafter the states themselves assumed responsibilities for licensure and, consequently, for establishing formal testing procedures. With this development, Boards of Examiners, or similar bodies, were appointed to examine officially all applicants for fitness to practice the medical profession. Today, all 50 states, as well as the District of Columbia and the Commonwealth of Puerto Rico, have official medical licensing agencies.

The usual means of measuring knowledge is the formal written examination, and it has an important place in all educational programs. ''Examination,'' the late President Eliot of Harvard once stated, ''is the most difficult of the educational arts and its influence on both students and teachers may be very great.'' Indeed, intelligently and thoughtfully prepared examinations can be made a most valuable educational exercise in any course of study. They not only force students to review and stimulate them to keep up with their work, but if the examinations are well designed and the results are interpreted carefully, they also may serve to test the quality of teaching.

How effective are formal written examinations in testing professional competence? Perhaps not as effective as they are in an educational program. Nevertheless, they are the only practical means of assessing the competence of large numbers of applicants for professional licensure. Although this practice is not ideal and does not test for such essential attributes as ethical and moral standards, carefully designed tests do play a definite role in separating the qualified practitioner from the unqualified and, in doing so, protect the public from the charlatan and the incompetent.

Examinations for licensure, however, have not always kept pace with the remarkable advances in medical knowledge and the resultant changes in methods of training for the practice of medicine. For this reason, many of the examination methods employed in former years have become inadequate. Thus, the purpose of the licensing examination is not so much to test the candidate's general knowledge in such individual subjects as anatomy, pathology, medicine, and surgery as to determine his or her ability to apply this knowledge to the diagnosis and treatment of disease and to determine the candidate's general fitness to practice the art and the science of medicine. In the past, unfortunately, most licensing examinations failed miserably in this last category.

The existence of separate licensing boards in all the states, the District of Columbia, and the Commonwealth of Puerto Rico, each setting its own type of qualifying examination for licensure, has led to great variation in the kind and quality of the examinations. This has worked against unity of procedures and standards and has made difficult the movement of physicians from one licensing jurisdiction to another. However, as will be described in more detail later, through the efforts of the Federation of State Medical Boards of the United States, a high-quality examination—the Federation Licensing Examination (FLEX)—prepared by a special Federation committee for administration twice a year, has been offered to any state medical board that wishes to use the examination as its own licensing test. A measure of its success is shown by the fact that it has been used by nearly all states since 1973. The prerequisites for licensure still vary from one state to another; any physician interested in licensure in any specific state should write directly to the State Board of Medical Licensure of that state for specific requirements and information.

Another confusing element in the licensing procedure has been added by the establishment in a number of states of separate boards of examiners in the basic sciences. These tests are designed to be given to candidates for admission to all branches of the healing professions, not only medicine but such other areas as chiropractic and neuropathy. In these jurisdictions certification by the basic science boards is required before admission to the specific professional examination is granted.

In most instances the members of these boards are teachers of such subjects as general chemistry, physics, biology, and anatomy. The tests therefore are not specifically prepared for physicians who have had intensive training in the basic medical sciences that form an integral part of medical education. The purpose of this examination is to determine whether the candidate has had adequate training in the fundamental sciences considered essential for admission to the licensing examination of the particular healing art the applicant wishes to practice. At best these tests are elementary when compared with the comprehensive training in the basic medical sciences given in schools of medicine. The consequent repetition, in part at least, of an examination in basic sciences by the medical licensing boards in these states has complicated still further the licensing of physicians. Fortunately, the number of these basic science boards is diminishing, and the time appears not far off when they will be done away with.

Thus, with all their defects and deficiencies, examinations are essential to the licensing procedure. They form not only an essential part of any well-planned program of education but are also, when well constructed, the only generally satisfactory method thus far devised for determining the professional competence and fitness to practice for a large number of candidates. They constitute a dependable measure of coordinated thinking as well as a test of knowledge not to be gained in any other way. Examinations are therefore here to stay, and the objective of all boards of medical licensure must be to administer examinations that are as fair, comprehensive, and valid tests of fundamental knowledge and clinical competence as it is possible to make.

TYPES OF EXAMINATIONS

Essay Examination

Many state boards of medical examiners employed the so-called essay examination in earlier years, but it is no longer generally used in licensing tests. In this test a limited number of questions is asked, and the candidate answers each one in a short composition or dissertation. The essay examination emphasizes description, definition, explanation, and discussion. Symptoms, signs, abnormalities in function, pathologic changes, etiology, and the diagnosis and treatment of disease conditions are described, and discussed by the candidate, sometimes at considerable length.

The advantages of the essay test are that it gives candidates an opportunity to consider thoughtfully each of a limited number of problems posed, to reveal their ability to organize their answers, to demonstrate their skill at description, and to present evidence of general scholarship, writing ability, penmanship, spelling, composition, and neatness of execution. All of these qualities are desirable accomplishments, but not all of them are the particular attributes that define a physician's overall competence to practice medicine.

Among the disadvantages are the relatively long time it takes to grade essay answers, the difficulty the examiner has of being uniformly fair in grading answers to the same question on different papers and the frequent quandary the examiner finds himself or herself in when, because of poor penmanship or a lack of knowledge of English on the part of the candidate, he or she cannot interpret an answer. The grading of essay examinations is therefore slow, subject to considerable subjective variation in evaluation of answers, and occupies an excessive amount of an examiner's time.

Finally, in view of the continued rapid expansion of medical knowledge in every field, it is now recognized that a limited number of essay questions does not permit as adequate testing of the candidate's general knowledge as is desired. Occasionally, therefore, oral or practical tests have been used to supplement the written test. With the additional information that such tests provide, the examining boards feel more secure in certifying a candidate for licensure. The great difficulty with this type of individual test, however, is that it cannot be given within a reasonable time, nor can adequate numbers of examiners be provided when great numbers of candidates must be examined. At present, if given at all, these individual tests are limited to those states where the number of candidates is small.

Multiple-Choice Examination

In recent years more and more State Boards of Examiners have been turning to the objective, or multiple-choice, examination. In this type of test each question is so prepared that the candidate is faced with a problem, the correct answer to which is included in the question and must be selected and indicated on the answer sheet by making a mark in the appropriate place. The characteristic feature of these tests is that candidates answer the questions by blackening, with a special pencil on the answer sheet, the space they believe to indicate the correct answer. Although this is considered a written examination, no actual writing of sentences is required. This kind of test has two important advantages: A great many more questions covering a much wider range of subjects can be asked in a given time than is possible in the essay examination; and the answers can be graded more objectively and with greater speed and accuracy than in any other type of examination. Thus, the number of questions that can be asked in an allotted period can be increased from 8 or 10, or at most 12, in an essay test, to 100, 150, or even more, in the objective test, thereby effectively broadening the scope of the examination.

At first the objective, or multiple-choice, examination met with considerable disapproval on the candidate's part because the technique was so new and different, and on the examiner's part because the construction of valid, unambiguous, and reliable questions proved to be so difficult (far more difficult, in fact, than the preparation of essay questions). But with the passage of time the objective examination has come into its own as a valid, comprehensive, and dependable test of a candidate's knowledge and, when applied effectively, of his or her competence and ability. Moreover, this type of examination seems to be the most searching, valid, and comprehensive type of test to administer to large groups of candidates.

Many different forms of objective, multiple-choice questions have been devised to test not only medical knowledge but those subtler qualities of discrimination, judgment, and reasoning. Certain types of questions may test an individual's recognition of the similarity or dissimilarity of diseases, drugs, and physiologic or pathologic processes. Other questions test judgment as to cause and effect or the lack of causal relationships. Case histories or patient problems are used to simulate the experience of a physician confronted with a diagnostic problem; a series of questions then tests the individual's understanding of related aspects of the case, such as associated laboratory findings, treatment, complications, and prognosis. In this type of examination each question has only one correct response among a number of possible choices—most often one correct response out of five choices, although the ratio may be somewhat less or considerably more.

Ambiguity of questions is exceedingly rare because of the intensive review process by the examination committees before they are used. The preparation of objective or multiple-choice examinations is extremely difficult, for the work of the examiners, instead of consisting of the time-consuming and usually tiresome reading and grading of essay-type answers, shifts to the preparation of the many questions included in the tests. Because generally the objective is to construct questions with only one correct answer, the preparation of an examination is best done by a group, usually an examination construction committee. The members of each group or committee should be skilled in one basic or clinical science discipline. Usually each member prepares questions in advance of a committee meeting, at which each question will be subjected to a critical review. Doubtful items are revised, modified, or discarded and new items may be developed. All items not approved unanimously are discarded. An examination prepared in this way, which is the method used by the National Board of Medical

Examiners, contains only material that has been thoroughly worked over and agreed upon as appropriate, free from ambiguity, and representative not only of important aspects of the subject but also of high standards of education.

SCORING OF MULTIPLE-CHOICE EXAMINATIONS

When objective multiple-choice examinations are used, the examinations are usually scored by electronic machines. To the casual observer, this machine scoring may look like a highly mysterious business. The answer sheets are loaded into the machine, a button is pressed, and the machine reads the sheets, matches the answers against an answer key, and punches the examinee's score into the automated machine data card. A manual check is also made to avoid the possibility of any technical error. Furthermore, these machines are not robots making their own decisions; they perform only in the way that they are programmed to perform. The responsible examiners determine whether an individual should pass or fail.

A grade of 75 has been established as the passing score for the examinations of the National Board. But it does not follow that it is necessary to respond correctly to 75% of the items in order to obtain this grade. Indeed, the scoring procedure is such that usually a score of about 50% to 60% of the questions answered correctly results in a passing grade of 75. In arriving at the passing score, the distribution curve of all those taking an examination is given consideration.

Examinations of the multiple-choice type have certain advantages over the time-honored essay tests. Although essay tests may probe more deeply into a limited number of subjects, multiple-choice examinations sample a much greater breadth of medical knowledge. Because the answer sheets can be scored by machine, the grading can be accomplished rapidly, accurately, and impartially. With this type of examination it becomes possible to determine the level of difficulty of each test and to maintain comparability of examination scores from test to test and from year to year for any single subject. Moreover, of even greater long-range significance is the facility with which the total test and the individual questions can be subjected to thorough and rapid statistical analysis, thus providing a sound basis for comparative studies and the continuing improvement in the quality of the test itself. Over the years, many different forms of objective questions have been devised to test not only medical knowledge but also those subtler qualities of discrimination, judgment, and reasoning. Certain types of questions may test an individual's recognition of the similarity or dissimilarity of diseases, drugs, and physiologic or pathologic processes. Other questions test judgment as to cause and effect or the lack of causal relationships. Case histories or patient problems are used to simulate the experience of a physician confronted with a diagnostic problem; a series of questions then tests the individual's understanding of related aspects of the case, such as signs and symptoms, associated laboratory findings, treatment, complications, and prognosis. Case-history questions are set up purposely to place emphasis on correct diagnosis within a context comparable with the experience of actual practice.

It is apparent from recent certification and board examinations that the examiners are devoting more attention in their construction of questions to more practical means of testing basic and clinical knowledge. This greater realism in testing relates to an increasingly interdisciplinary approach toward fundamental material and to the direct relevance accorded practical clinical problems. These more recent approaches to questions have been incorporated into this review series.

Of course, the new approaches to testing add to the difficulty experienced by the student or physician preparing for board or certification examinations. With this in mind, the author of this review is acutely aware not only of the interrelationships of fundamental information within the basic science disciplines and their clinical implications but also of the necessity to present this material clearly and concisely despite its complexity. For this reason, the questions are devised to test knowledge of specific material within the text and identify areas for more intensive study, if necessary. Also, those preparing for examinations must be aware of the inter-disciplinary nature of fundamental clinical material, the common multifactorial characteristics of disease mechanisms, and the necessity to shift back and forth from one discipline to another in order to appreciate the less than clear-cut nature separating the pedagogic disciplines.

The different types of questions that may be used on examinations include the completion-type question, where the individual must select one best answer among a number of possible choices, most often five, although there may be three or four; the completion-type question in the negative form where all but one of the choices is correct and words such as EXCEPT or LEAST appear in the question; the true-false type of question, which tests an understanding of cause and effect in relationship to medicine; the multiple true-false type in which the question may have one, several, or all correct choices; one matching-type question, which tests association and relatedness and uses four choices, two of which use the word, BOTH or NEITHER; another matching-type question that uses anywhere from three to twenty-six choices and may have more than one correct answer; and, as noted above, the patient-oriented question, which is written around a case and may have several questions included as a group or set.

Many of these question types may be used in course or practice exams; however, at this time the most commonly used types of questions on the USMLE exams are the completion-type question (one best answer), the completion-type negative form, and the multiple matching-type question, designating specifically how many choices are correct. Often included within the questions are graphic elements such as diagrams, charts, graphs, electrocardiograms, roentgenograms, or photomicrographs to elicit knowledge of structure, function, the course of a clinical situation, or a statistical tabulation. Questions then may be asked in relation to designated elements of the same. As noted above, case histories or patient-oriented questions are more frequently used on these examinations, requiring the individual to use more analytic abilities and less memorization-type data.

For further detailed information concerning developments in the evolution of the examination process for medical licensure (for graduates of both U.S. and foreign medical schools), those interested should contact the National Board of Medical Examiners at 3750 Market Street, Philadelphia, PA 19104, U.S.A; telephone number 215-590-9500.

Federation Licensing Examination (FLEX)

There have been many important developments in the field of medical qualifying examinations since 1968. The first significant achievement in the development of qualifying examinations was the introduction, in 1968, of the first Federation Licensing Examination (FLEX), prepared under the direction of the Examination Institute Committee of the Federation of State Medical Boards of the United States, Inc. Beginning in 1957, the Federation's Examination Institute Committee had held annual conferences designed to study examination procedures in the various states with the end in view of improving their quality and keeping them abreast of the continuing progress in medical education. As a result, there is general agreement to justify the continuation of this committee on a permanent basis.

At the present time this committee is charged: to provide state medical boards with high-quality, uniform, and valid examinations for purposes of evaluating clinical competence and qualification for licensure; to place licensure in a definite relation to modern medical education by updating state board examination procedures and providing flexibility; to establish uniform levels of examinations among the states; to create a rational basis for interstate endorsement; and to provide a basis for the management of the foreign medical graduate problem.

Following publication of their first complete report, in 1961, the Examination Institute Committee continued to hold special conferences and symposia at each annual Federation meeting, and to press forward in its efforts to develop an examination of high quality that would be acceptable to the various state medical boards. At first, it was believed that the Federation itself could set up an examination center, staffed by a medical director and a specialist in examination construction and preparation, that would be in competition with other examination centers, particularly the National Board of Medical Examiners, which had been functioning for more than 50 years. Since the cost was found to be prohibitive, the Examination Institute Committee consulted with the staff of the National Board of Medical Examiners, and the Federation Licensing Examination came into being. Thus, in 1967, the Federation of State Medical Boards gave the new examination its unanimous approval at its annual meeting; and in June 1968, candidates for licensure in six states took the first FLEX examinations. Since then, all but two states have accepted the FLEX examination as their own official licensing examination.

The FLEX is a uniform, valid, and reliable licensing examination, planned and prepared by FLEX Test Committees composed of Federation members and designed for use by any state medical licensing board. It is a 3-day examination given simultaneously by participating medical boards in the name of their own states twice a year, in June and December.

The arrangement with the National Board calls for making pools of already tested and validated objective questions in the six major basic medical science disciplines and the six major clinical fields available to the Test Committees composed of Federation members who represent the state medical boards that have decided to use the FLEX examination. From this collection of questions two subcommittees—one for the basic sciences and one for the clinical sciences—prepare the licensing examinations in these two fields. A third subcommittee selects the questions or problems to be given in the test of clinical competence.

This latter test is relatively new in licensing examinations in spite of the fact that such competence is the most essential requirement of a physician. A few state boards had attempted to solve the problem by requiring oral or practical tests in addition to the standard written tests, but for those boards that had a large number of applicants for licensure, individual tests of this kind were out of the question. The National Board of Medical Examiners had developed an ideal and unique practical test that had been used for some years with great success. This, the Federation's FLEX Committee (now called the FLEX Board) felt, met every need, and it was decided to add this practical test to those in the basic and clinical sciences. However, because of the many changes in the curricula of medical schools in this country, it was held that individual tests in anatomy, physiology, surgery, and so forth, were becoming outmoded. A comprehensive interdisciplinary examination that covered all basic medical science fields in one test and the clinical sciences in another was established. Questions in all of the important areas would be included in these tests; they would be "scrambled" without regard to discipline, but with all fields adequately represented. It was decided that about 90 questions each in anatomy, biochemistry, microbiology, pathology, pharmacology, and physiology would be mixed together in the basic sciences test, and about the same number of questions each in internal medicine, obstetrics and gynecology, pediatrics, preventive medicine and public health, psychiatry, and surgery would be mixed together in the clinical sciences test.

In each examination, the origin of the individual questions is known in the central office. Therefore, in spite of the scrambled character of the questions in the actual examination, it is possible to extract specific grades in each individual subject if these are needed. The FLEX Board felt, however, that each basic science and clinical science examination should be considered as a unit, with a single grade to be given for each entire test.

The examination in the basic sciences, given on the first day, is divided into three sections, A, B, and C, each lasting about 2½ hours, in which time some 180 questions must be answered, making a total of approximately 540 questions for the day. The clinical sciences examination, given on the second day, is presented in the same way.

On the third day the examination designed to test clinical competence is given. This test is divided into two sections that resemble in all details the two sections of Part III of the National Board examination. In the first section clinical material is presented in the form of pictures of patients or specimens, roentgenograms, electrocardiograms, and graphic or tabulated material about which searching questions are asked. In the second section a distinctive technique described as programmed testing is employed, the object being to assess the candidate's judgment in the sequential management of patients in a manner similar to that experienced in relation to his or her own patients in the course of studying their disease processes or injuries, evaluating findings, and planning treatment. A single overall grade is given to this entire part.

Because there will be many physicians who graduated from several to many years before appearing for this examination, the FLEX Board decided to provide, in addition to a single grade for each of the three parts (and of course, separate grades in each of the basic and clinical science subjects for those boards that might want them) a single overall grade for the entire examination, a grade that would give greater weight to the clinical, rather than the basic science, portion of the test. This is the so-called FLEX weight average. This average is developed by emphasizing the importance of the clinical parts of the examination, inasmuch as a weight of 1 is given to the basic sciences grade, a weight of 2 to the clinical sciences grade, and a weight of 3 to the clinical competence grade. How this weighted average is to be used will depend on the decision of each state medical board giving the FLEX examination. The FLEX Board recommends that a weighted average of 75 be the accepted passing grade.

Thus, there are now two important medical examinations for graduates of American and Canadian medical schools, those given by the National Board of Medical Examiners and those given under the auspices of the Federation of State Medical Boards of the United States. These two examinations do not conflict since their purposes are not exactly the same. The National Board examinations are designed to test the knowledge of students as they are learning medicine in medical schools today; these tests are focused on the student of today and the physician of tomorrow. The FLEX examination is designed to assess fundamental knowledge and, more especially, the clinical competence of the physician of today. A dual examination system has thus emerged, each examination important in its own right, each with a different objective and each aimed at its own clearly defined target.

Educational Council for Foreign Medical Graduates (ECFMG) Certification

The second significant achievement in the development of qualifying examinations was brought about as a result of the problems created by the ever increasing numbers of foreign-educated physicians, particularly from non-English-speaking countries, who were coming to the United States for further education and training, many of whom decided to remain in this country to practice. After a study by a committee representing the American Hospital Association, the American Medical Association, the Association of American Medical Colleges and the Federation of State Medical Boards of the United States, with the unofficial cooperation of the U.S. Department of State, the Educational Council for Foreign Medical Graduates (ECFMG) was created. The purpose of the Council is to develop and administer an evaluation procedure or qualifying examination that will effectively ascertain the fitness of foreign medical graduates to serve as interns and residents in hospitals in the United States or to come to the United States to otherwise practice medicine. Also included for those who come from countries where English is not the spoken language is a 1-hour examination designed to assess comprehension of English vocabulary and language structure (the ECFMG English test).

It was only natural that the Council should turn to the National Board of Medical Examiners for advice and help. The result was that the examinations, given twice each year, were, and continue to be, prepared and scored by the National Board. Indeed, so close became the association between these two organizations because of this relationship, that the home office of the Council, formerly in Evanston, Illinois, was moved to Philadelphia, Pennsylvania, where it is now located. This is the same city in which the home office of the National Board is located.

The Council on Medical Education of the American Medical Association has adopted rules providing that no approved hospital in the United States can now employ as interns or residents any foreign-educated physicians who do not hold the ECFMG Certificate unless they already have a valid state license. In spite of some criticism (most of it unwarranted) of the Council as well as its sponsoring agencies in the first few years, the Council, after giving more than 315,000 examinations in 48 centers in the United States and Canada and in over 105 foreign countries, has fully justified its existence. Indeed, at the present time practically every state that will accept foreign-educated physicians for licensure requires that all these applicants be certified before being admitted to the licensing examination in that state.

Foreign Medical Graduate Examination in the Medical Sciences (FMGEMS)

Until 1976, all foreign medical graduates desiring to undergo postgraduate medical training in the United States were required to take the ECFMG examination. This comprehensive clinical examination permitted certification by the ECFMG for acceptance into an accredited graduate medical education training program in the United States. In 1976, the United States Congress enacted amendments to the Immigration and Naturalization Act (INA) that required all foreign medical graduates who desire entrance into the United States for postgraduate training (or to practice medicine) to pass a new Visa Qualifying Examination (VQE). If this examination, a 2-day comprehensive test of preclinical (basic) and clinical knowledge, was passed, a certificate was issued by the ECFMG. This document was required to obtain the necessary visa to enter the United States. Thus, a passing grade on the VQE was deemed equivalent to passing Parts I and II of the National Board Examinations, provided the candidate also demonstrated competence in oral and written English. In 1977 (and in subsequent years), there was an extremely high rate of failure of the basic sciences (day 1) of the VQE in comparison to the ECFMG examination (that had much fewer questions in the basic sciences area).

The VQE examination is no longer given; it has been supplanted by the Foreign Medical Graduate Examination in the Medical Sciences (FMGEMS). In addition, all candidates from foreign medical schools must also pass the ECFMG English test. Passage of both examinations is therefore required for ECFMG certification.

A word of definition of a "foreign medical graduate" (FMG) is necessary before discussing the FMGEMS test. An FMG is any physician whose medical degree of qualification was conferred by any medical school located outside the United States, Canada, and Puerto Rico. That medical school, however, must be listed in the *World Directory of Medical Schools,* published by the World Health Organization. Citizens of the United States who have completed their medical education in schools outside the United States, Canada, and Puerto Rico are defined as "foreign medical graduates" (FMGs). Alternatively, foreign nationals who have graduated from United States, Canadian, or Puerto Rican medical schools are not FMGs.

Thus, the ECFMG certification provides assurance to all directors of training programs of the Accreditation Council for Graduate Medical Education (ACGME) that the FMG applicant has fulfilled the minimum standards for medical knowledge and mastery of the English language necessary to enter their programs. This ECFMG certification is also prerequisite for licensure to practice medicine in most states of the United States. (Some states may require that the candidate also pass the FLEX examination.)

English Language Examinations

Two English language examinations are approved by the ECFMG. The *ECFMG English test* is administered twice yearly (in January and July) in the morning of the second day (prior to the clinical science test) of the FMGEMS. The ECFMG states that examinees who take the clinical science component of the FMGEMS examination must also take the ECFMG English test that same day even if they have passed the English test at previous examinations. The only other English test that is acceptable to the ECFMG is an international or special administration of the *Test of English as a Foreign Language (TOEFL).* The ECFMG emphasizes that this testing is with the provision that applicants have previously taken an ECFMG English test. There are a number of important requirements concerning these English tests as well as details concerning the medical science examination and the registration procedures. The applicant for all examinations of this nature, therefore, should not assume that the information concerning any of the examinations described in this textbook is the final word. It is strongly recommended that the applicant communicate directly with the testing agencies.

Medical Science Examination

As indicated previously, the examination is formulated by the ECFMG and the NBME and is given twice yearly, in January and in July, as 2 half-day sessions on 2 successive days. The questions on the first day relate to preclinical (basic) sciences and on the second day to the clinical sciences. The overall examination consists of approximately 950 test items constructed in a multiple-choice format. The preclinical science questions, about 500 items in number, are derived from the areas of anatomy, biochemistry, behavioral sciences, microbiology, pathology, pharmacology, and physiology. The second-day examination in the clinical sciences is preceded by the English test, which is followed by 450 question items drawn in approximately equal numbers from the disciplines of internal medicine, obstetrics and gynecology, pediatrics, preventive medicine and public health, psychiatry, and surgery. As indicated above, this new 2-day examination replaces the VQE and ECFMG examinations.

United States Medical Licensing Examination (USMLE)

In August 1991 the Federation of State Medical Boards (FSMB) and the National Board of Medical Examiners (NBME) agreed to replace their respective examinations, the FLEX and NBME, with a new examination, the United States Medical Licensing Examination (USMLE). This examination will provide a common means for evaluating all applicants for medical licensure. It appears that this development in medical licensure will at last satisfy the needs for state medical boards licensure, the national medical board licensure, and licensure examinations for foreign medical graduates. This is because the 1991 agreement provides for a composite committee that equally represents both organizations (the FSMB and NBME) as well as a jointly appointed public member and a representative of the Educational Council for Foreign Medical Graduates (ECFMG).

As indicated in the USMLE announcement, ''It is expected that students who enrolled in U.S. medical schools in the fall of 1990 or later and foreign medical graduates applying for ECFMG examinations beginning in 1993 will have access only to USMLE for purposes of licensure.'' The phaseout of the last regular examinations for licensure was completed in December 1994.

The new USMLE is administered in three steps. Step 1 focuses on fundamental basic biomedical science concepts, with particular emphasis on ''principles and mechanisms underlying disease and modes of therapy.'' Step 2 is related to the clinical sciences, with examination on material necessary to practice medicine in a supervised setting. Step 3 is designed to focus on ''aspects of biomedical and clinical science essential for the unsupervised practice of medicine.''

Today Step 1 and Step 2 examinations are set up and scored as total comprehensive objective tests in the basic sciences and clinical sciences, respectively. The format of each part is no longer subject-oriented, that is, separated into sections specifically labeled Anatomy, Pathology, Medicine, Surgery, and so forth. Subject labels are therefore missing, and in each part questions from the different fields are intermixed or integrated so that the subject origin of any individual question is not immediately apparent, although it is known by the National Board office. Therefore, if necessary, individual subject grades can be extracted.

Step 1 is a two-day written test including questions in anatomy, biochemistry, microbiology, pathology, pharmacology, physiology, and the behavioral sciences. Each subject contributes to the examination a large number of questions designed to test not only knowledge of the subject itself but also ''the subtler qualities of discrimination, judgment, and reasoning.'' Questions in such fields as molecular biology, cell biology, and genetics are included, as are questions to test the ''candidate's recognition of the similarity or dissimilarity of diseases, drugs, and physiologic, behavioral, or pathologic processes.'' Problems are presented in narrative, tabular, or graphic form, followed by questions designed to assess the candidate's knowledge and comprehension of the situation described.

Step 2 is also a two-day written test that includes questions in internal medicine, obstetrics and gynecology, pediatrics, preventive medicine and public health, psychiatry, and surgery. The questions, like those in Step 1, cover a broad spectrum of knowledge in each of the clinical fields. In addition to individual questions, clinical problems are presented in the form of case histories, charts, roentgenograms, photographs of gross and microscopic pathologic specimens, laboratory data, and the like, and the candidate must answer questions concerning the interpretation of the data presented and their relation to the clinical problems. The questions are ''designed to explore the extent of the candidate's knowledge of clinical situation, and to test his [or her] ability to bring information from many different clinical and basic science areas to bear upon these situations.''

The examinations of both Step 1 and Step 2 are scored as a whole, certification being given on the basis of performance on the entire part, without reference to disciplinary breakdown. The grade for the examination is derived from the total number of questions answered correctly, rather than from an average of the grades in the component basic science or clinical science subjects. A candidate who fails will be required to repeat the entire examination. Nevertheless, as noted above, in spite of the interdisciplinary character of the examinations, all of the traditional disciplines are represented in the test, and separate grades for each subject can be extracted and reported separately to students, to state examining boards, or to those medical schools that request them for their own educational and academic purposes.

This type of interdisciplinary examination and the method of scoring the entire test as a unit have definite advantages, especially in view of the changing curricula in medical schools. The former type of rigid, almost standardized, curriculum, with its emphasis on specific subjects and a specified number of hours in each, has been replaced by a more liberal, open-ended curriculum, permitting emphasis in one or more fields and corresponding deemphasis in others. The result has been rather wide variations in the totality of education in different medical schools. Thus, the scoring of these tests as a whole permits accommodation to this variability in the curricula of different schools. Within the total score, weakness in one subject that has received relatively little emphasis in a given school may be balanced by strength in other subjects.

The rationale for this type of comprehensive examination as replacement for the traditional department-oriented examination in the basic sciences and the clinical sciences is given in the National Board Examiner:

> The student, as he [or she] confronts these examinations, must abandon the idea of ''thinking like a physiologist'' in answering a question labeled ''physiology'' or ''thinking like a surgeon'' in answering a question labeled ''surgery.'' The one question may have been written by a biochemist or a pharmacologist; the other question may have been written by an internist or a pediatrician. The pattern of these examinations will direct the student to thinking more broadly of the basic sciences in Step 1 and to thinking of patients and their problems in Step 2.

Until a few years ago, the Part I examination could not be taken until the work of the second year in medical school had been completed, and the Part II test was given only to students who had completed the major part of the fourth year. Now students, if they feel they are ready, may be admitted to any regularly scheduled Step 1 or Step 2 examination during any year of their medical course without prerequisite completion of specified courses or chronologic periods of study. Thus, emphasis is placed on the acquisition of knowledge and competence rather than the completion of predetermined periods.

Candidates are eligible for Step 3 after they have passed Steps 1 and 2, have received the M.D. degree from an approved medical school in the United States or Canada, and subsequent to the receipt of the M.D. degree, have served at least six months in an approved hospital internship or residency. Under certain circumstances, consideration may be given to other types of graduate training provided they meet with the approval of the National Board. After passing the Step 3 examination, candidates will receive their diplomas as of the date of the satisfactory completion of an internship or residency program. If candidates have completed the approved hospital training prior to completion of Step 3, they will receive certification as of the date of the successful completion of Step 3.

The Step 3 examination, as noted above, is an objective test of general clinical competence. It occupies one full day and is divided into two sections, the first of which is a multiple-choice examination that relates to the interpretation of clinical data presented primarily in pictorial form, such as pictures of patients, gross and microscopic lesions, electrocardiograms, charts, and graphs. The second section, entitled Patient Management Problems, utilized a programmed-testing technique designed to measure the candidate's clinical judgment in the management of patients. This technique simulates clinical situations in which the physician is faced with the problems of patient management presented in a sequential programmed pattern. A set of some four to six problems is related to each of a series of patients. In the scoring of this section, candidates are given credit for correct choices; they are penalized for errors of commission (selection of procedures that are unnecessary or are contraindicated) and for errors of omission (failure to select indicated procedures).

All parts of the National Board examinations are given in many centers, usually in medical schools, in nearly every large city in the United States as well as in a few cities in Canada, Puerto Rico, and the Canal Zone. In some cities, such as New York, Chicago, and Baltimore, the examination may be given in more than one center.

The examinations of the National Board have become recognized as the most comprehensive test of knowledge of the medical sciences and their clinical application produced in this country.

National Board of Medical Examiners

For years the National Board examinations have served as an index of the medical education of the period and have strongly influenced higher educational standards in each of the medical sciences. The Diploma of the National Board is accepted by 47 state licensing authorities, the District of Columbia, and the Commonwealth of Puerto Rico in lieu of the examination usually required for licensure and is recognized in the American Medical Directory by the letters DNB following the name of the physician holding National Board certification.

The National Board of Medical Examiners has been a leader in developing new and more reliable techniques of testing, not only for knowledge in all medical fields but also for clinical competence and fitness to practice. In recent years, too, a number of medical schools, several specialty certifying boards, professional medical societies organized to encourage their members to keep abreast of progress in medicine, and other professional qualifying agencies have called upon the National Board's professional staff for advice or for the actual preparation of tests to be employed in evaluating medical knowledge, effectiveness of teaching, and professional competence in certain medical fields. In all cases, advantage has been taken of the validity and effectiveness of the objective, multiple-choice type of examination, a technique the National Board has played an important role in bringing to its present state of perfection and discriminatory effectiveness.

Objective examinations permit a large number of questions to be asked, and approximately 150 to 180 questions can be answered in a 2½ hour period. Because the answer sheets are scored by machine, the grading can be accomplished rapidly, accurately, and impartially. It is completely unbiased and based on percentile ranking. Of long-range significance is the facility with which the total test and individual questions can be subjected to thorough and rapid statistical analyses, thus providing a sound basis for comparative studies of medical school teaching and for continuing improvement in the quality of the test itself.

Innovations in Formulating Test Questions

It is apparent from recent certification and board examinations that the examiners are devoting more attention in their construction of questions to more practical means of testing basic and clinical knowledge. This greater realism in testing relates to an increasingly interdisciplinary approach toward fundamental material and to the direct relevance accorded practical clinical problems. These newer approaches in testing will be incorporated into this text in the future. However, *Rypins' Questions and Answers for Basic Sciences Review*, 2nd edition, now includes questions that relate to these approaches.

Of course, the new approaches to testing add to the difficulty experienced by the student or physician preparing for board or certification examinations. The contributors to this book are acutely aware not only of the interrelationships of fundamental information with the basic science disciplines and their clinical implications but of the necessity to present their material clearly and concisely despite this complexity. For this reason, the questions provided at the end of each chapter are devised to test one's knowledge of specific material in that chapter. This permits the reader to identify areas for more intensive study. However, those preparing for examinations must be aware of the interdisciplinary nature of fundamental clinical material, the common multifactorial characteristics of disease mechanisms, and the necessity to shift back and forth from one chapter to another in order to appreciate the less than clear-cut nature separating the pedagogic disciplines.

Five Points to Remember

In order for the candidate to maximize chances for passing these examinations, a few commonsense strategies or guidelines should be kept in mind.

First, it is imperative to prepare thoroughly for the examination. Know well the types of questions to be presented and the pedagogic areas of particular weakness, and devote more preparatory study time to these weak areas. Do not use too much time restudying areas in which there is a feeling of great confidence and do not leave unexplored those areas in which there is less confidence. Finally, be well rested before the test, and if possible, avoid traveling to the city of testing that morning or late the evening before.

Second, know well the format of the examination and the instructions before becoming immersed in the challenge at hand. This information can be obtained from many published texts and brochures or directly from the testing service (National Board of Medical Examiners, 3750 Market Street, Philadelphia, PA 19104; telephone 215-590-9500). In addition, the many available texts and self-assessment types of examinations are valuable for practice.

Third, know well the overall time allotted for the examination and its components and the scope of the test to be faced. These may be learned by a rapid review of the examination itself. Then, proceed with the test at a careful, deliberate, and steady pace without spending inordinate time on any single question. For example, certain questions such as the "one best answer" (questions 1 to 3 of "Examples of Questions" below) probably should be allotted 1 to 1½ minutes each. The "matching" type of questions (numbers 4 to 18) should be allotted similar time. Multiple "true-false" type should be given about 1½ minutes; but these are rarely used now. This suggestion is still useful for this type of question because they are still offered in various educational institutions. Thus, each question of the five-component questions should be allotted approximately 20 seconds. With respect to the "recall" type of question, there is great need for logical judgment, for the candidate to infer an answer from the presentation of the data, and to discard illogical answers from the multiplicity of the choices. Further, the candidate should be aware that those questions containing the word *always* or *never* are unlikely to be wise choices; questions with words such as *may* and *could* are wiser selections.

Fourth, it follows that if a question is particularly disturbing, the candidate should note appropriately the question (put a mark on the question sheet) and return to this point later. Don't compromise yourself by so concentrating on a likely "loser" that several "winners" are eliminated because of inadequate time. One way to save this time on a particular "stickler" is to play your initial choice; your chances of a correct answer are always best with your first impression. If there is no initial choice, reread the question.

Fifth, allow adequate time to review answers, to return to the questions that were unanswered and "flagged" for later attention, and check every *n*th (e.g., 20th) question to make certain that the answers are appropriate and that you did not inadvertently skip a question in the booklet or answer on the sheet (this can happen easily under these stressful circumstances).

There is nothing magical about these five points. They are simple and just make common sense. If candidates have prepared themselves well and follow the preceding commonsense points, the chances are they will not have to return for a second go-round.

Examples of Questions

The following questions are presented as a guide to the physician preparing for examinations in the basic and clinical sciences. They offer the variety of types of multiple-choice questions that have been devised to provide objectivity in testing a large area of subject material that demands depth in knowledge and comprehension.

Objective Multiple-Choice Type

COMPLETION TYPE

The so-called completion-type item is the most common. Items of this type usually are placed together at the beginning of the test, as follows, with these directions:

Directions. *Each of the following questions or incomplete statements is followed by five suggested answers or completions. Select the one that is best in each case and blacken the corresponding space on the answer sheet.*

The following item illustrates this type, although obviously this question is rather easy.

QUESTION 1:

To which one of the following systems of the body does the heart belong?

(a) The digestive system
(b) The central nervous system
(c) The circulatory system
(d) The endocrine system
(e) The musculoskeletal system

The correct answer, of course, is (c). To make this question somewhat more difficult and avoid naming the correct system among the choice, the circulatory system can be omitted and an alternative choice, "None of the above," substituted for it. Then the question will appear as:

QUESTION 2:

To which of the following systems of the body does the heart belong?

(a) The digestive system
(b) The central nervous system
(c) The endocrine system
(d) The musculoskeletal system
(e) None of the above

The fifth choice, (e), now becomes the correct response. In this manner candidates are made to think of the various systems of the body and must know the right answer without its being suggested to them as one of the possibilities. In these examinations, the choice "None of the above" will appear and sometimes will be a correct and sometimes an incorrect response.

Another variant of the completion type of item is in the negative form, where all but one of the choices are applicable, and the candidate is asked to mark the one that does not apply. The following is an example:

QUESTION 3:

All of the following are associated with prerenal azotemia EXCEPT:

(a) Shock
(b) Dehydration
(c) Pernicious vomiting
(d) Gastrointestinal hemorrhage
(e) Multiple myeloma

The correct answer is (e).

ASSOCIATION AND RELATEDNESS ITEMS

Items of a somewhat different nature may be used effectively, as, for example, in determining the candidate's knowledge of the action and the use of closely related drugs or the distinguishing features of similar diseases. There follow specific directions for items of this type with a group of items taken from a pharmacology test and another group from a medicine test. As illustrated in this group of items, the candidate must have well-organized information about a number of related drugs and is required to demonstrate considerable understanding of the differential use of these drugs.

Directions. *Each group of questions below consists of five lettered headings followed by a list of numbered words or phrases. For each numbered word or phrase, select the one heading that is related most closely to it.*

QUESTIONS 4–9:

(a) Quinidine
(b) Theophylline
(c) Amyl nitrite
(d) Glyceryl trinitrate
(e) Papaverine

4. Relaxes smooth muscle of the arterial system; causes fall in arterial pressure; commonly administered in tablets sublingually *Answer:* (d)
5. An opium alkaloid; direct vasodilator action; used in instances of coronary occlusion and peripheral vascular disease *Answer:* (e)
6. Commonly effective in relieving symptoms of bronchial asthma *Answer:* (b)
7. The best for quick treatment of cyanide poisoning *Answer:* (c)
8. Increases the contractile force of the heart and is diuretic *Answer:* (b)
9. May be used in auricular fibrillation *Answer:* (a)

QUESTIONS 10–17:

(a) Coarctation of the aorta
(b) Patent ductus arteriosus
(c) Tetralogy of Fallot
(d) Aortic vascular ring
(e) Tricuspid atresia

10. Benefitted by systemic pulmonary artery anastomosis *Answer:* (c)
11. Most common type of congenital cyanotic heart disease *Answer:* (c)
12. Corrected surgically by resection and end-to-end anastomosis *Answer:* (a)
13. Possible cause of dysphagia in infants and children *Answer:* (d)
14. Wide pulse pressure *Answer:* (b)
15. Associated frequently with atrial septal defects *Answer:* (e)
16. A continuous murmur *Answer:* (b)
17. Hypertension in the arms and hypotension in the legs *Answer:* (a)

A further elaboration of association and relatedness items is considerably more searching and calls for a discriminatory understanding of a number of similar but distinguishable factors. For example, the following question reveals considerable information about the candidate's knowledge of the causes of hypoglycemia and the related functional disturbances: Four of the five situations in the numbered list below are common to one of the three functional disturbances designated by letters. The candidate is instructed to select one situation that is the exception and the functional disturbance common to the remaining four.

QUESTION 18:

(a) Clinically significant hypoglycemia
(b) Clinically significant hyperglycemia
(c) Clinically significant glycosuria

(1) Overdose of insulin
(2) Functional tumor of islet cells
(3) Renal glycosuria
(4) Hypopituitarism
(5) von Gierke's disease

If the candidate selects (a) and (3), the correct answer, he or she demonstrates knowledge that (1), (2), (4), and (5) may produce clinically significant hypoglycemia; that (3) does not; and that no combination of four of the five conditions is associated with hyperglycemia or glycosuria. In other words, the possession of both positive and negative information is probed. Specific directions for handling this form of discriminatory question read as follows:

Directions. *There are two responses to be made to each of the following questions. There are three lettered categories; four of the five numbered items are related in some way to one of these categories. (1) On the answer sheet blacken the space under the letter of the category in which these four items belong. (2) Then blacken the space under the number of the item that does not belong in the same category with the other four.*

Items of this type may be used to determine knowledge of disease symptomatology, laboratory findings, or therapeutic procedures, as shown by the following:

QUESTIONS 19–21:

19. (a) Multiple neurofibromatosis (von Recklinghausen's disease)
(b) Hemangioblastomas of the central nervous system
(c) Multiple sclerosis

(1) Neurofibromas of the skin
(2) Meningeal fibromas
(3) Congenital angiomas of the eye
(4) Lipomas of subcutaneous tissue
(5) Cystic disease of the pancreas

Answer: 1. (a)
2. (5)

20. (a) Contraindications to saddle-block anesthesia
(b) Contraindications to continuous caudal analgesia
(c) Contraindications to local anesthesia

(1) Deformity of the sacrum
(2) Cutaneous infections
(3) Perforated dura
(4) Decreased perineal resistance
(5) Prodromal labor

Answer: 1. (b)
2. (4)

21. (a) Eosinophilia of diagnostic significance
(b) Plasmacytosis of diagnostic significance
(c) Lymphocytosis of diagnostic significance

(1) Trichinosis
(2) Multiple myeloma
(3) Löffler's syndrome
(4) Hodgkin's disease
(5) Schistosomiasis

Answer: 1. (a)
2. (2)

Another variant of the association and relatedness type of question is demonstrated by the following example from a test in public health and preventive medicine:

Directions. *Each set of lettered headings below is followed by a list of words or phrases. For each word or phrase blacken the space on the answer sheet under:*

A if the word or the phrase is associated with (a) *only*
B if the word or the phrase is associated with (b) *only*
C if the word or the phrase is associated with *both* (a) and (b)
D if the word or the phrase is associated with *neither* (a) *nor* (b)

QUESTIONS 22–26:

(a) Maternal hygiene program
(b) School health program
(c) Both
(d) Neither

22. Periodic physical examination *Answer:* C—(a & b)
23. Audiometer test *Answer:* B
24. Nutritional guidance *Answer:* C—(a & b)
25. Serologic test for syphilis *Answer:* A
26. Immunization against rubella *Answer:* B

QUANTITATIVE VALUES AND COMPARISONS

In general, questions in this category will call for an understanding of quantitative values rather than rote memory of the quantities themselves. The test committees have agreed that these examinations should contain a minimum of questions calling for the memorizing of absolute quantitative amounts. Actual figures will be found only where the details of the information are considered to be of such importance that they should be a part of the working knowledge that a practicing physician should have in mind without recourse to a reference book. Knowledge of the comparative significance of quantitative values may be called for by items such as the following:

Directions. *The following paired statements describe two entities that are to be compared in a quantitative sense. On the answer sheet blacken the space under:*

A if (a) is *greater than* (b)
B if (b) is *greater than* (a)
C if the two are *equal or very nearly equal*

QUESTIONS 27–31:

27. (a) The usual therapeutic dose of epinephrine
(b) The usual therapeutic dose of ephedrine *Answer:* B
28. (a) The inflammability of nitrous oxide-ether mixtures *Answer:* A
(b) The inflammability of chloroform-air mixtures
29. (a) The susceptibility of premature infants to rickets *Answer:* A
(b) The susceptibility of full-term infants to rickets
30. (a) Life expectancy with glioblastoma of the occipital lobe
(b) Life expectancy with glioblastoma of the frontal lobe *Answer:* C
31. (a) The amount of glycogen in the cells of Henle's loop in a diabetic *Answer:* A
(b) The amount of glycogen in the cells of Henle's loop in a nondiabetic

Directions. *Each of the following pairs of phrases describes conditions or quantities that may or may not be related. On the answer sheet blacken the space under:*

A if increase in the first is accompanied by increase in the second or if decrease in the first is accompanied by decrease in the second
B if increase in the first is accompanied by decrease in the second or if decrease in the first is accompanied by increase in the second

C if changes in the second are independent of changes in the first

QUESTIONS 32–34:

32. (1) Urine volume
    (2) Urine specific gravity *Answer:* B
33. (1) Plasma protein concentration
    (2) Colloid osmotic pressure of plasma *Answer:* A
34. (1) Cerebrospinal fluid pressure
    (2) Intraocular pressure *Answer:* C

CAUSE AND EFFECT

A type of item that is especially applicable to some of the more elusive aspects of medicine and calls for an understanding of cause and effect is illustrated in the following type of questions:

Directions. *Each of the following sentences consists of two main parts: a statement and a reason for that statement. On the answer sheet blacken the space under:*

A if the statement and the proposed reason are *both true* and are *related* as cause and effect
B if the statement and the proposed reason are *both true* but are *not related* as cause and effect
C if the statement is *true* but the proposed reason is *an accepted fact or principle*
D if the statement is false but the proposed reason is *an accepted fact or principle*
E if the statement and the proposed reason are *both false*

Directions Summarized:
A = True True and related
B = True True and NOT related
C = True False
D = False True
E = False False

In situations that may be presented by this type of item, the right answer may sometimes be arrived at through good reasoning from an appreciation of the basic principles involved. The sample items are as follows:

QUESTIONS 35–39:

35. Herpes simplex usually is regarded as an autogenous infection BECAUSE patients given fever therapy frequently develop herpes. *Answer:* A
36. Cow's milk is preferable to breast milk in infant feeding BECAUSE cow's milk has a higher content of calcium. *Answer:* D
37. The corpus luteum of menstruation becomes the corpus luteum of pregnancy BECAUSE progesterone inhibits the activity of the anterior portion of the pituitary gland. *Answer:* B
38. The sinoauricular node serves as the pacemaker BECAUSE after its removal the heart fails to beat. *Answer:* C
39. A higher titer of antibody against the H antigen of the typhoid bacillus is a good index of immunity to typhoid BECAUSE any antibody to an organism can protect against disease caused by that organism. *Answer:* E

QUESTION 40:

A modification of the true-false type of question that calls for careful thought and discrimination is the "multiple true-false" variety. In this question a list of numbered items follows a statement for which several possible answers are given and the candidate is required to select the appropriate response from a list of answers designated by letters:

40. Live virus is used in immunization against:
    1. Influenza
    2. Poliomyelitis
    3. Cholera
    4. Smallpox

    Answers:
    A. Only 1, 2, and 3 are correct
    B. Only 1 and 3 are correct
    C. Only 2 and 4 are correct
    D. Only 4 is correct
    E. All are correct

STRUCTURE AND FUNCTIONS

Diagrams, charts, electrocardiograms, roentgenograms, or photomicrographs may be used to elicit knowledge of structure, function, the course of a clinical situation, or a statistical tabulation. Questions then may be asked in relation to designated elements of the same.

CASE HISTORIES

The most characteristic situation that confronts the practicing physician can be simulated by a clinical case history derived from a patient experience, which is followed by a series of questions concerning diagnosis, signs and symptoms, laboratory determinations, treatment, and prognosis. In answering these questions, much depends on arriving at the proper diagnosis, for, if an incorrect diagnosis is made, related symptoms, laboratory data, and treatment also will be wrong. These case history questions are set up purposely to place such emphasis on the correct diagnosis within a context comparable with the experience of actual practice.

Directions. *This section of the test consists of several case histories, each followed by a series of questions. Study each history, select the best answer to each question following it, and blacken the space under the corresponding letter on the answer sheet.*

The patient is a 21-year-old white man with a complaint of malaise, cough, and fever. The present illness had its onset 10 days prior to admission with malaise and a nonproductive cough, followed in 24 hours by a temperature varying from 100° F to 101° F that persisted up to the time of admission. On about the fourth day of illness the cough became more severe, producing scant amounts of white viscid sputum. Three days prior to admission, paroxysms of coughing began, followed sometimes by vomiting. Chilly sensations were noted but no frank shaking chills. Anterior parasternal pain on coughing has been present since the fifth day of illness.

On physical examination the temperature is 101° F; the pulse rate 110 beats per minute; the respiratory rate 32 per minute; and the blood pressure 108 mmHg systolic, 60 mmHg diastolic. The patient is well developed and well nourished, appears to be acutely but not chronically ill, and is dyspneic but not cyanotic.

Positive physical findings are limited to the chest and are as follows:

Vocal and tactile fremitus and resonance are within normal limits. In the left axilla a few fine rales are heard, and the bronchial quality of the sounds is increased, although the intensity is normal.

Blood findings are reported as follows:

White blood count, 3,400 (polymorphonuclears 30%, lymphocytes 62%, monocytes 5%, eosinophils 3%).

Roentgenogram of the chest reveals an increase in the density of the perihilar markings with ill-defined areas of patchy, soft, increased radiodensity at both bases and in the left upper lung field.

QUESTIONS 41–45:

41. Which one of the following is the most likely diagnosis?
    (a) Tuberculosis
    (b) Pneumococcal pneumonia
    (c) Primary atypical pneumonia *Answer:* (c)
    (d) Coccidioidomycosis
    (e) Bronchopneumonia
42. Which one of the following is the most likely additional physical finding?
    (a) Splenomegaly
    (b) Signs of meningeal irritation
    (c) Pleural friction rub
    (d) Frequent changes in distribution of chest findings *Answer:* (d)
    (e) Signs of frank lobar consolidation
43. Which one of the following laboratory findings is consistent with the diagnosis?
    (a) Elevation and further increase of cold agglutinins *Answer:* (a)
    (b) Positive blood culture
    (c) Marked leukocytosis with the beginning of recovery
    (d) Positive sputum examination
    (e) Positive skin test
44. Which one of the following is the therapy that should be given?
    (a) Bed rest and streptomycin
    (b) Bed rest and penicillin
    (c) Streptomycin and paraaminosalicylic acid
    (d) Bed rest and Aureomycin *Answer:* (d)
    (e) Psychotherapy and physical rehabilitation
45. Which one of the following is the probable outcome of this disease in this patient if untreated?
    (a) The fever will subside spontaneously by crisis
    (b) Recovery will be gradual, with relapse not unexpected. *Answer:* (b)
    (c) Empyema will develop
    (d) Residual fibrosis will appear with healing
    (e) Lung cavitation will not be unexpected

Objective examinations permit a large number of questions to be asked, for 150 to 180 in each subject can be answered in a 2½-hour period. Because the answer sheets are scorable by machine, the grading can be accomplished rapidly, accurately, and impartially. It is completely unbiased and percentile, since the human element is not a factor. Of long-range significance is the facility with which the total test and individual questions can be subjected to thorough and rapid statistical analyses, thus providing a sound basis for comparative studies of medical school teaching and for continuing improvement in the quality of the test itself. Furthermore, multiple-choice written examinations have certain advantages of real benefit to the candidate, to the medical school, and, ultimately, to state boards of medical examiners.

Review Questions

Following are examples of review questions. In those relating to the basic sciences in particular, an attempt has been made, in most of them at least, not merely to call for information based on recollection of past study but rather to relate the questions to practical clinical or patient problems. These questions are rhetorical in nature and would require an essay-type answer. The reviewer is presented these questions primarily as an overall suggestion of important areas for study and review.

QUESTIONS IN THE BASIC SCIENCES

Describe or diagram the conduction pathways of the heart. Indicate the sites of pathology or disturbances in the presence of:

(a) Paroxysmal tachycardia
(b) Adams-Stokes syndrome
(c) Heart block after myocardial infarction

Diagram the anatomy encountered in doing a tracheotomy.

What neurologic structures are found at the cerebellopontine angle, both within and outside of the brain, where pathology might be reflected in clinical symptoms?

A patient has sustained fractures of the lower left ribs posteriorly. What subjacent structures might be injured? What studies should be performed to determine the extent of the injury?

Diagram a cross section of the spinal cord at the level of L2, indicating major tracts. Indicate the blood supply to the cord at this level.

Name five congenital defects that may be detected at birth and give their embryologic derivation.

Diagram the abdominal aorta with its major branches. Indicate site of occlusion for Leriche syndrome.

Describe the embryologic development of the pituitary gland. Diagram its relationship to surrounding structures.

Diagram the relationship of the pancreas to the duodenum with its duct system. Describe its embryology.

Diagram the tracheobronchial tree, showing the major lung segments. Where will a foreign body aspirated into the tracheobronchial tree most frequently lodge?

Discuss the role of progesterone in pregnancy.

What is intermittent claudication? What is its cause?

What is meant by the specific dynamic action (SDA) of food? What is the significance of SDA in prescribing a diet for an obese patient?

Describe briefly the functions of the hypothalamus.

Define *each* of the following:

(a) Conditioned reflex
(b) Jaundice
(c) Orthopnea
(d) Emphysema
(e) Tidal air
(f) Heartburn

Name and discuss the factors responsible for the tonic activity of the respiratory center.

Explain why pulmonary edema develops first in dependent parts of the lungs.

Discuss the role of bile in fat digestion.

What is the origin of bilirubin found in the serum?

In a patient with jaundice and a mild anemia, what five *biochemical* determinations would, in your opinion, be most effective in the differential diagnosis? Explain your choices.

Define a vitamin.

Under what circumstances can hypervitaminosis develop? List the clinical and biochemical manifestations of any hypervitaminosis.

The following proteins may be found in human serum. Define four of the six listed below, list the methods by which they may be detected and explain their clinical significance:

(a) Cryoglobulin
(b) Myeloma protein
(c) Siderophilin (transferrin)
(d) Macroglobulin
(e) Cold agglutinin
(f) Haptoglobin

Define a *buffer system.* Give an example of a buffer system important in clinical medicine and explain the operation of the system in:

(a) Metabolic acidosis
(b) Respiratory alkalosis

What are the clinical manifestations of hypokalemia? What electrocardiographic changes are frequently associated with hypokalemia? List three clinical states in which hypokalemia is a common finding.

Define four of the following:

(a) Methemoglobin
(b) Thyroglobulin
(c) Respiratory quotient
(d) Pasteur effect
(e) Nitrogen balance
(f) Intrinsic factor

In advising a community hospital that is about to establish a clinical diagnostic radioisotope laboratory, what radioactive chemical compounds would you recommend? List the compounds (*not* just elements) and give at least *one* use for *each.*

Name three microorganisms sensitive to penicillin and three resistant to penicillin as it is administered in clinical practice.

Define the terms *anamnestic response* and *booster effect.* How are these principles applied to artificial immunization?

List three infections in which disease is caused primarily by the toxin of the infecting microorganism.

Name a vaccine in which the immunizing principle is a modified toxin.

Describe two laboratory tests for the diagnosis of syphilis. How may these tests be modified by antiluetic therapy?

Name two microorganisms that may induce cavitating

disease of the lung. Describe briefly the morphology and the staining characteristics of each.

What streptococcus is associated with "streptococcal" sore throat? What distinguishes this microorganism on blood agar culture? What are three possible sequelae of untreated streptococcal pharyngitis?

Name three bacteria that are frequently associated with meningitis. For each of the three types of meningitis, list an antimicrobial drug that is effective in its treatment.

What is the etiologic significance of a pneumococcus in the throat culture of an adult patient with pharyngitis? In the sputum of a patient with pneumonia? In the nasopharynx of a child with otitis media?

List three cultural or biochemical characteristics of pneumococcus.

What is Sabin's vaccine? Are its antigenic constituents living or dead? Name one constituent of the vaccine in addition to those that are intended for immunization. Does the vaccine prevent infection?

Classify the etiologic agent of "Asiatic influenza."

Which antimicrobial agents are effective in the treatment of uncomplicated influenza?

What is the most frequent cause of death in influenza?

Name two microorganisms frequently implicated in the fatal termination of influenza.

Describe three characteristics by which viruses differ from bacteria.

Identify three diseases caused by rickettsia.

What are selective media? Give the name of one such medium and its purpose. Of what value is penicillinase in diagnostic bacteriology?

Name two diseases that may be prevented or modified by the parenteral injection of antibody.

Name two diseases in which antibody must be used for optimal treatment.

What is the significance of:

(a) An elevated serum ASO (antistreptolysin O) titer
(b) An elevated serum heterophile antibody titer
(c) An elevated cold agglutinin titer in the serum

Compare infectious hepatitis and serum hepatitis with respect to:

(a) Etiologic agent
(b) Epidemiology
(c) Incubation period

Indicate for *each* of the following organisms whether it is sensitive or resistant *in vitro* to penicillin and tetracycline:

Streptococcus pyogenes
Neisseria gonorrhoeae
Neisseria meningitidis
Klebsiella pneumoniae
Hemophilus influenzae
Brucella abortus

Name three vaccines that contain living and three that contain dead infectious agents, listing also the microorganisms they contain. How would you test for the efficacy of immunization with any one of these agents (without exposing your patient to disease)?

List three gram-positive and three gram-negative bacteria. For *each* organism listed, give a brief description of its morphology.

Cite two laboratory characteristics of the staphylococci that are most commonly pathogenic for humans. What is the drug of choice for treating most staphylococcal infections acquired outside the hospital?

Name three diseases in humans caused by spirochetes. What are the names of the etiologic agents of these diseases?

Briefly discuss the most common gross pathology of an adenocarcinoma of the right hemicolon and contrast it with that most often seen in the descending colon. Correlate these gross findings with the usual initial symptom complex of each.

Which of the following is the most frequent site of carcinoma of the colon?

(a) The cecum
(b) The splenic flexure
(c) The sigmoid
(d) The rectum

Which of the following figures most nearly represents the percentage of carcinoma of the colon and the rectum that are detectable by digital rectal examination?

(a) 10%
(b) 2%
(c) 20%
(d) 50%

A 55-year-old woman is admitted to the hospital with complaints of tiredness, weakness, progressive enlargement of the abdomen and continuous mild generalized abdominal discomfort for "some time." No further reliable history is obtainable. Physical examination reveals a middle-aged woman with obvious recent wasting. The blood pressure is 130/80 mmHg; pulse 80 beats per minute and regular; temperature 97° F. The *only* other significant physical finding is an enlarged, tense abdomen exhibiting shifting dullness and fluid wave. (A routine urinalysis has revealed no significant abnormality, nor has an electrocardiogram.)

In the absence of other significant physical findings, what two conditions would you consider most probable in your provisional diagnosis?

What one simple and practical procedure, utilizing the

clinical laboratory, would best aid in the differential diagnosis between the two?

Indicate the characteristic clinical laboratory findings elicited by this procedure for *each* of the two conditions that you have mentioned.

Very briefly discuss cancer of the lip under the following headings:

(a) Sex incidence
(b) Location
(c) Gross pathology
(d) Microscopic pathology
(e) Spread
(f) Prognosis

In cases of pernicious anemia, name:

(a) The fundamental defect involved in the pathogenesis
(b) Three laboratory findings indispensable to a diagnosis of pernicious anemia
(c) Three accessory laboratory findings that confirm the diagnosis

The following phrases are descriptive of characteristics of certain neoplasms. In *each* case, name a neoplasm to which the phrase might correctly pertain:

(a) A tumor that has a high mortality but rarely, if ever, metastasizes
(b) A serotonin-secreting tumor that may produce spells of flushing of the skin
(c) An invasive tumor of the skin that rarely, if ever, metastasizes
(d) A neoplasm that may be mistaken for eczema
(e) A malignant neoplasm originating from the placenta
(f) A neoplasm associated with intermittent episodes of hypertension

A man, age 55 years, has had a recent myocardial infarction. Anticoagulant therapy is ordered.

What drug should be used for rapid anticoagulant effect, and what laboratory procedure should be used to check the result?

What drug should be used for long-term anticoagulant effect, and what laboratory test should be used for its control? Give the normal values for this test and the range of values optimal for the patient receiving anticoagulant therapy.

Discuss briefly the pathology of bronchogenic carcinoma, indicating usual sites of primary origin, histologic types, and method of spread.

List five common sites of metastasis of bronchogenic carcinoma, arranging them in order of frequency.

Following overindulgence in food and alcohol, a man, age 30, develops sudden severe epigastric pain with moderate rigidity and tenderness of the upper abdomen. There are nausea, vomiting, cyanosis, abdominal distention, rapid pulse, and shock.

Indicate two conditions that should be considered and laboratory findings that would aid in the differential diagnosis.

Describe clinical features that should suggest that a skin lesion is a malignant melanoma.

Describe briefly the histopathology of malignant melanoma.

Indicate method of spread and prognosis.

Name three diseases that can be transmitted by blood or blood products from donor to recipient.

What precautions should be taken to prevent such transmission?

QUESTIONS IN THE CLINICAL SCIENCES

A patient is admitted to a hospital unconscious immediately following an automobile accident. The neurologic examination is normal. Consciousness is not regained. Two hours later respirations are irregular, the left pupil is a little dilated, and the right arm is tonic. In another hour the right side of the face begins to twitch. The right arm is spastic, and the left pupil is fully dilated. Respirations are very irregular and slow. (Consider unmentioned phenomena to be normal.)

Write the letters *a* and *b* on your answer paper. After *each* letter write the *number* preceding the word or the expression that best completes the statement.

(a) At this time the diagnosis is:
 1. Depressed skull fracture
 2. Intracranial hematoma
 3. Subdural hematoma
 4. Epidural hematoma
(b) The immediate procedure should be:
 1. Lumbar puncture
 2. Neurologic consultation
 3. Electroencephalogram
 4. Angiogram
 5. Temporal trephine

Outline the procedure to be followed in the evaluation of a severe injury of the pelvis.

What basic information must you have to order and manage intelligently a patient's fluid intake for the few days following a major abdominal surgical procedure during which oral fluids cannot be taken in adequate amounts?

Following a cholecystectomy for gallstones but with no previous history of jaundice, a patient drains bile from the incision. This drainage gradually becomes less and finally ceases after 2 weeks. Concomitantly, the patient becomes jaundiced and develops periodic attacks of chills and fever. The stools become somewhat lighter in color but are not clay colored.

What conditions would you consider in the differential diagnosis?

What laboratory tests or diagnostic procedures, if any, would definitely confirm your diagnosis?

Should this patient be operated upon?

If operation is indicated, when should it be performed?

List the procedures you might employ if necessary to arrive at the diagnosis of a lesion of the lung that has been noted on an anteroposterior chest x-ray film.

What means would you use to manage the problem presented by the elderly, frail, weak individual who has great difficulty in getting rid of copious mucoid tracheobronchial secretions in the immediate postoperative period?

A 65-year-old man with chronic bronchitis and emphysema has a combined abdominal-perineal resection of the rectum and the sigmoid colon for carcinoma. During the immediate postoperative period he is being treated with an indwelling urethral catheter and an indwelling nasogastric tube. By the fourth postoperative day the patient's temperature has gradually risen since operation to 103° F by rectum.

What significance, if any, is the amount of fever?

What should be done in an attempt to explain it?

Peptic ulcers of the duodenum are treated surgically by a variety of procedures. Indicate the rational basis for the treatment of his lesion by:

(a) Vagotomy with pyloroplasty
(b) Subtotal gastric resection
(c) Gastroenterostomy

Outline your management of a patient presenting himself with a history of painless hematuria lasting for 1 day, 1 week ago.

Given a patient with severe hypertension, list some of the changes in the fundus of the eye that you would likely encounter in doing an ophthalmoscopic examination.

A 55-year-old woman with atrial fibrillation due to rheumatic heart disease experiences a sudden severe pain in the left leg. When she is seen at the hospital 4 hours later the pain is still present. The leg is cooler than the right from the knee down, and the skin is blanched. The toes can be moved, but sensation in the lower leg is decreased. Pulsation can be felt over the left common femoral artery at the level of Poupart's ligament on the left, but none below this level.

What is the clinical diagnosis?

At what specific point is the lesion most likely located?

What recommendations for management do you make?

A 32-year-old white man is found to have hypertension of 190 mmHg systolic and 100 mmHg diastolic on routine examination. What are the possible causes of this, and what clinical and laboratory findings would help in identifying these causes?

A 28-year-old Puerto Rican woman, the mother of children 6 and 8 years of age, complains of weakness, slight fever, anorexia, and hemoptysis. How should this situation be managed from the diagnostic and therapeutic standpoints? What is the most likely diagnosis, and what are the implications with respect to this patient's family?

Discuss the management of *each* of the following clinical situations:

(a) Congestive failure in a child with acute rheumatic pancarditis
(b) Paroxysmal ventricular tachycardia
(c) Premature ventricular beats in a patient with acute myocardial infarction

A 3-year-old child has a generalized convulsive seizure and is rushed to you in the emergency room of a hospital. Tabulate the common causes and give the clinical and laboratory findings of *each* cause mentioned.

Indicate briefly the clinical significance of *each* of the following:

(a) Bence Jones protein in the urine
(b) A positive heterophil agglutination test
(c) A high blood alkaline phosphatase
(d) A high blood acid phosphatase
(e) A positive porphobilinogen in the urine

A moderately obese middle-aged woman presents herself complaining of recurrent belching and a sense of a lump and burning in the substernal area. These symptoms occur especially when she stoops over or after a heavy meal, and when she goes to bed at night. Discuss differential diagnosis and treatment.

Outline the clinical and laboratory differential diagnosis of hematuria in an elderly male.

A middle-aged female patient with rheumatoid arthritis has been under long-term treatment with steroids. She now requires operation for acute appendicitis. What are the implications of the prior steroid therapy in such a situation, and how would you manage the medical aspects of the case?

Tabulate briefly the major indications and contraindications for use of each of the following:

(a) Oral hypoglycemic agents
(b) Nitrogen mustard
(c) Parenteral iron preparations
(d) Intravenous aminophylline
(e) Intravenous ACTH

A young adult man has anorexia, vomiting, and mild nausea for a few days and then notes dark urine and light stool. Discuss clinical and laboratory differential diagnosis and therapy.

Name one subjective complaint and one objective indication for estrogenic hormone in the management of a woman after her menopause.

A 9-year-old girl experiences prolonged vaginal bleeding. Examination reveals breast and vulvar development and a 6 cm by 9 cm tumor in the pelvis. What would you suspect?

What two complaints warrant a suspicion of gonococcal infection in the female? Indicate two procedures, either of which would confirm the diagnosis.

A 60-year-old nulliparous woman, 9 years postmenopausal, reports serous to bloody vaginal discharge on several occasions in the past month.

Indicate two probabilities.

How would you establish the diagnosis?

What two possibly predisposing factors would you consider when suspecting vaginitis is due to *Monilia?*

What would confirm that diagnosis?

What treatment would you prescribe?

A patient, gravida I, with uterus approximately term size, states that she cannot be more than 30 weeks pregnant. What three possibilities would you consider?

The child survived delivery by section when profuse antepartum bleeding was due to placenta previa. Name three possible causes if menstruation fails to occur by the sixth month postpartum.

What two observations noted during labor warrant a suspicion that defibrination of maternal blood may occur?

How can you determine if this is occurring?

If undetected, what could be the result?

Name three laboratory procedures that might be indicated repeatedly during the prenatal care of a normal patient.

Name three disadvantages inherent in ''deep'' general anesthesia for delivery at term.

List the activities of the U.S. Public Health Service.

What health hazards may be encountered in a boys' summer camp?

What voluntary agencies are active in the field of cardiovascular disease, and what are some of their activities?

What immunizations should be recommended for travelers to the Middle East and Africa?

What is meant by *each* of the following terms:

(a) Crude death rate
(b) Standardized death rate
(c) Infant mortality rate
(d) Birth rate

What services are offered by local health departments to the practicing physician?

Discuss health hazards in industry, and outline methods of preventing them.

Discuss health facilities provided by unions.

Rypins' Basic Sciences Review, 17th Edition,
edited by Edward D. Frohlich. Lippincott–Raven Publishers,
Philadelphia © 1997.

2

Anatomy

Neal E. Pratt, Ph.D., PT
Professor of Physical Therapy and
Neurobiology/Anatomy
Allegheny University of the Health Sciences
Philadelphia, Pennsylvania

Dennis M. De Pace, Ph.D.
Associate Professor of Neurobiology and Anatomy
Allegheny University of the Health Sciences
Philadelphia, Pennsylvania

Human anatomy is the study of the structure of the human body. This study is often subdivided into (1) ***gross anatomy,*** the study of structure as seen with the unaided eye; (2) ***microscopic anatomy (histology),*** the study of structure as seen with the aid of a microscope; (3) ***cytology,*** the study of the structure of cells; (4) ***embryology,*** the study of the origin, growth, and development of an organism from inception until birth; and (5) ***neuroanatomy,*** the structure of the nervous system.

The human body is organized into cells, tissues, organs, and organ systems. ***Cells*** are the smallest units of structure of the body that have, or had, the ability to carry on all of the vital functions of the body. ***Tissues*** are groups of cells and intercellular material that are specialized for the performance of specific functions. Each ***organ*** consists of certain arrangements of tissues that join in performing a specific bodily function or functions. An ***organ system*** is a group of organs that perform related functions. The major organ systems of the body are the integumentary, skeletal, muscular, nervous, circulatory (cardiovascular and lymphatic), respiratory, digestive, endocrine, urinary, and reproductive systems.

In the following review of human anatomy we will first discuss cell structure; this will be followed by a regional review of the back, upper extremity, lower extremity, head and neck, thorax, abdomen, and pelvis and perineum. The gross and microscopic anatomy, neuroanatomy, and embryology of the organ systems will be discussed as each region is reviewed.

CELL STRUCTURE

The cells of the body are composed of ***protoplasm,*** which is organized into two major components: the ***nucleus*** and the ***cytoplasm.*** The cytoplasm is separated from its surrounding environment by a plasma membrane and from the nucleus by a nuclear membrane (envelope).

NUCLEUS

Most cells possess one nucleus that in the interphase (nondividing) state consists of chromatin, one or more nucleoli, nucleoplasm, and an investing nuclear membrane. Some cells (*e.g.,* red blood cells) have no nuclei, whereas quite a few cells have more than one nucleus (*e.g.*, parietal cells of stomach, hepatocytes, osteoclasts).

Chromatin. Chromatin particles in the nucleus are the threads of deoxyribose nucleic acid (DNA) and proteins of the ***chromosomes.*** The DNA double helix of 20Å diameter that represents the genes of the chromosomes is coiled or folded back upon itself in forming each chromatin fibrillar thread of 100Å diameter. Chromatin material occurs in two forms: (1) ***heterochromatin,*** consisting of tightly coiled and condensed threads of DNA and protein, and (2) ***euchromatin,*** comprised of less-coiled, lighter staining, and more dispersed threads. The heterochromatin seems to represent the more inactive metabolic state, whereas euchromatin is more active in the synthesis of ribonucleic acid (RNA). Although the ratio of euchromatin to heterochromatin is different in various cells of the body, the chromatin content and chromosomal number are constant for somatic cells and for sex cells. Somatic cells contain 46 chromosomes (the diploid number), consisting of 22 pairs of autosomes and one pair of sex chromosomes (XX in females and XY in males). Sex cells contain 23 chromosomes (the haploid number) made up of one half of each pair of autosomal chromosomes and one of the pair of sex chromosomes (*i.e.*, an X or a Y).

Nucleolus. One nucleolus, or several nucleoli, are present in each cell. Most of each nucleolus is protein, 5% to 10% is RNA, and a small amount is DNA. The protein and RNA often appear as a meandering thick thread of ribonucleoprotein called a ***nucleolonema.*** The nucleolonema appears as fibrillar (pars fibrosa) and granular (pars granulosa) portions of the nucleolus. A chromosomal portion of intranucleolar chromatin (nucleolar organizer) contains the genes from which ribosomal RNA (rRNA) is transcribed and synthesized. The newly formed rRNA is packaged with proteins into ribosomal subunits; these pass from the pars fibrosa and pars granulosa before being transferred to the cytoplasm, where they are assembled into ribosomes.

Nucleoplasm. Nucleoplasm is an amorphous substance consisting of proteins, ions, and metabolites. Chromatin and nucleoli seem to be suspended in this substance.

Nuclear Membrane (Envelope). The nuclear membrane consists of two parallel unit membranes that are separated by a perinuclear space of about 20nm to 40nm. The ***unit membrane*** also is a component of the plasma membrane, Golgi apparatus, endoplasmic reticulum, lysosomes, mitochondria, coated vesicles, and secretion granules. With the electron microscope the basic unit membrane is seen as an 8nm-thick complex of an electron light area sandwiched between two electron dense areas. The dense areas seem to represent the membrane proteins and the polar ends of the phospholipid bilayers that make up the membrane. The light area represents the fatty acids of a bilayer of phospholipids. The *outer* unit membrane of the nuclear envelope is continuous with the endoplasmic reticulum. The *inner* unit membrane of the nuclear envelope is attached to the chromosomes by a fibrous network of three polypeptides called the nuclear lamina. Circular openings (nuclear pores), which are covered by thin membranes, occur at intervals throughout the nuclear envelope. The nuclear pores are important passageways for the transfer of substances between the cytoplasm and the nucleus.

CYTOPLASM

The cytoplasm contains dynamic ''living'' structural components of the cell (organelles) and ''nonliving'' metabolites or products of the cell (inclusions). The organelles include the plasma membrane, ribosomes, endoplasmic reticulum, Golgi apparatus, lysosomes, mitochondria, centrioles (centrosome), fibrils, filaments, microtubules, peroxisomes, and coated vesicles. Inclusions include stored gylcogen, lipid, protein, pigments, and secretion granules.

Plasma Membrane. The plasma membrane is a unit membrane 8nm thick consisting of a lipid bilayer in which there are membrane proteins. The lipid component consists of phospholipids, cholesterol, and glycolipids. The phospholipid molecules have their hydrophilic glycerol-phosphate heads oriented toward either the outer or the inner surface of the plasma membrane; the fatty acid tails of this double layer of phospholipid molecules meet in the center of the plasma membrane to form an intermediate hydrophobic zone. Cholesterol molecules stabilize the membrane, whereas glycolipids are located in the outer portion of the wall and seem to serve in cellular communication. Some membrane proteins extend through the plasma membrane (transmembrane proteins) and help to transport specific molecules into and out of the cell. Other membrane proteins extend only from the internal or external surface (*e.g.*, glycoproteins) of the membrane; these may serve as enzymes, attachment sites of the cytoskeleton or receptor sites. The membrane proteins can move around in the plasma membrane. A glycocalyx coats the outer surface of the cell. It consists of the carbohydrate components of glycolipids and glycoproteins of the membrane and also of glycoproteins and proteoglycans that have been absorbed on the cell surface.

Ribosomes. Ribosomes are rRNA plus protein. They occur as free ribosomes or as the granular component of the ***rough endoplasmic reticulum*** (RER). Generally, the free ribosomes are involved in the synthesis of structural proteins and enzymes that stay in the cell; the RER is necessary for the ***synthesis of proteins*** that are secreted from the cell and for producing lysosomal enzymes used in cellular digestion.

Endoplasmic Reticulum. The endoplasmic reticulum is a membranous network of tubules and flattened sacs that are often continuous with the outer layer of the nuclear membrane. That endoplasmic reticulum that does not have attached ribosomes is called ***smooth endoplasmic reticulum*** (SER); that with ribosomes is called rough endoplasmic reticulum or RER. SER is involved in steroid production in the adrenals and gonads, excitation-contraction mechanisms of muscle, absorption of fats in the intestine, and in cholesterol and lipid metabolism and drug detoxification in the liver. RER is involved in the production of protein products such as enzymes for secretion by the cell.

Golgi Apparatus (Golgi Complex). One or more Golgi apparatus may be found near the nucleus. Each consists of stacks of flattened smooth-surfaced saccules composed of unit membrane. The Golgi apparatus has an immature (forming, cis) face where new stacks are added, and a maturing (trans) face where secretory vesicles seem to bud off. Protein and sugar molecules manufactured in the RER pass to the forming face through transfer vesicles. In the Golgi apparatus the protein is condensed; sugars may be added to it and the product is packaged into secretory vesicles. The Golgi apparatus also is involved in cell membrane and lysosome production.

Lysosomes. Lysosomes are unit membrane-bound vesicles of digestive (hydrolyzing) enzymes. In the digestion of worn out parts of the cell, primary lysosomes fuse with autophagic vacuoles containing the dead part. In digesting endocytized (phagocytized, pinocytized) material, primary lysosomes fuse with the internalized membrane-bound substance forming a secondary lysosome. If the material is not completely digested, a membrane-bound residual body remains.

Mitochondria. Mitochondria are filamentous or granular structures that are comprised of a double unit membrane. The inner membrane, separated from the outer membrane by a space 6nm to 10nm wide, is thrown into many transverse folds (cristae) or tubules, which project into the fluid matrix in the interior of the mitochondrion. The inner surface of the cristae is studded with many ''elementary particles.'' Mitochondria are the sites where phosphate bond energy in the form of adenosine triphosphate (ATP) is produced.

Centrosome (Cell Center). The centrosome is located near the nucleus and consists of two ***centrioles*** surrounded by homogenous cytoplasm. The centrioles are cylindrical ($0.15\ \mu m \times 0.3$ to $0.5\ \mu m$) and lie perpendicular to each other. The wall of each centriole consists of nine parallel units, each of which is made up of three fused microtubules. Basal bodies, located at the base of cilia or flagella, are similar in structure to centrioles. Centrioles seem to be nucleation centers for microtubule formation; this is apparent in the formation of the spindle during cell division.

Microtubules. Microtubules are straight or wavy cylinders whose walls are made up of rows of tubulin. Microtubules function in maintaining cell shape, in intracellular transport, and in cell movement. Cilia and flagella are motile processes that extend from the free surfaces of many different cells. They consist of a core of microtubules, the axoneme, which is arranged as two central microtubules surrounded by nine peripheral doublets, each of which share a common wall of two or three protofilaments. Dynein arms possessing ATPase activity extend from one doublet toward an adjacent doublet. It is believed that motion of cilia and flagella is the result of doublets sliding within the axoneme as the dynein arms of one doublet walk along the adjacent doublet.

Filaments and Fibrils. Filaments are slender threads of protein molecules. Filaments less than 8nm in diameter are microfilaments, which are part of the cytoskeleton and are involved in cell contraction. Filaments between 8nm to 12nm in diameter are intermediate filaments (tonofilaments), which also lend skeletal support. Bundles of filaments comprise fibrils. Thus, myofibrils of skeletal muscle are comprised of small myofilaments (actin and myosin). Actin filaments also make up the core of microvilli, membrane modifications that project from the free surface of absorptive cells. The actin filaments of the microvilli intermingle with the filaments of the terminal web at the base of the microvilli.

Peroxisomes. Peroxisomes are small membrane-bound vesicles containing several oxidative enzymes involved in the production of hydrogen peroxide.

Coated Vesicles. The membranes of coated vesicles are coated on their cytoplasmic surface by several proteins (*e.g.,* clathrin). Coated vesicles are involved in intracellular transport or packaging of secretory material, or are specialized for the receptor-mediated endocytosis of macromolecules from the extracellular fluid. In the latter process the macromolecules are internalized when the coated plasma membrane to which it binds is pinched off as a coated vesicle. Cholesterol is internalized by this method. Coated vesicles join to form endosomes, before they fuse with lysosomes.

Inclusions. Glycogen, lipid droplets, and pigments (*e.g.,* lipofuscin, melanin, carotene) are stored in many of the cells of the body. Secretion granules are membrane-bound vesicles containing a protein or protein-carbohydrate secretory product.

Intercellular Junctions. Cells demonstrate variable degrees of cohesion and attachment. These junctions are particularly pronounced in epithelial and muscle tissues. ***Tight junctions*** (zonulae occludentes) form bands around the apical ends of epithelial cells. Since the outer leaflets of adjacent cell membranes fuse in a series of ridges in this type of junction, there is a relatively tight seal that prevents passage of materials from the lumen between the cells. The ***zonula adherens*** is a band that forms just deep to the tight junction. Microfilaments of the terminal web insert into a dense plaque on the cytoplasmic surface of the zonula membrane. This junction retains a 20-nm intercellular space. ***Desmosomes*** (maculae adherentes) are small spot junctions that are similar in structure to the zonula adherens, except that tonofilaments insert into the attachment plaque and there may be dense material in the intermediate space. The ***gap junction*** (nexus) is characterized as being an apposition of membranes of adjacent cells with a 2-nm intercellular space. This space is bridged by connexons that permit cells to communicate with each other through their 2-nm lumina.

PROTEIN SYNTHESES

The mechanisms for protein synthesis are important to understand because structural proteins comprise most of the important structures of the body and since most of the chemical reactions in the body are catalyzed by enzymes that are proteins. The general sequence of events in protein synthesis is the (1) activation of genes, (2) transcription of DNA to form messenger RNA (mRNA), (3) recognition of amino acids by their specific transfer RNA (tRNA) molecules, and (4) translation of the mRNA by the tRNA at the ribosomes (rRNA).

Activation of Genes. ***Structural genes*** (cistrons) are specific segments of the DNA molecule that provide coded messages essential for the assembly of certain amino acids in the production of specific structural proteins or enzymes. In order for different genes to exist, the double helix of DNA that comprises the chromosomes must possess structures whose variation in sequencing permits different proteins to be formed. These components of DNA are sequences of ***nucleotides.*** Each nucleotide is assembled so that one deoxyribose sugar unit and one unit of phosphoric acid provide part of the DNA strand while a nitrogenous base forms a side chain that pairs with the base of a nucleotide in the adjacent DNA strand of the double helix. The only four nitrogenous bases that exist in DNA are two purines, adenine (A) and guanine (G), and two pyrimidines, cytosine (C) and thymine (T). When the bases pair, adenine bonds only with thymine, and cytosine only with guanine. The sequence of the bases (*i.e.,* the sequence of genetic code letters A, T, C, and G) along a single strand of DNA determines which amino acids will be put together to form a particular protein. A sequence of three nitrogenous bases (codon) codes for each amino acid. Several codons in sequence form each cistron. Thus, the ***genetic code*** for protein synthesis is found in the nitrogenous base sequence of DNA.

Although each somatic cell contains all of the genes for that individual, relatively few genes are activated at any one time. A gene is activated only when a specific mRNA molecule is to be transcribed from the DNA. In this activation process, it appears that a specific gene regulatory protein acts as the activator by binding to the DNA and facilitating the binding of RNA polymerase to a promoter segment of the DNA. The latter binding promotes transcription of a specific mRNA when the specific RNA polymerase recognizes a starting point and moves down the gene to its termination signal. The affinity of the specific gene regulatory protein for the DNA may be increased or decreased by inducer and inhibitory ligands, respectively.

Transcription of Messenger RNA. Messenger RNA has a structure similar to a single strand of DNA, except that ribose sugar takes the place of deoxyribose, and thymine is replaced by uracil. When genes are activated, the DNA strands of the helix separate in the region of the involved cistron and the exposed nitrogenous bases serve as templates for the synthesis of a mRNA molecule. In this process adenine of the DNA pairs with uracil of the developing mRNA molecule, the thymine of DNA pairs with adenine of RNA, the guanine of DNA pairs with cytosine of RNA, and the cytosine of DNA pairs with guanine of RNA. The newly formed mRNA separates from the DNA strand, passes into the cytoplasm and becomes associated with tRNA.

Recognition and Transport of Amino Acids by Transfer RNA. Transfer RNA molecules are multipolar structures that are produced in the nucleus. Each tRNA molecule passes into the cytoplasm, where one of its poles recognizes and binds a specific amino acid. Another pole of each tRNA molecule contains a triplet of nitrogenous bases that is able to ''read'' the complementary codon of a mRNA molecule. A third pole recognizes ribosomes.

Translation of the Messenger RNA Message. Ribosomal RNA and tRNA play roles in translating the mRNA message. The small subunit of the ribosome attaches to a start codon on the mRNA molecule and then travels down the molecule from codon to codon. At each codon the appropriate tRNA that ''reads'' the codon attaches to the mRNA and deposits its amino acid. As each amino acid is assembled into a new protein molecule, the tRNAs are released and another ribosome may read the mRNA. When each ribosome reaches a stop codon, the translation is terminated. If the protein that is produced is a structural protein, the ribosomes used are free ribosomes. If the protein is to be a secretion product, the protein molecule passes through the ribosome, into the lumen of the rough (granular) endoplasmic reticulum, and through transfer vesicles to the region of the Golgi apparatus, where it is concentrated and packaged into secretory granules (storage vacuoles). When these membrane-bound granules fuse with the plasma membrane, the secretory product is elaborated by exocytosis. In some cells the concentration step is eliminated and the product is transferred directly to the plasma membrane from the endoplasmic reticulum and Golgi region.

CELL DIVISION

Somatic cells divide by the mitotic process of cell division, whereas sex cells divide by meiosis. Prior to both of these types of division the stem cell undergoes an interphase stage wherein the DNA is replicated during the S (synthesis) phase. In this replication process, the DNA strands separate (replication fork) when the bonds between nitrogenous bases are broken, and free nucleotides attach to their complementary bases. Thus, two new helices are formed of which one DNA strand in each helix has served as the template for the new chromatid. If mitosis occurs, the cell will divide into two daughter cells, each with the diploid number of 46 chromosomes. In meiosis two divisions (meiosis I and II) take place with no further replication of the DNA, thus producing four cells, each with the haploid (23) number of chromosomes.

Mitosis. After interphase the cell enters the ***prophase*** stage, where the chromosomal strands become coiled as they shorten and thicken. The two chromatids of each chromosome are joined by a centromere, the chromosomes are suspended in a spindle of microtubules that bridges between the two centrioles, and the nucleolus and nuclear envelope disappear. During ***metaphase*** the chromosomes align on a metaphase (equatorial) plate. In ***anaphase*** the chromosomes separate in the region of the centromeres, and each chromatid is pulled toward opposite poles of the cell. During ***telophase*** a cleavage furrow in the plasma membrane continues to separate the cytoplasm into two daughter cells while the nucleoli and nuclear envelope reappear.

Meiosis. In the first meiotic division (MI) cells undergo a lengthy prophase, and the homologous chromosomes come together in a synapsis. This configuration is called a tetrad of four chromatids. In metaphase these synapsed pairs line up on the equator, but they separate during anaphase and telophase so that the two new daughter cells will have only 23 chromosomes, each of which is represented by two chromatids. Thus, MI is a reduction division. In the second meiotic division (MII), the centromeres separate during metaphase so that each of the new daughter cells receives 23 chromatids, each of which becomes a new chromosome. The result of meiosis is the production of four sex cells from one stem cell, with each of the four cells having the haploid (23) number of chromosomes. In the female, three of the four daughter cells (polar bodies) die and do not become oocytes. In the male, all four daughter cells become spermatids, which transform into spermatozoa.

THE BACK AND THE HISTOLOGY OF BASIC TISSUES

Vertebral Column

INDIVIDUAL VERTEBRAE

Typical Vertebra. The component parts of the vertebral column, for the most part, are similar in construction. The two major portions are the anterior ***body*** and the posterior ***vertebral*** or ***neural arch.*** The body is in the form of a flattened cylinder that serves as the major weight-bearing portion of the vertebra. The vertebral arch is formed by the pedicles and laminae, has multiple projections, and together with the posterior aspect of the body forms the vertebral foramen. The paired ***pedicles*** project posteriorly from the posterolateral aspect of the upper half of each body, and the ***laminae*** project posteromedially (to join in the midline) from the posterior aspects of the pedicles. The ***transverse processes*** extend laterally from the arch; the ***single spinous*** process is directed posteriorly in the midline. The pairs of superior and inferior articular processes arise from the vertebral arch at about the junctions of the pedicles and laminae. Each articular process contains an articular facet, which is an articular surface of the zygapophyseal joint.

Regional Variation. The cervical region is unique because vertebra C1 and the upper aspect of C2 are anatomically and biomechanically different from the lower aspect of C2 and the rest of the cervical vertebrae. Vertebra C1 has no body but rather anterior and posterior arches that interconnect two lateral masses. Vertebra C2 is transitional in that it interconnects the upper and lower aspects of the cervical spine. The ***dens*** or ***odontoid process*** extends superiorly from the body of C2, and occupies the anterior area between the lateral masses of C1. Both the superior and inferior articular facets of C1, as well as the superior facets of C2, are positioned anterior to those of the rest of the cervical vertebrae. The delicate cervical vertebrae are distinguished by bifid spines and foramina in the transverse processes (C1–C6), which transmit the vertebral arteries. The bodies of vertebrae C3–C7 have prominent upward flares, ***uncinate processes,*** on their superolateral aspects. Thoracic vertebrae have articular facets or costal fovea (with which the ribs form synovial joints) on the posterolateral aspects of the bodies and the anterior aspects of the tips of the transverse processes, and very long spinous processes that are directed inferiorly so that they overlap the next lower vertebra. Lumbar vertebrae have very large heavy bodies and short strong spinous processes that are directed posteriorly. Their laminae are about half as high (superoinferiorly) as their bodies, and hence an interlaminar space exists between lumbar vertebrae.

CONNECTIONS BETWEEN ADJACENT VERTEBRAE

Joints. The vertebral arches are connected by the ***intervertebral*** or ***zygapophyseal articulations.*** These are synovial joints between the superior articular facets of the vertebra below and the inferior articular facets of the vertebra above. A thin joint capsule permits a limited amount of gliding motion between the articular surfaces. The orientation or plane of the joint space is a major determinant of the direction of motion that occurs between adjacent vertebrae.

The bodies are united (and separated) by a fibrocartilaginous ***intervertebral disk.*** This is a cartilaginous joint and thus permits limited motion. The disk is composed of a gelatinous core ***(nucleus pulposus)*** that is surrounded by a strong distensible envelope ***(anulus fibrosus)*** of fibrocartilage. The nucleus pulposus is separated from each vertebral body by a hyaline cartilage plate. Thus, the disk has all the physical properties of a closed fluid–elastic system; that is, any pressure within the disk is delivered equally and undiminished to all parts of the container, which in this case are the anulus fibrosus and the cartilaginous plates. The disk is also preloaded; it pushes the vertebral bodies apart and thus aids the alignment of adjacent vertebrae.

The ''joints of Luschka'' are found between the bodies of the lower cervical vertebrae (C2–C7), specifically between the uncinate processes of the lower vertebrae and the beveled inferolateral aspects of the bodies of the vertebrae above. These ''joints'' are thought to be clefts rather than true joints.

Ligaments. The ligaments of the vertebral column can be grouped into those that interconnect adjacent vertebrae and those that extend virtually the entire length of the vertebral column. The segmental ligaments include the ligamentum flavum, which connects the laminae, and the interspinous, supraspinous, and intertransverse ligaments, whose locations are self-explanatory. Two ligaments extend from the atlas to the sacrum. The anterior longitudinal ligament reinforces the anterior and anterolateral aspects of the vertebral bodies and intervertebral disks. The posterior longitudinal ligament attaches to the posterior aspects of the bodies and disks and is therefore within the vertebral canal. This ligament supports the posterior aspect of the disk in the midline but adds little support posterolaterally.

These ligaments are strong and tight and act to support the vertebral column as well as restrict motion. Spinal extension is limited by only the anterior longitudinal ligament while the rest of the above-named ligaments limit flexion. Side-bending is limited by the intertransverse ligaments. The intervertebral disk restricts motion in all directions.

VERTEBRAL COLUMN AS A WHOLE

Normal and Abnormal Curves. The anteroposterior curves of the vertebral column are compensatory adjustments to the bipedal posture. Normally each junctional area (lumbosacral, thoracolumbar, cervicothoracic, occipitocervical) is directly above the center of gravity of the body as a whole, and as a result little or no muscular activity is necessary to hold the spine upright during quiet standing. These curves are such that the lumbar and cervical regions present posterior concavities while the thoracic and sacral regions present posterior convexities. No lateral curvature normally exists. An exaggerated lumbar curve is called ***lordosis;*** an exaggerated thoracic curve, ***kyphosis.*** Any lateral curve is ***scoliosis.***

Motion of Vertebral Column. Motion of the vertebral column as a whole is the sum of the variable amount of motion that occurs between adjacent vertebrae. Although the intervertebral disk is easily distorted in any direction, and thus permits motion in any direction, its thickness is important in regulating the extent of motion. In addition, motion is limited by the tension of the vertebral column ligaments. The direction of motion is determined primarily by the orientation of the plane of the zygapophyseal joint. Motion in the upper portion of the cervical spine is limited because there are no intervertebral disks and because of the shapes of the vertebrae. Flexion and extension occur between the occipital condyles and C1; rotation is free between C1 and C2. In the lower cervical spine there are intervertebral disks and the planes of the zygapophyseal joints are obliquely oriented between the horizontal and coronal planes. As a result, flexion and extension, axial rotation, and lateral bending are quite free.

In the thoracic region the planes of the zygapophyseal joints are nearly coronal in orientation and thus permit flexion, extension, lateral bending, and rotation. However, all these motions are limited because of the thin intervertebral disks and the rigidity imposed by the rib cage.

The lumbar intervertebral disks are quite thick and the planes of the zygapophyseal joints are curved between the sagittal and coronal planes. The upper joints are more sagittal in orientation, the lower more coronal. This arrangement permits considerable flexion and extension, particularly between L5 and S1, but limits both lateral bending and rotation.

Integrity of the Vertebral Column. The static support of the normally aligned vertebral column is provided primarily by the ligaments discussed above as well as the intervertebral disk. As soon as motion occurs, the muscles become important in controlling the overall posture, but the relationship between adjacent vertebrae is still maintained by the ligaments. Bony support is a factor at only certain areas. The ***thoracic region*** is, of course, greatly reinforced by the thoracic cage; as a result vertebral dislocations seldom occur there. At other levels the only possible bony support is derived from the articular facets that form the zygapophyseal joints. The amount of this support, though, is dependent upon the orientation of the joint space. In the ***cervical region*** these joint spaces are nearly horizontal. As a result there is no bony block preventing one vertebra from sliding forward with respect to an adjoining vertebra. It follows that cervical dislocation can occur with only soft tissue damage (no fracture). On the other hand, the planes of the ***lumbar*** zygapophyseal joints are vertically oriented with the inferior articular facets overlapping the superior articular facets of the next lower vertebra. Any tendency toward dislocation is resisted by interlocking of the articular surfaces, and fracture usually accompanies dislocation.

The stability of the lower lumbar region (especially the ***lumbosacral junction***) is particularly dependent on bony support. The body of L5 is sitting on the anteriorly inclined superior aspect of the sacrum, and there is a natural tendency for this vertebra to slide anteriorly. This tendency is resisted by the zygapophyseal joints between L5 and the sacrum. Occasionally there is bony discontinuity of the lamina between the superior and inferior articular facets, a condition called ***spondylolysis.*** This means that the bony support normally provided by the zygapophyseal joint is lost, and anterior sliding of the L5 body is predisposed. Anterior subluxation of the vertebral body is referred to as ***spondylolisthesis.***

INTERVERTEBRAL FORAMEN

Normal Anatomy of the Intervertebral Foramen. The basic boundaries of this foramen are the same throughout the vertebral column. The superior and inferior aspects are the pedicles of the respective vertebrae. The anterior boundary consists of the intervertebral disk and portions of the adjacent vertebral bodies. Posteriorly the superior and inferior articular facets form the zygapophyseal joint. In addition, the ligamentum flavum blends with the medial aspect of the joint capsule of the zygapophyseal joint and thus forms the medial part of the posterior boundary. Although the specific anatomy of the foramen differs somewhat from region to region, pathology most commonly involves the more mobile cervical and lumbar regions; the following description is limited to those areas.

Pathology Involving the Intervertebral Foramen. In the ***cervical region*** the foramen is small, the intervertebral disk is positioned in the center of the anterior wall, and the relatively large spinal nerve practically fills the opening. Protrusion or rupture of the disk into the foramen will impinge on the nerve in the foramen; that is, rupture of the disk between cervical vertebrae 5 and 6 will involve spinal nerve C6. In addition, the size of the cervical intervertebral foramen can be reduced by inflammation of the zygapophyseal joint (arthritis) and by bony projections from the vertebral bodies. These bony spurs usually result from disk degeneration, which in turn causes irritation to ***Luschka's joints*** on the posterolateral aspects of the vertebral bodies. In the ***lumbar region*** the disk forms the lower half of the anterior wall of the foramen, and the upper vertebral body, the upper half. The opening is very large, and the relatively small spinal nerve exits in the upper part of the foramen opposite the vertebral body. Rupture of the disk at this level typically does not affect the spinal nerve in the same foramen but rather the spinal nerve that is descending in the anterolateral aspect of the vertebral canal (across the posterolateral aspect of the disk) to exit from the next lower intervertebral foramen. Thus, a rupture of the disk between lumbar vertebrae 4 and 5 will usually impinge on spinal nerve L5.

MICROSCOPIC STRUCTURE OF THE CONNECTIVE AND SUPPORTIVE TISSUES

The adult connective and supportive tissues are connective tissue proper, cartilage, and bone. ***Connective tissue proper*** is further classified into loose irregular (areolar) connective tissue and dense regular and irregular connective tissues. These tissues contain cells and a preponderance of intercellular fibers and ground substance.

Loose Irregular Connective Tissue. Loose connective tissue is found in the superficial and deep fascia and as the stroma of most organs. It is generally considered as the packing material of the body. Loose connective tissue contains most of the cell types and all of the fiber types found in the other connective tissues. The most common cell types are the fibroblast, macrophage, adipose cell, mast cell, plasma cell, and wandering cells from the blood. ***Fibroblasts*** contain the organelles that permit them to produce all of the fiber types and the intercellular material (see Table 2-1). In their production of these proteinaceous substances, mRNA, rRNA, and tRNA are produced in the nucleus and pass to the cytoplasm. Amino acids that have been taken into the fibroblast attach to specific tRNA and are translated on the mRNA in the region of the ribosomes of the RER. The polypeptides

TABLE 2-1. Secretory Cells and Their Products*

ORGAN SYSTEM: ORGAN, TISSUE, CELLS	PRODUCT
Skeletal (Connective tissue, cartilage, bone)	
Mast cells	Heparin, histamine
Fibroblasts, chondrocytes, osteocytes	Procollagen, elastin, GAGs
Osteoclasts	Hydrolytic enzymes
Plasma cells	Antibodies
Muscular	
Smooth muscle	Elastin
Nervous	
Neurons	Neurotransmitters (*e.g.*, epinephrine, norepinephrine, acetylcholine, GABA, dopamine, serotonin, substance P, oxytocin, ADH)
Schwann cells, oligodendroglia	Myelin*
Choroid plexus	Cerebrospinal fluid
Endocrine organs	
Pituitary gland and hypothalamus	(See Table 2-2.)
Thyroid	
Follicular cells	Thyroxine, triiodothyronine
Parafollicular cells	Calcitonin
Parathyroid chief cells	Parathyroid hormone
Suprarenal	
Zona glomerulosa	Mineralocorticoids (*e.g.*, aldosterone)
Zona fasciculata and zona reticularis	Glucocorticoids (*e.g.*, cortisol) and dehydroepiandrosterone
Medulla	Norepinephrine and epinephrine
(See below for reproductive endocrine cells.)	
Digestive	
Oral Cavity	
Von Ebner's and parotid glands	Serous secretion
Submandibular and sublingual	Serous and mucous secretions
Odontoblasts	Dentin
Ameloblasts	Enamel
Esophagus	
Mucosal and submucosal glands	Mucus
Stomach	
Lining epithelium, neck mucous cells, and cardiac glands	Mucus
Chief cells	Pepsin
Parietal cells	HCl, intrinsic antipernicious anemia factor
Enteroendocrine	Gastrin, glucagon
Pyloric glands	Alkaline glycoprotein secretion
Intestines	
Goblet cells	Mucus
Brunner's glands	Alkaline glycoprotein secretion
Paneth cells	Lysozyme
Enteroendocrine cells	Secretin, cholecystokinin, glucagonlike substance, somatostatin, gastric inhibitory polypeptide, motilin, serotonin, substance P, vasoactive intestinal polypeptide
Liver	
Hepatocytes	Bile, lipoprotein, prothrombin, albumin, fibrinogen, glucose
Pancreas	
Acinar cells	Protease, nuclease, amylase, lipase
Centroacinar and intercalated duct cells	Sodium bicarbonate
Islet alpha cells	Glucagon
Beta cells	Insulin
Delta cells	Somatostatin, gastrin(?)
Respiratory	
Bowman's glands	Serous secretion
Goblet cells	Mucus
Great alveolar (type II) cells	Surfactant

TABLE 2-1. *(continued)*

ORGAN SYSTEM: ORGAN, TISSUE, CELLS	PRODUCT
Cardiovascular (blood)	
Neutrophils and eosinophils	Hydrolytic enzymes
Basophils	Heparin and histamine
Platelets and megakaryocyte precursor	Serotonin, thromboplastin
Eye	
Tarsal glands	Sebum
Lacrimal glands	Tears
Ciliary body epithelium	Aqueous humor
Ear	
Stria vascularis of cochlea, cells of crista ampullares and maculae	Endolymph
Ceruminous glands	Cerumen (ear wax)
Integumentary	
Stratum germinativum	Tonofilaments, which become keratin*
Stratum granulosum	Interfilament matrix and membrane-coating substance of stratum corneum*
Melanocytes	Melanin
Sebaceous glands	Sebum
Sweat glands	Sweat
Mammary gland	Milk proteins and lipids
Urinary (kidney)	
Juxtaglomerular cells	Renin
Reproductive	
Male	
Seminiferous epithelium	Sperm
Sertoli cells	Androgen-binding protein, transferrin, inhibin, lactate
Interstial cells of Leydig	Testosterone
Seminal vesicle	Alkaline fluid rich in fructose
Prostate gland	Acid secretion rich in citric acid and acid phosphatase
Bulbourethral and urethral glands	Mucus
Female	
Theca interna cells	Androstenedione
Membrana granulosa cells	Estrogen, progesterone
Granulosa lutein cells	Estrogen, progesterone
Theca lutein cells	Estrogen(?)
Uterine glands	Glycogen-rich mucoid secretion
Cervical glands	Mucus
Cytotrophoblast cells	GnRH, Syncytial trophoblast
Syncytial trophoblast	Estrogen, progesterone, HCG, HPL (somatomammotropin, HCS), HCT

* This list is not complete; some cell products are also parts of cells.

GAGs = glycosaminoglycans
GnRH = gonadotropin-releasing hormone
HCG = human chorionic gonadotropin
HCS = human chorionic somatomammotropin
HCT = human chorionic thyrotropin
HPL = human placental lactogen

produced pass through the cisternae of the RER to the region of the Golgi complex where they are packaged into membrane-bound procollagen macromolecules that attach to the cell surface before discharge from the fibroblast. Outside the cell, the procollagen molecules are cleaved of their registration peptides forming tropocollagen, which is assembled into ***collagen*** (for a summary of most secretory cells of the body and their secretion, see Table 2-1). The Golgi complex also is responsible for adding the carbohydrate components to the glycosaminoglycans (GAGs) (mucopolysaccharides) of the ground substance. ***Macrophages*** are part of the reticuloendothelial system (mononuclear phagocyte system). They possess large lysosomes containing digestive enzymes, which are necessary for the digestion of phagocytized materials. ***Mast cells*** occur mostly along blood vessels and contain granules that represent the heparin and histamine produced by these cells. ***Plasma cells*** are part of the immune system in that they produce circulating antibodies. They are extremely basophilic because of their extensive RER. ***Adipose cells*** are found in varying quantities. When they predominate, the tissue is called adipose tissue.

Collagenous, reticular, and elastic fibers are irregularly distributed in loose connective tissue. Collagenous fibers are usually found in bundles of fibers and provide strength to the tissue. Each fiber is made up of fibrils, which are composed of staggered monomers of tropocollagen giving a 640Å periodicity to most normal collagen in the body. Many different types of collagen are identified on the basis of their molecular structure. Of the five most common types, collagen type I is the most abundant, being found in dermis, bone, dentin, tendons, organ capsules, fascia, and sclera. Type II is located in hyaline and elastic cartilage. Type III probably is the collagenous component of reticular fibers. Type IV is found in basal laminas. Type V is a component of placental basement membranes. Reticular fibers are smaller, more delicate fibers that form the basic framework of reticular connective tissue. Elastic fibers branch and provide elasticity and suppleness to connective tissue.

Ground substance is the gelatinous material that fills most of the space between the cells and fibers. It is composed of acid mucopolysaccharides (GAGs) and structural glycoproteins, and its properties are important in determining the permeability and consistency of the connective tissue.

Dense Connective Tissue. Dense irregular connective tissue is found in the dermis, periosteum, perichondrium, and capsules of some organs. All of the fiber types are present, but collagenous fibers predominate. Dense regular connective tissue occurs as aponeuroses, ligaments, and tendons. In most ligaments and tendons collagenous fibers are most prevalent and are oriented parallel to each other; fibroblasts are the only cell type present. The ligamenta flava are considered elastic ligaments because elastic fibers dominate.

Cartilage. Cartilage is composed of ***chondrocytes*** embedded in an intercellular matrix, consisting of fibers and an amorphous firm ground substance. Three types of cartilage (hyaline, elastic, and fibrous) are distinguished on the basis of the amount of ground substance and the relative abundance of collagenous and elastic fibers.

Hyaline cartilage is found as costal cartilages, articular cartilages, and cartilages of the nose, larynx, trachea, and bronchi. The intercellular matrix consists primarily of collagenous fibers and a ground substance rich in chondromucoprotein, a copolymer of a protein and chondroitin sulfates. The gel-like firmness of cartilage depends on the electrostatic bonds between collagen and the GAGs and the binding of water to the GAGs. The GAGs are composed of chondroitin and keratan sulfates covalently linked to core proteins, which are bound to hyaluronic acid molecules. Chondrocytes occupy lacunae. During the growth period of the cartilage these cells existed as chondroblasts, and they produced the intercellular matrix. All types of cartilage grow interstitially by the mitoses of cells in the center of the cartilage mass; most types also grow appositionally by the formation of chondroblasts from undifferentiated cells in the cellular layer of the perichondrium. Unlike the fibrous layer of the perichondrium, the cellular layer and the cartilage are avascular, so they receive nutriments and oxygen through diffusion from blood vessels in the fibrous layer of the perichondrium. Articular cartilages receive nutriments by diffusion from blood vessels in the marrow and from the synovial fluid. With old age, there is a decrease of acid mucopolysaccharides, an increase in noncollagenous proteins, and calcification may occur because of degenerative changes in the cartilage cells.

Elastic cartilage is found in the pinna of the ear, auditory tube and epiglottic, corniculate and cuneiform cartilages of the larynx. Elastic fibers predominate and thus provide greater flexibility to this cartilage. Calcification of elastic cartilage is rare.

Fibrous cartilage occurs in the anchorage of tendons and ligaments, in intervertebral disks, in the symphysis pubis, and in some interarticular disks and ligaments. Chondrocytes occur singly or in rows between large bundles of collagenous fibers. Compared with hyaline cartilage, only small amounts of hyaline matrix surround the chondrocytes of fibrous cartilage.

Bone. Bone tissue consists of ***osteocytes*** and an intercellular matrix that contains organic and inorganic components. The organic matrix consists of dense collagenous fibers and an osseomucoid substance containing chondroitin sulfate. The inorganic component is responsible for the rigidity of bone and is composed chiefly of calcium phosphate and calcium carbonate with small amounts of magnesium, fluoride, hydroxide, and sulfate. Electron microscopic studies show that these minerals are deposited in an orderly fashion on the surface of the collagenous fibrils in their interband areas. In the basic organization of bone tissue, osteocytes lie in lacunae and extend protoplasmic processes into small canaliculi in the intercellular matrix. The protoplasmic processes of adjacent osteocytes are in contact with one another and gap junctions are present. The matrix is organized into adjacent layers or lamellae. The number and arrangement of lamellae differ between compact and cancellous bone.

Compact bone contains haversian systems (osteons), interstitial lamellae and circumferential lamellae. ***Haversian systems*** consist of extensively branching haversian canals that are oriented chiefly longitudinally in long bones. Each canal contains blood vessels and osteogenic cells and is surrounded by 8 to 15 concentric lamellae and osteocytes. The collagenous fibers in adjacent lamellae run essentially at right angles to each other and spiral around the canal. Nutriments from blood vessels in the haversian canals pass through canaliculi and lacunae to reach all osteocytes in the system. Interstitial lamellae occur between haversian systems and represent the remains of parts of degenerating haversian and circumferential lamellae. Outer and inner circumferential lamellae occur under the periosteum and endosteum, respectively. Volkmann's canals enter through the outer circumferential lamellae and carry blood vessels and nerves that are continuous with those of the haversian canals and the periosteum. Sharpey's fibers are coarse perforating fibers that anchor the periosteum to the outer circumferential lamellae.

Bones are supplied by a loop of blood vessels that enter from the periosteal region, penetrate the cortical bone, and enter the medulla before returning to the periphery of the bone. Long bones are specifically supplied by arteries that pass to the marrow through diaphyseal, metaphyseal, and epiphyseal arteries. In the marrow cavity, some arteries end in sinusoids, and others branch and enter the haversian canals, where they supply fenestrated capillaries. The marrow sinusoids drain to veins that leave through nutrient canals. The capillaries of the haversian canals drain to veins that pass centrifugally to the periosteum and adjacent muscles.

Bone undergoes extensive remodeling, and haversian systems may break down or be resorbed in order that calcium can be made available to other tissues of the body. Bone resorption occurs by osteocytic osteolysis or by osteoclastic activity. In ***osteocytic osteolysis,*** osteocytes resorb bone that lies immediately around the lacunae. In ***osteoclastic activity,*** large multinucleated osteoclasts arise from osteoprogenitor cells and abut against an osseous surface. Here, their extensive ruffled surfaces and proteolytic enzyme secretions seem to be involved in the resorption of more extensive portions of bone than in osteocytic osteolysis. Osteoclasts are components of the mononuclear phagocyte system. In this way, portions of old haversian systems are resorbed, or longitudinal depressions are formed on the periosteal and endosteal surfaces of the bone. If new haversian systems are to be laid down in the gutters or tubes that remain after the resorptive process is complete, osteoblasts differentiate from osteogenic cells of the enlarged haversian canal or periosteum and begin to lay down a lamella at the periphery of the space. Successive new concentric lamellae are laid down inside this initial lamella.

Cancellous bone differs from compact bone in that the lamellae are organized into trabeculae or spicules. Few haversian systems are present, and most osteocytes are generally closer to the blood supply than in compact bone.

BONE DEVELOPMENT

Development of Vertebrae and Ribs. At the end of the second postfertilization week, the primitive streak gives rise to cells that migrate laterally between the ectoderm and entoderm, forming the intraembryonic mesoderm. At approximately the same time the notochord arises as a cranial midline migration from the primitive node. As development progresses, the intraembryonic mesoderm adjacent to the notochord thickens into longitudinal masses called the paraxial mesoderm. From the 21st to 30th days, the paraxial mesoderm differentiates into 42 to 44 paired segments called somites. This craniocaudal development of somites gives rise to four occipital, eight cervical, 12 thoracic, five lumbar, five sacral, and eight to ten coccygeal somites. Each somite further differentiates so that three distinct cellular regions are apparent. The ventromedial region, known as the sclerotome, eventually gives rise to supportive skeletal structures (*e.g.,* vertebrae and ribs); the dorsomedial part, called the myotome, forms the skeletal muscles; and the dorsolateral portion, called the dermatome, gives rise to the dermis of the skin and subcutaneous tissue.

During the fourth week the sclerotomic mesenchymal mass of each somite begins to migrate toward the midline to become aggregated about the notochord. In this migration, cells of the caudal half of each somite shift caudally to meet the cranially migrating cranial half of the adjacent sclerotome. From each of these joined masses, mesenchymal processes grow dorsally around the neural tube to form the neural arches of the vertebrae, and also give rise to rib primordia. Since a vertebra develops from parts of two pairs of adjacent sclerotomes the original intersegmental arteries will come to pass across the middle of the vertebral bodies. The segmental spinal nerves to the myotomes will come to lie at the level of the intervertebral disks and the myotomes. The notochord degenerates in the region of the vertebral bodies but persists in the center of the intervertebral disk as the nucleus pulposus. In the cervical region, the migration of sclerotome accounts for the formation of seven cervical vertebrae from eight somites. This is due to the cranial half of the first sclerotome becoming part of the occipital bone while the caudal half of the eighth sclerotome becomes part of the first thoracic vertebra. Thus, the first cervical nerve passes between the occipital bone and first cervical vertebra, while the eighth cervical nerve emerges between the seventh cervical and first thoracic vertebrae.

At 7 weeks separate ***chondrification centers*** develop in the bodies and the lateral half of each neural arch, and these subsequently fuse together. Later, ***ossification***

centers develop in the vertebral bodies, in each half of the neural arch and in each rib. These remain as separate centers throughout fetal life. The rib primordia give rise to ribs in the thoracic region, transverse processes of the lumbar vertebrae, parts of the transverse processes in the cervical region, and the alae of the sacrum. Rib primordia may become attached to either cervical or lumbar vertebrae, leading to cervical or lumbar ribs. In spondylolisthesis there is usually a defect in the formation of the pedicles due to nonunion of ossification centers. In this condition the spine, laminae, and inferior articular processes of the affected lower lumbar vertebra stay in place, while the body migrates anteriorly with respect to the vertebra below it. In spina bifida conditions there is failure of the neural arches to unite properly in the formation of the spinous process.

The Microscopic Development of Bone. There are two basic patterns of bone formation: intramembranous and endochondral. In both of these types of bone formation, the process of forming bone tissue and the histologic structure of the bone formed are identical. The major difference between these two types of development is the environment within which bone tissue is laid down.

Intramembranous bone formation occurs in flat bones of the skull and face as well as in the clavicle. In this type of development ectomesenchymal (mesenchyme derived from neural crest) cells differentiate into osteoblasts in a region where mesenchymal cells have produced a fine-fibered vascular membrane. The osteoblasts lay down lamellae of collagenous fibers and ground substance in the form of a meshwork of trabeculae within the membrane. Some osteoblasts become entrapped as osteocytes in this osteoid tissue. When organic ***osteoid tissue*** becomes impregnated with inorganic salts, it is called ***osseous tissue.*** Some intertrabecular spaces become marrow cavities when their mesenchyme differentiates into reticular connective tissue and blood-forming cells. Others become haversian canals as concentric lamellae are formed. At the periphery of the entire developing bone (*e.g.*, outer and inner surfaces of skull bones) the bone becomes quite compact in its development. This is accomplished by a mesenchymal condensation around the bone that differentiates into a periosteum. The inner cells of the periosteum become osteoblasts and lay down compact bone. Thus, the bone takes on an appearance of outer and inner tables of compact bone, between which is the diploe of spongy trabecular bone. Osteoclasts are associated with bone resorption, which takes place chiefly on the inner surfaces of the tables and trabeculae. The membranous junction between two developing flat bones is eventually ossified as a suture.

Endochondral bone formation is characterized by a cartilage model of the bone preceding bone histogenesis. In the formation of the cartilage model of a long bone, the oldest cartilage is found in the center of the shaft (diaphyseal) region. Cells in this region hypertrophy, produce phosphatase, and bring about calcification of the surrounding cartilaginous matrix. The result of this calcification is inhibition of diffusion of nutrient materials to the chondrocytes, and they die or they may become osteoprogenitor cells. While the cartilage in the center of the shaft is calcifying, the chondrogenic layer of the perichondrium is becoming vascularized. In this new environment, the undifferentiated mesenchymal cells of the chondrogenic layer start to differentiate into osteoblasts, which lay down a bony collar around the shaft of the cartilage model. The perichondrium is now a periosteum. Osteogenic tissue, containing osteoprogenitor cells and blood vessels from this osteogenic layer of the periosteum, pass between the trabeculae of the bony collar and penetrate into the degenerating calcified cartilage. This periosteal bud of tissue is instrumental in resorption of some of the smaller calcified cartilage spicules between lacunae and in the laying down of bone on remnants of the calcified cartilage. The center of the shaft now consists of bone marrow precursor cells, osteogenic tissue, and bony trabeculae that contain remnant cores of calcified cartilage. This area in the diaphysis is called the primary ossification center.

Since the newer cartilage lies toward the epiphyses, the ***metaphyses,*** (epiphyseal plates, physes) demonstrate the following developmental gradient as the diaphysis is approached: (1) a layer of tissue where cells are not dividing (zone of resting cartilage); (2) a layer where chondrocytes are dividing mitotically and interstitially in an axial orientation (zone of multiplication); (3) a layer where cells are enlarging (zone of cellular hypertrophy and maturation); and (4) a layer where the intercellular material is calcifying and cells are dying (zone of calcification). The shaft grows in length by the multiplication of cartilage cells at the zones of multiplication in each metaphyseal region and by osseous tissue being laid down on the remnants of calcified cartilage in the zone of calcification. This process also brings about an increase in length of the primary marrow cavity. An increase in width of the marrow cavity takes place by resorption of bone on the inner surface of the periosteal bony collar. Since this resorption is not as rapid as the appositional laying down of bone on the outer surface of the bony collar, the compact bone of the shaft increases in width.

Secondary ossification centers develop later in fetal life, or after birth, in the epiphyses. These are usually characterized by hypertrophy of chondrocytes and calcification of cartilage in the centers of the epiphyses where the older cartilage cells exist. Vascular and osteogenic buds of tissue enter the area from the metaphyseal region. A thin layer of dense bone is laid down on the surfaces of the epiphyses where a periosteum is present. On articular surfaces, no periosteum or perichondrium exists, and hyaline cartilage is retained as a covering to the underlying epiphyseal bone.

Muscles of the Back

SUPERFICIAL MUSCLES OF THE BACK

The superficial muscles of the back are found superficial to the thoracolumbar fascia. They represent most of the ***extrinsic muscles of the shoulder*** in that they interconnect the axial and appendicular portions of the skeleton, specifically extending from the vertebral column or rib cage to the scapula, clavicle, or humerus. Functionally, they are concerned with motion of the shoulder girdle and humerus. Innervation is supplied mainly by branches of the brachial plexus. The ***trapezius*** is innervated by the accessory (11th cranial) nerve and controls the position of the shoulder statically as well as during virtually any motion, especially when the arm is abducted or flexed. The ***latissimus dorsi*** is the major extendor of the humerus and shoulder depressor (the ''crutch-walking'' muscle), and is innervated by the thoracodorsal nerve. A plane of three muscles underlying the trapezius connects the vertebral column and scapula. The ***levator scapulae*** and the ***rhomboid major*** and ***minor*** are innervated by the dorsal scapular nerve and direct branches of the cervical plexus. The ***serratus anterior*** extends from the medial border of the scapula to the anterolateral thoracic wall. It functions to hold the medial surface of the scapula against the thorax and, working with the trapezius, is important in shoulder abduction and flexion. The long thoracic nerve innervates this muscle.

DEEP MUSCLES OF THE BACK

The deep or ***intrinsic muscles of the back*** consist of multiple groups of muscles that extend from the occipital bone to the sacrum, occupy the depression formed by the spinous and transverse processes, and are innervated segmentally by branches of the dorsal rami. Bilateral contraction of these muscles produces extension of the vertebral column; unilateral contraction causes side-bending and rotation. The ***spinotransversalis group*** consists of the ***splenius capitis*** and ***cervicis muscles,*** which are the most superficial muscles in the cervical and upper thoracic region. The ***erector spinae (sacrospinalis) group*** extends the entire length of the spine and consists of the laterally positioned ***iliocostalis,*** the medial ***spinalis,*** and the intermediate ***longissimus.*** The ***transversospinal group*** is deep to the erector spinae and consists of the obliquely oriented ***semispinalis, multifidi,*** and ***rotators.*** The deepest muscles are the ***segmental group,*** which consists of the ***interspinales*** and the ***intertransversarri muscles.*** The four ***suboccipital muscles*** occupy the interval between the occipital bone and vertebra C2. These muscles are the ***obliquus capitis superior*** and ***inferior,*** and the ***rectus capitis posterior major*** and ***minor.***

MICROSCOPIC STRUCTURE OF MUSCLE TISSUE

There are three types of muscle tissue: smooth, skeletal, and cardiac. All three types are comprised of muscle cells (fibers) that contain myofibrils possessing contractile filaments of actin and myosin.

Smooth Muscle. Smooth muscle cells are spindle-shaped and are organized chiefly into sheets or bands of smooth muscle tissue. This tissue is found in blood vessels and other tubular visceral structures. Smooth muscle cells contain both actin and myosin filaments, but the actin filaments predominate. The filaments are not organized into patterns that give cross striations as in cardiac and skeletal muscle. Filaments course obliquely in the cells and attach to the plasma membrane. Electron microscopy shows the plasma membrane as a ''typical'' trilaminar membrane. In specific regions where smooth muscle cells appose each other, leaving only narrow 2nm intercellular gaps, specialized zones of contact occur, which are known as nexuses or ''gap'' junctions. These junctions probably facilitate the transmission of impulses for contraction. In other intercellular regions a glycoprotein coat and a small amount of collagenous and reticular fibers are found.

Skeletal Muscle. Skeletal muscle fibers are characterized by their peripherally located nuclei and their striated myofibrils. The cross striations are due to the organization and distribution of actin and myosin filaments. These striations are organized within each muscle fiber into fundamental contractile units called ***sarcomeres,*** which are joined end to end at the Z lines (Fig. 2-1). The striations in a sarcomere consist of an A band bordered toward the Z lines by I bands. The I bands of a sarcomere are really half I bands that join at the Z lines with the other half I bands of adjacent sarcomeres. The midregion of the A band contains a variable light H band that is bisected by an M line. The light I band contains actin filaments that insert into the Z line. These filaments interdigitate and are cross bridged in the A band with myosin filaments, forming a hexagonal pattern of one myosin filament surrounded by six actin filaments. In the contraction of a muscle fiber a chemical reaction takes place in the region of the crossbridges, causing the actin filaments of the I band to move deeper into the A band, thus resulting in a shortening of the I bands.

Each skeletal muscle fiber is invested with a sarcolemma (plasmalemma) that extends into the fiber as numerous small transverse T tubules. These tubules ring the myofibrils at the A-I junction and are bordered on each

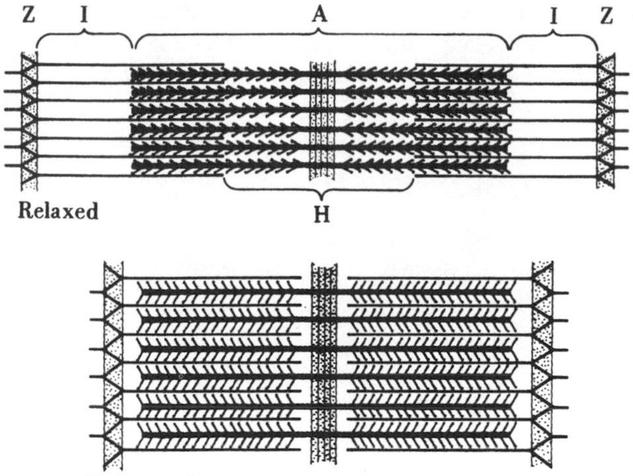

Fig. 2-1. Diagram of a sarcomere in the relaxed state *(top)* and contracted state *(bottom)*. During contraction the thin actin filaments of the I band are pulled into the A band by the myosin heads of the thick myosin filaments, thus reducing the length of the I bands and H zones. (Cormack DH: Ham's Histology, 9th ed, p 393. Philadelphia, JB Lippincott, 1987. Courtesy of E. Schultz and C. P. Leblond)

side by terminal cisternae of the sarcoplasmic (endoplasmic) reticulum. This arrangement of one T tubule with two terminal cisternae is called a triad. In excitation-contraction coupling, acetylcholine released from the motor end-plate causes depolarization of the muscle membrane, which is propagated to the T tubule-sarcoplasmic reticulum junction. This brings about release of calcium from the terminal cisternae of the sarcoplasmic reticulum, catalyzing the chemical reaction between the actin and myosin filaments in the region of the cross-bridges. In this process, calcium attaches to the TnC subunit of troponin, resulting in movement of tropomyosin and uncovering of the active sites for the attachment of actin to the cross-bridging heads of myosin. Because of this attachment, ATP in the myosin head hydrolyzes, producing energy, Pi and ADP, which results in a bending of the myosin head and a pulling of the actin filament into the A band. The actin-myosin bridges detach when myosin binds a new ATP molecule and when calcium returns to the terminal cisternae at the conclusion of neural stimulation.

Cardiac Muscle. Cardiac muscle contains striations and myofibrils that are similar to those of skeletal muscle. It differs from skeletal muscle in several major ways. Cardiac muscle fibers branch and contain centrally located nuclei and large numbers of mitochondria. Individual cardiac muscle cells are attached to each other at their ends by ***intercalated disks.*** These disks contain several types of membrane junctional complexes, the most important of which is the gap junction. This junction electrically couples one cell to its neighbor so that electrical depolarization is propagated through the heart by cell-to-cell contacts rather than by nerve innervation to each cell. The sarcoplasmic reticulum-T tubule system is arranged differently in cardiac muscle than in skeletal muscle. In cardiac muscle each T tubule enters at the Z line and forms a diad with only one terminal cisterna of sarcoplasmic reticulum.

DEVELOPMENT OF SKELETAL MUSCLES

Histogenesis of Skeletal Muscle. Skeletal muscle cells develop from mesenchyme that arises from the myotomes of somites or from the mesoderm of branchial arches. Stellate mesenchymal cells differentiate into elongated multinucleate myotubes containing peripherally located myofibrils and centrally located nuclei. Later in development, myofibrils will increase in size and number and the nuclei will migrate peripherally. In the limited regeneration of muscle, new fibers may be formed from satellite cells that lie between the skeletal muscle cell and its basement membrane.

Morphogenesis of the Skeletal Musculature. In the trunk and extremities, myotomes divide into a dorsally located epimere and a ventrally located hypomere. Dorsal and ventral rami develop from the segmental spinal nerves and innervate the epimere and hypomere, respectively. The epimere gives rise to the deep muscles of the back. Thus, these muscles, such as erector spinae, are innervated by the dorsal (primary) rami of spinal nerves. The hypomere develops into anterior and lateral body wall muscles of the cervical and thoracolumbar regions. Muscles of the extremities and those that attach the limbs to the trunk may arise from local somatic lateral mesoderm but are innervated by the ventral rami of spinal nerves. Subsequent migrations of segmental myoblasts, trailing their respective nerves, lead to the formation of complex nerve fiber plexuses from successive spinal cord levels. In addition to migration, five other basic processes occur in the establishment of muscles: (1) fusions of portions of successive myotomes (*e.g.,* erector spinae), (2) change from the original cephalocaudal direction of the fibers (*e.g.,* transversus abdominus), (3) longitudinal splitting of a myotomic mass to form more than one muscle (*e.g.,* rhomboideus major and minor), (4) tangential splitting (*e.g.,* intercostals), and (5) degeneration of parts or all of a myotome with conversion of the degenerated part to connective tissue (*e.g.,* serratus posterior inferior and superior).

Muscles of the head develop from eye (preotic) and tongue somites and from branchial arch mesenchyme. Some implicate neural crest cells in head muscle development.

Spinal Cord and Spinal Nerves

GROSS ANATOMY OF SPINAL CORD AND SPINAL NERVES

Basic Organization. The nervous system is composed of the central and peripheral nervous systems. The ***central nervous system (CNS)*** is enclosed within the cranial vault and vertebral canal and consists respectively of the brain and spinal cord. The ***peripheral nervous system*** is outside this bony encasement and is composed of peripheral nerves, which are branches of or continuations of the cranial and spinal nerves. The ***autonomic nervous system*** is anatomically a portion of both the central and peripheral nervous systems. The usual definition of this system is an anatomical one that includes the motor side of the system controlling smooth and cardiac muscle, glands, and viscera, and thus can be called the general visceral efferent system.

The spinal cord is a long cylindrical structure with a very small hollow core called the ***central canal.*** The central canal is a portion of the ***ventricular system.*** It is surrounded by the gray matter (cell bodies and terminal arborizations), which is in turn surrounded by the white matter (long ascending and descending pathways). The spinal cord is segmented, each segment corresponding to a specific portion of the body wall (including extremities) that it innervates. The diameter of the cord decreases from top to bottom with the exceptions of the low cervical and the lumbosacral regions, where enlargements include additional neurons for the innervation of the upper and lower extremities, respectively. The spinal cord terminates inferiorly at the inferior aspect of the first lumbar vertebra. This termination is in the form of an inverted cone and thus is called the ***conus medullaris.*** Vertical lines of nerve rootlets attach to the anterolateral and posterolateral aspects of the cord. The rootlets from a single segment coverge and form ***anterior*** and ***posterior roots.*** The two roots join in the intervertebral foramen to form the ***spinal nerve*** (Fig. 2-2). After exiting from the intervertebral foramen, the spinal nerve divides into ***ventral*** and ***dorsal rami*** whose muscular and cutaneous branches supply the body wall structures.

Both the brain and spinal cord are surrounded by three membranes that have both trophic and protective functions (see Fig. 2-2). For the most part the ***meninges*** of brain and cord are similar. The differences are outlined later in this chapter. The innermost layer of the meninges, the ***pia mater,*** is a thin membrane that conforms very closely to the contours of the spinal cord and brain and is firmly attached to the neural tissue. The vessels that supply the central nervous system are found in this membrane. The ***denticulate ligament*** is a series of pial extensions that project laterally and attach to the outermost meningeal covering, the ***dura mater.*** These ligaments serve to stabilize the spinal cord. The intermediate layer of the meninges is the ***arachnoid,*** a thin filmy membrane attached to the pia by numerous trabeculae. The area between the arachnoid and pia is the ***subarachnoid space,*** which is filled with cerebrospinal fluid. This fluid holds the arachnoid tightly against the outer dura mater; as a result, the ***subdural space*** is only a potential space. Together the pia and arachnoid are the soft coverings of the spinal cord and are called the ***leptomeninges.*** The dura mater is a strong thin membrane, the ***pachymeninx.*** It is

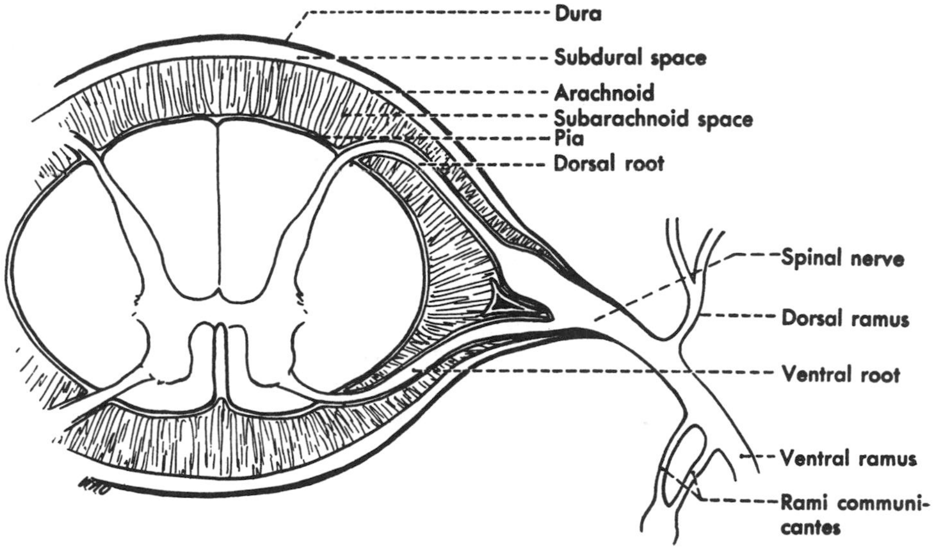

Fig. 2-2. Cross-sectional diagram of the spinal cord, nerve roots, and meninges. (Hollinshead WH: Anatomy For Surgeons, Vol 3, 3rd ed, p 175. Philadelphia, JB Lippincott, 1982)

separated from the bones and ligaments of the vertebral canal by the ***epidural space*** in which the epidural fat and ***internal venous plexus*** are found. This plexus is valueless and interconnects the body cavities and cranial vault. The dura, as well as the pia and arachnoid, extends laterally at the level of each spinal nerve and becomes continuous with the connective tissue coverings of the nerves. Inferiorly, the dural sac terminates at the second sacral vertebra. Since the arachnoid is so closely held against the inner aspect of the dura, the dural sac and subarachnoid space are co-extensive.

Relationship of Spinal Cord to Vertebral Column. The spinal cord extends from the foramen magnum to the lower border of the first lumbar vertebra. This means that only the very uppermost cervical cord segments are opposite the vertebra of the same name. Upper thoracic cord segments are one vertebral level higher than their correspondingly named vertebra, while the lumbar, sacral, and coccygeal cord segments lie opposite the last two thoracic and first lumbar vertebrae. Since each spinal nerve exits through its original intervertebral foramen, only the highest cervical spinal nerves are horizontally oriented, while each next lower spinal nerve is more obliquely oriented as it travels farther to its intervertebral foramen. As a result of this incongruity between spinal cord and vertebral column, the symptoms resulting from a spinal cord lesion do not usually correspond to the vertebral level of the lesion. For example, a lesion at vertebral level T12 could logically be accompanied by symptoms that correspond to cord segments L3 and below. The ***cauda equina*** is composed of lower lumbar, sacral, and coccygeal roots; these structures are the only neural elements in the subarachnoid space between the end of the spinal cord and the end of the dural sac. This area is the region of choice for spinal tap, as there is minimal risk to neural structures when a needle is inserted into the subarachnoid space. In addition, the interlaminar space between lumbar vertebrae allows easy access.

MICROSCOPIC STRUCTURE OF SPINAL NERVES AND THE SPINAL CORD

Spinal Nerves. The basic cell type of nerve tissue is the ***neuron.*** Each neuron consists of a nerve cell body (perikaryon) and one or more nerve processes (fibers). The cell body of a typical neuron contains a nucleus, Nissl material of rough endoplasmic reticulum, free ribosomes, Golgi apparatus, mitochondria, neurotubules, neurofilaments, and pigment inclusions. The cell processes of neurons occur as ***axons*** and ***dendrites.*** Dendrites contain most of the components of the cell body except the nucleus and Golgi apparatus, whereas axons contain the major structures found in dendrites except for the Nissl material. At the synaptic ends of axons, the presynaptic process contains vesicles from which are elaborated excitatory or inhibitory substances. The functional dendrites of some neurons, such as the sensory pseudounipolar neurons of spinal nerves, are structurally the same as axons. Unmyelinated fibers in peripheral nerves lie in grooves on the surface of neurolemma (Schwann) cells and are incompletely invested by the plasmalemma of these cells. Myelinated peripheral neurons are invested by numerous "jellyroll" layers of Schwann cell plasma membrane that constitute a myelin sheath. The Schwann cell cytoplasm and nucleus surround the myelin sheath. There are many Schwann cells along each myelinated fiber. In the junctional areas between adjacent Schwann cells there is a lack of myelin. These junctional areas along the myelinated process constitute the nodes of Ranvier.

Spinal nerves have an outer epineurial connective tissue investment and an inner more cellular perineurial covering that extends internally to surround nerve bundles. The cells of the perineurium form an epithelioid sheath wherein the cells are joined by occluding junctions and the layers of cells are separated by basal lamina material. This perineurial layer seems to be an effective barrier against material entering or leaving the nerve. A loose endoneurial connective tissue separates nerve processes and lies next to the basement membranes of the Schwann cells.

Spinal nerves contain the processes of neurons whose cell bodies are located in sensory dorsal root ganglia (pseudounipolar neurons), sympathetic ganglia (multipolar neurons), and in the gray matter of the spinal cord (multipolar neurons). Each spinal nerve contains myelinated and unmyelinated fibers that are invested by Schwann cells. In the ganglia, each cell body is surrounded by supportive satellite cells.

Spinal nerves contain neurons representing four functional components: (1) general somatic efferent (GSE) fibers to skeletal muscles, (2) general visceral efferent (GVE) fibers to smooth and cardiac muscle and glands, (3) general somatic afferent (GSA) fibers from the skin, muscle and tendon spindles, and joints, and (4) general visceral afferent (GVA) fibers from visceral structures.

Spinal Cord. The spinal cord consists of a central canal lined with ependymal cells and bounded by central gray matter and peripheral white matter. The H-shaped gray matter has anterior, posterior, and lateral horns. It consists of groups of nerve cell bodies (nuclei, cell columns), axons, dendrites, and glial cells that form a meshwork called ***neuropil.*** An architectural lamination permits classification of the gray matter into nine Rexed's layers, of which laminae I-VI are in the posterior horn, laminae VIII and IX are in the anterior horn, and lamina VII is intermediate to the two horns.

Glial cells are the supportive cells of the CNS. They consist of ependymal cells, two kinds of astrocytes, oligodendrocytes, and microglia. Protoplasmic astrocytes are found mostly in the gray matter, and fibrous astrocytes are located mostly in the white matter. Astrocytes provide structural support for nerve tissue and may help to isolate groups of nerve endings from each other. Since they are interposed between the capillaries and the neurons in the CNS, they may also serve a role in the nutrition of the neuron. Oligodendroglia invest nerve fibers to form the myelin of the CNS. One oligodendrocyte may envelope several fibers. Microglia, unlike the other glia, arise from mesodermally derived monocytes and are components of the mononuclear phagocyte system.

The ***anterior horn of gray matter*** contains the cell bodies of alpha and gamma motor neurons whose axons innervate extrafusal and intrafusal skeletal muscle fibers, respectively. These nerve cell bodies constitute the GSE cell column and are grouped into nuclei that supply axons to specific regions; for example, those most medial in the anterior horn go to the more axial musculature while those most lateral innervate the extremities and the lateral muscles of the trunk. The alpha motor neurons are in Rexed's layer IX, the gamma motor neurons are in layer VII, and mostly commissural neurons occupy layer VIII. Damage to alpha motor neurons results in a ***lower motor neuron (LMN) syndrome*** of flaccid paralysis, muscle atrophy, atonia, and loss of deep and superficial reflexes. If only some GSE neurons to a muscle are damaged then pareses, hypotonia, and hyporeflexia result.

The ***lateral horn of gray matter*** consists of preganglionic sympathetic neurons and is limited to all thoracic and the first two lumbar spinal cord segments. This lateral horn of gray matter constitutes the intermediolateral cell column. This GVE cell column is in Rexed's layer VII. Preganglionic parasympathetic cell bodies are scattered in layer VII of cord levels S2–S4 as well. Axons of preganglionic autonomics leave the cord by the ventral root and become part of the spinal nerve. Sympathetic preganglionics leave the nerve via the white rami communicantes and enter the sympathetic chain ganglia or become components of splanchnic nerves. They will synapse with postganglionic sympathetic neurons in the sympathetic chain or prevertebral ganglia. Unmyelinated postganglionic axons reentering the spinal nerve constitute the gray rami communicantes. Sacral parasympathetic preganglionics form pelvic nerves, which terminate on ganglia near, or in, the organs innervated.

The ***posterior horn of gray matter*** consists of several nuclear groups that constitute the GSA cell column. Most prominent of these nuclei are the posteromarginal nucleus of Rexed's layer I, substantia gelatinosa in layer II, the nucleus proprius mostly in layer IV, and nucleus dorsalis of Clarke in layer VII. These nuclei are "nuclei of termination" for incoming somatic afferents in the dorsal roots of spinal nerves, and they are involved in processing sensory information. First-order afferent pain and temperature neurons terminate on second-order neuron cell bodies in the posteromarginal nucleus, nucleus proprius, and deeper layers of the posterior horn. Axons of these second-order neurons transmit impulses contralaterally through the anterior white commissure and ascend in the lateral funiculus as the lateral spinothalamic tract. This tract synapses on third-order neurons in the ventral posterolateral (VPL) nucleus of the thalamus. Axons of VPL cells pass to the postcentral gyrus (areas 3, 1, 2; primary somesthetic area) of the parietal lobe and to an area of parietal cortex immediately above the lateral fissure (somatic sensory area II).

Sensory information from intrafusal fibers of neuromuscular spindles and tendon spindles is transmitted via IA and IB myelinated first-order neurons, respectively. These synapse on cells of the nucleus dorsalis (Clarke) at cord levels C8 to L3. Axons of these second-order neurons pass ipsilaterally to the cerebellum as the posterior spinocerebellar tract. IA and IB neurons entering the cervical cord above C8 ascend in the posterior white column to the medulla, where they synapse in the accessory cuneate nucleus. Cuneocerebellar and posterior spinocerebellar fibers pass through the inferior cerebellar peduncle to reach the anterior lobe and paravermal areas of the cerebellum. Incoming fibers for crude (light) touch synapse in cells of the posterior horn. Most of the axons of these second-order neurons cross in the anterior white commissure and ascend in the anterior funiculus as the anterior spinothalamic tract. This tract synapses in the VPL nucleus of the thalamus and the impulses are probably relayed to the postcentral gyrus. Visceral sensation (GVA) is probably received by nuclei of termination in the lateral portion of the posterior horn. Its transmission to higher centers is probably through multisynaptic ascending paths in the funiculus proprius lying adjacent to the gray matter. Collaterals from incoming neurons of the dorsal root enter the gray matter and synapse on internuncials and alpha motor neurons for reflex purposes. Those coming from spindle receptors and ending directly on alpha motor neurons are part of the monosynaptic stretch (myotatic) reflex. Terminals of association neurons interconnecting different segmental levels, as well as terminals of descending axons from suprasegmental levels, end on internuncials that synapse with gamma and alpha motor neurons.

The ***white matter*** is organized into posterior, lateral, and anterior white funiculi. Each funiculus contains both ascending and descending pathways (Fig. 2-3). In the posterior funiculus (posterior white column) the most prominent pathway is that concerned with two-point touch, vibratory and joint senses, and stereognosis. Spindle information by way of IA fibers from neuromuscular spindles and IB fibers from Golgi tendon organs also are

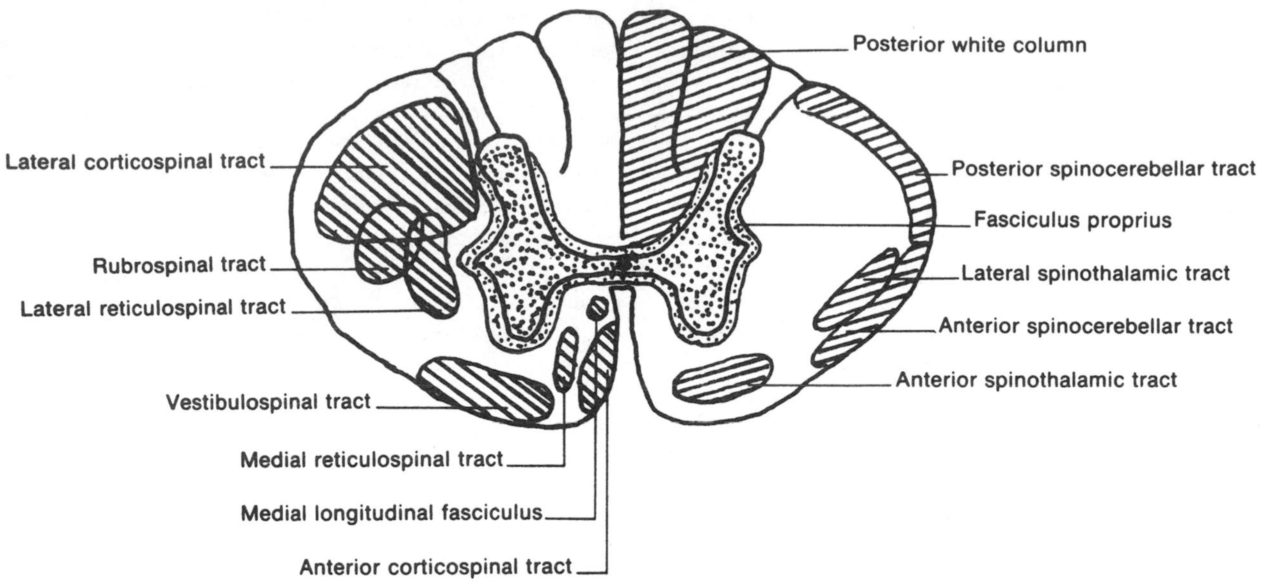

Fig. 2-3. Cross-sectional diagram of the spinal cord. The principal ascending pathways are indicated on the right. The principal descending pathways are shown on the left. The fasciculus proprius has both ascending and descending fibers of the spinospinal pathway.

transmitted in the posterior white column. Axons of these pathways in the posterior white column arise from cell bodies in the dorsal root ganglia, enter the cord in the medial bundle of the dorsal root, and ascend to the medulla, where they synapse on second-order neurons in the nuclei gracilis and cuneatus (see Fig. 2-22). Those axons entering dorsal roots below the T6 level constitute fasciculus gracilis and terminate in nucleus gracilis; those at and above T6 are in fasciculus cuneatus and terminate in nucleus cuneatus. Axons of the second-order neurons from the nuclei gracilis and cuneatus cross the midline as internal arcuate fibers and ascend as the medial lemniscus to the VPL nucleus of the thalamus where they synapse with third-order neurons whose axons go to the postcentral gyrus.

The most clinically prominent tracts of the lateral funiculus are the posterior spinocerebellar tract, the lateral spinothalamic tract, the lateral corticospinal tract (see Fig. 2-23), and the lateral reticulospinal tract (see Fig. 2-3). The posterior spinocerebellar tract is peripherally located beneath the posterolateral fasciculus at all levels of the spinal cord above L4. It conveys spindle information to the cerebellum. The lateral spinothalamic tract (see Fig. 2-21) is located ventrolaterally in the lateral funiculus and just deep to the anterior spinocerebellar tract. As previously mentioned, it represents the axons of second-order neurons of the pain and temperature pathway. The lateral corticospinal tract (see Fig. 2-3) is located just medial to the posterior spinocerebellar tract, mostly in the dorsal half of the lateral funiculus. This tract arises from pyramidal cells in the precentral gyrus and premotor area (areas 4 and 6) and postcentral (areas 3, 1, 2) gyrus (see Figs. 2-20, 2-23). From these gyri, axons descend in the brain stem, cross in the pyramidal decussation and descend in the contralateral lateral funiculus before terminating on internuncial neurons, which, in turn, synapse on alpha and gamma motor neurons. The lateral corticospinal tract constitutes the upper motor neurons of the pyramidal motor system. It is involved primarily in fine voluntary movements involving the more distal and phylogenetically "newer" musculature. It is facilitory to the antagonists of the antigravity muscles as well. The lateral reticulospinal tract arises from large cells (nucleus gigantocellularis) in the medial reticular formation of the medulla. Axons from these cells descend ipsilaterally in the lateral funiculus and are somewhat interspersed with axons of the lateral corticospinal tract. Stimulation of cells of the lateral reticulospinal tract inhibits alpha and gamma neurons innervating antigravity muscles (*i.e.*, extensors of the lower extremity and flexors of the upper extremity). Damage to these two tracts in the lateral funiculus results in the ***upper motor neuron (UMN) syndrome.*** This syndrome is discussed later in the section on somatic motor control mechanisms. Other pathways are found in the lateral funiculus. These are the rubrospinal pathway from the red nucleus, descending central autonomics from the hypothalamus, the spinotectal pathway to the superior colliculus of the mesencephalon, spinoreticular fibers to the brain stem reticular formation and interconnections between the spinal cord and inferior olivary nucleus.

In the anterior funiculus, the anterior spinothalamic tract, anterior corticospinal tract, lateral vestibulospinal tract, medial reticulospinal tract, and medial longitudinal fasciculus (MLF) are most prominent (see Fig. 2-3). The anterior spinothalamic tract is located just anterior to the ventral horn. Its origin, destination, and crude touch role were described previously. The anterior corticospinal tract has a similar origin and path to that of the lateral corticospinal tract, but it differs in that it is located near the anterior median fissure, it usually descends only to upper thoracic levels, and its axons have not crossed in the pyramidal decussation. These axons will cross, however, at the level where they terminate on internuncials that synapse with gamma and alpha motor neurons, supplying muscles of the upper extremity and neck. The vestibulospinal tract is interspersed with the anterior spinothalamic tract. It arises from cells in the lateral vestibular nucleus and descends ipsilaterally to end on internuncials that synapse with gamma and alpha motor neurons supplying antigravity muscles. Stimulation of this pathway results in facilitation of extensors of the lower extremity and of flexors of the upper extremity. The medial reticulospinal tract arises from nuclei in the medial portion of the pontine reticular formation. It descends ipsilaterally, lies lateral to the anterior corticospinal tract in the anterior funiculus and is involved in facilitation of antigravity muscles. The MLF lies in the most dorsal portion of the anterior funiculus next to the anterior median fissure. This composite tract contains axons arising from the mesencephalic tectum (tectospinal tract), vestibular nuclei (medial vestibulospinal tract), and the reticular formation of the brain stem (medial reticulospinal tract). Thus, unlike descending fibers of the lateral funiculus, which are facilitory to the antagonists of antigravity muscles and inhibitory to antigravity muscles, the descending fibers of the anterior funiculus are facilitory to antigravity muscles.

The spinal cord is supplied by descending branches from vertebral arteries and from radicular branches of segmental arteries. From these vessels paired posterior spinal arteries arise that descend dorsal to the posterior funiculus, while a single midline anterior spinal artery arises from the paired anterior spinal arterial branches of the vertebral. An arterial vasocorona plexus, lying in the pia adjacent to the lateral funiculus, interconnects the anterior and posterior radicular branches. The posterior spinal arteries supply the posterior funiculus, dorsal part of the dorsal horn of gray matter, and the posterolateral fasciculus (Lissauer). Sulcal branches of the anterior spinal artery supply all other parts of the spinal cord except the most peripheral portion of the lateral funiculus supplied by the arterial vasocorona. Spinal veins have a distribution that is generally similar to arteries. Sulcal and posterior veins empty into anteromedial, anterolateral, posteromedial, and posterolateral veins. These drain, in turn, to radicular veins that enter the epidural venous plexus.

Destruction of the posterior white column ipsilaterally results in astereognosis, in the inability to perceive the position of a limb in space, and in a loss of two-point touch and vibratory sense on the same side below the lesion. Damage to the lateral funiculus results in (1) a loss of pain and temperature contralaterally starting one segment below the lesion and extends caudally; (2) spastic paralysis, exaggerated deep reflexes, loss of superficial reflexes, and loss of fine distal motor activity ipsilaterally below the lesion; and (3) a Horner's syndrome of ptosis, pupillary constriction, and blanched and dry facial skin ipsilaterally if the lesion is above the upper thoracic intermediolateral cell column level.

DEVELOPMENT OF THE SPINAL CORD AND SPINAL NERVES

The CNS appears early in the third embryonic week of development as a thickened neural (medullary) plate of ectoderm. This plate is elongate, wider cephalically than caudally, and is located rostral to the primitive node of Hensen. It is continuous laterally with ectoderm that will give rise to the epidermis of the skin. With further development the lateral edges of the plate elevate to form ***neural folds*** that close the neural groove into a ***neural tube.*** The closure begins at the fourth somite and progresses cephalically and caudally, with the anterior neuropore closing on the 24th day of development and the posterior neuropore closing by the 26th day. Ectoderm arising at the junction of neural ectoderm with general surface ectoderm becomes segmentally arranged as the ***neural crest*** material lying dorsolateral to the neural tube. The cephalic enlargement of the neural tube differentiates into the brain and gives rise to motor components of cranial nerves. The caudal part becomes the spinal cord and also gives rise to the ventral roots of spinal nerves. Neural crest gives rise to sensory neurons comprising the dorsal root ganglia and some sensory cranial nerve ganglia, postganglionic autonomic ganglia of cranial and spinal nerves, Schwann cells, satellite cells, parenchyma of the adrenal medulla, pigment cells, and cartilage and bone cells in the head region.

Histogenesis of the Spinal Cord. The early neural tube consists of a neuroepithelium that differentiates into neuroblasts and spongioblasts (glioblasts). ***Neuroblasts*** differentiate into neurons whose cell bodies are localized into a mantle layer and whose axons contribute to a more peripheral marginal layer. Some of these axons ascend or descend in the marginal layer and become the association fibers of the tracts of the white matter. Others leave the white matter and become motor (efferent) nerve fibers of the ventral roots and spinal nerves. ***Spongioblasts*** lining the central canal differentiate into ependymal cells while others migrate into the marginal and mantle layers and become astrocytes and oligodendroglia.

The lateral walls of the neural tube are separated into dorsal alar plates and ventral basal plates by a longitudinally running sulcus limitans. The thin roof plate is obliterated in the fusions accompanying the formation of the posterior median septum; the floor plate remains as the anterior white and gray commissures. The mantle layer of the alar plate develops into the posterior horn of gray matter that contains the nuclei of termination for sensory neurons. Neurons of the posterior horn are internuncial, commissural and association neurons. The mantle layer of the basal plate becomes the anterior horn and lateral horn of gray matter. Neuroblasts of the anterior horn give rise to gamma and alpha motor neurons whose axons leave the cord in the ventral root and innervate intrafusal and extrafusal skeletal muscle fibers, respectively. Neuroblasts of the lateral horn give rise to preganglionic sympathetic neurons of the intermediolateral cell column at thoracic and L1–L2 levels. Preganglionic parasympathetic neurons arise in a similar position at S2–S4 levels.

Histogenesis of Spinal Nerves. Sensory neurons arise from neural crest material, and their cell bodies are located in dorsal root ganglia. Axons of the sensory cells either terminate in the posterior horn or ascend in the posterior white column as the fasciculus gracilis and fasciculus cuneatus. Somatic motor and preganglionic visceral efferent axons in spinal nerves arise from neuroblasts of the mantle layer as previously described. Postganglionic autonomic neurons differentiate from neural crest. Their cell bodies are aggregated into sympathetic and parasympathetic ganglia. Postganglionic axons are unmyelinated; those that traverse the spinal nerve enter it through the gray communicating rami. The myelin of all myelinated fibers in spinal nerves develops from neural crest material by the wrapping of differentiating Schwann cells around axons.

Nerve Degeneration and Regeneration. Injury to a nerve fiber leads to degeneration of the axon and myelin in the entire portion distal to the lesion (Wallerian or secondary degeneration) and also for a distance of one to two internodes in the proximal stump of the fiber (retrograde or primary degeneration). If injured neurons are components of ascending sensory pathways in the CNS, the sensory loss will be reflected as an anesthesia (loss of sensation), hypesthesia (diminished sensation), astereognosis (inability to identify an object held in the hand), hypalgesia (diminished sensitivity to pain), or analgesia (absence of pain) below the lesion. The degeneration, however, will be primarily in the entire distal stump above the lesion. Damage to the sensory levels (*e.g.*, dorsal roots) of reflexes can lead to hypotonia or atonia and hyporeflexia or areflexia at the level of the lesion. When injured neurons are components of descending motor pathways then the loss may be expressed as paresis, paralysis of movement or atrophy. Both the motor functional deficit and degeneration of the distal stump are below the lesion.

In degeneration of myelinated peripheral nerves, myelin in the distal stump and in the region of damage will retract from the nodes, break up into segments and will be phagocytized by Schwann cells. Most myelin has degenerated by 3 weeks after the injury, but some may remain for up to 3 months. The axon of the distal stump swells, fragments, and is phagocytized by the Schwann cells. Schwann cells of the distal stump, and for one to two internodes in the proximal stump, increase in size, divide and form longitudinal bands. These bands of Büngner move into the center of the nerve fiber as the myelin and axon degenerate, thus leaving a neurolemmal tubular space between the Schwann cells and their basement membrane. If the damage to the neuron is near the cell body, the whole neuron will degenerate. If the injury is farther away, the cell will not die but the cell body will swell, chromatolysis occurs, and the nucleus moves eccentrically to a position opposite the axon hillock. Chromatolysis is due to dispersion of RER and ribosomes and is not accompanied by loss of RNA, although it appears that Nissl is lost.

In regeneration of the peripheral nerve, Nissl material starts to reappear around the nucleus in the third week, the nucleus returns to its original position, and turgescence subsides. Schwann cells bridge the area of the cut, and the swelling axon tip splits into fine fibers that enter neurolemmal tubes. Of the new fibers that enter each tube, the one that is usually first to reach the nerve ending will be moved deeply into gutters on the surface of the Schwann cells while the others degenerate. If the regenerating neuron is to become myelinated, the Schwann cells will wrap it with their plasmalemma. If it is to remain unmyelinated, it will be incompletely invested in the Schwann cell gutters.

Degeneration and regeneration processes of the CNS are similar to those in peripheral nerves, but regeneration is seldom as complete or successful. Since Schwann cells are absent, oligodendroglia perform similar functions but have more limited capacities. Vascular and neuroglial elements respond more to trauma. Microglia and astrocytes proliferate and extend into the cut area and compete with neurolemmal tube formation in the damaged area. Thus, regenerating fibers in the CNS pass into poor neurolemmal tubes if they are not first blocked by extensive scar tissue formation.

UPPER LIMB

BONES AND JOINTS OF THE UPPER LIMB

The bones of the upper limb include the clavicle and scapula (which form the shoulder [pectoral] girdle), the humerus of the arm, the radius and ulna of the forearm, and the carpals, metacarpals, and phalanges of the hand.

Clavicle and Sternoclavicular and Acromioclavicular Articulations. The clavicle, through its articulations, is the only bony connection between the upper limb and the axial skeleton. As such, it keeps the limb away from the body, thereby enabling a large range of motion. Proximally directed force through the upper limb frequently causes clavicular fracture. These fractures are usually in the middle third of the bone because of its doubly curved shape; they are also easily diagnosed by palpation because of the clavicle's completely subcutaneous location.

The medial end of the clavicle articulates with the superolateral aspect of the manubrium at the ***sternoclavicular joint.*** The bones are separated by an intra-articular disk that both strongly supports the joint and usually forms two separate synovial cavities. The joint also is reinforced by the articular capsule and sternoclavicular, interclavicular, and costoclavicular ligaments.

The lateral end of the clavicle articulates with the acromion at the ***acromioclavicular joint.*** The synovial space is enclosed by a capsule, but the major supports for this joint are the components of the coracoclavicular ligament (conoid and trapezoid ligaments), which extend between the clavicle and the coracoid process.

Humerus. The humerus articulates with the scapula proximally and with the radius and ulna distally. The head forms a nearly hemispheric articular surface covered with articular cartilage; a slightly constricted anatomic neck marks the attachment of the capsule of the shoulder joint. The greater tubercle has three distinct facets where the supraspinatus infraspinatus and teres minor insert, and it is positioned lateral to the humeral head. The lesser tubercle lies anteriorly below the head and receives the subscapularis. The intertubercular groove is located anterolaterally between the tubercles and contains the tendon of the long head of the biceps. Immediately below the tubercles is the tapering surgical neck, so named because of the frequency of fracture in that area. The spiral groove curves around the posterolateral aspect of the midshaft of the humerus, passing inferior to the laterally placed deltoid tuberosity.

The distal end of the humerus has two articular surfaces: the ***trochlea*** medially and the rounded ***capitulum*** laterally. The trochlea articulates with the ***trochlear notch*** of the ulna and the capitulum with the ***radial head.*** Above the trochlea anteriorly the ***coronoid fossa*** receives the coronoid process of the ulna when the forearm is flexed. Above the trochlea posteriorly the ***olecranon fossa*** is occupied by the ***olecranon process*** of the ulna when the forearm is extended. The lateral epicondyle is smaller than the medial.

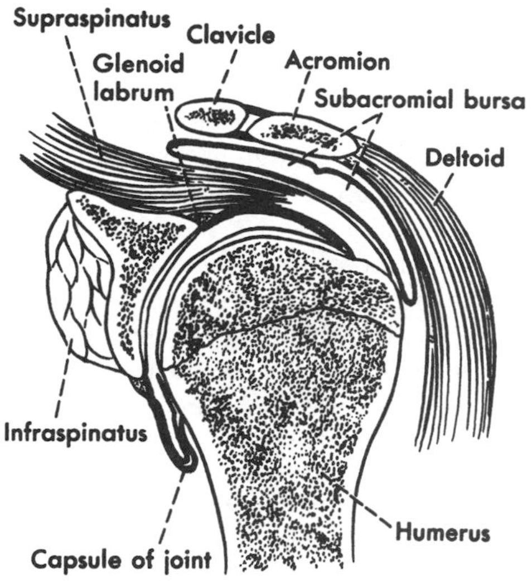

Fig. 2-4. Frontal section through the shoulder and suprahumeral space. (Hollinshead WH: Anatomy For Surgeons, Vol 3, 3rd ed, p 316. Philadelphia, JB Lippincott, 1982)

Shoulder Joint. The shoulder joint (Fig. 2-4) is a loose ball and socket joint formed by the articulation of the ***head of the humerus*** with the ***glenoid fossa*** of the scapula. In this joint maximal mobility is available at the expense of stability. The very loose articular capsule is redundant inferiorly when the joint is in the anatomic position. The glenoid cavity is deepened to a small degree by the glenoid labrum, a fibrocartilaginous wedge that attaches to the periphery of the glenoid fossa. The capsule extends from the rim of the glenoid fossa and the labrum to the anatomic neck of the humerus. It is reinforced anteriorly and inferiorly by the variable glenohumeral ligaments and by the coracohumeral ligament. The tendon of the long head of the biceps brachii ascends through the intertubercular groove and then passes across the superior aspect of the humeral head (between the fibrous and synovial portions of the capsule) to attach to the supraglenoid tubercle.

The major supports of this joint are the muscles of the ***rotator*** (musculotendinous) ***cuff:*** the subscapularis, supraspinatus, infraspinatus, and teres minor. The tendons of these muscles blend with the anterior, superior, and posterior aspects of the fibrous capsule and thus support the joint in those areas. The inferior aspect of the joint capsule, however, is loose and without muscular support.

Motion at the shoulder joint is very free and occurs

around an infinite number of axes. Although shoulder joint motion is a major factor in allowing the hand to assume innumerable locations and positions, proper function of the entire shoulder complex is absolutely necessary. Scapular motion as well as motion of the clavicle accompanies virtually every positional change of the upper limb. A loss of scapular, sternoclavicular, acromioclavicular, or glenohumeral range of motion can reduce the range of the entire upper limb. Scapular motion is controlled primarily by the trapezius and serratus anterior muscles. The motions listed below refer strictly to the shoulder joint, and the muscles indicated are the prime movers at that joint:

Flexion: anterior deltoid, pectoralis major, (especially the clavicular portion) coracobrachialis
Extension: latissimus dorsi, posterior deltoid, teres major
Abduction: middle deltoid, supraspinatus
Abduction: latissimus dorsi, pectoralis major (sternal portion)
Medial rotation: pectoralis major, latissimus dorsi, teres major, anterior deltoid, subscapularis
Lateral rotation: posterior deltoid, teres minor, infraspinatus

Suprahumeral Space. This is not a space in any sense but rather an area that is packed with structures of various types. The suprahumeral space (see Fig. 2-4) is between the head of the humerus and the arch formed by the acromion, coracoid, and the intervening coracoacromial ligament. The major structures within this space are the superior portion of the capsule of the shoulder joint, the tendon along with part of the supraspinatus muscle, the subdeltoid (subacromial) bursa, and the tendon of the long head of the biceps brachii muscle. Because humeral motion accompanies virtually every motion of the upper limb, the structures in this space are compressed continuously between the head of the humerus and the coracoacromial arch. This compression is more pronounced during flexion and abduction. Inflammation of any of these structures results in severe pain and thus loss of range of motion of the shoulder area.

Radius, Ulna, and Their Articulations. The radius is the lateral bone of the forearm. It has a small ***head*** proximally that is cylindrical in shape, and an expanded distal extremity, which is the major forearm contribution to the wrist joint. The ***ulnar notch*** is on the medial aspect of the expanded distal portion, and the lateral palpable ***radial styloid*** is the most distal bony prominence of the forearm. The ***dorsal radial tubercle*** (of Lister) is the most prominent bony landmark on the posterior aspect of the distal radius. The radial (bicipital) tuberosity is on the ventral proximal aspect of the radius.

The ulna is large proximally but narrows distally into the small round (but flat distally) head with the ***ulnar styloid*** extending past the head medially. The proximal portion of the bone has the deep ventrally directed ***trochlear notch*** The distal lip of the notch is the coronoid process; the proximal portion is the olecranon process and forms the point of the elbow. The lateral aspect of the proximal ulna is indented to form the ***radial notch.***

The ulna and radius are united through synovial joints both proximally and distally, with the interosseous membrane interconnecting the two shafts between these synovial joints. The ***proximal radioulnar joint*** is between the radial head and the radial notch of the ulna; the ***distal radioulnar joint*** is between the ulnar head and the ulnar notch of the radius. The proximal joint is stabilized primarily by the annular ligament of the radius, which attaches to the edges of the radial notch of the ulna and surrounds the head of the radius. The distal joint is reinforced primarily by an intra-articular disk that extends from the distal medial radius to the ulnar styloid. The proximal joint shares an articular capsule with the elbow joint; the distal joint has its own joint cavity.

Pronation and ***supination*** occur between the two bones of the forearm at the proximal and distal radioulnar joints. When the hand is supinated, the two bones are parallel. When the hand is pronated, the radius is wrapped around the ulna. Pronation is produced primarily by the pronator teres and pronator quadratus; supination by the biceps brachii and the supinator.

Elbow Joint. The elbow joint is formed between the trochlea of the humerus and the trochlear notch of the ulna medially, and between the capitulum of the humerus and the head of the radius laterally. The motion permitted at this joint—flexion and extension—is essentially determined by that part of the joint between the humerus and ulna. A common joint capsule encloses both the two portions of the elbow joint in addition to the proximal radioulnar joint. The capsule is thickened medially to form the ulnar collateral ligament and laterally to form the radial collateral ligament. The major flexors at the elbow are the brachialis, biceps brachii, and brachioradialis. The major extensor is the triceps brachii.

Bones of the Hand. The bones of the hand include the 8 carpal bones, 5 metacarpals, and 14 phalanges. The bones of the carpus are arranged in two rows. From lateral to medial, the proximal row consists of the ***scaphoid,*** the ***lunate,*** the ***triquetrum,*** and the ***pisiform*** bones. The distal row is composed of the ***trapezium,*** the ***trapezoid,*** the ***capitate,*** and the ***hamate*** bones. Each of the digits is composed of three phalanges except the thumb, which has only two. The phalanges are named by their position, that is, proximal, middle, and distal.

Wrist Joint and Joints of the Hand. The proximal articular surface of the wrist or ***radiocarpal joint*** is formed by the distal aspect of the radius and the medially placed intra-articular disk. This disk interconnects the ulnar styloid and the distomedial aspect of the radius. The distal articular surface is formed primarily by the scaphoid and lunate, with a small contribution from the triquetrum. The wrist joint has its own synovial cavity, which is separated from the distal radioulnar joint by the articular disk. The ***midcarpal articulation,*** which also has a separate joint cavity, is found between the two rows of carpal bones. The capsules of both joints are reinforced by collateral as well as dorsal and palmar ligaments. The motions that occur in the area of the wrist are contributed to by movement at both the radiocarpal and midcarpal joints. These motions and their major motors are:

Flexion: flexor carpi radialis, flexor carpi ulnaris
Extension: extensor carpi radialis longus, extensor carpi radialis brevis, extensor carpi ulnaris
Abduction or radial deviation: extensor carpi radialis longus and brevis, flexor carpi radialis, abductor pollicis longus, extensor pollicis brevis
Adduction or ulnar deviation: flexor carpi ulnaris, extensor carpi ulnaris

The ***carpometacarpal (CM) articulations*** of the four medial digits allow only minimal motion, even though they are synovial joints. The CM joint of the thumb is between the base of the first metacarpal and the trapezium. The shapes of its joint surfaces permit flexion, extension, abduction, adduction and, hence, circumduction. Rotation of the thumb is essential to opposition. Rotation occurs primarily at this joint and is provided by the action of the opponens pollicis.

The ***metacarpophalangeal (MP) joints*** are synovial in type and permit flexion, extension, abduction, adduction, and circumduction. Abduction and adduction are free only in extension as the collateral ligaments become taut in flexion and thereby reduce the side-to-side movement. Abduction and adduction are very limited at the MP joint of the thumb. The ***interphalangeal (IP) joints*** are all synovial articulations that permit only flexion and extension.

The muscles producing motion in the hand are:

MP flexion (not thumb): lumbricals, dorsal and ventral interossei, flexor digitorum profundus, flexor digitorum superficialis
MP extension (not thumb): extensor digitorum; extensor indicis, extensor digiti minimi
Digital abduction: dorsal interossei
Digital adduction: ventral interossei
Proximal IP (PIP) extension: lumbricals, dorsal, and ventral interossei
Distal IP (DIP) extension: lumbricals, dorsal, and ventral interossei
Proximal IP flexion: flexor digitorum superficialis, flexor digitorum profundus
Distal IP flexion: flexor digitorum profundus
NOTE: The combination of MP flexion and IP extention produces a functional position that is used in many activities requiring infinite control and gradation. These motions are the combined functions of the lumbricals and the interossei muscles.
Thumb flexion: flexor pollicis longus and brevis
Thumb extension: extensor pollicis longus and brevis
Thumb abduction: abductor pollicis longus and brevis
Thumb adduction: adductor pollicis
Opposition of the thumb: opponens pollicis, abductor pollicis brevis, and flexor pollicis brevis

COMPARTMENTATION OF THE UPPER LIMB

Arm. The arm is divided into anterior and posterior compartments by the medial and lateral intermuscular septa, which extend from the investing brachial fascia to the humerus. The muscles in the anterior compartment are the biceps brachii, brachialis, and coracobrachialis. These muscles are innervated by the musculocutaneous nerve and produce flexion at the elbow and supination of the forearm. Only the triceps brachii is found in the posterior compartment. This elbow extensor is innervated by the radial nerve.

Cubital Fossa. The cubital fossa is the depression anterior to the elbow and proximal part of the forearm. This fossa is bounded laterally by the brachioradialis muscle, medially by the pronator teres muscle, and proximally by a line interconnecting the medial and lateral epicondyles of the humerus. The tendon of the biceps brachii muscle disappears into this fossa as it passes toward the radial tuberosity; the bicipital aponeurosis (lacertus fibrosus) extends medially from the biceps tendon to the investing fascia of the forearm. This aponeurosis separates the superficially positioned median cubital vein from the deeper structures that pass through the fossa. The deeper structures are the brachial artery, which passes medial to the biceps tendon, and the median nerve, which is medial to the brachial artery.

Forearm. The forearm is separated into anterior and posterior compartments by the medial and lateral intermuscular septa, which extend from the antebrachial fascia to the ulna and radius, respectively, and by the interosseous membrane, which interconnects the radius and ulna. The muscles in the anterior compartment originate from the medial humeral epicondyle and the ventral aspects of the radius and ulna, and they function to pronate the forearm and flex the wrist and fingers. The pronator teres, flexor carpi radialis, palmaris longus, flexor digitorum superficialis, flexor pollicis longus, pronator quadratus, and the lateral half of the flexor digitorum profundus (to digits 2 and 3) are innervated by the median nerve. The flexor carpi ulnaris and medial half of the flexor

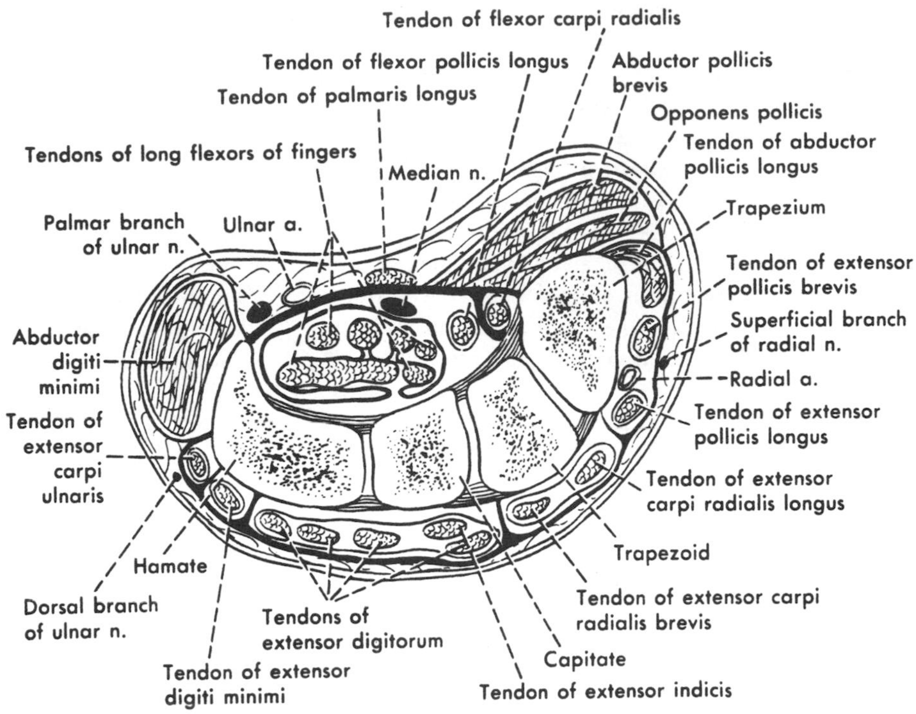

Fig. 2-5. Cross section at the wrist showing the carpal tunnel. (Hollinshead WH: Anatomy For Surgeons, Vol 3, 3rd ed, p 471. Philadelphia, JB Lippincott, 1982)

digitorum profundus (to digits 4 and 5) are innervated by the ulnar nerve. The muscles in the posterior compartment originate from the lateral humeral epicondyle and the dorsal aspects of the radius and ulna. These muscles, all innervated by the radial nerve, function to supinate the forearm and extend the wrist and digits at the MP joints. These posterior muscles are the brachioradialis, extensor carpi radialis longus, extensor carpi radialis brevis, extensor digitorum, extensor digit minimi, extensor carpi ulnaris, supinator, abductor pollicis longus, extensor pollicis brevis, extensor pollicis longus, and extensor indicis.

Carpal Tunnel. The carpal tunnel (Fig. 2-5) interconnects the anterior compartment of the forearm and the palm of the hand. It is a fibro-osseous canal, formed posteriorly and on both sides by the carpal bones and ventrally by the deep part of the flexor retinaculum (transverse carpal ligament). The structures that pass through this tunnel (canal) include the tendons of the flexor digitorium superficialis, flexor digitorum profundus, and flexor pollicis longus muscles, the synovial sheaths of those tendons, and the median nerve. Any of these structures, particularly the median nerve, can be compressed within the canal (carpal tunnel syndrome). The ulnar nerve and artery, tendon of the palmaris longus muscle, and palmar branch of the median nerve also cross the ventral aspect of the wrist but pass superficial to the deep part of the flexor retinaculum.

Hand. The ventral aspect of the hand is separated into thenar, hypothenar, and central compartments (Fig. 2-6). The antebrachial fascia continues into the hand and attaches along the first and fifth metacarpals. In the central region of the palm this fascia is greatly thickened to form the ***palmar aponeurosis.*** From the lateral border of this aponeurosis the thenar intermuscular septum extends into the palm and attaches to the first metacarpal. This septum together with the investing fascia around the lateral aspect of the palm delimits the ***thenar compartment,*** which contains the abductor pollicis brevis, flexor pollicis brevis, and opponens pollicis muscles. These muscles are innervated by the recurrent or thenar branch of the median nerve. The hypothenar intermuscular septum extends between the medial extent of the palmar aponeurosis and the fifth metacarpal and combines with the investing fascia on the medial aspect of the palm to form the ***hypothenar compartment.*** This compartment contains the abductor digiti minimi, flexor digiti minimi brevis, and opponens digiti minimi, all of which are innervated by the deep branch of the ulnar nerve. The ***central compartment*** is deep to the palmar aponeurosis in the center of the palm. It is bounded by the aponeurosis, the thenar and hypothenar intermuscular septa and a layer of fascia, the adductor interosseous or palmar interosseous fascia, that extends between the first and fifth metacarpals deep in the palm. Only the four small lumbrical muscles are found in this compartment. The two lateral lumbricals are innervated by the median nerve; the two medial ones, by the ulnar nerve. The long flexor tendons to the digits pass through this compartment. This compartment also

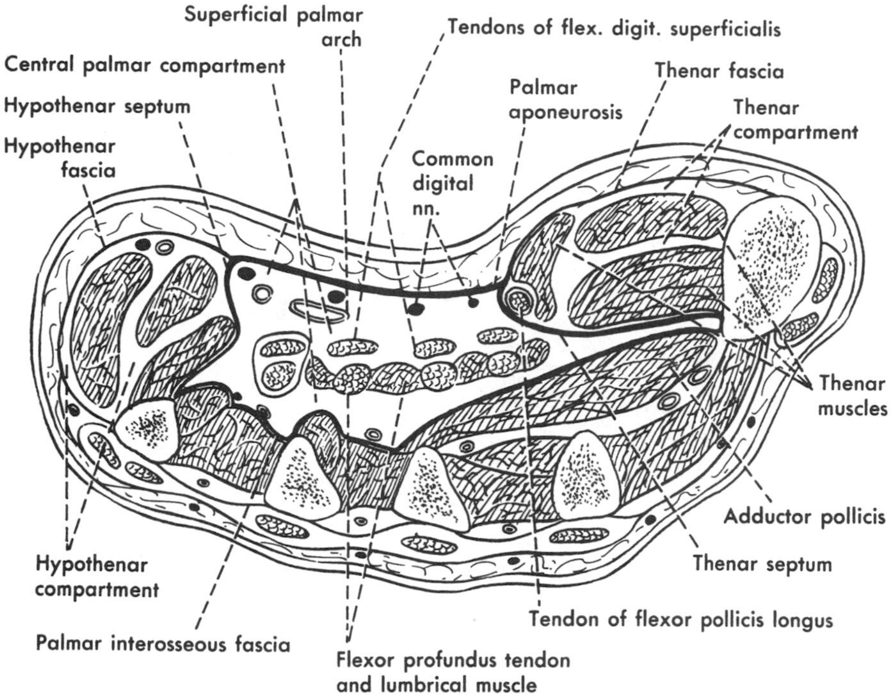

Fig. 2-6. Cross section of the hand. (Hollinshead WH, Rosse C: Textbook of Anatomy, 4th ed, p 236. Philadelphia, JB Lippincott, 1985)

contains the superficial palmar arterial arch, which is between the palmar aponeurosis and the long flexor tendons. The cutaneous branches of the median and ulnar nerves are distributed with the branches of the superficial arterial arch. The ***adductor interosseous compartment*** is essentially between the metacarpals. It is bounded dorsally by the dorsal interosseous fascia and ventrally by the adductor interosseous fascia. This space contains the dorsal and ventral interossei along with the adductor pollicis, all of which are innervated by the deep branch of the ulnar nerve.

Bursae and Spaces. The ***radial*** and ***ulnar bursae*** are synovial tendon sheaths that surround the long flexor tendons of the digits. They both start proximal to the wrist, pass through the carpal tunnel with the tendons, and extend either partially or completely through the palm and into the fingers. The radial bursa is associated only with the tendon of the flexor pollicis longus. The ulnar bursa surrounds all four tendons of both the flexor digitorum superficialis and profundus muscles. That part of this bursa associated with the little finger usually extends through the palm and into the digit while the others terminate at midpalmar levels. Thus, the synovial portions of the digital tendon sheaths of the index, middle, and ring fingers are not continuous with the ulnar bursa.

A pair of potential spaces (really fascial planes) exists at the approximate level of the adductor interosseous fascia, that is, in the plane just deep to the long digital flexor tendons in the central compartment. This plane is divided into a medial ***midpalmar space*** and a lateral ***thenar space*** by a septum that extends from the palmar aponeurosis to the third metacarpal. As indicated above, these are only potential spaces but can become actual spaces when filled with blood or inflammatory material.

NERVES OF THE UPPER LIMB

Brachial Plexus. Most of the muscles of the upper limb are supplied by branches of the brachial plexus (Fig. 2-7). The plexus is formed by the ventral rami of spinal nerves C5, C6, C7, C8, and T1. Ventral rami (commonly called the roots of the plexus) of C5 and C6 unite to form the ***superior trunk,*** C7 continues as the ***middle trunk,*** and the ***inferior trunk*** is formed by the union of C8 and T1. Each of the three trunks splits into anterior and posterior divisions. This separation into divisions determines the basic innervation pattern for the extremity; that is, the nerves formed from the anterior divisions innervate the muscles in the anterior compartments, and those from posterior divisions innervate posterior compartment muscles. The ***lateral cord*** is formed from the anterior divisions of the superior and middle trunks, and the anterior division of the inferior trunk continues as the ***medial cord.*** The posterior divisions of all three trunks unite to form the ***posterior cord.*** The cords of the plexus receive their names from their relationships with the second part of the axillary artery. The terminal peripheral nerves are formed in the axilla from the cords. The ***median nerve*** (C6–T1) is formed by contributions from both the medial and lateral cords. The remainder of the medial cord forms

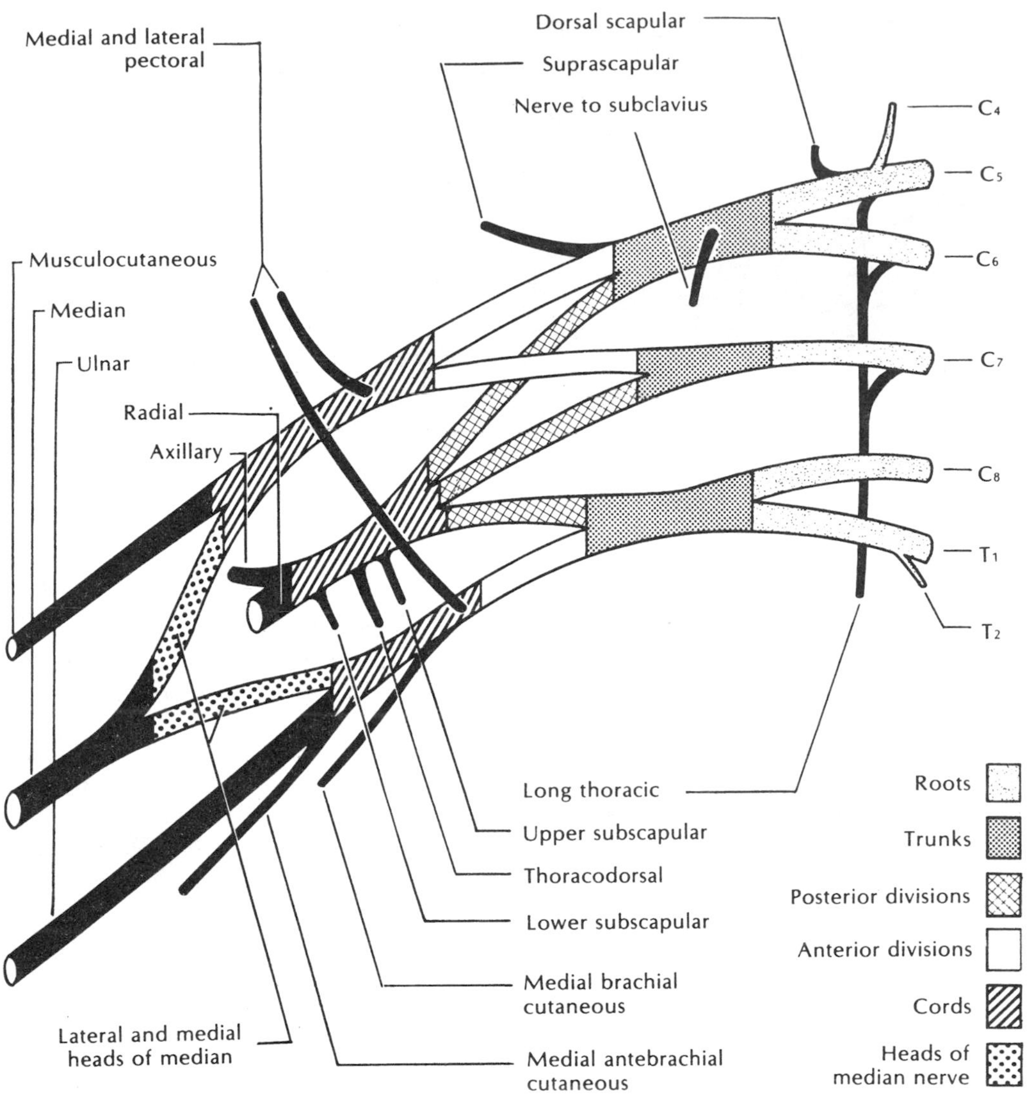

Fig. 2-7. Brachial plexus. (Christensen JB, Telford IR: Synopsis of Gross Anatomy, 5th ed, p 64. Philadelphia, JB Lippincott, 1988)

the ***ulnar nerve*** (C8–T1), and the termination of the lateral cord is the ***musculocutaneous nerve*** (C5, C6). The posterior cord gives rise to the ***radial*** (C5–C8) and ***axillary nerves*** (C5, C6).

Branches from the plexus proper are called ***collateral branches,*** and they supply most of the extrinsic and intrinsic muscles of the shoulder. (Extrinsic muscles extend from the axial skeleton to the scapula, clavicle, or humerus; intrinsic muscles connect the scapula or clavicle with the humerus.) The branches from the ventral rami are the ***dorsal scapular nerve*** (C5), which supplies both rhomboids and part of the levator scapulae, and the ***long thoracic nerve*** (C5–C7) to the serratus anterior. Two branches arise from the superior trunk: the ***nerve to the subclavius*** (C5) and the ***suprascapular nerve*** (C5, C6), which innervates the supraspinatus and infraspinatus muscles. The ***medial*** (C8, T1) and ***lateral*** (C5–C7) ***pectoral nerves*** branch from the medial and lateral cords, respectively. The medial pectoral nerve innervates the pectoralis major and minor; the lateral, only the major. The three ***subscapular nerves*** branch from the posterior cord. The ***upper*** and ***lower subscapular nerves*** (C5, C6) innervate the subscapularis and teres major muscles. The ***thoracodorsal nerve*** (middle subscapular) (C6–C8) innervates the latissimus dorsi muscle.

Median Nerve. The median nerve passes through the arm in the medial neurovascular bundle, which is located where the medial intermuscular septum joins the brachial fascia. In the distal part of the arm it inclines laterally and passes through the cubital fossa just medial to the brachial artery. The median nerve exits from the cubital fossa by passing through the pronator teres muscle and descends in the forearm deep to the flexor digitorum superficialis. The main trunk of the nerve supplies all of the superficial muscles except the flexor carpi ulnaris. The ***anterior interosseous branch,*** which arises in the proximal aspect of the forearm, supplies most of the deep muscles (flexor pollicis longus, pronator quadratus, lateral half of the flexor digitorum profundus). At the wrist the median nerve (see Fig. 2-5) is positioned deeply in the interval between the tendons of the flexor carpi radialis and the palmaris longus. It enters the hand by going through the carpal tunnel. Just distal to the deep part of the flexor retinaculum (transverse carpal ligament) the nerve branches into the ***thenar*** (recurrent) and ***digital*** (common and proper) ***branches.*** The thenar branch innervates the muscles in the thenar compartment. The digital branches supply the two lateral lumbricals and the skin on the entire ventral surfaces and the dorsal distal aspects of the lateral three and a half digits and some of the corresponding part of the palm. The lateral midpalmar skin is supplied by the ***palmar branch*** of the median nerve. This branch arises proximal to the wrist and does not pass through the carpal tunnel.

Musculocutaneous Nerve. From its origin in the axilla this nerve inclines laterally, going first through the coracobrachialis muscle and then between the biceps brachii and the brachialis. The nerve supplies these three muscles. It enters the subcutaneous tissue in the distal lateral arm, after which it continues into the forearm as the ***lateral antebrachial cutaneous.*** It supplies the skin of the lateral aspect of the forearm.

Ulnar Nerve. The ulnar nerve passes through the proximal half of the arm in the medial neurovascular bundle. It inclines posteriorly in the distal half of the arm, enters the posterior compartment and then passes behind the medial epicondyle of the humerus to enter the forearm. The nerve passes through the forearm under cover of the flexor carpi ulnaris, supplying this muscle and the ulnar half of the flexor digitorum profundus, and at the wrist it is deep to the tendon of the same muscle (see Fig. 2-5). It enters the hand by passing superficial to the deep part of the flexor retinaculum and lateral to the pisiform. Just distal to the pisiform it divides into ***deep*** and ***superficial branches.*** The superficial branch splits into common and proper digital nerves, which innervate the two medial lumbricals, the palmar skin of the medial one and a half digits, and the corresponding part of the palm. The deep branch passes through the hypothenar compartment and then sweeps laterally across the palm deep to the long flexor tendons. It innervates the muscles in the hypothenar compartment and the interossei as it crosses the palm and terminates in the adductor pollicis. The ulnar nerve also innervates the dorsal skin of the medial one and a half digits. This is accomplished by the ***dorsal cutaneous branch,*** which arises proximal to the wrist.

Radial Nerve. The radial nerve descends in the posterior compartment of the arm by curving obliquely around the posterior aspect of the midshaft of the humerus in the spiral groove. Its branches to the triceps brachii muscle arise both in the axilla and in the spiral groove. At about the midarm level, it enters the anterior compartment by piercing the lateral intermuscular septum and is positioned between the brachioradialis and the brachialis muscles. Just proximal to the elbow and deep to the brachioradialis it provides branches to the superficial muscles in the posterior compartment of the forearm and divides into ***superficial*** and ***deep branches.*** The superficial branch is cutaneous; it descends in the forearm under cover of the brachioradialis. It enters the subcutaneous tissue in the distal forearm and is cutaneous to the dorsal surface of the lateral three and a half digits and corresponding part of the dorsal hand. The deep branch is muscular (supplying the deep posterior muscles); it enters the posterior compartment of the forearm by wrapping around the neck of the radius in the substance of the supinator muscle. It then branches into its many muscular branches and continues through the forearm as the ***posterior interosseous nerve,*** which terminates at the level of the wrist.

Axillary Nerve. The axillary nerve passes anteroinferior to the shoulder joint (where it is occasionally stretched in an anterior shoulder dislocation) and then horizontally around the posterior aspect of the surgical neck of the humerus. It then enters the deep surface of the deltoid muscle. This nerve supplies both the teres minor and deltoid muscles.

PERIPHERAL NERVE LESIONS IN THE UPPER LIMB

Radial Nerve. When the radial nerve is interrupted in the axilla, the following symptoms are apparent:

1. Extension of the elbow and wrist is lost, and wrist drop results.
2. Extension of the thumb is lost; abduction is weakened.
3. Extension of the MP joints of the index, middle, ring, and little fingers is lost.
4. Grasp is weakened because of inability to extend and stabilize the wrist.
5. Supination of the forearm is weakened.
6. Radial and ulnar deviation of the wrist are weakened.
7. Sensation is lost on the dorsolateral aspects of the hand, arm, and the dorsal aspect of the forearm.

A radial nerve lesion at the level of the elbow would differ from that above primarily in that elbow extension would be unaffected; the severity of the other motor symptoms would depend upon the exact level of the involvement. Sensory loss would be limited to the dorsolateral hand.

Median Nerve. Paralysis of the median nerve at the wrist (as it passes through the carpal tunnel, resulting in a carpal tunnel syndrome) produces the following problems:

1. Flexion of the thumb is weakened.
2. Opposition of the thumb is lost, resulting in a derotated and adducted thumb (simian hand).
3. Flexion of the MP and extension of the PIP and DIP joints of the middle and index fingers are weakened, resulting in a slight clawing of these fingers.
4. Sensation is lost on the palmar surface and dorsal distal aspects of the lateral three and a half fingers and the corresponding portion of the distal palm.

Paralysis of the median nerve proximal to the elbow or in the axilla causes additional difficulties:

5. Flexion of the IP joints of the index and middle fingers is lost, resulting in an extension deformity, especially of the index finger.
6. Flexion of the PIP joints of the little and ring fingers is greatly weakened, resulting in slight clawing of those two fingers. (The combination of 5 and 6 produces a benediction attitude of the hand.)
7. Flexion of the IP joint of the thumb is lost.
8. Pronation of the forearm is lost.
9. Flexion of the wrist is weakened.
10. Sensation is lost on the entire lateral palm.

Ulnar Nerve. Paralysis of the ulnar nerve at the wrist results in the following difficulties:

1. Abduction and adduction of the fingers are lost.
2. Flexion of the MP joints and extension of the IP joints are weakened in the index and middle fingers and virtually lost in the ring and little fingers. As a result, clawing is severe in the little and ring fingers, and moderate in the middle and index fingers.
3. Adduction of the thumb is virtually lost.
4. Opposition of the little finger is lost.
5. Opposition of the thumb is somewhat difficult.
6. Palmar sensation of the medial one and a half digits and the corresponding portion of the palm is lost.

Paralysis of the ulnar nerve proximal to the elbow results in these additional problems:

7. Flexion of the DIP joints of the little and ring fingers is lost.
8. Flexion of the wrist is weakened and is accompanied by radial deviation.
9. Sensation of the dorsal aspects of the medial one and a half digits and corresponding portions of the hand is lost.

Combined Median–Ulnar Nerves. Interruption of both the median and ulnar nerves at the wrist results in the following:

1. Flexion of the MP joints and extension of the IP joints are lost; there is severe clawing of all four fingers.
2. Digital abduction and adduction are lost.
3. Thumb and little finger opposition are lost, hence a simian hand.
4. Sensation on the entire ventral surface of the hand and distal dorsal aspects of the digits is lost.

Blockage or lesion of the median and ulnar nerves proximal to the elbow causes the following additional difficulties:

5. Flexion of all joints distal to the elbow is lost.
6. Pronation of the forearm is lost.

Axillary Nerve. Paralysis of the axillary nerve as it leaves the posterior cord results in the following:

1. Virtual loss of useful shoulder joint abduction. Only a few degrees of abduction remain
2. Weakened shoulder flexion
3. Weakened medial and lateral rotation of the arm
4. Loss of sensation on the proximal lateral arm

Musculocutaneous Nerve. Paralysis of the musculocutaneous nerve at its origin results in:

1. Very weakened elbow flexion
2. Weakened supination of the forearm
3. Loss of sensation on the lateral forearm

BLOOD SUPPLY OF THE UPPER LIMB

Arteries. The blood supply of the upper limb is provided by the ***subclavian artery,*** which becomes the ***axillary artery*** as it crosses the first rib (Fig. 2-8). The first part of the axillary artery extends from the first rib to the pectoralis minor muscle, the second part is deep to the muscle, and the third part extends between the pectoralis minor and the lower border of the teres major muscle. The superior thoracic artery to the upper chest wall branches from the first part of the artery. There are two branches of the second part: the thoracoacromial trunk, which supplies the acromial, deltoid, pectoral, and clavicular regions, and the lateral thoracic branch, which descends along the anterolateral chest wall. The branches of the third part of the artery are the subscapular artery, which bifurcates into the circumflex scapular and thoraco-dorsal arteries, and the anterior and posterior humeral circumflex arteries, which arise at the level of the surgical neck of the humerus. The circumflex scapular artery forms potential anastomoses posterior to the scapula with

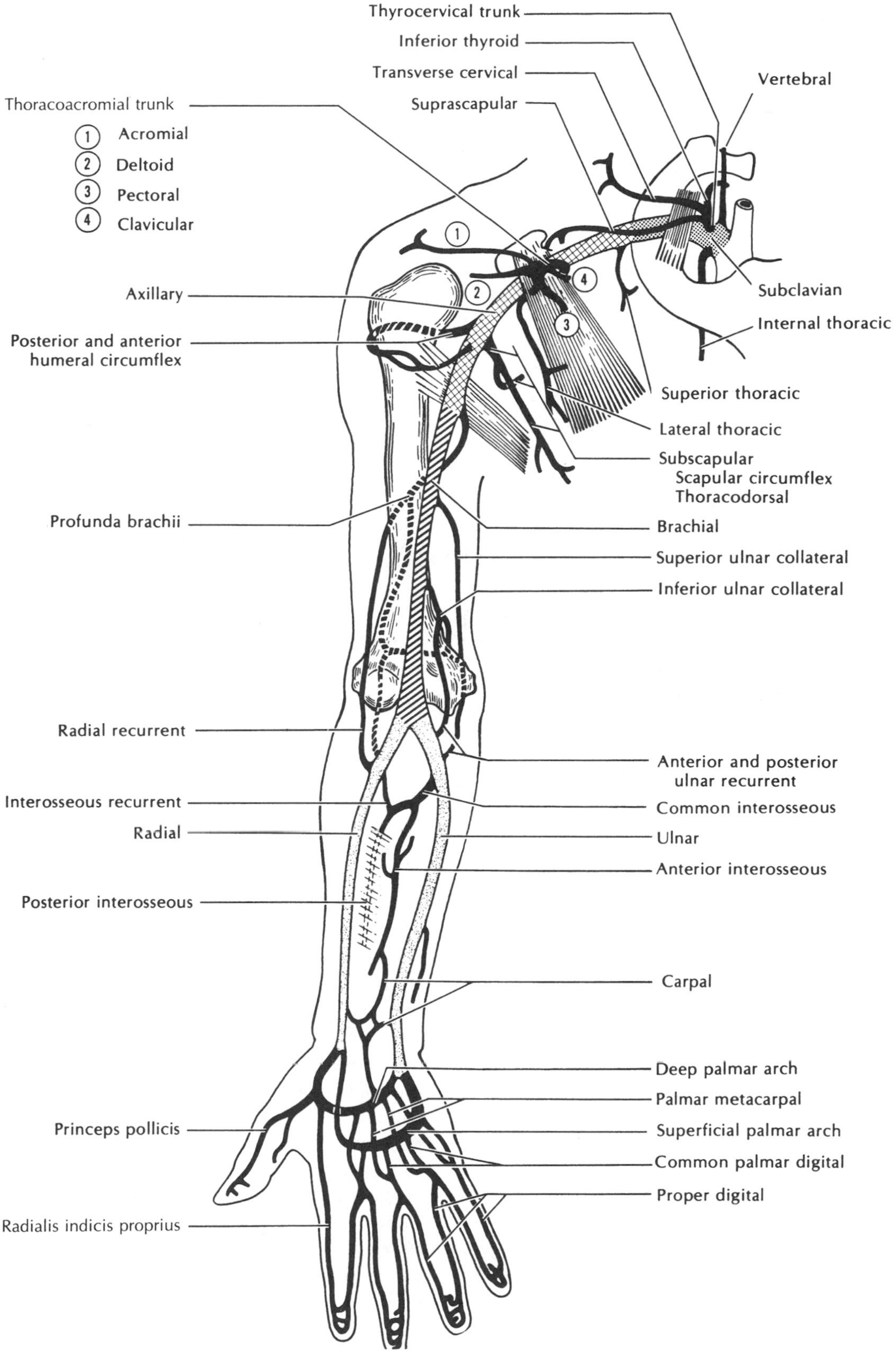

Fig. 2-8. Summary of arterial supply of the upper extremity. (Christensen JB, Telford IR: Synopsis of Gross Anatomy, 5th ed, p 86. Philadelphia, JB Lippincott, 1988)

branches of the subclavian artery. The posterior humeral circumflex artery accompanies the axillary nerve as it passes around the posterior aspect of the proximal humerus.

The ***brachial artery*** is the continuation of the axillary artery; it passes through the arm in the medial neurovascular bundle. It then inclines laterally in the distal half of the arm and crosses the elbow by passing through the cubital fossa. In the cubital fossa it is medial to the tendon of the biceps brachii muscle and lateral to the median nerve (between these two structures), and it is separated from the more superficial median cubital vein by the bicipital aponeurosis. It divides into the radial and ulnar arteries just opposite the radial head. Its largest branch is the deep brachial artery, which arises in the axilla and spirals around the humerus with the radial nerve.

The ***ulnar artery*** passes through the medial aspect of the forearm deep to the flexor carpi ulnaris muscle, and at the wrist it is just lateral to that muscle's tendon. It enters the hand by passing superficial to the deep part of the flexor retinaculum and lateral to the pisiform. Its largest branch is the common interosseous artery, which arises high in the forearm and immediately divides into the anterior and posterior interosseous arteries.

The ***radial artery*** descends through the lateral part of the forearm under cover of the brachioradialis muscle. Just proximal to the wrist it is lateral to the tendon of the flexor carpi radialis and readily palpable. It then inclines dorsally and enters the dorsum of the hand by passing through the ***anatomic snuff box.*** (The anatomic snuff box is bordered by the tendons of the abductor pollicis longus and extensor pollicis brevis laterally and the tendon of the extensor pollicis longus medially.)

The course of the ulnar artery in the hand is similar to that of the ulnar nerve in that it has a superficial and a deep branch. The superficial branch gives rise to the ***superficial palmar arch.*** This arch is at the level of the distal border of the extended thumb between the palmar aponeurosis and the long flexor tendons. The arch is completed by the superficial palmar branch of the radial artery, which branches proximal to the wrist and passes superficially through the thenar muscles. The arch has common digital branches to the fingers and a proper digital branch to the thumb. The radial artery passes through the snuff box and then between (passing dorsal to ventral) the first and second metacarpals. This course brings it into the deep part of the lateral palm where it gives rise to the ***deep palmar arterial arch.*** This arch, completed by the deep branch of the ulnar artery, accompanies the deep ulnar nerve. The position of this arch is proximal to the superficial arch and deep to the long flexor tendons. The palmar metacarpal branches of the deep arch communicate with branches of the superficial arch and the dorsal carpal arterial network.

Veins. The veins of the upper extremity consist of two sets: the ***deep*** and the ***superficial.*** The deep veins accompany the arteries and communicate frequently with the superficial veins, which are in the subcutaneous tissue.

The superficial veins are the basilic, cephalic, and median cubital. The ***basilic vein*** arises on the ulnar side of the dorsum of the hand and extends along the ulnar side of the forearm to the elbow. It crosses the anteromedial aspect of the elbow, pierces the brachial fascia, and empties into the brachial vein.

The ***cephalic vein*** begins at the radial side of the dorsal venous network and continues proximally through the lateral forearm and arm. At the shoulder it passes through the deltopectoral groove (separating the deltoid and pectoralis major muscles), after which it empties into the axillary vein.

The ***median cubital vein*** interconnects the cephalic and basilic systems superficial to the cubital fossa, and is commonly used for venipuncture.

LOWER LIMB

BONES AND JOINTS OF THE LOWER LIMB

Pelvis. The pelvis is composed of the two hip bones (os coxae) and the sacrum. The three bones are united at the two sacroiliac joints and the single symphysis pubis, thus forming the pelvic ring.

The ***os coxae*** is made up of three bones that fuse early in life: the pubis, ischium, and ilium. The ***pubis*** is located anteromedially. It consists of a body (which forms the symphysis with the body of the opposite side) and posterolaterally directed superior and inferior rami. The superior pubic ramus unites with the ilium; the inferior, with the ischium. The palpable pubic tubercle springs from the anterosuperior aspect of the body. The ***ischium*** is the posteroinferior portion of the hip bone. It has a heavy body, a palpable ischial tuberosity, and an ischial spine. The tuberosity is the inferiormost aspect of the hip bone and the point of origin of the hamstring muscles. The ischial spine projects posteromedially above the tuberosity and is palpable via rectal or vaginal examination. The ***ilium*** is the superiormost part of the os coxae, and its body is united with both the ischium and the pubis. The flattened and superiorly located iliac wing has a thickened crest that terminates anteriorly and posteriorly in the anterior and posterior superior iliac spines. The gluteal muscles attach to the lateral aspect of the iliac wing, and the iliacus muscle attaches medially. The posteromedial aspect of the iliac body presents the surface, the auricular surface, that articulates with the sacrum.

Inferiorly, portions of the pubis and ischium surround

the obturator foramen. Superior to the obturator foramen and on the lateral aspect of the os coxae, the three component bones form the socket of the hip joint, the acetabulum. Posteriorly and inferiorly, the area between the ischial tuberosity and ischial spine is the lesser sciatic notch; the area between the ischial spine and the posterior inferior iliac spine is the greater sciatic notch.

The ***sacroiliac joint*** is an unusual synovial joint in that it permits very little, if any, motion. It is formed by the highly irregular but congruent articular surfaces of the sacrum and ilium. These surfaces are bound tightly together by anterior and posterior sacroiliac ligaments as well as a large mass of interosseous ligaments. This joint commonly fuses in the fourth or fifth decade, particularly in males. The ***pubic symphysis*** is a cartilaginous joint between the pubic bodies, which permits only limited rocking motion.

The bones of the pelvis are involved in the formation of the walls of both the pelvic and abdominal cavities. The ***pelvic inlet*** separates the true pelvis below from the false pelvis (part of the abdominal cavity) above. The inlet is formed posteriorly by the sacral promontory, laterally by the arcuate line of the ilium and the iliopectineal line, and anteriorly by the superior aspects of the pubic bodies and symphysis.

Although there are many variations in pelvic architecture, the following classification has received general acceptance. Also, it must be stressed that although the following discussion considers four categories of pelvic shape, in reality most pelvises are mixtures of the various types. The ***gynecoid pelvis*** is regarded as the characteristic female pelvis. It is distinguished by an oval inlet with the transverse diameter exceeding the anteroposterior diameter. This pelvis is shallow with straight walls. The ischial spines are not prominent, and the subpubic arch is wide. It also has the appearance of being flattened from top to bottom, making it shorter and wider than the male pelvis. The ***android pelvis*** (male) has a heart-shaped inlet, is longer and heavier, and the angle of the subpubic arch is more acute. The ***anthropoid pelvis*** has an oval inlet with the long axis along the anteroposterior diameter. The ***platypelloid pelvis*** has a flattened oval inlet, which is caused by marked reduction in the anteroposterior diameter.

Femur. The femur is the largest and longest bone in the body. Proximally, the superomedially directed head is separated from the shaft by the neck, which joins the shaft at the trochanteric region. The head is slightly more than half of a sphere and is covered with articular cartilage, except in the region of the fovea. The angle between the neck and shaft is about 90 degrees in the female and greater than that in the male. The palpable greater trochanter is located superolaterally at this junctional area; the lesser is inferomedially. The long shaft inclines medially from above downward. The distal end of the femur has medial and lateral condyles, both of which are covered by articular cartilage. These articular surfaces come together anteriorly to form a groove for the patella. An intercondylar fossa separates the condyles inferiorly and posteriorly. The medial and lateral epicondyles are superior to the condyles on the medial and lateral aspects of the distal femur.

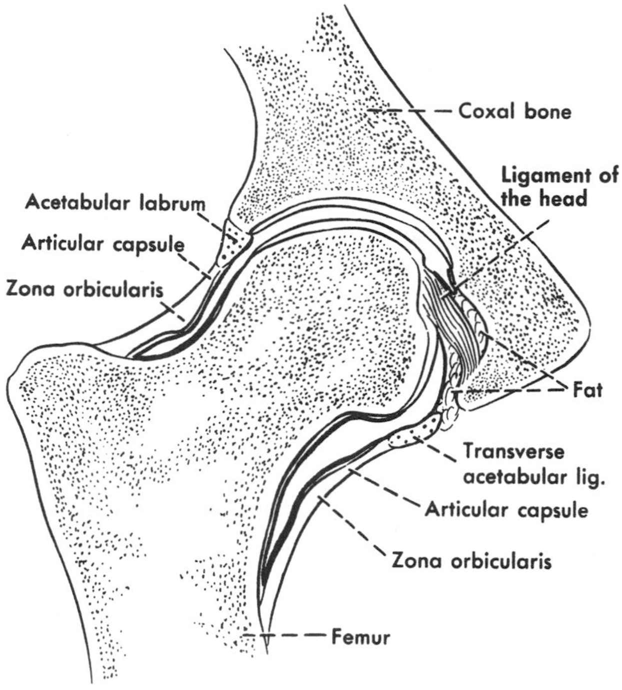

Fig. 2-9. A frontal section through the hip joint. (Hollinshead WH, Rosse C: Textbook of Anatomy, 4th ed, p 395. Philadelphia, JB Lippincott, 1985)

Hip Joint. The ***acetabulum*** is a deep socket with the horseshoe-shaped articular surface oriented so that its open end is directed inferiorly (Fig. 2-9). Therefore the articular surface is incomplete centrally and inferiorly. The head of the femur also has an area that is not covered by articular cartilage, the centrally located fovea. The two bony surfaces are quite congruent. The head of the femur is actually gripped by the fibrocartilaginous ***acetabular labrum,*** which, in addition to deepening the socket, also reduces its diameter and thereby holds the femur in place. That part of the labrum that bridges the inferior gap between the two limbs of the horseshoe-shaped acetabulum is the transverse acetabular ligament.

The ***capsule*** of the hip joint extends from the labrum and corresponding part of the os coxae across the joint and well down the femoral neck. Anteriorly it extends over the entire length of the neck and attaches to the area of the intertrochanteric line. Posteriorly it extends about two thirds of the way distally so that there is an extracapsular portion of the neck posteriorly. It is important to note that only the fibrous portion of the capsule is attached to the femur as just indicated. Where the fibrous layer attaches to the femur, the synovial layer passes from the fibrous layer to the bone and extends proximally along the neck to attach at the border of the articular suface of the head of the femur. Most of the blood vessels supplying the head and neck of the femur pass proximally along the neck of the femur deep to the synovial layer of the capsule. These vessels, called retinacular vessels, are firmly held against the bone and are vulnerable to laceration when the femoral neck is fractured. Again, it is important to note that the entire anterior aspect of the neck is intracapsular, but only the medial two thirds is intracapsular posteriorly.

A major amount of support of the hip joint is provided by three extracapsular ligaments that blend with the fibrous portion of the joint capsule. The ***iliofemoral ligament*** (Y ligament of Bigelow) extends from the anterior aspect of the body of the ilium across the front of the hip joint to the lower part of the intertrochanteric line. This ligament becomes taut as the hip is extended and is a major stabilizing force of the hip joint. The ***ischiofemoral ligament*** curves around the superior aspect of the joint. As the ligament tightens during hip extension, it forces the head of the femur into the acetabulum. The ***pubofemoral ligament*** crosses the joint inferiorly. The fovea of the head of the femur and the nonarticular portion of the acetabulum are connected by the ***ligament of the head of the femur*** (ligamentum teres), an intra-articular ligament that conveys a small blood vessel to the head of the femur and offers virtually no joint support.

Although the number of potential motions that can occur at the hip joint is infinite, it is convenient to describe those that correspond to the cardinal planes of the body. These motions and their major motors are as follows:

Flexion: psoas, iliacus, rectus femoris
Extension: biceps femoris, semitendinosus, semi-membranosus, posterior portion of the adductor magnus, gluteus maximus
Abduction: gluteus medius, gluteus minimus
Adduction: adductor magnus, adductor longus, adductor brevis, adductor minimus, gracilis
Lateral rotation: gluteus maximus, obturator internus and externus, gemelli, quadratus femoris
Medial rotation: gluteus medius and gluteus minimus, tensor fasciae latae

It should be noted that, based on the position of the hip (flexion or extension), certain adductors may rotate the thigh either medially or laterally.

Tibia and Fibula. The ***tibia*** is the weight-bearing bone of the leg and therefore is the major bone in the formation of both the ankle and knee joints. Superiorly it is expanded to form the flat tibial plateau, which is composed of the medial and lateral tibial condyles. These condyles are separated by the intercondylar area, which contains the intercondylar eminence. The anterior border of the shaft is subcutaneous throughout its length with an obvious protrusion superiorly where it begins as the tibial tuberosity. Inferiorly the tibia is expanded to form the articular surface for the ankle joint with the medialmost aspect extending distally as the medial malleolus.

The ***fibula*** is the lateral bone of the leg whose most apparent function is that of providing muscle attachments. This thin bone articulates with the tibia both proximally and distally. The interosseous membrane connects the two bones throughout most of their lengths. The inferior extent of the fibula is the lateral malleolus.

Knee Joint. The knee joint is formed between the rounded femoral condyles and the relatively flat tibial condyles. The length of the articular surface (front to back) of the femoral condyles greatly exceeds that of the tibial condyles; as a result, most knee motion is spinning and gliding of the femoral condyles on the tibial condyles. There is, however, some rocking motion between the two bones during the last few degrees of extension.

The poor congruency between the two sets of articular surfaces produces a dead space. This dead space is filled in part by the wedge-shaped articular disks, or ***menisci.*** Each of these is somewhat C-shaped and sits on the periphery of each tibial condyle and attaches centrally to the intercondylar area of the tibia. In addition to deepening the socket and increasing the congruency, the menisci absorb shock that is transmitted from femur to tibia and protect the capsule by keeping it from being pinched between the two bones. The lateral meniscus is almost a complete circle so that its central attachments are very close together. It is also loosely attached to the capsule, continuous with the posterior meniscofemoral ligament and thought to be connected to the popliteus muscle. Thus, the lateral meniscus is relatively movable; presumably this is why it is seldom injured. The medial meniscus is relatively immovable and therefore very frequently injured as it is caught between the medial tibial and femoral condyles. It is immovable both because it is C-shaped (and thus has wide central attachments) and it is attached firmly to the capsule and the medial collateral ligament.

The fibrous and synovial portions of the ***joint capsule*** do not correspond to one another. The fibrous portion encloses the entire joint area and is made up of the quadriceps tendon, patella, and patellar ligament anteriorly, the patella retinacula anteromedially and anterolaterally, and the iliotibial tract (band) laterally. Medially the tibial collateral ligament blends with the fibrous capsule. The synovial lining encloses the articular surfaces, but the intercondylar area is outside the joint space (but within the fibrous capsule). The volume of the joint space is largest when the knee is slightly flexed (approximately 20 to 30 degrees), and thus patients whose knees are effused will usually be most comfortable with their knees in that position.

The major ligamentous support of the knee is provided by the ***collateral*** and ***cruciate ligaments.*** The ***lateral*** (fibular) ***collateral ligament*** extends between the lateral femoral epicondyle and the head of the fibula and restricts medial displacement of the leg on the thigh. This ropelike structure is easily palpable and separated from the joint capsule. The ***medial*** (tibial) ***collateral ligament*** is a strong broad band, which connects the medial femoral epicondyle and the medial tibial condyle; it restricts lateral displacement of the leg on the thigh. It is palpable as a thickening in the joint space medially. The collateral ligaments are taut when the knee is extended but loosen somewhat when the knee is flexed, thus permitting rotation in that position. The collateral ligaments are obliquely oriented, and together they resist lateral rotation of the tibia on the femur. The cruciate ligaments occupy the intercondylar area and give the knee anteroposterior stabilization. From its anterior tibial attachment, the ***anterior cruciate ligament*** passes posteriorly, superiorly, and laterally to attach to the medial aspect of the lateral femoral condyle. It protects against posterior dislocation of the femur on the tibia. The ***posterior cruciate*** extends from its posterior tibial attachment anteriorly, superiorly, and medially to attach to the lateral aspect of the medial femoral condyle. It protects against anterior dislocation of the femur on the tibia. The cruciate ligaments are also obliquely oriented; together they resist medial rotation of the tibia on the femur. Although the cruciate ligaments are most taut in full flexion (posterior) and extension (anterior), portions of both are tense throughout the range of motion. And even though all of these ligaments are strong and reinforce the knee joint, the major stabilization of this joint is provided by the muscles (mainly quadriceps and hamstrings) that cross the joint.

The motions that occur at the knee and the major muscles that cause them are:

Extension: quadriceps femoris
Flexion: biceps femoris, semitendinosus, semimembranosus, gastrocnemius
Medial rotation: semimembranosus, semitendinosus, sartorius, popliteus
Lateral rotation: biceps femoris

Bones of the Foot. The bones of the foot are the ***tarsals, metatarsals,*** and ***phalanges.*** The seven tarsal bones are arranged in two rows with one bone between the rows. Proximally the talus sits on the calcaneus, and distally the bones (medial to lateral) are the medial, intermediate, and lateral cuneiforms and the cuboid. The navicular is essentially between the cuneiforms and the talus. The talus is the most superior bone in the foot and it receives all of the superincumbent weight from the leg. The metatarsals and phalanges are similar in number and position to the metacarpals and phalanges of the hand.

The bones of the foot are arranged to provide flexibility and stability, that is, they must perform the weightbearing function while providing for a soft landing and forceful takeoff. These requirements are met by the presence of several ***arches*** that are arranged so that weight hits the floor at the calcaneal tuberosity posteriorly and at the heads of the metatarsals anteriorly. The most important arch is the medial longitudinal arch, which consists of the calcaneus, talus, navicular, three cuneiforms, and the three medial metatarsals. The lateral longitudinal arch is made up of the calcaneus, cuboid, and two lateral metatarsals. A transverse arch exists at the level of the distal row of tarsals and bases of the metatarsals. The major static support of these arches (primarily the medial longitudinal arch) is provided by ligaments, which are the very important plantar calcaneonavicular (spring) ligament, the long plantar ligament, and the ligament-like plantar aponeurosis. Dynamic support is added by the intrinsic muscles of the foot. Three extrinsic muscles of the foot, the tibialis anterior and posterior and the peroneus longus, may provide additional dynamic support.

Ankle Joint. The ankle joint is formed superiorly by the tibia and fibula and inferiorly by the trochlea of the talus. The ***trochlea*** is a cylindrically shaped process with its long axis oriented from side to side and its articular surface located on both its rounded upper aspect and flat ends. The tibia articulates with the superior aspect and medial end (via the medial malleous) of the talus; the lateral malleolus, with the lateral end. The talus spins around in the mortise formed by the tibia and fibula. The anterior aspect of the trochlea is wider than the posterior. As a result, in dorsiflexion the widest portion of the trochlea is wedged between the malleoli (good bony stability). In plantar flexion this support is lost. Thus, most sprains occur when the ankle is plantar flexed. The distal tibia and fibula are lashed together by anterior and posterior tibiofibular ligaments. The major ligaments supporting the ankle joint are the medial (deltoid) and lateral collateral ligaments. The deltoid ligament is a broad band that connects the medial malleolus with the talus, navicular, and calcaneus. The lateral collateral ligament is composed of three distinct bands: the anterior and posterior talofibular ligaments and the calcaneofibular ligament. The anterior talofibular ligament is the most commonly injured ligament, accompanying the frequent plantar flexion-inversion sprain of the ankle.

The motions of the ankle and their major motors are as follows:

Plantar flexion: gastrocnemius, soleus, tibialis posterior
Dorsiflexion: tibialis anterior

Subtalar and Transverse Tarsal Joints. Although the motions of the foot (other than toe motion) are the sum totals of the individual amounts of motion that occur at each intertarsal joint, there are two areas (called functional joints) where most of this motion does occur. These functional joints are the subtalar and transverse tarsal (midtarsal) joints. The motions of the foot are ***inversion,*** which is a combination of adduction and supination, and ***eversion,*** which is a combination of abduction and pronation. The subtalar joint is inferior to the talus between the talus and the calcaneus. The two sets of articular surfaces that form this joint are separated by a strong interosseous ligament. The orientation of these joint spaces is an inclined plane that is directed anteriorly, medially, and inferiorly. The transverse tarsal joint consists of two joints that extend transversely across the foot. The medial articulation is between the talus and the navicular, the lateral between the calcaneus and the cuboid.

The motors of these foot motions are as follows:

Inversion: tibialis anterior, tibialis posterior, flexor hallucis longus, flexor digitorum longus
Eversion: peroneus longus and brevis

COMPARTMENTATION OF THE LOWER LIMB

Hip Region. Although there are no compartments per se around the hip, the muscles in this region can be placed in logical groups. The ***gluteal muscles*** are the lateral and posterolateral muscles of the hip. The gluteus maximus is innervated by the inferior gluteal nerve, and the gluteus medius and minimus and the tensor fascia lata are supplied by the superior gluteal nerve. Deep to the gluteus maximus there is a group of muscles called the short external rotators of the thigh. These muscles are innervated by direct branches of the lumbosacral plexus and consist of the piriformis, obturator internus, superior and inferior gemelli, and the quadratus femoris. Anteriorly, the iliopsoas (iliacus and psoas major muscles) extends from the abdominal cavity into the proximal thigh. This major hip flexor is supplied by direct branches of the lumbar plexus.

Thigh. The investing fascia of the thigh is the fascia lata. It is dramatically thickened laterally as the iliotibial tract or band. From its proximal attachment to the iliac crest, this band extends distally and crosses the anterolateral aspect of the knee before attaching to the anterolateral aspect of the lateral tibial condyle. Two intermuscular septa extend from this investing fascia to attach to the femur. Thus, these medial and lateral intermuscular septa separate the thigh into anterior and posterior compartments. The anterior compartment is actually anterolateral and the posterior compartment posteromedial. The muscles in the ***anterior compartment*** are innervated by the femoral nerve and consist of the sartorius and the four components of the quadriceps femoris—the rectus femoris, vastus medialis, vastus intermedius, and vastus lateralis. The posterior compartment has two groups of muscles—the medial femoral or adductors and the posterior femoral or hamstrings. The ***medial femoral muscles*** are mostly innervated by the obturator nerve and consist of the adductor longus, adductor brevis, adductor magnus, pectineus, gracilis, and obturator externus. The ***hamstrings*** are primarily innervated by the tibial portion of the sciatic nerve and consist of the biceps femoris, semitendinosus, and semimembranosus.

Femoral Triangle. The femoral triangle is the anterior junction region between the abdomen and thigh, and it contains important structures that supply the lower limb. The triangle is defined by the inguinal ligament above, the sartorius muscle laterally, and the medial border of the adductor longus muscle medially. The floor is formed by the adductor longus, pectineus, and iliopsoas muscles. The superficial and deep inguinal lymph nodes are found respectively superficially and deep to the investing fascia in this area. In addition to receiving superficial lymphatics from the lower extremity, the superficial nodes drain the lower abdominal wall, buttock, perineum, and lower portions of the anal canal and vagina. From lateral to medial the following structures descend through the triangle: the femoral nerve, the femoral artery, and the femoral vein. The femoral artery is midway between the anterior superior spine of the ilium and the pubic tubercle. The femoral sheath is an extension of transversalis fascia that forms a sleeve around the femoral vessels as they enter the thigh. The area just medial to the vein is within the sheath and is called the femoral canal, and it is the usual path of a femoral hernia. After leaving the triangle, the femoral vessels pass through the thigh just deep to the sartorius muscle, an area called the ***adductor*** (subsartorial) ***canal.***

Popliteal Fossa. The popliteal fossa is a deep diamond-shaped area behind the knee. It is bounded superomedially by the tendons of the semitendinosus and semimembranosus muscles, superolaterally by the tendon of the biceps femoris, and inferiorly by the heads of the gastrocnemius muscle. Its floor is the posterior (supracondylar or popliteal) portion of the distal femur. The popliteal vessels pass vertically through this fossa with the artery closest to the bone and thereby vulnerable to laceration when this part of the femur is fractured. The tibial nerve passes through the center of this fossa superficially, and the common peroneal nerve follows the tendon of the biceps femoris muscle. This space is packed with loose connective tissue.

Leg. The leg has anterior, lateral, and posterior compartments. The major partition consists of the subcutaneous tibia, the interosseous membrane, the fibula, and the posterior intermuscular septum, which separates the posteromedially situated posterior compartment from an anterolateral region. This anterolateral area is subdivided into anterior and lateral compartments by the anterior intermuscular septum. The ***anterior compartment*** is just lateral to the tibia and contains the tibialis anterior, extensor hallucis longus, extensor digitorum longus, and peroneus tertius muscles, all of which are innervated by the deep peroneal nerve. These muscles dorsiflex the ankle, invert the foot, and extend the toes. The ***lateral compartment*** is superficial to the fibula and its muscles are primarily everters of the foot. The two muscles in this compartment—the peroneus longus and brevis—are innervated by the superficial peroneal nerve. All ***posterior compartment*** muscles are innervated by the tibial nerve and function to plantar flex and invert the foot and flex the toes. The posterior compartment muscles are the gastrocnemius, soleus, and plantaris superficially; the flexor hallucis longus, flexor digitorum longus, tibialis posterior, and popliteus form the deep group.

Foot. The organization of the foot is similar to that of the hand, but the compartmentation is less complete in the foot. There is a definitive compartment associated with the small toe and a deep one more or less between the metatarsals. However, fascial separations complete the formation of neither a central compartment nor one associated with the great toe.

For the most part the muscles of the foot are similar to those of the hand but are usually described in layers rather than in compartments. All of the plantar muscles are innervated by either the medial or lateral plantar nerves, both branches of the tibial nerve. The ***superficial layer*** consists of the abductor hallucis (medial plantar), flexor digitorum brevis (medial plantar), and abductor digiti minimi (lateral plantar). The ***intermediate layer*** is limited to the central area of the foot and is formed by the tendon(s) of the flexor digitorum longus and related muscles, that is, the quadratus plantae (lateral plantar) and lumbricals (medial and lateral plantar nerves). The ***deep layer*** consists of the flexor hallucis brevis (medial plantar), adductor hallucis (lateral plantar), and flexor digiti minimi (lateral plantar). A fourth layer is usually described; it consists of both the plantar and dorsal interossei, all of which are supplied by the lateral plantar nerve. The foot differs from the hand also in that it has dorsal intrinsic muscles. These muscles, the extensor hallucis brevis and extensor digitorum brevis, extend the toes and are innervated by the deep peroneal nerve.

NERVES OF THE LOWER LIMB

Lumbosacral Plexus. Branches of the lumbosacral plexus (Fig. 2-10) supply most of the lower extremity. The ***lumbar plexus*** is formed in the substance of the psoas major muscle from the ventral rami of L1 through L4. All of L1 and part of L2 give rise to cutaneous nerves that supply the lower abdominal wall, the anterior part of the perineum and the proximal portion of the lower limb. The rest of the plexus forms major nerves of the lower extremity. The ***sacral plexus*** (L4 through S4) is formed in the pelvis on the ventral aspect of the piriformis muscle. The combined contribution of L4 and L5 to the sacral plexus is the lumbosacral trunk, which enters the pelvis by passing just lateral to the sacral promontory.

Femoral Nerve. The femoral nerve (L2–L4) emerges from the lateral aspect of the psoas major muscle and enters the thigh by passing deep to the inguinal ligament. Upon entering the femoral triangle, it immediately branches into its many muscular branches. Its terminal branch, the cutaneous saphenous nerve, continues through the thigh in the adductor canal. It enters the subcutaneous tissue in the distal thigh and supplies the skin on the medial aspect of the knee, leg, and foot.

Obturator Nerve. This nerve (L2–L4) emerges from the medial aspect of the psoas major muscle just above the pelvic brim. It then enters the pelvic cavity and passes anteriorly and ventrally toward the obturator canal, through which it enters the medial aspect of the thigh. It ends there by dividing into its terminal muscular and cutaneous branches. The cutaneous branches of this nerve supply the medial thigh and knee.

Gluteal Nerves. The superior gluteal nerve (L4–S1) arises in the pelvis but immediately exits by passing above the piriforms muscle and through the greater sciatic notch. It passes anteriorly between the gluteus medius and minimus muscles (supplying both) and terminates by supplying the tensor fasciae latae muscle. The inferior gluteal nerve (L5–S2) also arises in the pelvis and exits immediately by passing below the piriformis and through the greater sciatic notch directly into the substance of the gluteus maximus muscle.

Sciatic Nerve. The sciatic nerve is the largest nerve in the body. It consists of the tibial and common peroneal nerves, which are enclosed in a common connective tissue sheath. The sacral plexus essentially terminates as the sciatic nerve. This nerve leaves the pelvis by passing below the piriformis (usually) and through the greater sciatic notch. Its course through the gluteal region is curved, first passing midway between the ischial tuberosity and the posterior inferior iliac spine and then between the greater trochanter and the ischial tuberosity. It descends through the middle of the posterior thigh between the medial and lateral hamstring muscles, and typically divides into the common peroneal and tibial nerves in the distal thigh as it enters the popliteal fossa.

The ***common peroneal nerve*** passes superficially through the popliteal fossa just medial to the biceps femoris muscle and its tendon. It passes superficial to the lat-

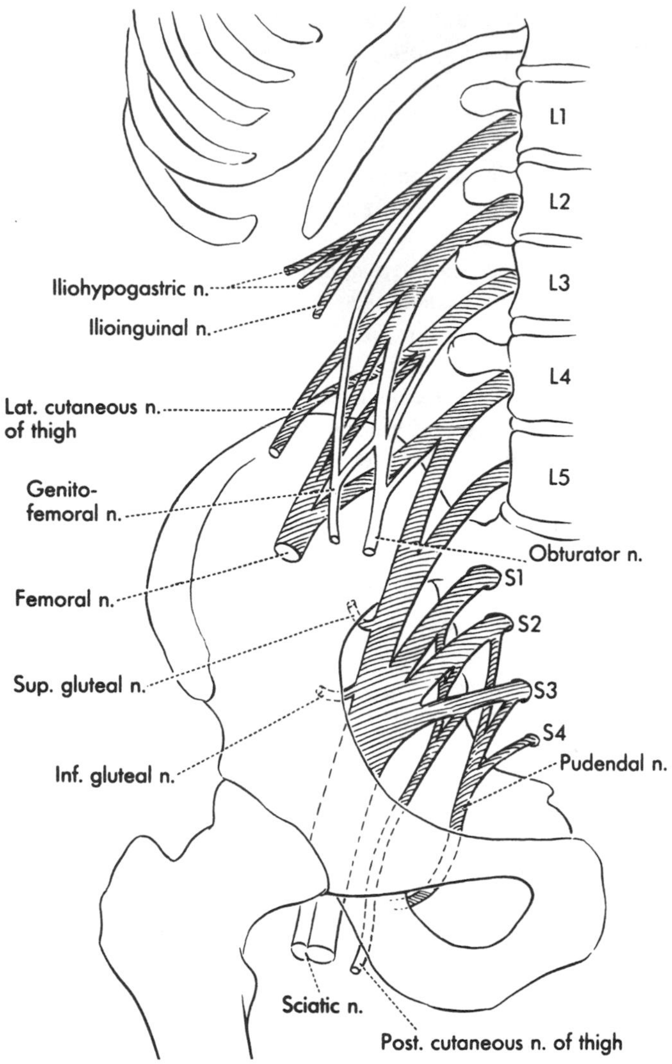

Fig. 2-10. Diagram of the lumbosacral plexus. (Hollinshead WH, Rosse C: Textbook of Anatomy, 4th ed, p 338. Philadelphia, JB Lippincott, 1985. After a figure from Sections of Neurology and the Section of Physiology, Mayo Clinic and Mayo Foundation: Clinical Examinations in Neurology, 2nd ed. Philadelphia, WB Saunders, 1963. Reprinted by permission of the Mayo Foundation)

eral femoral condyle and then wraps around the lateral aspect of the neck of the fibula. The nerve divides into its terminal branches, the superficial and deep peroneal nerves, as it passes the neck of the fibula. In the thigh the common peroneal innervates only the short head of the biceps femoris. The ***superficial peroneal nerve*** enters the lateral compartment of the leg, supplies the peroneus longus and brevis muscles, and then descends to innervate the skin on the dorsum of the foot. The ***deep peroneal nerve*** passes through the lateral compartment into the anterior compartment. It descends through this compartment, supplies the muscles in this compartment, and then enters the dorsum of the foot, where it supplies the extensor digitorum brevis and the extensor hallucis brevis muscles. It has a very small cutaneous distribution to the web space between the great and second toes.

The ***tibial nerve*** descends superficially through the center of the popliteal fossa. It enters the posterior compartment of the leg by passing between, and then deep to, the two heads of the gastrocnemius muscle. It descends through the leg between the superficial and deep groups of muscles and enters the foot by passing behind the medial malleolus. The tibial nerve supplies all the muscles in the posterior compartment of the leg. As it enters the foot, it divides into the ***medial*** and ***lateral plantar nerves.*** The medial plantar nerve is homologous with the median nerve of the hand. It passes into the medial aspect of the foot and divides into muscular branches as well as cutaneous branches (plantar digital nerves) that supply the skin on the plantar surface of the medial three and a half toes and corresponding part of the ball of the foot. The lateral plantar nerve is similar in course and distribution to the ulnar nerve in the hand. It passes diagonally across the plantar aspect of the foot by going through the abductor hallucis and then between the flexor digitorum brevis and quadratus plantae muscles. It then terminates by dividing into superficial and deep branches. The superficial branch has muscular branches, and is cutaneous to the plantar aspect of the lateral one and one half toes and corresponding part of the sole in that area. The deep branch dives deeply and passes medially across the foot deep to long flexor tendons and terminates by supplying the adductor hallucis.

PERIPHERAL NERVE LESIONS IN THE LOWER LIMB

The lower limb is used almost exclusively as a means of locomotion. The muscles are concerned with both weight-bearing and forward propulsion of the entire body. Therefore, in analyzing peripheral nerve lesions, it is only reasonable to evaluate the disturbances in the normal gait pattern that are caused by nerve damage.

Superior Gluteal Nerve. The abductors of the hip maintain the coronal balance during the stance phase of gait; that is, when an individual is standing on one foot, the hip abductors on the weight-bearing side prevent dropping of the pelvis to the opposite side (hip adduction). A patient with a superior gluteal nerve injury will exhibit a positive ***Trendelenburg sign*** during the stance phase of gait or when asked to stand on one foot; that is, his pelvis will drop to the non-weight-bearing side, and he will shift his trunk laterally to the weight-bearing side in order to bring the center of gravity over the supporting limb.

Inferior Gluteal Nerve. At heel-strike there is a tendency for the trunk to bend forward, that is, hip flexion. This is counteracted by the gluteus maximus. If this nerve is totally severed, the patient will compensate by throwing the trunk backward at heel-strike, thus preventing the line of gravity from moving anterior to the hip joint.

Femoral Nerve. At heel-strike and continuing through most of the stance phase, the quadriceps muscles maintain knee extension and thus support the body weight. With a loss of quadriceps function the patient must lock the knee and keep the line of gravity well in front of the joint. As a result this patient will whip his leg into extension by forceful thigh flexion followed by a rapid halt of this flexion (by way of the gluteus maximus), which snaps the knee into extension by pendulum action. As soon as the knee is extended he plants the heel on the floor, extends his hip (to hold the knee extension), and flexes his trunk (to get the line of gravity ahead of the knee joint). He then ***vaults*** over a rigidly extended knee. External rotation of the femur commonly accompanies the preceding maneuvers; in this position the medial collateral ligament of the knee is positioned to help maintain knee extension.

Deep Peroneal Nerve. During gait the anterior compartment muscles of the leg shorten the length of the limb during the swing phase by dorsiflexing the ankle; they also prevent plantar flexion (foot-slap) at heel-strike. When a patient with a deep peroneal nerve lesion (total paralysis) takes a step, he must lift his leg high so the plantar flexed foot can clear the ground ***(steppage gait).*** There is no heel-strike because the ball of the foot hits the ground before the heel. If there is partial paralysis of the deep peroneal nerve (the tibialis anterior is weakened), the foot can be dorsiflexed during the swing phase, but at heel-strike the weakened muscle cannot prevent plantar flexion and the ball of the foot hits the ground with a ***slap.***

Tibial Nerve. The forward momentum for locomotion is provided by the foot pushing down and back against the ground (plantar flexion). This function is lost with a tibial nerve lesion. The result is a noticeable lag in forward momentum at the point of push-off.

BLOOD SUPPLY OF THE LOWER LIMB

Arteries. Most of the lower extremity is supplied by the ***femoral artery*** (Fig. 2-11). The gluteal region receives the ***superior*** and ***inferior gluteal arteries*** from the internal iliac, and the ***obturator artery*** (also a branch of the internal iliac) supplies a portion of the medial thigh. The femoral artery is the continuation of the external iliac artery, which enters the thigh by passing deep to the inguinal ligament. It descends through the femoral triangle and adductor canal. As it enters the popliteal fossa by passing through the adductor hiatus, its name changes to the popliteal artery. A femoral pulse is taken about midway between the anterior superior spine of the ilium and the pubic tubercle. The largest branch of the femoral is the ***deep femoral artery,*** which arises in the femoral triangle and descends just medial to the femur. The ***medial and lateral circumflex arteries*** arise from the deep femoral soon after it arises. The deep femoral also has perforating branches that pass into the posterior compartment of the thigh.

The ***popliteal artery*** passes through the deepest portion of the popliteal fossa, where it has several genicular branches. When a popliteal pulse is taken the artery must be compressed against the femur. This is done with the knee flexed to remove the tension on the fascia covering the fossa. The artery terminates by dividing into the anterior and posterior tibial arteries as it enters the posterior compartment of the leg.

The ***anterior tibial artery*** immediately enters the anterior compartment of the leg by passing above the superior margin of the interosseous membrane. It descends through the anterior compartment and enters the foot by crossing the anterior aspect of the ankle; there it becomes the ***dorsalis pedis artery.*** On the dorsum of the foot—where the dorsalis pedis pulse is best taken—the artery is between the tendons of the extensor hallucis longus and the extensor digitorum longus. The dorsalis

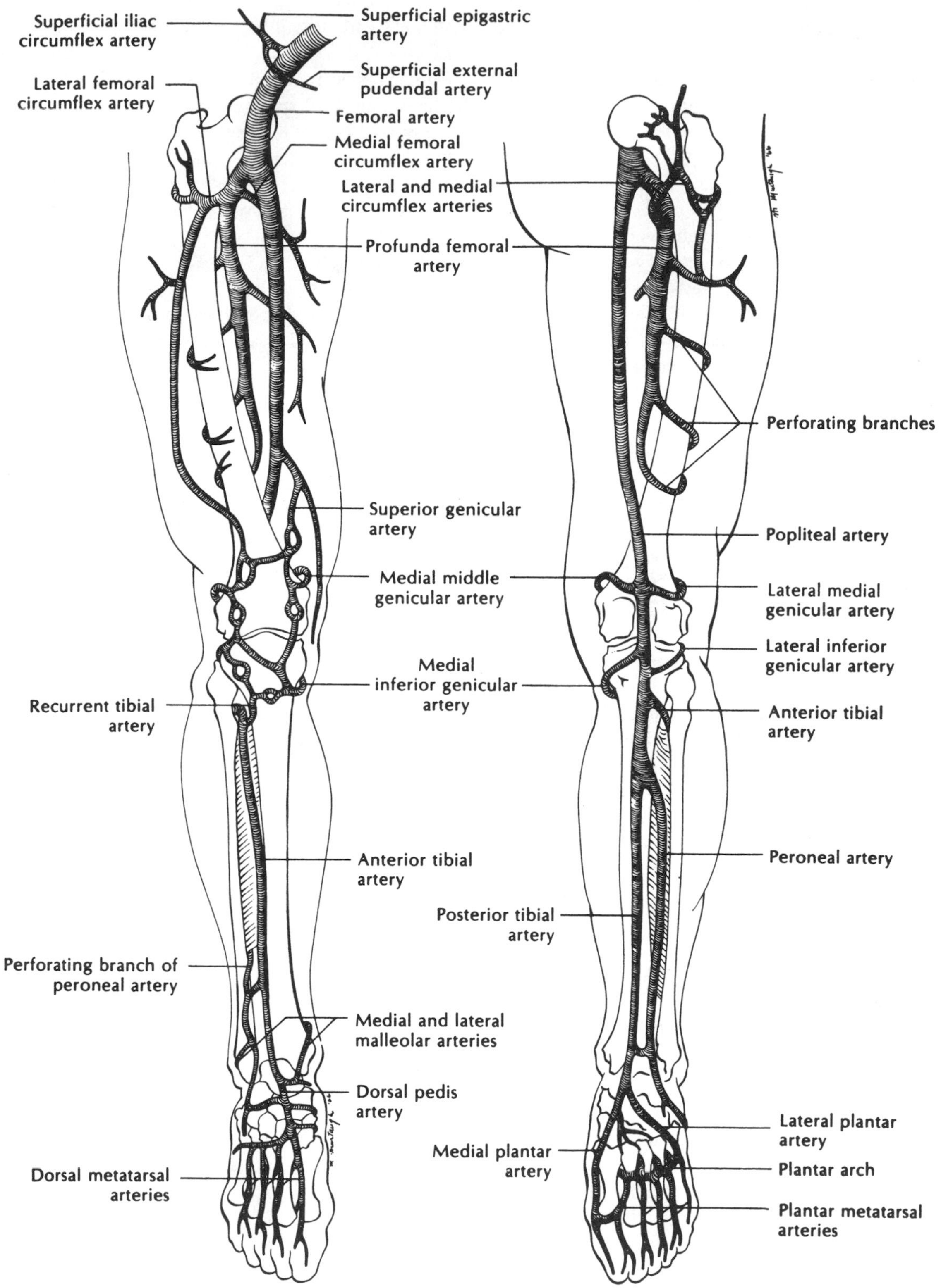

Fig. 2-11. Arteries of the lower limb. (Christensen JB, Telford IR: Synopsis of Gross Anatomy, 5th ed, p 278. Philadelphia, JB Lippincott, 1988)

pedis artery terminates into branches, most of which supply the dorsum of the foot. One of these branches, the deep plantar branch, passes into the plantar aspect of the foot by going between the first and second metatarsals and there helps form the ***plantar arterial arch.***

The ***posterior tibial artery*** descends through the deep portion of the posterior compartment of the leg, inclining medially as it descends. It enters the foot behind the medial malleolus where a posterior tibial pulse can be taken. It terminates as it passes around the medial malleolus by dividing into ***medial and lateral plantar arteries.*** It has a large peroneal branch high in the posterior compartment, the ***peroneal artery,*** which descends in the lateral part of the posterior compartment and terminates around the ankle.

The medial and lateral plantar arteries correspond in course and distribution to the medial and lateral plantar nerves. There is only one arterial arch in the foot, which corresponds to the deep arch of the hand, and is formed by the deep branch of the lateral plantar artery and the deep plantar branch of the dorsalis pedis artery.

Veins. The veins of the lower extremity consist of deep and superficial veins. The deep veins correspond rather closely to the pattern of the arteries. The two saphenous veins are the main superficial veins. The ***greater saphenous vein*** begins on the dorsomedial aspect of the foot and ascends along the anteromedial aspect of the leg and thigh. It terminates by passing through the saphenous opening of the fascia lata and emptying into the femoral vein just distal to the inguinal ligament. The greater saphenous vein passes just anterior to the medial malleolus, where it is commonly secured for venous cutdown. The ***lesser saphenous vein*** begins as a network on the dorsolateral aspect of the foot. It ascends behind the lateral malleolus and through the middle of the calf, and it terminates by emptying into the popliteal vein in the popliteal fossa.

HEAD AND NECK

SUPERFICIAL STRUCTURES OF THE HEAD AND NECK

Major Surface Landmarks and Regions. The anterolateral aspect of the neck is divided into anterior and posterior triangles by the prominent sternocleidomastoid muscle. The ***anterior triangle*** is in front of this muscle and extends to the inferior margin of the mandible and to the midline. Behind the sternocleidomastoid the ***posterior triangle*** is also delimited by the superior border of the trapezius muscle and the middle third of the clavicle. The face can be divided into several areas that include the orbit, nose, forehead, temporal region, maxillary region, and mandibular region. It is convenient to start with the well-defined orbit, which is protected and delimited by the prominent supraorbital and infraorbital margins, which meet laterally. Extending posteriorly at the level of the infraorbital margin, the zygomatic arch separates the temporal region above from the mandibular or lower jaw region below. The mandibular region extends inferiorly and then anteromedially to join the same region of the opposite side. The maxillary or upper jaw region is inferior to the infraorbital margin and lateral to the nose. The posterior part of the head is the occipital region.

Microscopic Structure of the Skin and Scalp. The skin consists of an outer ***epidermis*** of stratified squamous keratinized epithelium and an underlying ***dermis*** of dense irregularly arranged fibroelastic connective tissue. Beneath the dermis is a ***subcutaneous layer*** of loose connective tissue. The epidermis varies in structure and thickness, depending on the region of the body. On the palmar surface of the hand and on the soles of the feet the epidermis consists of four layers. These are, from the dermis to the surface, the stratum germinativum, stratum granulosum, stratum lucidum, and stratum corneum.

The stratum germinativum is further divisible into a stratum basale and stratum spinosum. Epidermal cells in both of these layers are capable of mitoses. Cells of the stratum spinosum (prickle cells) are joined at numerous desmosomes (macula adherens) where many tonofilaments converge toward the plasma membrane. Desmosomes are dense bodies where plasma membranes of adjacent cells appear thickened because of a dense layer on their cytoplasmic surfaces. A thin intermediate lamina occurs in the intercellular space at a desmosome. Tonofilaments will give rise to the fibrous protein keratin. Melanin granules are found in the deeper cells of the stratum germinativum in caucasians and in more cells of the deeper epidermal layers in colored races. Melanin is produced in melanocytes, which arise from neural crest. The melanin granules are distributed to the epidermal cells by a process of cytocrine secretion. The color of the skin is dependent on the amount of melanin, carotene, and the vascularity of the skin.

The stratum granulosum represents cells that are older and further differentiated in the keratinization process than those of the deeper layers. Keratohyalin granules predominate and will give rise to the interfilamentous amorphous matrix that will be prevalent in cells of the stratum corneum. Membrane-coating granules in the granulosal cells provide the intercellular ''sealing'' cement between cells of the stratum corneum. The stratum lucidum contains flattened translucent cells that have lost their nuclei; the cytoplasm contains an orderly array of tonofilaments. Cells of the stratum corneum also have lost their organelles and contain soft keratin, which consists of tightly packed filaments embedded in an amorphous matrix.

The dermis is divisible into papillary and reticular layers. The papillary layer is immediately underneath the epidermis and contains dense fine collagenous fibers, blood vessels, and free and encapsulated (e.g., Meissner's tactile corpuscles) nerve endings. The reticular layer contains coarser bundles of collagenous fibers. Smooth muscle can be found in this layer in the nipple and scrotum. Hair follicles, arrector pili smooth muscles, sebaceous glands, and the ducts of sweat glands are located in the reticular layer. The secretory portions of simple tubular sweat glands, the roots of hairs, and pacinian corpuscles (deep pressure receptors) are constituents of the subcutaneous layer. Extensive accumulations of fat in this layer determine it as the panniculus adiposus.

Secretory portions of sweat glands consist of a high cuboidal epithelium invested by contractile myoepithelial cells. Since no part of the cell is lost in the secretory process, it is classified as a merocrine type of secretion. The ducts are stratified cuboidal, except for the intraepidermal portion, which is lined by the epidermal epithelium.

Sebaceous glands have short ducts that empty into hair follicles, except for those in the labia minora and glans penis, where they open directly to the surface. The secretory portion of the sebaceous gland is stratified cuboidal; the lumen is generally filled with rounded cells containing numerous fat droplets. The secretion of sebum involves the holocrine discharge of sebaceous cells. New cells proliferate and differentiate from more basal regions of the gland.

Hairs are most prevalent in the scalp and are lacking in such areas as the palms of the hands and soles of the feet. Each hair consists of a root and a shaft. The root is enclosed by a tubular hair follicle that consists of inner and outer epithelial root sheaths, both derived from epidermis, and an outer connective tissue root sheath that corresponds to the dermis. At its lower end the follicle and root expand into a hair bulb, which is indented by a connective tissue hair papilla. The hair, consisting of an inner medulla, a cortex, and outer cuticle, grows upward from the differentiation of matrix cells in the hair bulb. Pigment in the cortical layer and air in the cortex and medulla determine the color of the hair. Arrectores pilorum of smooth muscle run in the obtuse angle between the follicle and epidermis, and they attach to the follicle deep to the sebaceous glands. Contraction causes erection of the hair and dimpling of the skin (goose flesh) at the smooth muscle attachment in the dermis. In the scalp and face, skeletal muscles are found in the superficial fascia.

Organization of the Blood Vessels to the Head and Neck. The common carotid arteries are the major arteries to the head and neck. The external carotid supplies most of the head and neck structures outside the cranial cavity; the internal carotid supplies the orbit and (along with the vertebral artery) cranial cavity. On the right the common carotid is one of the main terminal branches of the brachiocephalic trunk, while on the left it is a direct branch from the arch of the aorta. In a plane deep to the sternocleidomastoid muscle each artery ascends along a line that passes behind the sternoclavicular joint and through the midpoint between the angle of the mandible and the mastoid process. It terminates by dividing into the internal and external carotids between the levels of the hyoid bone and prominence of the thyroid cartilage (laryngeal prominence or Adam's apple). The carotid body and sinus are located at this bifurcation. The ***internal carotid*** has no branches in the neck and passes directly toward the carotid canal, through which it enters the cranial cavity.

The ***external carotid*** artery ascends to the neck of the mandible where it divides into its terminal branches: the ***maxillary artery,*** which passes deep to the neck of the mandible into the infratemporal fossa, and the ***superficial temporal artery,*** which ascends into the temporal region to supply that region and the anterior part of the scalp. Six other branches commonly arise from the external carotid artery. The ***superior thyroid artery*** supplies primarily the thyroid gland and larynx. The ***lingual artery*** passes deeply toward the tongue. The ***facial artery*** crosses the inferior margin of the mandible just anterior to the angle (where a facial pulse can be taken). From this point the facial artery follows a tortuous course obliquely across the face toward the angle between the nose and medial aspect of the eye. It supplies the superficial structures of the face as it winds superficial and deep to them. The ***ascending pharyngeal artery*** supplies the pharyngeal and palatal regions. The ***occipital*** and ***posterior auricular branches*** supply primarily the superficial regions designated by their names.

The ***jugular system of veins*** drains most of the head and neck. The main vessel is the internal jugular vein, which begins at the base of the skull where it receives most of the venous blood from the cranial cavity. It descends through the neck in company with the carotid arteries, receiving multiple tributaries from outside the cranial cavity, and terminates by joining the subclavian vein to form the brachiocephalic vein.

Cutaneous Nerves. The cutaneous innervation is easily defined if the head and neck are divided into three areas (Fig. 2-12). The first includes the entire face and the anterior part of the scalp, extending posteriorly to a line across the top of the head that connects the two external auditory meatuses (interauricular line). The skin of this area is innervated by the three divisions of the fifth cranial (trigeminal) nerve. The ophthalmic nerve innervates the bridge of the nose, upper eyelid and cornea, forehead, and scalp. The maxillary division covers the

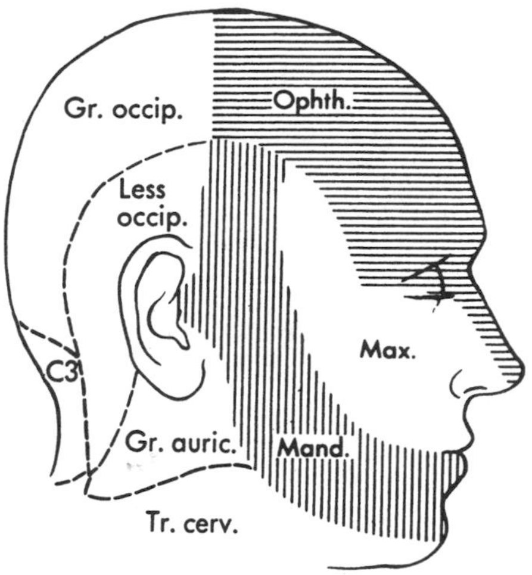

Fig. 2-12. Approximate cutaneous distribution of the three divisions of the fifth nerve and of cervical nerves to the face and scalp. (Hollinshead WH: Anatomy For Surgeons, Vol 1, 3rd ed, p 317. Philadelphia, JB Lippincott, 1982)

lateral aspect of the nose, cheek, and anterior temporal region. The mandibular innervation corresponds to the area overlying the mandible and the posterior temporal region. The second area includes the posterior neck and the corresponding part of the occipital region, which extends anteriorly to the interauricular line. This area is supplied by cutaneous branches of the dorsal rami of cervical spinal nerves. The third area includes the anterolateral neck, posterior triangle and shoulder pad region, and the skin surrounding the ear posteriorly. This third area is innervated by the cutaneous branches of the cervical plexuses (lesser occipital, great auricular, transverse cervical, and supraclavicular nerves).

Facial Muscles. The muscles of facial expression are found in the subcutaneous tissue of the face, neck (platysma), and scalp (epicranius). They function to move the skin and regulate the shapes of the openings on the face. Many muscles are associated with the muscle surrounding the mouth (orbicularis oris) and those surrounding the eyes (orbicularis oculi). The buccinator muscle is deeply located in the cheek and represents the only muscle in the interval between the maxilla and mandible. All of these muscles are innervated by the seventh cranial (facial) nerve.

Parotid Gland. The largest of the salivary glands is located anteroinferior to the ear and extends inferiorly to the level of the angle of the mandible. It has a deep portion that extends posterior and then medial to the ramus of the mandible. The main trunk of the facial nerve enters the posterior aspect of the gland and divides into its main divisions within the substance of the gland. The parotid duct passes anteriorly around the masseter muscle and empties into the oral cavity just opposite the second upper molar.

Microscopic Structure of Major Salivary Glands. The parenchyma of the parotid gland consists of ***serous acini*** and ducts. The acini are grouped into lobules and lobes by connective tissue septa. Pyramid-shaped cells with apical accumulations of zymogen granules and basal concentrations of RER line the small lumina of the serous acini. Myoepithelial cells lie between the acinar cells and the basal lamina. The serous secretion of the acinar cells passes into ***intercalated ducts,*** which empty into ***striated ducts.*** Both of these ducts are intralobular ducts. Intercalated ducts have small lumina and are lined by simple cuboidal epithelium. Striated (salivary) ducts are larger and are lined by a simple columnar epithelium whose cells have extensive infoldings of the plasma membrane on their basal surfaces. These basal striations with their interposed mitochondria are like those in cells of the distal convoluted tubules of the kidney and perform similar functions in the reabsorption of sodium and water from the luminal fluid. After reabsorption, the secretion in the striated ducts passes successively to interlobular, interlobar, and the main excretory (Stensen's) ducts. The simple columnar epithelial lining of the ducts gets taller as the main duct is approached. Stensen's duct is lined by pseudostratified columnar epithelium that contains some goblet cells. At the opening of the duct into the oral cavity, the epithelium becomes stratified squamous nonkeratinized epithelium.

The submandibular gland is a mixed seromucous gland whose acini are preponderantly serous. ***Mucous alveoli*** are frequently capped by ***serous demilunes*** or have some serous cells lining their terminal portions. The secretion from serous demilunes passes between mucous cells to reach the lumen. Mucous cells contain basally flattened nuclei, RER, and apical membrane-bound mucigen droplets. The ducts of the submandibular gland are microscopically similar to those of the parotid, but striated ducts are longer and more numerous. The main duct (Wharton's) opens into the mouth beneath the tongue.

The sublingual gland is a mixed gland, but the mucous alveoli predominate. Striated (salivary) ducts and intercalated ducts are few in number. The main excretory ducts open into the mouth at the side of the frenulum and, like the main ducts of the parotid and submandibular gland, are lined by pseudostratified columnar epithelium.

FASCIAL PLANES AND COMPARTMENTS OF THE NECK

Fascial Planes. The ***superficial layer*** (investing layer) of cervical fascia encircles the neck and encloses the sternocleidomastoid and trapezius muscles (Fig. 2-13). The ***prevertebral fascia*** surrounds the vertebral

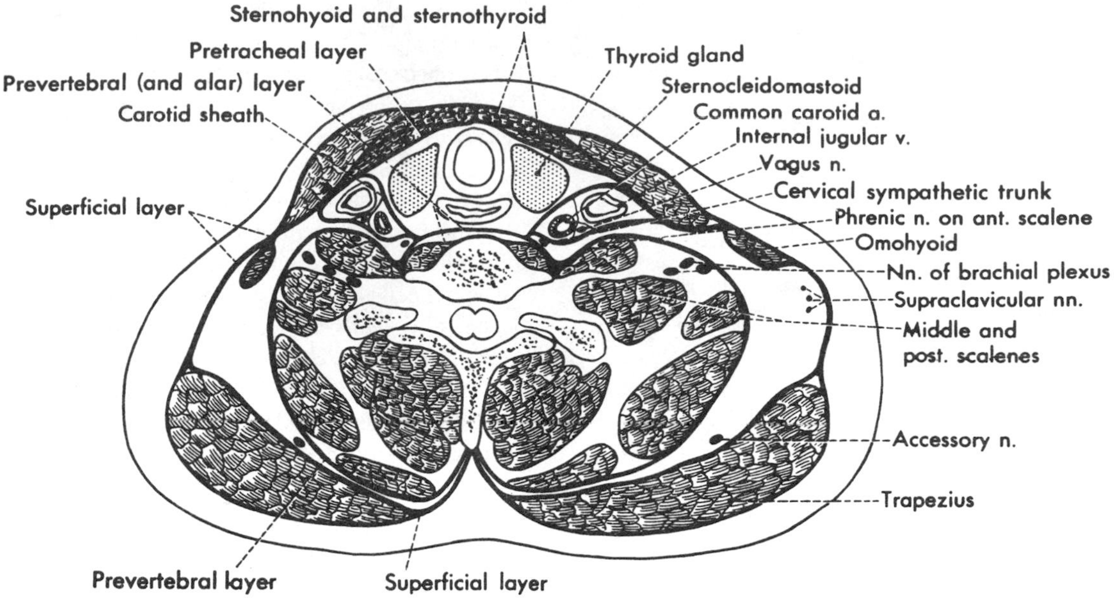

Fig. 2-13. Chief layers of the cervical fascia below the hyoid bone. (Hollinshead WH: Anatomy For Surgeons, Vol 1, 3rd ed, p 271. Philadelphia, JB Lippincott, 1982)

column and its associated muscles, that is, the longus capitis and colli, the scalenes, and the deep muscles of the back in the cervical region. The visceral structures of the neck are enclosed in a sleeve of fascia called the ***pretracheal fascia*** anteriorly and laterally and the ***buccopharyngeal fascia*** (between the pharynx or esophagus and the vertebral column) posteriorly. The infrahyoid muscles have their own fascia, which is between the investing and pretracheal layers of cervical fascia. In the lateral part of the neck and deep to the plane of the sternocleidomastoid muscle, the several layers of cervical fascia meet and contribute to the formation of the vertically oriented ***carotid sheath.***

Anterior Triangle. Many surgical approaches to the viscera of the neck are made through this area, which is bounded by the midline, inferior margin of the mandible and the sternocleidomastoid muscle. The part of the anterior triangle above the digastric muscle is the submandibular triangle, and the area below the digastric is sometimes divided into the carotid triangle above the omohyoid muscle and muscular triangle below. The carotid sheath structures—the vagus nerve, the carotid artery, and the internal jugular vein—pass vertically through this area, located deep to the sternocleidomastoid muscle. The cervical sympathetic chain is deep in the triangle on the anterolateral aspects of the cervical vertebrae. The lateral lobes of the thyroid gland are immediately adjacent to the lateral aspects of the trachea and lower larynx, while the isthmus of the thyroid crosses the midline in front of the upper rings of the trachea. The parathyroids are related to the posterior surface of the upper and lower aspects of the lateral lobes of the thyroid. The esophagus lies behind the trachea and larynx.

The submandibular triangle contains the submandibular gland, the facial artery and vein, the mylohyoid vessels and nerves, and the hypoglossal nerve.

Posterior Triangle. The posterior triangle is bounded by the superior border of the trapezius, the posterior border of the sternocleidomastoid, and the middle third of the clavicle. This area is easily visualized by asking the patient to hunch his shoulder anteriorly and turn his head to the opposite side. Several major structures supplying the upper limb are accessible through this triangle.

The cutaneous branches of the cervical plexus enter the subcutaneous tissue after curving around the posterior middle third of the sternocleidomastoid muscle. The accessory nerve emerges from beneath the middle of the posterior border of the sternocleidomastoid, passes obliquely across the triangle and dives deep to the superior border of the trapezius about 3 cm above its clavicular attachment. The inferior belly of the omohyoid muscle crosses the inferior aspect of the triangle a few centimeters above the clavicle.

The floor of the posterior triangle is muscular, consisting of the splenius capitis, levator scapulae, and the scalene muscles. The anterior and middle scalene muscles attach inferiorly on the first rib. These two muscles, together with a small portion of the first rib, form a narrow triangle (***scalene triangle*** or scalene groove) through which the roots (ventral rami) of the brachial plexus and the subclavian artery enter the posterior triangle. Any of these structures can be compressed as they pass through this narrow opening. This neurovascular compression can be caused by muscle hypertrophy, the occurrence of a cervical rib, and so forth. Since the posterior border of the anterior scalene muscle corresponds to the lower part of the posterior border of the sternocleidomastoid muscle, the scalene groove is readily palpable. The roots of the plexus are palpable as hard cords, and the subclavian pulse can be taken by compressing the subclavian artery against the first rib. In addition, the inferior deep cervical lymph nodes are associated with the anterior scalene. These ***anterior scalene nodes***—the final sentinel nodes for the thoracic duct on the left and the right lymphatic duct on the right—are palpated in the same area.

Although only a portion of the ***subclavian artery*** is in the posterior triangle, it is included here. This artery is divided into three parts on the basis of its relationship to the anterior scalene muscle (see Fig. 2-8). The first part arises from the arch of the aorta on the left and the brachiocephalic trunk on the right. It passes superolaterally to the medial margin of the anterior scalene. The branches of the first part are the ***vertebral artery,*** which ascends deep to the anterior scalene to enter the transverse foramen of C6; the ***thyrocervical trunk,*** which has suprascapular, transverse cervical, and inferior thyroid branches; and the ***internal thoracic artery,*** which descends deep to the costal cartilages just lateral to the sternum. The second part of the subclavian lies posterior to the anterior scalene. Its only branch is the ***costocervical trunk,*** which gives rise to the deep cervical and highest intercostal arteries. The third part extends from the lateral border of the anterior scalene to the first rib. The ***dorsal scapular artery*** may arise from this part.

VISCERAL STRUCTURES OF THE NECK

Larynx. The larynx (Fig. 2-14) is a tubular organ composed of nine cartilages that are connected by elastic membranes and synovial joints. It is lined by a mucosa that covers the vocal cords and is innervated by branches of the vagus nerve. The cartilages of the larynx consist of three single ones: epiglottis, thyroid, and cricoid; and three pairs: arytenoids, corniculates, and cuneiforms.

The larynx is that portion of the airway between the pharynx and the trachea. It is anterior to cervical vertebrae 4 through 6, and related anteriorly to the infrahyoid muscles and laterally to the inferior constrictor muscle of the pharynx and the lobes of the thyroid gland.

The vocal apparatus ***(glottis)*** consists of the true vocal folds and the opening ***(rima glottidis)*** between the folds. The area above the true folds, extending to the laryngeal additis (entrance), is the ***vestibule*** or ***supraglottic portion.*** The false vocal folds are above the true folds, and the area extending laterally between the true and false folds is the ***ventricle.*** The vocal fold (true vocal cord) contains the thin cranial edge of the conus elasticus. This free edge is the so-called vocal cord. The ***vocal fold*** is divided into anterior ***intramembranous*** and posterior ***intracartilaginous portions.*** The intramembranous portion stretches between the thyroid and arytenoid cartilages and is capable of tension changes and vibration. The intracartilaginous portion is formed by the arytenoid cartilage. The numerous intrinsic muscles moving the laryngeal cartilages lie deep to the thyroid cartilage except the cricothyroid, which alone is innervated by the external branch of the superior laryngeal nerve, and which functions to tense the vocal cords. The others are innervated by the inferior laryngeal (recurrent) branch of the vagus. These muscles include the posterior cricoarytenoid, which abducts the vocal cords; the transverse arytenoid and lateral cricoarytenoid, which adduct the vocal cords; and the thyroarytenoid and vocalis muscles, which relax the vocal cords. The internal branch of the superior laryngeal nerve is sensory to the supraglottic portion of the larynx and the adjacent part of the pharynx. The recurrent laryngeal nerve innervates the infraglottic mucosa of the larynx. The blood supply is provided by the superior and inferior thyroid arteries.

Pharynx. The pharynx extends from the base of the skull to the beginning of the larynx and esophagus. Posteriorly it is in contact with the upper six cervical vertebrae; laterally it is related to the internal and the common carotid arteries, the internal jugular vein, the sympathetic trunk, and the last four cranial nerves. Anteriorly it communicates with the nasal cavity and the oral cavity; inferiorly it communicates with the larynx and esophagus.

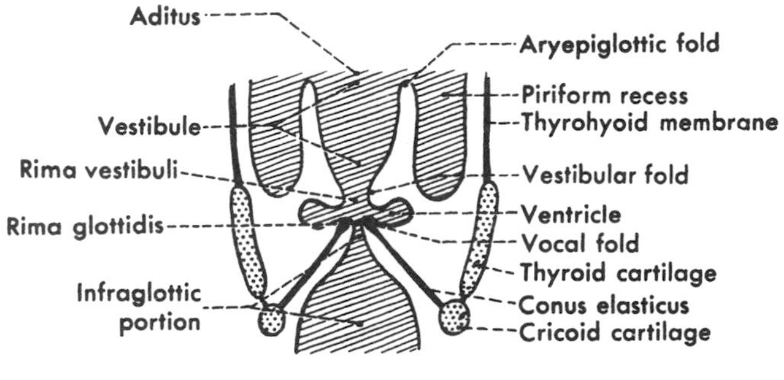

Fig. 2-14. Cavity of the larynx and its subdivisions in a frontal section. (Hollinshead WH: Anatomy For Surgeons, Vol 1, 3rd ed, p 420. Philadelphia, JB Lippincott, 1982)

That portion of the pharynx above the soft palate is the ***nasopharynx.*** The auditory (eustachian) tube opens on the lateral wall of the nasopharynx. The projecting cartilage of the auditory tube produces a marked elevation (the torus tubarius) around the opening, and the pharyngeal recess is the fossa behind the posterior lip of the torus. The pharyngeal tonsil (''adenoid'') is found on the posterior wall of the nasopharynx. The ***oropharynx*** is posterior to the oral cavity, and it is limited above by the soft palate and below by the superior aspect of the epiglottis. The oral pharynx communicates with the oral cavity through the ***fauces*** (throat), which is below the soft palate and above the root of the tongue. Laterally the fauces are bounded by two mucosal-covered muscular columns (pillars of the fauces): anteriorly the palatoglossal fold and posteriorly the palatopharyngeal fold. The lateral area between the folds is the tonsillar fossa, which contains the palatine tonsil. The ***laryngopharynx*** extends from the superior edge of the epiglottis inferiorly to the lower border of the cricoid cartilage, essentially surrounding the larynx laterally and posteriorly. The vertical groove between the lateral aspect of the larynx and the pharyngeal wall is the piriform recess.

The ***muscles of the pharynx*** are the three constrictors and the stylopharyngeus, the latter passing downward between the superior and the middle constrictors. The constrictors overlap each other from below upward and surround the pharynx, and all three are inserted into a fibrous raphe in the posterior midline. Between muscles and mucous membrane is the pharyngobasilar fascia, which is especially strong above where it is attached to the basilar process of the occipital bone and the petrous portion of the temporal bone. The inferior constrictor arises from the cricoid cartilage and the oblique line of the thyroid cartilage and encircles the pharynx. The middle constrictor arises from the greater and the lesser horns of the hyoid bone. The superior constrictor arises from the lower end and the hamulus of the medial pterygoid plate, the pterygomandibular ligament and the posterior end of the mylohyoid line on the inner surface of the mandible. The constrictor muscles are innervated by the tenth cranial nerve and the stylopharyngeus by the ninth cranial nerve. The ninth cranial nerve is also a major sensory nerve innervating the pharyngeal mucosa. As a result, the sensory limb of the gag reflex is the ninth cranial nerve and the motor limb the tenth cranial nerve.

Microscopic Structure of the Thyroid and Parathyroid Glands. The thyroid gland is invested by a thin capsule of connective tissue that projects into its substance and divides it imperfectly into lobes and lobules. The parenchyma consists of ***follicles*** that are closed epithelial sacs lined by simple cuboidal or simple columnar epithelium, the cells being low when the gland is underactive and taller when the gland is overactive. Follicles vary from 50 μ to 500 μ in diameter, and the size of each follicle is somewhat dependent on the degree of distention by the stored colloid in the lumen of the follicle. In the production of thyroxine and triiodothyronine the follicular cells receive iodide and amino acids from extensively distributed fenestrated capillaries lying adjacent to the basement membrane. Through the mechanisms of a basally located RER and apically oriented Golgi apparatus, a glycoproteinaceous thyroglobulin is produced. This substance is discharged at the apical end of the cell into the follicular lumen where it is stored along with nucleoproteins and proteolytic enzymes as colloid. Under the influence of thyroid-stimulating hormone (TSH), portions of thyroglobulin are taken into the apex of the follicular cell by pinocytosis, and the droplets are hydrolyzed by lysosomal activity into thyroxine and triiodothyronine. These substances are then secreted from the basal aspect of the cell into the surrounding capillaries. ***Parafollicular cells*** located between follicle cells and the basement membrane, and also found between follicles, differ structurally from follicle cells by being larger and lighter staining. They produce calcitonin.

A connective tissue capsule separates parathyroid glands from the thyroid gland. Fine connective tissue septa penetrate the parathyroid glands and divide the parenchyma into irregular cords of chief (principal cells) and oxyphil cells. ***Chief cells*** produce parathyroid hormone and are found in two functional states as light and dark chief cells. Dark chief cells contain membrane-bound argyrophilic secretory granules, a relatively large Golgi complex, and large filamentous mitochondria. Light cells have a smaller Golgi complex and few secretory granules. Oxyphilic cells are very acidophilic, are engorged with mitochondria and have a small nucleus, and do not appear until the end of the first decade of life. Their function is unknown.

Microscopic Structure of the Larynx and Trachea. As previously mentioned, the tubular larynx is composed of nine cartilages connected by elastic membranes and intrinsic skeletal muscles. It is lined with a mucosa whose folds form the true and false vocal folds. The mucosa of each ***true vocal fold*** covers the vocal ligament (free margin of the conus elasticus) and vocalis muscle. The lining epithelium of the true vocal fold and of most of the epiglottis is stratified squamous nonkeratinized epithelium. Some taste buds may be found in the epiglottic epithelium. The rest of the lining is pseudostratified ciliated columnar epithelium that contains goblet cells and is underlain by a lamina propria containing mixed seromucous glands. Inhaled particulate matter is entrapped in the sticky mucous secretion, which is transported to the pharynx by ciliary movement in the more fluid serous medium. There are no glands in the true vocal folds, but the surface is kept moist by the secretions that arise from numerous glands lining the ventricles. Lymphatic tissue in the ventricles may constitute the laryngeal tonsil. The thyroid, cricoid, and most of the arytenoid cartilages are hyaline cartilage. The epiglottis, cuneiform, corniculate, and tips of the arytenoid cartilages are elastic cartilage.

The trachea is a tubular structure whose wall, from the luminal surface outward, consists of a mucosa, submucosa, and adventitia. The mucosa is similar to that of most of the larynx in that it is comprised of a pseudostratified ciliated columnar epithelium with goblet cells, the most prominent basement membrane in the body, and a lamina propria that contains many longitudinally directed elastic fibers. The indistinct submucosa contains seromucous glands that also extend between the C- and Y-shaped hyaline cartilage rings in the adventitial layer. The open interval of the C-shaped cartilages faces the esophagus and is bridged with fibroelastic tissue and a trachealis smooth muscle that runs circularly, attaching at the inner surface of each cartilage end.

Microscopic Structure of the Pharynx. The wall of the pharynx consists of a mucosa, muscularis, and fibrosa. A submucosal layer exists only in the superior lateral region and near the junction with the esophagus. The epithelium of the nasopharynx is pseudostratified ciliated columnar epithelium with goblet cells; that of the oropharynx and laryngopharynx is stratified squamous nonkeratinized epithelium. The lamina propria contains many elastic fibers that constitute a dense elastic layer immediately adjacent to the muscularis. Mucous glands are found beneath the stratified squamous epithelium, whereas mixed glands occupy the lamina propria under the pseudostratified ciliated columnar epithelium. Aggregations of lymphatic nodules in the posterior nasopharyngeal mucosa constitute the pharyngeal tonsils (adenoids). The superior, middle, and inferior constrictor muscles and the stylopharyngeus and salpingopharyngeus muscles constitute the skeletal muscles of the muscularis layer. The fibrosa layer is a tough fibroelastic layer that attaches the pharynx to surrounding structures.

TEMPORAL AND INFRATEMPORAL REGIONS

Osteology. The ***temporal fossa*** is superficial to those areas of the frontal, parietal, and squamous portions of the temporal and greater wing of the sphenoid bones that are bounded superiorly and posteriorly by the temporal lines. It extends inferiorly to the zygomatic arch and anteriorly to the frontal process of the zygomatic bone.

The ***infratemporal fossa*** is deep to the ramus of the mandible and the zygomatic arch. It is limited above by the infratemporal crest of the sphenoid, medially by the lateral pterygoid plate, anteriorly by the maxilla, and inferiorly by the alveolar border of the maxilla. The infratemporal fossa is continuous medially with the pterygopalatine fossa via the pterygomaxillary fissure. It communicates with the middle cranial fossa by openings in its roof: the foramen ovale and foramen spinosum. Connections with the orbit are established through the inferior orbital fissure.

Temporomandibular Joint. The temporomandibular articulation is formed between the anterior portion of the mandibular fossa and the articular tubercle of the temporal bone above and the condyle of the mandible below. The articular surfaces are covered by fibrocartilage and are separated by an articular disk. This disk separates the joint space into two compartments. The joint capsule is rather loose between the temporal bone and articular disk but tighter and stronger between the disk and mandibular condyle. As a result, different types of movement occur between the temporal bone and disk and between the disk and condyle. The disk and condyle slide as a unit relative to the mandibular fossa, and the condyle rotates as a hinge on the disk. For example, opening the mouth (depression of the mandible) involves anterior translation of the disk and condyle as well as rotation between the condyle and disk.

Muscles of Mastication. The muscles of mastication are the masseter, the temporalis, and the medial and lateral pterygoids. They are found both in the temporal and infratemporal fossae and superficial to the ramus of the mandible.

The ***masseter*** extends from the zygomatic arch to the outer surface of the ramus of the mandible, and it is an elevator of the mandible. The ***temporalis*** muscle arises from the temporal fossa of the skull and inserts on the borders and the inner surface of the coronoid process. It elevates and retracts the mandible. The ***medial pterygoid*** arises from the inner surface of the lateral pterygoid plate and inserts on the angle and the inner surface of the ramus of the mandible. The ***lateral pterygoid*** arises from the zygomatic surface of the greater wing of the sphenoid and the outer surface of the lateral pterygoid plate. It inserts in the depression in front of the neck of the mandible and the articular disk. Both pterygoid muscles (especially the lateral) cause deviation of the mandible to the opposite side and are thereby responsible for the grinding action of chewing. In addition, the medial pterygoid is an elevator and the lateral pterygoid is a protruder of the mandible. Mandibular depression is produced by the lateral pterygoid and floor of the mouth muscles. All muscles of mastication are innervated by the mandibular division of the trigeminal nerve.

Contents of the Infratemporal Fossa. In addition to the pterygoid muscles, the infratemporal fossa contains the proximal portion of the maxillary artery, the mandibular division of the trigeminal nerve, and the pterygoid plexus of veins.

The ***maxillary artery*** is the larger of the two terminal branches of the external carotid. It arises in the substance of the parotid gland and enters the infratemporal fossa by passing deep to the ramus of the mandible. It passes obliquely through the fossa (either deep or superficial to the lateral pterygoid muscle) on its course to the pterygopalatine fossa via the pterygomaxillary fissure. While in the infratemporal fossa it gives off the anterior tympanic, deep auricular, middle meningeal, inferior alveolar, pterygoid, masseteric, buccal, and deep temporal branches. The ***middle meningeal artery*** enters the middle cranial fossa through the foramen spinosum and is the major arterial supply to the cranial dura mater.

The ***mandibular nerve*** enters the infratemporal fossa through the foramen ovale. The main trunk of this nerve is short (1 cm) so that it branches high in the fossa. It has muscular branches to the muscles of mastication, and the mylohyoid, tensor tympani, and tensor veli palatini. Its sensory branches are the buccal nerve to the cheek, the auriculotemporal nerve to the posterior temporal region, the lingual nerve to the oral cavity, and the inferior alveolar nerve to the mandibular dentition and the skin covering the chin.

Parasympathetics are distributed in certain branches of this nerve. The otic ganglion is located medial to the main trunk of the nerve just inferior to the foramen ovale. The preganglionic input to this ganglion is from the lesser petrosal nerve, whose fibers exit the brainstem in cranial nerve IX. (Between cranial nerve IX and the lesser petrosal these fibers pass through the tympanic nerve and the tympanic plexus.) The postganglionic fibers from the otic ganglion are distributed with the auriculotemporal branch to the parotid gland. The other source of preganglionic fibers is the chorda tympani branch of the seventh cranial nerve, which enters the infratemporal fossa through the petrotympanic fissure and joins the lingual nerve high in the fossa. The lingual nerve transports these preganglionic fibers to the submandibular ganglion (located in the submandibular triangle) where they synapse and are then distributed to the submandibular, sublingual, and lingual glands.

The ***pterygoid plexus of veins*** surrounds the pterygoid muscles. It receives blood from the face, nasal cavity, orbit, palate, cranial cavity, pharynx, and infratemporal fossa. It drains into the maxillary vein, which joins the superficial temporal vein to form the retromandibular vein.

PTERYGOPALATINE FOSSA

Osteology. The pterygopalatine fossa is between the maxilla in front and the pterygoid portion of the sphenoid behind. Medially it is bounded by the perpendicular plate of the palatine bone. It communicates laterally with the infratemporal fossa by the pterygomaxillary fissure, medially with the nasal cavity by the sphenopalatine foramen, inferiorly with the oral cavity by the palatine canal and the greater and lesser palatine foramina, posterosuperiorly with the middle cranial fossa by the foramen rotundum, anterosuperiorly with the orbit by the inferior orbital fissure, and posteromedially with the pharynx by the pharyngeal canal. The pterygoid canal is a canal through the pterygoid portion of the sphenoid that opens onto the posterior wall of the pterygopalatine fossa.

Contents of the Pterygopalatine Fossa. This fossa contains the terminal portion of the maxillary artery, the maxillary division of the trigeminal nerve, and the ***pterygopalatine parasympathetic ganglion.*** The preganglionic parasympathetic fibers that synapse in this ganglion exit the brain stem in the facial nerve. From the facial nerve the course of these fibers is in the greater petrosal nerve, which passes into the middle cranial fossa by the hiatus of the facial canal and then out of the fossa by a small foramen in the region of the foramen lacerum. The greater petrosal nerve then joins the deep petrosal nerve (which contains postganglionic sympathetic fibers), and together they pass through the pterygoid canal as the nerve of the pterygoid canal. This nerve terminates in the ganglion, the parasympathetics synapsing, and sympathetics merely passing through. Both fiber types are then distributed with branches of the maxillary nerve. The parasympathetic secretomotor fibers are thus distributed to the mucosa of the nasal cavity, palate, pharynx, and paranasal sinuses and to the lacrimal gland. The course of these fibers to the lacrimal gland is circuitous; they pass sequentially in the infraorbital nerve, its zygomatic branch, a communicating branch between the zygomatic and lacrimal nerves, and the lacrimal nerve to the gland.

The ***maxillary nerve*** continues as the infraorbital nerve, which passes into the floor of the orbit and eventually terminates on the face by the infraorbital foramen. The branches of the maxillary nerve and the proximal portion of the infraorbital nerve are the palatine (greater and lesser) to the palate, the nasopalatine and lateral nasal branches to the nasal cavity, the pharyngeal nerve to the nasopharynx, the zygomatic nerve to the skin of the zygomatic region of the face, and the superior alveolar nerves to the maxillary sinus and dentition.

The branches of the ***pterygopalatine artery*** (third part of the maxillary artery) are the posterior superior alveolar to the maxillary sinus and maxillary dentition, the infraorbital artery, the descending palatine artery to the palate, the pharyngeal artery, and the sphenopalatine artery to the nasal cavity.

ORAL CAVITY

The mouth or oral cavity consists of a vestibule and the mouth proper. The vestibule of the mouth lies between the lips and cheeks externally and the gums and teeth internally. It receives the parotid duct opposite the second upper molar tooth.

The ***mouth proper*** is bounded laterally and in front by the alveolar arches and the teeth; behind, it communicates with the pharynx through the fauces. It is roofed by the hard and the soft palates. The floor is composed of the tongue and the reflection of its mucous membrane to the gum lining the inner aspect of the mandible; the midline reflection is elevated into a fold called the frenulum linguae. On each side of this fold is the caruncula sublingualis containing the openings of the submandibular (Wharton's) ducts. Behind these are the openings of the ducts of the sublingual glands.

Lips and Cheeks. The lips are muscular folds covered externally by skin and internally by mucosa (mucous membrane). The upper lip extends to the nasolabial sulcus and contains a vertical midline groove, the philtrum. The mentolabial sulcus separates the lower lip from the skin of the chin. The lips receive their blood supply from labial branches of the facial artery. Their sensory nerve supply is by infraorbital branches of the trigeminal nerve to the upper lip and mental branches to the lower lip; the facial nerve supplies the orbicularis oris muscle. Microscopically the cutaneous surface consists of a thin skin, which possesses hairs, and sweat and sebaceous glands. The vestibular surface consists of stratified squamous nonkeratinized epithelium, lamina propria, and a submucosa rich in mucous and mixed seromucous labial glands. The orbicularis oris muscle lies between the dermis and submucosal layers. The red area of the lip lies in the free margin of the lip at the junction between skin and mucosa. It is covered by stratified squamous epithelium containing variable degrees of keratinization and deeply indenting vascular papillae. No glands are present, and the epithelium is kept moist by licking of the lips.

The cheeks are similar in structure to the lips. Thick submucosal fibers tightly bind the mucosa to the buccinator muscle, thus reducing the chance of chewing on mucosal folds. Mixed buccal glands occupy the submucosa.

Tongue. The tongue is a muscular organ whose bilateral muscle masses are separated in the midline by a fibrous septum. Extrinsic muscles interconnect the tongue and the hyoid bone (hyoglossus), styloid process (styloglossus), mandible (genioglossus), and palate (palatoglossus). Portions of the genioglossus function in protrusion of the tongue; the styloglossus and palatoglossus elevate the tongue; the hyoglossus depresses the sides; and the styloglossus and other portions of the genioglossus serve in retraction of the tongue. Intrinsic muscles are oriented in vertical, longitudinal, and transverse bundles and function to control the shape of the tongue. Both intrinsic and extrinsic muscles, with the exception of the palatoglossus (which is innervated by the vagus nerve), are innervated by the hypoglossal (12th) nerve. At its root the tongue is connected to the pharynx, palate, and epiglottis; the glossoepiglottic folds attach the root to the epiglottis and bound the vallecula.

The tongue is divisible into an anterior two thirds and a posterior one third by a V-shaped sulcus terminalis on the dorsum of the tongue. The apex of the V points posteriorly and ends in the foramen cecum, which marks the site of the embryonic thyroid diverticulum.

The mucosa over the anterior two thirds is characterized by filiform and fungiform papillae. ***Filiform papillae*** are the most numerous and uniformly distributed. They have a slender vascular core of connective tissue and are covered by a partially keratinized epithelium. ***Fungiform papillae*** are knoblike projections that are larger and more scattered than the filiform papillae. Their epithelium is mostly stratified squamous nonkeratinized and contains taste buds. ***Vallate papillae*** are the largest and least numerous of the papillae. They are oriented parallel to the sulcus terminalis and are 9 to 12 in number. Each papilla is surrounded by a trench into which underlying serous glands of von Ebner empty. The sides of the papillae and trench contain many ***taste buds,*** which extend intraepithelially from the basement membrane to the surface. Taste buds contain spindle-shaped neuroepithelial cells that receive sensory nerve endings. Anterior lingual glands are located near the tip of the tongue and are mixed seromucous glands.

The mucosa over the root of the tongue is stratified squamous nonkeratinized epithelium overlying connective tissue, lymphatic nodules, and mucous glands. Aggregations of lymphatic nodules around single crypts constitute lingual tonsils.

The tongue and floor of the mouth receive their blood supply from branches of the lingual artery. Branches of the lingual vein drain the tongue. The 5th, 7th, 9th, 10th, and 12th cranial nerves supply the tongue. The hypoglossal nerve (12th) supplies SE fibers to the skeletal muscles. Temperature, pain, and touch receptors are supplied in the anterior two thirds of the tongue by GSA fibers of the lingual nerve from the mandibular branch of the trigeminal nerve (5th), while GVA fibers of the glossopharyngeal (9th) nerve subserve the same function in the posterior one third of the tongue. Taste buds in the anterior two thirds are supplied by special visceral afferent (SVA) fibers of the facial nerve (7th) that reach the tongue via the chorda typmani and lingual nerves. Taste buds of the vallate papillae are supplied by SVA fibers of the glossopharyngeal nerve. Taste buds and general sensations near the epiglottis are supplied by the superior laryngeal branch of the vagus nerve.

Teeth. Teeth, gums, and alveolar bone provide a wall between the vestibule and the mouth proper. Twenty deciduous teeth and 32 permanent teeth are equally distributed between the upper and lower jaws. Each tooth consists of a free crown, a root buried in an alveolus (socket) of the jaw, and a neck between the crown and root at the gum margin. Dental pulp of connective tissue, vessels, and nerves occupies a pulp chamber in the crown and root. The root is suspended in the alveolar bone by a periodontal membrane. The wall of the tooth consists of enamel, dentin, and cementum. ***Enamel*** is the hardest structure in the body, and it covers the crown. It consists of radially arranged rodlike enamel prisms that were elaborated by ameloblasts before the tooth erupted. Ameloblasts developed from the enamel organ, which differentiated from a dental ledge of oral ectoderm. Each of the enamel prisms is invested by a prism sheath, which is rich in organic matter. Adjacent prism sheaths are cemented together by interprismatic substance. ***Dentin*** lines the pulp chamber and lies internal to enamel in the crown and internal to cementum in the root. Dentin consists of a meshwork of collagen fibers oriented parallel to the surface of the tooth, and a calcified ground substance composed of GAGs and mineral salts. This dentin matrix is permeated by radially arranged dentinal tubules containing dentinal fibers (of Tomes), which are processes of odontoblasts lining the pulp chamber. These cells are necessary for the production of the dentin matrix. ***Cementum*** is like a bony covering of the dentin; it is more acellular and avascular than bone, but collagen lamellation and bone cells (cementocytes) are present. Cementocytes and odontoblasts arise from ectomesenchyme of neural crest origin.

The sensory nerves to the maxillary teeth are branches of the maxillary division of the fifth nerve. The posterior superior alveolar nerve supplies the molars, the middle superior alveolar innervates the bicuspids, and the anterior superior alveolar supplies the canine and incisor teeth. These branches and palatine branches of the maxillary nerve also supply the gums. The lower teeth are supplied by the inferior alveolar nerve from the mandibular branch of the trigeminal nerve. Blood supply is by way of the superior alveolar branches of the maxillary artery and the inferior alveolar artery.

Palate, Isthmus of the Fauces, and Palatine Tonsil. The palate forms the roof of the mouth and consists of hard and soft portions. The ***hard palate*** is formed by the palatine processes of the maxillae and the horizontal portions of the palatine bones. An incisive canal penetrates it anteromedially, and greater and lesser palatine foramina lie posterolaterally. The bony palate is covered inferiorly by a mucoperiosteum that is much like that of the gums in that it consists of a stratified squamous epithelium that demonstrates keratinization, parakeratinization, or nonkeratinization in different regions. Parakeratinized epithelia are similar to keratinized epithelia, except the surface cells retain their nuclei. An accumulation of fat is found anteriorly in the submucosa; mucous glands are plentiful in the submucosa of the posterior two thirds of the hard palate. Transverse corrugations of the mucosa in the anterior region and a median raphe also are characteristic features.

The ***soft palate*** is a muscular organ that extends posteriorly from the hard palate. It is lined on the nasopharyngeal side by pseudostratified ciliated columnar epithelium and on the oral side and free margin by stratified squamous nonkeratinized epithelium. The submucosa contains mucous glands on the oral side and mixed seromucous glands on the nasal side. Most of the skeletal muscles of the soft palate insert into either the palatine aponeurosis, which is continuous with the pharyngobasilar fascia, or are continuous with their opposite partner in the midline. The most anterior layer of muscle is the palatoglossal muscle. As indicated previously, this muscle and the mucosa covering it constitute the anterior pillar of the fauces (glossopalatine arch). The most posterior layer of muscle is formed by the palatopharyngeus muscle, which with its mucosa constitutes the posterior pillar of the fauces (palatopharyngeal arch). The uvular muscles extend from the hard palate to the tip of the uvula.

The levator veli palatini and the tensor veli palatini are the major muscles of the palate. The tensor veli palatini arises from the scaphoid fossa at the root of the pterygoid plate; its tendon passes around the hamulus, spreads just above the glossopalatine muscle, and attaches to the palatine aponeurosis. The levator veli palatini arises from the under surface of the petrous bone behind the tensor and spreads out in the soft palate above the tensor. These two muscles elevate the soft palate.

All of the muscles of the soft palate except the tensor are supplied by the vagus nerve; the tensor veli palatini is supplied by the mandibular division of the fifth cranial nerve. The principal artery of the hard palate is the greater palatine branch of the maxillary artery. It enters through the greater palatine foramen and runs forward toward the incisive canal where it anastomoses with branches of the sphenopalatine artery. The soft palate is supplied by the lesser palatine artery, ascending palatine branches of the facial artery, and branches of the ascending pharyngeal artery. Palatine veins are tributaries to the pterygoid plexus.

The isthmus of the fauces is the communication between the oral cavity proper and the oral pharynx. It is bounded above by the soft palate, below by the tongue, and laterally by the glossopalatine arch.

The palatine tonsil is located between the anterior and posterior pillars. It bulges into this depression and is covered by a mucosal fold of the anterior pillar; there is a depressed supratonsillar fossa above the tonsil. The free surface of the tonsil, lined by stratified squamous nonkeratinized epithelium, dips into the underlying lymphatic nodular aggregation as 10 to 20 branching primary and secondary crypts. Lymphocytes from the underlying diffuse and nodular lymphatic tissue often heavily infiltrate the epithelium. The tonsils produce lymphocytes; the presence of plasma cells indicates that tonsils are involved in antigen-antibody reactions. The presence of many neutrophils is characteristic of tonsillar inflammation. Each tonsil is partially invested basally by a connective tissue capsule that sends septa around the aggregations of nodules that invest each crypt. Some mucous glands and the superior pharyngeal constrictor and styloglossus muscles lie peripheral to the capsule. Efferent lymphatic vessels penetrate the pharyngeal wall and pass to superior deep cervical nodes, especially the jugulodigastric node. The arterial supply to the palatine tonsil is by the ascending palatine branch of the facial artery, tonsillar branch of the facial artery, palatine branch of the ascending pharyngeal artery, dorsal lingual branch of the lingual artery, and descending palatine branch of the maxillary artery. The nerves innervating the tonsil are branches of the maxillary division of the trigeminal nerve and the glossopharyngeal nerve.

NASAL CAVITY AND PARANASAL SINUSES

Nasal Cavity. The nasal cavity (Fig. 2-15) extends from the base of the anterior cranial fossa to the roof of the mouth (palate) and is divided into right and left sides by the ***nasal septum.*** The septum is formed by the perpendicular plate of the ethmoid, the vomer, and the septal cartilage. The nasal cavity is related superiorly to the anterior cranial fossa; laterally to the ethmoid air cells, maxillary sinus, and orbit; inferiorly to the oral cavity; and posterosuperiorly to the sphenoid sinus. It opens anteriorly on the face by way of the vestibule and nares and is continuous posteriorly by the choanae with the nasopharynx. The superior, middle, and inferior ***conchae*** divide the cavity into superior, middle, and inferior ***meatuses.*** The area posterosuperior to the superior concha is the sphenoethmoidal recess.

Most of the nasal cavity is lined by a mucoperiosteum consisting of a pseudostratified ciliated columnar epithelium, seromucous glands, and an extensive blood supply. The venous plexuses of the conchae and septum can become engorged with blood, thus restricting the nasal passage by swelling of the mucosa. The rostral direction of the arterial blood flow in the mucosa aids in warming the air. The superior portion of the nasal cavity constitutes the ***olfactory mucosa,*** whose pseudostratified columnar olfactory epithelium consists of modified bipolar neuroepithelial cells and basal and supporting cells. Nonmotile cilia of the bipolar cells are considered to be the olfactory receptor mechanism of the functional dendrite, and its axon passes to the olfactory bulb. Serous glands of Bowman empty to the olfactory surface, where their secretion washes the cilia and prepares them to respond to new stimuli.

The GSA fibers to the mucosa of the nasal cavity are from the anterior and posterior ethmoidal nerves (ophthalmic V), and the lateral nasal and nasopalatine nerves (maxillary V). The olfactory epithelium in the upper part of the nasal cavity is innervated by SVA fibers from the olfactory (first cranial) nerve. All parasympathetic (GVE) fibers are from the pterygopalatine ganglion and distributed by branches of the maxillary division of the trigeminal nerve. The blood supply to the nasal cavity is provided by three arteries: the maxillary, ophthalmic, and facial arteries. The anterosuperior portions of the lateral wall and septum are supplied by the anterior and posterior ethmoidal branches of the ophthalmic artery. Most of the lateral wall (posteroinferior portion) is supplied by the lateral nasal branches of the maxillary artery, and the same area of the septum is supplied by the sphenopalatine branch of the maxillary. The area around the external nares is supplied by the superior labial branches of the facial artery.

Paranasal Sinuses. The ***maxillary sinus*** is related to the orbit above, the nasal cavity medially, the posterior maxillary teeth inferiorly, the infratemporal fossa posterolaterally, and the cheek anterolaterally. The sinus empties into the middle meatus by way of the hiatus semilunaris and is best drained when lying on the opposite side. Since the opening is well above the inferior extent of the sinus, the top of the head should be lower than the lower jaw for complete drainage to be accomplished.

The ***frontal sinus*** is in the frontal bone deep to the superciliary ridge. It is related anteriorly to the forehead, posteriorly to the anterior cranial fossa, and inferiorly to the orbit, ethmoid air cells, and the nasal cavity. It empties into the middle meatus and is best drained in the upright position.

The ***ethmoid air cells*** are interposed between the upper portion of the nasal cavity and the orbit. They are related superiorly to the anterior cranial fossa and inferiorly to the maxillary sinus. These sinuses drain into the superior and middle meatuses. The locations of these openings are variable, and hence the optional drainage position varies between upright and lying on the opposite side.

The ***sphenoid sinus*** is in the body of the sphenoid bone. It is inferior to the sella turcica, the hypophysis and the optic nerve, and bounded laterally by the cavernous sinus. The pterygoid canal is in the floor of the sinus. This sinus empties into the sphenoethmoidal recess. It drains best with the head flexed more than 90 degrees.

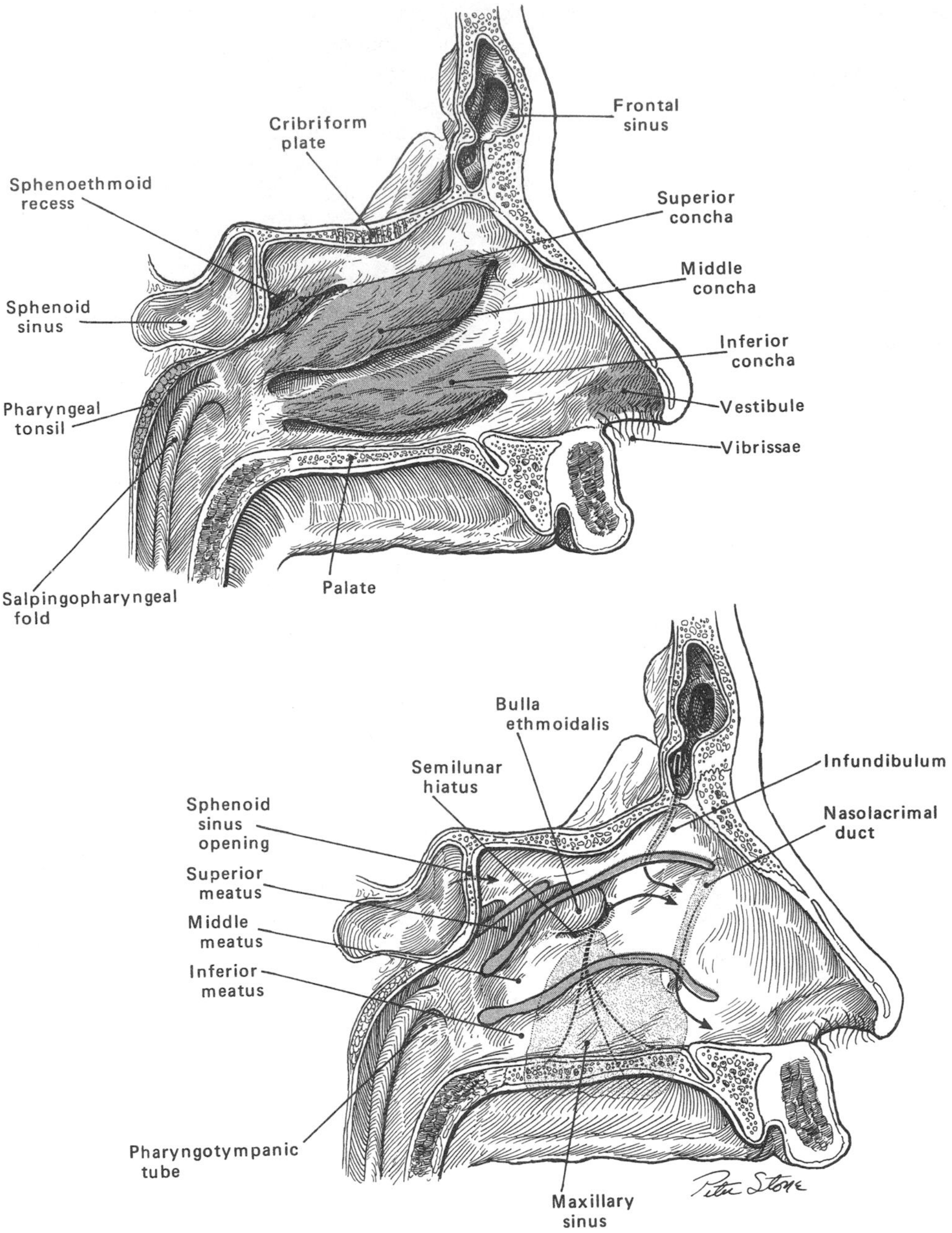

Fig. 2-15. Nasal cavity. *(Top)* Structures of the lateral wall. *(Bottom)* Drainage pathways of the paranasal sinuses and the nasolacrimal duct, with conchae removed. (Christensen JB, Telford IR: Synopsis of Gross Anatomy, 5th ed, p 395. Philadelphia, JB Lippincott, 1988)

The mucosa of the paranasal sinuses is continuous with that of the nasal cavity but contains a thinner pseudostratified columnar epithelium and sparser glands whose mucus flows toward the nasal cavity. The secretomoter fibers to the mucosa are postganglionic parasympathetics from the pterygopalatine ganglion that are distributed primarily with branches of the maxillary nerve.

ORBITAL REGION

Osteology. The orbital cavities are four-sided pyramids. The roof of each is formed by the orbital plate of the frontal bone and the lesser wing of the sphenoid. The floor is formed by the orbital surface of the maxilla, the orbital process of the zygoma, and the orbital process of the palatine bone. The medial wall is formed by the nasal process of the maxilla, the lacrimal, the ethmoid, and the sphenoid bones. The lateral wall is formed by the orbital process of the zygomatic bone and the greater wing of the sphenoid. The orbit is related superiorly to the frontal sinus and anterior cranial fossa; medially to the nasal cavity, ethmoid air cells, and sphenoid sinus; inferiorly to the maxillary sinus; and laterally to the temporal fossa and the middle cranial fossa. The orbit communicates with the cranial cavity by way of the superior orbital fissure and the optic canal, with the infratemporal and pterygopalatine fossae by way of the inferior orbital fissure, and with the sphenoid sinuses and nasal cavity by way of the anterior and posterior ethmoidal foramina.

Contents of the Orbit. The contents of the orbit are enclosed in a tough, conically shaped layer of fascia, the ***periorbita.*** The periorbita is only loosely attached to the walls of the orbit (in reality it is the periosteum of these bones), and it is continuous at the apex of the orbit through the optic canal and the superior orbital fissure with the periosteal layer of cranial dura. The meningeal layer of cranial dura forms a tubular sleeve around the optic nerve; this layer blends with the sclera of the eyeball. As the arachnoid and pia also follow the optic nerve to the eyeball, the subarachnoid space surrounds the optic nerve and extends the same distance. Within the confines of the periorbita the extraocular structures are embedded in fat.

The ***extraocular eye muscles*** control the movements of the eyeball and the upper eyelid. The inferior oblique, levator palpebrae, and the superior, medial, and inferior rectus muscles are all innervated by the oculomotor (third) nerve. The lateral rectus is supplied by the abducens (sixth) nerve and the superior oblique by the trochlear (fourth) nerve. Since the orbital and visual axes do not coincide, only the medial (adduction) and lateral rectus (abduction) muscles produce single motions. The superior and inferior rectus muscles are both adductors; the inferior rectus also produces depression and extorsion while the superior causes elevation and intorsion. The superior oblique produces abduction, depression, and intorsion; the inferior oblique causes abduction, elevation, and extorsion. Rotation of the eye is based on the 12 o'clock point on the eyeball moving medially (intorsion) or laterally (extorsion).

The ***optic nerve*** enters the orbit through the optic canal and passes through the center of the orbital cone toward the eyeball. The ***oculomotor, trochlear, ophthalmic,*** and ***abducens nerves*** enter by way of the superior orbital fissure. The oculomotor nerve has two divisions: the superior supplies the superior rectus and levator palpebrae muscles, and the inferior provides the motor root (preganglionic parasympathetics) to the ciliary ganglion and innervates the medial and inferior rectus muscles and the inferior oblique. The trochlear nerve is very small and passes superomedially to the superior oblique muscle. The ophthalmic nerve divides into the lacrimal nerve, which supplies the lacrimal gland; the frontal nerve, which terminates as the supratrochlear and supraorbital nerves; and the nasociliary nerve, which has ethmoidal and infratrochlear branches. The abducens nerve passes through the lateral part of the orbit to the lateral rectus.

The ***ciliary ganglion*** is a parasympathetic ganglion located in the posterior third of the orbit just lateral to the optic nerve. Preganglionic fibers reach this ganglion through the motor root of the oculomotor nerve and after synapsing reach the eyeball by way of the short ciliary nerves. These fibers innervate the ***sphincter pupillae*** and the ***ciliary muscle.*** Sensory (GSA) fibers to the eyeball are provided by the nasociliary branch of the ophthalmic nerve. These fibers reach the bulb via the long ciliary nerves, which are branches of the nasociliary. In addition, the nasociliary nerve provides a sensory root to the ciliary ganglion through which sensory fibers reach the bulb by way of the ganglion and the short ciliary nerves. Sympathetic fibers reach the bulb through either long or short ciliary nerves as well as with various arteries. The ***sympathetics*** innervate the ***dilator pupillae*** muscle and the ***superior tarsal muscle.***

The ***ophthalmic artery*** arises from the internal carotid artery as the latter passes the optic nerve. The ophthalmic artery then enters the orbit by passing inferior to the optic nerve and through the optic canal. The ***central artery of the retina*** enters the optic nerve about halfway along the orbital course of the nerve. It travels to the retina within the substance of the nerve (with the central vein of the retina) and is therefore surrounded by the subarachnoid space and is vulnerable to any pressure changes in that system. Other major branches of the ophthalmic artery are the ciliary branches to the eyeball, the lacrimal artery, and the ethmoidals. The superior and inferior ophthalmic veins drain primarily into the cavernous sinus, although there are communications with the pterygoid plexus and the veins of the face.

Eyelid. The upper and lower eyelids are movable folds that are separated by a palpebral fissure at their free margins. Each lid is covered by thin skin that is modified posteriorly into a mucous membrane called the palpebral conjunctiva. The palpebral conjunctiva consists of a lamina propria and a stratified epithelium whose surface cells fluctuate in various regions between squamous and columnar. The palpebral conjunctiva is continuous with the bulbar conjunctiva at the fornix. The lamina propria of the palpebral conjunctiva is firmly attached to the ***tarsal plate*** of dense connective tissue that contains the sebaceous tarsal (meibomian) glands. The tarsal glands open onto the free border of the lid. In the upper lid the superior tarsal muscle and tendinous slips of the levator palpebrae superioris attach to the tarsal plate. Ptosis of the eye can occur in (1) Horner's syndrome, in which there is damage to the sympathetic innervation of the involuntary superior tarsal muscle; or (2) oculomotor nerve damage, in which the innervation to the skeletal superior levator palpebrae muscle is compromised. The tarsal plate is attached laterally to the zygomatic bone and medially to the frontal process of the maxilla by lateral and medial palpebral ligaments. Anterior to the tarsal plate is the palpebral portion of the orbicularis oculi muscle. A subcutaneous tissue, which seldom contains fat, lies between the skin and the orbicularis oculi muscle. Cilia (eyelashes) are large hairs arranged in two or three irregular rows on the free margins of the eyelids. Large sebaceous glands (Zeis) and large spiral sweat glands (Moll) are closely associated with the cilia.

Lacrimal Apparatus. The lacrimal apparatus consists of the lacrimal gland, lacrimal ducts, lacrimal sac, and the nasolacrimal duct. The lacrimal gland is situated near the front of the lateral roof of the orbit. Its main ducts open onto the upper lateral half of the conjunctival fornix. Microscopically this gland resembles the parotid in that it is comprised of serous acini. Tears from the lacrimal gland move across the eyeball to the medial angle of the eye where they enter the lacrimal canaliculi. The canaliculi arise on the medial margins of the upper and lower lids at the lacrimal puncta on the lacrimal papillae. The lacrimal ducts carry the lacrimal secretion medially to the lacrimal sac, which is an upward expansion of the nasolacrimal duct. The nasolacrimal duct is lined by columnar epithelium and passes downward, backward, and slightly laterally to enter the nasal cavity at the inferior meatus.

Eyeball. The eyeball consists of three layers: (1) an outer fibrous tunic composed of the sclera and cornea; (2) a vascular coat (uvea) of choroid, ciliary body, and iris; and (3) the retina formed of pigment and sensory (nervous) layers (Fig. 2-16). The anterior chamber lies between the cornea anteriorly and the iris and pupil posteriorly; the posterior chamber lies between the iris anteriorly and the ciliary processes, zonular fibers, and lens posteriorly. Both chambers possess aqueous humor, which is produced in the region of the ciliary processes and exits through the uveal meshwork and canal of Schlemm at the lateral iris angle of the anterior chamber. The canal of Schlemm drains into the anterior ciliary veins. The vitreous body occupies the space between the lens and the retina.

In embryonic development the optic nerve and retina developed as an evagination of the diencephalon, the pigment layer of the retina arising from the outer layer, and the nervous layer arising from the inner layer of the optic cup formed by indentation of the optic vesicle. The lens developed from a lens vesicle that took origin from a thickened lens placode of general surface ectoderm. The outer epithelium of the cornea also developed from surface ectoderm. The other investing tunics of the eyeball developed from head mesenchyme, while the extrinsic eye muscles arose from eye (preotic) somites.

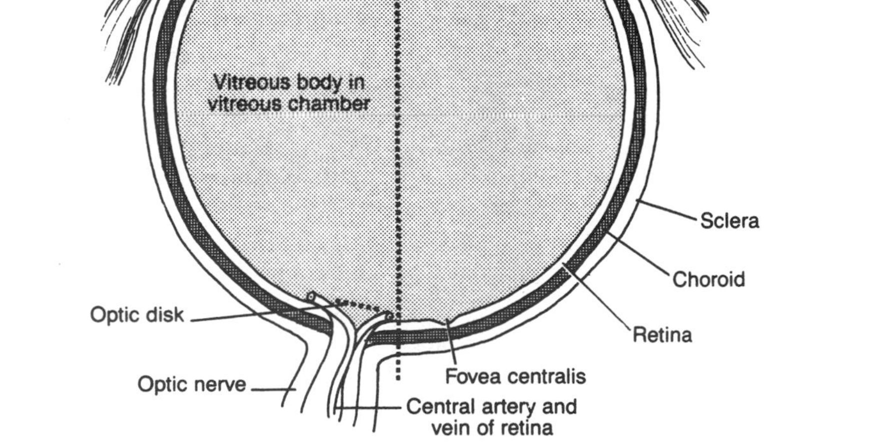

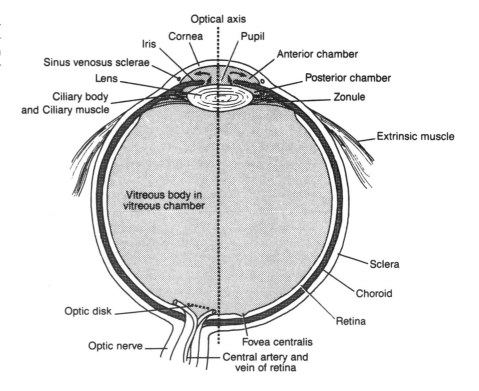

Fig. 2-16. Diagram of a horizontal section of the eye. (Cormack DH: Ham's Histology, 9th ed, p 680. Philadelphia, JB Lippincott, 1987)

The ***cornea*** constitutes the anterior one sixth of the eye. Its front free surface is lined with stratified squamous nonkeratinized epithelium, and its posterior surface is lined with endothelium that is continuous with the spaces of the uveal meshwork. Underlying the endothelium is a prominent basement membrane called Descemet's membrane; below the anterior epithelium is a thin connective tissue membrane (Bowman's membrane). Between both membranes is the substantia propria comprising the bulk of the cornea. This layer consists of many lamellae of collagenous fibrils held together by a glycoprotein ground substance. The collagen fibrils of adjacent layers run perpendicular to each other and may interweave from layer to layer.

The ***sclera*** forms the posterior five sixths of the fibrous tunic and is composed of dense fibrous connective tissue. Although continuous with the cornea, it is delimited from the cornea by internal and external scleral sulci. Nerve fibers of the optic nerve perforate it posteromedially at the optic disc, forming the lamina cribrosa. Extrinsic eye muscles insert into the sclera, and the loose outer scleral layer is continuous with the loose tissue of Tenon's space investing the eyeball. Ciliary vessels and nerves perforate the sclera around the entrance of the optic nerve; other emissaria, which transmit venae vorticosae from the choroid layer, occur midway between the sclerocorneal junction and the optic nerve.

The ***choroid*** layer consists of vascular loose connective tissue; it is separated externally from the sclera by a potential perichoroidal space and firmly attached internally to the pigment layer of the retina. The vessel and capillary layers of the choroid are the most prominent layers. The capillary layer supplies the outer layers of the retina and is the only portion of the choroid not continued forward into the ciliary body.

The ***ciliary body*** is bounded posteriorly at the ora serrata by the retina and choroid; laterally by the sclera; medially by the posterior chamber, vitreous body, and lens; and anteriorly by the iris. The posterior two thirds of the ciliary body is smooth on its inner surface, whereas the anterior one third bears radially arranged ***ciliary processes.*** The forward continuation of the choroid forms the ciliary muscle layer, vessel layer, and lamina vitrea. The forward continuation of the retina gives rise to the outer pigment and inner ciliary epithelial layers and to the internal limiting membrane. The smooth muscle of the ciliary body is oriented in meridional, radial, and circular directions. Its action is to relax the tension on the suspensory zonular ligaments, thus allowing the lens to become more convex due to its elasticity. It is supplied by parasympathetic fibers of the oculomotor nerve. Preganglionic fibers arise in the Edinger-Westphal complex of the mesencephalon, course through the oculomotor nerve and short motor root of the ciliary ganglion, and synapse with postganglionic cell bodies in the ciliary ganglion. Myelinated postganglionic nerves traverse the 12 short ciliary nerves and choroid layer to reach the ciliary body.

The vascular layer is thick in the ciliary processes, contains fenestrated capillaries, and is covered by the pigment and ciliary epithelia. The ciliary epithelium, over the summits of the processes, is modified by basal infoldings of the plasmalemma for transport. This epithelium is involved in aqueous humor formation. Occluding junctions between ciliary epithelial cells may be a major site of a blood–aqueous barrier.

The ***iris*** is attached peripherally to the anterior end of the ciliary body. The anterior surface of the iris demonstrates an inner pupillary zone separated from an outer ciliary zone by a collarette (iris frill). The iris is lined anteriorly by a discontinuous layer of fibroblasts and melanocytes, and posteriorly by pigment epithelium. Underlying the anterior surface layer is an anterior border layer formed principally of chromatophores; deep to this is a vascular stromal layer containing the sphincter pupillae muscle. These layers are an anterior continuation of the uvea. The vascular stroma is bordered posteriorly by the pigment epithelium and the more deeply lying dilator pupillae muscle; these two layers are a forward continuation of the retina. The color of the iris depends on the thickness of the anterior border layer and on the pigmentation of its cells. If the layer is thick and heavily pigmented, the eyes are seen as brown; if the layer is small and little pigment is present, the light passes through the vascular stroma and is reflected off of the pigment epithelium as blue. The arterial supply to the iris is by way of long ciliary and anterior ciliary arteries from the ophthalmic division of the internal carotid arteries. These vessels form a major arterial circle in the vessel layer of the attached margin of the iris. Radial branches from this circle pass toward the pupillary margin, forming a minor arterial circle. The sphincter pupillae and dilator pupillae muscles arise from the pigment epithelium and thus are of neural ectodermal origin. The sphincter pupillae is innervated by parasympathetic fibers of the oculomotor nerve by a pathway that is similar to that for the ciliary muscle. The dilator pupillae muscle is supplied by postganglionic sympathetic fibers that arise from cell bodies in the superior cervical ganglion, follow the internal carotid artery to the cavernous plexus, pass through the nasociliary and its long ciliary branch, and traverse the choroid to reach the iris. The preganglionic sympathetic neurons arise in the intermediolateral cell column of T1 and T2 spinal cord segments, and their axons traverse the ventral roots, white communicating rami, and sympathetic trunk to attain the superior cervical ganglion.

The ***retina*** is divisible into ten layers: (1) pigment epithelium, (2) layer of rod and cone outer and inner segments, (3) external limiting membrane, (4) outer nuclear layer, (5) outer plexiform layer, (6) inner nuclear layer, (7) inner plexiform layer, (8) ganglion cell layer, (9) nerve fiber layer, and (10) internal limiting membrane. The simple cuboidal cells of the pigment epithelium have melanin-containing cytoplasmic processes that interdigitate with the rod and cone outer segments. Layers 2 to 5 contain the ***rod*** and ***cone*** receptors of the light pathway. The outer segments of rods and cones contain numerous stacked membranous discs derived from the plasma membrane and containing visual pigments. The outer discs of the rods differ from cones in that they lose their plasma membrane continuity and are discharged from the cell. Pigment cells phagocytize these extruded discs and also supply vitamin A to the receptor cells. The outer segment of cones and rods is connected to the inner segment by a connecting stalk containing a cilium. The inner segment contains the protein-producing endoplasmic reticulum and Golgi complex necessary for the replacement of rod discs and the nurturing of cone discs. The cell bodies and nuclei of rods and cones constitute the outer nuclear layer. The axons (pedicles) of these cells pass into the outer plexiform layer where they synapse with dendrites of bipolar cells and processes of horizontal cells. ***Bipolar cells*** are the second-order neuron in the visual pathway. Their nuclei are in the inner nuclear layer, and their axons synapse with dendrites of the third-order neuron ganglion cells in the inner plexiform layer. The cell bodies of midget and diffuse ***ganglion cells*** constitute the ganglion cell layer, and their axons form the nerve fiber layer. By these arrangements of cells one cone may synapse with one bipolar cell, which in turn synapses with one midget ganglion cell, or several rods or cones may synapse with one bipolar cell, which synapses with a diffuse ganglion cell. Horizontal interconnections are accomplished between rods and cones by horizontal cells and between ganglions cells by amacrine cells. The outer and inner limiting membranes are formed by the ends of processes of supporting Müller's cells whose nuclei, like those of bipolar, horizontal, and amacrine cells, are located in the inner nuclear layer.

All of the retinal layers external to the inner nuclear layer receive nourishment from choroid capillaries. The rest of the retina is supplied by capillaries derived from branches of the central retinal artery of the optic nerve. The retinal arteries enter at the optic disc and branch into superior and inferior nasal and superior and inferior temporal arteries, the larger branches of which run in the nerve fiber layer. The veins accompany the arteries. Diagnostically the arteries are bright red; the veins are wine colored. The arterial "reflex" from the bloodstream is broader and brighter than the venous "reflex." Choroidal vessels are pinker, flatter, and more bandlike than the retinal vessels.

In examination of the fundus of the eyeball, a macula lutea is seen in the visual axis about 2½ disc diameters to the temporal side of the optic disc. It is a darker oval area in the retinal field that has a central depression called the ***fovea centralis.*** The ***fovea*** is relatively devoid of retinal vessels. The fovea is a site for acute central vision where cones predominate and most retinal layers have been "moved aside" for more immediate access of light rays to the cones.

The ***lens*** is a biconvex body whose posterior surface has a greater convexity. It consists of a capsule, anterior epithelium, and lens substance. The capsule ensheaths the lens and is the site where zonular fibers insert. It consists of basal and reticular laminae. The anterior epithelium contains simple cuboidal cells that become elongate at the equator of the lens where they give rise to new lens fibers. The lens substance consists of prismatic lens fibers that are meridionally arranged, with older fibers more centrally located than the newer ones. Desmosome junctions are present between the newer cells; sutures mark the junction of fibers in the central part of the lens.

EAR

Temporal Bone. The temporal bone houses the middle ear cavity, contains a network of interconnected canals that form the internal ear, and participates in the formation of various cranial and extracranial fossae. It is composed of squamous, mastoid, petrous, and tympanic parts. The ***squamous portion*** forms part of the mastoid process, external auditory meatus, and the mandibular fossa and has the zygomatic process, which forms part of the zygomatic arch. It helps define the middle cranial fossa. The ***mastoid portion*** forms most of the mastoid process and part of the wall of the posterior cranial fossa. The ***tympanic part*** forms most of the external auditory meatus and all of the styloid process. The ***petrous portion*** projects anteromedially toward the dorsum sellae where it ends. Its petrous ridge separates the anterior face from the posterior face. The anterior face forms the posterior portion of the floor of the middle cranial cavity. The posterior face is the anterolateral aspect of the posterior cranial fossa and contains the opening of the internal auditory meatus.

External Ear. The external ear is composed of the external cartilaginous portion; the pinna, or auricle; and the external auditory meatus. The external auditory meatus is about 3 cm in length, connects the auricle and the middle ear cavity, and consists of a lateral cartilaginous and a medial osseous portion. In the infant the osseous meatus is merely a bony ring; in the adult it is about 2 cm long. It is narrowest at the isthmus about 0.5 cm from the tympanic membrane. The entire external auditory meatus is S-shaped. The convexity of the outer cartilaginous portion is directed upward and posteriorly, while that of the inner osseous portion is directed downward and anteriorly.

Middle Ear. The middle ear, or tympanic cavity, is generally shaped like a flat cigar box. Its long axis parallels the tympanic membrane so that it is obliquely oriented, sloping medially from above downward and from behind forward. The cavity is divided into three regions: the middle ear cavity proper at the level of the tympanic membrane; the attic, or epitympanum, above the membrane; and the hypotympanum below the membrane. The cavity communicates posterolaterally with the mastoid air cells by way of the attic and mastoid antrum, and anteromedially with the nasopharynx by way of the auditory tube.

The ***lateral wall*** is formed primarily by the tympanic membrane. This membrane is angularly concave with its apex—the umbo—directed medially. It is composed of a fibrous stratum covered laterally by skin and medially by mucous membrane. The greater part of the periphery of the membrane is a thickened fibrocartilaginous ring that attaches to the bony tympanic sulcus. Superiorly the sulcus and fibrous stratum are deficient, and thus the membrane is lax (pars flaccida). The rest of the membrane is called the pars tensa.

The ***medial wall*** of the middle ear cavity separates that cavity from the inner ear. Prominent on that wall are (1) the promontory, which corresponds to the first turn of the cochlea; (2) the oval window, which contains the foot plate of the stapes and lies a little above and behind the promontory; (3) the round window below the oval window; and (4) the pyramid containing the stapedius muscle.

The ***roof*** is the ***tegmen tympani,*** a thin portion of the petrous temporal bone, which forms part of the floor of the middle cranial fossa. The ***floor*** of the middle ear is formed by the roof of the jugular foramen. The ***anterior wall*** is formed below by the roof of the carotid canal; above it is deficient where the auditory tube opens into the tympanic cavity. The ***posterior wall*** is formed inferiorly by the descending portion of the facial canal; superiorly the attic is in communication with the mastoid antrum.

The ***ossicles*** of the middle ear are the malleus, incus, and stapes. The manubrium of the malleus attaches to the umbo of the tympanic membrane, the foot plate of the stapes fits into the oval window, and the incus interconnects the stapes and malleus.

The ***chorda tympani*** nerve branches from the facial nerve and passes between the incus and malleus as it crosses the medial surface of the tympanic membrane. The chorda tympani conveys taste and preganglionic parasympathetic fibers to the lingual nerve, which it joins in the infratemporal fossa. The ***tympanic plexus*** is located on the promontory. It contains sympathetics (by way of the caroticotympanic branch of the internal carotid plexus), and sensory and preganglionic parasympathetic fibers (both by way of the tympanic branch of the glossopharyngeal nerve).

The ***auditory (eustachian) tube*** is about 3.8 cm to 4 cm in length, extending from the tympanum obliquely forward, downward and inward. Its posterolateral third is bony; the pharyngeal two thirds are cartilaginous.

The air cells of the mastoid process communicate with the middle ear by means of the antrum and the attic. Up to the age of 5 years there is usually only one cell, the antrum, after which the mastoid consists of a large number of cells communicating with one another and the antrum. This area is lined with a continuation of the mucous membrane of the tympanum.

Inner Ear or Labyrinth. The inner ear is contained in the petrous portion of the temporal bone and consists of an osseous labyrinth containing a membranous labyrinth. Between the bony and membranous labyrinth is perilymph. Within the membranous labyrinth is endolymph.

The ***osseous labyrinth*** is a series of cavities in bone consisting of a central vestibule that is continuous with three semicircular canals posterolaterally and the cochlea anteromedially. The vestibule is separated from the laterally situated middle ear cavity by a bony wall containing the fenestra ovalis. This oval window is closed by the foot plate of the stapes. In the posteromedial wall of the vestibule is the opening of the vestibular aqueduct, which extends to the posterior wall of the petrous portion of the temporal bone. The three ***semicircular canals*** are oriented at right angles to each other. The anterior (superior) and posterior canals are vertically oriented; the lateral (horizontal) canal is horizontally positioned. The positioning of the semicircular canals is such that the anterior canal of one osseous labyrinth runs parallel to the posterior canal of the other side. The anterior canal runs transverse to the long axis of the petrous bone. Its anterior limb is dilated into an ampulla just before its entrance into the vestibule; the posterior limb joins the anterior limb of the posterior canal to enter the vestibule as a crus commune. The posterior canal runs parallel to the posterior wall of the petrous bone, and its posterior limb enters the vestibule just beyond the ampulla. Both limbs of the lateral canal enter the vestibule, and an ampulla is located on the anterior limb. The ***cochlea*** is conical, has two and one half turns, and its apex is directed forward, outward, and downward. Mesenchymal epithelium lines the periosteum of the osseous labyrinth.

The ***membranous labyrinth*** consists of an interconnected series of fibrous sacs lined by simple squamous epithelium. The epithelium is derived from an otic vesicle that developed from an otic placode of general surface ectoderm. With the exception of the vestibule, the membranous labyrinth conforms generally to the contour of the osseous labyrinth. The larger membranous portion in the upper posterior part of the vestibule is the utricle; that in front of the utricle is the saccule. The utricle receives the openings of the membranous semicircular canals. The saccule communicates with the membranous cochlear duct by the ductus reuniens. An utriculosaccular duct interconnects the utricle and saccule and continues backward through the vestibular aqueduct as the endolymphatic duct. The latter duct terminates as an endolymphatic sac under the dura lining the posterior surface of the petrous portion of the temporal bone. There are six neuroepithelial receptor areas in each labyrinth: (1) macula utriculi, (2) macula sacculi, (3–5) one crista ampullaris in each ampulla, and (6) organ of Corti in the cochlear duct. The organ of Corti is supplied by the cochlear division of the eighth nerve; the maculae and cristae are innervated by the vestibular division.

The ***cristae ampullares*** are thickened ridges of epithelium and connective tissue placed transversely to the long axis of each semicircular canal. The epithelium of each crista consists of sustentacular cells and two configurations (types I and II) of neuroepithelial cells called ***hair cells.*** Each hair cell contains one kinocilium and many stereocilia that project into an overlying gelatinous mass called the cupula. In the horizontal canals the kinocilia are on the utricular side of the hair cells; in the superior (anterior) and posterior canals the kinocilia are located away from the utricle. Displacement of the stereocilia toward the kinocilia increases the rate of discharge from the hair cells, while movement in the opposite direction decreases the rate of discharge in the vestibular nerve. Thus, movement of ***endolymph*** toward the utricle in the ampullary end of the horizontal semicircular canal causes an increased rate of discharge in that crista. Thus, when an individual is first rotated while the lateral canals are in a horizontal position, the endolymph flow in the horizontal canal on the side of direction of rotation would be essentially ampullopetal, resulting in increased rate of discharge, while the endolymph in the horizontal canal of the opposite ear is ampullofugal, and there is a decreased rate of discharge. In postrotation the opposite occurs. If the head is positioned so that the horizontal canals are vertically oriented, and warm water is added to one ear, then convection currents produce an ampullopetal flow in that ear resulting in a rate of discharge that exceeds that from the unstimulated ear. The use of cold water produces an opposite direction of endolymph flow; thus, the results are opposite to those for warm water. Both the type I and type II hair cells are innervated by the dendritic terminals of bipolar cells of the vestibular ganglion. Some cells receive efferent neurons. The vestibular ganglion lies in the upper part of the outer end of the internal auditory meatus. Axons from the vestibular ganglion pass medially in the internal auditory canal as the vestibular portion of the vestibulocochlear nerve and enter the brain stem at the pons-medulla junction.

The ***maculae*** are similar to the cristae in that they are local thickenings of the membrane, they contain hair cells and sustentacular cells, and their hair cells penetrate a gelatinous membrane. The macular gelatinous membrane contains calcium carbonate crystals called otoliths (otoconia) and is called the otolithic membrane. The hair cells in various regions of the macula utriculi have their kinocilia placed on different sides so that the macula can detect linear acceleration and the position of the head in respect to gravitational forces. The macula of the saccule also is involved with equilibratory action.

The ***organ of Corti*** is located on the basilar membrane of the membranous cochlear duct. The ***cochlear duct*** (scala media) is filled with endolymph, runs throughout most of the cochlea, and is separated from the upper scala vestibuli by the vestibular membrane and from the lower scala tympani by the basilar membrane. The basilar membrane is suspended between the centrally located osseous spiral lamina of the modiolus and the peripherally located periosteal thickening called the spiral ligament. On the lateral wall of the cochlear duct is the stria vascularis. It is lined with pseudostratified columnar epithelium, which is highly vascularized, and is involved in endolymph production. The organ of Corti is an arrangement of supportive and hair cells on the upper border of the basilar membrane. The neuroepithelial hair cells are arranged into inner and outer hair cells by their relationship to an inner tunnel (of Corti) formed by inner and outer pillar cells. The hair cells are supported by outer and inner phalangeal cells whose phalangeal processes form a firm reticular lamina at the peripheral surfaces of the hair cells. The microvillous hairs of the hair cells are in contact with the overlying gelatinous tectorial membrane, thus establishing a mechanism wherein vibrating movement of the basilar membrane will cause stimulation of hair cells by bending of the microvilli. This mechanical stimulus is transduced into electrical energy by the hair cells and transmitted to the terminal dendritic endings of the special somatic afferent (SSA) cells of the spiral cochlear ganglion. Axons of these bipolar nerve cells pass into the axis of the modiolus, course upward into the internal acoustic meatus, become the cochlear portion of the vestibulocochlear nerve, and synapse in the dorsal and ventral cochlear nuclei at the pons-medulla junction of the brain stem.

The blood supply of the labyrinth is by way of the internal auditory (labyrinthine) and stylomastoid arteries. The stylomastoid is a branch of the posterior auricular. The internal auditory arises from the basilar artery, or in common with the anterior inferior cerebellar artery, and traverses the internal acoustic meatus before branching into cochlear and vestibular branches. The veins accompany the arteries and drain as internal auditory veins into the superior petrosal or transverse sinuses.

PITUITARY GLAND

The pituitary gland, or hypophysis (Fig. 2-17), is located in the sella turcica of the body of the sphenoid bone. It is attached to the hypothalamus by its pituitary stalk, which penetrates the diaphragma sellae, a dural covering to the sella turcica. The hypophysis is in relation laterally to the internal carotid artery and the other contents of the cavernous sinus; it is bounded rostrally and superiorly by the optic chiasma. It is composed of an adenohypophysis and a neurohypophysis. The gland is about 1.5 cm in its greatest diameter and about 1 cm in its rostrocaudal extent.

The ***adenohypophysis*** consists of a pars tuberalis, which forms an anterolateral cuff to the infundibulum (infundibular stalk), a ***pars distalis*** (anterior lobe), which produces most adenohypophyseal hormones, and a pars intermedia, which is interposed between the pars distalis anteriorly and the pars nervosa posteriorly. The parenchyma of the pars distalis is comprised of cords of cells that are closely apposed to fenestrated sinusoidal capillaries constituting a secondary capillary plexus. The latter receive venous trunks originating from capillary loops (primary capillary plexus) within the hypothalamus that extend into the pars tuberalis and infundibular stalk; this vascular arrangement constitutes the hypophyseal portal system. The primary capillary plexus is supplied by superior hypophyseal arteries, which arise from the internal carotid and posterior communicating arteries. The cell cords of the pars distalis are comprised of chromophils and chromophobes. Chromophobes are considered to be degranulated chromophils. Chromophils are divisible by the staining reaction of their secretion granules into various types of ***basophils*** and ***acidophils*** which produce the hormones of the pars distalis (Table 2-2). The release of these hormones into the adjacent capillaries is controlled by releasing and inhibiting hormones produced in hypothalamic neurons and released into the portal system in the infundibular stalk, as well as by direct feedback from the organs that are targets of pituitary secretions. Here the factors are taken up in primary capillaries and traverse

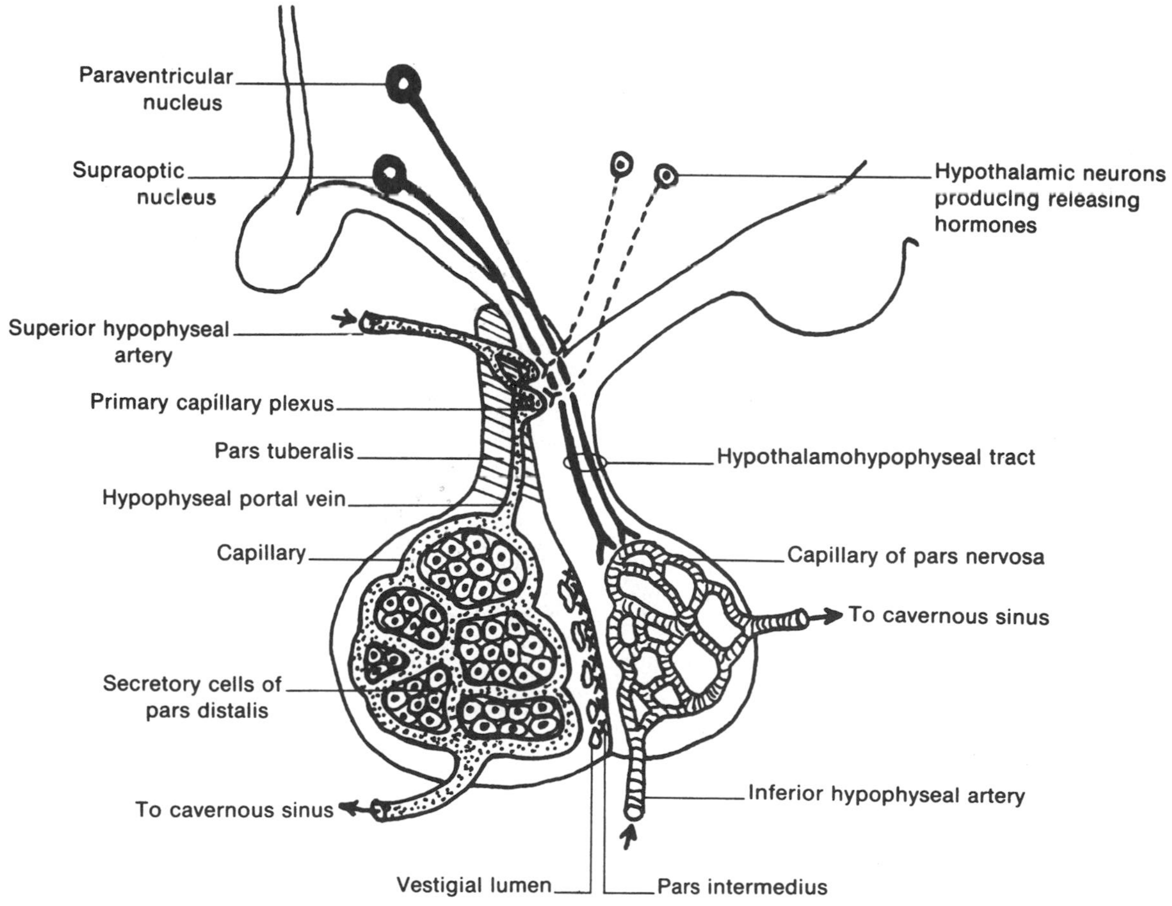

Fig. 2-17. Diagram of the pituitary gland, its vascularity, and the hypothalamo-hypophyseal pathways.

TABLE 2-2. Hormones of the Pituitary Gland

HORMONES	CELLS OF ORIGIN	RELEASING AND INHIBITING HORMONES
Pars distalis		
Growth hormone (GH)	Acidophils	Growth hormone-releasing factor (GRF) Somatostatin (growth-inhibiting hormone, GIH)
Prolactin (PRL)	Acidophils	Prolactin-releasing factor (PRF) Prolactin-inhibiting factor (PIF)
Thyroid-stimulating hormone (TSH)	Basophils	Thyrotropin-releasing hormone (TRH)
Follicle-stimulating hormone (FSH)	Basophils	Gonadotropin-releasing hormone (GnRH)
Luteinizing hormone (LH)	Basophils	Gonadotropin-releasing hormone (GnRH)
Adrenocorticotropic hormone (ACTH)	Basophils	Corticotropin-releasing factor (CRF)
Pars intermedia		
Melanocyte-stimulating hormone (MSH)	Basophils	MSH-releasing factor (MRF) MSH-inhibiting factor (MIF)
Pars nervosa		
Oxytocin	Paraventricular neurons	
Antidiuretic hormone (ADH, vasopressin)	Supraoptic and paraventricular neurons	

venous trunks and the secondary capillary plexus where the factors leave the capillaries to bring about hormone release or inhibition by the cells of the pars distalis. The pars intermedia and pars tuberalis consist mainly of basophils.

The ***neurohypophysis*** consists of the infundibular stalk and pars nervosa, and by some definitions includes the median eminence and secretory neurons of the hypothalamus. The secretory cells of the neurohypophysis are hypothalamic neurons. Cell bodies in the supraoptic and paraventricular nuclei of the hypothalamus give rise to unmyelinated axons that help make up the ***hypothalamo-hypophyseal tract*** of the infundibular stalk. The axons of this tract terminate adjacent to fenestrated capillaries in the pars nervosa. Glial supportive cells of the pars nervosa are called pituicytes. The hormones produced and transported in the neurons (Table 2-2), their binding protein (neurophysin), and ATP constitute a neurosecretory material that may accumulate in the axons and their endings as Herring bodies before discharge into the capillaries. Secretory neurons from other hypothalamic nuclei (*e.g.*, preoptic, arcuate, dorsomedial) send axons to the infundibular stalk where they empty their releasing or inhibitory hormones into the primary capillary plexus of the portal system. The neurohypophysis is supplied by inferior hypophyseal arteries from the internal carotid. The veins of the hypophysis are the lateral hypophyseal veins, which drain to the cavernous and intercavernous sinuses.

DEVELOPMENT OF THE HEAD AND NECK

Development and Fate of the Branchial Arches. During the third and fourth weeks of development the embryo develops head and tail folds that result in the incorporation of the dorsal portions of the primitive yolk sac entoderm as foregut, midgut, and hindgut. The rostral portion of the ***foregut*** (primitive pharynx) develops five lateral pairs of ***pharyngeal pouches;*** these and the floor of the pharynx give rise to the tongue, pharynx, trachea, larynx, lungs, eustachian (auditory) tube, middle ear cavity, thyroid gland, parathyroid glands, and thymus gland. The more caudal portions of the foregut will develop into the esophagus, stomach, part of the duodenum, and the liver and pancreas.

While the pharyngeal pouches are forming internally, five pairs of branchial (pharyngeal) arches appear externally. These are numbered 1, 2, 3, 4, and 6 (5). They are separated by branchial (pharyngeal) grooves, which are aligned with the pharyngeal pouches to form branchial (pharyngeal) membranes consisting of outer ectodermal and inner entodermal layers. Each groove is numbered according to the arch that lies rostral to it. Each branchial arch is comprised of an outer ectodermal layer and an inner entodermal lining with a vertical bar of mesoderm and a cranial nerve interposed between the two layers.

The first arch is divisible into mandibular and maxillary processes. The surface ectoderm of these arches will become the epidermis of the upper and lower jaws, the epithelium of most of the oral cavity, the parenchyma of the major salivary glands, and the enamel of the teeth. The mandibular and maxillary divisions of the trigeminal nerve course in these arches and supply the skin of the face with sensory nerves (GSA) and the muscles of mastication with motor (SVE) nerves. The muscles developing from the mandibular arch are the temporalis, masseter, medial and lateral pterygoids, mylohyoid, anterior belly of the digastric, tensor veli palatini, and tensor tympani. Mesenchyme and neural crest of the mandibular arch develop into a transitory Meckel's cartilage before forming a mandible, malleus and incus; mesenchyme of the maxillary arch forms the maxilla, premaxilla, zygomatic bone, and part of the temporal bone. The first branchial groove gives rise to the external acoustic meatus. The first branchial membrane develops into the tympanic membrane, and the first pharyngeal pouch presages part of the auditory (eustachian) tube and middle ear cavity.

The second (hyoid) arch grows back over arches 3 to 6 and will fuse with them, obliterating branchial grooves 3 to 6 and a transitory cervical sinus that was formed in this caudal growth. Improper obliteration of the cervical sinus can result in a cervical cyst in the adult. Cervical (branchial) fistulas may remain if communications are retained externally and/or internally through the branchial membranes. Since the ectoderm of the second arch gives rise to the epidermis of much of the neck, the openings of external branchial fistulas occur in the neck along the anterior margin of the sternocleidomastoid muscle. Internal fistulas most often occur into the second pouch. Since the tonsil develops in the region of the second pouch, internal fistulas of the second pouch open into the tonsillar region. Mesenchyme of the second arch gives rise to the muscles of facial expression, the stapedius, posterior belly of the digastric and stylohyoid muscles. It, along with neural crest, also gives rise to the stapes, styloid process, stylohyoid ligament, and lesser cornua and upper part of the body of the hyoid bone. The facial nerve runs in the second arch and supplies SVE innervates to the muscles developing from this arch.

The third pharyngeal arch gives rise to the stylopharyngeus muscle supplied by the glossopharyngeal nerve and to the lower part of the body and greater cornua of the hyoid bone. The entoderm of the dorsal part of the third pharyngeal pouch gives rise to parathyroid III, which will develop further into the parenchyma of the inferior parathyroid gland the ventral part of the third pharyngeal pouch becomes the thymus gland.

The fourth and sixth arches give rise to the laryngeal cartilages and the pharyngeal, palatal, and laryngeal muscles. All of these, except the tensor palatini and stylopharyngeus, are innervated by the vagus nerve, with the superior laryngeal branch supplying the fourth arch and the recurrent laryngeal branch passing through the sixth arch. The dorsal part of the fourth pharyngeal pouch gives rise to the superior parathyroid gland; the ventral part of the fourth pharyngeal pouch unites with the fifth (sixth) pharyngeal pouch to give rise to the ultimobranchial body, which probably forms the calcitonin-producing parafollicular cells of the thyroid gland.

Aortic arches arise from the aortic bulb and enter each branchial arch, where they run chiefly caudal to the cranial nerve of each arch. Although the aortae of the first and second arches largely disappear, a small portion of the first aortic arch contributes to the maxillary artery while the second aortic arch contributes to the hyoid and stapedial arteries (see Fig. 2-27). The third aortic arch becomes part of the internal carotid and common carotid arteries. The right fourth arch becomes part of the right subclavian artery, and the left fourth arch becomes the arch of the aorta. The proximal portions of both sixth aortic arches become parts of the pulmonary arteries; the left distal part becomes the ductus arteriosus. Since the recurrent laryngeal is caudal to the sixth aortic arch, retention of the ductus arteriosus as the ligamentum arteriosum accounts for the left recurrent laryngeal looping around the arch of the aorta caudal to the ligament, whereas the right loops higher around the subclavian artery.

The tongue develops from elevations in the floor of the primitive pharynx and by forward migration of developing muscle from occipital somites. The body of the tongue arises from two lateral swellings and a median tuberculum impar in the floor of the mandibular arch. The root of the tongue develops from a copula of mesenchyme of the second, third, and fourth arches. The epiglottic swelling also comes from mesenchyme of the fourth arch. The muscles of the tongue develop from occipital somites and are innervated by the hypoglossal nerve. Since the oral membrane, demarcating the ectodermally lined stomodeum from the entodermal primitive pharynx, existed just in front of the fauces, most of the epithelium of the body of the tongue arose from ectoderm while the root and foramen cecum area developed from entoderm. Thus, general sensation from the anterior two thirds of the tongue is carried by branches of the trigeminal nerve, whereas the posterior one third is innervated by the glossopharyngeal nerve. The thyroid gland develops as an evagination from the floor of the pharynx at the level of the first pharyngeal pouch. It migrates caudally to the region of the larynx, leaving the foramen cecum as the site of original evagination and often leaving thyroglossal duct cysts along its migratory course. Thyroglossal duct cysts can be found in the root of the tongue, along the neck, and in or behind the hyoid bone.

Development of the Face, Nasal Cavity, and Oral Cavity. By the sixth week of embryonic development a frontal prominence overhangs the cephalic end of the stomodeum. It is bounded laterally by nasal pits surrounded by horseshoe-shaped elevations. The medial portion of the horseshoe-shaped elevation is the ***nasomedial process;*** the lateral portion is the ***nasolateral process.*** The nasolateral process is delimited from the maxillary process by the naso-optic (nasolacrimal) furrow. The developing oral cavity is bounded inferiorly by distal fusion of the mandibular processes of the first branchial arch. As the maxillary processes become more prominent they fuse with the nasomedial processes and push them toward the midline; this displaces the frontal prominence upward and leads to fusion of the nasomedial processes in the midline. The fused nasomedial processes (intermaxillary segment) give rise to the medial part of the upper lip, distal nose, incisor teeth and associated upper jaw, and the primary palate (median palatine process). The ***maxillary process*** gives rise to the rest of the upper lip, teeth, and jaw and the palatine shelves forming the secondary palate. The lower lips, jaw, and teeth are formed from the ***mandibular processes.*** The nasolacrimal duct is formed at the point of obliteration of the naso-optic furrow by fusion of the nasolateral and maxillary processes. Inability of these processes to fuse leads to an oblique facial cleft. The nasolateral processes give rise to the alae of the nose.

The ***nasal pits*** become deeper and break through the bucconasal membrane into the primitive oral cavity. Toward the end of the second embryonic month the ***palatine shelves*** (lateral palatine processes) of the maxillary processes grow medially and fuse with the primary palate, rostrally, and with each other and with the inferiorly growing nasal septum caudally. The lateral palatine processes thus give rise to a secondary palate, which separates the nasal cavity above from the definitive oral cavity below. The caudal free borders of the palatine shelves project as the soft palate into the pharynx, dividing it into an upper nasopharynx and lower oropharynx. Incomplete degeneration of the bucconasal membrane can lead to choanal atresia. Failure of the palatine shelves to fuse in the midline, or to fuse with the primary palate, produce cleft palate. Such clefts can be divided into three groups: (1) those occurring between the palatine shelves and the primary palate (anterior, primary palate types); (2) those occurring posterior to the incisive foramen at the point of fusion of the palatine shelves with each other (posterior, secondary palate types); and (3) those involving defects in both the anterior and posterior palate (complete unilateral or bilateral types). The anterior and complete types may be associated with cleft lip if the nasomedial and maxillary processes fail to merge (fuse). Median cleft of the upper lip and jaw is due to the lack of fusion of the nasomedial processes with each other.

Development of the Hypophysis. The hypophysis arises from two sources: Rathke's pouch and the infundibulum. Rathke's pouch arises as an evagination of stomodeal ectoderm that pinches off from the stomodeum and migrates toward the diencephalon where it becomes adherent to the rostral surface of the infundibulum. The infundibulum develops as an outgrowth of neural ectoderm from the hypothalamus of the diencephalon. The infundibulum gives rise to the neurohypophysis; Rathke's pouch develops into the adenohypophysis.

CENTRAL NERVOUS SYSTEM AND CRANIAL NERVES

The structure and localization of the spinal cord and spinal nerves were covered previously in the section on the back.

Cranial Cavity. The cranial cavity (Fig. 2-18) is formed by a roof (calvaria) and a floor. The calvaria is formed by the single frontal and occipital bones, the paired parietal bones, portions of the greater wings of the sphenoid, and the squamous parts of the temporal bones. The parietal bones are united by the sagittal suture and with the frontal bone at the coronal suture. Posteriorly the occipital and parietal bones are united at the lambdoidal suture.

The floor of the cranial cavity is divisible into three cranial fossae: anterior, middle, and posterior. The ***anterior cranial fossa*** is formed medially by the cribiform plate of the ethmoid and the crista galli, and laterally by the orbital plate of the frontal bone. Posteriorly both the body of the sphenoid and its lesser wing participate in the formation of this fossa, which is related anteromedially to the frontal sinus and inferiorly to the nasal cavity, ethmoid sinuses, and the orbit. The multiple openings in the cribiform plate transmit the rootlets of the olfactory nerve into the superior aspect of the nasal cavity. The foramen cecum is anterior to the crista galli and may transmit an emissary vein between the nasal cavity and the superior sagittal sinus. The anterior cranial fossa houses the frontal lobes of the brain and the olfactory bulbs and tracts.

The ***middle cranial fossa*** has a central and two lateral portions. The ***central part*** is formed by the body of the sphenoid and consists of the sella turcica posteriorly and the chiasmatic groove anteriorly; it houses the hypophysis (pituitary) and optic chiasm. This part of the fossa is related inferiorly (and anteriorly) to the sphenoid sinus and laterally to the cavernous sinus. The optic canals convey the optic nerves open into the orbits.

The ***lateral part of the middle cranial fossa*** houses the temporal lobe of the brain and is formed by the greater wing of the sphenoid and parts of both the squamous and petrous portions of the temporal bone. This part of the fossa is related inferiorly to the infratemporal fossa and middle ear cavity, laterally to the temporal fossa, anteriorly to the orbit, and medially to the sphenoid sinus. There are a number of openings in this fossa. The superior orbital fissure (containing the ophthalmic division of the trigeminal, oculomotor, trochlear, and abducens nerves, and the ophthalmic veins) opens into the orbit; the foramen rotundum (containing the maxillary division of the trigeminal nerve) opens into the pterygopalatine fossa; the foramen ovale (containing the mandibular division of the trigeminal nerve) and the foramen spinosum transmitting the middle meningeal artery) open into the infratem-

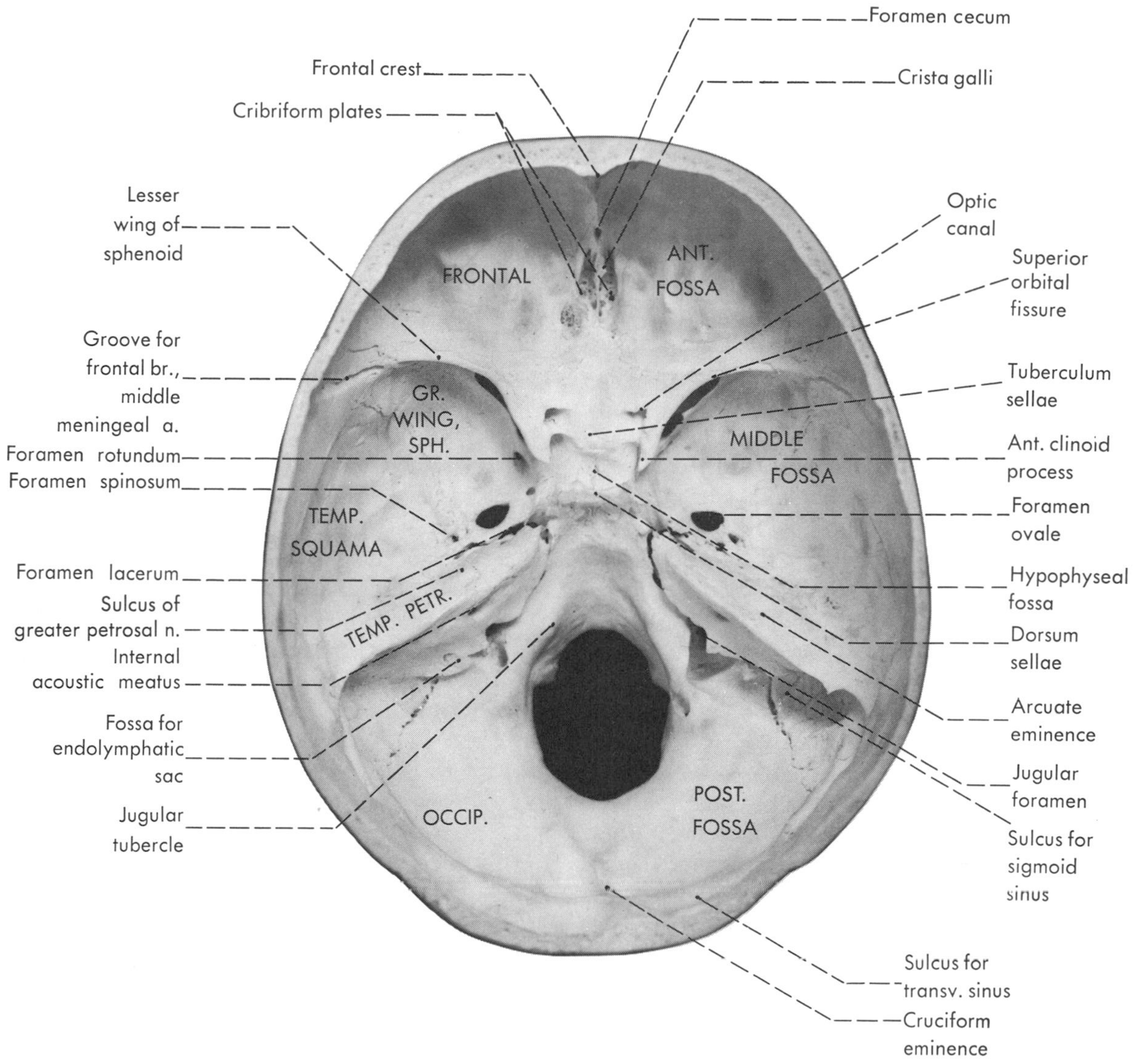

Fig. 2-18. Interior of the base of the skull. GR. WING, SPH. is the greater wing of the sphenoid; TEMP. SQUAMA and TEMP. PETR. are the squamous and petrous portions of the temporal bone; and OCCIP. is the occipital bone. (Hollinshead WH: Anatomy For Surgeons, Vol 1, 3rd ed, p 57. Philadelphia, JB Lippincott, 1982)

poral fossa. The foramen lacerum is an irregularly shaped opening at the apex of the petrous pyramid; in life, this opening is filled by fibrous tissue and is the floor of the carotid canal and thus nothing passes through the opening.

The ***posterior cranial fossa*** is formed by the posterior aspect of the body of the sphenoid, a portion of the petrous portion of the temporal bone, and the occipital bone. Anteriorly in the midline the inclined plane formed by the sphenoid and the basilar portion of the occipital bone is occupied by the brain stem; the midbrain is surrounded by the notch of the tentorium cerebelli. The cerebellum occupies the rest of the posterior fossa. The foramen magnum, the large single opening in this fossa, transmits the spinal cord–brain stem junction and its meningeal coverings, the accessory nerve, the vertebral and the anterior and posterior spinal arteries, and the communication between the dural venous sinuses and the internal vertebral venous plexus. The hypoglossal canal transmits the hypoglossal nerve, and the jugular foramen contains the glossopharyngeal, vagus, and accessory nerves, and the continuity between the dural venous sinuses and the internal jugular vein. The internal acoustic meatus is an opening on the posterior face of the petrous pyramid, which transmits the facial and vestibulocochlear nerves and the labyrinthine artery.

Gross Brain Topography. The brain consists of three basic parts, the cerebral hemispheres (telencephalon), the brain stem, and the cerebellum. The cerebral hemispheres and cerebellum cover much of the superior and lateral surface of the brain stem. From the cerebral hemispheres to the spinal cord the brain stem consists of (1) the diencephalon, (2) the mesencephalon, (3) the metencephalon (pons), and (4) the myelencephalon (medulla). In relation to the skull the frontal and temporal lobes of the cerebral hemispheres lie in the anterior and middle cranial fossae, respectively; the cerebellar hemispheres are in the posterior cranial fossa. The diencephalon, mesencephalon, and pons rest on the superior surface and clivus of the body of the sphenoid bone, while the medulla occupies a groove on the basilar part of the occipital bone extending from the sphenoid to the foramen magnum. The brain is invested by dura, arachnoid, and pia mater.

The ***dura*** serves as the periosteum of the skull and also reflects between the cerebral hemispheres in the longitudinal cerebral fissure as the falx cerebri. The falx is continuous posteriorly with another dural reflection, the tentorium cerebelli, lying in the transverse cerebral fissure between the occipital lobes of the telencephalon above and the cerebellum below. Important venous sinuses are found in the dura. The superior sagittal sinus in the attached margin of the falx cerebri drains to the transverse sinuses at the periphery of the tentorium cerebelli. These in turn drain to the internal jugular veins via the sigmoid sinuses. An inferior sagittal sinus in the free margin of the falx cerebri and the great vein of Galen from the brain drain to the straight sinus running in the junction of the falx and tentorium. The straight sinus drains to the transverse sinus. An anterior group of sinuses includes the cavernous, intercavernous, superior and inferior petrosal sinuses and basilar plexus.

The ***arachnoid*** does not project into the sulci of the telencephalon, and it is separated from the pia by a subarachnoid space. This space is enlarged into subarachnoid cisterna at the cerebellum–medulla junction (cisterna magna), between the cerebral peduncles (interpeduncular cistern), superior and lateral to the midbrain (cisterna ambiens), and at several other areas. Arachnoid granulations, projecting into the superior sagittal sinus, serve as a mechanism for the flow of cerebrospinal fluid from the subarachnoid space into the venous system. The ***pia*** is vascular, and the underlying glial membrane blends with the walls of pial blood vessels as they penetrate the brain substance. Tight junctions of the nonfenestrated brain capillaries provide the chief component of the ***blood–brain barrier.***

The ***cerebral hemispheres*** are interconnected by a corpus callosum, an anterior commissure, and by the lamina terminalis, which lies rostral to the third ventricle. Each cerebral hemisphere consists of an outer gray ***cortex*** (pallium), underlying white matter, a deeply located nuclear mass called the ***basal ganglia,*** and a lateral ventricle. The cortex and its underlying white matter are thrown into a fairly consistent localization of gyri and sulci that make it possible to define frontal, parietal, temporal, occipital, insular, and limbic lobes. The more rostral ***frontal lobe*** is separated from the parietal lobe by the central sulcus (of Rolando). In the frontal lobe the precentral gyrus (motor area) borders the central sulcus and is demarcated from the more rostral superior, middle, and inferior frontal gyri by the precentral sulcus (see Fig. 2-20). On the basal surface the frontal lobe is comprised of an olfactory bulb and tract lying between the gyrus rectus and the orbital gyri. The ***parietal lobe*** consists of the more rostral postcentral gyrus (somesthetic area) and the posteriorly located superior and inferior parietal gyri. On the medial aspect the parietal and occipital lobes are divisible by the parieto-occipital sulcus; laterally the boundary is less precise. The lateral fissure (sulcus) helps to form an inferior boundary to the frontal and parietal lobes. It terminates caudally where the inferior parietal gyrus caps it as the supramarginal gyrus. The rest of the inferior parietal gyrus abuts against the posterior extent of the superior temporal sulcus and is called the angular gyrus.

The lateral surface of the ***occipital lobe*** consists of lateral occipital gyri. The medial surface is divided by the calcarine fissure into a cuneus above and a lingual gyrus below. That portion of the cortex immediately bordering the calcarine fissure is the striate (visual) cortex. The lateral surface of the ***temporal lobe*** is comprised of superior, middle, and inferior temporal gyri. The transverse temporal gyri (of Heschl) lie medial to the superior temporal gyrus in the floor of the lateral fissure. It is the primary receptive area for hearing. The insula lies deep in the lateral fissure and constitutes a cortical cover to the lenticular nucleus. On the basal surface of the temporal lobe the occipitotemporal gyrus and parahippocampal gyri lie medial to the inferior temporal gyri. The more medial parahippocampal gyrus ends rostrally as the uncus, is bounded laterally by the collateral fissure and medially by the hippocampal fissure, and is continuous around the caudal end (splenium) of the corpus callosum with the cingulate gyrus. The rostral part of the parahippocampal gyrus, the uncus, and the lateral olfactory stria and gyrus (which project from the olfactory trigone and tract) comprise the primary olfactory receptive area. The ***limbic lobe*** includes the subcallosal, cingulate, and parahippocampal gyri, as well as the dentate gyrus and hippocampus, which lies deep to the hippocampal fissure.

The ***diencephalon*** contains the third ventricle and is divisible into four parts: the roof, or epithalamus; the dorsolaterally located thalamus; the floor and ventromedially oriented hypothalamus; and the ventrolateral subthalamus. The diencephalon is bounded above by the transverse cerebral fissure. While this fissure extends caudally between the occipital lobe and cerebellum and is occupied by the tentorium cerebelli, rostrally it lies between the corpus callosum and fornix above and the epithalamus (tela choroidea, pineal body, habenula) and thalamus below. It extends laterally and ventrally as the choroid fissures adjacent to the choroid plexuses of the lateral and third ventricles, respectively. Rostrally, the transverse cerebral fissure ends blindly behind the interventricular foramen (of Monro) where the choroid plexus of the third ventricle is continuous with that of the lateral ventricle. The diencephalon is bounded laterally by the internal capsule and the cerebral peduncles. Basally the surface shows anteroposteriorly the optic chiasm, infundibular stalk and pituitary gland, and mammillary bodies.

The ***mesencephalon*** lies between the diencephalon and pons. Its dorsal surface consists of two superior colliculi, two inferior colliculi, the brachia of these colliculi, which connect to the lateral and medial geniculate nuclei of the diencephalon, respectively, and the emerging trochlear (fourth) nerve. Ventrally the mesencephalon demonstrates cerebral peduncles, interpeduncular fossa, and emerging oculomotor (third) nerves. An iter (cerebral aqueduct of Sylvius) connects the third ventricle of the diencephalon with the fourth ventricle in the pons.

The ***pons*** is bounded dorsally by the attached cerebellum. The lateral surface is made up of the middle cerebellar peduncle with its emerging root of the trigeminal (fifth) nerve. Ventrally the basis pontis forms a bridge between the middle cerebellar peduncles. On the superior aspect the superior medullary velum, superior cerebellar peduncles, and cerebellum form the roof of the fourth ventricle. The tegmentum forms the floor of the ventricle and demonstrates a facial colliculus in the medial eminence located medial to the sulcus limitans.

The ***cerebellum*** overlies the posterior surface of the pons and upper medulla. It consists of a midline vermis and two lateral hemispheres. The surface of the cerebellum has elevations called folia, which are separated by sulci. On the superior surface a primary fissure separates an anterior lobe (paleocerebellum) from the posterior lobe (neocerebellum). On the inferior surface a posterolateral fissure demarcates the posterior lobe from the flocculonodular lobe (archicerebellum). There is another phylogenetic division of the cerebellum into a vermis (archicerebellum), paravermis (paleocerebellum), and lateral hemispheres (neocerebellum). The cerebellum is attached to the brain stem by paired inferior, middle, and superior cerebellar peduncles—which basically connect the cerebellum to the medulla, pons, and mesencephalon, respectively. The substance of the cerebellum consists of a cortex of gray matter, a medullary core called the arbor vitae, and four pairs of deep nuclei. Afferent neurons to the cerebellum enter primarily by way of the inferior and middle cerebellar peduncles and ascend in the arbor vitae to synapse on cells of the granular layer of the cortex. Axons of granular cells ascend to the molecular layer where they run parallel to the folia and synapse with dendrites of Purkinje cells, which send axons to the deep nuclei. Of these Purkinje axons, those from the neocerebellum synapse on cells of the dentate nuclei, those from the paleocerebellum synapse in the emboliform and globose nuclei, and those from the archicerebellum synapse in the fastigial nuclei. Axons from cells in the dentate, emboliform, and globose nuclei project to the thalamus and red nucleus by way of the superior cerebellar peduncles, while those from the fastigial nuclei pass by way of the inferior cerebellar peduncle (juxtarestiform body) to terminate in vestibular nuclei.

The upper part of the ***medulla*** (open medulla) contains a portion of the fourth ventricle. A tela choroidea of pia and ependyma form the roof of this part of the fourth ventricle. The floor is divisible into a medial eminence and a more lateral vestibular area. At the junction of the pons and medulla the fourth ventricle is open laterally to the subarachnoid space through the foramen of Luschka. A midline opening, the foramen of Magendie, is located at the caudalmost tip of the tela choroidea. The dorsal surface of the more inferior closed part of the medulla represents an enlarged upward continuation of the fasciculus cuneatus and fasciculus gracilis of the spinal cord. These areas are referred to as the tuberculum cuneatum and tuberculum gracilis (clava). They lie caudal and lateral to the fourth ventricle.

The ventral surface of the medulla, from the midline laterally, consists of pyramids and pyramidal decussation, preolivary sulcus, olivary eminence, and postolivary sulcus. The abducens (sixth) nerve exits at the pons-medulla junction in line with the hypoglossal (twelfth) nerve rootlets, which emerge from the preolivary sulcus. The glossopharyngeal (ninth), cranial accessory (eleventh), and vagus (tenth) nerves exit from the postolivary sulcus. The facial (seventh) and vestibulocochlear (eighth) nerves emerge below the lateral recess of the fourth ventricle at the pons-medulla junction. They are in close anatomic relationship to the inferior cerebellar peduncle (restiform body), which courses anterior to the lateral recess in passing from the medulla to the cerebellum.

Blood Supply to the Brain. The brain is supplied by the vertebral and internal carotid arteries. The ***vertebral arteries*** enter the foramen magnum and give off posterior inferior cerebellar and anterior and posterior spinal arteries. The vertebral arteries unite at the pons-medulla junction to form the basilar artery. The basilar artery runs in the basilar sulcus of the pons and terminates at the level of the mesencephalon by branching into posterior cerebral arteries. The basilar gives off the anterior inferior cerebellar, labyrinthine, paramedian, short and long circumferential and superior cerebellar arteries. Branches of the vertebral and basilar arteries supply the cerebellum, mesencephalon, pons, medulla, medial portion of the occipital lobe, and part of the temporal lobe and diencephalon.

The ***internal carotid artery*** courses through the cavernous sinus and emerges from the sinus medial to the anterior clinoid process. It gives off the ophthalmic artery to the orbit; the posterior communicating artery to the posterior cerebral artery; and the anterior choroidal artery, which supplies the optic tract, choroid plexus of the lateral ventricle, basal ganglia, posterior part of the internal capsule, and the hippocampus. Lateral to the optic chiasm the internal carotid bifurcates into the middle cerebral and anterior cerebral arteries. The anterior cerebral arteries, connected by an anterior communicating artery, supply the medial surface of the frontal and parietal lobes. The middle cerebral artery passes into the lateral fissure and supplies the insula, lateral surface of the cerebral hemisphere, and part of the inferior surface of the temporal lobe. The basal ganglia and part of the internal capsule are supplied by the lenticulostriate branches of the middle cerebral artery. The internal carotid and vertebral arterial supplies are interconnected, forming the ***circle of Willis,*** which consists of the anterior communicating, anterior cerebral, posterior communicating, and posterior cerebral arteries. Central branches from the circle of Willis supply the basilar portion of the diencephalon and basal ganglia and give rise to the hypophyseal portal arterial system of the adenohypophysis.

Lesions resulting in vascular deficiency of the anterior cerebral artery result in contralateral UMN paralysis or paresis of the leg and foot and loss of two-point touch and vibratory sense in the leg and foot region. Compromise of the posterior cerebral artery leads to contralateral homonymous hemianopsia and may damage portions of the thalamus and cerebral peduncles. Middle cerebral artery damage can give UMN and sensory losses to the contralateral upper extremity trunk and face. It may also result in aphasia, agnosia, and apraxia. Posterior inferior cerebellar artery occlusion can result in Horner's syndrome, a contralateral loss of pain and temperature on the extremities and trunk, an ipsilateral loss of pain and temperature on the face, and a loss of functions mediated by way of the glossopharyngeal and vagus nerves.

Superficial and deep cerebral veins drain to the dural venous sinuses. The great cerebral vein (Galen) receives the internal cerebral veins and drains to the straight sinus. Superior, middle, and inferior superficial veins drain to the superior sagittal or basal sinuses. The midbrain, pons, and medulla drain by small veins into the sinuses at the base of the brain. The cerebellum is drained by superior and inferior cerebellar veins into adjacent dural venous sinuses.

Circulation of Cerebrospinal Fluid. Cerebrospinal fluid is formed by the choroid plexuses of the lateral, third, and fourth ventricles. Cerebrospinal fluid passes from the lateral ventricle through the interventricular foramen (of Monro) to the third ventricle and thence through the iter into the fourth ventricle. It exits through the foramina of Luschka and Magendie into the subarachnoid space (cisterna magna) and diffuses into the superior longitudinal sinus through the arachnoid granulations. Internal hydrocephalus may result from blockage of the ventricular pathway and most commonly occurs in the iter. Hydrocephalus that occurs from blockage of the foramina of Luschka and Magendie results in the enlargement of all of the ventricles.

Development of the Brain. By the fourth week of embryonic development the neural tube of the cephalic region appears as three vesicles: the prosencephalon, mesencephalon, and rhombencephalon. The prosencephalon enlarges into two lateral telencephalic hemispheres and a midline diencephalon by the fifth week. The mesencephalon does not subdivide further, but the rhombencephalon differentiates into a more cephalic metencephalon and a caudal myelencephalon. With the extensive growth of the brain at this period the brain flexes in its confined space. The cephalic flexure occurs between the mesencephalon and metencephalon, the pontine flexure at the metencephalon–myelencephalon junction, and the cervical flexure at the junction of the myelencephalon and spinal cord. The metencephalon develops into the pons and cerebellum; the myelencephalon differentiates into the medulla.

In later development, the telencephalic hemispheres enlarge greatly, flex into C-shaped structures and fuse with the lateral wall of the diencephalon at a point that will be occupied later by the posterior limb of the internal capsule. The pontine flexure will become more pronounced and a metencephalic rhombic lip of alar plate material will grow dorsally and develop into the cerebellum. The mantle layers of both the cerebral hemispheres and cerebellum give rise to deep nuclei and migrate peripherally to form the cortical gray material. The deep nuclei of the cerebral hemispheres are the basal ganglia consisting of amygdaloid, caudate, lenticular (putamen and globus pallidus), and claustrum nuclear complexes.

In the brain stem, the differentiation of mantle and marginal layers does not result in as distinct a layering of gray and white matter as in the cerebral hemispheres, cerebellum, and spinal cord. Individual nuclei and fiber tracts are identifiable, but in many areas nuclei and fibers are interspersed and constitute a ***reticular formation.*** In addition to this major organizational difference between the spinal cord and brain stem, the structure of the latter also differs from the cord as a result of (1) the expansion and thinning out of the roof plate in those areas that develop ventricles, (2) the development of phylogenetically newer structures, (3) the acquisition of cell columns for three new functional components of cranial nerves, and (4) the specialization and lack of segmentation that leads to cranial nerves that do not all have the same functional components.

The ***cell columns*** of the brain stem develop from the mantle layer. Those developing from the basal plate are nuclei of origin for motor (efferent) neurons whose axons leave the brain stem in cranial nerves. Those developing from the alar plate are nuclei of termination on which incoming sensory (afferent) axons will synapse; these nuclei of termination represent cell bodies of association and internuncial neurons. Seven functional components are formed, but no cranial nerve contains all seven. These functional components are (1) SE to skeletal muscles of occipital and eye somite origin, (2) SVE to skeletal muscles of branchial arch origin, (3) GVE to postganglionic parasympathetic ganglia, (4) GVA receiving sensory neurons from visceral structures, (5) SVA receiving neurons from taste and olfactory receptors, (6) GSA from exteroceptive neurons, and (7) SSA receiving neurons from the eye and ear.

The cell columns of the brain stem are more discontinuous in their cephalocaudal extent than those of the spinal cord, and their localization corresponds generally to the emergence of the cranial nerves. A notable exception to this is the GSA cell column, which continues upward from the dorsal horn of the spinal cord (as the spinal and chief nuclei of cranial nerve V) to the midpons level, receiving trigeminal nerve fibers throughout its extent. A mesencephalic nucleus of V represents an upward extension of the GSA column but involves proprioceptive neurons. There are no cell columns for the olfactory and optic nerves. Thus, the cell columns are limited to the mesencephalon, pons, and medulla. The cross-sectional localization of brain stem cell columns differs markedly from those of the spinal cord. Most of this difference is due to the development of the ventricles. It is recalled that in the spinal cord the gray matter, as seen in cross section, is oriented vertically into a dorsal horn (alar plate) and ventral horn (basal plate) lying lateral to the central canal. With the expansion of the central canal into the ventricles of the brain, the roof plate becomes stretched out as the tela choroidea (ependyma plus pia), and the alar plate is displaced lateral to the basal plate. Consequently in the pons and medulla the nuclei of termination transmitting sensory input are located lateral to the nuclei of origin for motor output. The basic sequential localization from the midline laterally is SE, SVE, GVE, GVA, SVA, GSA, SSA. All of the nuclei of these columns in the pons and medulla lie in the floor of the fourth ventricle or near the central canal, with the exception of the SVE column, which migrates ventrolaterally into the reticular formation.

In the phylogenetic development of the brain stem, the older systems dealing with crude sensibilities and gross axial movements are retained centrally, while the phylogenetically newer structures dealing with discriminatory sensation and with the regulation of finer and more discrete movements are added more ventrolaterally.

The complex topography of the diencephalon and telencephalon and their interrelationships are better appreciated through an understanding of their development. As the ventricles of the diencephalon and telencephalon form, the roof plate of each becomes attenuated as the tela choroidea. Vascularized portions of this pia and ependyma extend into the ventricles as the choroid plexuses of the third and lateral ventricles. These choroid plexuses are continuous with each other at the interventricular foramen. The diencephalon may arise entirely from the alar plate; the optic nerve and retina develop as an evagination of the diencephalon.

The lamina terminalis arises as the most rostral wall of the telencephalon. As the telencephalic hemispheres grow tremendously in size, they grow forward, then backward, circumscribing a C-shaped growth pattern terminating at the temporal pole. The forward growth leaves the lamina terminalis displaced posterior to the frontal pole; the anterior commissure and corpus callosum develop in the lamina terminalis.

The C-shaped growth pattern is reflected in the formation of the anterior horn, body, and inferior horn of the lateral ventricle. The caudate nucleus follows this path with its head in the ventral–lateral floor of the anterior horn and its tail extending into the dorsal–lateral wall of the inferior horn of the lateral ventricle. The caudate nucleus ends near the amygdaloid nucleus located just rostral to the inferior horn of the lateral ventricle. The caudate nucleus grows around the lenticular nucleus, which is anchored at its point of fusion with the diencephalon. The internal capsule develops in this point of fusion. The insular cortex, anchored to the lenticular nucleus, is overgrown by the extensive peripheral growth of the C-shaped hemisphere. The C-shaped growth is also reflected by the fornix. This structure is a fiber pathway that extends from the hippocampal formation in the temporal lobe to the mammillary bodies in the hypothalamus; it forms the anterior boundary of the interventricular foramen in its route.

Internal Topography of the Brain Stem. The brain stem is an upward continuation of the spinal cord. As each of the higher brain stem and cortical centers was added to the nervous system in its phylogenetic development, connections between each of the levels were established, older centers at each level were retained, and many parts were traversed by tracts interconnecting the cerebral cortex with the spinal cord. In addition to these pathways and centers, central connections with cranial nerves also can be localized at the various brain stem levels.

Medulla. The lower part of the closed medulla is similar to the spinal cord in that it has a central canal, fasciculus gracilis, fasciculus cuneatus, lateral and anterior spinothalamic tracts, posterior and anterior spinocerebellar tracts, lateral reticulospinal tracts, and anterior corticospinal tracts in essentially the same locations as in the spinal cord. The substantia gelatinosa, the posteromarginal nuclei, and the posterolateral fasciculus continue upward as the spinal nucleus and tract of cranial nerve V, respectively. The major difference between the low medulla and spinal cord is that the lateral corticospinal tract is just forming by the decussation of fibers from the ***pyramids*** of the medulla. At this and higher levels there will be more of an admixture of gray matter and fibers in that area that corresponds to the gray matter of the spinal cord.

At higher regions of the closed medulla the ascending axons of the posterior funiculus synapse on cell bodies in the nucleus gracilis and nucleus cuneatus. Since these nuclei are displaced at higher levels by the expanding fourth ventricle, axons from these nuclei arch ventrally around the central canal as the internal arcuate fibers and decussate to form the ***medial lemniscus.*** This bundle of ascending fibers represents the axons of second-order neurons for the stereognosis—two-point touch pathway that will traverse the medulla, pons, and mesencephalon before synapsing in the ventral posterior lateral nucleus of the thalamus. In the medial lemniscus, fibers carrying impulses from sacral levels are localized just above the pyramid, while fibers representing cervical levels are located more dorsally just below the MLF.

The inferior olivary nucleus occupies the ventral part of the medulla lateral to the medial lemniscus and pyramids. The vestibulospinal (lateral) tract runs dorsal to this nucleus. The spinothalamic and spinocerebellar tracts lie along the lateral margin of the medulla in the postolivary sulcus region.

The ***hypoglossal nucleus*** (SE) extends throughout most of the medulla and lies dorsal to the MLF. Lateral to it is the dorsal motor nucleus (GVE) of the vagus. Axons from the hypoglossal nucleus pass ventrally and exit in the preolivary sulcus. Axons from the ***dorsal motor nucleus*** course laterally and exit from the postolivary sulcus. GVA and SVA fibers, which enter the brain stem in the vagus nerve and at higher levels in the glossopharyngeal and facial nerves, descend in the fasciculus solitarius and terminate on the cells of the ***nucleus solitarius*** and dorsal sensory nucleus of the vagus lying adjacent to the fasciculus. In the closed medulla the fasciculus and nucleus solitarius lie dorsal to the dorsal motor nucleus of cranial nerve X, and at open-medulla levels they lie lateral to the motor nuclei.

In the open medulla the hypoglossal and vagal nuclei form prominences in the floor of the fourth ventricle medial to the sulcus limitans. The sensory nuclei, that is, the nucleus solitarius (GVA and SVA), vestibular nuclei (SSA), and spinal nucleus of cranial nerve V (GSA), lie lateral to the sulcus limitans. At high-medulla levels the ***vestibular nuclei*** (SSA) lie dorsomedial to the spinal nucleus and form a vestibular area in the floor of the fourth ventricle lateral to the sulcus limitans. At the level of the lateral recess, ***cochlear nuclei*** (SSA) form the most lateral prominence in the floor of the fourth ventricle. The ***nucleus ambiguus*** (SVE) is located in the reticular formation halfway between the spinal nucleus of cranial nerve V and the inferior olivary nucleus. Axons from this nucleus loop dorsomedially before exiting laterally in the vagus, accessory, and glossopharyngeal nerves. Lateral to the spinal tract of cranial nerve V is the ***inferior cerebellar peduncle.*** It consists of the posterior spinocerebellar tract, olivocerebellar fibers from the contralateral inferior olivary nucleus, cuneocerebellar fibers from the accessory cuneate nucleus, and some other ascending and reticular connections. The reticular formation is divisible into medial and lateral groups of nuclei. The lateral groups are basically sensory in that they receive ascending sensory information. The lateral small-celled area is associated with respiratory responses and is where the pressor center is located. The medial gigantocellular nucleus gives rise to the lateral reticulospinal tract and is inhibitory to antigravity muscles. This and adjacent medial nuclei constitute centers involved in respiratory and depressor circulatory responses. An ascending reticular activating system of multisynaptic connections arises primarily from the medial nuclei of the reticular formation.

Pons. The pons is divisible into a dorsal tegmentum and a ventral phylogenetically newer basis pontis. The ***tegmentum*** is an upward continuation of the medulla. It differs from the medulla in that the inferior olivary nucleus disappears and a central tegmental tract and superior olivary nucleus are located in its place; the medial lemniscus is oriented horizontally in the basal part of the tegmentum; the spinothalamic tracts are located at the lateral tip of the medial lemniscus; the corticospinal tracts are in the basis pontis and not in pyramids; cell columns and pathways relating to cranial nerves V to VIII are present.

At the pons-medulla junction the inferior cerebellar peduncle passes ventral to the lateral recess of the fourth ventricle before entering the cerebellum. At this location dorsal and ventral cochlear nuclei lie dorsolaterally and ventrally, the spinal tract and nucleus of cranial nerve V are medial, and the vestibular nuclei are dorsomedial to the inferior cerebellar peduncle. The cochlear nuclei receive axons of the bipolar neurons of the spiral cochlear ganglion. Axons from the cochlear nuclei pass medially through the tegmentum to ascend contralaterally and ipsilaterally just lateral to the spinothalamic tracts as the lateral lemniscus. Some of the axons of this pathway synapse in the superior olivary nucleus and nucleus of the lateral lemniscus before terminating in the inferior colliculus. The superior olivary nucleus lies dorsal to the spinothalamic tracts in the ventrolateral tegmentum. The vestibular nuclei receive axons from bipolar neurons of the vestibular ganglion and from the cerebellum. They send axons to the cerebellum, to the center for lateral gaze, to the oculomotor nuclei and spinal cord via the MLF, and into the spinal cord as the lateral vestibulospinal tract.

The ***basis pontis*** contains the corticospinal (pyramidal) tract, corticobulbar (corticonuclear) fibers to cranial nerve motor nuclei, and corticopontine fibers that terminate on pontine nuclei. Axons of the pontine nuclei cross the midline and pass laterally and dorsally into the cerebellum as the ***middle cerebellar peduncle.***

In lower pontine levels the ***facial*** (SVE) ***nucleus*** occupies the ventrolateral tegmentum. Axons from this nucleus course dorsomedially and superiorly and loop around the ***abducens nucleus*** before passing ventrolaterally and inferiorly to exit at the pons-medulla junction. The loop (internal genu) of the facial nerve and the adjacent abducens nucleus form an abducens (facial) colliculus in the floor of the fourth ventricle. Axons from the abducens (SE) nucleus pass ventrally and inferiorly to exit at the pons-medulla junction. A parabducens group of cell bodies representing a center for lateral gaze lies inferior to the MLF in the paramedian pontine reticular formation (PPRF). Superior and inferior salivatory nuclei, containing the cell bodies of parasympathetic preganglionic nerves of the facial and glossopharyngeal nerves respectively, occupy the tegmentum but are not sharply localized.

At mid-pons levels, the trigeminal nerve penetrates the middle cerebellar peduncle and runs to the lateral tegmentum. GSA fibers of this nerve, whose cell bodies are located in the trigeminal ganglion, terminate in the ***principal (chief, main) sensory nucleus*** and ***spinal nucleus of cranial nerve V*** (Fig. 2-19). The principal sensory nucleus is the upward continuation of the spinal nucleus and receives touch fibers. Axons from this nucleus cross and ascend in the ventral secondary tract of cranial nerve V, running adjacent to the medial lemniscus, and terminate in the ventral posterior medial (VPM) nucleus of the thalamus. Some axons from the principal sensory nucleus ascend uncrossed to the VPM nucleus as the dorsal secondary tract of cranial nerve V running lateral to the MLF. Some entering touch fibers of the trigeminal nerve bifurcate and send descending branches to the upper part of the spinal nucleus of cranial nerve V. Pain fibers enter in the trigeminal nerve, descend as the spinal tract of cranial nerve V and terminate on cell bodies in the caudal portion of the spinal nucleus of cranial nerve V. Axons from the spinal nucleus of cranial nerve V cross the midline and ascend in the ventral secondary tract of cranial nerve V. The ***motor*** (SVE) ***nucleus of cranial nerve V*** lies medial to the chief sensory nucleus of cranial nerve V. Its axons emerge from the pons in the motor root (portio minor) of the trigeminal nerve. A ***mesencephalic nucleus of cranial nerve V*** of unipolar neurons extends into the mesencephalon from midpons levels. It lies next to the lateral portion of the central gray material and represents the first-order neurons of a proprioceptive (GSA) pathway of the fifth nerve. Thus, these cells are unique in that they are sensory ganglion cells that did not end up in ganglia but were retained in the brain stem during development of the neural tube.

At upper pons levels, the fourth ventricle narrows as the isthmus region of the pons-mesencephalon junction is approached. The superior medullary velum and ***superior cerebellar peduncles*** form the roof and lateral walls of the ventricles. In the region of the isthmus, the superior cerebellar peduncles move ventrally into the tegmentum. The fibers of these peduncles will decussate in the tegmentum of the mesencephalon and will ascend to the red nucleus and ventral lateral nucleus of the thalamus.

The reticular formation of the pons is an upward continuation of that in the medulla. The caudal and oral pontine reticular nuclei give rise to the pontine (medial) reticulospinal tract, which is facilitory to antigravity muscles. The main ascending pathway of the reticular formation is the central tegmental tract.

Mesencephalon. The mesencephalon is divided at the level of the cerebral aqueduct into a dorsal ***tectum*** and into two ventral ***cerebral peduncles.*** The tectum consists of two superior colliculi and two inferior colliculi. Each cerebral peduncle is subdivided by the substantia nigra into a dorsal tegmentum and a ventral crus cerebri.

At the inferior colliculus level axons of the lateral lemniscus terminate in the ***inferior colliculus.*** Fibers from this relay nucleus of the hearing pathway pass laterally into the brachium of the inferior colliculus and synapse on cells of the medial geniculate body, which, in turn, send axons to the transverse temporal gyri (of Heschl). The mesencephalic nucleus and root and the nucleus pigmentosus (locus ceruleus) lie ventral to the inferior colliculi in the lateral extent of the central gray. In the dorsomedial limits of the tegmentum the ***trochlear nucleus*** nestles in the dorsal surface of the MLF. Below the MLF fibers of the superior cerebellar peduncle decussate before passing upward toward the red nucleus; the medial lemniscus, secondary tracts of cranial nerve V and spinothalamics lie ventral and lateral to this decussation. Axons from the trochlear nucleus course dorsally in the central

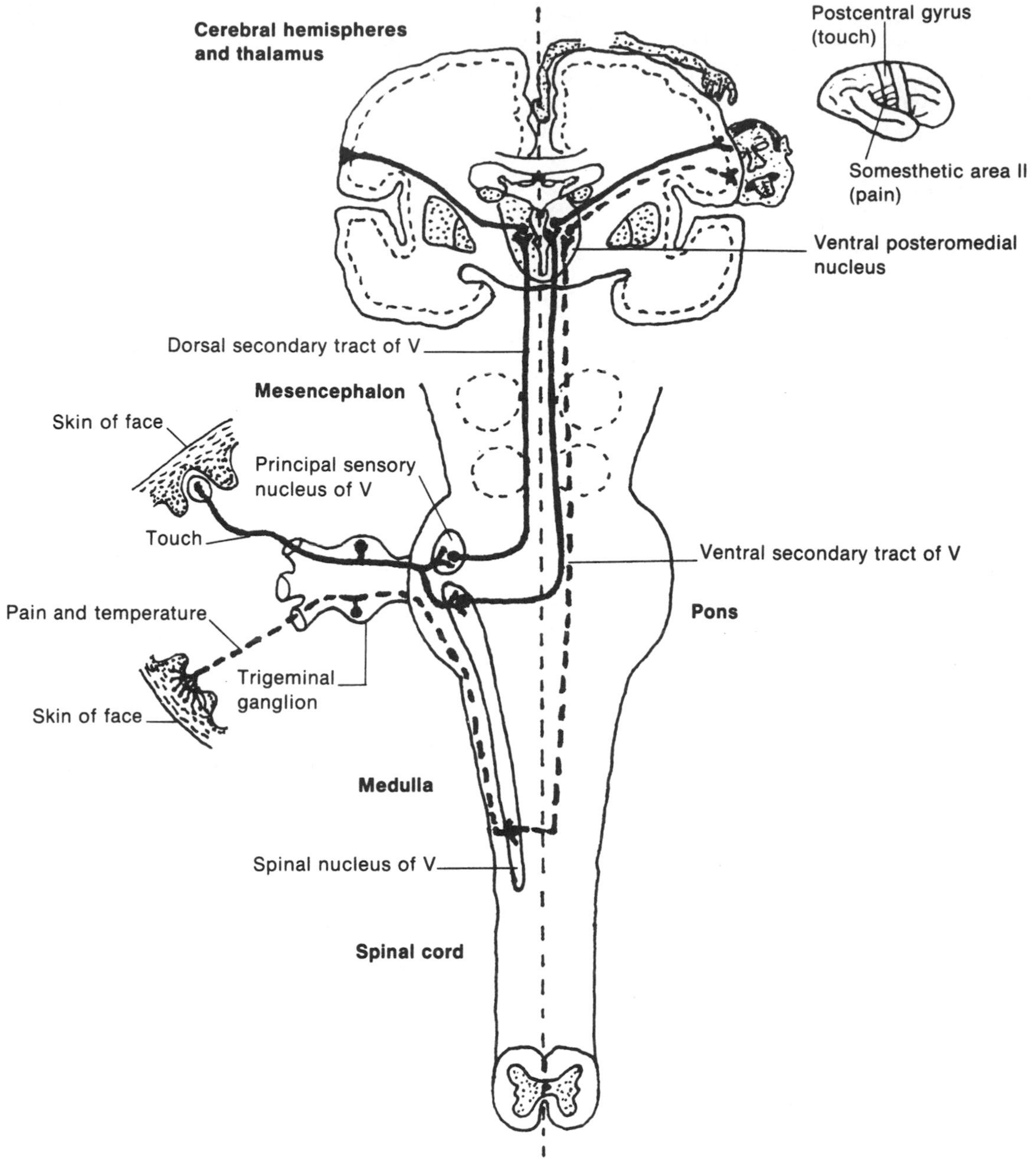

Fig. 2-19. The trigeminal nerve pathways for pain and temperature *(dashed line)* and touch *(solid lines)* from the face.

gray, decussate in the superior medullary velum and exit below the inferior colliculi. The crus cerebri contains the corticopontine, corticobulbar, and corticospinal pathways. Corticobulbar and corticospinal fibers occupy the middle third of the crus.

The most significant features of the superior colliculus levels are the superior colliculi, oculomotor nuclear complex and nerves, and the red nucleus. The ***superior colliculus*** receives optic fibers from the optic tract and occipital cortex by way of the brachium of the superior colliculus. The superior colliculus is involved in aligning the fovea on a visual target (fixation reflex). The oculomotor nuclear complex consists of the ***oculomotor*** (SE) and ***Edinger-Westphal*** (GVE) ***nuclei,*** which are located medial to the MLF. The oculomotor nerve passes ventrally to exit medial to the crus cerebri in the interpeduncular fossa. SE axons innervate the levator palpebrae superioris, medial rectus, superior and inferior recti, and inferior oblique muscles. Preganglionic parasympathetic axons from the Edinger-Westphal nucleus run to the ciliary ganglion where they synapse on postganglionic neurons that innervate the sphincter pupillae and ciliary muscles. The ***red nucleus*** lies in the ventromedial tegmentum and is surrounded by dentatothalamic axons of the superior cerebellar peduncle that are going to the ventral lateral nucleus of the thalamus. Some axons of the superior cerebellar peduncle synapse on cells of the red nucleus. The red nucleus also receives corticorubral fibers. Major efferent paths from the red nucleus are the rubroreticular and the rubrospinal tracts.

The ***pretectal area*** at the junction with the diencephalon is considered part of the mesencephalon. Features of this area are the pretectal nuclei, posterior commissure, and subcommissural organ. Pretectal nuclei lie rostral to the superior colliculi, receive optic tract axons by way of the brachium of the superior colliculi and send crossed and uncrossed axons to the Edinger-Westphal nucleus. The pretectal nuclei constitute the association limb of the pupillary light reflex. The crossing fibers of this reflex either pass through the posterior commissure or decussate in the central gray below the cerebral aqueduct. The posterior commissure lies dorsal to the cerebral aqueduct at the level where it joins the third ventricle. The subcommissural organ is modified ependyma located beneath the posterior commissure. The columnar ciliated cells of this organ may secrete aldosterone and may serve as a volume receptor.

The ***reticular formation*** consists of many nuclei whose cells release a variety of neurotransmitters. A median (raphe) group of nuclei contains serotonergic neurons. A medial group, which includes the cells of origin of the medial reticulospinal (nucleus pontis oralis and caudalis) and lateral reticulospinal (nucleus gigantocellularis) tracts, produces serotonin and possibly substance P. A lateral group of nuclei (*e.g.,* locus ceruleus) constitutes a norepinephrine and epinephrine system. A dopaminergic system of neurons includes cells of the substantia nigra.

Diencephalon. The diencephalon consists of an epithalamus, thalamus, hypothalamus, and subthalamus. The ***epithalamus*** is in the roof of the third ventricle and is composed of the tela choroidea, striae medullares, habenular trigones, and pineal gland. The stria medullares convey fibers from the septal and preoptic area to the habenular nuclei. Axons from the habenular nuclei pass to the mesencephalon through the paired fasciculus retroflexus.

The ***thalamus*** is bounded laterally by the posterior limb of the internal capsule and medially by the third ventricle. It extends anteroposteriorly from the interventricular foramen to the pretectal area, and it lies above the hypothalamus and subthalamus. The thalamus is separated into medial, lateral, and anterior nuclear groups by the internal medullary lamina. The medial group nuclei are the midline and dorsomedial nuclei. The midline nuclei make connections with the hypothalamus. The dorsomedial nucleus receives afferents from the amygdaloid nucleus, hypothalamus, and temporal cortex and sends axons to the prefrontal cortex. Intralaminar nuclei receive spinothalamic fibers and reticulothalamics from the reticular activating system. The centromedian nucleus is an intralaminar nucleus that receives fibers from the motor cortex (area 4) and globus pallidus and sends axons to the putamen. The lateral group of thalamic nuclei are divisible into a ventral tier and a dorsal tier. The ventral tier consists of the ventral anterior, ventral lateral, and ventral posterior (VPL and VPM) nuclei. All of these ventral tier nuclei are relay nuclei. The VPL nucleus receives the medial lemniscus and spinothalamics. The VPM receives secondary ascending trigeminal pathways. Axons from both the VPM and VPL nuclei pass into the posterior limb of the internal capsule and terminate in the great somesthetic area (postcentral gyrus, area 3, 1, 2), those from VPM terminating closer to the more ventral portion of the postcentral gyrus than those from the VPL. Some axons conveying nociceptive information from the VPL and VPM nuclei terminate in somatic sensory area II located in the parietal lobe above the lateral fissure. The ventral lateral nucleus receives dentatothalamic fibers and pallidothalamic fibers and sends axons to the precentral gyrus (motor cortex). The latter fibers arise from cells in the medial aspect of the globus pallidus and pass through the fasciculus lenticularis to reach the prerubral field. From here they loop laterally over the zone incerta to enter the thalamus via the thalamic fasciculus. The ventral anterior nucleus receives pallidothalamic fibers by this same pathway and projects axons to the premotor cortex. The dorsal tier nuclei are the lateral dorsal, lateral posterior, and pulvinar. These nuclei are association nuclei and have interconnections with the parietal cortex. The pulvinar receives fibers from the metathalamus (medial and lateral geniculate bodies) and sends axons to the parastriate (area 18) and peristriate (area 19) areas in the occipital cortex and also to the inferior parietal cortex. The anterior nucleus of the thalamus relays mammillothalamic impulses from the mammillary bodies to the cingulate gyrus.

The ***subthalamus*** lies ventral to the thalamus between the hypothalamus and posterior limb of the internal capsule. It consists of the subthalamic nucleus, zona incerta, fasciculus lenticularis, prerubral field (of Forel), and the fasciculus thalamicus. The subthalamic nucleus lies on the internal capsule and substantia nigra and is separated from the zona incerta above by the fasciculus lenticularis. It has interconnections with the globus pallidus. Lesions of this nucleus produce hemiballism contralaterally.

The ***hypothalamus*** consists of groups of nuclei in the floor of the third ventricle. The nuclei are divided into medial and lateral groups by the fornix as it passes through the hypothalamus on its way to the mammillary body. The lateral group includes the lateral and tuberal nuclei. The medial group is subdivided anatomically into three groups: (1) anterior group, which includes the preoptic, anterior, supraoptic, and paraventricular nuclei; (2) middle group, containing the dorsomedial and ventromedial nuclei; and (3) posterior group of posterior and mammillary nuclei.

The hypothalamic nuclei can also be grouped on the basis of their functional connections into autonomic, neuroendocrine, and olfactory groups. The anteromedial hypothalamic group of nuclei generally are concerned with parasympathetic regulation, whereas the posterolateral group is more involved in sympathetic regulation. Both nuclear groups receive ascending GVA, GSA, and SVA (taste) input from the reticular formation and send out descending central autonomics to preganglionic neurons by way of reticulospinal and reticuloreticular pathways. These regions also receive olfactory input from the amygdaloid and septal areas and have interconnections with the thalamus, prefrontal cortex, and limbic lobe.

The neuroendocrine nuclei are the supraoptic and paraventricular group, which produce posterior pituitary hormones, and a hypophysiotrophic group, which produce adenohypophyseal releasing and inhibiting factors. These nuclei and their manner of secretion have been discussed previously.

The mammillary, preoptic, and lateral hypothalamic nuclei receive input from the olfactory cortex. These nuclei have reciprocal connections with the limbic lobe and also project to other hypothalamic and brain stem nuclei.

Telencephalon (Cerebral Hemispheres). The ***primary receptive areas*** of each cerebral hemisphere (Fig. 2-20) are the postcentral gyrus (areas 3, 1, 2) for two-point touch, joint sense, and vibratory sense; the striate cortex (17) for vision; the transverse temporal gyri (41 and 42) for hearing; the base of the postcentral gyrus (43) for taste; and the periamygdaloid region (34) for smell. The gyri adjacent to these areas constitute the ***unisensory association areas,*** where sensory information is recognized as that perceived before (gnosis). These unisensory areas are the adjacent postcentral gyrus (5), superior parietal gyrus (7), and supramarginal gyrus (40) for areas 3, 1, 2; the peristriate (19) and parastriate cortex (18) for area 17; the adjacent superior temporal gyrus (42 and 22) for 41 and 42; areas 5 and 40 for area 43; and the parahippocampal gyrus (42 and 22) for area 34. The angular gyrus (39) and adjacent areas 19 and 22 constitute ***multisensory association areas,*** where one can recognize an object through perception of one sense and can recall what the other sensations would be for that object (*e.g.*, seeing and recognizing a chicken and recalling what it would feel, taste, sound, and smell like). This multisensory area of the parietotemporal cortex is an area for language and the formulation of complex motor activities, especially in the dominant hemisphere (usually the left). Thus, damage to the angular gyrus on the left side may result in receptive aphasia and apraxia. Lesions of unisensory areas in the dominant hemisphere result in agnosia (*e.g.*, visual agnosia, astereognosis). Lesions of the right posterior and inferior parietal lobe may lead to extinction and denial of one's contralateral body parts or environment.

Fibers from the parietal-temporal-occipital cortex by way of the arcuate, superior longitudinal, and inferior occipitofrontal fasciculi connect with the prefrontal, premotor, and motor cortex of the frontal lobe. The ***prefrontal cortex*** is for initiative, judgment, and creativity. Broca's area in the inferior frontal gyrus of the dominant hemisphere is the motor speech area. Lesions of this area result in expressive aphasias. The frontal eye fields (8) and Exner's writing center (8) are located in the posterior part of the middle frontal gyrus. Destructive lesions of the former lead to transient conjugate gaze to the side of the lesion, whereas lesions of the latter result in a writing apraxia. The ***motor cortex*** (area 4) in the precentral gyrus and the ***premotor cortex*** (6 and 8) in front of area 4 control motor activity, especially of the contralateral extremities.

The cerebral cortex receives and projects fibers from and to lower centers by way of the ***internal capsule.*** The anterior limb of the internal capsule between the head of the caudate and lenticular nucleus contains connections with the prefrontal cortex. The posterior limb of the internal capsule between the thalamus and lenticular nucleus contain corticospinal fibers from the frontal lobe and receive projections to the parietal and temporal lobes. The genu of the internal capsule at the level of the interventricular foramen transports corticobulbar fibers. Sublenticular fibers of the internal capsule are auditory and optic radiations. Retrolenticular fibers are also optic radiations.

Summary of Cranial Nerves. The ***first (olfactory) nerve*** is comprised of the central processes of bipolar olfactory cells (SVA) whose cell bodies are located in the olfactory epithelium on the upper part of the nasal septum and the lateral nasal wall. These unmyelinated fibers (fila olfactoria) pass into the anterior cranial fossa through the lamina cribrosa of the ethmoid bone and enter the olfactory bulb. After synapse with the mitral cells of the bulb the impulses travel in the olfactory tract to the lateral olfactory stria and terminate in the pyriform lobe. The pyriform lobe is the cortical receptive area for olfaction; it consists of the lateral olfactory stria, the uncus (periamygdaloid area), and the anterior part of the parahippocampal gyrus.

The ***second (optic) nerve*** is formed by the central processes of the retinal ganglion cells (SSA), which converge at the optic papilla. After piercing the sclera, the optic nerve passes through the orbital fat, traverses the optic canal, and joins with its opposite fellow to form the optic chiasma. The visual pathway from retina to occipital cor-

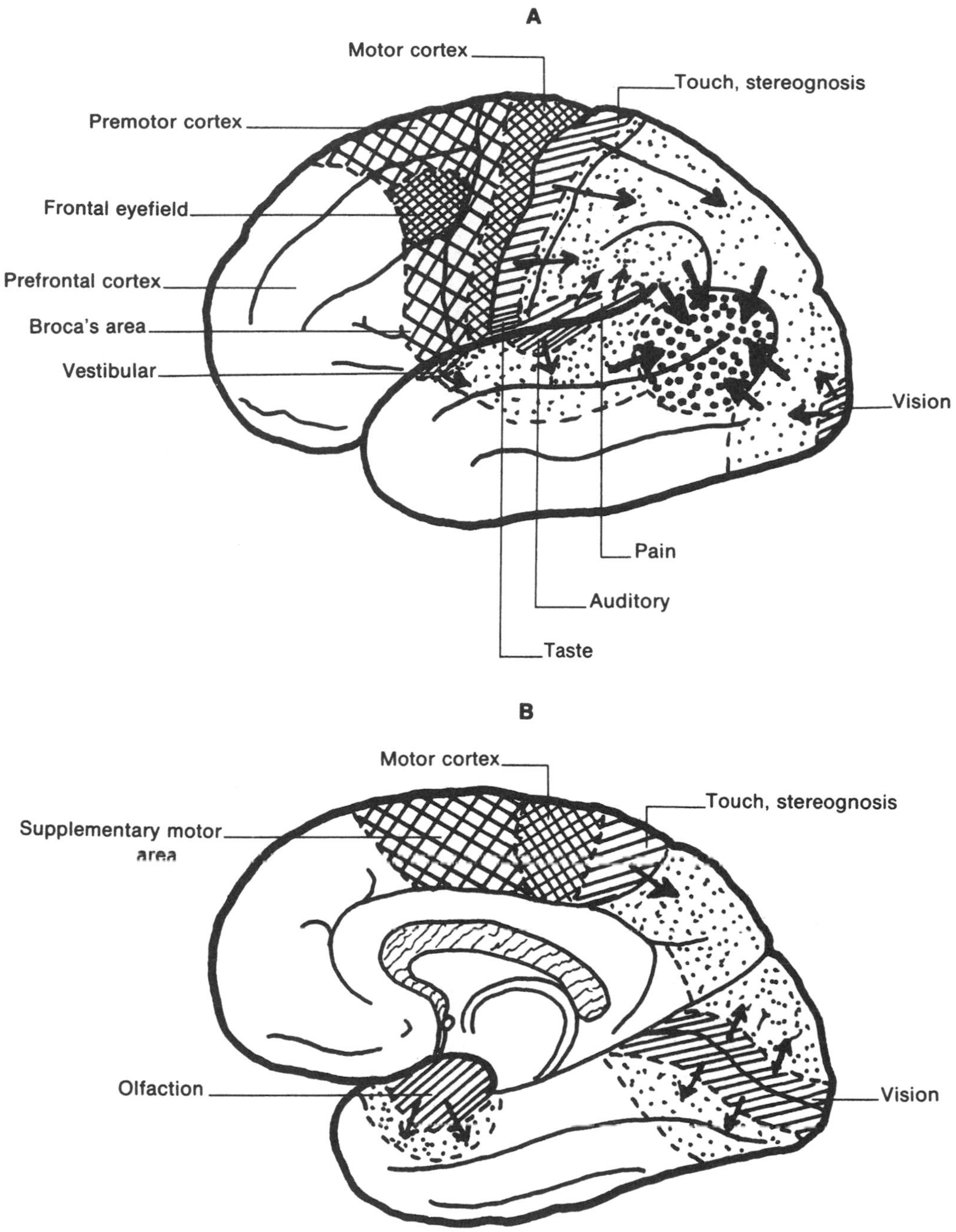

Fig. 2-20. Functional areas of the cerebral cortex as shown in lateral view *(A)* and in medial view *(B)*. The primary receptive areas are shown in diagonal lines. The unisensory association areas are shown in small dots. The multisensory association area is shown in large dots. The motor areas are crosshatched.

tex consists of four orders of neurons. The first-order neurons are the rods and cones. The second-order neurons are bipolar cells, and the third-order neurons are ganglion cells. The cell bodies of all three orders of neurons are located in the retina. Axons of the ganglion cells comprise the optic nerve, chiasm, and tract and terminate in the lateral geniculate body except for 20% of the axons, which continue directly to the pretectal area. Those axons from the nasal half of the retina decussate in the optic chiasm; those from the temporal half of the retina remain uncrossed. Thus the optic tract consists of axons from the temporal half of the ipsilateral eye and the nasal half of the contralateral eye. The fourth-order neurons are located in the lateral geniculate nucleus. Axons of these cells pass into the sublenticular and retrolenticular portion of the internal capsule, loop over the roof of the inferior horn of the lateral ventricle, and course posteriorly as the optic radiations to the striate cortex (area 17) located above and below the calcarine fissure in the occipital lobe. This pathway is also referred to as the ***geniculocalcarine tract.*** The pathway from the upper retina projects to the cuneus while that from the lower retina projects to the lingual gyrus below the calcarine fissure.

Lesions in the visual pathway give rise to deficits in the visual fields and some loss of visual reflexes. Since light rays from specific portions of the visual field project to opposite parts of the retinal fields, lesions in the nasal retinal field will result in loss of vision in the temporal visual field, while damage to the upper retinal field will demonstrate blindness in the lower visual field. In recalling the topographic distribution of fibers in the pathway, it is readily apparent that (1) lesions in front of the chiasma lead to blindness (anopsia), or partial blindness, on the side of the damaged optic nerve or retina; (2) midline lesions of the optic chiasm result in bitemporal heteronymous hemianopsia; and (3) lesions of the pathway posterior to the chiasm give homonymous hemianopsias (or quadrantic anopsias) to the side opposite to that of the lesion. Because of the topography of optic radiations and terminations in the striate cortex, lesions in the rostral portion of the temporal lobe or below the calcarine fissure can give upper quadrantic anopsias to the opposite side.

When light is shone into one eye, the ipsilateral pupil will constrict (direct response) and the contralateral pupil will constrict (consensual response). The afferent limb of this pupillary light reflex consists of rods and cones → bipolar cells → ganglion cells whose axons pass through the brachium of the superior colliculus to the pretectal area. The association limb is comprised of neurons of the pretectal nucleus that send axons ipsilaterally, and contralaterally (by way of the posterior commissure or central gray) to the Edinger-Westphal nucleus. The efferent limb of the pupillary light reflex involves innervation of the sphincter pupillae muscles by a pathway involving the preganglionic neurons of both Edinger-Westphal nuclei and oculomotor nerves, and the postganglionic neurons of both ciliary ganglia. Section of one optic nerve results in blindness in that eye and loss of direct and consensual pupillary light response when light is shone into the blind eye. When light is shown into the other eye, the direct and consensual responses are intact. Damage to an oculomotor nerve results in loss of pupillary constriction in that eye regardless of which eye is stimulated.

When a person focuses on a near object after focusing on a far object, three responses take place: (1) convergence of the eyes by contraction of the medial recti muscles, (2) pupillary constriction by contraction of the sphincter pupillae muscles, and (3) rounding of the lens because of constriction of the ciliary muscle. This reflex is referred to as the near reflex (accommodation-convergence-pupillary reflex). There are two notable distinctions between this reflex and the pupillary light reflex: (1) the pathway involves cortical connections, and (2) the efferent limb involves both SE and GVE parasympathetic components. The afferent limb involves rods and cones → bipolar cells → ganglion cells → lateral geniculate nucleus → area 17. The association limb consists of connections from area 17 → area 18 (parastriate) → area 19 (peristriate) and its corticomesencephalic axons to the oculomotor complex. The efferent limb involves the oculomotor and Edinger-Westphal nuclei, the oculomotor nerves, and the ciliary ganglia and nerves.

In the reflexes involving the turning of the head and eyes in response to visual impulses, there are cortical connections that project to a center for convergence in the midbrain tegmentum, the rostral interstitial nucleus of the MLF for vertical gaze in the midbrain and diencephalon, and the paramedian pontine reticular formation for lateral gaze in the pons. The lateral conjugate gaze center and pathways will be discussed further in the section on the abducens nerve. The association limb for reflex turning of the head probably relays through the superior colliculus and tectospinal tract to anterior horn cells and spinal accessory neurons in the cervical cord.

The ***third (oculomotor) nerve*** contains both SE and GVE parasympathetic fibers. These fibers arise from the oculomotor (SE) and Edinger-Westphal (GVE) nuclei of the midbrain, run ventrally through the tegmentum, and emerge on the medial aspect of the cerebral peduncles. The third nerve traverses the cavernous sinus and enters the orbital cavity through the superior orbital fissure. Preganglionic neurons terminate on postganglionic cells of the ciliary ganglion. Axons of the postganglionic cells run as short ciliary nerves and innervate the sphincter pupillae and ciliary muscles. SE fibers supply the levator palpebrae superioris, the superior, inferior, and medial recti, and the inferior oblique muscles.

Damage to the oculomotor nerve results in several characteristic symptoms. Ptosis (drooping of the upper eyelid) occurs as a result of denervation of the levator palpebrae superioris; the pupil is dilated, since the dilator pupillae is unopposed by the sphincter pupillae; and the direct and consensual responses of the pupillary light reflex are lost. The ciliary muscle is paralyzed and accommodation is impaired. Denervation of the extrinsic muscles results in external strabismus because of unopposed action of the lateral rectus and superior oblique muscles.

The upper motor neurons to the third, fourth, and sixth cranial nerve nuclei arise in the occipital lobe (areas 18 and 19) for smooth pursuit movements and in frontal eye fields (area 8) in the caudal portion of middle frontal gyrus for saccadic (jerky) eye movements. The latter movements are used in reading or ''searching out'' an object. Both UMN (corticobulbar) neurons for smooth pursuit and saccades work through LMN via the conjugate gaze centers.

The ***fourth (trochlear) nerve*** arises from the trochlear nucleus (SE) at the inferior colliculus levels. Axons of these cells pass dorsally around the cerebral aqueduct, decussate with fibers of the opposite side, and emerge as the fourth nerve at the superior medullary velum. The fourth nerve passes ventrally around the brain stem, traverses the cisterna basalis and the cavernous sinus, and enters the orbit through the superior orbital fissure. It supplies the superior oblique muscle, which intorts the eye when abducted, and depresses the eye when adducted.

The ***fifth (trigeminal) nerve*** contains both general somatic afferent fibers and special visceral efferent fibers. The motor fibers arise from the motor nucleus of cranial nerve V in the pons and emerge laterally from the middle cerebral peduncle in the motor root of the trigeminal nerve. The motor root passes beneath the trigeminal ganglion, exits the skull through the foramen ovale, and joins sensory fibers to form the mandibular nerve. Motor branches of the mandibular nerve innervate the muscles of mastication and tensor tympani and tensor veli palatini muscles. Sensory pseudounipolar neurons have their cell bodies located in the trigeminal ganglion. They distribute their functional dendrites over the ophthalmic, maxillary, and mandibular nerves and send axons to the pons as the sensory root of cranial nerve V. Upon entering the pons, the fibers from pain and temperature receptors descend as the spinal tract of cranial nerve V to terminate in its spinal nucleus. Touch fibers end in the principal sensory nucleus and in the upper part of the spinal nucleus of the fifth nerve. Crossed secondary fibers for pain, temperature, and touch ascend as the ***ventral secondary tract of the fifth nerve*** to the VPM nucleus. Some touch fibers ascend ipsilaterally in the ***dorsal secondary tract*** to the VPM nucleus. Third-order neurons of the VPM nucleus send axons to the postcentral gyrus.

The first-order cell bodies of proprioceptive pathways are located in the mesencephalic nucleus of cranial nerve V. The location of secondary pathways to the cerebral cortex and cerebellum from this nucleus has not been completely established.

The ***ophthalmic nerve*** passes from the trigeminal (semilunar) ganglion in the wall of the cavernous sinus through the superior orbital fissure. In the superior orbital fissure it breaks up into three terminal branches: (1) the frontal nerve with supraorbital, frontal, and supratrochlear branches; (2) the lacrimal nerve; and (3) the nasociliary nerve.

The ***maxillary nerve*** arises from the anterior border of the trigeminal ganglion, traverses the wall of the cavernous sinus, and passes into the pterygopalatine fossa through the foramen rotundum. From the pterygopalatine fossa the nerve enters the orbit through the inferior orbital fissure and becomes the infraorbital nerve. This nerve passes into the infraorbital canal, where it gives off superior alveolar nerves, and emerges at the infraorbital foramen to supply the face through inferior palpebral, external nasal, and superior labial branches. Major branches in the pterygopalatine fossa are (1) zygomatic nerve, which supplies the skin of the side of the forehead and cheek, and communicates postganglionic parasympathetic fibers from the pterygopalatine ganglion to the lacrimal nerve, and (2) pterygopalatine nerves, which supply the posterior superior nasal cavity, nasopharynx, palate, orbit, and posterior upper teeth. A middle meningeal nerve arises from the maxillary nerve near its origin and passes with the middle meningeal artery to the dura mater.

The ***mandibular division*** supplies the muscles of mastication and is sensory to the lower teeth, gums, mandible, tongue, lower lip, lower part of the face, and the skin of the auricula and temporal region. Just outside the foramen ovale it gives off a meningeal branch, which enters the skull through the foramen spinosum, and a medial pterygoid nerve supplying the medial pterygoid muscle and otic ganglion. Beyond these branches, the mandibular nerve divides into anterior and posterior divisions. The anterior division gives off motor branches to the temporalis, masseter, and lateral pterygoid muscles and gives off a sensory buccal branch to the mucous membrane and skin of the cheek. The posterior division is mainly sensory and has several major branches: (1) the auriculotemporal whose roots encircle the middle meningeal artery and carry sensory fibers to the temporal and ear regions as well as postganglionic parasympathetic fibers to the parotid gland from the otic ganglion; (2) the inferior alveolar supplying the mylohyoid muscle, lower teeth, lower lip, and chin; and (3) the lingual nerve supplying the mucosa of the anterior two thirds of the tongue with GSA exteroceptive fibers of the fifth nerve and with SVA taste fibers of the facial nerve, the latter entering the lingual nerve by way of the chorda tympani nerve.

Lesions of the trigeminal nerve result in exteroceptive deficits of pain, temperature, and touch in the areas supplied by the damaged components. Lesions of the ophthalmic division result in loss of the afferent limb of the corneal blink reflex. Damage to one ophthalmic nerve produces loss of the direct and consensual blink. If the efferent limb, mediated by the facial nerve, were damaged and the ophthalmic was intact then stimulation of the cornea would result in blink of only that eye that had an intact seventh nerve innervating the orbicularis oculi muscle. Lesion to the mandibular nerves could result in deviation of the jaw to the affected side upon opening of the jaws due to the unopposed action of the contralateral external pterygoid muscle.

The ***sixth (abducens) nerve*** leaves the brain at the posterior border of the pons, traverses the cavernous sinus, enters the orbit through the superior orbital fissure, and innervates the ipsilateral lateral rectus muscle. This nerve arises from SE cell bodies in the floor of the fourth ventricle at the facial colliculus level of the pons. The abducens nucleus receives afferents from the ipsilateral ***lateral gaze center*** (parabducens nucleus, PPRF) located near the abducens nucleus below the MLF. Some axons from the abducens nucleus cross the midline and ascend in the contralateral medial longitudinal fasciculus to reach cells of the oculomotor nucleus that innervate the contralateral medial rectus muscle. Thus, stimulation of neurons in the PPRF results in conjugate deviation of the eyes to the side stimulated, since the ipsilateral abducens and lateral rectus, and contralateral oculomotor and medial rectus are activated. The abducens and oculomotor nuclei also are supplied by fibers that course through the MLF from vestibular nuclei and superior colliculi.

Section of the abducens nerve may lead to medial deviation (strabismus) of the affected eye since the medial rectus is unopposed. There is diplopia and inability to turn the eye laterally. Lesion of the abducens nucleus area often involves both the abducens and lateral gaze center. In this type of lesion there is inability for both eyes to look laterally toward the side of the lesion, and there is a tendency for persistent conjugate deviation toward the opposite side.

The ***seventh (facial) nerve*** contains GSA, SVA (taste), GVA, SVE, and GVE functional components. GSA fibers arise from receptors in a small area near the external ear, pass to pseudounipolar cell bodies in the geniculate ganglion, and course into the pons at the pons-medulla junction to terminate in the spinal nucleus of cranial nerve V. SVA fibers arise from taste buds in the anterior two thirds of the tongue and traverse the lingual nerve and chorda tympani to reach the geniculate ganglion. Axons of these cells enter the pons and descend in the fasciculus solitarius to end in the upper part of the solitary (gustatory) nucleus. GVAs arise from the submandibular, sublingual, lacrimal, nasal, and minor salivary glands. Their cell bodies are in the geniculate ganglion, and their axons terminate in the nucleus solitarius. GVE preganglionic parasympathetic neurons arise in the superior salivatory nucleus of the pons and are distributed (1) to the pterygopalatine ganglion by way of the greater petrosal nerve, and (2) to the submandibular ganglion by way of the chorda tympani and lingual nerves. Postganglionic fibers from the pterygopalatine ganglion supply the lacrimal gland and the small glands of the pharynx, palate, paranasal sinuses, and nasal cavity. Postganglionics leaving the submandibular ganglion supply the submandibular, sublingual, and minor oral salivary glands. SVE neurons arise in the facial motor nucleus, form an internal genu around the abducens nucleus, emerge in the facial nerve at the pons-medulla junction and are distributed through numerous branches to the muscles of facial expression, the stapedius muscle, posterior belly of the digastric muscle, and stylohyoid muscle.

The facial nerve leaves the pons as two roots: (1) the motor root, and (2) the nervus intermedius. The latter nerve contains taste and parasympathetic fibers. Both roots enter the internal acoustic meatus with the vestibulocochlear nerve. At the fundus of the meatus, the facial nerve enters the facial canal in the petrous portion of the temporal bone. Near the tympanic cavity it bends (external genu) posteriorly above the oval window and descends to exit at the stylomastoid foramen. The geniculate ganglion is located at the bend, and the greater superficial petrosal nerve branches from this region. The nerve to the stapedius muscle and chorda tympani arise from the nerve while it is in the facial canal. The chorda tympani courses through the bone, enters the posterior wall of the tympanum, and passes deep to the mucous membrane and medial to the tympanic membrane and manubrium of the malleus. It exits anteriorly from the tympanum, emerges from the skull, and joins the lingual nerve. That portion of the facial nerve exiting from the stylomastoid foramen divides into posterior auricular, digastric, stylohyoid, temporal, zygomatic, buccal, mandibular, and cervical branches.

Lesions of the facial nerve (such as in Bell's palsy) result in weakness to all of the facial muscles ipsilateral to the lesion. This is distinct from lesions of the UMNs (corticobulbar tract), which bilaterally innervate that part of the facial nucleus supplying the upper facial muscles but only contralaterally supply cells to the lower face. Thus, in UMN lesions there is weakness to the contralateral lower face. Peripheral nerve lesions also may result in (1) loss of taste in the anterior two thirds of the tongue, (2) impaired lacrimation, and (3) hyperacusis due to loss of the dampening effect of the stapedius muscle.

The ***eighth (vestibulocochlear) nerve*** is a SSA nerve arising from receptors for hearing in the cochlear duct and arising from the maculae and cristae of the vestibular apparatus. It is comprised of the processes of bipolar cells whose cell bodies lie in the spiral cochlear ganglion and vestibular ganglion. Axons of these cells run in the internal acoustic meatus and enter the pons at the pons-medulla junction.

Cochlear fibers synapse in the dorsal and ventral cochlear nuclei. From these nuclei axons pass bilaterally, synapsing in the superior olivary nucleus, nucleus of the lateral lemniscus, and inferior colliculus. From the inferior colliculus axons pass to the medial geniculate nucleus, where impulses are relayed to the transverse temporal gyrus (of Heschl). Lesions of one nerve result in deafness to that ear. Unilateral lesions of the central pathway lead only to a diminution in hearing due to the bilateral representation.

Entering ***vestibular fibers*** may pass directly to the flocculonodular lobe of the cerebellum or synapse on vestibular nuclei. The vestibular pathway to consciousness is not known. There are reflex connections from vestibular nuclei to the spinal cord (by way of the MLF and vestibulospinal tract), to the center for lateral conjugate gaze and to motor nuclei of the brain stem reticular formation. Some of these connections are better appreciated when the pathways involving reflex activities that accompany angular rotation of the head are considered. When the head is inclined 30 degrees forward and is first rotated to the right the endolymph of both horizontal semicircular canals does not move initially as fast as the cristae ampullares. This gives a relative displacement of endolymph to the left, although endolymph is actually moving to the right. After rotation the cristae stop moving, but there is continued brief movement of endolymph to the right in the direction of rotation. Since stimulation of cristae of the horizontal canal toward the utricle results in depolarization of the hair cells, an imbalance occurs during rotation and postrotation between the two canals. In postrotation to the right the left vestibular nerve is stimulated while the right vestibular nerve is being inhibited. This results in rapid alternating eye movements (nystagmus). The pathway for the slow component of nystagmus to the right in postrotation to the right involves the left vestibular nerve, left vestibular nuclei, right lateral gaze center, right abducens nucleus and nerve, left MLF, and oculomotor nucleus and nerve. In this pathway axons from vestibular nuclei may ascend in the MLF to reach the oculomotor nucleus and cross to the opposite abducens nucleus, or they may go to the opposite lateral gaze center, which in turn, makes connections with the abducens and oculomotor nuclei. Accompanying past-pointing and a tendency to fall to the right are mediated through connections of the left vestibular nucleus with the cerebellum and through connections of the left vestibulospinal tract with anterior horn cells of antigravity muscles, thus causing a thrust to the right. Nausea, increased salivation, and vomiting are mediated through connections of the vestibular nuclei with such motor nuclei as the dorsal motor nucleus of cranial nerve X, the nucleus ambiguus, the salivatory nuclei, and other reticular nuclei.

The ***ninth (glossopharyngeal) nerve*** contains GSA, SVA (taste), GVA, SVE, and GVE functional components. GSA fibers arise from skin receptors in the posterior part of the external auditory meatus and auricula. These fibers are distributed in the auricular branch of the vagus. They pass to the glossopharyngeal near the jugular foramen and the pseudounipolar cell bodies of these GSA neurons are located in the superior ganglion in the jugular foramen. Axons of these cells enter the upper medulla, in the postolivary sulcus, and synapse on cells of the spinal nucleus of cranial nerve V.

SVA fibers arise from taste buds in the posterior one third of the tongue. They pass through lingual branches and their cell bodies are in the inferior ganglion. Axons terminate in the solitary (gustatory) nucleus. GVA fibers arise in the mucosa and glands of the posterior tongue, fauces, and pharynx. Their cell bodies are located in the inferior ganglion, and their axons terminate in the solitary nucleus. The carotid sinus nerve of the glossopharyngeal conveys GVA fibers from the carotid sinus to the nucleus solitarius. Axons from this nucleus course to the dorsal motor nucleus of cranial nerve X, where they synapse on neurons whose fibers pass into the vagus nerve and constitute the efferent limb of the carotid sinus reflex.

SVE fibers arise in the nucleus ambiguus and pass through the glossopharyngeal nerve to innervate the stylopharyngeus. GVE preganglionic parasympathetics have their cell bodies in the inferior salivatory nucleus. Axons of these neurons pass into the tympanic nerve. This nerve arises from the inferior ganglion, courses through the temporal bone, runs on the promontory, and helps to form the tympanic plexus in the middle ear cavity. The preganglionics leave the plexus in the lesser superficial petrosal nerve and synapse on postganglionics in the otic ganglion. Postganglionic axons run in the auriculotemporal branch of the trigeminal nerve and are distributed to the parotid gland.

In the gag reflex, the afferent limb is by way of GVA fibers from the oropharynx to the association limb in nucleus solitarius. Axons of the latter nucleus are both crossed and uncrossed to the hypoglossal nucleus for tongue movements and to the nucleus ambiguus for pharynx, larynx, and soft palate movements. Lesions of the glossopharyngeal can result in some loss of taste in the posterior third of the tongue and in a loss of the gag reflex when the affected side is stimulated.

The ***tenth (vagus) nerve*** contains the same five functional components as do the facial and glossopharyngeal nerves. The small GSA component travels from the external ear in the auricular branch of the vagus and has its cell bodies located in the superior (jugular) ganglion lying in the posterior part of the jugular foramen. Axons from this ganglion enter the medulla in the postolivary sulcus and end in the spinal nucleus of cranial nerve V. The SVA fibers arise from taste buds in the region of the epiglottis. SVA cell bodies are in the inferior (nodose) ganglion, located inferior to the jugular foramen, and their axons terminate in the gustatory part of the nucleus solitarius. GVA fibers arise in the mucosa and walls of the intestine (as far as the splenic flexure), the stomach, esophagus, pharynx, larynx, trachea, lungs, heart, carotid body, and kidney. Their cell bodies are located in the inferior ganglion, and their axons terminate in the nucleus solitarius.

SVE nerves arise from the nucleus ambiguus and are distributed to the skeletal muscles of the pharynx, soft palate, larynx, and esophagus. Pharyngeal branches supply the pharyngeal plexus that gives branches to the pharyngeal constrictor muscles and all of the palatine muscles except the tensor veli palatini. The external branch of the superior laryngeal nerve supplies the cricothyroideus and part of the inferior pharyngeal constrictor muscles. The internal branch of the superior laryngeal supplies sensory and parasympathetic secretomotor fibers to the larynx and epiglottis. All of the laryngeal muscles, except the cricothyroideus, are supplied by the recurrent (inferior) laryngeal nerve. The right recurrent arises in the root of the neck and arches under the subclavian. The left recurrent arises in the upper thorax, loops around the arch of the aorta just below the ligamentum arteriosum, and ascends to the larynx.

The GVE fibers arise from the dorsal motor nucleus of cranial nerve X. These preganglionics are distributed through numerous branches of the vagus to the terminal parasympathetic ganglia in or on the heart, larynx, trachea, lungs, and digestive system from the pharynx to the splenic flexure. The terminal ganglia of most of the gastrointestinal tract are the myenteric and submucosal nerve ganglia and plexi. Postganglionic axons from terminal ganglia supply smooth and cardiac muscle and glands.

The peripheral branches of the vagus nerve are extensive. In the jugular fossa, the vagus gives off auricular and meningeal nerves. In the neck it gives off pharyngeal, superior laryngeal, right recurrent laryngeal, and the superior cardiac nerves. In the thorax the vagus gives off the left recurrent, inferior cardiac, anterior and posterior bronchial, and esophageal nerves. The right and left vagus form an esophageal plexus around the esophagus from which most of the left vagus enters the abdomen as the anterior vagus; most of the right contributes to the posterior vagus. Vagal branches in the abdomen are the gastric, hepatic, and celiac.

A unilateral lesion of the vagus nerve or its nuclei produces paresis of the ipsilateral vocal cord, resulting in abnormal phonation and hoarseness. In addition, the affected side of the soft palate is lower than the normal side. Upon phonation, the uvula points toward the normal side. Lesions of the vagus also demonstrate abnormal gag and swallowing reflexes since the vagus constitutes the efferent limbs of those reflexes.

The ***eleventh (accessory) nerve*** consists of two parts, a cranial and a spinal part. The cranial part arises in the nucleus ambiguus (SVE), exits from the postolivary sulcus of the medulla, passes through the jugular foramen, and merges with the vagus near the inferior vagal ganglion. The spinal part arises from anterior horn cells of the upper five cervical segments. Axons of these cells pass laterally through the lateral funiculus, ascend between the dentate ligament and the dorsal roots, and pass as a nerve trunk through the foramen magnum into the cranial cavity. This nerve trunk communicates with the cranial part of the accessory and the vagus and exits from the jugular foramen to distribute fibers to the sternocleidomastoid and trapezius muscles.

Lesions of the spinal accessory produce weakness in shoulder shrugging on the affected side, and the arm cannot be raised to the vertical plane because of paresis of the trapezius. In addition, there may be weakness in rotating the head and face to the opposite side.

The ***twelfth (hypoglossal) nerve*** is an SE nerve that arises from the hypoglossal nucleus and emerges from the preolivary sulcus of the medulla. It passes through the hypoglossal canal, loops ventrally and anteriorly above the hyoid bone, and innervates the tongue musculature.

Unilateral lesions of the hypoglossal nerve or nucleus result in deviation of the tongue to the affected side upon protrusion. This is due to the action of the unopposed genioglossus of the normal side. There may be fasciculations and wasting on the affected side. Since corticobulbar fibers are crossed, damage to these fibers causes the tongue to deviate away from the lesion upon protrusion.

Major Ascending and Descending Pathways. The following outline is a summary of some of the major clinically significant ascending and descending pathways that course through the spinal cord and brain stem. Lesions of the ascending pathways produce loss of sensation ipsilaterally if the lesion occurs below the decussation, and contralaterally if the lesion is above the crossing second-order neurons.

Ascending Pathways of the Spinal Cord

1. ***Pain and temperature pathway*** (Fig. 2-21)
   Neuron I: Cell bodies in dorsal root ganglion and axon in dorsal root.
   Neuron II: Cell bodies in the posteromarginal nucleus and nucleus proprius. Axons cross to the opposite side in the anterior white commissure and ascend as the lateral spinothalamic tract.
   Neuron III: Cell bodies in the VPL nucleus of the thalamus. Axons ascend in the posterior limb of the internal capsule to the postcentral gyrus and to a region of the parietal lobe bordering the lateral fissure (somesthetic area II).
2. ***Two-point touch, stereognosis, vibratory sense pathway*** (Fig. 2-22)
   Neuron I: Cell bodies in dorsal root ganglion. Axons of dorsal root ascend in the posterior white column. Those entering below T6 ascend in the fasciculus gracilis; those entering above T6 ascend in fasciculus cuneatus.

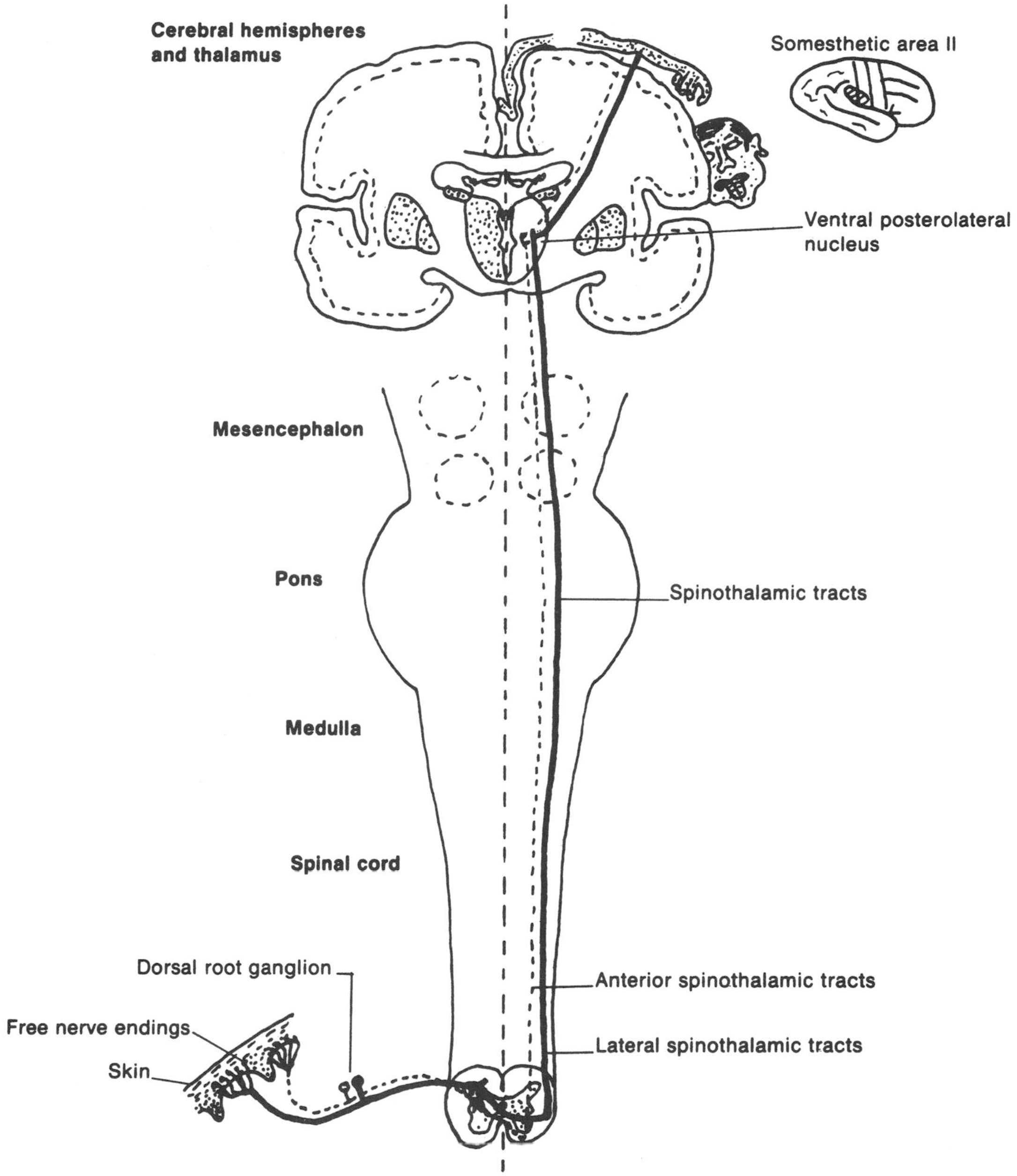

Fig. 2-21. Lateral spinothalamic tract *(solid lines)* for pain and temperature and anterior spinothalamic tract *(dashed lines)* for light touch.

Neuron II: Cell bodies in nucleus gracilis and cuneatus. Axons cross and ascend as the medial lemniscus.

Neuron III: Cell bodies in the VPL nucleus of the thalamus. Axons to the postcentral gyrus by way of the posterior limb of the internal capsule.

3. ***Crude (light) touch pathway*** (see Fig. 2-21)

Neuron I: Cell bodies in the dorsal root ganglion. Axons of the dorsal root enter the dorsal horn.

Neuron II: Cell bodies in the dorsal horn. Axons are mostly crossed and ascend as the anterior spinothalamic tract.

Neuron III: In the VPL nucleus of the thalamus; send axons to the postcentral gyrus.

4. ***Posterior spinocerebellar and cuneocerebellar pathways***

Neuron I: Dendrites arise in neuromuscular spindles and Golgi tendon organs as IA and IB fibers, respectively. Cell bodies in the dorsal root ganglia. Axons enter via dorsal roots; those below L3 as-

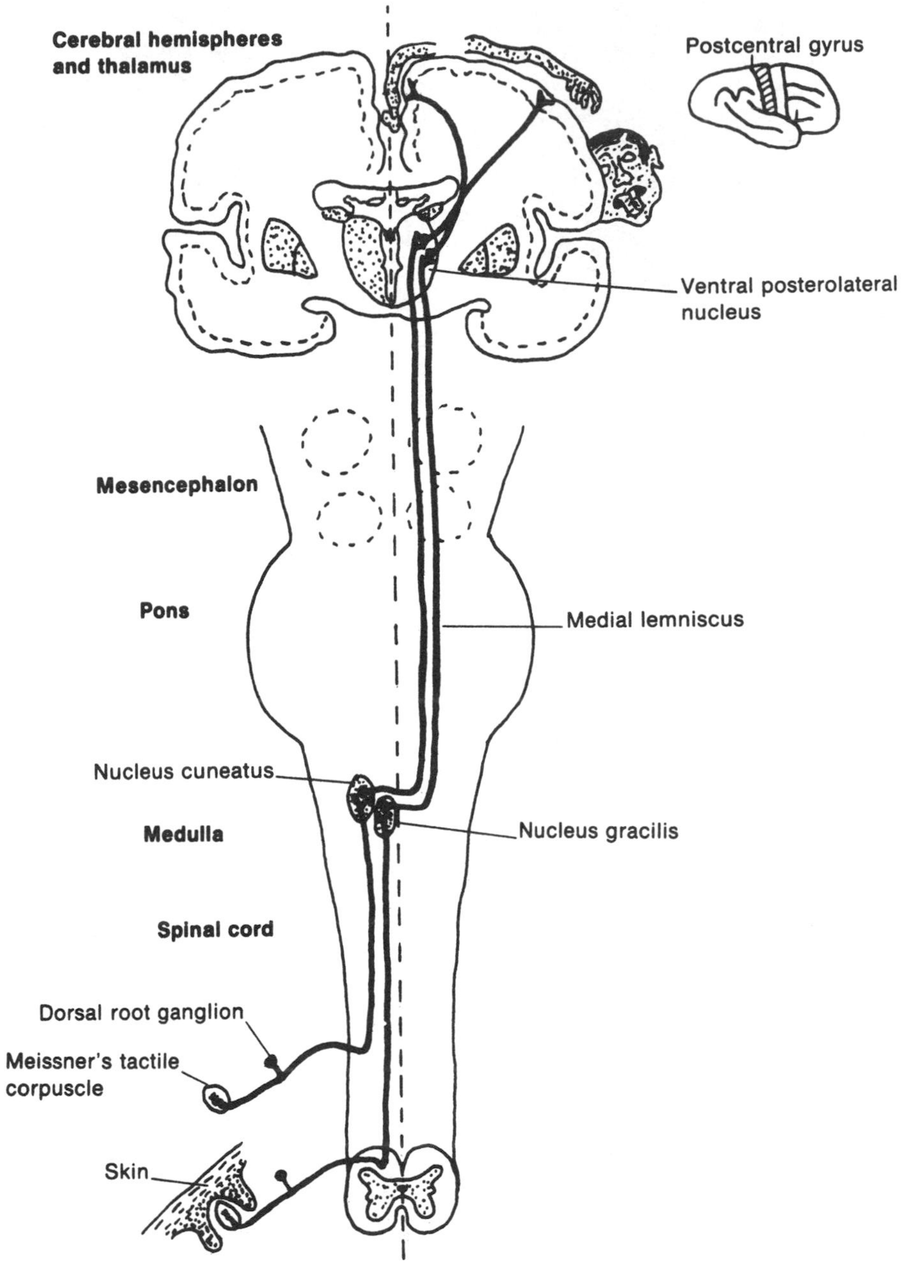

Fig. 2-22. Posterior white column pathway for two-point touch, joint sense, vibratory sense, and stereognosis. The pathway utilizing the nucleus gracilis originates at foot and leg levels, whereas the pathway synapsing in the nucleus cuneatus arises in the upper extremity.

cend in the posterior white column to the nucleus dorsalis, while those above C8 ascend to the accessory cuneate nucleus. The rest will enter the nucleus dorsalis near the level of entry.

Neuron II: Cell bodies in the nucleus dorsalis (Clarke's column) receive first-order neurons from below the C8 cord level. Axons of these cells ascend ipsilaterally as the posterior spinocerebellar tract to the cerebellum. Cell bodies in the accessory cuneate nucleus of the medulla receive ascending first-order neurons from levels above C8. Axons from this nucleus form the cuneocerebellar tract, which becomes part of the inferior cerebellar peduncle.

Ascending Pathways Arising at Brain Stem Levels

1. ***Pain and temperature pathway*** (see Fig. 2-19)

Neuron I: Dendrites in the maxillary, mandibular, and ophthalmic division of the trigeminal nerve. Cell bodies in the trigeminal ganglion. Axons enter the pons and descend to the low medulla as the spinal tract of cranial nerve V. Some first-order neurons from the posterior ear region are part of the facial, glossopharyngeal, and vagus nerves. Their axons enter the spinal nucleus of cranial nerve V.

Neuron II: Cell bodies in the spinal nucleus of cranial nerve V. Axons cross and ascend as the ventral ascending secondary tract of cranial nerve V.

Neuron III: Cell bodies in the VPM nucleus. Axons to the postcentral gyrus and somesthetic area II via the posterior limb of the internal capsule.

2. ***Touch pathways*** (see Fig. 2-19)

Neuron I: Cell bodies in the trigeminal ganglion. Axons to the principal sensory nucleus and to the upper part of the spinal nucleus of cranial nerve V.

Neuron II: Cell bodies in the principal sensory nucleus and spinal nucleus of cranial nerve V. Axons from both nuclei cross and ascend as the ventral secondary ascending tract of cranial nerve V. Some axons from the principal sensory nucleus of cranial nerve V ascend ipsilaterally as the dorsal secondary ascending tract of cranial nerve V.

Neuron III: Cell bodies in the VPM nucleus of the thalamus; axons go to the postcentral gyrus.

3. ***Hearing pathway***

Neuron I: Dendrites from the hair cells of the organ of Corti to bipolar cells in the spiral cochlear ganglion; axons to the pons-medulla junction.

Neuron II: Cell bodies in the dorsal and ventral cochlear nuclei; axons are both crossed and uncrossed and ascend as the lateral lemniscus to the inferior colliculus. There may be relays through the superior olivary nucleus, nucleus of the lateral lemniscus, and nucleus of the trapezoid body in this ascent.

Neuron III: Cell bodies in the inferior colliculus. Axons pass into the brachium of the inferior colliculus.

Neuron IV: Cell bodies in the medial geniculate body. Axons pass in the sublenticular limb of the internal capsule to the transverse temporal gyri of Heschl.

4. ***Visual pathway***

Neuron I: Rods and cones

Neuron II: Bipolar cells of the retina

Neuron III: Cell bodies are the ganglion cell layer of the retina. Axons course as the optic nerve, optic chiasm, and optic tract. Axons from the nasal half of the retina cross in the optic chiasm.

Neuron IV: Cell bodies in the lateral geniculate body. Axons pass in the sublenticular and retrolenticular limbs of the internal capsule and in the geniculocalcarine tract (optic radiations) to the calcarine striate cortex (area 17).

Descending Pathways of the Brain and Spinal Cord

1. Pyramidal system (see Fig. 2-23)

a. By way of corticospinal tract

UMN: Cell bodies are in the precentral gyrus (area 4) and in the postcentral gyrus and premotor cortex. Axons descend in the posterior limb of the internal capsule, the crus cerebri, basis pontis, and pyramids. Most cross at the pyramidal decussation and descend in the lateral corticospinal tract. They synapse on internuncials at the level of the lower motor neuron innervated.

LMN: Cell bodies in the anterior horn of the spinal cord as alpha motor neurons to extrafusal muscle fibers and as gamma efferent neurons to intrafusal muscle fibers. This pathway tonically facilitates the antagonists of antigravity muscles and phasically controls the distal muscles in fine movements.

b. By way of corticobulbar pathways

UMN: Cell bodies located near the lateral fissure in the precentral and postcentral gyri and in the premotor cortex. Axons pass through the genu and posterior limb of the internal capsule and crus cerebri. Those from frontal eye fields to the lateral gaze center (PPRF) for saccadic eye movements, to that portion of the hypoglossal nucleus that supplies the genioglossus nuclei, and to that portion of the facial motor nucleus that supplies muscles of the lower face are crossed. Those that supply the lateral gaze center for smooth pursuit movements and those that terminate on the spinal accessory nucleus are uncrossed. All other corticobulbar fibers are both crossed and uncrossed.

LMN: Cell bodies in the SE and SVE nuclei of cranial nerves III through VII and IX through XII.

2. Major extrapyramidal tracts (see summary of tracts in Fig. 2-3)

a. By way of vestibulospinal tract

UMN: Cell bodies are located in the lateral vestibular nucleus. Axons of this tract are uncrossed and located in the anterior funiculus and end on internuncial neurons.

LMN: Gamma and alpha motor neurons to antigravity muscles are facilitated.

b. By way of lateral reticulospinal tract

UMN: Cell bodies are in the gigantocellular nucleus in the reticular formation of the medulla. Axons of this tract are uncrossed and are located in the lateral funiculus.

LMN: Gamma and alpha motor neurons to antigravity muscles are inhibited.

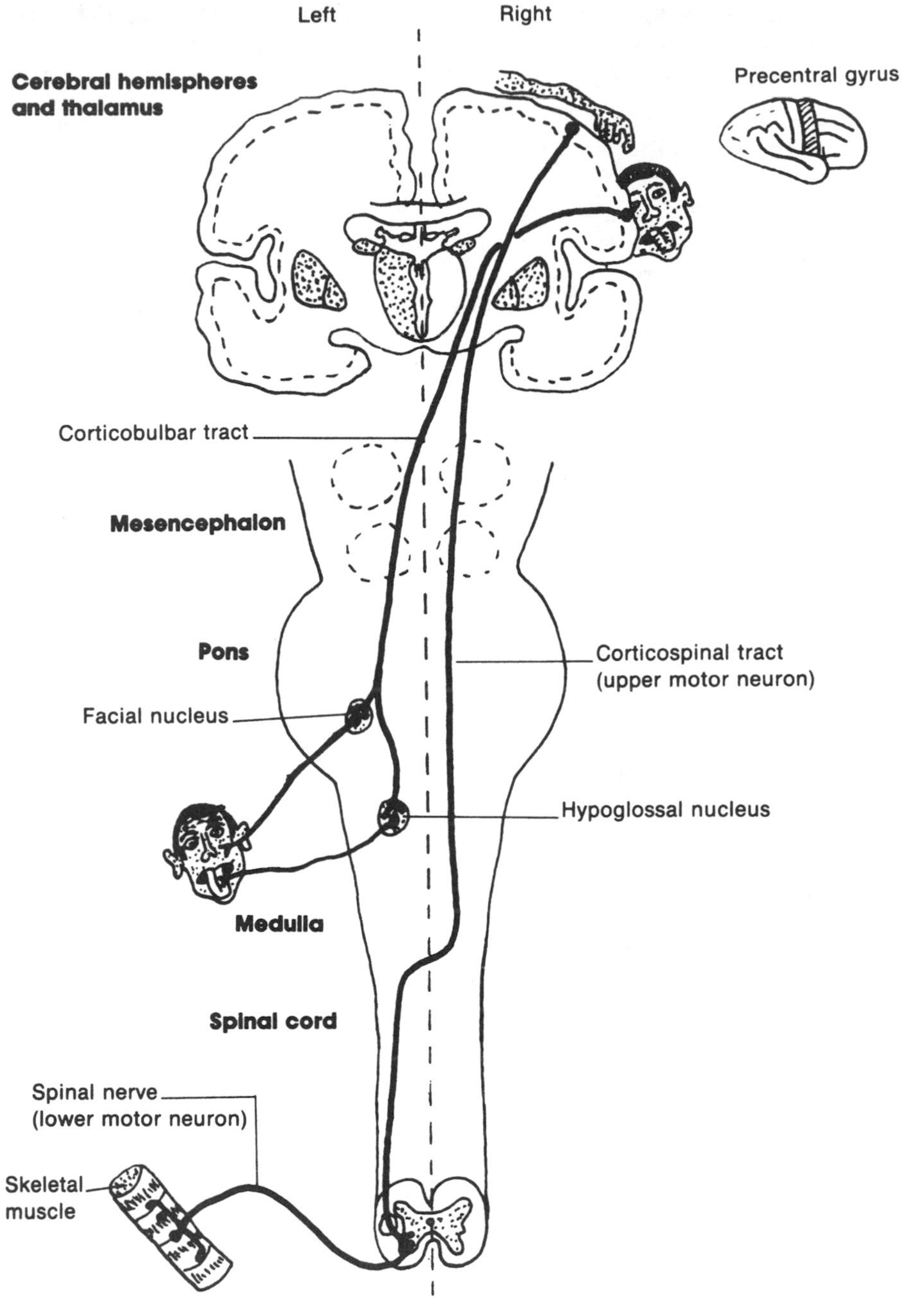

Fig. 2-23. Corticospinal and corticobulbar tracts. Only the crossed corticospinal pathway to upper extremity muscles and crossed cortical bulbar pathways to the lower face and genioglossus muscles are shown.

c. By way of medial reticulospinal tract

UMN: Cell bodies are in the oral and caudal pontine reticular nuclei. Axons of this tract descend mostly uncrossed in the reticular formation of the brain stem and in the anterior funiculus.

LMN: Gamma and alpha motor neurons of antigravity muscles are facilitated.

d. By way of rubrospinal tract

UMN: Cell bodies are in the red nucleus. Axons cross in the ventral segmental decussation and descend in the rubrospinal tract. This tract is located in the lateral reticular formation of the brain stem and in the lateral funiculus of the spinal cord. Axons end on internuncials.

LMN: Gamma and alpha motor neurons probably facilitate the antagonists of antigravity muscles.

e. By way of central descending autonomics

UMN: Cell bodies are in the hypothalamus and in the reticular formation. Axons descend in the lateral reticular formation of the brain stem and lateral funiculus of the spinal cord.

LMN: Preganglionic sympathetic neurons in the intermediolateral cell column of the lateral horn at thoracic, lumbar, and sacral levels of the spinal cord.

Somatic Motor Control Mechanisms. The somatic motor anterior horn cells of the spinal cord and the SE (nuclei 3, 4, 6, and 12) and SVE (nucleus ambiguus and motor nuclei of 5 and 7) neurons of the brain stem are regulated by afferent and association fibers from all levels of the CNS. Afferent and internuncial neurons innervating anterior horn cells within one level of the spinal cord constitute a segmental level of motor control. An example of this is the myotatic stretch reflex where IA fibers from the muscle spindle of a stretched muscle convey impulses monosynaptically at the level of entry of the dorsal root, with an alpha motor neuron supplying the extrafusal muscle fibers of that muscle.

Intersegmental connections of afferent and association neurons within the spinal cord constitute a mechanism for intersegmental regulation of motor activity. Such connections may involve collaterals from long ascending and descending pathways or shorter spinospinal fibers of the fasciculus proprius. An example of this is the pain withdrawal reflex wherein pain fibers are stimulated. The impulse is carried to several levels of the cord by way of the fasciculus proprius in order that motor neurons involved in the body adjustment of withdrawal can be stimulated.

Suprasegmental control pathways involve connections of the spinal cord with higher centers of the CNS. This constellation of numerous suprasegmental connections can best be appreciated if they are divided into phylogenetically older and newer systems. Such a scheme can include older antigravity and vestibular regulation, the next oldest regulation of the more stereotyped grosser movements involving the more axial musculature and the newer fine discrete movements.

Antigravity and vestibular connections involve input from muscle spindles and the vestibular apparatus. These afferents make connections through the spinocerebellar tracts and vestibular nuclei with the cerebellum; the vestibular fibers end in the flocculonodular lobe, while spindle information is conveyed to vermal and paravermal areas of the anterior and posterior lobes of the cerebellum. Cerebellar efferents, through dentatorubral fibers of the superior cerebellar peduncle, synapse in the red nucleus with cells of the rubrospinal tract, which bring about the facilitation of antagonists of the antigravity muscles. Cerebellar efferents from the flocculonodular lobe arise from the fastigial nuclei and terminate in the lateral vestibular nuclei. Axons from the lateral nucleus constitute the lateral vestibulospinal tract, which is facilitory to antigravity muscles. The medial and lateral reticulospinal tracts receive input from all levels of the CNS and are facilitory and inhibitory, respectively, to the antigravity muscles.

The regulation of *gross stereotyped movements* involves the basal ganglia and their ascending connections with the cortex and their descending connections through the reticular formation. In these circuits the premotor cortex and centromedian nucleus of the thalamus receive ascending afferent input and relay this information to the caudate and putamen. The neostriatum (putamen and caudate) also receives input from the substantia nigra. The neostriatal nuclei send axons to the globus pallidus and probably have a regulatory effect on it. The efferent outflow from the basal ganglia (lenticular nucleus) is from the globus pallidus to (1) the motor and premotor cortex by way of the ventral anterior and ventral lateral nuclei of the thalamus, and (2) the motor neurons of the spinal cord and brain stem by way of the subthalamus, prerubral field, red nucleus and the reticulospinal, rubrospinal, and reticuloreticular pathways. Pallidal efferents to the thalamic nuclei course through the internal capsule and then pass between the subthalamic nucleus and zona incerta in the fasciculus lenticularis to reach the prerubral field (of Forel). From the prerubral field, axons loop laterally toward the thalamus in the fasciculus thalamicus, or they descend in the reticular formation to contralateral motor nuclei. Other pallidal efferents loop around the internal capsule in the ansa lenticularis in their pathway to the thalamus.

Lesions of the basal ganglia, subthalamus, and substantia nigra are associated with disturbances in involuntary movements (dyskinesias) and in muscle tone. Lesions of the subthalamic nucleus can lead to hemiballism on the opposite side due to release of the globus pallidus from the inhibitory control of the subthalamus. Parkinsonism (paralysis agitans) is characterized by a decrease of dopamine in the substantia nigra and neostriatum (caudate and putamen). The tremor at rest and rigidity of this disorder may be due to inability of the neostriatum to regulate the globus pallidus. Lesions producing chorea and athetosis are probably in the striatum but are not as clearly localized as the other basal ganglia disorders.

The pathways involved in the initiation and performance of a *fine coordinated movement* involve (1) input to the cortex, (2) a feedback loop between the cerebral cortex and the cerebellum, (3) corticospinal and corticobulbar pathways, and (4) alpha and gamma motor neurons of the spinal cord and brain stem. In these pathways ascending exteroceptive input is relayed through the thalamus to the primary receptive areas of the cortex (areas 3, 1, 2; 41 and 42; 43; 17). Projections from the primary receptive areas go to unisensory association areas lying adjacent to the primary receptive areas (see Fig. 2-20). The specific sensation for each receptive area is "recognized" in each unisensory association area. Projections

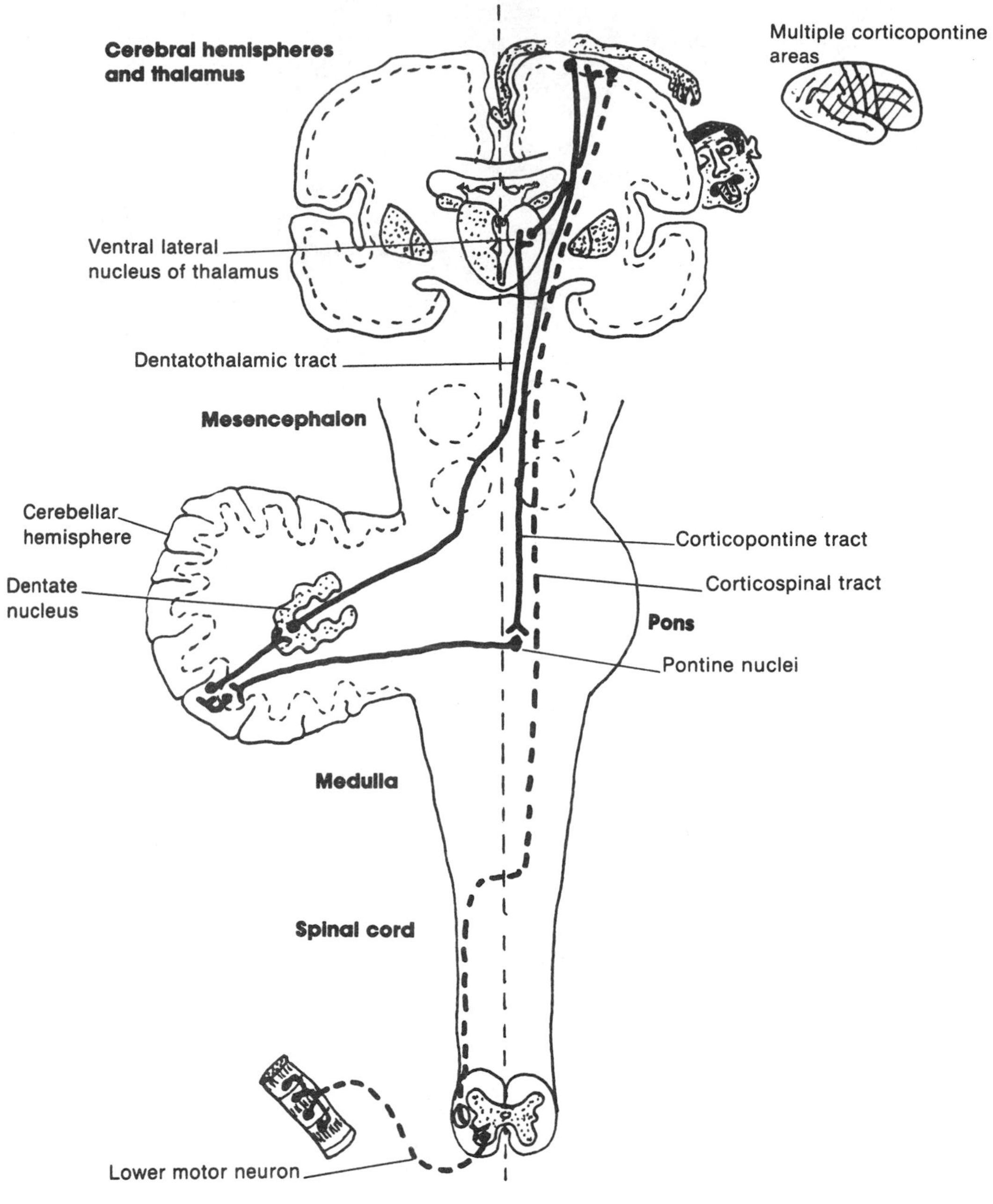

Fig. 2-24. The neocerebellar circuit *(solid lines)* for the coordination of skilled motor activities are carried out by way of the corticospinal tract and lower motor neurons *(dashed lines).*

from the unisensory association areas congregate in multisensory association areas in the junctional area of the inferior parietal gyrus (areas 39 and 40), superior temporal gyrus (area 22), and lateral occipital gyri (area 19). In these areas gnosis from more than one sensation is utilized in the initiation and formulation of learned complex motor activity.

Axons from these parietal, occipital, and temporal regions, as well as axons from the prefrontal cortical center for initiative and judgment and from premotor and motor regions, descend as corticopontine pathways to pontine nuclei (Fig. 2-24). Frontopontine fibers descend through the anterior limb of the internal capsule and medial portion of the crus cerebri. The other corticopontine fibers descend in the posterior limb of the internal capsule and lateral part of the crus cerebri. After they synapse on cells of the pontine nuclei, axons of the latter cells carry impulses across the midline of the basis pontis and ascend to the cerebellar cortex in the middle cerebellar peduncle. These pontocerebellar fibers are mossy fibers that end in the granule cell layer. From here impulses spread through the molecular layer of the neocerebellar cortex of the posterior lobe and are transmitted to Purkinje cells. Axons of Purkinje cells pass to the dentate nucleus, where they synapse on cells whose fibers cross the midline in the decussation of the superior cerebellar peduncle and ascend to the ventral lateral nucleus of the thalamus. From the ventral lateral nucleus axons ascend to the motor cortex.

The ultimate descending pathway for fine discrete movements is by way of the corticospinal and corticobulbar tracts to anterior horn cells and brain stem SE and SVE neurons. In this complex pathway, which involves a double crossing of fibers in the cerebral cortex-cerebellar loop and a single crossing of the corticospinal tract, the cerebellum acts as a computer coordinating the activity of numerous neurons.

Lesions of the cerebellum may demonstrate deficits in motor activity. Neocerebellar lesions produce a lateral cerebellar syndrome in which the symptoms are on the same side of the body as the involved cerebellar hemisphere. This syndrome demonstrates an asynergia of voluntary skilled activity characterized by hypotonia and postural fixation defects, especially of the limbs. Some clinical signs and abnormal reflexes of neocerebellar disease are dysmetria, intention tremor, rebound phenomenon, disdiadochokinesis, explosive speech, decomposition of movement, and tendency to fall to the side of the lesion. Flocculonodular syndrome is primarily a disorder of locomotion and equilibrium. This is characterized by truncal ataxia with the patient falling, or walking on a wide base or with a drunken gait.

Lesions of various portions of the cerebral cortex lead to deficits in motor activity. Immediately after partial or complete lesions of the precentral gyrus, there is flaccid paralysis of the contralateral limbs and loss of superficial and deep reflexes, and hypotonus and exaggerated deep reflexes may occur. Involvement of the premotor area and corticoreticular fibers may lead to spastic paralysis. Lesions of Broca's area in the inferior frontal opercular and triangular areas of the dominant hemisphere may result in expressive aphasia. Sensory aphasias are more often associated with lesions of the posterior temporoparietal region. Ideomotor and ideational apraxias appear to be associated with lesions of the dominant parietal lobe in the region of the inferior parietal gyrus. Ablative lesions of the frontal eye fields in the posterior part of the middle frontal gyrus interfere with voluntary conjugate eye movements to the opposite side. Corticobulbar lesions can result in contralateral lower facial paralysis, a deviation of the tongue to the opposite side upon protrusion, and ipsilateral weakness in shoulder shrugging. Damage to the corticospinal tract in the spinal cord will give an ipsilateral UMN complex of symptoms within several weeks of the onset of the injury. This constellation of symptoms includes: (1) increased segmental muscle tone (hypertonus), especially in extensors of the lower extremity and in flexors of the upper extremity because of loss of lateral reticulospinal fibers; (2) increased deep tendon reflexes (hyperreflexia); (3) absence of or diminished superficial reflexes; (4) presence of pathologic reflexes such as the Babinski reflex; and (5) loss of fine movements. Lesions of LMNs produce flaccid paralysis or paresis, loss of deep and superficial reflexes, and denervation atrophy.

Visceral Motor Control Mechanisms. The hypothalamus is the highest subcortical center for the regulation of visceral activity. It receives ascending information from the spinal and cranial nerves by way of the reticular formation. In addition to these spinoreticular and reticuloreticular pathways, the hypothalamus receives input from the thalamus, basal ganglia, and cerebral cortex. Efferents from the hypothalamus descend to the brain stem and spinal cord and also terminate in the thalamus, cortex and hypophysis.

As previously indicated, hypothalamic nuclei are structurally divisible into medial and lateral groups by the columns of the fornix. The lateral group includes lateral and tuberal nuclei. The medial group is further subdivided into anterior, middle, and posterior groups. The anterior group includes the preoptic, anterior, supraoptic, paraventricular, and periventricular nuclei. The dorsomedial and ventromedial nuclei comprise the middle group; the posterior and mammillary nuclei make up the posterior group.

Functional classification of nuclei into autonomic and endocrine neurosecretory groups makes the hypothalamic regions easier to appreciate. An anteromedial group of nuclei are involved in parasympathetic regulation. A posterolateral group of posterior, tuberal, and lateral nuclei regulate sympathetic activity. Outflow from the hypothalamus to preganglionic parasympathetic and preganglionic sympathetic cells of the brain stem and spinal cord is by way of periventricular fibers that multisynaptically utilize the dorsal longitudinal fasciculus or the reticuloreticular and reticulospinal pathways.

The endocrine neurosecretory nuclei are the supraoptic and paraventricular and the hypophysiotrophic area of nuclei. The supraoptic and paraventricular nuclei produce antidiuretic (vasopressin) and oxytocin hormones that are secreted in the pars nervosa. The hypophysiotrophic nuclei include several hypothalamic nuclei (*e.g.*, ventromedial, arcuate, preoptic) whose axons terminate in the infundibular stalk adjacent to capillary loops of the hypophyseal portal vascular system. Releasing and inhibiting factors produced in neurons of the hypophysiotrophic area pass into these capillary loops and are transported by way of venous trunks of the pituitary stalk and capillaries of the pars distalis to the chromophobes and chromophiles of the anterior pituitary.

Visceral motor activity is influenced by descending pathways from the olfactory cortex and the limbic system. Olfactohypothalamic fibers course from the pyriform cortex to the hypothalamus. Impulses from the amygdala course in a ventral path and also in the stria terminalis to reach the hypothalamus and septal nuclei. Basal olfactory regions and the septal area are connected through the hypothalamus with the mesencephalic reticular formation by way of the medial forebrain bundle. The septal region is also in communication with the mesencephalic reticular formation through a pathway that includes the stria medullaris, habenular nucleus, habenulopeduncular tract (fasciculus retroflexus), interpeduncular nucleus, and tegmental nuclei.

The ***limbic cortex*** is phylogenetically ''older'' cortex that forms a ring around the corpus callosum and diencephalon. It includes the subcallosal area, cingulate gyrus, isthmus (retrosplenial area), parahippocampal gyrus, and hippocampal formation (hippocampus and dentate gyrus). All of these regions are connected through an association bundle called the cingulum. Axons from the hippocampal formation pass as the fimbria and fornix to the mammillary bodies and septal region. The mammillary bodies are linked to the cingulate gyrus through the mammillothalamic tract and its relay through the anterior nucleus of the thalamus. The mammillotegmental tract is a descending pathway from the mammillary bodies to the reticular formation of the brain stem.

In addition to the interconnections of the hypothalamus and amygdala with the phylogenetically older olfactory and limbic cortex, there are neocortical connections in the limbic lobe. An important circuit is that between the prefrontal cortex and the hypothalamus through a relay in the dorsomedial nucleus of the thalamus.

Lesions of the hypothalamus affect visceral activity. Damage to the lateral hypothalamic nucleus may abolish appetite and lead to weight loss, whereas lesions of the satiety center in the ventromedial nucleus may lead to obesity through excessive eating. Lesions of the supraoptic nuclei can lead to diabetes insipidus. Bilateral temporal lobe lesions involving the pyriform cortex, amygdala, and hippocampal formation may produce disturbances in olfaction, emotional behavior, and recent memory.

THORAX

The thorax is bounded posteriorly by the thoracic vertebrae and the ribs, laterally by the ribs and the intercostal spaces, and anteriorly by the sternum, the costal cartilages, and ribs. The sternal angle (of Louis) is formed by the junction of the manubrium and the body of the sternum. It marks the level of the second costal cartilages, the bifurcation of the trachea, and the lower aspect of the fourth thoracic vertebra.

SURFACE MARKINGS

Lungs and Pleura. The boundaries of the lungs and pleura may be mapped on the surface of the body as follows: The apex of the pleura extends about 2.5 cm above the medial third of the clavicle. Its border then passes medially behind the sternoclavicular joint, and the two pleura meet in the midline behind the sternal angle. The medial edge passes inferiorly to about the seventh costal cartilage, where it inclines laterally. The medial edge of the left pleura inclines laterally at the level of the fourth costal cartilage because of the heart. This indentation of the medial edge of the pleura on the left is the cardiac notch. In the midclavicular line (below the middle of the clavicle), the lower border of the pleura is at the level of the eighth rib and in the midaxillary line is at the tenth rib. Posteriorly at the scapular line (vertebral border of the scapula), the level of the pleura corresponds to the twelfth rib. The surface projection of the superior aspect of the lung corresponds to that of the pleura. The lung does not extend quite as far medially as the pleura so that the costal and mediastinal layers of parietal pleura are in contact, thus forming the ***costomediastinal recess.*** The inferior border of the lung inclines laterally at the sixth costal cartilage. At the midclavicular line it is at the level of the sixth rib, at the midaxillary line the eighth rib, and at the scapular line the tenth rib. The area of pleural cavity below the inferior margin of the lung, where the parietal layers of costal and diaphragmatic pleura are in contact during quiet breathing, is called the ***costodiaphragmatic recess.*** During deep inspiration the lung descends into this recess.

The ***interlobar fissures*** separating the lobes of the lungs can also be approximated on the surface. The ***oblique fissure*** of the left lung divides the superior lobe from the inferior lobe; that of the right lung separates the inferior lobe below from the superior and middle lobes above. The oblique fissure is at the level of the fourth rib posteriorly (base of the spine of the scapula), the fifth rib in the midaxillary line, and the sixth rib in the midclavicular line. A ***horizontal fissure*** separates the superior lobe from the middle lobe of the right lung. This fissure is at the level of the fourth costal cartilage next to the sternum, and at the level of the fifth rib in the midaxillary line where it joins the oblique fissure.

Surface Projections of the Heart. The heart may be mapped on the anterior thoracic wall by lines connecting four points. Point 1 is at the level of the second left costal cartilage, 1 cm to 2 cm lateral to the edge of the sternum. Point 2 lies 1 cm to 2 cm lateral to the edge of the sternum at the level of the third costal cartilage on the right. Point 3 is located at the level of the right sixth costal cartilage, 1 cm to 2 cm from the sternal margin. Point 4 lies 7 cm to 8 cm from the midline in the left fifth intercostal space, and marks the location of the apex of the heart. The ***lower (diaphragmatic) border*** corresponds to a line drawn from the apex through the xiphisternal articulation to point 3. The ***right border*** is indicated by a slightly convex line running from the right third costal cartilage to the right lower border. It is formed by the right atrium below and the superior vena cava above. The ***left border*** is formed by the left ventricle and the left auricular appendage. It curves from the second left costal cartilage to the apex. The ***posterior surface*** or base of the heart is formed largely by the left atrium and a portion of the right atrium. All of the great veins—pulmonary and venae cavae—enter this portion of the heart. Most of the ***anterior*** (sternocostal) ***surface*** of the heart is formed by the right ventricle, with smaller portions of the left ventricle to the left, and the right atrium to the right. The ***inferior*** or diaphragmatic ***surface*** is formed predominantly by the left and right ventricles.

The pulmonary and aortic orifices lie opposite the upper and lower margins of the third costal cartilage along the left margin of the sternum. The aortic valve lies behind the left side of the sternum at the level of the third interspace. The pulmonary valve is located to the left of the third chondrosternal articulation. The right atrioventricular (tricuspid) valve is in the midsternal line at the level of the fifth intercostal space. The left atrioventricular (mitral) valve lies at the left fourth sternochondral articulation.

Surface Projections of the Major Vessels. The ***thoracic aorta*** may be mapped on the surface of the body as follows: The ascending aorta extends from the aortic orifice on the left sternal margin to a point on the right margin of the sternum at the upper border of the second costal cartilage. The arch of the aorta curves to the left and backward, and its upper convexity lies about 2 cm below the suprasternal notch. The descending thoracic aorta extends from the left side of the lower border of the fourth thoracic vertebra to the aortic hiatus of the diaphragm located in front of the body of the twelfth thoracic vertebra. The branches arising from the aortic arch are the brachiocephalic trunk in the midline, the left common carotid a little to the left, and the left subclavian still farther to the left and on a more dorsal plane.

The right and the left brachiocephalic veins unite to form the ***superior vena cava*** behind the first right chondrosternal junction. Posterior to the right sternoclavicular joint the brachiocephalic artery divides and the right brachiocephalic artery divides and the right brachiocephalic vein begins. Posterior to the left sternoclavicular joint, the left common carotid and the left subclavian join to form the left brachiocephalic vein.

MEDIASTINUM

The mediastinum contains all the thoracic viscera except the lungs. It is located between the pleural cavities and between the sternum and vertebral column. It is divisible into superior, anterior, posterior, and middle regions.

Superior Mediastinum. The superior mediastinum is that part of the mediastinum located above the sternal angle. It contains the aortic arch and its branches, the superior vena cava and its tributaries, the vagus, recurrent laryngeal and phrenic nerves, trachea, esophagus, thoracic duct, left highest intercostal vein, the remains of the thymus, and some lymph nodes.

Anterior Mediastinum. The anterior mediastinum is the area in front of the pericardial cavity. It contains the thymus, internal thoracic vessels, lymph nodes, and surrounding connective tissue.

Posterior Mediastinum. The posterior cavity behind the heart and the great vessels contains the thoracic aorta, esophagus, vagus nerves, thoracic duct, azygos and hemiazygos veins, lymph nodes, and sympathetic trunks.

Middle Mediastinum. The middle mediastinum contains the heart and the pericardium.

HEART

Gross Structure of the Heart. The heart is a four-chambered organ consisting of the two ventricles and two atria. An interatrial septum separates the two atria; an interventricular septum lies between the left and right ventricles. Anterior and posterior interventricular sulci on the sternocostal and diaphragmatic surfaces of the heart mark the location of the interventricular septum. The coronary (atrioventricular) sulcus encircles the heart at the atrioventricular (A-V) junction. The sulci are occupied by the vessels that supply the heart.

The borders of the heart were discussed previously in the section on surface markings. The ***apex*** of the heart is part of the left ventricle, and it points downward and to the left. It is located deep to the left fifth intercostal space about 4 cm below and 2 cm medial to the left nipple, and it is overlapped by an extension of the pleura and lungs. The ***base*** of the heart faces upward, to the right and toward the back. It consists mainly of the left atrium, part of the right atrium, and proximal parts of the great vessels. Its superior boundary is at the bifurcation of the pulmonary artery, and its inferior boundary is at the coronary sulcus. The left boundary of the base is at the oblique vein of the left atrium, and the right boundary is at the sulcus terminalis. The base is separated from the bodies of T5–T8 vertebrae by the thoracic aorta, esophagus, and thoracic duct. The ***sternocostal surface*** of the heart is formed by the right atrium, right ventricle, and a small part of the left ventricle. The ***diaphragmatic surface*** is comprised of the two ventricles.

The ***right atrium*** is larger than the left and is comprised of two parts: (1) a principal cavity (sinus venarum), and (2) an auricula. The smooth-surfaced sinus venarum is that part of the atrium between the ostia of the superior and inferior venae cavae and the right A-V opening. The superior vena cava opens into the upper and posterior part of the sinus venarum; the inferior vena cava opens into the lowest part of the sinus venarum near the interatrial septum. The coronary sinus opens between the ostium of the inferior vena cava and the A-V foramen. Rudimentary valves guard the openings of the inferior vena cava and coronary sinus. The auricula is rough surfaced because of muscular ridges (musculi pectinati). It is demarcated externally from the sinus venarum by the sulcus terminalis and internally by the crista terminalis.

The dorsal wall of the right atrium consists of the interatrial septum. The fossa ovalis, representing the embryonic foramen ovale, is an oval depression in the septal wall located above the openings of the coronary sinus and inferior vena cava. It is bounded above and at its sides by the limbus fossa ovalis representing the embryonic free margin of septum secundum.

The ***right ventricle*** is bounded on the right by the coronary sulcus and on the left by the anterior interventricular sulcus. Its superior part, the conus arteriosus (infundibulum), is continuous with the pulmonary trunk. Inferiorly, its wall forms the acute margin of the heart. The wall of the right ventricle is about one third the thickness of the left ventricle, but the capacity (85 ml) of both ventricles is the same. The internal surface is quite irregular because of ridges of muscle called trabeculae carneae. Some of these project from the wall of the ventricle and insert through chordae tendineae on the apices, margins, and ventricular surfaces of cusps of the right A-V valve.

The right A-V (tricuspid) valve has anterior (infundibular), posterior (marginal), and medial (septal) cusps. The anterior cusp is the largest, the posterior is the smallest. These leaflets are composed of strong fibrous tissue that is continuous at their bases with the annuli fibrosi of the fibrous skeleton separating the atria from the ventricles. The anterior papillary muscle arises from the anterior and septal walls and is attached to the anterior and posterior cusps by chordae tendineae. The septomarginal trabecula (moderator band) extends from the interventricular septum to the base of the anterior papillary muscle. The posterior papillary muscle arises from the posterior wall, and its chordae tendineae insert on the posterior and septal cusps.

The ***conus arteriosus*** has a smooth inner surface. It is limited from the rest of the ventricle by a ridge of muscular tissue called the crista supraventricularis. At the summit of the conus is the orifice of the pulmonary trunk. The pulmonary valve consists of three cusps: anterior, right, and left. Each cusp has a sinus between it and the wall of the pulmonary trunk, and its convexity is directed toward the ventricle. Adjacent cusps attach at a common commissure. A thin marginal lunula portion of each cusp runs from each commissure to a thickened nodule in the central free margin of the cusp. When the valve is closed, the lunulae and nodules of the cusps are in contact.

The ***left atrium*** consists of a principal cavity (sinus venarum) and an auricula. The smooth-walled sinus venarum receives the four pulmonary veins. The interatrial septum covering the fossa ovalis of the right atrium constitutes a valve of the foramen ovale. The left auricula is longer than that of the right atrium. It curves ventrally around the base of the pulmonary trunk, and it lies over the proximal portion of the left coronary artery.

The ***left ventricle*** is longer, more conical and thicker than the right. It forms the apex of the heart and is separated from the right ventricle by the muscular and membranous parts of the interventricular septum. It has two openings, the left A-V (mitral), which is regulated by the mitral valve, and the aortic, which has the aortic valve. The left A-V valve consists of a large anterior (aortic) and a smaller posterior cusp. Each cusp receives chordae tendineae from both the anterior and posterior papillary muscles. The aortic opening is anterior and to the right of the mitral valve. The portion of the ventricle below the aortic orifice is called the ***aortic vestibule.*** The aortic valve consists of three cusps, posterior, right, and left. The cusps are similar in structure to those of the pulmonary valve, but they are bigger and stronger. The right and left coronary arteries originate from the right and left aortic sinuses (of Valsalva), respectively.

The ***skeleton of the heart*** consists of a series of fibrous rings (annuli fibrosi) and fibrous trigones. Fibrous rings surround each A-V orifice, the aortic opening, and the pulmonary orifice. The cusps of each of the associated valves are attached to the rings. The membranous part of the interventricular septum also is continuous with the fibrous tissue of these annuli. At the junction of the A-V rings with the aortic ring a right fibrous trigone is formed. A left fibrous trigone occurs between the aortic and left A-V rings.

Microscopic Structure of the Heart. The heart wall consists of three layers: (1) an inner endocardial layer, (2) a middle myocardial layer, and (3) an outer epicardial layer. The ***endocardium*** consists of endothelium and a subendothelial connective tissue layer of fine collagenous and elastic fibers and some smooth muscle fibers. The endocardium of the atria is thicker than that of the ventricles. A subendocardial layer of loose connective tissue and blood vessels binds the endocardium to the myocardium. This layer in the ventricles contains the specialized muscle fibers of the conduction system.

The ***myocardium*** consists of spiraling bundles of cardiac muscle that take origin from the annuli fibrosi. In the atria the myocardium is a thin layer of fibers with a simple arrangement. The muscle of the ventricles is more complex and consists of several layers. The ventricular bands of muscle originate from the fibrous anulus and course in a helical manner from right to left and toward the apex. Some of the more superficial fibers can be traced in a mantle covering both ventricles. Some intermediate fibers weave from ventricle to ventricle by way of the septum. The more numerous deeper fibers pass into either of the ventricular walls and end by piercing deeply and becoming the papillary muscles. The microscopic structure of cardiac muscle was reviewed with skeletal muscle tissue in the section on the back.

The ***epicardium*** consists of mesothelium and an underlying connective tissue layer. A subepicardial layer of loose connective tissue containing blood vessels, nerves and fat binds the epicardium to the myocardium. The epicardium is the visceral pericardium.

The A-V valves consist of a core of dense connective tissue, which is continuous with the annuli fibrosi, and an outer layer of endocardium. The endocardium on the atrial surface of the valves is thicker than that on the ventricular side. Chordae tendineae are composed of dense regularly arranged connective tissue. The aortic and pulmonary semilunar valves resemble the atrioventricular valves, but they are much thinner.

Recent work indicates that the atrial myocytes contain granules which have been identified as one or several polypeptides called atriopeptin(s), which are responsible for a profound natriuresis.

Conduction System of the Heart. This system is composed of specialized cardiac muscle found in the sinoatrial (S-A) node and in the A-V node and bundle. The heart beat is initiated in the ***S-A node (pacemaker of the heart)*** located in the right atrium in the upper part of the crista terminalis just to the left of the opening of the superior vena cava. Cells of the S-A node are slender and fusiform. From the S-A node the cardiac impulse spreads throughout the atrial musculature to reach the ***A-V node*** lying in the subendocardium of the atrial septum directly above the opening of the coronary sinus. The A-V node has small irregularly arranged branching fibers that contain few myofibrils. Thereafter the impulse is conducted to the ventricles by passing through the specialized tissue of the A-V bundle (of His). This bundle consists of a crus commune and right and left bundle branches. The common bundle travels from the A-V node into the membranous part of the interventricular septum. It divides into right and left bundle branches that pass in the subendocardium along the muscular part of the septum and distribute to the ventricles as Purkinje tissue. ***Purkinje cells*** are large specialized cardiac muscle cells that usually are binucleate and contain much centrally located sarcoplasm.

The innervation of the heart is from both the parasympathetic and sympathetic divisions of the autonomic nervous system. Right and left thoracic cardiac branches from the vagus nerves pass to the deep cardiac plexus where they synapse on postganglionic parasympathetic neurons. The vagus nerves also give rise to superior and inferior cervical cardiac nerves. The left inferior cervical cardiac nerve ends in the superficial cardiac plexus; the rest end in the deep plexus. Superior, middle, and inferior cervical cardiac nerves arising from sympathetic ganglia also descend to cardiac plexi. The left superior cervical cardiac sympathetic nerve ends in the superficial cardiac plexus; the rest end in the deep plexus. The deep cardiac plexus also receives thoracic cardiac branches from the upper five thoracic sympathetic ganglia. The coronary and pulmonary plexi and the right and left atria are supplied by branches from the superficial and deep plexi. The right vagal and sympathetic branches end chiefly in the region of the S-A node while the left branches end chiefly in the region of the A-V node.

Heart rate and force of contraction appear to be controlled mainly through the inhibitory action of the vagus nerves. Reflex slowing of the heart results from stimulation of the carotid sinus and the special pressure end organs in the carotid body. Impulses ascend in the carotid branch of the glossopharyngeal nerve to the inferior ganglion, thence to the solitary nucleus, and finally to the dorsal motor nucleus of the vagus in the medulla. Efferent cardioinhibitory impulses pass down the vagi to the cardiac plexus to synapse there with postganglionic fibers that terminate at the S-A node.

Cardiac pain impulses arise in free nerve endings, in the cardiac connective tissue and adventitia of the cardiac blood vessels. They then travel in visceral sensory fibers through the cardiac plexus, the middle and the inferior cervical cardiac and thoracic cardiac nerves, and the sympathetic chain ganglia of the neck and the upper thorax. All the pain fibers continue through the white rami communicantes of spinal nerves T1 and T5 and traverse the corresponding dorsal roots and their ganglia. Their cell bodies are located in the dorsal root ganglia, and the central fibers pass from these spinal ganglia to the dorsal horns of the upper thoracic cord segments.

Cardiac pain is referred to cutaneous areas that supply sensory impulses to the same segments of the cord that receive the cardiac sensation. Thus, they involve mainly the region of C7 through T5 and lie predominantly on the left side. The C8 and T1 segments are responsible for referred pain along the medial side of the arm and the forearm.

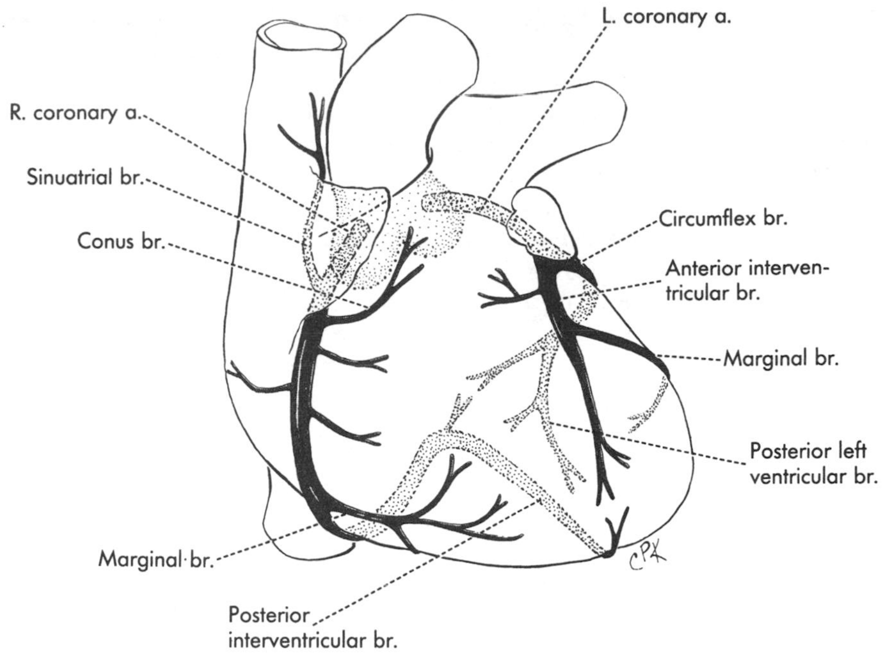

Fig. 2-25. The coronary arteries shown from an anterior view of the heart. (Hollinshead WH, Rosse C: Textbook of Anatomy, 4th ed, p 535. Philadelphia, JB Lippincott, 1985)

Blood Vessels of the Heart. The arterial supply of the heart (Fig. 2-25) is provided by right and left coronary arteries. Venous drainage is chiefly through cardiac veins, which empty into the coronary sinus.

The ***right coronary artery*** originates from the right aortic sinus and courses ventrally between the pulmonary trunk and the right atrium. It descends in the right part of the A-V groove, passing onto the posteroinferior aspect of the heart. It terminates by dividing into two branches: the posterior interventricular artery, which passes toward the apex in the posterior interventricular sulcus where it anastomoses with the anterior interventricular branch of the left coronary, and a short continuation of the main trunk which anastomoses with the circumflex branch of the left coronary. Its marginal branch passes along the lower border of the right ventricle.

The ***left coronary artery,*** which is usually larger than the right, originates from the left aortic sinus. It passes posterior and then to the left of the pulmonary trunk, branching into the circumflex and anterior interventricular arteries as it emerges from behind the pulmonary trunk. The circumflex artery passes to the left in the left A-V sulcus and anastomoses with the right coronary artery on the posteroinferior aspect of the heart. The anterior interventricular artery descends toward the apex in the anterior interventricular sulcus and passes onto the diaphragmatic surface, where it anastomoses with the posterior interventricular branch of the right coronary.

For the most part, the ***cardiac veins*** accompany the coronary arteries and open into the coronary sinus, which empties into the right atrium. The remainder of the drainage occurs by means of small anterior cardiac veins that drain much of the anterior surface of the heart and terminate directly into the right atrium.

The ***coronary sinus*** is located in the posterior A-V sulcus and drains into the right atrium at the left of the mouth of the inferior vena cava. It receives three veins: (1) the great cardiac vein, which runs in the anterior interventricular sulcus; (2) the middle cardiac vein, located in the posterior interventricular sulcus; and (3) the small cardiac vein, which accompanies the marginal branch of the right coronary artery.

PERICARDIUM

The pericardium consists of two parts, an outer fibrous layer and an inner serous layer that adheres to the inner surface of the fibrous pericardium and reflects onto the outer surface of the heart.

Fibrous Pericardium. This tough connective tissue membrane surrounds the entire heart. Posteriorly and superiorly it blends with the adventitia of the great vessels. Inferiorly, it blends with the central tendon of the diaphragm. It is attached to the manubrium by a superior pericardiosternal ligament and to the xiphoid process by an inferior pericardiosternal ligament. In the area between these two ligamentous attachments, most of the anterior surface of the pericardium is separated from the thoracic wall by the lungs and pleural cavities. Only a small portion of the pericardium is intimately related to the lower left portion of the sternum and the medial ends of the fourth through the sixth costal cartilages. In this region no lungs or pleura intervene between the chest wall and fibrous pericardium. This small portion of the pericardium corresponds to the cardiac notch in the left lung and underlies the left fourth and fifth intercostal spaces. This relation permits needle entry to the pericardial cavity without traversing the pleural cavity. The fibrous pericardium is in contact posteriorly with the bronchi, esophagus, and descending thoracic aorta. The lateral outer surfaces of the fibrous pericardium are in close contact with the adjacent parietal pleura. The phrenic nerve and the pericardiocophrenic vessels descend between these two layers.

Serous Pericardium. This is a thin membrane comprised of mesothelium and an underlying connective tissue lamina. This membrane lines the pericardial cavity with a smooth glistening surface that facilitates cardiac movement. The serous pericardium, by its location, is divisible into two layers, parietal and visceral. The parietal layer lines the deep surface fibrous pericardium. At the points where the fibrous pericardium blends with the walls of the great vessels entering and leaving the heart, the parietal layer of the serous pericardium is reflected onto the vessels and then the heart muscle to form the visceral layer (epicardium) of the serous pericardium. These reflections are in the form of two tubular sheaths, one sheath for the aorta and pulmonary trunk (arterial mesocardium), and the other for the pulmonary veins and venae cavae (venous mesocardium). That portion of the pericardial cavity passing horizontally between the two tubular sheaths remains as the ***transverse pericardial sinus.*** The reflection of the visceral pleura over the veins forms an inverted U-shaped cul-de-sac dorsal to the heart that is referred to as the ***oblique pericardial sinus.***

MAJOR VESSELS OF THE THORAX

The great vessels entering and leaving the heart are constituents of either the pulmonary or systemic vascular circuits. The pulmonary circulation is represented by the (1) pulmonary trunk originating from the right ventricle and branching into left and right pulmonary arteries, and (2) four pulmonary veins returning blood from the lungs to the left atrium. The systemic circulation is represented by the aorta, which originates from the left ventricle, and the superior and inferior venae cavae, which return blood to the right atrium. Lymphatic drainage from the thorax is by way of the thoracic duct and right lymphatic duct.

Pulmonary Trunk. This vessel arises from the infundibulum of the right ventricle and ascends obliquely and dorsally to the level of the sternal end of the second left costal cartilage where it divides into the left and right pulmonary arteries. In its course it passes in front of and then to the left of the ascending aorta. Anteriorly the pulmonary trunk is separated from the sternal end of the second left intercostal space by the left lung, pleura, and pericardium. At its origin it is related on the left to the left auricle and the left coronary artery, on the right to the right auricle and occasionally the right coronary artery.

Pulmonary Arteries. The right pulmonary artery is longer and wider than the left. It passes horizontally to the right and enters the hilus of the lung immediately below the upper lobe (eparterial) bronchus. In its course it passes dorsal to the ascending aorta, the superior vena cava, and the superior right pulmonary vein and lies ventral to the esophagus, right bronchus, and anterior pulmonary plexus. The left pulmonary artery passes laterally and posteriorly toward the root of the left lung, passing anterior to the left bronchus and the descending aorta. The ligamentum arteriosum connects the arch of the aorta above with the left pulmonary artery below. The superior left pulmonary vein lies at first ventral and then inferior to the left pulmonary artery.

Pulmonary Veins. These vessels emerge from each of the five lobes of the lungs. Upon entering the lung root, however, those from the superior and middle lobes of the right lung unite. Thus, four terminal pulmonary veins course from the roots of the lungs to the left atrium. The superior right pulmonary vein passes dorsal to the superior vena cava, and the inferior right pulmonary vein passes behind the right atrium before both enter independently through the dorsal and right wall of the left atrium. The superior and inferior left pulmonary veins course anterior to the descending aorta and enter separately through the posterior wall of the left atrium near its left border. Fusion of the left pulmonary veins into a common trunk is not uncommon.

Aorta. This vessel is the main arterial trunk of the systemic circulation. It ascends from the left ventricle, arches to the left and dorsally over the root of the left lung, descends within the thorax on the left side of the vertebral column and enters the abdominal cavity through the aortic hiatus of the diaphragm. Thus, the parts of the aorta are the ascending aorta, the arch of the aorta, and the thoracic and abdominal portions of the descending aorta.

The ***ascending aorta*** arises from the base of the left ventricle at the caudal level of the third left costal cartilage. It passes obliquely upward to the right as far as the level of the second right costal cartilage. Initially, it is related anteriorly to the pulmonary trunk and the right auricle; more superiorly, it is separated from the sternum by the pericardium, variable portions of the right pleura, ventral margin of the right lung, loose areolar tissue, and the remains of the thymus. The coronary arteries arise from the ascending aorta.

The ***arch of the aorta*** lies in the superior mediastinum. It begins at the upper border of the second right sternocostal articulation. It curves cranially and dorsally to the left and then descends along the left side of the vertebral column to the level of the intervertebral disk between the fourth and fifth thoracic vertebrae where it continues as the descending aorta. In its course it passes at first ventral to the trachea and then to the left of this structure and the esophagus. Arising from the superior aspect of the aortic arch are three large vessels: the brachiocephalic artery (innominate), the left common carotid artery, and the left subclavian artery.

The ***brachiocephalic artery*** is the first branch from the arch of the aorta. It arises behind the middle of the manubrium sterni and courses obliquely upward toward the right sternoclavicular joint where it divides into the right subclavian and common carotid arteries.

The ***left common carotid artery*** arises from the arch of the aorta behind and immediately to the left of the brachiocephalic artery. Its thoracic portion extends up to the level of the left sternoclavicular joint. In its course it passes in front of the trachea, left recurrent laryngeal nerve, esophagus, thoracic duct, and left subclavian artery.

The ***left subclavian artery*** arises from the arch of the aorta about 2.5 cm distal to the left common carotid. It ascends almost vertically on the left side of the trachea to the root of the neck where it arches upward and laterally. It lies behind the left vagus nerve, left phrenic nerve, left superior cardiac sympathetic nerve, and left brachiocephalic vein. It passes in front of the left lung, pleura, esophagus, and thoracic duct.

The ***thoracic portion of the descending aorta*** lies in the posterior mediastinum. It extends downward from the upper border of the body of the fifth thoracic vertebra to the aortic opening in the diaphragm at the level of the twelfth thoracic vertebra. It has branches that supply the walls and viscera of the thorax. The thoracic descending aorta is related posteriorly to the left pleura and lung, the vertebral column, and the hemiazygous veins. Anteriorly, from above downward, it is related to the root of the left lung, pericardium, esophagus, and diaphragm. On its right side are the azygos vein and thoracic duct, while on the left side are the left lung and pleura.

Superior Vena Cava. The vessel returns blood to the right atrium from the upper half of the body. It arises from the junction of the right and left brachiocephalic veins at the level of the lower border of the first right costal cartilage and enters the right atrium at the level of the third right costal cartilage. The superior vena cava is related posteromedially to the trachea and anteromedially to the ascending aorta. The phrenic nerve is positioned between the superior vena cava and the parietal layer of mediastinal pleura on the right. The superior vena cava receives the ***azygos vein*** on its posterior surface at the level of the second costal cartilage. The azygos vein enters the thorax through the aortic hiatus in the diaphragm, ascends along the right side or anterior aspect of the vertebral column, receives the hemiazygos vein at the T9 level (and possibly the accessory hemiazygos vein at the T8 level), and finally passes posterior to the root of the right lung before arching anteriorly over the root to enter the superior vena cava.

Both ***brachiocephalic veins*** are formed by the union of the internal jugular and subclavian veins. The right brachiocephalic vein arises dorsal to the sternal end of the clavicle and passes almost vertically downward in front of the trachea and vagus nerve and behind the sternohyoid and sternothyroid muscles and right lung and pleura. The left brachiocephalic vein is longer than the right. It courses obliquely downward and to the right from its origin deep to the medial end of the clavicle, and it joins the right brachiocephalic vein to form the superior vena cava at the lower border of the right first costal cartilage. The thoracic portion of each brachiocephalic vein receives an internal thoracic and often an inferior thyroid vein. In addition, the left receives the left highest intercostal vein.

Inferior Vena Cava. This vessel returns blood to the right atrium from the caudal half of the body. It enters the thorax by piercing the diaphragm (vertebral level T8) between the middle and right leaflets of the central tendon. It ascends in a slightly anteromedial direction in the middle mediastinum and pierces the fibrous pericardium. The inferior vena cava is separated, in its extrapericardial course, from the right pleura and lung by the right phrenicopericardiac ligament. In its short intrapericardial course it is invested on its right and left sides with a reflection of the serous paricardium.

Thoracic Duct. The thoracic duct is the common trunk of all lymphatics of the body except those that drain to the right lymphatic duct from the upper right quadrant of the body. It originates in the cistena chyli of the abdomen at the second lumbar vertebra, enters the thorax through the aortic hiatus of the diaphragm, and ascends through the posterior mediastinum between the aorta and azygos vein, and posterior to the esophagus. At the level of the T5 vertebra it crosses the midline to the left side, enters the superior mediastinum and ascends between the esophagus and pleura to enter the venous system at the junction of the left subclavian and internal jugular veins.

Right Lymphatic Duct. This duct receives lymph from several lymphatic vessels: from the right side of the head and neck through the right jugular trunk; from the right upper extremity by way of the right subclavian trunk; and from the right side of the thorax, right lung, and part of the convex surface of the liver through the right bronchomediastinal trunk.

Microscopic Structure of Vessels. Blood and lymphatic vessels generally consist of three tunics: tunica intima, tunica media, and tunica adventitia. These tunics are most pronounced in the larger vessels and vary with the type and size of vessels as to their constituents. Capillary walls consists of an endothelium, basal lamina, pericytes, and surrounding connective tissue. The endothelium may be continuous and contain no pores, or it may be fenestrated with pores closed by a thin membrane. Either type of endothelium contains tight intercellular junctions. Fenestrated capillaries can be found in the kidney and endocrine organs. In larger arteries and veins the three tunics are more pronounced. The ***tunica intima*** consists of endothelium, subendothelial connective tissue with smooth muscle, and an internal elastic membrane. In larger arteries the internal elastic membrane is fenestrated, often doubled and highly developed. The ***tunica media*** is more pronounced in arteries than in veins. In medium-sized (muscular, distributing) arteries it contains mostly circularly arranged smooth muscle and some elastic fibers. In large arteries (elastic, conducting) elastic lamellae predominate, but smooth muscle is present. The media of arterioles consists of several layers of circularly arranged smooth muscle. The adventitia of arteries is not as pronounced as the tunica media. It is comprised of elastic and collagenous fibers and, in larger vessels, vasa vasorum that supply the outer layers.

Veins have a poorly defined tunica media, but the ***tunica adventitia*** is well developed. In medium-sized veins this outer layer contains mostly collagenous fibers. In the adventitia of large veins are longitudinally running smooth muscle fibers. Venous valves are local foldings of the intima. Venules have relatively thinner walls than arteries of similar diameter.

Lymphatic vessels are microscopically similar to veins. Lymphatic capillaries appear as endothelium-lined clefts in connective tissue and have very thin walls. The thoracic duct has a thick tunica media consisting of longitudinal and circular smooth muscle bundles. Its tunica intima is prominent, but the adventitia is poorly defined.

DEVELOPMENT OF THE HEART AND MAJOR VESSELS

The heart and major vessels arise from blood islands of hemangioblastic tissue that were derived from mesoderm. The heart begins to form in the third embryonic week. One embryonic and two extraembryonic (umbilical and vitelline) vascular circuits are completed by the end of the first month of development.

Early Development of the Heart and Vascular Circuits. Two ***endocardial tubes*** are formed deep to the epimyocardial (myocardial mantle) thickening of splanchnic mesoderm by the coalescence of blood islands. These tubes run longitudinally and are deep to the horseshoe-shaped prospective pericardial cavity. With the lateral folding and forward growth of the embryo, the endocardial tubes are shifted ventrocaudally and fuse in the midline. The adjacent epimyocardium fuses in the midline around the fused endocardial tubes, forming a single hollow heart tube that is suspended in the primitive pericardial cavity by the dorsal mesocardium.

The coalescence of other blood islands in the embryo forms blood vessels that are in continuity with the heart tube. In the ***embryonic circulation,*** paired anterior and posterior cardinal veins drain the embryo cranial and caudal to the heart, respectively, and join to form the paired common cardinal veins (ducts of Cuvier); the latter veins drain into the caudal extent of the endocardial tube at the sinus venosus. Blood leaves the cranial extent of the endocardial tube and is distributed into five paired aortic arches that pass dorsally around the foregut in the branchial arches to empty into the paired dorsal aortae. Blood then circulates through branches of the aortae to capillaries that are in continuity with tributaries of the cardinal veins.

Blood vessels developing in the placenta (chorion) are linked to the embryonic circuit to form an ***umbilical*** (allantoic, placental) ***circuit.*** In this circuit umbilical arteries arise from the aorta, pass through the body stalk and go to capillaries of the placenta. Oxygenated and nutritive blood returns by the left umbilical vein to the sinus venosus. The right umbilical vein disappears soon after it is developed.

The ***vitelline circuit*** involves vascular channels in the yolk sac. Vitelline (omphalomesenteric) arteries arise from the abdominal aorta and pass along the yolk stalk to capillaries in the yolk sac. Blood returns to the sinus venosus by vitelline (omphalomesenteric) veins.

After birth the umbilical arteries will remain, in part, as a portion of the internal iliac and superior vesical arteries and the medial umbilical ligaments. The umbilical vein persists as the round ligament of the liver. Portions of the vitelline veins become the portal vein. The vitelline arteries fuse with each other and give rise to the superior mesenteric artery.

Folding and Partitioning of the Heart. With fusion of the endocardial tubes, several dilations become apparent. These are, from cephalic to caudal, the bulbus cordis (truncus arteriosus plus the conus arteriosus), ventricle, atrium, and sinus venosus. Arteries leave the cephalic end of the bulbus cordis from a swelling called the aortic bulb (aortic sac). Veins enter at the sinus venosus. With the loss of the dorsal mesocardium, except where the veins and arteries enter and leave, the heart begins to flex into an S-shaped structure. The first flexure occurs at the junction of the bulbus cordis and ventricle. The second flexure causes the sinus venosus and atrium to shift dorsally. The adjacent bulboventricular walls disappear, and this part of the bulbus and primitive ventricle become part of a common ventricular chamber. The atrium becomes sandwiched between the pharynx dorsally and the rest of the conus and truncus ventrally, causing the atrium to bulge laterally into right and left swell-

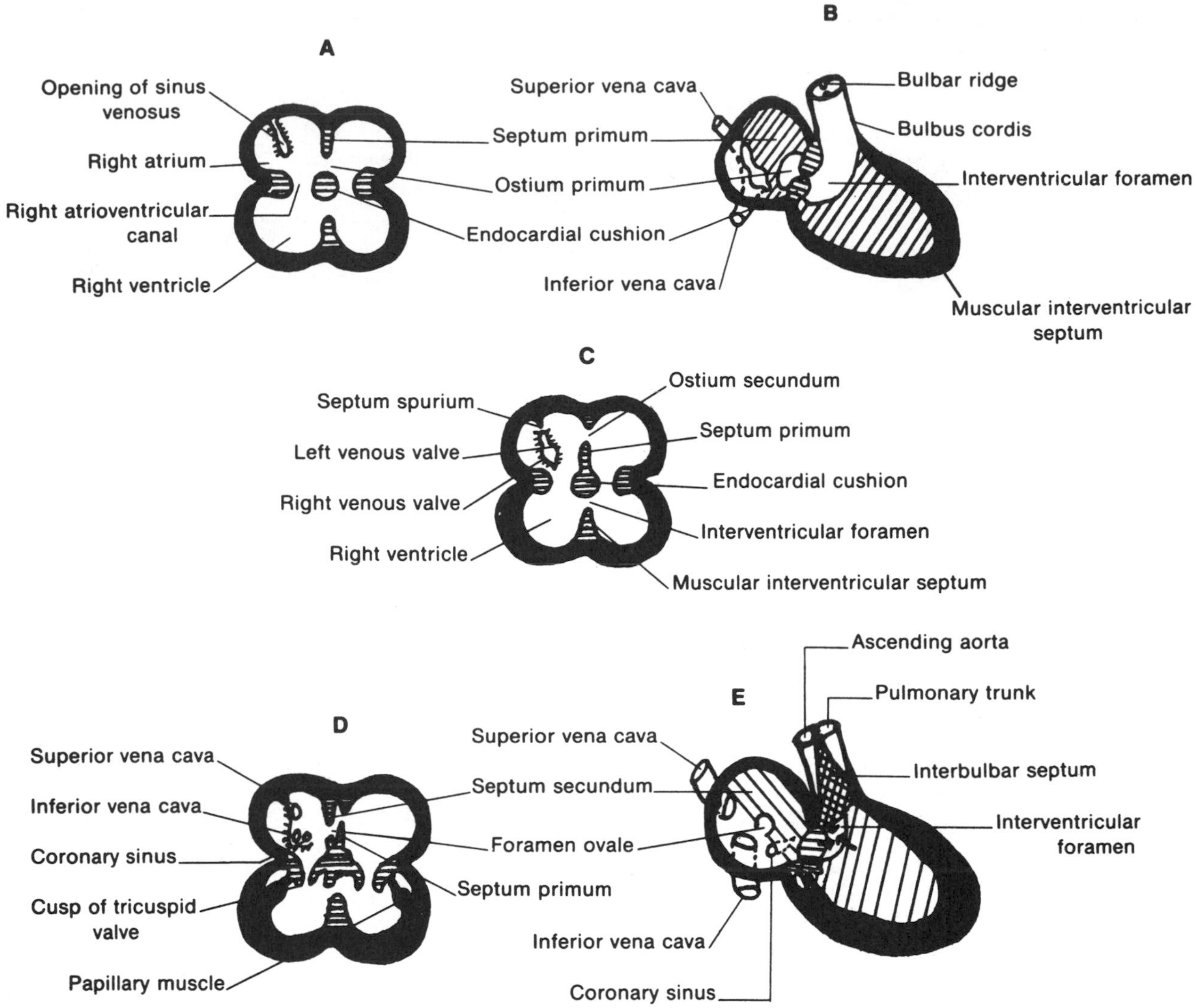

Fig. 2-26. The partitioning of the heart and the bulbus cordis. *(A)*, *(C)*, and *(D)* are frontal views. *(B)* and *(E)* are lateral views as seen from the right side. *(A)* and *(B)* represent the development in a 4-week-old embryo, and *(D)* and *(E)* represent development in a 6.5-week-old embryo.

ings. The sinus venosus becomes shifted to the right and eventually is incorporated into the primitive right atrial swelling. The pattern of blood flow is from veins to common atrium, to common ventricle, to conus, to truncus, to aortic bulb, and then to aortic arches.

During the second month of development the heart is partitioned into four chambers (two atria and two ventricles), A-V valves are formed, and the conus, truncus, and aortic bulb are partitioned into ascending aorta and pulmonary trunk (Fig. 2-26).

In ***partitioning of the atrium*** endocardial tissue from the dorsal and ventral walls fuses into an endocardial cushion that separates the A-V communication into right and left A-V canals. While this is taking place an endocardial septum primum grows toward the endocardial cushion from the dorsal wall of the atrium. Before fusing with the cushion, an ostium primum exists temporarily between the free margin of the septum primum and the cushion. This ostium will not disappear before an ostium secundum arises from the degeneration of septum primum cephalically. In the seventh week a septum secundum grows dorsocaudally to the right of septum primum and leaves a crescentic free area covered only by septum primum. The communication from the right to the left atrium through the crescentic opening and ostium secundum is the foramen ovale. The valve of the foramen ovale is part of septum primum. The interatrial septum thus arises from septum primum and septum secundum.

The sinus venarum of the right atrium is formed by the incorporation of the sinus venosus into the right atrium so that the developing great veins enter independently. The smooth-surfaced portion of the left atrium arises after the absorption of the common trunk of the pulmonary veins, thus leaving four pulmonary veins entering at the boundaries of this area.

In ***partitioning of the ventricle*** a muscular interventricular septum grows toward the endocardial cushion. Just caudal to the cushion an interventricular foramen remains for a short time before it is closed by endocardial tissue from the free margin of the interventricular septum, the endocardial cushion and the conal septum.

In ***septation of the aortic bulb, truncus arteriosus, and conus arteriosus*** a ridge of endocardial tissue develops on opposite walls of each of these structures. These ridges fuse in the middle of the lumen to form a bulbar (aortic, conal, truncal) septum. This septum spirals about 180 degrees as it descends from the aortic bulb into the conus, thus establishing a pulmonary trunk that intertwines with the ascending aorta. Semilunar valves develop in these vessels as localized swellings of endocardial tissue. The conal septum eventually descends to help close the interventricular septum.

In ***development of A-V valves,*** subendocardial and endocardial tissues project into the ventricle just below the A-V canals. These bulges of tissue are excavated from the ventricular side and invaded by muscle. Eventually all of the muscle, except that remaining as papillary muscles, disappears, and three right cusps of the right A-V valve and two cusps of the left A-V valve remain as fibrous structures.

Development of Major Arterial Vessels. Five pairs of aortic arches develop cephalocaudally in branchial arches (Fig. 2-27A,B). They bridge from the ventral aortic roots to the dorsal aortae. In comparative studies the five aortic arches represent the first, second, third, fourth, and sixth aortic arches. In humans the first, second, and distal part of the right sixth aortic arches (fifth) disappear. The remaining aortic arches, ventral aortic roots, and dorsal aortae give rise to major arteries. The internal carotid arteries develop from the third aortic arches and the dorsal aortae cephalic to the third arches. The common carotids arise from the ventral aortic roots and the proximal part of the third arches. The external carotids arise in a similar position to the ventral aortic roots lying cephalic to the third arch. The right subclavian artery arises from the right fourth arch, the seventh dorsal intersegmental artery, and the intervening portion of the right dorsal aorta. The left subclavian artery arises from the left seventh dorsal intersegmental artery. The arch of the aorta develops from the left fourth aortic arch and some septation of the aortic bulb. The pulmonary arteries arise from the proximal portions of the sixth arches along with some new vascular buds. The ductus arteriosus, linking the pulmonary trunk with the aorta, is the distal portion of the left sixth arch. The brachiocephalic artery originates from the right ventral aortic root between the fourth and sixth arches. The right dorsal aorta caudal to the right seventh dorsal intersegmental arteries disappears down to the embryonic low thoracic region where the paired dorsal aortae had fused into one midline vessel. The dorsal aortae between the third and fourth arches degenerate.

Development of Major Venous Channels. The superior and inferior caval systems and the portal vein arise from early embryonic vessels (Fig. 2-27C,D).

The ***superior vena cava*** forms from the right common cardinal vein and a caudal portion of the right anterior cardinal vein up to the entrance of the left brachiocephalic (innominate) vein. The latter vessel arises from a thymicothyroid anastomosis of veins. The right brachiocephalic develops from the right anterior cardinal vein between this anastomotic venous attachment and the right seventh intersegmental vein (right subclavian). The left common cardinal vein and part of the left horn of the sinus venosus become the coronary sinus that drains the heart wall into the right atrium.

The ***inferior vena cava,*** from heart to common iliacs, arises from (1) a small portion of the right vitelline vein, (2) a new vessel in the mesenteric fold of the degenerating mesonephros, (3) the right subcardinal vein, and (4) a sacrocardinal vein joining the caudal extent of the posterior cardinal veins. The subcardinals and their anastomosis, which developed to drain the mesonephros, also give rise to the renal, gonadal, and suprarenal veins.

The ***azygos venous system*** arises mostly from the supracardinal veins and their anastomosis. The most cephalic portion of the azygos vein is derived from the right posterior cardinal vein.

The ***portal and hepatic veins*** arise from the vitelline (omphalomesenteric) veins and their anastomoses.

Fetal Circulation. The circulation of the blood in the embryo results in the shunting of well-oxygenated blood from the placenta to the brain and the heart while relatively desaturated blood is supplied to the less essential structures.

Blood returns from the placenta by way of the (left) umbilical vein, is shunted in the ductus venosus through the liver to the inferior vena cava and thence to the right atrium. There is relatively little mixing of oxygenated and deoxygenated blood in the right atrium because the valve overlying the orifice of the inferior vena cava directs the flow of oxygenated blood from that vessel through the foramen ovale into the left atrium, while the deoxygenated stream from the superior vena cava is directed through the tricuspid valve into the right ventricle. From the left atrium the oxygenated blood and a small amount of deoxygenated blood from the lungs passes into the left

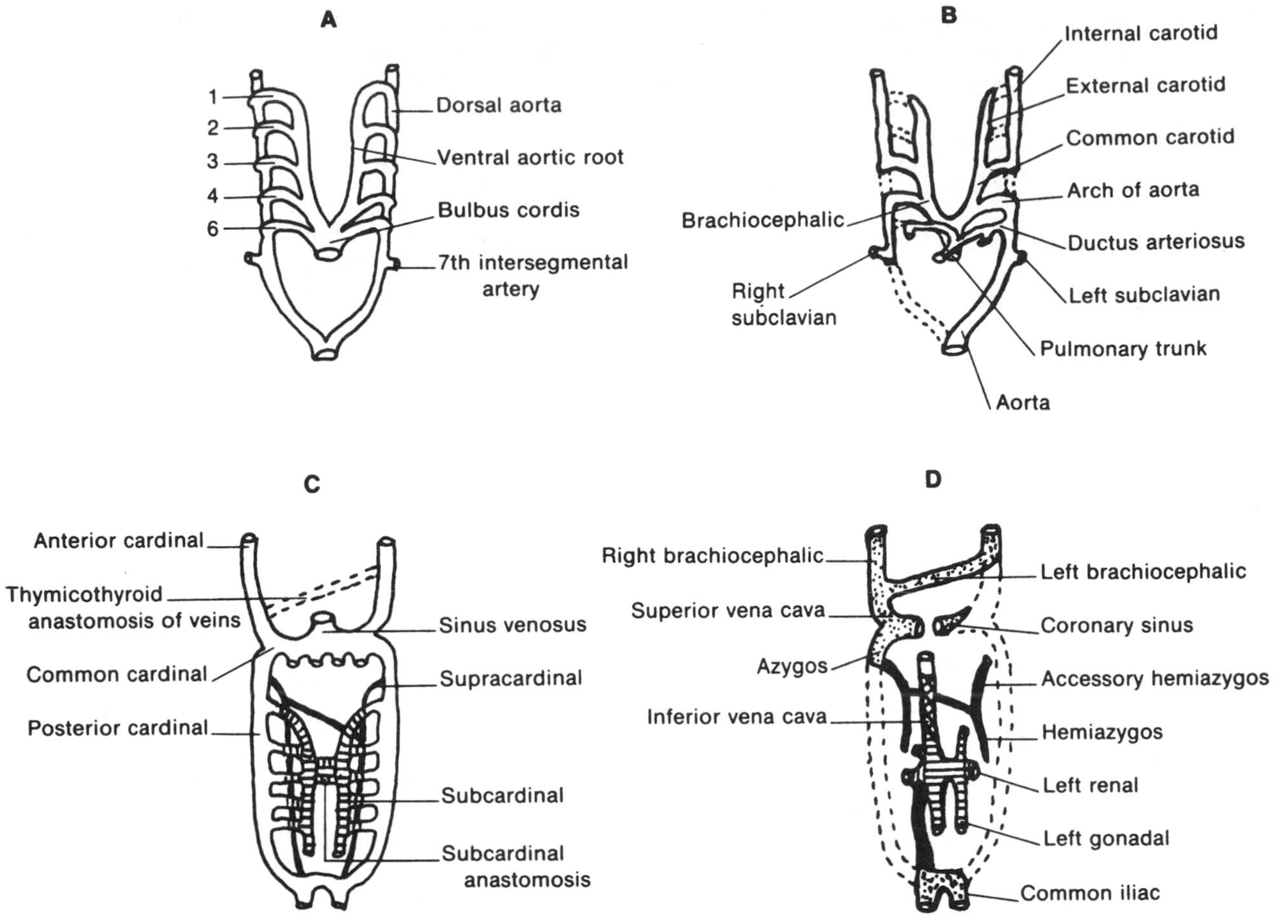

Fig. 2-27. Schematic ventral views of developing major blood vessels. *(A)* represents early aortic arch development. *(B)* shows the fate of the aortic arches. The dashed lines represent degenerating arteries. *(C)* represents early formation of the cardinal system of veins. The thymicothyroid anastomosis of veins *(dashed lines)* is a later acquisition. *(D)* shows the fate of the cardinal system of veins in the development of the superior and inferior venae cavae and the azygos system of veins.

ventricle and thence into the ascending aorta from which it is supplied to the brain and the heart through the vertebral, the carotid and the coronary arteries.

Because the lungs of the fetus are inactive, most of the deoxygenated blood from the right ventricle is shunted by way of the ductus arteriosus from the pulmonary trunk into the descending aorta. This blood supplies the abdominal viscera and the inferior extremities and is carried to the placenta, for oxygenation, through the umbilical arteries arising from the aorta.

Circulatory Changes at Birth. When respiration begins, the lungs expand, resulting in increased blood flow through the pulmonary arteries and a pressure change in the left atrium. This pressure change brings the septum primum and the septum secundum together and causes functional closure of the foramen ovale. Simultaneously, active contraction of the muscular wall of the ductus arteriosus results in its functional closure. Several months later it will become ligamentous as the ligamentum arteriosum. The ductus venosus functionally closes and becomes the ligamentum venosum. The fate of the umbilical arteries and veins was described previously in the section on extraembryonic circuits.

CONGENITAL ABNORMALITIES OF THE HEART AND GREAT VESSELS

The complicated sequence of development in the heart and the major arteries accounts for the many congenital abnormalities that alone or in combination may affect these structures.

Septal defects include patent foramen ovale (incidence of about 10%) and other atrial or ventricular septal defects. An ostium secundum (foramen ovale) defect lies in the interatrial wall and is relatively easy to close surgically. An ostium primum defect lies directly above the A-V boundary and is often associated with a defect in the membranous part of the interventricular septum and in the A-V valves. A high interatrial septal defect may result, which probably is an improper shifting and incorporation of the sinus venosus into the right atrium.

Interventricular septal defects usually involve the membranous part of the interventricular septum and are due mostly to improper formation of the conal septum. Rarely the septal defect is so large that the ventricles form a single cavity, giving a trilocular heart (cor triloculare biatriatum). The latter is due to improper development of the primitive muscular interventricular septum. Failure of closure of the interventricular foramen also may be due to defective development of the septum membranaceum contribution from the fused endocardial cushions.

Congenital pulmonary stenosis may involve the trunk of the pulmonary artery and its valve or the infundibulum of the right ventricle. If this is combined with an interventricular septal defect, the compensatory hypertrophy of the right ventricle develops sufficiently high pressure to shunt blood through the defect into the left side of the heart; this mixing of blood results in the child's being cyanosed at birth.

Fallot's tetralogy is the most common congenital abnormality causing cyanosis. It is comprised of pulmonary stenosis, right ventricular hypertrophy, an interventricular septal defect with an overriding aorta, the orifice of which lies cranial to the septal defect and receives blood from both ventricles.

Transposition of the great vessels is due to improper spiraling of the bulbar septum in the formation of the great vessels. This results in either complete transposition, where the aorta is from the right ventricle and the pulmonary trunk is from the left ventricle, or in incomplete transposition where both vessels are reversed but both exit from the right ventricle.

Aortic stenosis is due to either bulbar septum displacement or localized improper growth in supravalvular, valvular, and subvalvular regions of the aorta.

Patent ductus arteriosus is a relatively common developmental abnormality. If not corrected it causes progressive work hypertrophy of the right heart and pulmonary hypertension.

Aortic coarctation may be due to abnormal retention of the fetal isthmus of the aorta or to incorporation of smooth muscle from the ductus into the wall of the aorta. The constriction may occur from the level of the left subclavian artery to the ductus arteriosus (preductal type), the latter being widely patent and maintaining the circulation to the lower part of the body. In other cases the coarctation may involve a segment below the entrance of the ligamentum arteriosum (postductal type), and the circulation to the lower limb is maintained by collateral arteries around the scapula that anastomose with the intercostal arteries.

Dextrorotation of the heart is the most spectacular of the abnormalities. The heart and its emerging vessels lie as a mirror image to the normal anatomy. It may be associated with reversal of all the intraabdominal organs in situs inversus.

Abnormal development of the aortic arches may result in the arch of the aorta lying on the right or actually being double. Rarely an abnormal right subclavian artery arises from the dorsal aorta and passes behind the esophagus and thus causes difficulty in swallowing (dysphagia lusoria). Double aorta is due to retention of the right dorsal aorta between the seventh dorsal intersegmental artery and the point of fusion of the aortae. If this portion remains and the right fourth aortic arch disappears, then the right subclavian arises from the aorta.

TRACHEA AND LUNGS

Gross Structure of the Trachea and Lungs. The trachea extends from the cricoid cartilage (vertebral level C6) to the level of the upper border of T5, where it bifurcates into left and right bronchi. It is related posteriorly to the esophagus and anteriorly to the thyroid gland and vessels, the sternohyoid and sternothyroid muscles, the thymus, the manubrium sterni, the major arteries and veins, and the deep cardiac plexus.

The right bronchus is both shorter and wider and diverges from the midline less than the left bronchus. Each bronchus enters the hilus of the lung at the mediastinal surface along with the pulmonary and bronchial arteries and veins, lymphatic vessels and lymph nodes, and autonomic nerve fibers. The right bronchus divides into three lobar bronchi: the superior, middle, and inferior. The left bronchus divides into a superior and inferior lobe bronchus. Each of the lobar bronchi in turn subdivides to supply bronchopulmonary segments. In the right lung these segments are (1) the apical, posterior, and anterior of the superior lobe; (2) the medial and lateral of the middle lobe; and (3) the superior, medial basal, lateral basal, anterior basal, and posterior basal of the inferior lobe. In the left lung these bronchopulmonary segments are (1) the apical-posterior, anterior, superior, and inferior of the superior lobe; and (2) the superior, anteriormedial basal, lateral basal, and posterior basal of the inferior lobe. The segmental bronchi further subdivide to smaller bronchi and bronchioles in the substance of the lung.

The lungs project laterally from the mediastinum and are invested by visceral pleura, which is continuous at the hilum with the parietal pleura. The pleural cavity lies between the visceral and parietal pleura, and it surrounds the lung. The pleura is a moist serous membrane, and under normal circumstances its surfaces do not adhere to one another. Based on location, the parietal pleura is subdivided into costal, mediastinal, and diaphragmatic portions.

Each lung is conical in shape and has an apex and base; three borders, the inferior, posterior, and anterior; and three surfaces, the costal, diaphragmatic (base), and mediastinal. The apex extends approximately 2.5 cm into the root of the neck (superior to the clavicle), while the base rests on the convex surface of the diaphragm. The costal surface faces the ribs. The mediastinal surface is in contact with mediastinal pleura and bears impressions of the structures in the mediastinum. The posterior border is in the concavity on either side of the vertebral column. The anterior border is sharp and projects into the costomediastinal recess, except on the left in the cardiac notch region where the pericardium is not overlapped anteriorly by the lung. The inferior border is sharp and projects into the costodiaphragmatic recess. The right lung is divided into superior, middle, and inferior lobes by two interlobar fissures; the left lung is divided into superior and inferior lobes by one interlobar fissure. The surface projections of these fissures are described previously in the section on surface markings.

The ***afferent and the efferent innervation*** of the lung is derived from the anterior and the posterior pulmonary plexuses, which receive branches from the vagus and the thoracic sympathetic trunk. Stimulation of the vagi brings about constriction of bronchioles, while stimulation of the sympathetic fibers causes dilation. The visceral afferents transmit pain and reflex activity, and return to the CNS by way of both the vagal and sympathetic pathways.

Microscopic Structure of the Lungs. The ***conducting portion*** of the respiratory system includes the nasal cavity, nasopharynx, laryngopharynx, trachea, bronchi, and bronchioles down to and including the terminal bronchioles. The oropharynx is shared with the digestive system. All but the bronchioles and oropharynx are characterized by (1) a mucosa of pseudostratified ciliated columnar epithelium with goblet cells and an underlying connective tissue containing mixed seromucous glands, and (2) usually a cartilaginous or bony support. The ***respiratory portion*** consists of respiratory bronchioles, alveolar ducts, alveolar sacs, and alveoli. A respiratory bronchiole and its branches constitute a lobule. All respiratory portions contain alveoli in their walls.

The microscopic structure of the larynx and trachea was described in the section on the head and neck. The main bronchi and segmental bronchi are similar to the trachea. The smaller bronchi have cartilaginous plates instead of rings. In bronchioles the cartilage disappears, circular smooth muscle becomes more prominent, and the ciliated epithelium becomes simple columnar and simple cuboidal. Glands are no longer present in the terminal bronchioles.

Respiratory bronchioles have simple cuboidal epithelium except at those sites where alveoli are present (Fig. 2-28). Alveolar ducts are completely lined by alveolar sacs and alveoli, and their lumina are marked by spiraling bundles of smooth muscle. Alveoli are separated from each other by interalveolar septa that contain an extensive capillary net, reticular and elastic fibers, blood cells, macrophages and lymph nodes and nodules. The alveolus is lined by an extremely attenuated simple squamous epithelium. Blood in the capillaries is separated from the air in the alveoli by nonfenestrated endothelial cells and their basal lamina and the simple squamous ***(alveolar type I)*** cells and their basal lamina. The basal laminae of the alveolar and endothelial epithelia are fused in the thinnest blood–air transport regions. ***Great alveolar (septal, type II)*** cells bulge between the squamous cells into the alveolar lumen and produce surfactant. Alveolar phagocytes (dust cells) migrate into alveolar spaces and engulf debris.

Bronchial arteries, carrying nourishment to the lungs, course along the bronchi to the respiratory bronchioles. Venous return of this blood is mainly through pulmonary veins, but some blood returns by way of the bronchial veins to the azygos system. Pulmonary arteries branch and follow the air tubes to the capillary plexi in the alveoli. Oxygenated blood is returned through pulmonary veins that travel in the interlobular connective tissue septa.

ESOPHAGUS

Gross Structure of the Esophagus. The esophagus extends from the pharynx at the C6 level to the stomach. It passes in front of the bodies of the vertebrae in the superior and posterior mediastinum and penetrates the diaphragm at the esophageal hiatus (vertebral level T10). It is supplied by the vagal and sympathetic fibers that form an esophageal plexus around the esophagus. In the lower thorax, anterior and posterior vagal trunks accompany the esophagus through the diaphragm to the stomach. Parasympathetic preganglionic fibers penetrate the wall and synapse on postganglionic neurons in the myenteric (Auerbach's) and submucosal (Meissner's) plexi.

Microscopic Structure of the Esophagus. The esophagus demonstrates well the general microscopic plan of the gastrointestinal system. The wall consists of four layers: (1) mucosa, (2) submucosa, (3) muscularis externa, and (4) adventitia or serosa. The ***mucosa*** consists of stratified squamous nonkeratinized epithelium, a lamina propria with some mucous glands at the upper and lower extents of the esophagus, and a well-developed muscularis mucosae of smooth muscle. The ***submucosa*** contains some mucous glands and the autonomic submu-

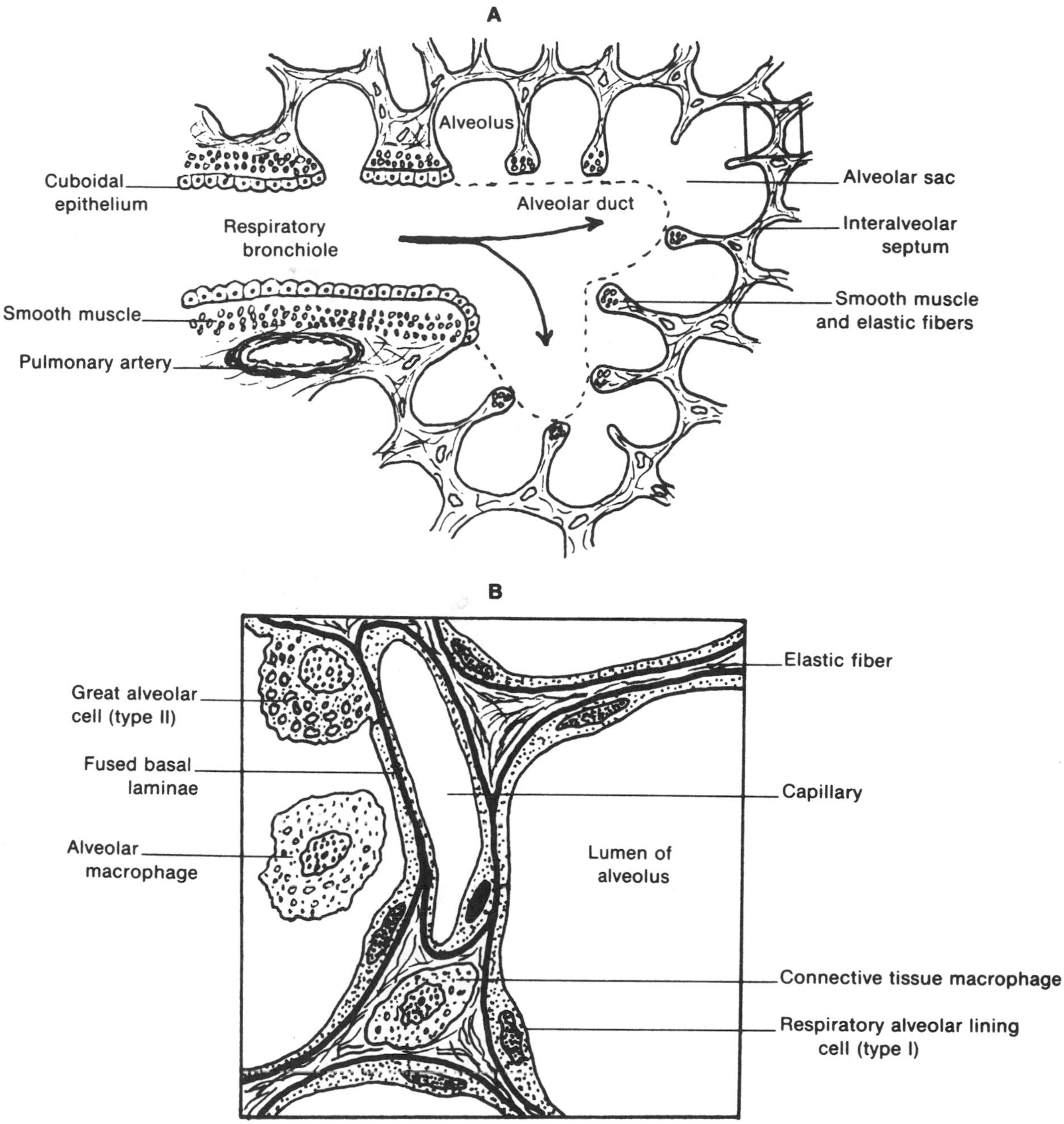

Fig. 2-28. *(A)* shows a respiratory bronchiole opening into two alveolar ducts whose lumina are outlined by the knobs of smooth muscle that border the openings into alveoli and alveolar sacs. *(B)* is an enlargement of the interalveolar septum area outlined in *(A)*. The simplest blood–air barrier consists of the cytoplasm of alveolar lining cells and endothelial cells and their fused basal laminae.

cosal nerve plexus. The ***muscularis externa*** consists of an outer longitudinal and inner circular layer of muscle with the myenteric plexus sandwiched between the two layers (Fig. 2-29). The submucosal and myenteric plexi contain postganglionic parasympathetic neurons and in some configurations cells of the enteric nervous system. In the upper esophagus the muscle is skeletal; in the lower portion it is smooth muscle, and in the middle it is mixed. The ***adventitia*** is connective tissue that merges imperceptibly with that of the surrounding mediastinum. In the short abdominal portion of the esophagus, the outer layer is peritoneum and thus consists of mesothelium and underlying connective tissue and is called a serosa.

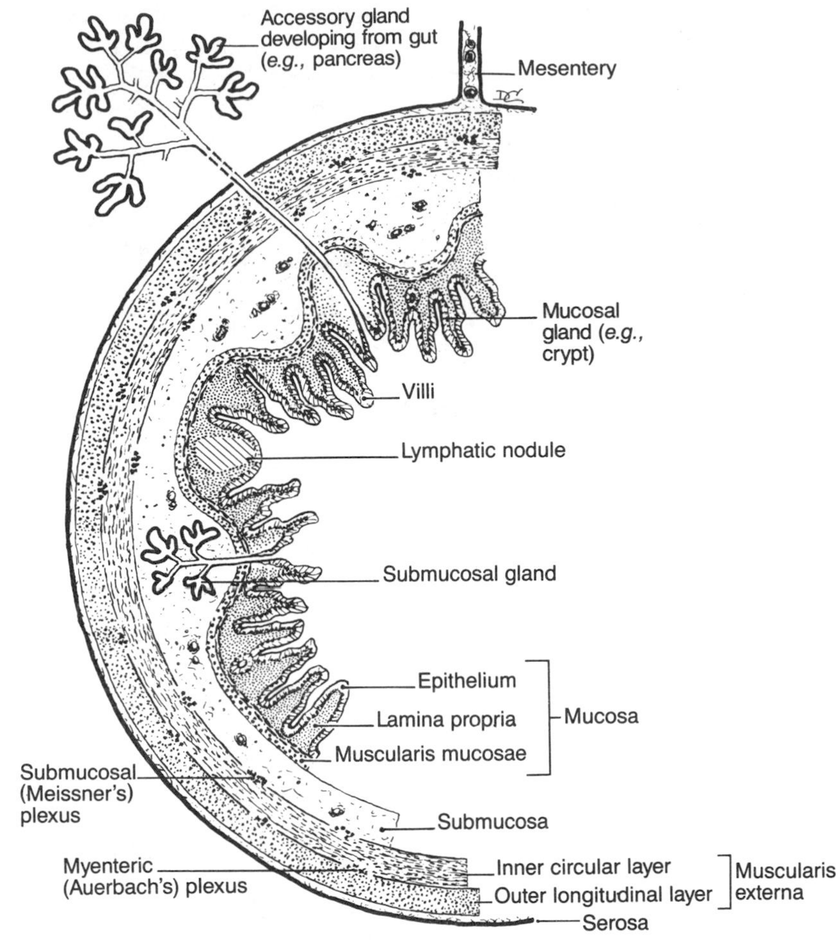

Fig. 2-29. General plan of the gastrointestinal tract. (Cormack DH: Ham's Histology, 9th ed, p 492. Philadelphia, JB Lippincott, 1987)

DEVELOPMENT OF THE TRACHEA, LUNGS, ESOPHAGUS, AND DIAPHRAGM

An ***entodermal respiratory diverticulum*** develops from the floor of the foregut just caudal to the last pharyngeal pouch. The larynx, trachea, bronchi, and lungs develop from this diverticulum. The esophagus differentiates from the foregut caudal to this outgrowth. In the development of the larynx, the opening is constricted into a narrow T-shaped laryngotracheal orifice by underlying mesodermal arytenoid swellings. There is a transitory period when the opening is completely obliterated by an overgrowth of epithelium. Persistence of portions of this may lead to webs that obstruct the laryngeal opening.

All cartilage, muscle, and connective tissue of the larynx, trachea, and lungs arise from splanchnic mesoderm. The epithelium and glands develop from branching of the entodermal diverticulum. The main bronchi divide dichotomously through 17 generations of subdivisions by the end of the sixth month. An additional seven divisions will occur by early childhood.

As the bronchial buds divide, the lung increases in size, and it bulges laterally into the embryonic coelom. The early coelom consists of a more ventral prospective pericardial cavity in continuity with a more dorsal pleural cavity, which is continuous caudally with the prospective peritoneal cavity via the pericardioperitoneal canals. The presumptive thoracic cavity is separated from the presumptive peritoneal cavity by the septum transversium. Right and left pleuropericardial folds project from the lateral body wall and septum transversum, grow medially between the heart and lungs, and fuse with the primitive mediastinum. Thus, these folds form the pericardial sac and become part of the definitive mediastinum and thus separate the pleural from the pericardial cavities. Pleuroperitoneal folds grow from the septum transversum at right angles to the pleuropericardial membranes. These folds invest the esophagus and, along with the septum transversum, contribute to the formation of the diaphragm and obliterate the pericardioperitoneal canals, thus separating the thoracic from the abdominal cavities. In addition, the definitive diaphragm receives a major contribution of muscle in its development from the lateral body wall.

Tracheoesophageal fistulas may develop from improper separation of the respiratory diverticulum from the foregut, by malformation of the esophagotracheal septum, or by secondary fusion of the esophagus with the trachea. In the most usual fistula the upper part of the esophagus ends blindly, while a lower portion is connected to the trachea by a narrow canal. This may result from dorsal deviation of the esophagotracheal septum in its caudal growth.

Diaphragmatic hernias can arise from improper formation of either the septum transversum, the pleuroperitoneal folds, or the muscular component from the body wall.

LYMPHATIC ORGANS OF THE THORAX

Thymus. The thymus is larger in the infant than it is in the adult. It consists of two lateral lobes invested by a connective tissue capsule that sends septa into the gland and divides it into lobules. The gland lies in the anterior part of the superior mediastinum and it extends from the fourth costal cartilage to the lower border of the thyroid gland. It lies anterior to the great vessels and fibrous pericardium. Microscopically the thymus is divisible into a central medulla and an outer cortex. The reticular cell meshwork contains lymphocytes (thymocytes) and differs from the other lymphatic tissues in that the reticular cells are derived from entoderm (of the third pharyngeal pouch). The cortex contains more lymphocytes and is less vascular than the medulla. Thymic (Hassall's) corpuscles in the medulla are concentric arrangements of flattened, and often hyalinized, cells. The corpuscles vary in size and occurrence and seem to be indicative of degeneration of reticular cells of the thymus.

Branches of the internal thoracic and thyroid arteries pass through thymic septa and enter the corticomedullary junction as arterioles. Here, the arterioles give off direct branches to the medulla and also feed capillaries that loop into the cortex before draining into postcapillary venules of the medulla and corticomedullary junction. Macromolecules cannot pass through the walls of the capillary loops, since the endothelial cells have a thick basement membrane that is bounded by reticular cells. Thus, the cortical lymphocytes seem to be protected from circulating antigens by a ***blood–thymus barrier.*** Large numbers of lymphocytes pass through the walls of the postcapillary venules and drain by way of thymic veins into the left brachiocephalic, inferior thyroid, and internal thoracic veins. The thymus is essential for the production of thymus-dependent (T) lymphocytes that are involved in cell-mediated immunologic responses and that also assist B-lymphocytes in humoral responses.

Lymph Nodes of the Thorax. The lymphatic nodes of the thorax are divided into parietal and visceral groups. The ***parietal nodes*** include the sternal, intercostal, and diaphragmatic nodes. The ***sternal nodes*** are located along the internal thoracic artery and receive afferents from the breast, the deeper structures of the anterior thoracic wall, and the upper surface of the liver. Their efferents pass as a trunk to the junction of the subclavian and internal jugular veins. The ***intercostal nodes*** occupy the posterior parts of the intercostal spaces. They receive afferents from the posterolateral chest area. Efferents from the lower intercostal nodes carry lymph to the cisterna chyli, while the upper nodes send efferents to the thoracic duct and right lymphatic duct. ***Diaphragmatic nodes*** located anteriorly drain toward the sternal nodes, whereas those in the middle and posterior drain to the posterior mediastinal nodes. Superficial lymphatic vessels of the thoracic wall ramify beneath the skin and converge toward the axillary nodes. Lymphatic vessels of the mammary glands drain toward the surface along the interlobular septa and empty into a plexus located deep to the areola. This plexus also receives lymph from the areola and skin over the gland. It drains in two trunks to the axillary lymph nodes. Some drainage from the medial portion of the gland goes to the sternal nodes, while some efferents pass to interpectoral glands deep to the pectoralis major muscle, and others pass inferiorly toward abdominal nodes.

The ***visceral lymph nodes*** consist of anterior and posterior mediastinal and tracheobronchial nodes. The anterior mediastinal nodes are located in front of the great vessels and receive afferents from the thymus, pericardium and sternal nodes. Their efferents unite with those of the tracheobronchial nodes to form the right and left bronchomediastinal nodes. The posterior mediastinal nodes lie behind the pericardium and along the esophagus and descending aorta. Their afferents come from the liver, esophagus, and pericardium. Most efferents from these nodes go to the thoracic duct. The tracheobronchial nodes filter lymph from the trachea, bronchi, lungs, and heart.

Microscopically, lymph nodes are bean shaped, possess a hilum, and are surrounded by a capsule that sends trabeculae into a stroma of reticular tissue containing lymphocytes. Nodules of dense lymphatic tissue are located peripherally in the cortical region. If the node is in the "active" stage, the nodules contain germinal centers that consist of medium-sized lymphocytes and larger undifferentiated lymphocytes. These areas produce small lymphocytes that are pushed peripherally in the nodule and then into surrounding lymphatic sinuses. Nodes receive lymph peripherally through afferent vessels that penetrate the capsule and drain into a subcapsular sinus. This sinus drains along cortical peritrabecular sinuses to medullary sinuses (which lie between trabeculae and medullary cords of lymphatic tissue) before exiting from the lymph node at the hilum through efferent lymphatic vessels. Reticular cells and macrophages lining the sinuses perform a filtering function by phagocytizing dead cells and particulate matter and by offering antigens to the lymphocytes.

Lymph nodes play a major role in the immune responsc. The B lymphocytes are found in the subcapsular cortical tissue, in germinal centers, and in medullary cords. In bacterial infections, antigens pass to the B-lymphocytes and trigger them to form blast cells in the germinal centers that proliferate and differentiate into antibody-producing lymphocytes and plasma cells. These cells pass to the medullary cords where antibodies and B-lymphocytes pass into efferent lymphatic vessels and are transported by the circulatory system to the site of infection. T-lymphocytes are located in deep cortical (paracortical) areas known as the ***thymus-dependent zone.*** This zone contains many postcapillary venules, whose cuboidal endothelium permits a recirculating pool of T-lymphocytes, and some B-lymphocytes, to enter the lymph node. It is thought that uncommitted lymphocytes from the thymus and bone marrow enter the lymph nodes through these venules and react with antigens from foreign cells. In this response, T-lymphocytes in the deep cortex become blast cells, proliferate, and form small long-lived memory cells and short-lived effector (killer) cells which enter the circulation.

MUSCLES, NERVES, AND VESSELS OF THE THORACIC WALL

Muscles. The major muscles are the external and internal intercostals, the subcostal, and the transversus thoracis. The ***intercostal muscles*** fill the intercostal spaces, the external sloping medially from above downward and the internal sloping laterally from above downward. ***Subcostal muscles*** are fasciculi of the internal intercostals that extend over two or more intercostal spaces near the angles of the ribs. The ***transversus thoracis muscle*** arises from the dorsal surface of the lower sternum and xiphoid process and extends upward and laterally to insert on the second through the sixth costal cartilages. In respiration, the intercostals apparently maintain both size and rigidity of the intercostal spaces, while the entire rib cage is elevated by the scalene muscles.

Nerves. The intercostal muscles are innervated by ***intercostal nerves,*** which are the continuations of the ventral rami of thoracic spinal nerves. The intercostal nerves and vessels occupy the costal grooves (on the inferior aspects of the ribs), with the nerves inferior to the intercostal arteries and veins. Each intercostal nerve has two cutaneous branches: the lateral cultaneous nerve in the midaxillary line and the anterior cutaneous nerve just lateral to the sternum.

Arteries and Veins. Posterior intercostal arteries arise from the aorta and, in the upper spaces, from the costocervical trunk of the subclavian artery. They supply the deep muscles of the back, contents of the spinal canal and most of the intercostal space, and end by anastomosing with the anterior intercostal arteries, which are branches of the internal thoracic artery. The posterior intercostal veins are tributaries to the azygous system while the anterior intercostal veins empty into the internal thoracic veins. Both systems—the arterial and the venous—represent potential collateral vascular routes.

CIRCULATING BLOOD

Blood cells (formed elements) constitute 45% of the total volume of circulating blood; plasma comprises the remaining 55%. Of the 45% cell volume, erythrocytes (red blood corpuscles, RBCs) make up 44%, and the remaining 1% is composed of leukocytes (white blood cells). The plasma, minus its bloodclotting factors, is called ***serum.***

Plasma acts as a medium for metabolic substances and circulating cells. Like tissue fluid, its primary components are water, inorganic salts, and a number of proteins. Albumin, the most abundant plasma protein, maintains the colloid blood pressure. Gamma globulins are also important since they include the circulating antibodies. Beta globulins transport lipids, hormones, and metal ions. Prothrombin and fibrinogen are products of the liver that are essential components of the clotting process. Chylomicrons are microscopic particles of fat that are especially prominent in the plasma after a fatty meal.

Erythrocytes, when mature, are anucleate biconcave discs approximately 8 μm in diameter and 2-μm thick. There are about 4.8 and 5.5 million erythrocytes per cubic millimeter of blood in the normal female and normal male, respectively. Erythrocytes lack the usual complement of organelles, and they do not have the capacity for protein synthesis. Each RBC exists for about 120 days, and it lacks the mechanism to reproduce itself. About 17% of the erythrocytes possess some residual ribosomal material and, due to their stained appearance, are called ***reticulocytes;*** they are considered to be immature erythrocytes. The reticulocyte count provides a rough index of the rate of erythrocyte development.

Leukocytes are divisible into granular leukocytes and nongranular leukocytes. The granular leukocytes are further classified as eosinophils, basophils, and neutrophils on the basis of the affinity of their granules for different stains. The nongranular leukocytes are the lymphocytes and monocytes.

Neutrophils are about twice the size of erythrocytes and make up about 60% to 70% of the white blood cells. Their nuclei consist of three to five lobes that are interconnected by fine filaments of nuclear material. Two types of granules are present in the cytoplasm: the specific granules, which stain with neutral dyes, and nonspecific granules, which are azurophilic. Both types of granules contain hydrolytic enzymes that are used by the cell in the digestion of phagocytized materials.

Eosinophils are about the size of neutrophils but constitute only 1% to 3% of the total leukocyte population. The nucleus is usually bilobed and the chromatin is dense. The eosinophilic granules are membrane-bound vesicles containing lysosomal enzymes.

Basophils are about the same size as the other granular leukocytes. They constitute only 0.5% of the white blood cells. The nucleus is usually S-shaped and its chromatin is less dense than that of the other granular leukocytes. The basophilic membrane-bound cytoplasmic granules contain histamine and heparin.

Lymphocytes constitute 20% to 35% of the white blood cell population. Most of the mature lymphocytes are the size of erythrocytes, but larger cells traditionally called large and medium lymphocytes are occasionally seen in circulating blood. The small lymphocyte has a relatively large round or slightly indented nucleus of dense chromatin. The nucleus is surrounded by a thin rim of cytoplasm containing a few ribosomes and some nonspecific azurophilic granules. The small lymphocytes are further designated as T- and B-lymphocytes. ***T-lymphocytes*** are cytotoxic cells of the cell-mediated response that "kill" foreign cells and sensitizing agents that enter the body. They also assist the ***B-lymphocytes*** (and their subsequent plasma cells) in their humoral antibody response to such invasive organisms as bacteria and viruses.

Monocytes range from 9 μm in diameter and make up 3% to 8% of the circulating leukocytes. The nucleus is oval, kidney shaped, or horseshoe shaped. The cytoplasm is more abundant than that of lymphocytes; it contains a few azurophilic granules, a Golgi complex, polyribosomes, and some glycogen. Monocytes give rise to macrophages when they pass into connective tissues.

Platelets (thrombocytes) are small, irregular disk-shaped structures that are 1 μm to 2 μm in diameter. They are basophilic fragments of large cells located in the bone marrow and known as megakaryocytes. There are 250,000 to 300,000 platelets in a cubic millimeter of blood. They have a natural tendency to cling to each other and to all wettable surfaces they contact when blood is shed. Platelets contain serotonin, which helps to constrict small blood vessels during vascular injury. They also contain thromboplastin, a substance released by platelets and injured endothelial cells. Thromboplastin helps convert prothombin of the plasma to thrombin. The thrombin then converts plasma fibrinogen to fibrin which forms a network trapping blood cells and platelets. Thus, a blood clot, or thrombus, is formed.

BLOOD CELL FORMATION (HEMOPOIESIS)

The main hemopoietic tissue in the body is bone marrow. Since all of the erythrocytes, platelets, and granular leukocytes are produced in bone marrow, these blood components are called the ***myeloid elements.*** The specific development of these elements is referred to as myelopoiesis. Although the nongranular elements are produced in both lymphatic tissues and bone marrow, they are referred to as ***lymphoid elements;*** their development is termed lymphopoiesis.

The first blood cells develop in the third embryonic week from yolk sac and body stalk mesoderm. During the second month of development hemopoietic sites arise in the liver, spleen, and mesonephric kidneys. In later months of fetal development, bones are established, and the bone marrow becomes the dominant hemopoietically active tissue. ***Red bone marrow*** consists of a reticular fiber meshwork, which contains and supports reticular cells, myelopoietic (blood forming) cells, adipose cells, and thin-walled sinusoids. The myelopoietic cells occur in many stages. Some are relatively undifferentiated stem cells from which all myeloid elements arise. Some are mature erythrocytes, granular leukocytes, and nongranular leukocytes, which are about ready to leave the bone marrow through the sinusoids and veins. The majority of cells, however, are in the numerous stages of differentiation that stem cells go through during erythropoiesis, granulopoiesis, and thrombopoiesis.

Erythropoiesis is the formation of erythrocytes from stem cells. In this process pluripotent stem cells, which have the potential to give rise to any blood cell type, differentiate into proerythroblasts. The latter cells divide and differentiate into basophilic proerythroblasts, which contain free polyribosomes, a condensed nucleus, and no nucleoli. Without nucleoli the cells cannot produce ribosomes. Thus, when they divide into smaller polychromatophilic erythroblasts, their basophilia disappears and their acidophilia increases due to accumulating hemoglobin. When these cells have acquired their full amount of hemoglobin and their nuclei become very small and concentrated, they are called normoblasts (orthochromatic erythroblasts). When the nuclei are extruded they become erythrocytes. Erythropoietin, produced by the kidney, regulates proerythroblast formation. The maturation of erythrocytes is regulated by the extrinsic factor (vitamin B_{12}) and the intrinsic factor (a mucoprotein produced in the stomach).

Granulopoiesis is the formation of basophils, eosinophils, and neutrophils from stem cells that differentiate through myeloblast, promyelocyte, myelocyte and metamyelocyte stages. The myeloblast has a large nucleus with several prominent nucleoli; its cytoplasm is basophilic. When these cells acquire azurophilic granules, they are called promyelocytes. As promyelocytes mature into myelocytes, their nuclei become more dense, nonspecific azurophilic granules increase in number, and specific granules make their appearance. If the latter are neutrophilic, then the cell is a neutrophilic myelocyte; if basophilic or eosinophilic granules are present, the cell is a basophilic myelocyte or eosinophilic myelocyte. All of the cells from myeloblast through myelocyte are capable of mitosis. This ceases when the myelocyte nucleus becomes dense and more deeply indented as a metamyelocyte is formed. During maturation of the metamyelocyte into a mature granulocyte, the nucleus becomes more deeply indented and then becomes lobated or S-shaped. As this takes place, certain juvenile forms of cells are detected. In neutrophil formation the horseshoe-shaped nucleus often designates the cell as a band or stab cell. Since the life span of granular leukocytes is considerably shorter (about 14 hours) than that of erythrocytes (120 days), there are more developmental forms of granular leukocytes in the marrow than there are of erythrocytes.

Thrombopoiesis is the formation of blood platelets from megakaryocytes. In this process, plasma membranes of megakaryocytes partition off cytoplasmic fragments, which are released from the cell and pass into the blood stream as platelets. The megakaryocyte may then die and is replaced by a stem cell in the marrow. Megakaryocytes are very large cells with multilobed nuclei. Blood platelets live for only about 8 to 11 days.

Lymphopoiesis is the formation of lymphocytes from a stem cell. In this process a stem cell differentiates into a large lymphocyte (lymphoblast) that further divides and matures into medium lymphocytes and then into small lymphocytes. The sites of these lymphopoietic changes are in the bone marrow and in the lymphatic tissues of the spleen, thymus, lymph nodes, tonsils, and mucous membranes of the body. The theory that the small lymphocyte is an end point of differentiation is questioned, for it appears that the small lymphocyte can be the stem cell for large lymphoblasts that produce other small lymphocytes and antibody-producing plasma cells. In the establishment of the immune system, stem cells are sent to the thymus, the mucous membrane of the gut, and return to the bone marrow. In the thymus the stem cells become T-lymphocyte precursors, which pass to other tissues and become small cytotoxic ''killer'' lymphocytes. Stem cells that return to the bone marrow become lymphocytes that develop into antibody-producing B-lymphocytes.

Monopoiesis is the formation of monocytes from stem cells. Monocytes seem to develop in the marrow from pluripotent stem cells. After a few days developing in the marrow, monocytes pass into the circulation for 1 or 2 days before entering the connective tissue and becoming macrophages.

MAMMARY GLAND

The mammary glands are integumentary glands located from the level of the second to sixth or seventh rib on the anterior of the thorax. In fetal development they first appear as ectodermal thickenings along a milk line extending between the upper and lower extremities. As development proceeds, 15 to 20 ectodermal invaginations branch and hollow out to give rise to the 15 to 20 lobes of the mammary gland, which are arranged in a radial fashion deep to the nipple. Thus, each lobe has a single excretory duct opening on the nipple. Each of these ducts diverges at the base of the nipple and increases in size to form an ampulla (lactiferous sinus). Deep to the ampulla the ducts branch into intralobular ducts. In the male and nonpregnant female gland there are few ducts present, and the epithelium changes from stratified to simple cuboidal epithelium in proceeding from larger to smaller ducts. In the lactating female, the gland has ducts that have proliferated, and their terminal portions develop into secretory alveoli lined by a simple pyramidal epithelium invested by myoepithelial cells. The lining epithelium secretes milk proteins by the exocytosis of secretion granules (merocrine type of secretion); milk lipids in the membrane-bound lipid vacuoles are externalized by the apocrine type of secretion. The lobes of the gland are supported by a dense connective tissue sheath, between the interstices of which are large accumulations of fat. Suspensory ligaments (of Cooper) run through the gland, attaching the deep layer of the superficial fascia to the dermis. The areola is covered by a thin, delicate pigmented skin. Underlying glands (of Montgomery) open on its surface. Smooth muscle fibers also lie deep to the nipple and areola.

The nerves to the mammary gland are the intercostals (second to sixth), by way of lateral and anterior cutaneous branches. Sympathetic fibers accompany these nerves or the vessels supplying the gland. The arteries are the second and third perforating branches of the internal thoracic and the two external mammary branches of the lateral thoracic artery. Additional twigs from the intercostal arteries may enter the deep surface of the gland.

DIAPHRAGM

The diaphragm is a thin dome-shaped muscle consisting of a series of radial fibers that arise from the inner side of the thoracic outlet (subcostal margin) and insert into a central aponeurosis or tendon. On the right its dome reaches to the fifth rib; on the left, to the fifth interspace.

The diaphragm arises from three areas: (1) a small sternal part that attaches to the posterior aspect of the xiphoid process, (2) an extensive costal portion that attaches to the subcostal margin, and (3) a lumbar portion. The lumbar portion consists of the right and left crura, which arise from the anterior aspects of the lumbar vertebra and surround the aortic hiatus (T12), through which pass the aorta and thoracic duct. The esophageal hiatus (T10) is anterior to the aortic hiatus; and the opening for the inferior vena cava (T8) is more anterior and to the right. The diaphragmatic muscle is supplied by the phrenic nerves; the peripheral part of the diaphragm receives sensory fibers from the intercostal nerves. The diaphragm flattens as it contracts and thus draws the central tendon downward. This movement increases the thoracic volume and decreases the pressure within the thoracic cavity.

The phrenic nerve arises from the ventral rami of spinal nerves C3–C5. It descends over the cupula of the pleura, in front of the root of the lung, and between the pericardium and pleura, to reach the diaphragm. Referred pain from the diaphragm occurs in the shoulder because both structures are innervated by sensory fibers to the C4 level of the spinal cord.

CROSS SECTIONS OF THE THORAX

The following cross sections are included to demonstrate relationships and emphasize the importance of cross-sectional anatomy in the interpretation of cross-sectional images. The orientation of all cross sections corresponds to that used clinically in displaying the various types of cross-sectional images; for example, the reader is viewing the inferior aspect of the section with the patient's left on the right of the page.

Figure 2-30 is a section approximately through the junction of the superior and inferior parts of the mediastinum. The plane passes through the junction of thoracic vertebrae four and five, the lower aspect of the manubrium of the sternum, and includes ribs one through five. The arch of the aorta is passing posterolaterally to the left and is cut so that the origins of its three branches are apparent. From proximal to distal, these are the brachiocephalic, left common carotid, and left subclavian arteries. The fourth opening in this section is a slice through a slightly abnormal arching of the aorta. The left brachiocephalic vein is passing to the right in front of the aorta, just superior to the level, where it joins the right brachiocephalic vein to form the superior vena cava. The trachea, just superior to its bifurcation, is separated from the vertebral column by the esophagus, which is somewhat to the left at this level. The thoracic duct is posterolateral to the esophagus. The internal thoracic arteries are posterior to the lateral aspects of the sternum. The lungs are sectioned superior to the hilar regions. Thus, the pleural cavities are seen completely surrounding the lungs. The oblique fissure of the left lung separates the anteriorly located superior lobe from the more posteriorly positioned inferior lobe.

The plane of Figure 2-31 is through vertebra T8, the junction of the fourth rib with the sternum, and the middle mediastinum. The oblique fissure clearly separates the superior and inferior lobes of the left lung. On the right, both oblique and horizontal fissures are present so the superior, middle, and inferior lobes are partially demarcated.

The heart is sectioned so that all four chambers are visible. The posterior surface is formed almost entirely by the left atrium while the right atrium forms the right border.

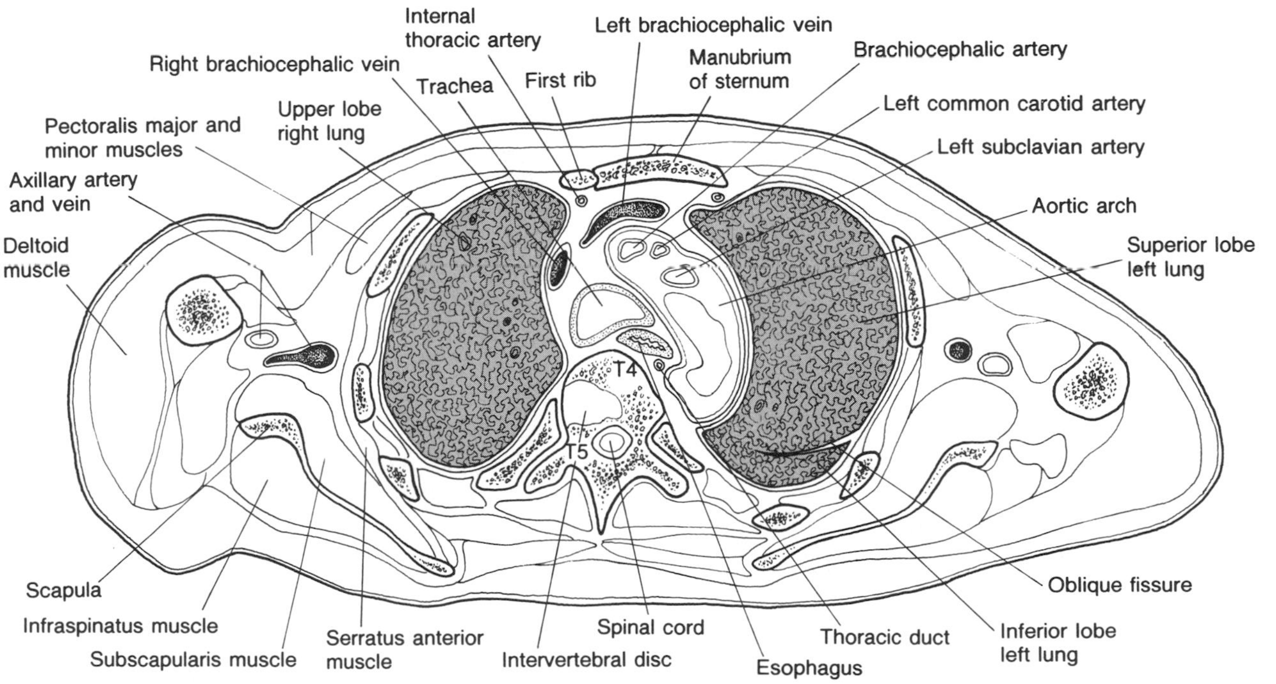

Fig. 2-30. A section through the junction of the superior and inferior parts of the mediastinum. (Courtesy of Ms. Carolyn Volpe)

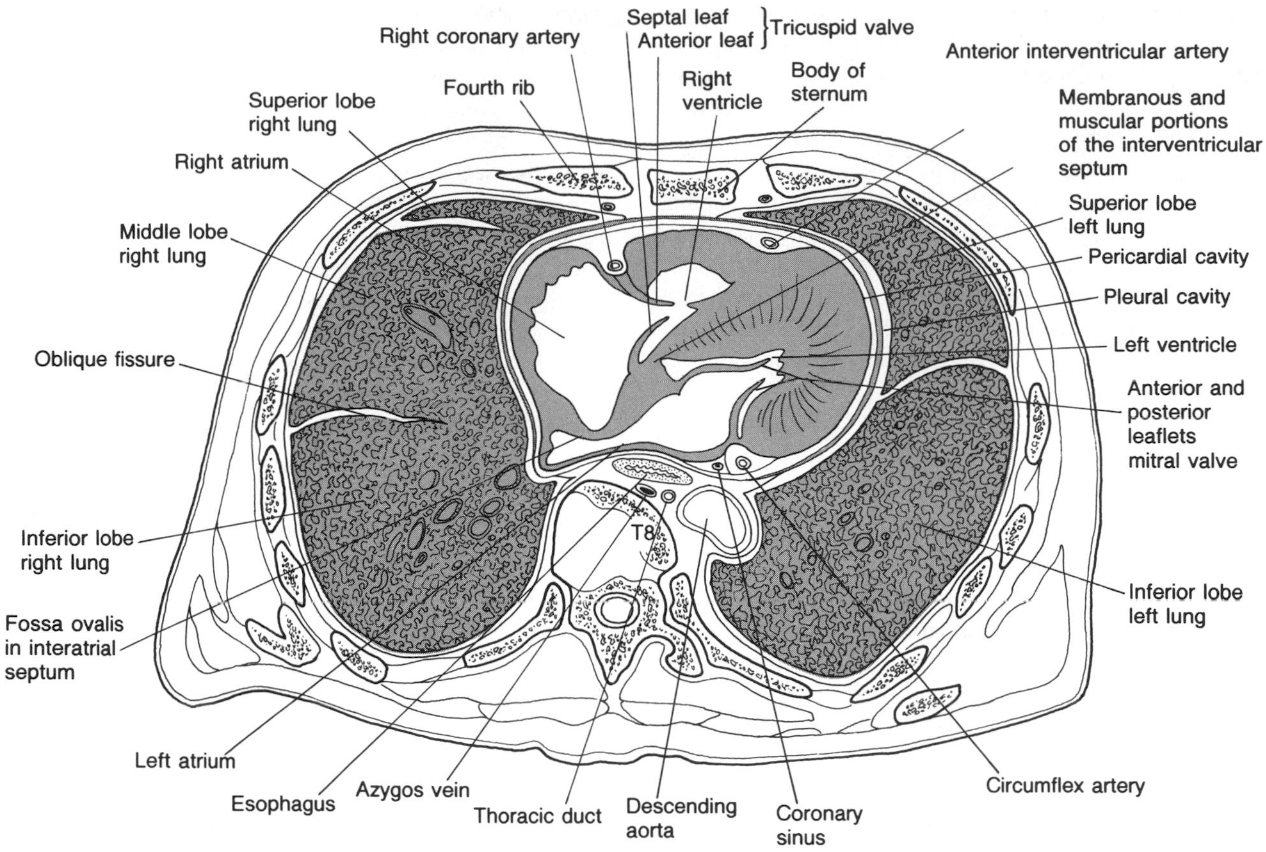

Fig. 2-31. A section through the eighth thoracic vertebra, the junction of the fourth rib with the sternum and the middle mediastinum. (Courtesy of Ms. Carolyn Volpe)

Note that the interatrial septum is essentially in the coronal plane. The right and left ventricles form the anterior and right borders respectively. The latter two chambers are separated by the obliquely oriented interventricular septum; both its muscular and membranous portions are visible. The tricuspid valve is anterior and somewhat to the right of the mitral valve. The coronary (A-V) sulcus houses the right coronary artery anteriorly and the coronary sinus and circumflex branch of the left coronary posteriorly. The anterior interventricular sulcus is not easily seen, but its location is marked by the anterior interventricular artery.

In the posterior mediastinum the esophagus descends directly posterior to the right atrium. The azygous vein and thoracic duct are essentially between the esophagus and vertebral column, with the azygous vein to the right of the thoracic duct. The descending portion of the thoracic aorta is anterolateral (on the left) to the vertebral bodies.

ABDOMEN

SURFACE ANATOMY

Regions. The regions of the abdomen may be defined by two horizontal and two vertical lines. The right and left ***semilunar lines*** correspond to the lateral edges of the rectus abdominis muscles. The ***transpyloric plane*** is a horizontal line through a point halfway between the suprasternal notch and the upper border of the pubic symphysis; this plane is also midway between the xiphisternal joint and the umbilicus. The ***transtubercular plane*** is a lower horizontal line at the level of the top of the iliac crest. These four lines subdivide the abdomen into the following nine regions (superior to inferior): in the center the epigastric, the umbilical, and the pubic regions; on the sides the right and the left hypochondriac, lumbar, and inguinal regions.

The abdomen may also be divided into four areas by a vertical line and a horizontal line that pass through the umbilicus. The division establishes right and left upper and lower quadrants.

The transpyloric plane is at the level of the pylorus, the body of the first lumbar vertebra, the tip of the ninth costal cartilage on each side, and the fundus of the gallbladder on the right side. The semilunar line is the lateral border of the sheath of the rectus abdominis muscle and is a slightly curved line extending from the tip of the ninth costal cartilage to the pubic tubercle. The linea alba is the vertical median line between the rectus abdominis muscles.

Stomach. The stomach varies considerably in size and position, but its cardiac and pyloric portions are relatively fixed. The cardiac orifice is opposite the seventh costal cartilage about 2.5 cm to the left of the xiphisternal joint. The pyloric orifice is on the transpyloric plane about 1.5 cm to the right of the midline. The lesser curvature is indicated by a curved line that passes downward and to the right and connects these two points. The fundus reaches the fifth interspace in the left semilunar line. The greater curvature may extend to the level of the umbilicus or lower. The pregastric space (Traube) overlies the stomach, is semilunar in outline, and is bounded by the lower edge of the left lung, the anterior border of the spleen, the left costal margin, and the lower edge of the left lobe of the liver.

Small Intestine. The duodenum may be mapped by four continuous lines: (1) a transverse line from the pylorus to the junction of the transpyloric and the right semilunar lines, (2) a descending line passing inferiorly to the lowest level of the subcostal margin (subcostal line at L3), (3) another transverse line passing from right to left and ending about 3.0 cm to the left of the midline, and (4) an ascending line for one to two vertebral levels that terminates at the duodenojejunal flexure. The rest of the small intestine occupies a large amount of the abdominal cavity. The coils of the jejunum are predominantly in the upper left quadrant and those of the ileum in the lower right quadrant. The ileocolic junction is slightly below and medial to the intersection of the right semilunar and transtubercular lines.

Large Intestine and Vermiform Appendix. The cecum lies in the right iliac and hypogastric regions. The middle of its lower border is located about one third (5 cm) of the distance along a line from the right anterior superior iliac spine to the umbilicus. This point (McBurney's) is where tenderness can be elicited when the appendix is inflamed. The right colic flexure is on a level just below the transpyloric plane 2.5 cm lateral to the right semilunar line. The left colic flexure lies just above the transpyloric plane 2.5 cm lateral to the left semilunar line.

Liver. The upper border of the liver corresponds to a horizontal line passing just below the nipples. The inferior border of the liver rather closely parallels the right inferior costal margin, which it leaves at the tip of the ninth costal cartilage, extending from this point obliquely across the subcostal angle to just below the left nipple.

Pancreas. The head of the pancreas occupies the curve of the duodenum and is bounded accordingly. The neck is in the midline at the transpyloric line. The body extends to the left and slightly superiorly, and the tail is in contact with the spleen.

Spleen. The spleen is situated posteriorly beneath the left ninth, tenth, and eleventh ribs. The upper pole lies about 3 cm lateral to the left of the tenth thoracic spine. The lower pole extends as far forward as the midaxillary line at the level of the eleventh rib.

Kidney. The kidneys are about 10 cm long, with about one third of their length being above the transpyloric plane, and the left kidney is about 1 cm to 1.5 cm higher. The upper pole is about 5 cm from the midline; the lower pole, 7.5 cm from the midline. Both kidneys extend above the level of the twelfth rib. The hilum is 5 cm from the midline at the level of L1. On the dorsal aspect of the body the position of the kidneys may be indicated by a parallelogram. Two vertical lines are drawn 2.5 cm and 10 cm from the midline, and the parallelogram is completed by two horizontal lines at the levels of the tips of the spinous processes of T11 and L3.

Ureter. The location of the ureter is indicated by a line from the hilum of the kidney to the bifurcation of the common iliac artery where the ureter enters the pelvis. This vertical line is 3 cm to 4 cm lateral to the midline and is anterior to the transverse processes of the lumbar vertebrae.

ABDOMINAL WALL

Superficial Fascia. This fascia is composed of superficial and deep layers. The superficial or fatty layer ***(Camper's fascia)*** is continuous with the superficial fascia of adjacent areas, for example, thigh and perineum. The deep or fibrous layer ***(Scarpa's fascia)*** attaches to the deep fascia of the thigh but continues into the perineum as the superficial perineal fascia. Thus, fluid collecting in the superficial perineal space can extravasate into the abdominal wall (between the fibrous layer of the superficial fascia and the fascia of the external abdominal oblique muscle) but not into the thigh.

Muscles. The interval between the inferior costal margin and the superior aspect of the pelvis (pubis, inguinal ligament, iliac crest) contains four major muscles, all of which are segmentally innervated by thoracic and lumbar nerves. The external abdominal oblique, internal abdominal oblique, and transversus abdominis are lateral to the semilunar line; the rectus abdominis is medial. The most superficial muscle is the external oblique whose fibers are directed anteriorly, medially, and inferiorly. The fibers of the internal oblique are perpendicular to those of the external oblique. The transversus abdominis fibers are transversely oriented. The aponeuroses of all three muscles extend medially, and together they form the rectus sheath. The rectus abdominis is the only vertically oriented muscle, and it extends between the superomedial aspect of the pubis and the medial aspect of the inferior costal margin and the xiphoid process. Its tendinous inter-

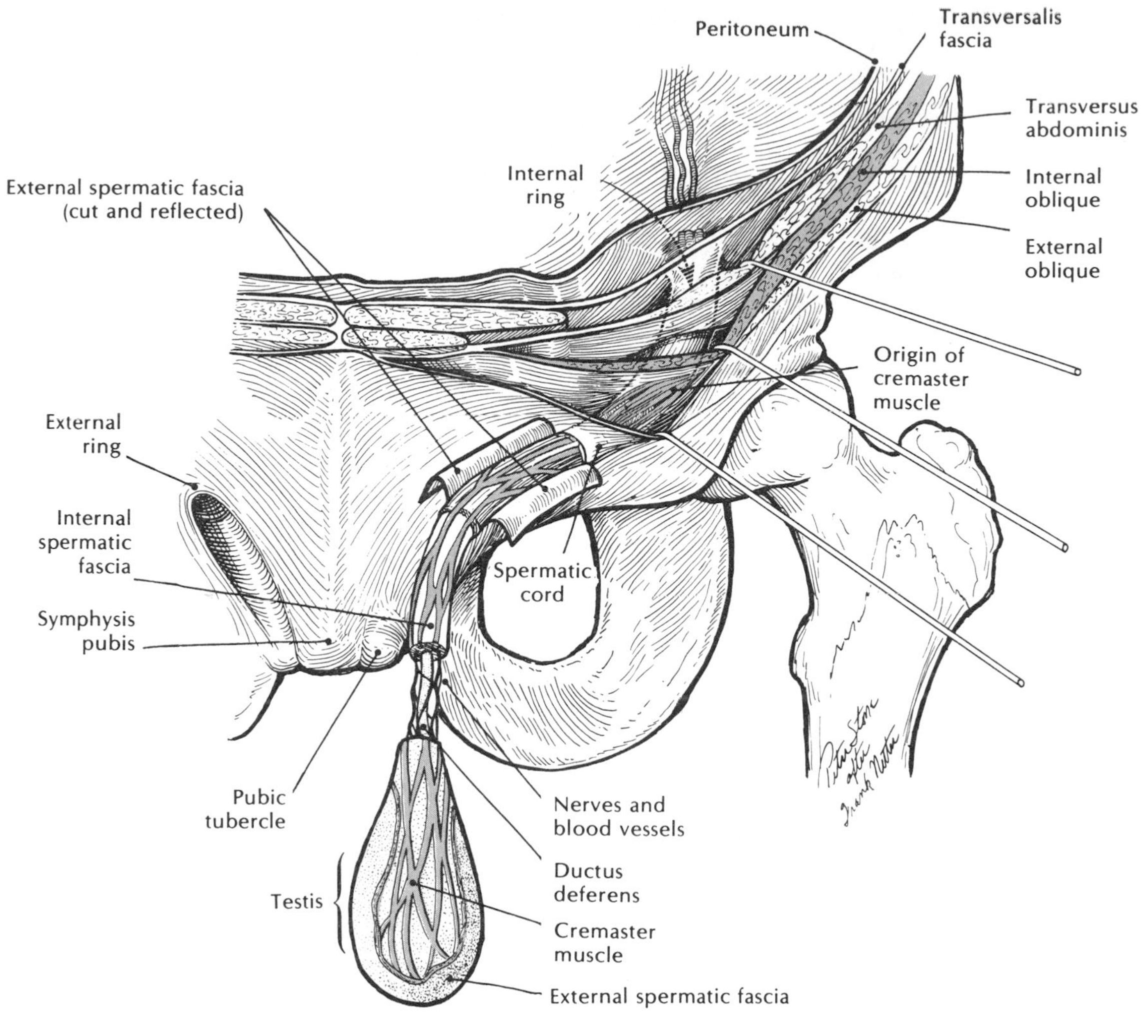

Fig. 2-32. Inguinal canal and spermatic cord. (Christensen JB, Telford IR: Synopsis of Gross Anatomy, 5th ed, p 151. Philadelphia, JB Lippincott, 1988, Langley LL, Telford IR, Christensen JB: Dynamic Anatomy and Physiology, 5th ed. New York, McGraw Hill, 1980)

sections account for the ''ripples'' seen on the surface of the abdomen.

Inguinal Region. The inferior aspect of the abdominal wall is composed primarily of the aponeuroses of the abdominal muscles. The inferior margin of the external oblique aponeurosis forms the ***inguinal ligament*** as it stretches between the anterior superior iliac spine and the pubic tubercle. This tough band also is an attachment for some of the other abdominal muscles, and it participates in the formation of the inguinal canal.

The ***inguinal canal*** is an obliquely oriented pathway through the abdominal wall (Fig. 2-32). It stretches between the superficial (external) and deep (internal) inguinal rings and is directed inferomedially just above the inguinal ligament. The ***superficial ring*** is a split in the external oblique aponeurosis just superolateral to the pubic tubercle. The medial and lateral edges of the ring are called the medial (superior) and lateral (inferior) crura. The ***deep ring*** is the beginning of a sleeve of transversalis fascia that extends along the spermatic cord. This ring is located about halfway between the anterior superior iliac spine and the pubic tubercle.

The boundaries of the inguinal canal are as follows: (1) floor: inguinal ligament; (2) anterior wall: external oblique aponeurosis; (3) posterior wall: medially the conjoined tendon (falx inguinalis), which is composed of the arching medial attachments of the internal oblique and the transversus abdominis, and laterally the transversalis fascia; and (4) roof: conjoined tendon as it arches over the contents of the canal.

The spermatic cord consists of the vas deferens and its artery, the pampiniform plexus of veins, lymphatics, sympathetic nerve fibers, the ilioinguinal nerve, the nerve and artery to the cremasteric muscle, and the testicular artery. Most of these structures are enclosed within the (1) ***internal spermatic fascia,*** which is derived from the transversalis fascia; (2) the ***cremasteric muscle*** and ***fascia,*** which are derived from the internal oblique; and (3) the ***external spermatic fascia,*** which is derived from the aponeurosis of the external oblique.

Inguinal hernias are either direct or indirect, based on the path of the herniating sac. The ***indirect hernia*** follows the course of the testis during development, that is, it passes into the canal through the internal opening and then through the canal. After exiting through the superficial ring, it usually passes into the scrotum. The neck of this type of hernia is found lateral to the inferior epigastric vessels, and the hernial sac is covered with peritoneum and the three fascial coverings of the spermatic cord. A ***direct hernia*** passes through Hesselbach's triangle, that is, the triangular area defined by the lateral border of the rectus abdominis, the inferior epigastric vessels, and the inguinal ligament. The neck of this type of hernial sac is medial to the inferior epigastric vessels and covered by a layer of peritoneum and transversalis fascia. Since this hernia will pass through the superficial ring, it is also covered by the external spermatic fascia.

CONTENTS OF THE ABDOMINAL CAVITY PERITONEUM AND MESENTERIES

The peritoneum is similar to the pleura in that it consists of a parietal layer that lines the abdominopelvic cavity and a visceral layer that is reflected over organs. It is also similar in that the peritoneal cavity contains nothing other than a small amount of lubricating fluid and in reality is a potential space. It differs from the pleura in that its visceral layer reflects in varying degrees over multiple organs. Some organs—jejunum and ileum—are almost completely covered by peritoneum and attached to the posterior body wall by a mesentery and thus are said to be (completely) peritonealized. Other organs (kidneys) are essentially outside the peritoneum and covered by peritoneum on only one side. These organs are extraperitoneal or, if located on the posterior body wall, retroperitoneal. Those organs that are neither peritonealized nor extraperitoneal, but are somewhere in between, are partially peritonealized.

The ***peritoneal cavity*** is separated into greater and lesser peritoneal sacs. The ***lesser sac*** (omental bursa) is posterior to the stomach, lesser omentum, and caudate lobe of the liver. The ***greater sac*** is the rest of the peritoneal cavity. The two areas are connected only through the ***epiploic foramen*** (of Winslow), which is small. The anterior border of this foramen is the right free margin of the lesser omentum, which is formed by the hepatoduodenal ligament and contains (1) the common bile duct, (2) the portal vein, (3) the proper hepatic artery, and (4) lymphatics and nerves.

Within the peritoneal cavity there are areas where inflammatory material can accumulate and become sequestered. These areas are as follows: In the abdomen there are the subphrenic and subhepatic spaces, and the paravertebral gutters. The ***subphrenic spaces*** are found between the liver and the diaphragm, being separated into right and left portions by the coronary and falciform ligaments and lesser omentum. The subhepatic spaces are inferior to the visceral surface of the liver, the right being inferior to the right and caudate lobes of the liver, and the left (omental bursa) inferior to the quadrate lobe. These ***subhepatic spaces*** are connected through the epiploic foramen. The ***paravertebral gutters*** are vertically oriented and on either side of the lumbar vertebral bodies. Each is subdivided into two gutters by the ascending and descending portions of the colon. Thus, each paravertebral gutter consists of a ***medial*** and a ***lateral paracolic gutter.*** When a person is in the supine position, material in the paracolic gutters tends to move superiorly into the subphrenic and subhepatic spaces. In the pelvis of both the male and female there are ***pararectal fossae*** on either side of the rectum. In the male the ***rectovesical pouch*** is found between the rectum and the bladder. In the female the uterus and broad ligament divide that area into two pouches, the ***vesicouterine pouch*** anteriorly and the ***rectouterine pouch*** (of Douglas) posteriorly.

Folds and fossae of the peritoneum occur on the lower part of the anterior abdominal wall. These consist of the single median umbilical fold, and the medial and lateral umbilical folds. The median fold overlies the remains of the urachus; the medial folds are formed by the obliterated umbilical arteries and the lateral by the inferior epigastric vessels. The ***supravesical fossae*** are between the median and medial folds; the ***medial*** and ***lateral inguinal fossae*** are medial and lateral respectively to the lateral fold. Indirect hernias pass through the lateral inguinal fossa, whereas direct hernias pass through either the supravesical or medial inguinal fossa.

The specific peritoneal relationships of each organ are covered with the discussion of that organ.

Stomach. This organ extends from the cardiac opening of the esophagus to the pylorus. It consists of a fundus, a body, and a pyloric portion, the latter made up of the pyloric antrum, canal, and sphincter. Its right or upper border forms the lesser curvature, to which the lesser omentum attaches. The lower and left border forms the greater curvature and gives attachment to the greater omentum and gastrolienal ligament. Posteriorly the stomach is in contact with the spleen, the splenic artery, the diaphragm, the left kidney and suprarenal, the pancreas, and the transverse mesocolon; anteriorly it is in contact with the liver, the diaphragm, and the abdominal wall.

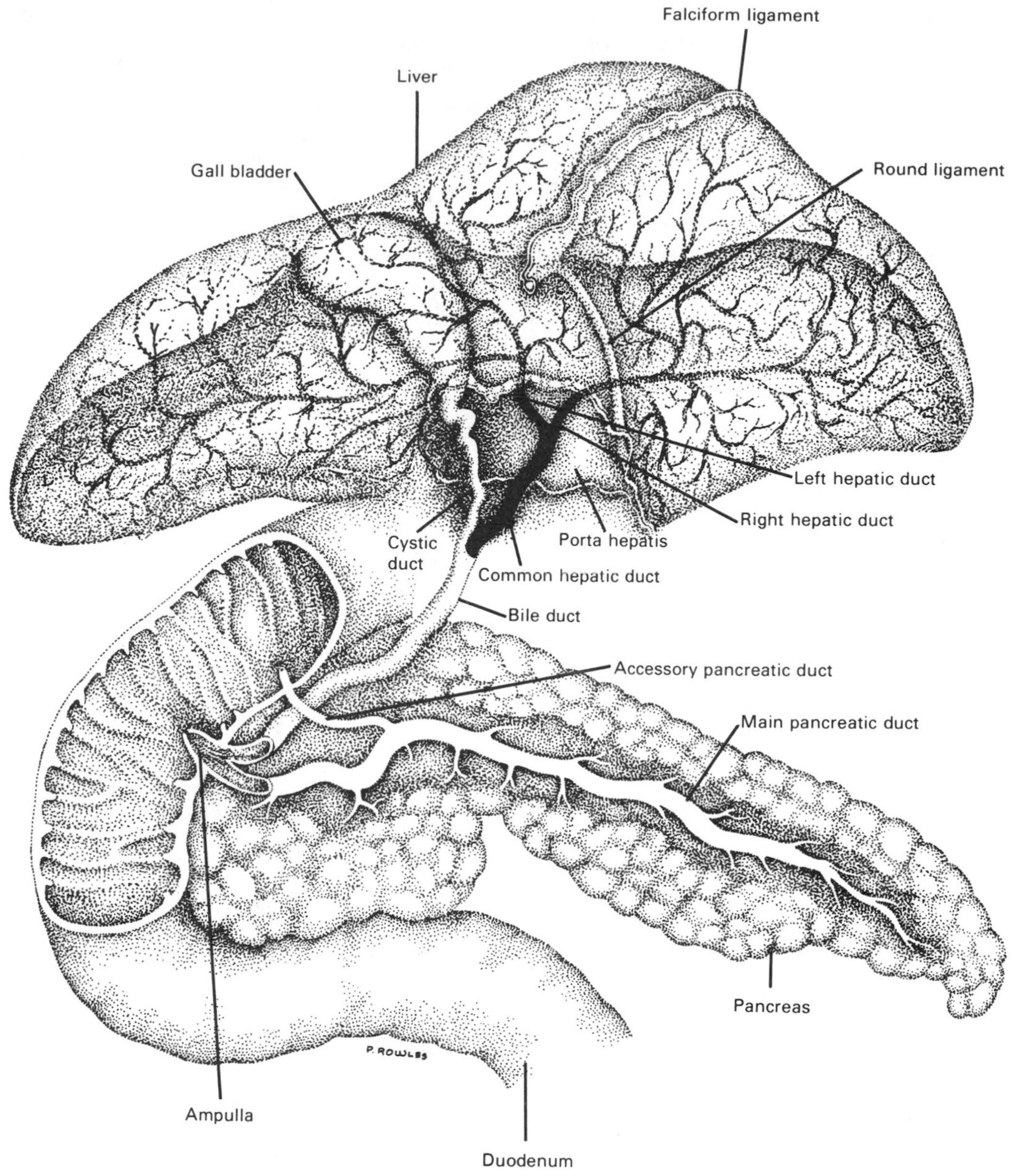

Fig. 2-33. Duct systems of the liver, pancreas, and gallbladder. (Christensen JB, Telford IR: Synopsis of Gross Anatomy, 5th ed, p 168. Philadelphia, JB Lippincott, 1988)

The blood supply to the stomach is provided by the three main branches of the celiac trunk: the common hepatic, left gastric, and splenic arteries. Each of these main branches has branches that pass along the greater or lesser curvatures of the stomach. Venous and lymphatic drainage parallels the arterial supply. The veins are tributaries of the portal vein, and the lymphatics all eventually pass to the celiac group of aortic lymph nodes.

Small Intestine. The ***duodenum*** is a C-shaped tube surrounding the head of the pancreas (Fig. 2-33). It is divided into four parts, most of which are retroperitoneal. The first part is short and ascends slightly from the gastroduodenal junction. It is related anteriorly to the gallbladder and liver and posteriorly to the portal vein, common bile duct, gastroduodenal artery, and the inferior vena cava. The second part descends in the right medial paracolic gutter. Posteriorly it is related to the right kidney and suprarenal gland while anteriorly it is crossed by the transverse colon. The common bile duct and main pancreatic duct empty into it posteromedially. The third part passes from right to left in front of the vena cava, the body of the third lumbar vertebra and the aorta; it passes behind the superior mesenteric vessels. The fourth part is short and curves superiorly and then anteriorly at the duodenojejunal junction. It is suspended from the area of the right crus of the diaphragm by a peritoneal fold called the suspensory ligament of Treitz.

The mesenteric portion of the small intestine is divided into the proximal ***jejunum*** and distal ***ileum.*** The ***mesentery*** is a fan-shaped double layer of peritoneum continuous with the serosa of the jejunum and ileum and enclosing their vessels. The root of the mesentery is about 15 cm long, and its attachment to the posterior body wall extends from the duodenojejunal junction obliquely down and to the right, crossing the third part of the duodenum, the inferior vena cava, and the right ureter. The mesentery contains the intestinal and ileocolic branches of the superior mesenteric vessels as well as lymphatics and autonomics. The transition from jejunum to ileum is not abrupt, but certain differences do exist. The amount of mesenteric fat tends to increase from above downward, as does the number of arcades formed by the vessels in the mesentery. However, the blood supply to the jejunum is greater, so that its pink color is more intense than that of the ileum. The jejunum has a thicker wall as the plicae circulares are higher and more numerous.

Large Intestine. This portion, the ***colon,*** extends from the ileocecal valve to the anus. It is characterized by sacculations (haustra), which are produced by three longitudinal muscle bands (taenia) that converge at the appendix. Between the sacculations are the semilunar folds, and along the free surface of the colon there are pouches containing fat (appendices epiploicae).

The ***cecum*** is a cul-de-sac of the colon below the entrance of the ileum. It is found in the right iliac fossa and is most often almost entirely enveloped in peritoneum. The ileocecal valve is formed by two liplike folds projecting into the medial aspect of the cecum.

The ***vermiform appendix*** is a blind tube that attaches to the posteromedial aspect of the cecum about 2.5 cm below the ileocecal valve. It is most commonly found behind the cecum (retrocecal), although it may be in a variety of positions including extending into the pelvis. It has a slight valve and, although variable, is usually about 10 cm in length. It has no true mesentery but is covered with a peritoneal fold and is supplied by an appendicular branch of the ileocolic artery.

The ***ascending colon*** is the continuation of the cecum that passes superiorly against the posterior body wall and the right kidney. Just below the right lobe of the liver, it makes a sharp bend to the left. This bend is the right colic or hepatic flexure. The ***transverse colon*** extends between the hepatic and the splenic flexures and is suspended from the posterior abdominal wall by the transverse mesocolon. The attachment of the mesocolon crosses the second part of the duodenum and the pancreas, then attaches to the greater curvature of the stomach. The transverse colon is related to the liver, gallbladder and stomach anteriorly, and to the spleen superiorly on the left side of the body. The ***descending colon*** extends from the splenic flexure to the left iliac fossa, passing along the lateral aspect of the left kidney and posterior body wall before becoming the ***sigmoid colon.*** Both the ascending and descending portions of the colon are typically partially peritonealized and therefore fixed in place, as opposed to the peritonealized, mobile transverse colon.

Liver. The anterior, superior, and posterior surfaces of the liver form a dome that is related to the respiratory diaphragm. Through the diaphragm the liver is related to the lungs, pleura, heart, and pericardium. Its posteroinferior or visceral surface is related to the hepatic flexure of the colon, right kidney and suprarenal gland, gallbladder, duodenum, esophagus, and stomach. The visceral surface has an H-shaped configuration in which the center bar of the H is the ***porta hepatis*** where the portal vein, autonomics, and hepatic artery enter, and the common hepatic duct and lympathics exit. The limb of the H extending anteriorly on the right contains the gallbladder; posteriorly on the right is the inferior vena cava; anteriorly on the left is the ligamentum teres; and posteriorly on the left is the ligamentum venosum. That part of the liver between the two anterior limbs is the ***quadrate lobe;*** that portion between the two posterior limbs is the ***caudate lobe.*** Functionally the liver is separated into a large right lobe and a smaller left lobe, which includes the quadrate and caudate lobes.

The liver is partially enclosed within a complicated system of peritoneal folds (Fig. 2-34). The ***falciform ligament*** reflects from the anterior belly wall to the liver and contains the ligamentum teres in its inferior border. Anteriorly the falciform ligament reflects over the right and left lobes of the liver. On the superior and posterior aspects of the dome of the liver the two layers of this ligament initially diverge toward the sides of the liver. At the most lateral extents of these reflections, each layer turns sharply medially and posteriorly; the two layers converge toward one another in the region of the ligamentum venosum. As the two layers of the falciform ligament diverge and then converge in this pattern, they reflect onto the diaphragm. This crown-shaped pattern of peritoneal reflections between the posterosuperior surface of the liver and the under surface of the diaphragm is termed the ***coronary ligament.*** It surrounds the bare area of the liver, an area in which no peritoneum separates the liver and the diaphragm. The right and left extents of the coronary ligament are called the right and left ***triangular ligaments,*** respectively. The lesser omentum extends from the visceral surface of the liver to the lesser curvature of the stomach. The free edge of the lesser omentum is formed as the peritoneum surrounds the portal vein, hepatic artery, and common bile duct. This free edge extends between the first part of the duodenum and the porta

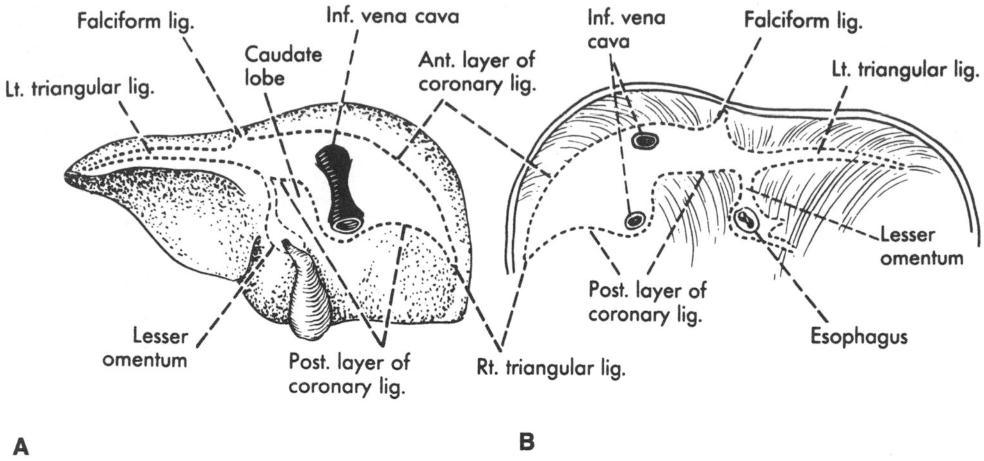

Fig. 2-34. Posterior view of the liver and its peritoneal attachments, illustrated schematically. *(A)* shows the posterior diaphragmatic and visceral surfaces, with lines of reflexion of peritoneum and ligaments indicated; *(B)* shows attachments to the diaphragm. (Hollinshead WH, Rosse C: Textbook of Anatomy, 4th ed, p 646. Philadelphia, JB Lippincott, 1985)

hepatis and forms the anterior boundary of the epiploic foramen (of Winslow), which is the entrance to the lesser omental sac.

The ***portal system*** includes all of the veins that drain the blood from the abdominal part of the digestive tube (except for the lower part of the rectum) and from the spleen, the pancreas, and the gallbladder. The portal vein is formed behind the neck of the pancreas by the union of the superior mesenteric and the splenic veins. It enters the porta of the liver and there, with the hepatic artery, divides into right and left lobar branches. These branches supply the liver lobules and eventually drain to the inferior vena cava by way of hepatic veins. At the porta hepatis, the hepatic artery and the common bile duct are in front of the portal vein with the artery to the left, the duct to the right.

In ***portal obstruction*** there are several alternate routes that blood may take to get from the portal venous system into the systemic circulation without going through the liver. These potential communications are between (1) the superior rectal veins with the middle and inferior rectal veins (which are tributaries of the internal iliac and internal pudendal respectively); (2) esophageal branches of the left gastric with esophageal tributaries of the azygous systems of veins; (3) portal tributaries in the mesenteries with body wall (retroperitoneal) tributaries of the lumbar, renal, and phrenic veins; (4) portal tributaries in the liver with tributaries to the abdominal wall veins in the falciform ligament; and (5) portal tributaries in the liver with phrenic veins across the bare area of the liver.

Gallbladder and Ducts. The ***bile passages*** include the gallbladder, the cystic duct, the hepatic duct, and the common bile duct (see Fig. 2-33). The gallbladder is a pear-shaped viscus lying below the liver between the right and the quadrate lobes. It has a broad fundus, a body, and a neck that narrows into the cystic duct. The body of the gallbladder is related superiorly to the liver, inferiorly to the transverse colon, and posteriorly to the duodenum or pyloric end of the stomach. The fundus of the gallbladder is at the tip of the ninth costal cartilage.

The cystic duct unites with the hepatic duct to form the common bile duct. The common bile and the main pancreatic duct unite just proximal to the point at which they empty into the second part of the duodenum at the major duodenal papilla. This common opening is protected by the sphincter of Oddi.

Pancreas. The pancreas (see Fig. 2-33) lies between the stomach and the posterior abdominal wall, and extends from the duodenum to the spleen. It is completely retroperitoneal. It is divided into a head, lying within the concavity of the duodenum; a neck, which is constricted posteriorly by the portal vein; a triangular body; and a tail that rests upon the spleen. The secretions of the neck, body, and tail portions of the pancreas are carried through the main pancreatic duct, through which they enter the duodenum. The accessory pancreatic duct of Santorini traverses the head of the pancreas and enters the duodenum 2 cm above the major duodenal papilla.

The main arteries supplying the pancreas are the superior and the inferior pancreaticoduodenal and the splenic, the latter running behind the upper part of the body and the tail of the pancreas.

Spleen. This organ occupies the left hypochondrium and the epigastrium under the ribs. Its parietal surface is in relation to the dome of the diaphragm. Its visceral surface is related to the stomach, left kidney, splenic flexure of the colon, and the tail of the pancreas. It is completely peritonealized and connected by peritoneal reflections to the posterior body wall in the region of the left kidney by the lienorenal ligament and to the stomach by the gastrolienal ligament. Its blood supply is provided by the splenic artery.

Kidney. The kidneys are surrounded by perirenal fat and supported by the renal fascia. They extend from the last thoracic to the third lumbar vertebrae, the right kidney being lower than the left. The kidneys are entirely retroperitoneal and are partially separated from the peritoneum by the duodenum on the right and the pancreas on the left.

The kidneys occupy the most dorsal position of all the abdominal organs. Each kidney lies against the diaphragm and the 12th rib above and against the psoas major and the quadratus lumborum below. The anterior relationships of the left kidney are the spleen, stomach, pancreas, left colic flexure, and the small intestine. The anterior surface of the right kidney is related to the liver, second part of the duodenum, and the right colic flexure.

The renal hilus is directed anteromedially and is the concave aspect of the kidney. The renal artery enters the kidney through this area, while the renal vein and ureter exit at this site. The final collecting cistern for urine is the ***renal pelvis.*** The pelvis occupies a large percentage of the hilus and is usually at the level of the body of L1. The pelvis narrows rapidly to form the ***ureter,*** which conducts the urine to the bladder. The ureter is retroperitoneal and descends through the abdominal cavity almost vertically on the anterior aspect of the psoas major muscle. The right ureter is related anteriorly to the duodenum, the vessels to the ascending colon, the root of the mesentery, and the testicular or ovarian vessels. The left ureter is related anteriorly to the left colic vessels, testicular or ovarian vessels, and the sigmoid colon. At roentgenographic examination in which the ureters are filled with contrast medium, they are seen to cross the transverse processes of the lumbar vertebrae. As the ureters enter the pelvis, they incline medially and usually cross the termination of the common iliac arteries (or their branches). Their pelvic courses are inferomedial to the posterior aspect of the bladder. The ureters have three natural constrictions: at the junction of the renal pelvis and the ureter, where they cross the common iliac arteries, and as they pass through the wall of the bladder.

Generally, each kidney is supplied by a single large renal artery that is a direct branch from the abdominal aorta. A common variation, though, is two or three renal arteries on one or both sides.

Suprarenal Glands. The retroperitoneal suprarenal (adrenal) glands sit on the superior poles of each kidney. Both glands are related posteriorly to the diaphragm. The right suprarenal is related anteriorly to the liver and medially to the inferior vena cava. The anterior aspect of the left gland forms part of the posterior wall of the omental bursa and may be related to the splenic artery and the pancreas. Each gland receives a rich blood supply by way of branches from the renal and inferior phrenic arteries and from the aorta.

BLOOD SUPPLY OF THE ABDOMEN

The abdominal aorta (Fig. 2-35) enters the abdomen through the aortic hiatus (T12) and extends to the lower portion of the fourth lumbar vertebral body where it terminates by dividing into the large ***common iliac arteries*** and into its true continuation, the rudimentary ***median sacral artery.*** The aorta descends vertically along the anterior (or slightly to the left) aspect of the lumbar vertebral bodies.

Its branches are as follows:

Inferior phrenic

This pair of arteries arises just below the diaphragm or from the celiac trunk and distributes to the inferior surface of the diaphragm.

Celiac trunk

The highest of the unpaired vessels, it arises at vertebral level T12. This artery is very short; it passes anteriorly behind the peritoneum and above the pancreas, where it divides into its three branches: the left gastric, splenic, and common hepatic. The ***left gastric*** passes to the left, distributes to the lesser curvature of the stomach, and has esophageal and hepatic branches. The ***splenic*** passes to the left along the upper surface of the pancreas. It forms part of the floor of the lesser omental sac and supplies the pancreas and spleen and has the short gastric and left gastroepiploic branches to the greater curvature of the stomach. The ***common hepatic artery*** runs anterolaterally to the right toward the upper aspect of the first part of the duodenum. Its gastroduodenal branch descends behind the duodenum and has anterior and posterior superior pancreaticoduodenal, and right gastroepiploic branches. The continuation of the common hepatic after the gastroduodenal branch is the proper hepatic artery. This artery passes to the right and ascends to the porta hepatis through the lesser omentum. The right gastric artery usually branches from the proper hepatic soon after its beginning; the cystic artery branches where the proper hepatic passes the cystic duct.

Middle suprarenal

These vessels are usually single, one passing directly to each suprarenal gland.

Superior mesenteric

This single artery branches from the anterior aspect of the aorta just inferior (L1) to the celiac trunk and passes

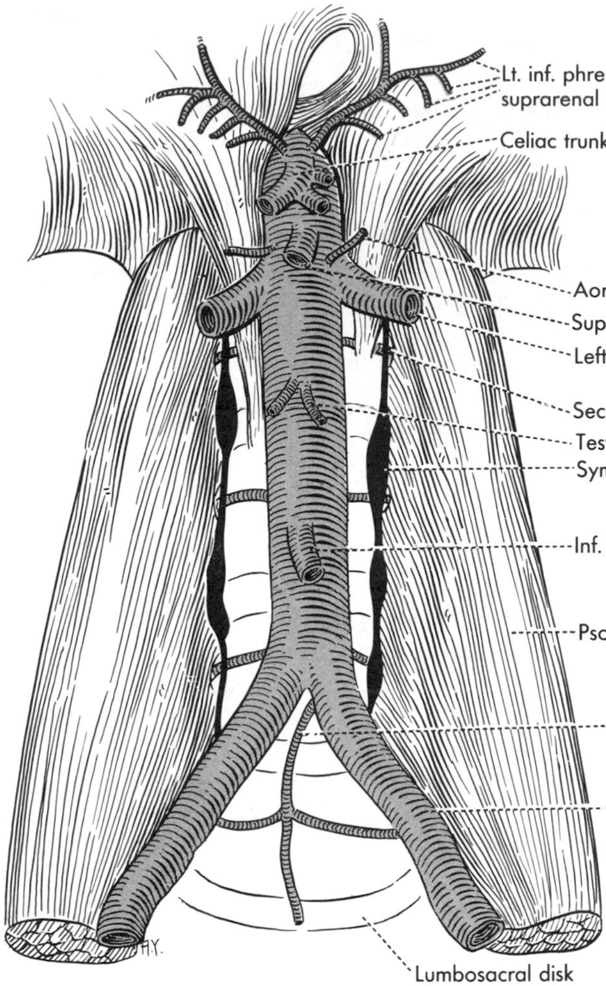

Fig. 2-35. The abdominal part of the aorta and its branches. (Hollinshead WH, Rosse C: Textbook of Anatomy, 4th ed, p 686. Philadelphia, JB Lippincott, 1985)

between the pancreas and the third part of the duodenum. Its branches supply the gastrointestinal tract from the middle of the duodenum through the transverse colon. One of its branches, the inferior pancreaticoduodenal artery, divides into anterior and posterior branches that form the pancreaticoduodenal arcades with the anterior and posterior superior pancreaticoduodenal arteries. The other branches are the intestinal arteries, the ileocolic artery, the right colic artery, and the middle colic artery.

Renal artery

Arising at about the level of the second lumbar vertebra, these two large arteries pass across the crura of the diaphragm and the psoas major muscles in their transverse courses to the hila of the kidneys. The right is longer than the left, and it passes posterior to the inferior vena cava.

Testicular or ovarian arteries

These small arteries arise just inferior to the renal arteries. The retroperitoneal testicular arteries descend obliquely toward the deep inguinal ring where they become part of the spermatic cord. The ureteric branches arise as the testicular arteries cross the ureters. The abdominal course of the ovarian arteries is similar to that of the testiculars. As they reach the pelvic brim, the ovarian arteries swing medially and pass through the suspensory ligament of the ovary to the ovary.

Inferior mesenteric

Arising just below the third part of the duodenum (L3), this artery passes obliquely downward and to the left, behind the peritoneum. Its left colic, sigmoid, and superior rectal branches supply the descending colon, the sigmoid colon, and the upper portion of the rectum.

Lumbar arteries

The four lumbar arteries supply primarily the body wall and those structures within the vertebral canal.

Common iliac arteries.

The large terminal branches of the aorta, the common iliacs, arise slightly to the left of the midline in front

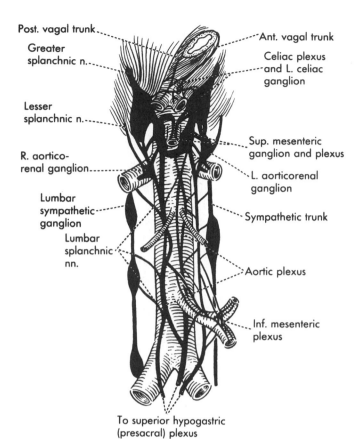

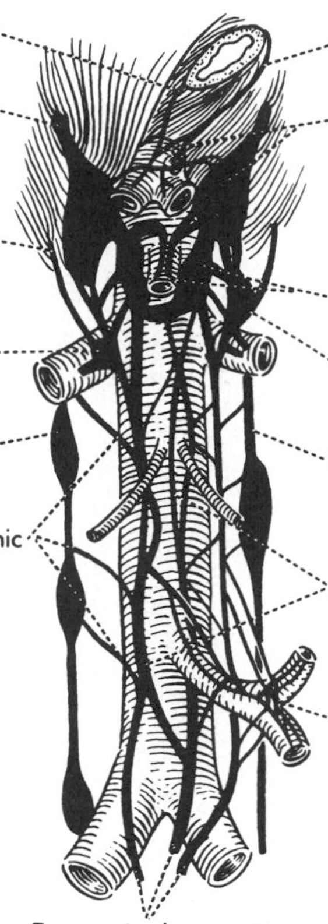

Fig. 2-36. The autonomic nerve plexuses and ganglia associated with the aorta. (Hollinshead WH, Rosse C: Textbook of Anatomy, 4th ed, p 697. Philadelphia, JB Lippincott, 1985)

of the body of the fourth lumbar vertebra. The common iliacs divide into the internal and external iliac arteries just lateral to the sacral promotory. Each internal iliac enters the pelvis to supply pelvic and perineal structures. The external iliac passes under the inguinal ligament where it becomes the femoral artery.

Middle sacral artery.

The true caudal continuation and termination of the aorta, this vessel arises from the posterior aspect of the aorta just above its bifurcation. It passes inferiorly on the ventral aspect of the lumbar vertebrae, enters the pelvis, and descends on the anterior surface of the sacrum and coccyx. It gives rise to parietal branches in its course.

NERVE SUPPLY OF THE ABDOMEN

Body Wall. The skin of the abdominal wall is innervated by the anterior and lateral cutaneous branches of intercostal nerves seven through eleven (T7–T11), the subcostal nerve (T12), and the iliohypogastric branch of the first lumbar nerve. The underlying muscles of the abdominal wall are innervated segmentally by muscular branches of the same nerves.

Viscera. Autonomic innervation of the viscera of the abdominal cavity is provided by sympathetic fibers from spinal cord segments T5 through L1 or L2 and parasympathetic fibers from the vagus nerve and spinal cord segments S2 through S4. These fibers generally are distributed in periarterial plexuses that are associated with the abdominal aorta and its branches. The aortic (preaortic) plexus is a continuous plexus (Fig. 2-36) found on the ventral aspect of the aorta and associated with the three large unpaired arteries. It is divided into the celiac, superior mesenteric, and inferior mesenteric plexuses, with the intermesenteric plexus connecting the superior and inferior mesenterics and the inferior mesenteric plexus continuing inferiorly as the superior hypogastric plexus. Continuations of these plexuses follow various other branches of the aorta to their respective destinations and bear the names of the arteries, for example, the renal plexus.

The sympathetic input into the celiac and superior mesenteric plexuses is from the ***greater*** (T5–T10), ***lesser*** (T10–T12), and ***least*** (T12) ***splanchnic nerves.*** These nerves arise in the thorax and enter the abdomen by passing through the crura of the diaphragm.

The intermesenteric, inferior mesenteric, and superior hypogastric plexuses receive additional sympathetic fibers from the ***lumbar splanchnic nerves,*** which are branches of the lumbar portion of the sympathetic trunk. The fibers in the thoracic and lumbar splanchnic nerves

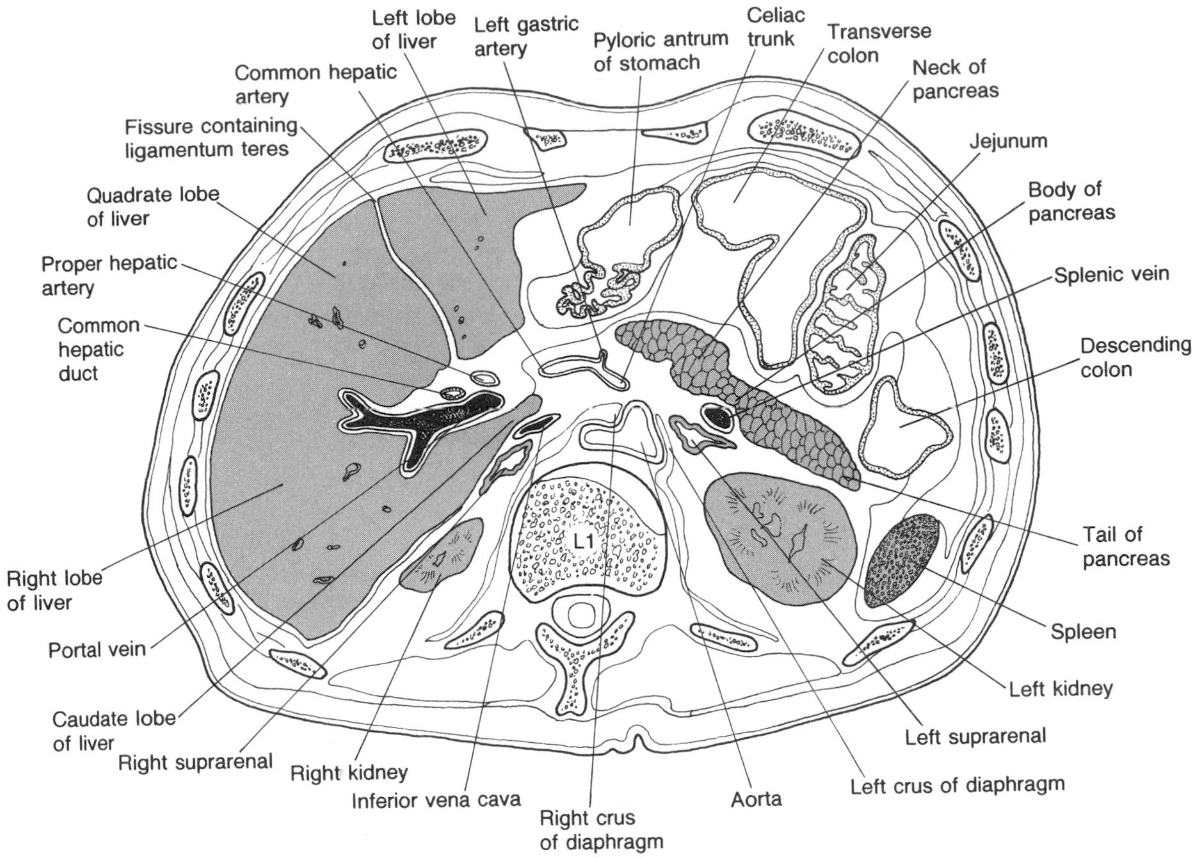

Fig. 2-37. A section through the upper portion of the first lumbar vertebra. (Courtesy of Ms. Carolyn Volpe)

are preganglionic. They synapse with postganglionic fibers in ganglia associated with the aortic plexuses. The largest and most demonstrable of these is the celiac ganglion.

Vagal (parasympathetic) ***fibers*** supply the organs of the abdomen and the gastrointestinal tract as far distally as the splenic flexure of the large intestine. The vagus nerves enter the abdomen with the esophagus as the anterior and posterior vagal trunks. The trunks distribute on the anterior and posterior aspects of the stomach and enter the celiac plexus.

The ***pelvic splanchnics*** (parasympathetic fibers from spinal cord segments S2–S4) provide direct retroperitoneal branches to the descending and sigmoid portions of the large intestine.

The fibers in both the vagus and pelvic splanchnic nerves are preganglionic. They synapse with postganglionic fibers either in or very near the organ innervated.

Afferent fibers from the abdominal viscera reach the CNS through both the vagus and splanchnic nerves. Those sensory fibers in the vagus are concerned with muscular and secretory reflexes. Most pain fibers are thought to be carried in the splanchnic nerves.

CROSS SECTIONS OF THE ABDOMEN

Figure 2-37 represents a section through the upper portion of the first lumbar vertebra. The liver occupies most of the right half of the abdomen, with the left lobe extending to the left and anterior to the stomach. The left and quadrate lobes are separated by the fissure containing the ligamentum teres, and the right lobe is most of the large portion on the right. The caudate lobe is posterior (and superior) to the porta hepatis. In the porta hepatis the portal vein is posterior to both the common hepatic duct and the proper hepatic artery, with the duct being to the right of the artery. The superior pole of the right kidney is related anteriorly to the right lobe of the liver and the right suprarenal gland. The right suprarenal gland is bounded anteriorly by the inferior vena cava, posteriorly by the right kidney, laterally by the right lobe of the liver, and medially by the right crus of the diaphragm. The celiac trunk passes anteriorly from the aorta and branches into the left gastric artery, which passes anteriorly, and the common hepatic artery, which passes to the right. The left kidney is related laterally to the spleen and anteriorly to the body and tail of the pancreas, the left suprarenal, and the descending colon. The left suprarenal is postero-

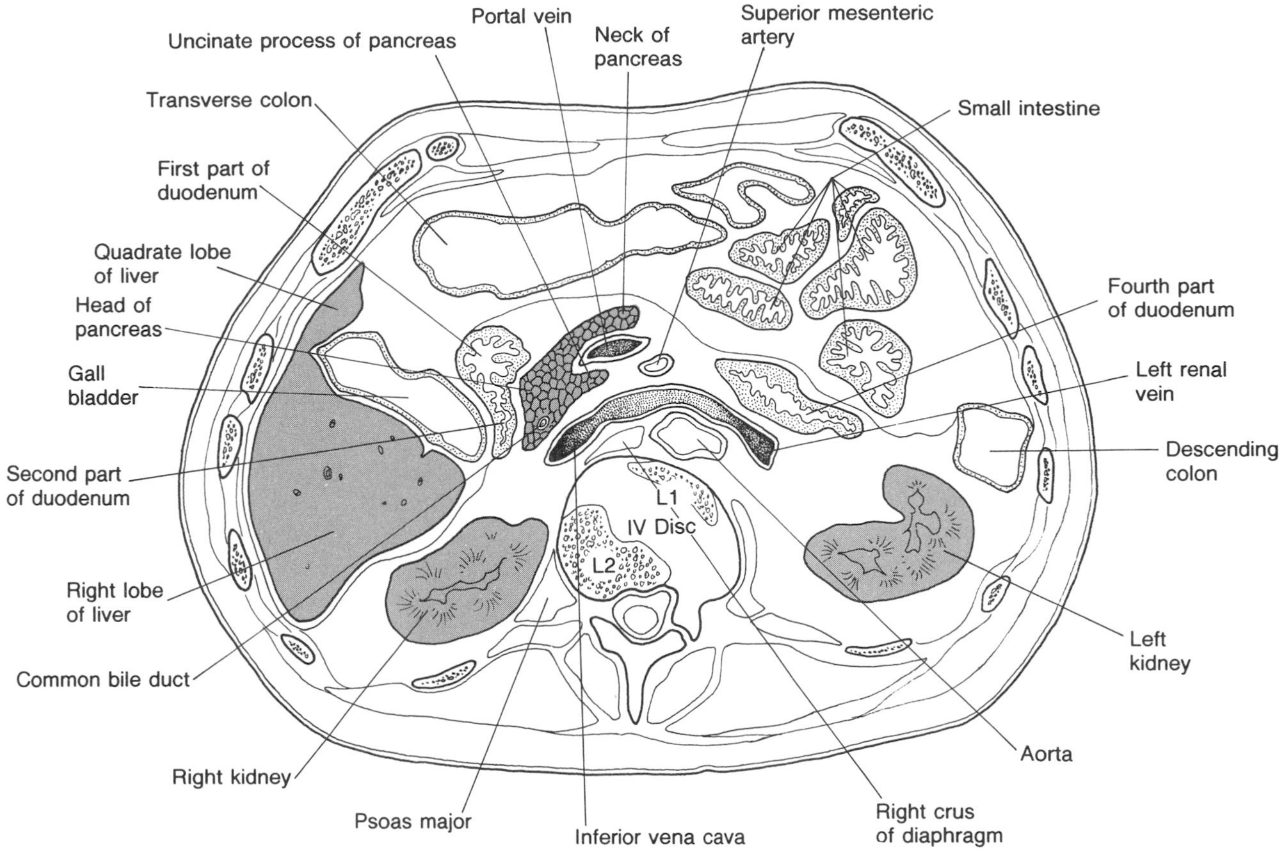

Fig. 2-38. A section through the intervertebral disc between the first and second lumbar vertebrae. (Courtesy of Ms. Carolyn Volpe)

medial to the splenic vein and body of the pancreas, anteromedial to the left kidney, and lateral to the left crus of the diaphragm. The splenic vein is positioned between the pancreas anteriorly and the left suprarenal posteriorly. The splenic vein would be displaced (splenic vein sign) anteriorly by a mass in the left suprarenal and posteriorly by a pancreatic mass. The pyloric antrum of the stomach is posterior to the left lobe of the liver and anterior to the pancreas.

Figure 2-38 represents a section that passes through the intervertebral disc between lumbar vertebrae one and two. Only portions of the right and quadrate lobes of the liver are found at this level, with the gallbladder found in the groove between the two. The inferior vena cava is positioned slightly to the right of the vertebral column; the left renal vein passes to the right anterior to the aorta and posterior to the superior mesenteric artery on its way to the inferior vena cava. The portal vein is seen where it is formed, posterior to the neck of the pancreas and anterior to the uncinate process. The first and second parts of the duodenum are continuous, the second passing posteriorly from the first. The head of the pancreas is related to the first and second parts of the duodenum and has the common bile duct embedded in its posterior aspect. The transverse colon passes from right to left, crossing the duodenum and the pancreas. The descending colon descends along the posterior abdominal wall, passing anterior to the left kidney.

Figure 2-39 represents a section through the third lumbar vertebra. The inferior vena cava is anterior and somewhat to the right of the vertebral column; the aorta is anterior and somewhat to the left. The third part of the duodenum passes from right to left across the vertebral column, anterior to the great vessels and posterior to the superior mesenteric artery. The hepatic flexure of the colon is related laterally to the inferior tip of the right lobe of the liver. The right kidney, which is still present at this level, is related anteriorly to the hepatic flexure of the colon and the second part of the duodenum. The ureters descend across the anterolateral aspects of the psoas major muscles. The superior mesenteric artery occupies the root of the mesentery.

MICROSCOPIC STRUCTURE OF ABDOMINAL ORGANS

Gastrointestinal Tract. The general histologic plan of the gastrointestinal tract consists of four layers:

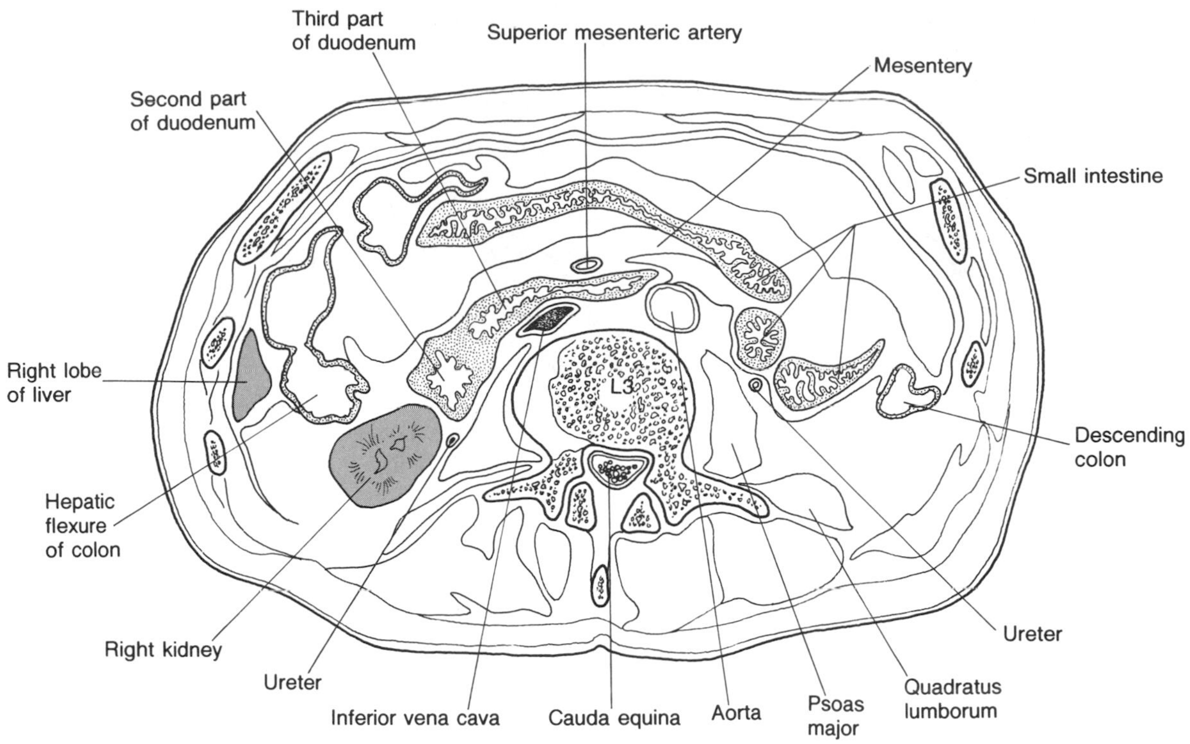

Fig. 2-39. A section through the third lumbar vertebra. (Courtesy of Ms. Carolyn Volpe)

an inner mucosa, a submucosa, a muscularis externa, and an outer serosa (see Fig. 2-29). These were reviewed in the section on the esophagus. Different parts of the gastrointestinal tract retain the basic plan but differ as to their internal configuration of the mucosa, epithelial lining, type and extent of mucosal and submucosal glands, and by their thickness and configuration of muscle.

The ***stomach*** is structurally modified for the production of hydrochloric acid and pepsin and for the mixing of food with these substances. In the empty stomach the mucosa is thrown into longitudinal folds called ***rugae.*** Throughout the stomach the simple columnar lining epithelium produces mucus and indents into the mucosa as gastric pits. One or more mucosal glands empty into the base of each pit. The length of glands and pits and the glandular cell types differ in the cardiac, body (fundus), and pyloric regions of the stomach. Gastric glands of the body and fundus are the most prevalent and contain the most diverse cell types. In this type of gland, chief cells are located mostly in the base (fundus), parietal cells are located in the neck and isthmus region, mucous neck cells are in the neck, and argentaffin (enteroendocrine, enterochromaffin, amine precursor uptake [and] decarboxylation [APUD]) cells are scattered. Undifferentiated columnar cells in the neck region of the gland differentiate and move upward to replace the lining epithelium, which turns over every 3 to 7 days. Other undifferentiated cells move into the glands where they differentiate into the gland cells.

Chief cells produce pepsin and are typical enzyme-secreting cells in that they contain much RER, a well-established Golgi apparatus, and membrane-bound zymogen granules. In these cells, amino acids attached to tRNA are carried to rRNA of the RER where the pepsinogen code is translated from mRNA. The protein product passes into the cisterna of the RER and is carried to transfer vesicles near the Golgi apparatus. In this region the membrane-bound pepsinogen granule is formed. The granule passes to the apical surface of the cell where the product is discharged when the membrane of the granule fuses with the plasma membrane and then opens to the lumen (exocytosis, merocrine secretion). ***Parietal cells*** produce HC1 and seem to produce the intrinsic antipernicious anemia factor. They are rounded, or pyramidal, cells whose apices open to the lumen through an intercellular canal between adjacent chief cells. An extensive infolding of the surface membrane forms intracellular canaliculi into which microvilli project. SER and mitochondria are prevalent, and the cells are often binucleate. In the production of HC1, sodium chloride probably passes to the intracellular canaliculi where hydrogen ion, supplied by carbonic acid in the cell, is exchanged for sodium. Thus,

HCl passes into the lumen of the gland while bicarbonate passes from the cell into the blood. Mucous neck cells produce mucus of a different nature than that of the surface epithelium. Argentaffin cells are sandwiched between the other gland cells and the basement membrane. Some of these produce serotonin while other types of these cells produce cholinesterase; both of these secretions are discharged into the bloodstream. Other ***enteroendocrine*** (APUD) ***cells*** seem to produce a glucagonlike substance, while still others produce gastrin.

Pyloric and cardiac glands contain only cells that are similar to the neck mucous cell. In the pyloric region the gastric pits are deep, and the glands are very tortuous and appear shorter.

The muscularis externa layer of the stomach, unlike other portions of the GI tract, contains three layers of smooth muscle, an outer longitudinal, a middle circular, and an inner oblique layer. The two inner layers are thickened in the pylorus as the pyloric sphincter muscle. The serosa is continuous at the greater curvature with the two layers of the greater omentum and at the lesser curvature with the two layers of the lesser omentum.

The ***small intestine*** is structurally modified for the absorption of nutritive substances. The absorptive surface is large because of (1) mucosal and submucosal folds called plicae circulares, (2) mucosal projections called villi, and (3) microvilli forming a striated border on the simple columnar lining epithelium. Mucus is secreted by goblet cells in the lining epithelium. These cells increase in number at progressively lower levels of the gastrointestinal tract where drier wastes are accumulating. ***Crypts of Lieberkühn*** are mucosal glands that are found throughout the intestine; they empty at the bases of the villi. Their cells replace the lining cells of the villi every 7 to 8 days and thus show mitoses and gradations of differentiation. Some of the enteroendocrine gland cells produce secretin and cholecystokinin. Argentaffin cells and Paneth's cells are present in the crypts of Lieberkühn. In the upper part of the duodenum, Brunner's glands occupy the submucosa and empty into the crypts or the bases of intervillous spaces. Their cells are similar to those in the pyloric glands and produce an alkaline glycoprotein secretion. The lower ileum contains aggregations of lymphatic nodules called Peyer's patches. These are located opposite the mesentery attachment, chiefly in the mucosa. The muscularis externa consists of inner circular and outer longitudinal smooth muscle layers. Myenteric and submucosal nerve plexi containing autonomic postganglionic cell bodies and cells of the enteric nervous system are present throughout the intestine and stomach.

The absorption of fats, carbohydrates, proteins, and water in the small intestine takes place through the simple columnar lining cells of the villi since the tight junctions (zonula occludens) of the ***junctional complexes*** (zonula occludens, zonula adherens, and macula adherens) do not permit intercellular passage. Thus, carbohydrates, fats, and proteins must be broken down in the lumen before absorption can take place. Some of this is accomplished by pancreatic enzymes and liver bile salts. Intestinal juices produced by crypt glands and the lining epithelium are also involved in the terminal hydrolytic digestion of carbohydrates and proteins. The active sites of much of this activity seem to be in the microvillus region near the glycoprotein "fuzz" coat of the plasma membrane. Substances absorbed through the surface epithelium pass to capillaries or the central lacteal of the villi for distribution in the portal vein or thoracic duct, respectively. In fat absorption, bile salts and lipase produce micelles of fatty acids and monoglycerides which passively enter the cell. In the cytoplasm, the SER resynthesizes triglycerides and the RER produces proteins in the production of chylomicrons; these are discharged into the intercellular space, where they pass mostly to the lacteals.

The ***large intestine*** absorbs much water and produces mucus that lubricates the feces. No villi are present, and the crypts open directly on the surface. The lining epithelium is simple columnar with a striated border, and it contains many goblet cells. The outer longitudinal layer of the muscularis externa has three longitudinally running thickened bands of smooth muscle (taenia coli).

The ***appendix*** is microscopically similar to the colon except that it is smaller, does not have taenia, and possesses a prominent ring of lymphatic nodules that occupy most of the lamina propria and the submucosa.

The ***anal canal*** functions to retain and eliminate wastes. The colonlike mucosa of the upper portion forms longitudinal anal columns just above the horizontally oriented anal valves. Epithelium over the anal valves is stratified squamous nonkeratinized epithelium. It becomes keratinized about 2.5 cm below the valves. The lamina propria contains large internal hemorrhoidal veins and circumanal glands. The inner circular layer of the muscularis becomes the internal anal sphincter. The outer longitudinal layer disappears and is replaced in position by skeletal muscle of the external anal sphincter.

Liver and Gallbladder. The liver is surrounded by a tough connective tissue capsule that penetrates it at the porta to produce many septa. These septa provide support for the parenchyma and divide it into lobes and lobules. Branches of the portal vein and hepatic artery further subdivide within the septa and supply the lobules. These vessels and bile ducts constitute portal triads (portal canals, spaces) at the junction of adjacent lobules.

The ***hepatic lobules*** consist of a central vein from which anastomosing hepatic plates of cells, usually one cell thick, radiate toward the periphery (Fig. 2-40). Between the plates are hepatic sinusoids that connect the portal vein and hepatic artery peripherally with the central vein centrally. Blood drains from the central vein to sublobular veins and leaves the liver by way of the hepatic

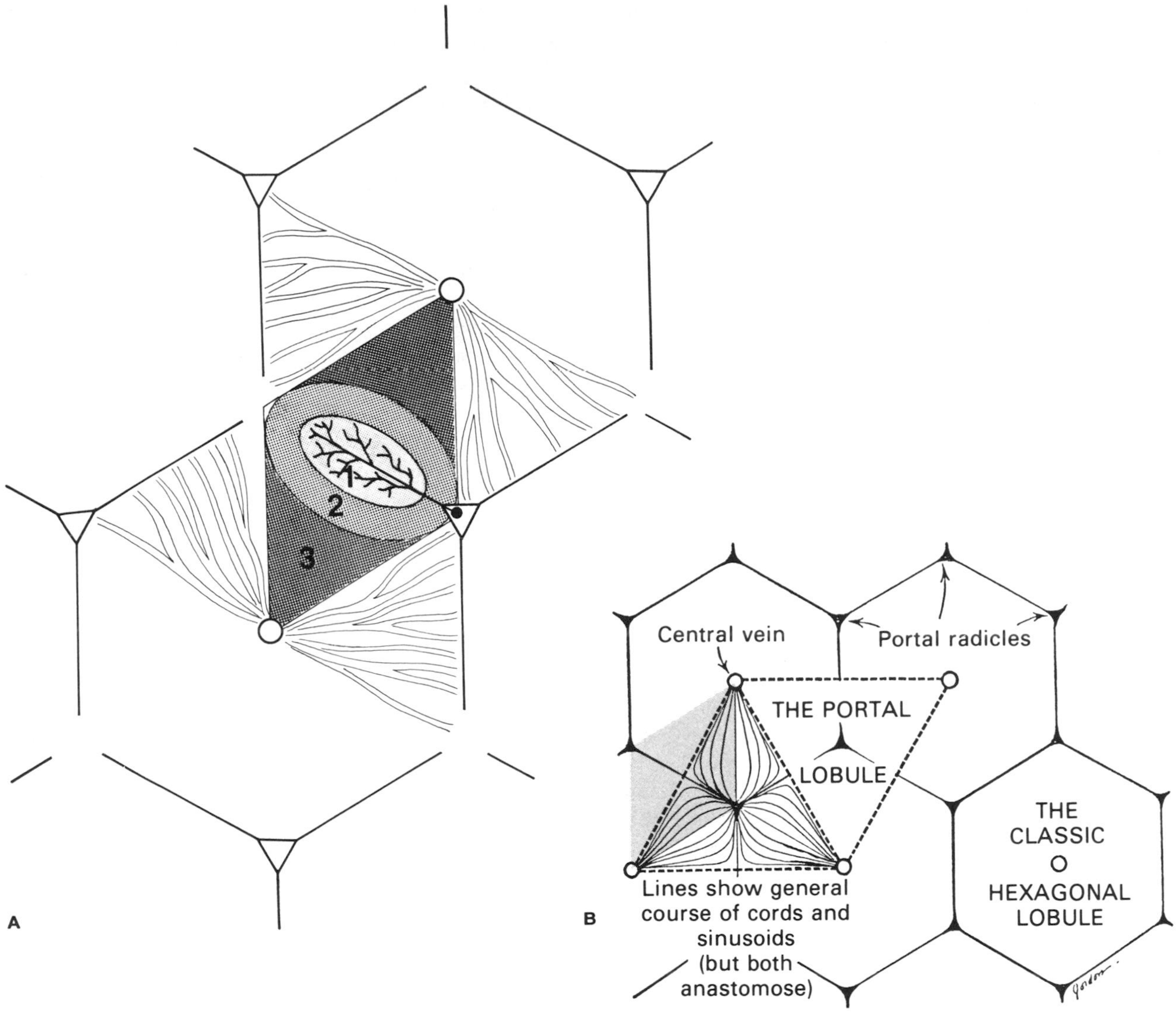

Fig. 2-40. Diagrammatic representation of *(A)* the liver acinis and *(B)* the classic lobule and portal lobule. In *(A)* the numbers indicate the distance of zones from the blood supplied by the vascular backbone extending from the portal area. In *(B)* the portal area is the center of the portal lobule, whereas the central vein is the center of the classic lobule. (Cormack DH: Ham's Histology, 9th ed, p 527. Philadelphia, JB Lippincott, 1987)

veins. The sinusoids are discontinuously lined by endothelial cells and phagocytic Kupffer cells (stellate macrophages) of the reticuloendothelial system. The lining cells abut against microvilli of the hepatocytes, leaving a space (of Disse) between the base of the endothelial cell and the hepatocyte; this space is continuous with the sinusoids, thus providing for efficient interchange between blood in the sinusoid and the hepatocyte. Bile canaliculi lie between adjacent hepatocytes in the hepatic plates and are expansions of the intercellular spaces between the cells. They are separated from the rest of the intercellular space by occluding junctions; microvilli of the hepatic cells extend into the canalicular lumen. These canaliculi receive bile produced by the hepatocytes and conduct it peripherally into small ducts that open into the bile ducts of the portal triad. Bile is transported out of the liver in hepatic ducts; it then traverses the cystic duct and is stored and condensed in the gallbladder. Bile is discharged from the gallbladder through the cystic duct and common bile duct and empties at the sphincters of Oddi and Boyden into the duodenum. The epithelium lining the bile ducts grades from low cuboidal to high columnar with the increasing caliber of the ducts. ***Hepatocytes*** are polyhedral, with one or more large rounded nuclei. They contain a wide range of organelles that are consistent with the many and diverse functions these cells perform. The SER is involved in the synthesis of glycogen, in the inactivation and detoxification of drugs, in the synthesis of bile acids, and in the production of water-soluble bilirubin glucuronide. The RER synthesizes lipoproteins, prothrombin, albumin, and fibrinogen. Hepatocytes also store lipids, carbohydrates, and vitamins; recirculate bile acids; and can carry out gluconeogenesis. Kupffer cells, like other cells of the mononuclear phagocyte system, assist hepatocytes by producing bilirubin by the breakdown of hemoglobin from phagocytized worn-out erythrocytes.

Two methods of classification of liver lobules are used other than the classic hepatic lobule mentioned above (Fig. 2-40). The ***portal lobule*** has a portal triad at the center, with the periphery of the lobule being those adjacent portions of hepatic plates that drain into the bile duct of the portal triad. The ***hepatic*** (Rappaport) ***acinus*** is a diamond-shaped area that drains into an interlobular vein between adjacent hepatic lobules; the periphery of the acinus extends to the central veins of the two adjacent lobules.

The ***gallbladder*** is lined by a mucous membrane that is thrown into folds. It possesses a simple columnar epithelium whose sodium pump transports sodium chloride through the epithelium and extensive lateral intercellular spaces to underlying capillaries; this leads to the passive reabsorption of water and the concentration of bile. A circularly arranged smooth muscle layer is present and is surrounded by a prominent connective tissue layer.

Pancreas. The pancreas is divided into lobules by connective tissue septa. The lobules are packed with serous acini consisting of enzyme-secreting pyramidal cells and centroacinar cells. The serous-secreting cells are similar in structure to other protein-secreting cells (*e.g.*, chief cells of the stomach). The cells are arranged in acini with small centroacinar cells lining the lumen. The pyramidal secretory cells are regulated by cholecystokinin, which causes secretion of proteases, nucleases, amylase, and lipase. The centroacinar and intercalated duct cells, when stimulated by secretin, produce high concentrations of sodium bicarbonate. The intercalated ducts drain acini to larger intralobular ducts, which empty successively to interlobular ducts and the main pancreatic duct (of Wirsung) or accessory duct (Santorini). The larger ducts have simple columnar epithelium, goblet cells, and mucous glands; the smaller ducts are lined with simple cuboidal epithelium.

Islets of Langerhans are heavily vascularized groups of cells scattered throughout the pancreas. There are several cell types present in the islets. The most common type is the insulin-producing beta cell. Absence or malfunction of these cells leads to diabetes mellitus. Another prominent cell type of the islets is the alpha cell which produces glucagon, a hyperglycemic-glycogenolytic factor. Delta cells in the islets produce somatostatin and possibly gastrin, while PP cells may help regulate acinar cell secretion.

Spleen. The spleen is the largest lymphoid organ in the body, and it is specialized for filtering blood. The spleen consists of white pulp (splenic nodules) and red pulp. The ***white pulp*** is dense lymphatic tissue; the ***red pulp*** is looser and consists of lymphatic splenic cords of tissue and venous sinusoids. Arterial blood enters the spleen at the hilum in the splenic artery. Branches of this artery pass in connective tissue trabeculae that radiate from the capsule at the hilar region. These are trabecular (interlobular) arteries. At the ends of the trabeculae the adventitia of the arteries takes on the character of reticular tissue and becomes infiltrated with lymphocytes forming splenic nodules (white pulp). These arteries are eccentrically located in the nodules and are called central arteries. After numerous branchings these arterioles leave the white pulp and enter the reticular connective tissue of the red pulp that surrounds the splenic nodules. In the red pulp the pulp arterioles divide into sheathed arterioles that empty into sinusoids via terminal arterial capillaries or empty first into the pulp reticulum and then filter between the lining cells of the sinusoids. Many macrophages of the reticuloendothelial (mononuclear phagocytic) system lie outside the walls of the sinusoids and phagocytize worn-out RBCs. The venous sinuses empty into pulp veins that pass to trabecular veins before blood is emptied by way of the splenic vein. In addition to the filtering of blood, the spleen controls the blood volume by storing RBCs and by periodically discharging the blood through the contraction of smooth muscle and the action of elastic fibers in the capsule and trabeculae. The spleen also produces lymphocytes, monocytes, plasma cells, and antibodies. Most of the lymphocytes that leave the spleen are from the recirculating pool of lymphocytes; relatively few new lymphocytes are formed in the spleen. The spleen is involved in both the cell-mediated and humoral responses to antigens. In the white pulp, T-lymphocytes are located in the periarterial sheath with B-lymphocytes being located more peripherally. When B cells are activated, they move to the germinal center and give rise to plasma cells, which elaborate antibodies in the red pulp. Activated B cells also return to the general circulation by way of the red pulp sinuses. In the secondary responses to antigens by memory cells, the spleen is one of the most active organs in antibody secretion.

Suprarenal (Adrenal) Glands. The suprarenal glands are divisible into two parts: a mesodermally derived cortex and a neural ectodermally derived medulla. A thick connective tissue capsule sends radially directed trabeculae of reticular fibers into the underlying cortex. The ***cortex*** consists of an outer zona glomerulosa, a middle zona fasciculata, and an inner zona reticularis. Columnar cells of the zona glomerulosa are arranged in arches. They produce mineralocorticoids (*e.g.*, aldosterone). The zona fasciculata consists of cords of cells that radiate inward from the zona glomerulosa. These cords are two cells thick, contain cuboidal cells that are often binucleate, and are separated from adjacent cords by fenestrated capillaries that radiate inward from the capsule. Fasciculata cells often contain much lipid and appear vacuolated. The zona reticularis consists of irregularly arranged cords of cells that may contain lipofuscin pigment. Fasciculata and reticularis cells are under the control of adrenocorticotropic hormone (ACTH) from the adenohypophysis; they produce glucocorticoids (*e.g.*, cortisol, corticosterone) and the sex hormone dehydroepiandrosterone. The most prominent organelle in adrenal cortical cells is an extensive SER, which is indicative of steroid-secreting cells.

The ***suprarenal medulla*** produces epinephrine and norepinephrine in its polyhedral basophilic cells. These cells receive terminations of preganglionic sympathetic nerve fibers, and each cell is located between a venule and a capillary. The cells exhibit the chromaffin reaction. The blood supply of the suprarenal gland is by branches of the suprarenal arteries that (1) go directly to the medulla from the capsule, and (2) go indirectly to the medulla through capsular arterioles and their radiating capillary plexuses that pass between the cortical cords of cells before reaching the medulla.

Kidney, Ureter, and Bladder. The ***kidney*** is divisible into an outer cortex and an inner medulla (Fig. 2-41). The ***medulla*** consists of renal pyramids, with the broad base of each pyramid facing the cortex, while the apex (renal papilla) opens into a minor calyx. The 10 to 16 minor calyces open into two or three major calyces, which in turn empty into the funnel-shaped renal pelvis

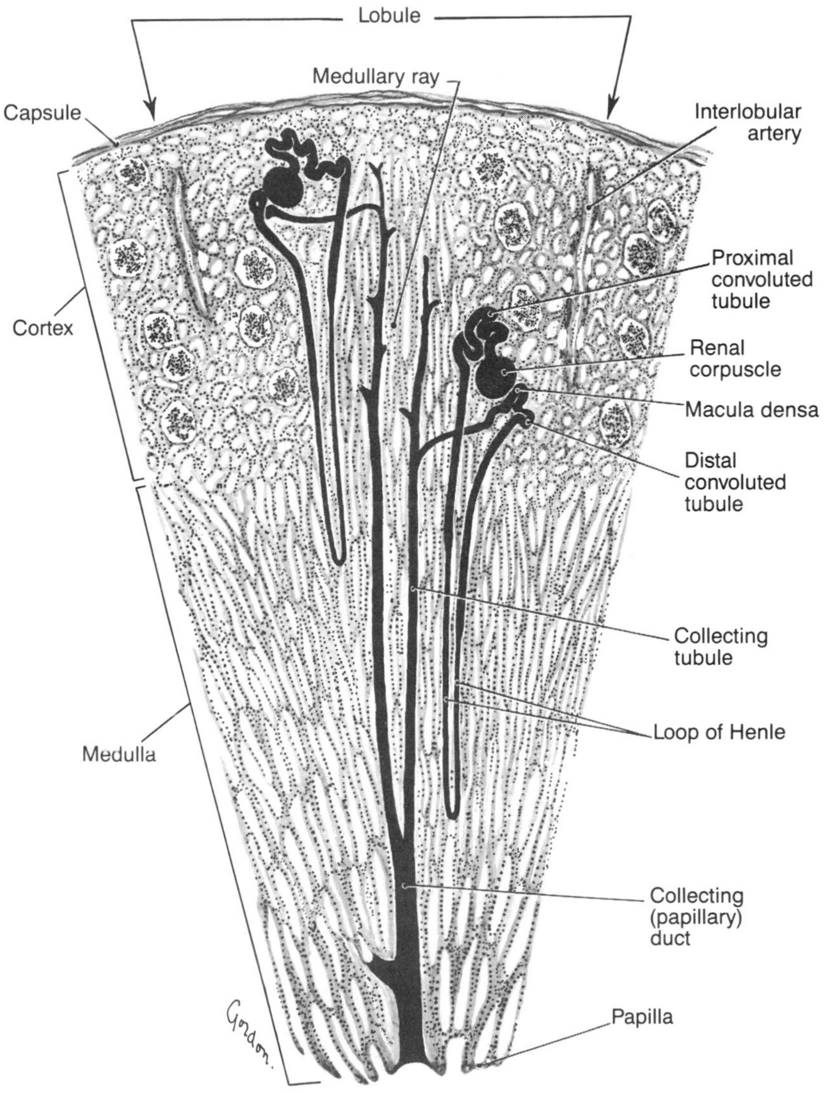

Fig. 2-41. Diagrammatic representation of a kidney lobule. Two nephrons emptying into collecting tubules are represented in black. (Cormack DH: Ham's Histology, 9th ed, p 569. Philadelphia, JB Lippincott, 1987)

at the hilus of the kidney. The ***cortex*** lies peripheral to the medulla and extends between the pyramids as renal columns. The cortex consists of medullary rays (pars radiata) and cortical labyrinths (pars convoluta). The medullary rays are parallel accumulations of collecting tubules and thick and thin limbs of the loop of Henle, which radiate toward the medulla. Each of these is surrounded by cortical labyrinth tissue of glomeruli and convoluted tubules that empty into the tubules of the medullary ray. A medullary ray and its surrounding cortical labyrinth constitutes a lobule. A kidney lobe is a renal pyramid with its overlying cortex and renal columns.

The functional unit of the kidney is the ***uriniferous tubule,*** which consists of a nephron and collecting tubule. (Note: Some authors define the uriniferous tubule as the nephron.) The nephron is comprised of the renal corpuscle (of glomerulus and Bowman's capsule), the proximal convoluted tubule; the thick descending limb, thin portion of descending limb, loop of Henle, thin portion of ascending limb, thick ascending limb; and the distal convoluted tubule (see Fig. 2-41). The glomerulus is a tuft of fenestrated capillaries fed by an afferent arteriole and drained by a smaller efferent arteriole. It is invested by podocytes of the visceral layer of Bowman's capsule. The podocytes have pedicles that interdigitate with those from adjacent podocytes and attach to a basal lamina between the podocyte and the capillary endothelium. Filtration slits 25nm wide exist between pedicles and communicate with the lumen of Bowman's capsule. At the basal lamina surface these slits are connected by a thin slit membrane. The podocytes, basal lamina, and fenestrated endothelium constitute the ***filtration barrier.*** Mesangial phagocytic (stalk) cells in the glomerulus probably remove filtration residues from the basal lamina, which is the main filter for large molecules. The parietal layer of Bowman's capsule consists of simple squamous epithelium.

The ***proximal convoluted tubule*** is the longest and widest portion of the nephron. It is comprised of a simple pyramidal epithelium possessing a brush border (microvilli) and indistinct lateral borders. The proximal convoluted tubule is located in the cortical labyrinth. It is continuous with, and histologically similar to, the thick descending limb of Henle's loop that courses in the medullary ray. Both the proximal and straight descending tubules resorb 85% or more of the water and sodium chloride of the glomerular filtrate. Glucose and amino acids also are resorbed by the epithelium of these tubules. The ***thin portion of Henle's loop*** is comprised of simple squamous epithelium. Its descending and ascending portions function similarly to the thick descending and ascending portions, respectively.

The thick ascending and ***distal convoluted tubules*** have a low cuboidal epithelium with scattered microvilli and an extensive infolding of the basal plasma membrane. In these tubules sodium is transported out of the cells, and the filtrate becomes hypotonic and acidic. Where the distal tubule abuts against the afferent glomerular arteriole the epithelium is columnar and constitutes the macula densa. The muscle cells of the adjacent afferent glomerular arteriole are replaced by large pale juxtaglomerular cells containing granules. These cells produce renin and along with cells of the macula densa and some interposed cells constitute the ***juxtaglomerular complex.*** Renin acts on its substrate, angiotensinogen, producing angiotensin I, which is converted to angiotensin II; the latter brings about increased secretion of aldosterone by the adrenal cortex. Aldosterone acts on the distal convoluted tubule to bring about reabsorption of sodium and thus reduce sodium loss in the urine.

The ***collecting tubules*** consist of pale, clear simple cuboidal epithelium with distinct lateral boundaries. These tubules join to form papillary ducts lined by simple columnar epithelium. Under the influence of antidiuretic hormone from the neurohypophysis, the epithelium of the collecting tubules becomes more permeable to water, and the latter is passively removed from the urine.

Arterial blood is carried to the hilar region of the kidney by the renal artery. This artery branches into interlobar branches that give rise to arcuate arteries passing along the corticomedullary junction. Interlobular arteries arise from the arcuate arteries and pass peripherally in the cortical labyrinths to give rise to afferent glomerular arterioles supplying the glomeruli. From the glomeruli, efferent arterioles supply the capillary plexi around the tubules. Capillaries of the medulla are supplied by arteriolae rectae from the efferent arterioles. Venous drainage is by venae rectae, and interlobular, arcuate, interlobar, and renal veins that accompany the arteries.

The ***ureters*** are lined with transitional epithelium. External to the lamina propria is a muscularis layer consisting of inner longitudinal and outer circular smooth muscle layers. Near the bladder an additional outer longitudinal layer is added.

The ***urinary bladder*** is histologically similar to the lower part of the ureter in that it has a mucosa with transitional epithelium, a three-layered muscularis layer, and an outer connective tissue layer. The superficial (facet) transitional cells have a luminal plasma membrane of thick plates separated by thinner membrane. During contraction of the bladder the thick areas invaginate and form vesicles of reserve membrane.

DEVELOPMENT OF ABDOMINAL ORGANS

The development of the urogenital system will be covered in the section on the pelvis and perineum.

Development of the Digestive System. The entodermal ***foregut*** gives rise to the pharynx, esophagus, stomach, liver, pancreas, and part of the duodenum. The ***midgut*** gives rise to the rest of the small intestine, ascending colon, and proximal two thirds of the transverse colon. The ***hindgut*** develops into the rest of the large intestine as far as the upper part of the anal canal. The lower part of the rectum and much of the anal canal is established by the separation of the cloaca into a dorsal anorectal canal and ventral urogenital sinus by the urorectal septum. The rest of the anal canal develops from an ectodermally lined anal pit.

The ***stomach*** appears in the fourth embryonic week as a dilation of the foregut. As it shifts caudally from its position above the septum transversum, it rotates so that its original left surface faces anteriorly and its dorsal greater curvature extends to the left.

The ***intestines*** develop from the caudal part of the foregut and the cephalic and caudal limbs of a midgut loop that extend into the belly stalk. The cephalic limb extends from the upper duodenum to the yolk stalk. It gives rise to the rest of the small intestine, except the last 40 cm to 50 cm of the ileum. The caudal limb extends from the yolk stalk to the hindgut and it gives rise to the rest of the ileum, the cecum, the ascending colon, and the proximal two thirds of the transverse colon. As the loop develops, it rotates counterclockwise (in an AP view) around the omphalomesenteric (vitelline) artery, the latter becoming the superior mesenteric artery (Fig. 2-42A,B). This rotation places the transverse colon above the jejunum and ileum, anterior to the duodenum, and just below the stomach. By the tenth week the abdomen enlarges, and the gut loop reenters the abdomen. The cephalic limb enters first, crowding the descending colon to the left. Partial persistence of the yolk stalk may remain as a Meckel's diverticulum attached to the ileum 40 cm to 50 cm from the ileocolic junction.

The ***liver*** arises in the fourth embryonic week as a ventral diverticulum of the foregut. This diverticulum grows through the ventral mesentery and into the caudal face of the septum transversum. The more proximal part of the hepatic diverticulum gives rise to the common bile duct, cystic duct, gallbladder, and hepatic ducts. The more distal portions differentiate into the hepatic plates and the smaller bile ducts. Since the liver grows in the septum transversum and bulges from its caudal face, it is covered by peritoneum lining the septum transversum, except at the bare area of the liver where it abuts directly against the septum (diaphragm).

The ***pancreas*** forms from dorsal and ventral entodermal buds located at the level of the duodenum. The dorsal bud grows into the dorsal mesentry. The proximal portion of the ventral bud joins with the common bile duct, whereas the distal portion grows into the dorsal mesentery and fuses with the dorsal bud as the anterior portion of the duodenum grows more extensively than the dorsal part. The main pancreatic duct (of Wirsung) develops from the ventral bud and the distal part of the dorsal primordium. The proximal portion of the dorsal bud may give rise to the accessory duct (of Santorini).

Development of the Abdominal Mesenteries and Spleen. The abdominal mesenteries develop primarily from the embryonic dorsal mesentry. The ventral mesentery may give rise to the lesser omentum and the falciform ligament; although the latter probably forms from a ''shearing'' of peritoneum covering the anterior body wall. The peritoneum covering the liver reflects at the bare area of the liver to form the coronary and triangular ligaments of the liver. Much of the dorsal mesogastrium suspending the stomach fuses with the dorsal body wall to form the dorsal lining of the lesser sac. The rest of the dorsal mesogastrium fuses with the embryonic transverse mesocolon to form the definitive mesentery of the transverse colon and then drapes over the small intestine to become the greater omentum (Fig. 2-42C,D). The spleen develops from mesoderm of the dorsal mesogastrium. Most of the dorsal mesentery of the duodenum fuses with the dorsal body wall, making it and the pancreas secondarily retroperitoneal. The dorsal mesentery of the jejunum and ileum becomes the mesentery proper. The dorsal mesentery of the ascending and descending colon mostly fuses with the dorsal body wall, making these organs secondarily retroperitoneal. The dorsal mesentery of the sigmoid colon becomes the sigmoid mesocolon.

PELVIS AND PERINEUM

GROSS BOUNDARIES OF THE PELVIS AND PERINEUM

Pelvis. The osteology of the bones that form the pelvis and the basic types of pelvic architecture are discussed in the section on the lower extremity. The discussion here includes a definition of the pelvic cavity and the various planes of the pelvis.

The ***pelvic cavity proper*** (minor or true pelvis) is below the pelvic inlet and above the pelvic diaphragm or pelvic floor. The inlet is defined by the sacral promontory, arcuate line of the ilium, pecten pubis, and the upper aspect of the symphysis pubis. The area above this plane is the major or false pelvis and is part of the abdominal cavity. The ***floor of the pelvis*** is a muscular sling composed of the levator ani and coccygeus muscles. This trough-shaped sling slopes inferiorly from lateral to medial and from posterior to anterior. Its lateral attachment extends along a tendinous arch from the symphysis pubis to the ischial spine. The levator ani attaches to this arch and, after descending toward the midline, attaches to the levator ani of the opposite side along a median raphe. The coccygeus fills the gap between the ischial spine and the

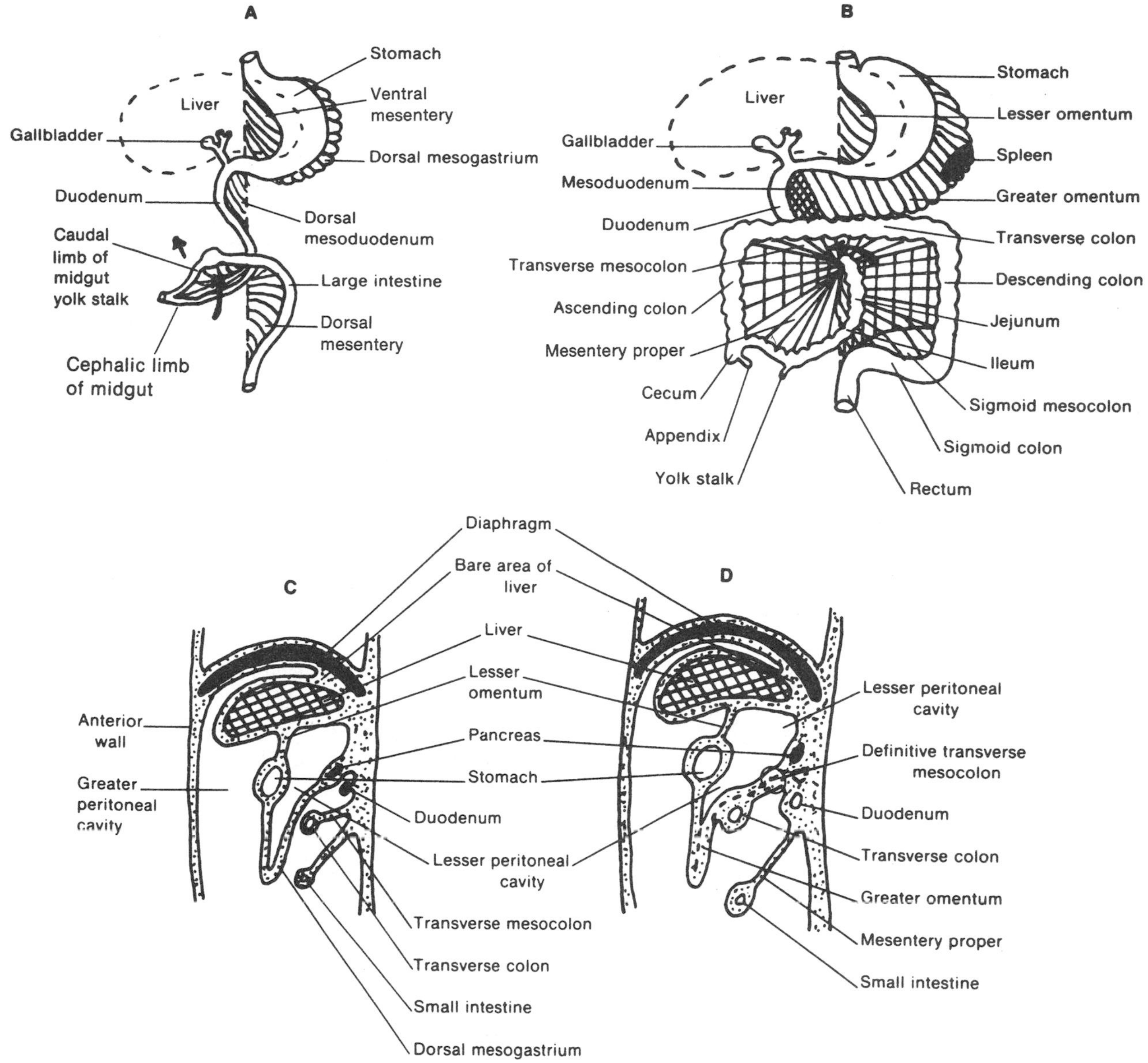

Fig. 2-42. Rotation of the gut and development of the mesenteries. *(A)*, early, and *(B)*, late, are anterior views of the rotation of the stomach and gut. The crosshatched areas of the mesentery are areas where it has become secondarily fused to the dorsal body wall. *(C)*, early, and *(D)*, late, are sagittal sections of the abdomen showing the greater and lesser peritoneal cavities, the formation of the definitive greater omentum and transverse mesocolon, and the secondarily retroperitoneal formation of the duodenum and pancreas.

sacrum and coccyx. The lateral wall of the pelvic cavity consists of the obturator internus and piriformis muscles along with the corresponding portions of the hip bone.

The ***plane of the pelvic inlet*** is the plane that has the greatest dimensions. In the female, the transverse diameter exceeds the AP diameter by a considerable amount. The distance between the sacral promontory and the uppermost aspect of the symphysis pubis is the anteroposterior diameter of the inlet or the ***conjugate*** vera (true conjugate). Not strictly part of the pelvic inlet but important obstetrically is the ***obstetric conjugate,*** the distance between the promontory and the most posterior aspect of the symphysis pubis, which is the part of the symphysis closest to the promontory. The ***diagonal conjugate*** can be measured by vaginal exam and is the distance between the promontory and the inferior aspect of the symphysis pubis. The transverse diameter of the inlet is the greatest distance between the arcuate lines.

The ***plane of the pelvic outlet*** is defined by the inferior aspect of the symphysis pubis, the ischiopubic rami, the ischial tuberosites, the sacrotuberous ligaments, and the tip of the sacrum. The AP diameter extends from the inferior aspect of the symphysis pubis to the tip of the sacrum. The transverse diameter of the outlet is the distance between the inner edges of the ischial tuberosities.

The ***plane of the midpelvis*** is the plane of least dimensions. The AP diameter of this plane extends from the inferior aspect of the symphysis to the sacrum, at the level of the ischial spines. The transverse diameter of the midpelvis is the distance between the ischial spines, which is the smallest diameter of the pelvis.

Perineum. The perineum (Fig. 2-43) is best defined as the region of the pelvic outlet below the pelvic floor. It is a diamond-shaped area that is defined by the inferior aspect of the symphysis pubic anteriorly, the ischiopubic rami anterolaterally, the ischial tuberosities laterally, the sacrotuberous ligaments posterolaterally, and the coccyx posteriorly. An imaginary line between the two ischial tuberosities separates the perineum into two triangular areas: the anterior urogenital triangle and the posterior anal triangle. The roof of the perineum is the floor of the pelvis, that is, the pelvic sling that is formed by the levator ani and coccygeus muscles.

In the ***urogenital triangle*** (Fig. 2-44) the urogenital diaphragm is a horizontal musculofascial shelf that stretches between the ischiopubic rami. It is formed by superior and inferior layers of fascia that enclose the sphincter urethrae and deep transverse perineal muscles. In the male it contains the bulbourethral glands (Cowper's glands). This diaphragm is penetrated by the membranous urethra in both sexes and the vagina in the female. The area between the superior and inferior fasciae of the urogenital diaphragm encloses the ***deep perineal space*** or pouch.

The ***superficial perineal space*** is inferior or superficial to the inferior fascia of the urogenital diaphragm. It is limited externally or superficially by Colles' fascia, which attaches to the posterior edge of the urogenital diaphragm and is continuous with the membranous (fibrous) layer of subcutaneous tissue (Scarpa's fascia) of the abdomen. This limiting layer also attaches to the isochiopubic ramus and the fascia lata of the thigh so that urine from a ruptured urethra or blood from hemorrhage may extravasate up into the abdominal wall (but not into the thigh) from the superficial perineal space. In the male the superficial perineal space contains the crura of the corpora cavernosa and related ischiocavernosus muscles, the corpus spongiosum and bulb of the penis with the

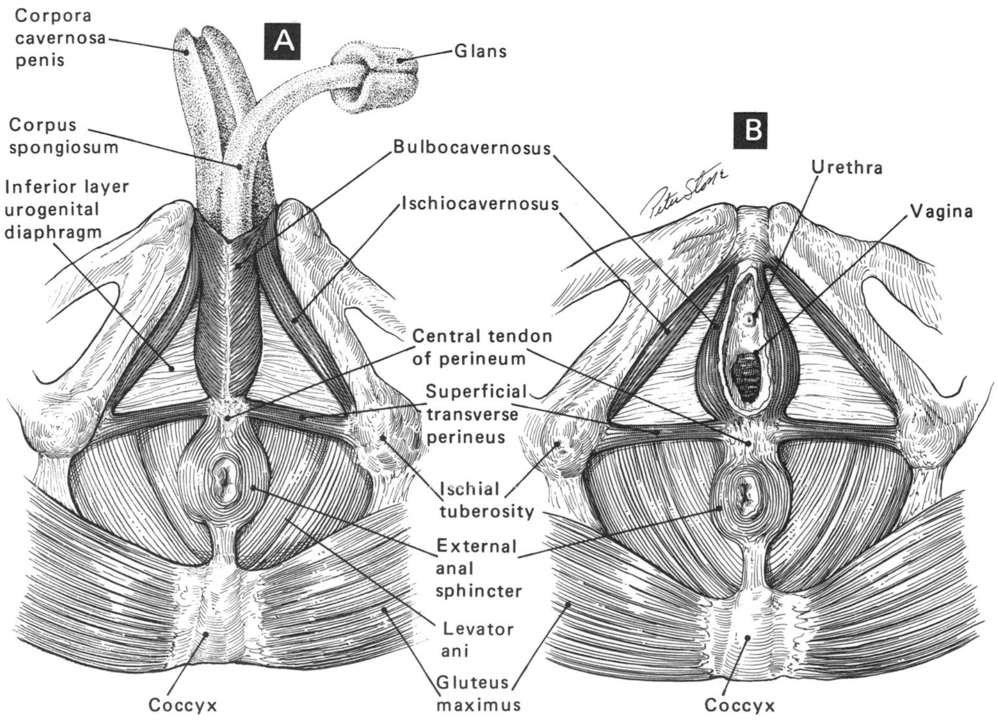

Fig. 2-43. Perineum: *(A)* male; *(B)* female. (Christensen JB, Telford IR: Synopsis of Gross Anatomy, 5th ed, p 203. Philadelphia, JB Lippincott, 1988)

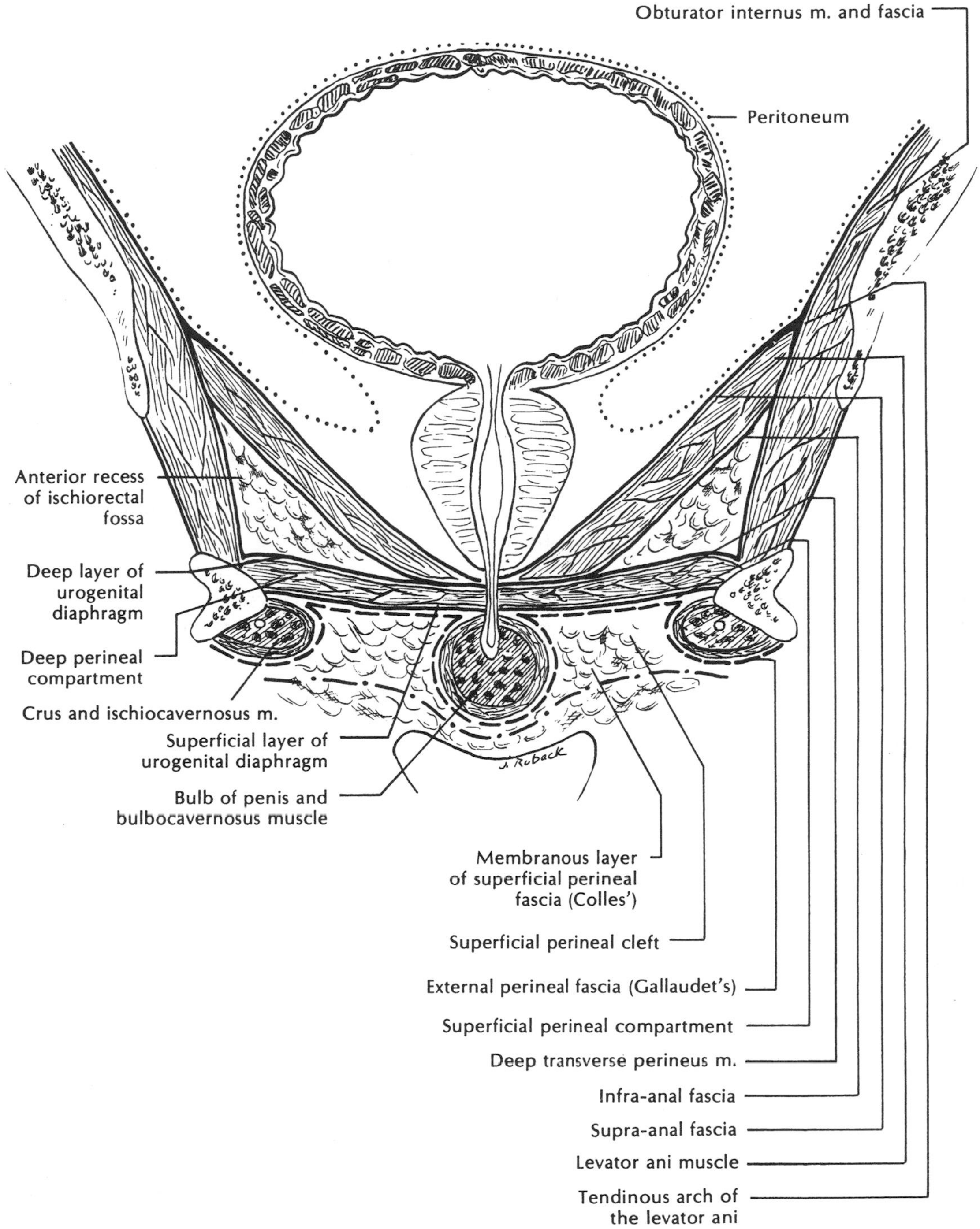

Fig. 2-44. A coronal section through the urogenital triangle of the male perineum. (Christensen JB, Telford IR: Synopsis of Gross Anatomy, 5th ed, p 217. Philadelphia, JB Lippincott, 1988)

related bulbospongiosus muscle, and the superficial transverse perineal muscle. In the female this space contains the crura of the clitoris and related ischiocavernosus muscles, the bulbus vestibuli and related bulbospongiosus muscle, the superficial transverse perineal muscle, and the greater vestibular glands (Bartholin's glands). The urethral opening is approximately 2.5 cm posterior to the clitoris.

The ***ischiorectal fossa*** is the fat-filled, wedge-shaped area that is inferolateral to the pelvic sling and medial to the lower portions of the obturator internus muscle and the os coxae. In the region of the anal triangle, the floor of the fossa is the subcutaneous tissue and skin. The posterior recess of this fossa extends posterolaterally under the inferior margin of the gluteus maximus muscle. The anterior recess extends into the urogenital triangle above the urogenital diaphragm. The pudendal (Alcock's) canal is a slit in the obturator internus fascia along the lateral wall of this fossa in the anal triangle. The internal pudendal vessels and the pudendal nerve traverse this canal as they pass anteriorly into the urogenital triangle. The inferior rectal arteries and nerves branch from the parent structures in the pudendal canal and pass through the ischiorectal fossa toward the rectum and anal canal.

The nerve supply to the perineum is provided primarily by the pudendal nerve (S2–S4). Its branches are the inferior rectal, perineal, and posterior scrotal (labial) nerves. These branches supply all of the muscles and most of the skin of the perineum. The skin of the anterior part of the perineum is supplied by the anterior scrotal (labial) branches of the ilioinguinal nerve. Autonomics to the perineum are apparently distributed through the pudendal nerve.

VISCERA OF THE PELVIS AND PERINEUM

Gastrointestinal Tract. The ***sigmoid colon*** begins at the pelvic rim, descends to the left pelvic wall, traverses the pelvis from left to right, and bends upon itself to join the rectum in the midline. It is supported by the sigmoid mesocolon. The sigmoid and its mesocolon are extremely variable in length, exceeding by far the variability in other parts of the gastrointestinal system.

The ***rectum*** is that portion of the bowel below the midsacral region where the sigmoid mesocolon ceases. The lowest part of the infraperitoneal portion presents a dilated ampulla. Anteriorly the upper two thirds of the rectum is in contact with the coils of the ileum. In the male the lower third is related anteriorly to the trigone of the bladder, the seminal vesicles, the ductus deferens, and the prostate. In the female the lower third is in contact anteriorly with the vagina and the cervix. Posteriorly it is related to the sacrum in both sexes.

The upper third of the rectum is covered anteriorly and laterally by peritoneum; the middle third, only anteriorly; and the lower third passes below the peritoneum.

The ***anal canal,*** which is sometimes called the second portion of the rectum, is 2.5 cm to 3.5 cm in length. It turns dorsally, making a right angle as it passes through the pelvic floor to the anus, and is surrounded by internal and external sphincters.

The following structures can be palpated during a rectal examination in the normal male: the anorectal ring, anteriorly the prostate, posteriorly the coccyx and sacrum, and laterally the ischiorectal fossa and the ischial spines. The normal female presents the same structures with the exception of anteriorly, where the perineal body and the cervix of the uterus are palpable.

Urinary System. The pelvic portion of the ***ureter*** passes in front of the sacroiliac joint and medial to the internal iliac artery. In the male it passes posterior and inferior to the ductus deferens. In the female it passes inferior to the uterine artery and lateral to the cervix of the uterus. The vesical portion runs obliquely downward and medially through the bladder about 20 mm to 25 mm from its counterpart.

The empty ***bladder*** is posterior to the pubic symphysis and totally within the pelvic cavity below the pelvic inlet. The fully distended bladder of the adult projects well into the abdominal cavity. The bladder is extraperitoneal with its superior and posterosuperior surfaces covered with peritoneum. Laterally it is related to the levator ani and the obturator internus muscles. In the male the bladder is related superiorly to coils of small intestine and the sigmoid colon; posteriorly to the rectovesical pouch, the rectum, the seminal vesicles, and termination of the vas deferens; and inferiorly to the prostate gland. In the female it is related superiorly to coils of the small intestine and the body of the uterus, posteriorly to the vagina and supravaginal portion of the cervix, and inferiorly to the pelvic fascia and the urogenital diaphragm.

The ***male urethra*** extends from the bladder to the glans penis, traversing (1) the prostate gland, (2) the urogenital diaphragm, and (3) the length of the corpus spongiosum. The prostatic portion contains the numerous small openings of the prostatic ducts and the crista urethralis, with the colliculus seminalis containing the openings of the ejaculatory ducts. As the urethra passes through the urogenital diaphragm, it is somewhat narrowed and is surrounded by the sphincter. In the cavernous portion the urethra is dilated at the openings of the Cowper's glands and also terminally at the fossa navicularis.

The ***female urethra*** is short and it passes through the urogenital diaphragm, where it is surrounded by the sphincter urethrae. It ends shortly thereafter, opening about 1 inch posterior to the clitoris.

Male Reproductive System. The testis and the epididymis lie in the scrotum and are separated from those of the opposite side by the scrotal septum. The epididymis lies along the posterior border of the testis. It is enlarged above to form a head and tapers to a body and small tail below. It is formed predominantly by the greatly contorted duct of the epididymis, which empties into the beginning of the ductus deferens.

The ductus deferens ascends toward the inguinal canal, which it traverses. At the internal abdominal ring it leaves the spermatic cord, passes downward and backward over the lateral surface of the bladder and medially to the ureter, penetrates the prostate gland, and opens into the prostatic portion of the urethra through the ejaculatory duct. Just before it enters the prostate, it is joined by the club-shaped seminal vesicles.

The prostate gland surrounds the urethra between the inferior surface of the bladder and the superior surface of the urogenital diaphragm. It is related anteriorly to the symphysis pubis, laterally to the levator ani muscles, inferiorly to the urogenital diaphragm, and posteriorly to the rectum.

Female Reproductive System. The ***ovaries*** lie against the lateral pelvic walls just below the pelvic inlet and posteroinferior to the lateral aspect of the uterine tubes. Each ovary is enclosed in a mesovarium, a posterior reflection of peritoneum from the broad ligament. The ovary is suspended from the lateral pelvic wall by the suspensory ligament of the ovary, through which the ovarian vessels, nerves, and lymphatics pass to the gland. Each ovary is connected to the uterus just below the uterine tube by the ovarian ligament.

The ***uterus*** consists of the fundus, body, and cervix. The cavity of the uterus is continuous superolaterally with the narrow lumina of the uterine tubes and inferiorly with the cavity of the vagina. The fundus is the superior domed portion that projects above the cavity of the body. The body is the major portion of the uterus, and the cervix is the inferior portion, part of which projects into the vagina. The uterine cavity is largest within the body. It narrows abruptly at the body–cervix junction to form the internal os. The lumen of the cervix (cervical canal) is narrow and ends inferiorly as the narrow external os, which is readily palpated during a rectal examination. The normally positioned uterus rests on the posterosuperior aspect of the bladder so that the uterovesical pouch is usually empty. The rectouterine pouch (of Douglas) separates the uterus from the rectum posteriorly. Laterally the uterus is related to the broad ligament and the ureter; the latter passing just lateral to the supravaginal portion of the cervix and inferior to the uterine artery.

The ***uterine*** (fallopian) ***tubes*** extend laterally from the superolateral aspects of the uterus. Each tube consists of a narrow-lumened isthmus, a dilated and long ampulla, and the terminal infundibulum, which is composed of numerous fingerlike fimbriae. The tubes curve posteriorly near the lateral pelvic walls where their fimbriae partially cover the ovaries. The uterine tubes are the most superior structures in the broad ligament.

The normal uterus is both anteflexed and anteverted. Anteflexion is a forward bend within the uterus itself at the level of the internal os. Anteversion is a forward bend of about 90 degrees at the junction of the uterus and the vagina. This places the uterus in approximately the horizontal plane with its anterior surface resting on the posterosuperior surface of the bladder. Malposition usually involves one of the following: (1) turning of the entire organ, retroversion (backward turning) or anteversion (forward turning); (2) bending of the body on the cervix, retroflexion (backward bending) or anteflexion (anterior bending); or (3) shifting in the position of the entire organ, retrocession, anteposition, prolapse or procidentia, the latter is the extreme degree of prolapse in which the cervix extrudes from the introitus. This results from extreme relaxation of the pelvic floor, the urogenital diaphragm, and the uterine ligaments.

The ***vagina*** extends from above the inferior extent of the cervix of the uterus to its external opening in the vestibule. From above downward it is inclined anteriorly as it passes through the pelvic floor and the urogenital diaphragm. The upper portion of the vagina, which surrounds the inferior part of the cervix, is divided into anterior, lateral, and posterior fornices. The vagina is related anteriorly to the base of the bladder and the urethra; posteriorly through the very thin wall of the posterior fornix, to the rectouterine pouch, rectum and anal canal; and laterally to the levator ani muscle and the ureter, which passes near the lateral fornix.

In a ***vaginal examination*** the urethra, bladder, and symphysis pubis are palpable anteriorly; the rectum and rectouterine pouch posteriorly; the ovary, uterine tube, and lateral pelvic wall laterally; and the cervix in the apex of the vagina.

The vestibule is surrounded by the labia minora and receives the vagina, urethra, and major and minor vestibular glands.

The ***broad ligament*** is a reflection of peritoneum that passes over the uterus and related structures from front to back and extends laterally to the lateral pelvic walls. As such it forms a curtain across the pelvis from side to side; the broad ligament has an anterior and a posterior layer. Lateral to the uterus the most superior structure in the broad ligament is the uterine tube; below and behind that is the ovarian ligament; and below and anterior is the round ligament. The mesovarium is the reflection of the posterior layer that suspends the ovarian ligament and ovary. That part of the broad ligament above the mesovarium that suspends the uterine tube is called the mesosalpinx. That part of the broad ligament below the mesovarium is the mesometrium. At the base of the broad ligament posteriorly, the posterior layer of mesometrium is elevated over the underlying uterosacral ligament as the rectouterine fold. The extraperitoneal connective tissue found between the layers of the broad ligament is the parametrium. The parametrium in the base of the broad ligament is thickened and forms the cardinal ligaments.

BLOOD SUPPLY TO THE PELVIS AND PERINEUM

The blood supply to the pelvic viscera and to the perineum is provided by branches of the internal iliac artery. The umbilical artery gives rise to the artery of the ductus deferens and the superior vesical artery, which supplies the bladder. The inferior vesical artery also supplies the bladder and the prostate and seminal vesicles in the male. The uterine artery (homologue to the artery of the ductus deferens) usually arises separately and passes medially to supply the uterus, uterine tube, and upper part of the vagina. The vaginal artery supplies most of the vagina. The middle rectal artery supplies the middle portion of the rectum and anastomoses with the superior and inferior rectal arteries. The internal pudendal artery exits the pelvis through the greater sciatic foramen, passes around the ischial spine, and then enters the perineum through the lesser sciatic foramen. It supplies the somatic and visceral structures of the perineum. Other branches of the internal iliac artery are the superior and inferior gluteal arteries, which supply the gluteal region; the iliolumbar and lateral sacral arteries, which supply the posterior body wall; and the obturator, which passes into the medial thigh.

MICROSCOPIC STRUCTURE OF PELVIC CONTENTS

Male Reproductive System. The *testis* is ovoid and surrounded by a thick connective tissue capsule, the tunica albuginea. This capsule penetrates the testis at the mediastinum and sends radiating septula into it, dividing the testis into lobules. Within the lobules are seminiferous tubules and a loose fibrous stroma. The stroma contains interstitial cells of Leydig, which are characterized by rod-shaped crystalloids (of Reinke), much SER, and mitochondria with tubular cristae. Under the influence of luteinizing hormone (LH), also known as interstitial cell-stimulating hormone (ICSH), these cells produce testosterone; the SER and tubular cristae are characteristic of steroid-secreting cells. The seminiferous tubules consist of contorted loops that join by straight tubules with the rete testis. The convoluted portions in the viable male are lined by a germinal (seminiferous) epithelium resting on a basal lamina that is bounded by peritubular myoid cells that probably produce a peristaltic action. The seminiferous epithelium contains supportive ***Sertoli cells*** and ***sex cells*** in various stages of spermatogenesis. The Sertoli cells are connected to each other by occluding and gap junctions. These cells support, protect, and nurture the sex cells; they also phagocytize excess cytoplasm in spermatozoan production, and, under the influence of follicle-stimulating hormone (FSH), they secrete androgen binding protein (ABP), which serves to concentrate testosterone needed for spermatogenesis. They also secrete transferrin, inhibin, and produce lactate needed by the germ cells. The developing sex cells are located between the Sertoli cells. Spermatogonia are located next to the basal lamina in a basal (extratubular) compartment formed by the tight junctions of the Sertoli cells. These tight junctions contribute to the formation of a restrictive blood–testes barrier. The primary spermatocytes and secondary spermatocytes lie nearer the lumen in the adluminal (intratubular) compartment between Sertoli cells. Spermatids are embedded in the apices of the Sertoli cells where they transform into spermatozoa. A cross section of a tubule may show several of six stages of development. This is due to different timing in the proliferation and division of stem cells.

Spermatogonia are the only sex cells present until the time of puberty when two different types are present. These are the A or stem cell and the B or derivative cell. A cells may divide into A cells or into two B cells. B cells grow and differentiate into primary spermatocytes. Each primary spermatocyte undergoes the reduction division of meiosis and gives rise to two secondary spermatocytes containing the haploid number (23) of chromosomes. Each secondary spermatocyte divides quickly into two spermatids. When each spermatid undergoes transformation into a spermatozoa the nucleus condenses, an acrosome vesicle is formed by the Golgi complex, the acrosome vesicle collapses as a lysosomal head cap over the nucleus, an axial filament (flagellum) grows from the proximal centriole, and mitochondria form a helix around the proximal flagellum of the middle piece. Most of the cytoplasm is cast off, leaving only a thin cytoplasmic investment to the head, neck, middle piece, and tail of the spermatozoon. In the principal piece of the tail the cytoplasm forms a fibrous sheath that does not extend into the end piece of the tail.

Sperm are transported through straight tubules, rete testis, and efferent ductules to be stored in the tail of the epididymus, where they mature and become motile. At ejaculation sperm pass from the head of the epididymus into the ductus deferens, ejaculatory ducts, and urethra.

Straight seminiferous tubules and ***rete testis*** are lined by simple cuboidal to columnar epithelium. These empty into 10 to 15 ***efferent ductules*** that are lined by alternating cuboidal and tall ciliated columnar epithelium. A basal layer of rounded cells is surrounded by a lamina propria and some circular smooth muscle fibers. The cilia of the efferent ductules move spermatozoa into the ***ductus epididymidis*** (epididymus). This duct contains pseudostratified columnar epithelium containing basal cells and principal cells with long microvilli (stereocilia). This duct supplies nutritive substances to the sperm and absorbs excess fluid accompanying the sperm. The epithelium is invested by a circular smooth muscle layer.

The ***vas (ductus) deferens*** has a mucosa that is similar to that of the ductus epididymidis. The muscular layer is highly developed into inner longitudinal, middle circular and outer longitudinal layers. This duct is invested in the spermatic cord by the cremasteric muscle and the pampiniform plexus of veins. The ductus deferens dilates into an ampulla before terminating as the short slender ejaculatory duct, which pierces the prostate and opens into the urethra at the urethral crest. The mucosa of these structures is folded and the epithelium is not as tall as in the rest of the ductus deferens. The supporting wall of the ejaculatory duct is made up of fibrous tissue. Muscular contraction of the ductus deferens and the ductus epididymidis propel the spermatozoa to the urethra during the ejaculatory process.

The ***seminal vesicle*** consists of a mucosa folded into a complex system of elevations, a prominent muscularis and an adventitia. The epithelium is low pseudostratified columnar epithelium, and it secretes a viscid alkaline fluid rich in fructose.

The ***prostate*** is an aggregation of 30 to 50 tubulosaccular glands. The glandular epithelium is simple cuboidal to columnar, with patches of pseudostratified columnar. The cells have apical secretion granules that contribute to the formation of the faintly acid secretion that is rich in citric acid and acid phosphatase. The lumina may contain lamellated prostatic concretions (corpora amylacea). The stroma between the tubules contains smooth muscle fibers.

The ***male urethra*** has three parts, the prostatic, membranous, and cavernous (penile) or spongy portions. The prostatic urethra is lined mostly with transitional epithelium. The membranous and penile portions are lined with pseudostratified and stratified columnar epithelium, except at the meatus where the epithelium is stratified squamous. The prostatic urethra has a crest on its posterior wall. The paired ejaculatory ducts and prostatic utricle open on this crest. The ducts of the prostatic gland open into the prostatic urethra. The membranous urethra is encircled by a sphincter of skeletal muscle fibers from the deep transverse perineal muscle. The cavernous urethra extends throughout the penis. It occupies the corpus spongiosum and receives the ducts of the bulbourethral glands and the branching mucous urethral glands (of Littre).

The ***bulbourethral glands*** (Cowper's) are variably tubular, alveolar, or saccular mucous glands that are enclosed in the membranous urethral sphincter. Their ducts, containing mucous areas of epithelium, open into the cavernous urethra about 2.5 cm in front of the urogenital diaphragm.

The ***penis*** consists of three cylinders of erectile tissue: two dorsal corpora cavernosa and one ventral corpus spongiosum. The latter terminates distally as the glans penis, and it contains the cavernous urethra. A dense fibrous tunica albuginea surrounds the cavernous bodies and separates the corpora from one another by an incomplete median (pectiniform) septum. The three corpora are enclosed in a common loose irregularly arranged connective tissue layer that underlies the investing skin. The skin folds over the glans as the prepuce. The skin of the glans adheres firmly to the erectile tissue since the loose connective tissue layer is lacking. The epithelium of the inner surface of the prepuce and that of the glans is stratified squamous and is characteristic of that lining a moist surface. It is continuous at the urethral orifice with the epithelium lining the urethra.

The ***erectile tissue*** of the corpora cavernosa consists of endothelium lined lacunae that are separated by fibrous trabeculae containing smooth muscle. The lacunae are large centrally but are narrow peripherally where they communicate with a venous plexus underlying the tunica albuginea. In the corpus spongiosum the arrangement is similar except for an elastic tunica albuginea, thinner trabeculae, and uniform lacunae. The corpora cavernosa are supplied by two branches of the penile artery: the dorsal artery and the deep arteries. The branches of the dorsal arteries supply capillaries of the trabeculae that drain through the lacunae to the venous plexus. The deep arteries are the chief vessels for filling the lacunae during erection. These vessels run in the cavernous bodies and give off trabecular branches that empty directly to the lacunae through helicine arteries. The latter vessels have a thick circular muscle layer and an intima with longitudinal thickened cushions. During erection the smooth muscle in the cavernous trabeculae and helicine arteries relaxes under parasympathetic influence, the helicine arteries become patent, and the lacunae are engorged with more blood than can be rapidly drained by the compressed peripheral lacunae and venous plexus. At the end of erection, smooth muscle contraction due to sympathetic control shuts off the blood supplied by helicine arteries and forces blood into the peripheral venous plexus.

Female Reproductive System. The ***ovary*** is an exocrine organ secreting secondary oocytes, and it is an endocrine organ producing estrogens and progesterone. It is divided into an outer cortex and inner medulla. The cortex basically consists of a rather cellular connective tissue stroma, ovarian follicles, and a simple cuboidal surface epithelium (germinal epithelium). The medulla consists of loose connective tissue, blood vessels, lymphatics, nerves, some smooth muscle, and a few vestigial tubular structures called rete ovarii.

An ***ovarian follicle*** consists of a developing ovum and an investment of follicle cells and connective tissue. Follicles originate in the embryo and undergo extensive changes during the childbearing years when they are under the influence of adenohypophyseal hormones. In the embryo, primordial sex cells develop into oogonia, which differentiate into primary oocytes; the latter go through the prophase of the first meiotic division before they enter an arrested dictyotene stage. Each cell is surrounded by a single layer of follicle cells from the germinal epithelium. Many of these embryonic primordial follicles die, but 70,000 to 400,000 survive in the cortex of the ovary until the time of puberty.

At puberty, hypothalamic nerve cells produce gonadotropin-releasing hormone (GnRH). This hormone stimulates FSH release by basophils of the anterior pituitary gland. Under the influence of FSH and other factors, ovarian follicles develop periodically. In this process, some oocytes emerge from the arrested dictyotene stage and start to complete the first meiotic division. Coincident with this, follicle cells enlarge and proliferate to form a stratified cuboidal epithelial layer around the oocyte, thus forming a primary follicle. As the follicle enlarges, spaces between follicle cells coalesce to form an antrum filled with liquor folliculi. The growing follicle is now called a secondary (vesicular) follicle. As this follicle differentiates, the follicular cells around the antrum form a stratified epithelial membrana granulosa that sits on a prominent basal lamina. This in turn is surrounded by an inner richly vascular theca interna and an outer more fibrous theca externa. The cells of the theca interna contain much SER and produce androstenedione under the influence of LH; the androstenedione, a weak androgen (testosterone), is converted to estrogen by granulosa cells under the influence of FSH. The oocyte is surrounded by a protein-polysaccharide layer called the zona pellucida. Cytoplasmic processes of the oocyte and of the immediate surrounding follicle cells of the corona radiata are closely aligned in the substance of the zona pellucida. The combined oocyte, zona pellucida, and corona radiata project into the antrum of the follicle as the cumulus oophorus.

The mature vesicular follicle occupies much of the thickness of the cortex, and it causes a bulge (stigma) on the surface of the ovary. Its primary oocyte completes the first meiotic division and becomes a secondary oocyte. The secondary oocyte is relatively metabolically inactive, but it possesses more extensive protein producing mechanisms than are found in the primary oocyte. It starts its second meiotic division and reaches the metaphase stage at about the time it is ovulated from the ovary along with the zona pellucida and corona radiata of granulosa cells. Just prior to ovulation large amounts of estrogen and small amounts of progesterone are produced by the follicle, and more luteinizing hormone is produced by the adenohypophysis.

After ovulation a small amount of blood accumulates in the collapsed follicular remains, and a clot is formed in the antrum region. Under the influence of LH the granulosa and theca interna cells enlarge, accumulate lipid, and become lutein cells of a ***corpus luteum.*** The granulosa lutein cells constitute the bulk of the corpus luteum and produce progesterone and estrogen. The theca lutein cells are smaller, less in number, more deeply staining, found at the periphery, and may produce estrogens. Lutein cells possess major characteristics of steroid-secreting cells in that they have relatively more SER and have mitochondria containing "tubular" lamellae rather than cristae. After clot formation the thecal connective tissue penetrates into the developing corpus luteum and replaces the blood clot in the central core.

If the ovulated secondary oocyte is fertilized and implantation takes place the corpus luteum will survive for about 6 months under the influences of human chorionic gonadotropin (HCG) from the placenta before it starts to regress. If the secondary oocyte is not fertilized, the corpus luteum will last for about 14 days. When a corpus luteum degenerates the lutein cells become swollen, then pyknotic, and a hyalinized scar of connective tissue replaces the dead lutein cells. This white scar is called the ***corpus albicans.***

Usually only one follicle reaches maturity and is involved in ovulation during each cycle. The other maturing follicles are no longer supported by the waning levels of FSH after ovulation and they degenerate. In small follicles the oocyte degenerates and the stroma invades the follicle, leaving no trace of the follicle. In larger follicles, cells of the theca interna enlarge, and the basement membrane becomes a distinct glassy membrane before coarser stromal fibers penetrate the degenerating follicle, giving the atretic follicle the appearance of a small corpus albicans.

The ***uterine tube (oviduct, fallopian tube)*** has four regions: infundibulum, ampulla, isthmus, and interstitial (intramural) portion. The wall of each of these parts consists of a mucosa, muscularis, and serosa. The mucosa of the trumpet-shaped infundibulum, and to a lesser extent that of the ampulla, is characterized by many elongate fimbriae. The epithelium of all parts of the uterine tube is simple columnar and is comprised of ciliated cells and peg-shaped secreting cells. These cell types may be different functional states of the same cell. The relative numbers of these cell types vary, depending on the estrogenic or progesteronic influences. The muscularis consists of inner circular and outer longitudinal smooth muscle layers. These layers are relatively thicker in passing from the infundibulum to the interstitial portion. The serosa is lined by mesothelium and is a continuation of the peritoneal covering of the broad ligament.

The ***uterus*** is comprised of a body, fundus, and cervix. The body and fundus are histologically similar, and their walls consist of three layers: perimetrium (serosa), myometrium (muscularis), and endometrium (mucosa). The perimetrium is the serosal continuation of the broad ligament. The myometrium is composed of an inner layer of longitudinal smooth muscle, a thick middle layer of circular smooth muscle and large blood vessels, and an outer layer of longitudinal and circular smooth muscle. These smooth muscle cells undergo hyperplasia and hypertrophy during pregnancy. The basic constituents of the endometrium are simple columnar epithelium that is partly ciliated; a lamina propria stroma containing mesenchymelike cells, reticular fibers, and varying amounts of leukocytes; simple tubular glands; and two sets of arteries. One set of arteries (basal arteries) supplies the glands and stroma of the deepest part of the lamina propria. The other set (coiled, spiral arteries) supplies the rest of the endometrium.

The endometrium is under the influence of ovarian progesterone and estrogen. It reflects this influence in the marked structural changes characteristic of the ***menstrual cycle.*** Four uterine stages of the cycle are recognized: menstrual, proliferative (follicular, estrogenic), secretory (luteal, progesteronic), and premenstrual (ischemic). The menstrual stage takes place from days 1 to 5 of the cycle. The proliferative occurs from days 5 to 14, the secretory from days 14 to 27, and the premenstrual from days 27 to 28. These are approximate times.

During the proliferative stage the endometrium grows from a height of 0.5 mm to 2 mm to 3 mm. In this process, epithelial cells of the gland remnants form a new epithelial lining and straight glands. The stroma develops from the deep (basal) layer. Spiral arteries grow into this new functional layer. In the secretory stage, under the influence of estrogen and progesterone, the endometrium grows another 2 mm in height. An increase in interstitial fluid in part of the functional layer divides it into an inner edematous spongy layer and an outer compact layer. The uterine glands grow, become corkscrew-shaped, and produce a glycogen-rich mucoid secretion. Coiled (spiral) arteries elongate and empty into venous sinusoids by way of capillaries. The premenstrual stage is the result of a decrease of progesterone and estrogen production by the corpus luteum. In this stage the coiled arteries kink, there is a drop in the blood supply to the functional layer, the edema decreases, and the glands begin to fragment. During the menstrual stage the functional layer becomes anemic and ischemic. Arteries and veins break down, and blood oozes into the uterine cavity through the degenerating glands and surface epithelium. The entire functional layer is sloughed off during this stage. The basal arteries are not affected, so the basal layer is retained.

The ***placenta*** consists of a maternal component (decidua basalis) and a fetal component (chorion frondosum). Since the embryo implants into the compacta layer of the endometrium, the ***decidua basalis*** is that portion of the functional layer that lies deep to the embryo. Glands and blood vessels of this layer empty into intervillous spaces. The stromal cells swell markedly, accumulate glycogen, and are called decidual cells. The ***chorion frondosum*** consists of a chorionic plate off of which anchoring villi arise and attach to the endometrium. Free villi extend from the anchoring villi into the intervillous spaces. In the first third of pregnancy the villi have cores of fetal connective tissue containing fetal capillaries with nucleated RBCs. This core of tissue is covered by an inner cytotrophoblastic and an outer syncytial trophoblastic epithelial layer. Later in pregnancy, the fetal vessels contain nonnucleated RBCs, the cytotrophoblast disappears, and the syncytial trophoblast is thin except for clumps of syncytial knots where the nuclei are located. An acidophilic fibrinoid material accumulates over the syncytial trophoblast in late pregnancy. The "placental barrier" in the late placenta consists of the syncytial trophoblast, the endothelium of the fetal vessels, and the intervening basal laminae of these epithelia, which are fused into one basal lamina in the thinnest portions of the barrier. In the first trimester, the cytotrophoblast and fetal connective tissue are added layers in this barrier. The cells of the cytotrophoblast produce the syncytial trophoblast and probably a GnRH. The syncytial trophoblast cells produce estrogen, progesterone, HCG, human placental lactogen (HPL) or human chorionic somatomammatropin (HCS), and human chorionic thyrotropin (HCT).

The ***cervix*** consists of a mucosa, muscularis, and adventitia. It does not undergo the extensive cyclic changes of the endometrium, although some changes in structure are seen in pregnancy. The portio vaginalis of the cervix projects into the vagina. The mucosa of the cervix is thrown into folds (plicae palmatae). It consists of simple columnar epithelium with some cilia, extensive forked mucus-secreting glands, and a firm stroma that is rich in collagenous and elastic fibers. The epithelium changes to stratified squamous at the portio vaginalis. During pregnancy the cervical glands become larger and secrete a mucous plug that seals the cervical canal. At the time of parturition the lamina propria becomes more edematous, looser, and cellular. The muscularis layers are similar to those in the uterine body and fundus except that there is no inner longitudinal muscular layer. The adventitia contains collagenous fibers that are continuous with surrounding structures.

The ***vagina*** also is comprised of a mucosa, muscularis, and adventitia. The lining epithelium of the mucosa is stratified squamous nonkeratinized, but keratohyaline granules may be found in some of the cells. Under the influence of estrogen the epithelium accumulates glycogen, and many pyknotic surface cells appear. When estrogen levels are low a basal layer of cells is prominent. The lamina propria contains many elastic fibers and some large blood vessels. No glands are present. The muscularis consists of a thin inner circular layer and thicker outer longitudinal layer of smooth muscle. A sphincter of skeletal muscle is found at the lower end of the vagina.

The ***hymen*** has the same structure as the vaginal mucosa. It is a thin fold at the opening of the vagina into the vestibule.

The *clitoris* corresponds to the dorsal penis in the male. It has two small cavernous bodies of erectile tissue that end in the glans clitoridis. It is covered by stratified squamous epithelium. Specialized nerve endings, such as Meissner's and Pacinian corpuscles, are located in the subepithelial stroma.

The *labia minora* flank the vestibule. They have a vascularized connective tissue core that is covered by stratified squamous epithelium possessing a thin keratinized layer. Sebaceous glands, not associated with hairs, are located in the stroma.

The *labia majora* are folds of skin that cover the labia minora. The inner surface is like that of the labia minora. The outer surface is covered by skin containing hairs, sweat glands, and sebaceous glands. The interior of these folds contains much adipose tissue.

The *vestibule* is lined by partially keratinized stratified squamous epithelium. Minor vestibular glands, placed chiefly near the clitoris and opening of the urethra, secrete mucus. The longer major vestibular glands are analogous to the bulbourethral glands of the male. They are located in the lateral wall of the vestibule. Their ducts open close to the attachment of the hymen.

DEVELOPMENT OF THE UROGENITAL SYSTEM

The urinary and reproductive systems take origin from the urogenital sinus and the intermediate mesoderm.

Development of the Kidney and Ureter. Three pairs of embryonic kidneys develop in humans. These are the pronephros, mesonephros, and metanephros. The pronephros and mesonephros will degenerate, but their development is essential for the establishment of the metanephros, which becomes the definitive kidney.

The *pronephros* arises at the C3–T1 vertebral levels by the dorsal proliferation of cords of cells from the intermediate mesoderm. These cords become pronephric tubules. They grow caudally and link up with the other pronephric tubules, forming a common pronephric duct that extends caudally toward the cloaca. The pronephric kidney does not function, but the pronephric duct is important for the normal formation of the mesonephric kidney.

The *mesonephros* develops by the formation of mesonephric tubules from the intermediate mesoderm of the C6–L3 vertebral levels. Unlike the pronephric tubules, these tubules do not communicate with the coelom but receive a capillary glomerulus from the aorta, which is encapsulated by the proximal blind end of the tubule. The distal end of the mesonephric tubules tap into the pronephric duct and contribute to its caudal growth. This enlarged pronephric duct taps into the cloaca, and its name is changed to the mesonephric (Wolffian) duct. The extensive growth of the mesonephros produces a large urogenital ridge projecting from the dorsal body wall.

The *metanephros* arises from two sources: the ureteric bud (metanephric diverticulum) and the metanephrogenic intermediate mesoderm of the L4–S1 vertebral levels. The ureteric bud arises as a tubular outgrowth from the mesonephric duct near its entrance into the cloaca. It grows toward the intermediate mesoderm where its blind end becomes capped by metanephrogenic tissue. The ureteric bud elongates as the ureter, and its blind end enlarges as the renal pelvis and undergoes a series of branchings. These branchings give rise to the major and minor calyces and the collecting tubules. The metanephrogenic condensations capping the blind ends of the collecting tubules develop into nephrons. One end of the blind nephron forms a Bowman's capsule around a glomerulus of capillaries. The other end taps into the collecting tubule.

Development of the Urinary Bladder and Urethra. The urinary bladder and urethra develop from the entoderm of the urogenital sinus and allantois. In early development the allantois is a diverticulum of the cloaca. A urorectal septum of mesoderm arises between the allantois and hindgut, grows caudally, and divides the cloaca into a dorsal rectum and ventral urogenital sinus. With this division, the mesonephric duct empties into the urogenital sinus. As the urogenital sinus and a small adjacent portion of the allantois enlarge to form the urinary bladder, portions of the mesonephric and metanephric (ureter) ducts are incorporated into the wall of the urogenital sinus. This results in the ureters entering the bladder and the mesonephric ducts entering more caudally into the less dilated portion of the urogenital sinus. This distal portion of the urogenital sinus will become the urethra of the male and the urethra, vestibule, and part of the vagina of the female.

Development of the Reproductive System. Even though the sex of the embryo is determined at fertilization, the gonads, ducts, and external genitalia pass through an indifferent stage of development in which male and female components have the same appearance. This stage lasts until about the sixth week of development.

In the *indifferent stage,* gonads form on the medial wall of the urogenital ridges. Starting in the third week, primordial sex cells migrate from the entoderm of the yolk sac to the urogenital ridge. By the sixth week the coelomic epithelium has proliferated, invaginated, and surrounded the primordial sex cells to form primitive gonadal (primary sex) cords in the underlying mesoderm of the gonad.

In the indifferent stage of genital duct formation, both mesonephric and Müllerian (paramesonephric) ducts are present. The Müllerian ducts arise as longitudinal invaginations of the coelomic epithelium on the lateral wall of the urogenital ridge. Cranially this duct remains open to the coelom. Caudally it opens through the dorsal wall of the urogenital sinus. In its craniocaudal course it lies at first lateral to the mesonephric duct, then passes anterior to it, and finally fuses with the opposite müllerian duct medial to the mesonephric ducts. During this fusion the urogenital ridges of the two sides are brought together to form a genital cord (septum) between the developing bladder anteriorly and the rectum posteriorly.

In the indifferent stage of the development of the external genitalia, mesoderm invades the lateral walls of the external opening of the urogenital sinus producing elevations called urogenital (urethral) folds (Fig. 2-45C). These folds unite anterior (cephalic) to the urogenital opening at the genital tubercle. Labioscrotal swellings develop lateral to the urogenital folds.

In the development of the ***male reproductive system*** the gonadal cords become testis cords that differentiate into seminiferous tubules and rete testis. The primordial sex cells become spermatogonia, whereas ingrowing coelomic epithelial cells give rise to supportive (Sertoli) cells. Leydig cells develop from mesenchyme. Efferent ductules develop from adjacent mesonephric tubules (Fig. 2-45A). The developing testis produces müllerian-inhibiting hormone (MIH) and androgens, which lead to the degeneration of the müllerian duct and to the differentiation of the mesonephric duct into the ductus epididymidis, vas (ductus) deferens, and ejaculatory duct. The seminal vesicle arises as an outgrowth of the mesonephric duct. The urogenital sinus gives rise to the urethra and the prostate, bulbourethral, and urethral glands. The genital tubercle enlarges and carries with it inferiorly a urethral plate of entoderm. This plate is transformed into the penile (cavernous) urethra after the lateral urogenital folds fuse ventrally (Fig. 2-45D). The urethral plate, urogenital folds and genital tubercle (phallus) give rise to the definitive penis. The scrotum is formed by the ventral fusion of the labioscrotal swellings. The testes descend late in gestation from their retroperitoneal abdominal location. They are ''anchored'' in the scrotum by the gubernaculum testis, which is derived from mesoderm of the urogenital ridge caudal to the testis. The path of descent is indicated by the inguinal canal. This follows the embryonic pathway of the processus vaginalis evaginating from the peritoneum.

In the development of the ***female reproductive system*** the initial gonadal cords degenerate and a second series of ovarian cords develop from primordial sex cells and coelomic epithelium. This second set of cords splits into groups of follicles near the surface of the developing ovary. Each primitive ovarian follicle consists of a developing sex cell surrounded by a flattened layer of follicular cells. The sex cells complete the prophase of the first meiotic division and are in the arrested dictyotene stage by the time of birth. From the sixth month until parturition there is a tremendous rate of degeneration of primitive follicles, the number decreasing from about 6 million to about 400,000 or less.

The unfused portions of the müllerian ducts develop into the uterine tubes (Fig. 2-45B). The fused portion give rise to the uterus and part of the vagina. The genital cord remains as the broad ligament of the uterus. The proper ligament of the ovary and the round ligament of the uterus probably arise from the mesoderm of the urogenital ridge caudal to the ovary. The mesonephric duct and tubules degenerate, but some remain as the paroophoron (tubules), epoophoron (tubules and duct), and Gartner's duct (duct). Where the fused müllerian ducts empty into the urogenital sinus, some entodermal tissue forms a vaginal plate that eventually hollows out as the lower two thirds of the vagina; the upper one third is thought to arise from the müllerian ducts. The urogenital sinus caudal to the vaginal opening becomes enlarged as the vestibule.

In the female the genital tubercle remains relatively small as the clitoris (Fig. 2-45E). The urethral folds become the labia minora, and the labioscrotal swellings develop into the labia majora. The hymen probably forms from the entoderm of the vaginal plate.

Congenital Malformations of the Urogenital System. ***Horseshoe kidney*** is usually due to fusion of the caudal ends of the two kidneys across the midline. This probably occurs as they are approximated in their cranial migration out of the pelvis over the umbilical arteries. The fused caudal poles become entrapped between the inferior mesenteric artery and aorta, and the continued ascent of the kidneys results in their elongation and horseshoe shape. ***Bifid ureter*** is usually the result of a premature division of the ureteric bud. When this occurs it may result in double pelvis or double kidney. ***Exstrophy of the bladder*** is caused by failure of mesoderm to invade the area anterior to the developing bladder. This results in improper development of the anterior abdominal wall and bladder with exposure of the posterior mucosal wall to the outside. ***Congenital hydrocoele*** is a collection of fluid in a remnant of the processus vaginalis. In ***hypospadias*** the external meatus of the urethra is on the ventral surface of the penis or scrotum. This may be caused by improper closure of the urogenital folds or labioscrotal swellings and by failure of the outer ectodermal cells to grow into the glans and join the penile urethra.

Improper fusion of the müllerian ducts leads to many different abnormalities of the uterus. These range from uterus didelphys with its two bodies (bicornis) and two cervices bicollis to uterus arcuatus in which there is a minor degree of imperfect fusion in the fundus. ***Double vagina*** is due to a defect in the canalization of the paired sinovaginal bulbs that give rise to the vaginal plate.

Pseudohermaphroditism is a condition in which the

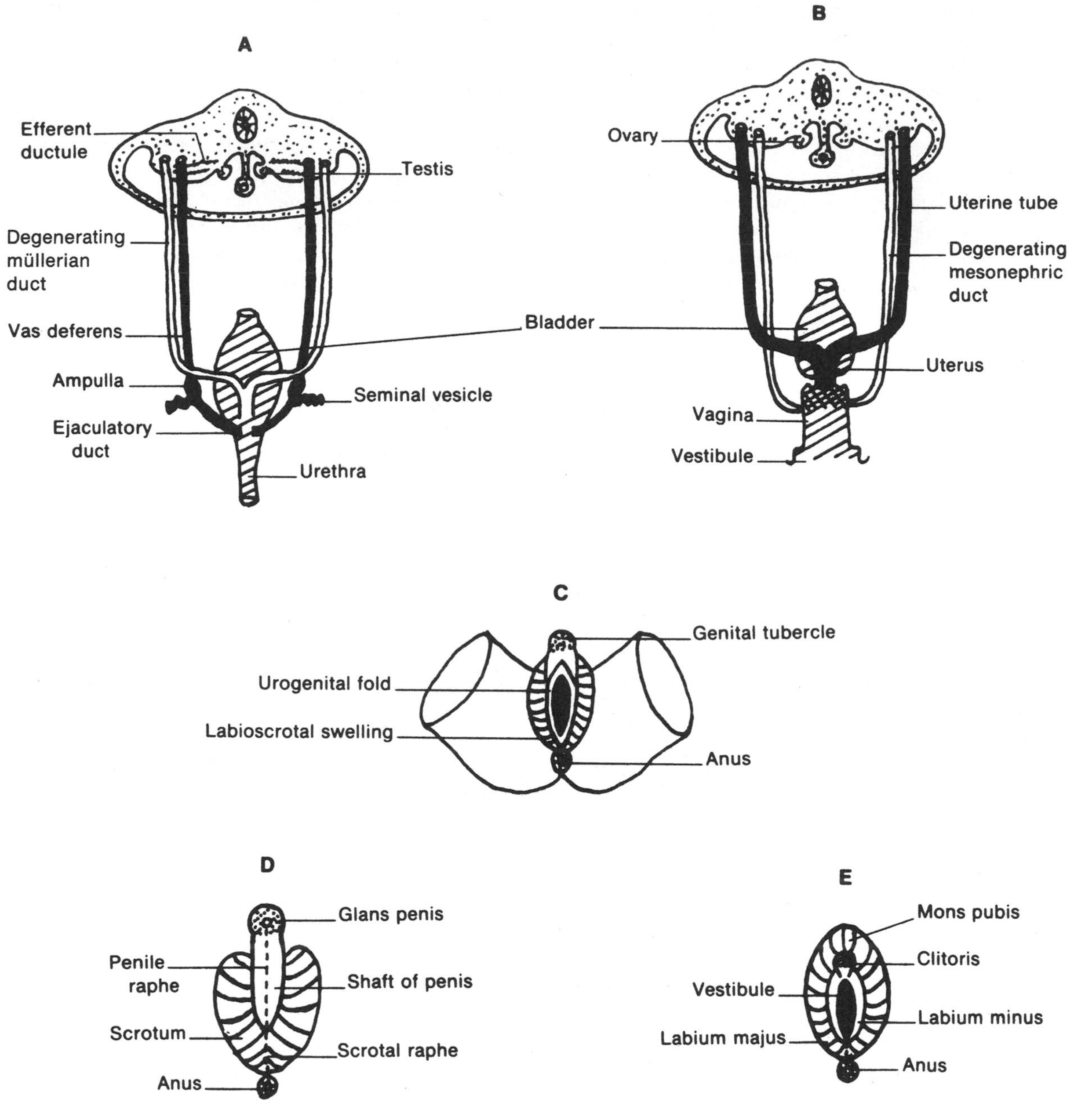

Fig. 2-45. Development of the urogenital system. *(A)* The male reproductive ducts are shown in black developing from the mesonephric tubules (efferent ductules) and mesonephric duct; the urethra develops from the urogenital sinus (hatched). *(B)* The female reproductive ducts develop from the müllerian ducts (black) and urogenital sinus (hatched). The upper one third of the vagina (cross-hatched) may develop from the müllerian ducts. *(C)* The indifferent stage of external genitalia development. *(D)* and *(E)* Male and female external genitalia, respectively, developing from the genital tubercle (stippled), urogenital folds (white), and labioscrotal swellings (hatched). The vestibule (black) is lined by entoderm of the urogenital sinus.

individual has either testes (male pseudohermaphrodite) or ovaries (female pseudohermaphrodite) but possesses external genitalia of the opposite sex. In hermaphroditism, both ovarian and testicular tissue are present. In ***testicular feminization*** the male duct system and external genitalia are not induced to develop. An immature female duct system and female external genitalia remain. In ***adrenogenital syndrome*** a genetic abnormality results in absence of an enzyme necessary for the production of hydrocortisone. This leads to an excess of ACTH, which causes overproduction of adrenal androgens. In females the excessive androgen causes hypertrophy of the clitoris and fusion of the labia majora, thus producing female hermaphroditism. In males the overproduction may cause precocious secondary sexual characteristics.

EARLY EMBRYOLOGY AND DEVELOPMENT OF THE PLACENTA

Fertilization. At ovulation a secondary oocyte, zona pellucida, and corona radiata of follicle cells are discharged from the ovary and drawn into the infundibulum of the uterine tube where a spermatozoan can penetrate the zona pellicuda and secondary oocyte (Fig. 2-46). In this process, acrosome enzymes aid in penetration of the corona radiata and zone pellucida, while a cytoplasmic response of the secondary oocyte leads to a zonal reaction that prohibits penetration by other spermatozoa. The union of the spermatozoan and secondary oocyte in the process of fertilization brings about the following major physical consequences: (1) reactivation of the secondary oocyte, (2) completion of the second meiotic division with formation of the second polar body, (3) establishment of a zygote (fertilized ovum) with the diploid number (46) of chromosomes, and (4) establishment of the mitotic spindle for the first cleavage division.

Cleavage and Blastodermic Vesicle Formation. During cleavage a series of mitoses occur in the zygote that result in successive 2, 4, 8, and 16 cell stages. These divisions take place over a period of about 3 days as the developing conceptus passes down the uterine tube. At about the time the 16-cell morula reaches the uterine cavity, fluid penetrates between some of the cells and produces a cavity in the solid ball of cells. The conceptus is now called a blastodermic vesicle (blastocyst). It consists of an outer layer of cells called the trophoblast, a cavity of the blastodermic vesicle (blastocoele), and an inner cell mass. After 3 days in the uterine cavity, the conceptus "hatches" from the zonal enclosure, and the sticky trophoblastic cells adhere to the endometrium.

Establishment of Ectoderm, Entoderm, and Mesoderm. In the eighth day of development the inner cell mass cavitates to form an ectodermally lined amniotic cavity. The ectoderm of the embryonic disk will eventually give rise to the neural tube, neural crest, and epidermis. An inner entodermal layer of cells also differentiates from the inner cell mass. These cells proliferate to form the yolk sac. The dorsal portion of the yolk sac later will become incorporated into the embryo as the primitive gut. Embryonic mesoderm arises from an elongate mass of cells called the primitive streak. The mesodermal cells turn inward along the midline and move

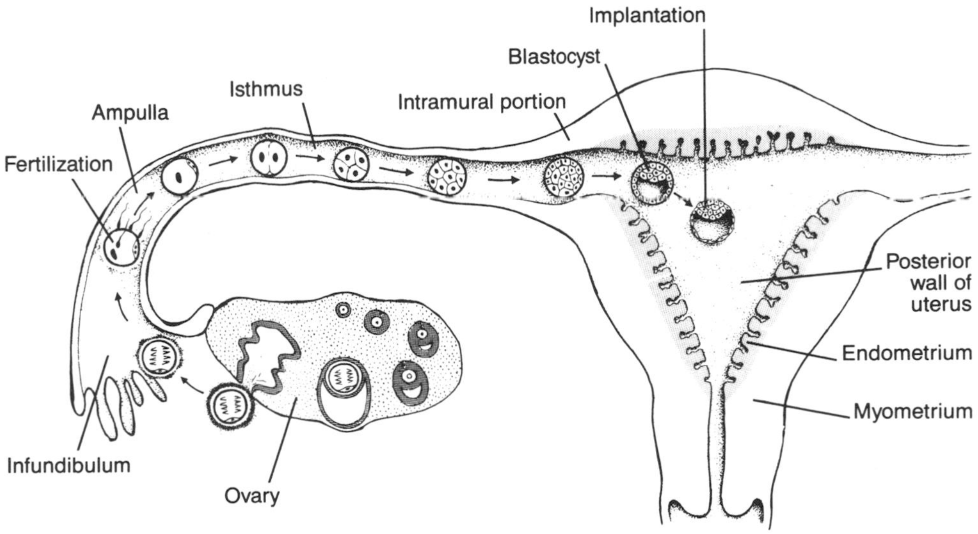

Fig. 2-46. Diagram illustrating ovulation, fertilization, cleavage, and blastocyst formation. (Cormack DH: Ham's Histology, 9th ed, p 633. Philadelphia, JB Lippincott, 1987. After Moore KL: The Developing Human. Clinically Oriented Embryology, 4th ed. Philadelphia, WB Saunders, 1988; modified with permission)

laterally, insinuating themselves between the ectoderm and entoderm. In its forward, caudal, and lateral movement, the embryonic mesoderm eventually joins the extraembryonic mesoderm that arises from the trophoblast. The notochord arises as a midline forward growth of cells from the primitive (Hensen's) node. In the third week of development, the embryonic mesoderm will have differentiated into paraxial (somite, dorsal), intermediate, and lateral mesoderm. The paraxial mesoderm will develop further into paired somites whose sclerotome eventually give rise to vertebrae and ribs, whose myotome will give rise to skeletal muscle, and whose dermatome will develop into connective tissues. The intermediate mesoderm will differentiate into much of the urogenital system. The lateral mesoderm, like the extraembryonic mesoderm, splits to form a coelom. That lateral mesoderm adjacent to the ectoderm is somatic mesoderm, while that next to entoderm is splanchnic mesoderm. Somatic mesoderm later will give rise to body wall tissues. Splanchnic mesoderm further differentiates into the cardiovascular system; smooth muscle and connective tissues in the walls of most visceral structures; mesenteries; and the spleen.

Development of the Placenta. After the attachment of the blastodermic vesicle to the uterus at about the sixth postfertilization day, the trophoblast proliferates rapidly, and the conceptus begins to implant into the compacta layer of the endometrium. It is completely embedded in the uterine stroma by the eleventh postfertilization day (see Fig. 2-46). In the rapid proliferation of cytotrophoblastic cells, fusion of the outer cells forms an outer syncytial trophoblast over the single inner layer of cytotrophoblast. The coalescence of lacunae formed in the syncytial trophoblast leads to the formation of primary stem villi and intervillous spaces. The villi are most extensive in the trophoblast that faces the deeper layers of the endometrium. It is in this region where most of the nutriments are being supplied to the trophoblast from invaded uterine glands and blood vessels. The primary stem villi consist of a core of cytotrophoblast surrounded by syncytial trophoblast. Later, mesoderm invades these villi, and they become secondary stem villi containing a core of connective tissue. By the end of the third week, blood vessels start to form in the secondary villi, and they are designated as tertiary villi. With the vascularization of the trophoblast, it is called the chorion. That part of the chorion that is the deepest in the uterine wall becomes the chorion frondosum portion of the placenta; the rest of it loses its villi and is called the chorion laeve. An anchoring villus and its free-floating villi constitute a cotyledon. Septa formed from the cytotrophoblastic coating and decidual tissue of the intervillous space project from the decidua and incompletely separate the cotyledons from each other. The functional layer of the endometrium deep to the chorion frondosum is the decidua basalis; that adjacent to the chorion laeve is the decidua capsularis; and the rest is the decidua parietalis. As the embryo enlarges the uterine cavity is obliterated, and the decidua capsularis and decidua parietalis fuse into a much compressed layer. After birth of the newborn, the decidual layers, placenta, chorion laeve, and amnion will be discharged as the afterbirth.

QUESTIONS IN ANATOMY

Both essay and multiple-choice questions are presented in this section. The answers to the multiple-choice questions are at the end of this chapter. The answers to the essay questions are in the text.

Essay Questions

Contrast the five principal regions of the vertebral column, giving the characteristics of typical vertebrae and curvatures and the exact movements permitted in each region.

Draw the normal curves of the spine.

Describe a typical thoracic vertebra.

List the various factors that permit movement of the vertebral column. Why do lumbar dislocations usually involve fracture while cervical dislocations do not?

Why does a rupture of the disk between lumbar vertebrae 4 and 5 usually impinge on spinal nerve L5?

How do cartilage and bone differ in their vascularity and in the mode of their nutritional supply?

How do seven cervical vertebrae develop from eight pairs of cervical sclerotomes? What is the embryologic basis of spondylolisthesis? spina bifida?

Describe the major components of the growing epiphyseal disk. How does a long bone grow in length and width?

What are the major functions of the superficial muscles of the back? the deep muscles of the back? What is the innervation to these muscles?

Describe a sarcomere. Are actin and myosin found in both the A and I bands? What is the T tubular system? What are the functions of intercalated disks?

What motor functional components of nerves innervate skeletal muscle of branchial arch origin? skeletal muscle of somite origin? smooth muscle of splanchnic mesoderm origin?

Draw a cross section of the thoracic cord, indicating the principal ascending and descending tracts.

Describe the formation of a typical spinal nerve.

Describe the contents and extent of the cauda equina. What area is the region of choice for a spinal tap? Why?

Give the extent and the relationships of the spinal cord

and its meninges. Into which space is an anesthetic injected through the inferior aperture of the sacral canal as in caudal analgesia?

List the functional components of a spinal nerve. Which of these is a component of the autonomic nervous system? Where are preganglionic and postganglionic autonomic neurons located?

Name the nuclei of termination for incoming GSA fibers of spinal nerves.

Where would chromatolysis take place in hemisection of the spinal cord at the T3 level? What would be the sensory loss from this lesion? What would be the motor loss?

What is the fate of neural crest material? What cells are responsible for the formation of myelin in the CNS? in the PNS?

Describe the events of degeneration and regeneration of a peripheral nerve.

What would be the functional loss if the sulcal arteries supplying the C7 level were thrombosed? What area of the cord is supplied by the posterior spinal arteries?

Name the one bony link between the upper extremity and the axial skeleton.

What is the major support of the acromioclavicular joint?

Where is the surgical neck of the humerus?

Describe the articular capsule of the shoulder joint; its attachment.

What are the major supports of the shoulder joint?

What motions occur at the shoulder joint?

What muscles cause each of the motions at the shoulder joint?

Name the structures found in the suprahumeral space. What is the importance of the suprahumeral space?

At what joints do pronation and supination occur?

Describe the articular surfaces that form the elbow joint? What motions occur at this joint? What muscles cause the motions?

Between what bones is the wrist joint formed? What motions occur at the wrist joint? What muscles cause each of these motions?

What motions are available at the four medial carpometacarpal joints? How do the motions of the CM joint of the thumb differ from those of the other four?

List the motions that can occur at the metacarpophalangeal joints and the major motors of each.

Contraction of the muscles in the anterior compartment of the arm causes what motions? in the posterior compartment?

What nerve innervates the muscles in the anterior compartment of the arm? in the posterior compartment?

The muscles in the anterior compartment of the forearm are innervated by what nerves? in the posterior compartment?

What motions are caused by contraction of the muscles in the anterior compartment of the forearm? in the posterior compartment?

Describe the compartmentalization of the ventral aspect of the hand. What nerve(s) innervate(s) the muscles of each compartment?

Describe the radial and ulnar bursae.

Describe the locations of the midpalmar and thenar spaces.

Describe the organization of the brachial plexus.

Name the collateral branches of each part of the plexus.

Specifically define the locations of the ulnar and median nerves at the wrist.

What physical problems result following an injury to the radial nerve? musculocutaneous nerve? ulnar nerve? median nerve?

Trace the course of the brachial artery through the arm, and the radial and ulnar arteries through the forearm and hand.

Where exactly are radial and ulnar pulses taken?

Which artery terminates as the major contributor to the superficial palmar arterial arch? deep palmar arterial arch?

Describe the location and courses of the cephalic and basilic veins. Where does each empty into the deep veins?

What three bones form the os coxae? Describe the location of the acetabulum, obturator foramen, ischial spine, ischial tuberosity, greater sciatic notch, lesser sciatic notch, iliac crest with its anterior and posterior superior spines, and the pubic tubercle.

Compare the articular surfaces that form the hip joint with those that form the shoulder joint.

Compare the acetabular labrum with the glenoid labrum.

Define the extent of the articular capsule of the hip joint. What parts of the femoral neck are intracapsular and what parts are extracapsular?

Describe in general the blood supply to the femoral neck and head. What is unique about the courses of some of these vessels?

Describe the extracapsular ligaments of the hip joint. What are the functions?

What motions can occur at the hip joint? What are the muscles involved in each motion?

Describe the articular surfaces that form the knee joint.

What motions are available at the knee joint? What muscles cause these motions?

Describe the menisci. What are their functions?

Against what types of forces do the cruciate ligaments protect the knee? the collateral ligaments?

List the bones of the foot. Which of these form the medial longitudinal arch? the lateral longitudinal arch?

What ligament is the most important support of the longitudinal arches of the foot?

Describe the formation of the ankle joint.

What motions are available at the ankle joint? What muscles cause each of the motions?

What ligament is usually injured in an inversion-plantar flexion sprain?

At what joints do inversion and eversion occur primarily? These motions are produced by the contraction of what muscles?

Describe the location of the gluteal muscles; innervation; functions.

Name the muscles of the anterior compartment of the thigh; innervation; functions.

List the medial and posterior femoral muscles; innervation; functions.

Describe the femoral triangle. What structures pass through the triangle and what are their relationships?

Describe the popliteal fossa and the relationships of the structures within the triangle.

List the muscles found in each of the compartments of the leg; innervations; functions.

Describe the compartmentation of the foot. What nerves innervate the muscles in each compartment?

Fibers from which spinal cord segments are found in the lumbosacral plexus? Where is the lumbar portion of the plexus formed? the sacral portion?

Describe the courses of the medial and lateral plantar nerves and compare each with its homologous nerve in the hand.

Describe the limp that would accompany an injury of the superior gluteal, inferior gluteal, femoral, deep peroneal, and tibial nerves.

Describe the course of the femoral artery through the thigh. How does it begin? Where exactly is it located in the femoral triangle?

At what point does the femoral become the popliteal artery? Where is the artery in the popliteal fossa? How can a popliteal pulse be taken?

Describe the courses of the main arterial trunks through the leg.

Compare the arterial supply of the foot with that of the hand.

Describe the exact location of the greater saphenous vein as it crosses the ankle joint.

Which nerves leave the anterior cranial fossa?

Which structures are found in the posterior cranial fossa? What are the important foramina of this region? Name the structures passing through each foramen.

Which structures pass through the foramen magnum?

Name the structures passing from the middle cranial fossa to the orbit through: (1) the optic foramen, (2) the superior orbital fissure, (3) the foramen rotundum, (4) the foramen ovale, and (5) the foramen lacerum.

List the contents of the infratemporal fossa. Where does this fossa communicate with the cranial cavity?

Describe the important relationships of the mastoid air cells.

Describe the location and the extent of the pharynx, the parts into which it is usually divided, the structure of its walls, and the location of its various openings.

Describe the site and boundaries of the opening of the eustachian tube into the pharynx.

Describe the temporomandibular joint. In which direction does this joint usually become dislocated?

What are the structures and the spaces found just external to each part of the bony wall of the orbit? Indicate where each is related to the orbital wall.

Describe the extraocular muscles and give their nerve supply.

Describe the relationships of the palatine tonsil. Which artery is most commonly in close relation to the palatine tonsil? State the course of this artery and its relationships to the tonsil.

Give the relations of the branches of the external carotid artery? the internal carotid artery?

Describe the layers of the scalp. What are its blood and nerve supply?

Describe the meninges of the brain. In what parts of the brain are ventricles and choroid plexuses located?

Trace the pathway of the cerebrospinal fluid from its origin in the choroid plexus of the lateral ventricle to the superior sagittal sinus. What happens if the iter is occluded? At what other sites is the flow likely to be obstructed?

What are the principal fissures and lobes of the cerebrum?

Describe the internal and external topography of the medulla. Which cell columns extend into the medulla from the spinal cord?

Which cranial nerves arise from the medulla?

From what nuclei of origin in the brain stem do preganglionic parasympathetic fibers arise? Where do these fibers synapse and what organs do they supply?

Give, in general, the distribution of the vagus nerve. What are its functional components?

Give the origin, course, and distribution of the hypoglossal nerve.

What cranial nerves convey the afferent and efferent nerves (limbs) of the cough reflex? carotid sinus reflex? gag reflex? corneal blink relex? pupillary light reflex? What are the nuclei of termination and origin of these reflexes?

What nerves supply general somatic afferent, special visceral afferent, and somatic efferent fibers to the tongue? How is the tongue mucosa modified to carry out the functions of the tongue?

If the uvula points to the right on phonation, which nerve is most likely damaged?

What is the relation of the facial nerve to the middle

ear? the jugular vein? Describe the bony and the membranous labyrinths. Describe the middle ear and the mastoid. What is the anatomic basis for paralysis of only the lower contralateral face in corticobulbar lesions compared to paralysis of the whole ipsilateral side in facial nerve lesions?

Why do unilateral lesions of the auditory pathway within the CNS rarely result in deafness?

Describe the possible pathway for postrotational nystagmus starting with stimulation of the hair cells in the crista of the lateral semicircular canal.

Give the location within the central nervous system of the nuclei that directly innervate the voluntary ocular muscles. Where do afferent fibers to these nuclei originate and in which tracts do they travel to reach the nuclei? What are the necessary nerve connections for lateral conjugate gaze?

If the right fifth nerve is damaged, will the left eye blink if the right cornea is stimulated? If the right facial nerve is damaged and the fifth nerve is intact, will any eye blink if the right cornea is stimulated?

Describe the orbit and its contents.

Describe the eyeball.

Describe the normal anatomy of the fundus of the eye as seen with the ophthalmoscope. How are the arteries and the veins differentiated from each other?

What is the vascular supply of the retina? What nutritive pathway is compromised in detachment of the retina?

Describe the autonomic innervation of the eyeball and eyelid. Ptosis can occur following injury to what two nerve pathways? What are the symptoms of Horner's syndrome, and where might a lesion be located that could lead to this?

Describe the circulation of aqueous humor. In what area might blockage of the pathway lead to glaucoma?

Trace the flow of tears from their origin to their arrival in the nasal cavity. Where are the tarsal glands located and what types of glands are these?

What is the nerve pathway involved in the near reflex (accommodation, convergence, and pupillary reflex)?

Describe the optic nerve, its termination, and point of emergence from the skull.

Outline the visual pathway. Trace light rays from a point in the upper right quadrant of the visual field to the retina; then trace the impulses from the rods and cones stimulated to the specific site in the occipital cortex where the impulses would be received.

Contrast the effects of the destruction of the right optic nerve and of the left optic tract on the retina and the field of vision.

Describe the olfactory nerve, including its origin, termination, and exit from the skull.

Locate the lamina cribrosa.

Give the course and function of the pyramidal (corticospinal) tract. What is its relation to the cerebral motor cortex?

Describe the course of the medial lemniscus. Where do these fibers originate and terminate? What is the functional significance of this pathway?

Where are the primary receptive cortical areas for two-point touch, vision, hearing, and olfaction? Which relay nuclei of the diencephalon send fibers to these areas?

Where would be a likely site for a lesion that would give contralateral paralysis to the extremities and trunk and would also give paralysis of lateral gaze of the ipsilateral eye to the side of the lesion? Where would the lesion be if there was contralateral paralysis of the extremities, ipsilateral paralysis of medial gaze, ptosis, and dilated pupil?

Which functional components or pathways make up the internal capsule of the brain? Where in this structure is each component found?

Describe the paralysis resulting from a destructive lesion that involves the posterior limb of the internal capsule.

Where do the principal afferents to the cerebellum originate? Describe the course that each follows to reach its termination in the cerebellum.

What is the major output of the cerebellum? Where do the efferent pathways from the neocerebellum go? Where do the efferent pathways from the flocculonodular lobe terminate? What is the function of the cerebellum?

What is the major outflow of the lenticular nucleus? What connections are made with the subthalamic nucleus and what is the effect of this nucleus on the globus pallidus?

Which structures receive their blood supply from the internal carotid artery?

What blood vessels comprise the arterial circle of Willis?

Which major ascending and descending pathways could be compromised if there was occlusion of the anterior spinal artery where it arises from the vertebral artery?

What deficits would occur if the posterior inferior cerebellar artery were occluded?

Give the position, relationships, attachments, innervation, and embryonic origin of the pituitary gland. Into what parts is the pituitary gland divided and what are the characteristics of the cells in the various parts? What is the functional significance of each of the cell types?

Describe the pathway of hypothalamic-releasing hormones from their production in the hypothalamus to their site of action on chromophils of the adenohypophysis. How does this pathway differ from the neurosecretory tracts that terminate in the neurohypophysis?

Which structures are most susceptible to injury when the pituitary gland undergoes enlargement? Where are these structures found in relation to the pituitary?

Describe the major efferent pathways of the hypothalamus. What is the relationship between the hypothalamus and autonomic nervous system? the limbic system?

What are the two main divisions of the autonomic nervous system? Discuss the origins of these two divisions from the central nervous system. Where, in general, are the peripheral adrenergic and cholinergic fibers found within these two systems?

To which structures are the nerve fibers from the superior cervical ganglion distributed? What would be the results of destruction of this ganglion?

Describe the microscopic structure of the salivary glands. Where do their ducts open into the oral cavity?

Which of the major salivary glands are mixed seromucous glands? Both the pancreas and parotid can be affected in mumps. Compare the exocrine portions of these two glands. How are the cells of the striated (salivary) ducts of the parotid similar to the cells of the distal convoluted tubule of the kidney?

What are the major contents of the anterior triangle of the neck? the posterior triangle? In which triangle of the neck could you palpate the anterior scalene nodes? the roots of the brachial plexus?

Describe the carotid sheath, its contents, and its relation to the cervical sympathetic trunk.

Describe the cervical plexus and give the structures innervated by it.

Which anatomic structures are traversed in tracheotomy?

What comprises the true vocal fold? What nerves regulate the muscles of the larynx? What would be the motor and sensory loss if the superior laryngeal nerve were severed?

Give the gross and the microscopic structures of the thyroid gland and its important relations. What is its blood supply? Where may ectopic and accessory thyroids be found? Explain their location on the basis of the embryonic development of the thyroid.

Give the number, the position, and the relationships of the parathyroid glands. Describe briefly the origin and the development of these glands.

Give the position, relationships, and microscopic structure of the thymus. Explain the occasional inclusion of parathyroid tissue in the thymus. Compare the thymus gland at birth and at puberty.

If there is a complete branchial fistula at the second pharyngeal pouch and cleft, where will it open internally and externally?

Describe the development of the face. What is the embryologic basis for cleft lip? cleft palate? choanal atresia?

Outline the boundaries of the lungs and pleura on the chest wall.

Name the lobes and the fissures of each lung and explain how they can be mapped out on the chest wall.

Give the outline of the heart as projected on the surface of the anterior thoracic wall. Which structures of the heart form the boundaries described above? Which chambers lie directly beneath the anterior chest wall?

Locate the heart valves as projected into the anterior chest wall. Which of these valves lie near the surface and which are placed more deeply? If sounds from the more deeply placed valves are projected in the direction of blood flow through these valves, where would be the areas of maximum audibility for each?

What are the boundaries of the mediastinum? Give the contents of the anterior, the middle, and the posterior portions.

Give the positions and the relationships of the trachea in the thorax. At what level does it branch into the right and left bronchi? In which of these bronchi is a foreign body most likely to lodge? Explain.

How many bronchopulmonary segments are there in each lung and lobe?

Describe the right pleural sac. Why does the lung collapse when an opening forms from the air passages of the lung into the pleural sac?

Describe the innervation of the lungs. Indicate the functional significance of the nerve fibers involved.

Describe the changes in the histology of the walls of the respiratory tract as one proceeds from the trachea to the alveoli. How far down the conducting pathways do cartilage, glands, and ciliated epithelium extend?

Describe the lining epithelium of the alveoli. What structures constitute a blood–air barrier?

Give the location and microscopic structure of the valves of the heart. What are the functions of the chordae tendineae and the papillary muscles? How are these structures arranged to subserve their functions? Compare the right and the left atrioventricular orifices and their valves. Why is one valve larger than the other?

Contrast the right and left ventricles of the heart as to structure of the walls, volume of the cavities, and valvular arrangements.

Describe the development of the interatrial septum. Where is the foramen ovale? What is the embryologic basis of the foramen ovale defect and the foramen primum defect? What embryologic structures contribute to the development of the membranous part of the interventricular septum?

Describe the arch of the aorta, including its important relationships.

Describe the fate of the five pairs of aortic arches. What is the developmental reason for a right subclavian artery arising from the arch of the aorta? How does transposition of the aorta and pulmonary artery arise?

What embryologic vessels are retained and which fail to form in the formation of double superior venae cavae? What postnatal structures arise from the left umbilical vein, vitelline veins, vitelline arteries, and umbilical arteries?

Describe the blood supply to the heart.

Describe the efferent innervation to the heart, including the location of the cell bodies of the various neurons involved.

Give the anatomic arrangements that provide for reflex slowing of the heart on stimulation of the carotid sinus.

The stellate ganglion has been removed for the relief of anginal pain. What effects other than the relief of anginal pain may result? Explain the anatomic basis for each of these additional effects.

Describe in detail the anatomic arrangement of the structures in the heart responsible for the initiation and transmission of the heart beat.

Describe in detail the anatomic modifications in the heart and the resultant changes in the circulation of the blood in a normal infant following birth. What results if these normal changes do not take place? Explain.

Describe the composition, the extent, and the attachments of the pericardial sac. Where can it be opened for drainage without going through the pleura?

Describe the diaphragm, including its origin, structure, attachments, and orifices. Give the mechanism of its action. Where is referred pain from the diaphragm commonly experienced and how is this related to its innervation?

What are the roles in inspiration of the diaphragm, abdominal muscles, intercostal muscles, and scalene muscles?

Contrast the gross and the histologic features of the esophagus and the trachea as related to the functions of each of these tubes.

What is a possible embryologic reason for tracheoesophageal fistula? for diaphragmatic hernia?

Where does the thoracic duct empty and what does it drain?

Describe the lymphatics of the thoracic cavity. What is the effect, if any, of blocking the thoracic duct at the point at which it empties into the venous system?

Describe the pathway of lymph through a lymphatic node. What is the function of the reticuloendothelial (mononuclear phagocyte) system? What is the function of a lymph node?

Compare the microscopic structure of the thymus with that of a lymph node. What is the gross relationship of the thymus to the great vessels?

Discuss the lymphatic drainage of the breast, mentioning all possible pathways and connections.

Describe the normal gross and microscopic structure of the mammary gland.

Describe the origin, the course, and the termination of the splanchnic nerves. What is the functional nature of the various fibers running in these nerves, and where are the cell bodies of these fibers located? What would be the vascular effects in the abdomen on section of the splanchnic nerves?

Divide the abdomen into nine surface regions and name them. What structures do the horizontal dividing lines represent?

Divide the abdomen into four regions.

Locate the stomach on the surface, including the cardiac orifice and the pyloric orifice.

On the surface locate the duodenum, the ileocolic junction, the cecum, and the right and left colic flexures.

On the surface outline the liver and indicate the exact location of the gallbladder.

On the surface locate the pancreas, spleen, kidneys, and ureter.

What muscles form the anterior abdominal wall?

What abdominal muscle or its aponeurosis forms the superficial inguinal ring, the deep inguinal ring, and the floor, roof, anterior and posterior walls of the inguinal canal?

Differentiate between the pathway of a direct versus an indirect inguinal hernia.

Differentiate between organs that are retroperitoneal, partially peritonealized and ''completely'' peritonealized. Give specific examples of each.

Describe the location of the lesser peritoneal sac.

Name the three structures in the free edge of the lesser omentum.

Describe the parts of the stomach.

What are the four parts of the duodenum?

Where are the jejunum and ileum normally located? How does the jejunum differ grossly and microscopically from the ileum?

How does the large intestine differ grossly and microscopically from the small intestine?

With what organs are the ascending, transverse and descending parts of the colon related?

With what organs is the liver related? Where is the gallbladder found with respect to the liver? With what organs is the gallbladder related?

Describe the bare area of the liver.

Describe the peritoneal relationships of the liver.

What is the relationship between the inferior vena cava and the liver?

Where are the caudate and quadrate lobes of the liver?

What organs are drained by the portal vein? What alternate pathways may blood take when the normal path for portal blood through the liver is obstructed?

Describe the bile duct system of the liver and gallbladder.

Describe the relationships of the pancreas. Into what does the main pancreatic duct empty?

Describe the peritoneal relationships of the spleen.

At what vertebral levels are the kidneys found?

What structures form the kidney bed? What structures are related to the anterior surfaces of each kidney?

Describe the course of the ureters. To what structures is each ureter related? At what locations are the ureters naturally constricted?

Describe the location and relationships of each suprarenal gland.

At what vertebral level does the aorta pass through the thoracic diaphragm? At what vertebral level does the abdominal aorta bifurcate? Where is the abdominal aorta with respect to the lumbar vertebrae?

Name the three large unpaired branches of the aorta and give the distribution of each.

What general areas are supplied by the common iliac arteries?

The sympathetic fibers that innervate the abdominal viscera originate from what spinal cord segments? Where do the synapses occur between the preganglionic and postganglionic sympathetic and parasympathetic fibers that supply the abdominal viscera?

What part of the gastrointestinal tract is supplied by the vagus nerve?

Describe the system of nerve plexuses along the ventral aspect of the aorta.

What nerves innervate the skin and muscle of the abdominal wall?

What are the major differences in character in the normal mucosa of the alimentary canal, beginning with the esophagus, and terminating at the anus? What are the associated changes in function?

Describe the stomach. Give its relations and describe the microscopic structure of gastric glands. What cells produce HCl? pepsin? mucus? serotonin?

Describe the modifications of the small intestine for the function of absorption. What structures accentuate the absorptive surface area. Locate Brunner's glands. What do they produce?

Describe the histologic structure of the vermiform appendix.

What is the microscopic structure of the liver? Describe the circulation of the blood through the liver. Explain on an anatomic basis why certain ingested poisons cause damage initially to the periphery of the liver lobules. In case of portal obstruction, what collateral venous circulation might be established?

Give the contents of the portal areas (canals, triads).

How is the mucosa of the gallbladder structurally adapted to the functions it performs?

Describe the histologic structure of the pancreas. Give the functional significance of its various structures. What are the most prominent ultrastructural characteristics of cells of the exocrine secretory units?

What is the microscopic structure of the spleen? Describe the flow of blood through the spleen. Describe the position, relationships, and peritoneal attachments of the spleen.

Describe the microscopic structure of the adrenal gland. What is the nerve and blood supply to the cortex and medulla? Locate the cell bodies of neurons that supply the medulla.

Describe the histologic structure of the kidney. What is the blood supply to the various components of the renal cortex and medulla? How are the different parts of the nephron structurally adapted to carry out their functions?

What constitutes the filtration barrier of the renal corpuscle?

What are the histologic features of the ureter and urinary bladder that permit them to readily accommodate large quantities of water?

Describe the rotation of the gut. What are the fates of the cephalic and caudal limbs of the gut loop?

How does the lesser peritoneal sac develop? What embryologic structures contribute to the formation of the greater omentum? What is the fate of the vitelline (omphalomesenteric) artery?

Locate the following structures and give their embryologic significance: (1) ligamentum arteriosum, (2) ligamentum venosum, (3) round ligament of the liver, (4) Meckel's diverticulum, and (5) lateral umbilical ligaments.

Compare the peritoneal arrangements of the various parts of the large intestine. Explain the manner in which a structure that in early development is suspended by peritoneum becomes secondarily retroperitoneal.

Describe the origin of the pancreas.

Compare the suprarenal medulla with a sympathetic ganglion as to its origin, structure, and function. Describe the development of the suprarenal gland.

How does the bare area of the liver reflect the development of the liver in the caudal face of the septum transversum? From what embryonic germ layer do the epithelium and glands of most of the digestive system arise?

Differentiate the true from the false pelvis.

Define the pelvic inlet and the pelvic outlet.

What muscles form the pelvic diaphragm? Describe their lateral attachments.

Define the AP and transverse diameters of the pelvic inlet, pelvic outlet, and midpelvis.

Define the boundaries of the urogenital and anal triangles.

Describe the boundaries of the ischiorectal fossa, including its anterior and posterior recesses and its contents.

What is the pudendal canal and what are its contents?

Describe the deep perineal space. What are its contents in the male and the female?

Define the superficial perineal space. What are its contents in the male and the female?

What nerves innervate the skin of the perineum?

What structures are palpable in the male and female via rectal examination?

Define the location of the urinary bladder and name the organs to which it is related in both the male and female.

Trace the course of the urethra in both the male and female.

To what structures is the prostate gland related?

Describe the course of the ductus (vas) deferens.

Describe the location of the ovaries.

How are the ovaries related to the uterine tubes?

Define the parts of the uterus.

How is the uterus related to the vagina?

What is the normal position of the uterus? To what structures is it related?

What structures are normally palpable by a vaginal examination?

How is the broad ligament related to the uterus?

What are the mesometrium, mesovarium, mesosalpinx, parametrium, and the cardinal ligaments?

Name the visceral branches of the internal iliac artery and describe their general distributions.

Describe the origin, migration and fate of primordial sex cells in the formation of the indifferent stage of the gonad and in the formation of the testis and ovary.

Describe the histologic structure of the testis. Where and how does spermatogenesis take place?

Describe the histologic structure of the epithelium lining the rete testis, efferent ductules, ductus epididymidis, and ductus deferens.

Describe the male urethra, its parts, their characteristics and relationships. Explain on an anatomic basis where in the course of the urethra difficulty might be experienced in passing a rigid catheter.

What ducts empty into the urethra, and what is the nature of the substances being delivered to the urethra?

Describe the histologic characteristics of the penis. What structures are adapted for the function of erection? Why is the urethra not completely compressed during erection?

What is the origin of the vesicular ovarian (graafian) follicle? What is ovulation? When does it occur in relation to the menstrual cycle? When does it occur in relation to oogenesis?

Describe the development and histology of the corpus luteum.

If fertilization and implantation do not take place, when during the menstrual cycle will the corpus luteum degenerate? What is a corpus albicans?

Describe the histologic structure of the uterine (fallopian) tube. What is the function of the ciliated epithelium?

Describe the histologic structure of the uterus. State the major endometrial changes that take place during the menstrual cycle and during pregnancy. What is the effect of estrogen on the uterus? of progesterone?

Describe the mucosa of the cervix. What changes take place in the cervix during the menstrual cycle? during pregnancy?

Describe the histology of the vagina. How does its epithelium change during the menstrual cycle?

Compare the histology of the clitoris and penis.

What are the fates of the mesonephric ducts, müllerian ducts, and urogenital sinus in the male? in the female?

What is the difference in origin of the nephrons and collecting tubules?

What is the embryologic basis of double vagina? uterus didelphys? bipartite uterus?

What is the normal fate of the processus vaginalis in the male? What is hydrocoele?

What is the fate of the urethral folds and labioscrotal swellings in the male? in the female? What embryologic structures are involved in the formation of hypospadias? What causes, and what is the effect of, congenital adrenal hyperplasia?

What series of events immediately follows penetration of a secondary oocyte by a spermatozoon? Where does fertilization usually occur?

For what period of time is the developing conceptus in the uterine tube? in the uterine cavity? On what postfertilization day does implantation occur?

Into what layers of the endometrium does the embryo implant?

Describe the development of the placenta. When are both cytotrophoblast and syncytial trophoblast present? When are nucleated red blood cells normally found?

Describe the histologic structure of the placenta. What is the chorion frondosum? What is a cotyledon? Where are decidual cells found? What is the decidua basalis?

Describe the placental barrier. Describe the flow of blood through the placenta.

What is the fate of the primitive streak and primitive (Hensen's) node?

What is the developmental relation of the allantois to the urinary bladder?

What is the fate of the primitive yolk sac? How are the respiratory and digestive systems related to the yolk sac?

What is the fate of the neural plate?

What is the fate of the sclerotome? myotome? intermediate mesoderm?

Multiple-Choice Questions

ONE-ANSWER TYPE

Select the *one* statement that most accurately completes the sentence or answers the question. Answers are at the end of this chapter.

1. In a cell with especially high energy (ATP) requirements, which of the following organelles would you expect to be most highly developed?
   (a) Rough endoplasmic reticulum
   (b) Mitochondria
   (c) Centrioles
   (d) Peroxisomes
2. Cells with large amounts of rough endoplasmic reticulum are most likely to:
   (a) Produce steroids
   (b) Line the lumen of blood vessels
   (c) Produce structural proteins that remain in the cell
   (d) Synthesize a proteinaceous secretory product
3. Regarding the nucleus:
   (a) Chromosomes in areas of euchromatin are probably less functionally active than in areas of heterochromatin.
   (b) The nucleolar membrane separates the nucleolus from the chromosomes.
   (c) The nuclear envelop consists of two membranes, and is penetrated by pores to allow passage of material between the nucleus and the cytoplasm.
   (d) Chromosomes and the nuclear envelop are most prominent during the metaphase stage of mitosis.
4. Assuming a person had received enough exposure of x rays to the whole body to destroy cells as they attempt to divide, which one of the following functions would survive best?
   (a) Hair growth
   (b) Red blood corpuscle production
   (c) Intestinal absorption of fat
   (d) Cardiac contraction
5. Choose the correct statement regarding the free surface specializations of epithelial cells.
   (a) Cilia contain a core of nine peripheral and two central microfilaments.
   (b) Microvilli contain a core of microfilaments.
   (c) Microvilli insert into centrioles (basal bodies).
   (d) Stereocilia contain a core of microtubules that inserts into centrioles (basal bodies).
6. Which of the following is *not* used in classifying the various types of epithelia?
   (a) The number of layers of cells
   (b) The shape of the cells at only the free surface
   (c) The terminal specialization or modification at the free surface
   (d) The relative amount of intercellular material to the cellular content
7. The specific intercellular junctional mechanism through which cells are electrically coupled is the:
   (a) Desmosome
   (b) Tight junction
   (c) Zonula adherens
   (d) Gap junction
8. Which of the following fibers or fibrils is most like collagen in its chemical composition?
   (a) Muscle fibers
   (b) Elastic fibers
   (c) Neurofibrils
   (d) Reticular fibers
9. Tendons are composed of:
   (a) Dense irregularly arranged connective tissue
   (b) Dense regularly arranged connective tissue
   (c) Large elastic fibers with fibroblasts lying between the fibers
   (d) Large collagenous fibers with fibroblasts lying in lacunae between the fibers
10. In which of the following organs would you be most likely to find elastic cartilage?
   (a) Lungs
   (b) Developing long bone
   (c) Larynx
   (d) Inner ear
11. The stiffness of cartilage is due primarily to the presence of:
   (a) Chondroitin sulfate
   (b) Collagen fibers
   (c) Hyaluronic acid
   (d) The perichondrium
12. Bone remodelling normally:
   (a) Involves removal of existing bone by osteoblasts
   (b) Involves deposition of calcified cartilage on existing trabeculae of bone
   (c) Can occur in response to mechanical stress and fluctuations in the blood calcium level
   (d) Occurs during the "growing years," but ceases by the age of 50
13. Which statement is true for muscle tissue?
   (a) Cardiac and smooth muscle cells both branch and have central nuclei.
   (b) Cardiac and smooth muscle tissue both possess gap junctions.
   (c) Skeletal muscle satellite cells lie outside the basement membrane of the muscle and are connective tissue cells.
   (d) Cardiac and smooth muscle tissue are each more vascular than skeletal muscle tissue.
14. Neurons:
   (a) Of the central nervous system have Nissl material that extends into both dendrites and axons
   (b) Of the central nervous system are invested by myelin produced by Schwann cells

(c) And glial cells in the gray matter of the spinal cord make up a meshwork called neuropil
(d) Of sympathetic ganglia are unipolar or pseudounipolar

15. Which of the following is *not* produced by a neuron?
(a) Antidiuretic hormone (ADH)
(b) Luteinizing hormone-releasing hormone (LHRH)
(c) Epinephrine
(d) Calcitonin

16. Neuromuscular spindles:
(a) Contain both afferent and efferent nerve fibers
(b) Contain infrafusal fibers which are usually larger than extrafusal fibers
(c) Are located in the myenteric plexus of the intestine
(d) Regulate the state of contraction of cardiac muscle

17. Which of the following cells is morphologically closest to the earlier ''blast'' stage?
(a) Promyelocyte
(b) Platelet
(c) Neutrophilic metamyelocyte
(d) Reticulocyte

18. Which of the following cell types is most numerous in a normal blood smear?
(a) Neutrophil
(b) Eosinophil
(c) Lymphocyte
(d) Monocyte

19. Myelocytes:
(a) Have an indented nucleus
(b) Are incapable of division
(c) Have ''specific'' granules
(d) Arise from metamyelocytes

20. In the heart:
(a) Purkinje fibers are modified nerve fibers constituting part of the cardiac conduction system.
(b) The endocardium of the atria is thicker than that of the ventricles.
(c) Papillary muscles are involuntary smooth muscle tissue that insert into chordae tendinae.
(d) The sinoatrial (S-A) node is modified connective tissue of the cardiac skeleton.

21. Afferent lymphatic vessels are found supplying:
(a) Peyer's patches
(b) The spleen
(c) Lymph nodes
(d) The thymus

22. Which one of the following does *not* transport blood through its sinusoids?
(a) Bone marrow
(b) Spleen
(c) Lymph node
(d) Liver

23. Which of the following organs is least likely to demonstrate mucus-secreting cells or glands?
(a) Vagina
(b) Esophagus
(c) Cervix
(d) Colon

24. Which of the following is a component of the mucosa (mucous membrane)?
(a) Enteroendocrine cells of the stomach
(b) Hair follicle
(c) Auerbach's myenteric nerve plexus
(d) Sweat gland

25. Which of the following is *not* correct for the small intestine?
(a) Monoglycerides and fatty acids diffuse through the absorptive cell plasma membrane.
(b) The nodules of Peyer's patches may extend into the submucosal layer.
(c) Chylomicrons are often found in the intercellular spaces between absorptive cells.
(d) The outer longitudinal layer of the muscularis externa is thickened into taenia coli.

26. In the kidney:
(a) As much as 80% of the amino acids and glucose of the ultrafiltrate are reabsorbed by the thin portion of the loop of Henle.
(b) Renin, produced by the juxtaglomerular apparatus, acts directly on arterial smooth muscle to cause vasodilation.
(c) Antidiuretic hormone causes the collecting tubules to become more permeable to water, thus concentrating the urine.
(d) Interlobular arteries arise from arcuate arteries and pass into the cortex via the medullary rays.

27. During the differentiation of a spermatozoan (spermiogenesis) the acrosome arises by accumulation of material in:
(a) Mitochondria
(b) The nucleus
(c) The Golgi complex
(d) The nuclear envelope

28. In the male reproductive system:
(a) Spermatozoa pass in order through efferent ductules, rete testis, and ductus epididymidis.
(b) The ductus deferens, seminal vesicle, and prostate all have smooth muscle in their walls.
(c) The seminal vesicle is the main source of acid phosphatase in the semen.
(d) The prostate gland is a site where spermatozoa are stored and become mature.

29. In the female reproductive system:
(a) Uterine glands secrete a carbohydrate-rich

substance and also are necessary for regeneration of the surface epithelium of the uterus during the menstrual cycle.
(b) The cytotrophoblast of the placenta is most prominent during the third trimester of pregnancy.
(c) Theca externa cells of ovarian follicles secrete most of the ovarian estrogen.
(d) Ovulation occurs at the time when progesterone has reached its highest level in the blood plasma.

30. Which one of the following ''structure-secretory product'' combinations is correct?
(a) Syncytiotrophoblast–progesterone and estrogen
(b) Acidophils of the pars distalis–follicle-stimulating hormone (FSH)
(c) Beta cells of the islets of Langerhans–glucagon
(d) Zona glomerulosa of the suprarenal gland–cortisone

31. Which of the following is characteristic of the 27th day of the menstrual cycle?
(a) Stasis of blood in the basal straight arteries of the endometrium
(b) Constriction of the coiled spiral arteries
(c) Increased proliferation of the endometrium
(d) Increased edema of the functional spongy layer of the endometrium

32. Which one of the following organs possesses all of these characteristics: has both an exocrine and endocrine organ; is under the influence of hypophyseal hormones; has cells completing the second meiotic division?
(a) Ovary
(b) Liver
(c) Testis
(d) Pancreas

33. Which one of the following organs possesses all of these characteristics: serous acini, intercalated ducts, striated ducts, no mucous alveoli?
(a) Sebaceous gland
(b) Pancreas
(c) Sublingual gland
(d) Parotid gland

34. Which one of the following organs possesses all of these characteristics: stratified squamous nonkeratinized epithelium, serous and mucous glands, skeletal muscle, special visceral afferent nerve fibers?
(a) Esophagus
(b) Tongue
(c) Vagina
(d) Anal canal

35. Three sites where substances readily pass between the vascular system and a surface lining epithelium are in the lung alveoli, renal corpuscles, and chorionic villi. Which one of the following is found in all three structures?
(a) Lining cells that secrete lipoidal or steroidal substances
(b) Macrophages
(c) Fenestrated endothelial cells
(d) Angiotensin-producing cells

36. In the ear:
(a) Endolymph fills the scala tympani and scala vestibuli.
(b) The organ of Corti contains hair cells, each of which possesses one true cilium.
(c) Bipolar neurons in the spiral cochlear ganglion each have a peripheral process that ends on hair cells, and a central process that is a component of the cochlear nerve.
(d) The stapes is located in the round window of the scala tympani.

37. In the eye:
(a) Visual pigments are located in discs of the outer segments of cells of the pigmented layer of the retina.
(b) Accommodation (focusing on a near object) involves the relaxation of ciliary smooth muscle, resulting in release of tension on the ciliary zonule and rounding of the lens.
(c) The blind spot produced by the optic disc is medial to the visual axis.
(d) The pupil gets larger in response to parasympathetic nerve stimulation.

38. Which of the following primary afferent or efferent fibers of medullary cranial nerves is paired with an *incorrect* nucleus of termination or origin?
(a) General somatic afferent (GSA) fibers of IX-nucleus solitarius
(b) Special visceral efferent (SVE) fibers of XI-nucleus ambiguus
(c) General visceral efferent (GVE) fibers of X-dorsal motor nucleus
(d) Special visceral afferent (SVA) fibers of IX-gustatory nucleus

39. After a peripheral lesion of the abducens nerve in the orbit, one might expect to find all of the following *except:*
(a) Chromatolysis in the facial colliculus of the pons
(b) Loss of myelin in the abducens nerve distal to the lesion
(c) Degenerating fibers in the contralateral medial longitudinal fasciculus (MLF)
(d) Paralysis of the ipsilateral lateral rectus muscle

40. Which one of the following structures is *not* supplied by direct branches of the artery with which it is matched?
   (a) Spinal tract of the trigeminal nerve–posterior inferior cerebellar artery
   (b) Medial lemniscus–anterior spinal artery
   (c) Corticospinal tract–posterior cerebral artery
   (d) Visual (striate) cortex–anterior cerebral artery
41. Bilateral injury to the facial nerves at their emergence from the pons-medulla junction could result in:
   (a) Hyperacusis because of impaired stapedius muscle activity
   (b) Loss of taste from the posterior one third of the tongue
   (c) Loss of all flow of saliva
   (d) Ptosis in both eyes
42. After a right upper motor neuron lesion of the facial nerve there is a:
   (a) Loss of the sense of taste on the right anterior portion of the tongue
   (b) Loss of the corneal reflex on the right side
   (c) Loss of ability to wrinkle the forehead on the left side
   (d) Paralysis of lower facial muscles on the left side
43. If there is a destructive lesion of the crista ampullaris in the left horizontal semicircular canal all of the following are likely to be present *except:*
   (a) A tendency to fall to the left
   (b) Past-pointing to the left
   (c) A sense of the room rotating to the right
   (d) Nystagmus with a fast component to the right
44. A destructive tumor in the cerebellopontine angle could result in all of the following *except:*
   (a) Deafness in the ipsilateral ear
   (b) Lateral strabismus ipsilaterally
   (c) Impaired corneal reflex
   (d) Absence of normal vestibular responses
45. All of the following result in constriction of the left pupil *except:*
   (a) Focusing the eye on a near object after focusing on a far object
   (b) Shining light in the right eye of a normal person
   (c) Shining light on only the nasal half of the retina of the right eye of a person whose optic chiasm has been totally destroyed
   (d) Shining light in the right eye of a person whose left optic nerve was destroyed
46. Which of the following eye movements and reflexes would be *least* affected by bilateral destruction of the parastriate (18) and peristriate (19) areas of the cerebral cortex?
   (a) Smooth eye pursuit of a moving object
   (b) The near (synkinetic, accommodation-convergence) reflex
   (c) The pupillary light reflex
   (d) Saccadic movements occurring in the shift of gaze from one object to another
47. Destruction of which of the following would *most likely* result in a deficit of memory for recent events?
   (a) Cingulate gyrus
   (b) Parietal lobe
   (c) Anterior—medial region of the temporal lobe
   (d) Medial dorsal nucleus of the thalamus
48. The intervertebral foramen is bounded:
   (a) Superiorly and inferiorly by the lamina of the involved vertebrae
   (b) Posteriorly by the zygopophyseal joint
   (c) Posteriorly by the posterior longitudinal ligament
   (d) Anteriorly by the intervertebral disc and the anterior longitudinal ligament
49. The shoulder joint is least reinforced by muscles of the rotator cuff:
   (a) Anteriorly
   (b) Inferiorly
   (c) Posteriorly
   (d) Superiorly
50. The major origin of the superficial group of anterior forearm muscles is the:
   (a) Lateral epicondyle of the humerus
   (b) Proximal ventral aspects of the radius and ulna
   (c) Olecranon process of the humerus
   (d) Medial epicondyle of the humerus
51. Which of the following intrinsic thumb muscles is *not* found in the thenar compartment?
   (a) Adductor pollicis
   (b) Flexor pollicis brevis
   (c) Abductor pollicis brevis
   (d) Opponens pollicis
52. The muscles in the adductor–interosseous compartment of the hand are innervated by the:
   (a) Median nerve
   (b) Median and ulnar nerves
   (c) Radial nerve
   (d) Ulnar nerve
53. The anterior cruciate ligament of the knee:
   (a) Is most taut when the knee is flexed
   (b) Attaches to the anterior intercondylar region of the tibia
   (c) Protects against posterior dislocation of the tibia on the femur
   (d) Protects against anterior dislocation of the femur on the tibia

54. Palpable just medial to the patellar ligament in the interval between the femur and tibia is the:
   (a) Anterior cruciate ligament
   (b) Fibular collateral ligament
   (c) Tendon of the popliteus muscle
   (d) Medial meniscus
55. Due to bony support, the most stable position of the ankle joint is:
   (a) Dorsiflexion
   (b) Inversion
   (c) Plantar flexion
   (d) Eversion
56. The major blood supply to the posterior femoral muscles is provided by:
   (a) The obturator artery
   (b) The perforating branches of the deep femoral artery
   (c) The medial and lateral femoral circumflex vessels
   (d) The superior gluteal artery
57. On the dorsum of the foot the dorsalis pedis pulse can be taken:
   (a) Medial to the tendon of the tibialis anterior muscle
   (b) Between the tendons of the tibialis anterior and extensor hallucis longus muscles
   (c) Between the tendons of the extensor hallucis longus and extensor digitorum longus muscles
   (d) Between the tendons of the extensor digitorum longus and peroneus tertius muscles
58. The posterior tibial pulse is taken:
   (a) Posterior to the medial malleolus
   (b) Anterior to the medial malleolus
   (c) Posterior to the lateral malleolus
   (d) Between the calcaneal tendon and the lateral malleolus
59. Which of the following functions of the muscles of mastication is incorrect?
   (a) Masseter: elevation of the mandible
   (b) Medial pterygoid: elevation of the mandible
   (c) Temporalis: retraction of the mandible
   (d) Lateral pterygoid: deviation of the mandible to the same side
60. Most of the muscle of the pharyngeal wall is innervated by cranial nerve:
   (a) IX
   (b) X
   (c) XI
   (d) XII
61. The parasympathetic fibers that innervate the sphincter pupillae muscle *do not* pass through the:
   (a) Short ciliary nerves
   (b) Cranial nerve III
   (c) Long ciliary nerves
   (d) Cavernous sinus
62. Laceration of the facial nerve immediately distal to the geniculate ganglion would *least likely* cause:
   (a) An inability to close the ipsilateral eye
   (b) Loss of taste on the anterior two thirds of the tongue
   (c) Loss of lacrimation
   (d) Loss of submandibular salivation
63. The common carotid artery bifurcates:
   (a) At the level of the cricoid cartilage
   (b) Between the levels of the cricoid and thyroid cartilage
   (c) Between the levels of the thyroid cartilage prominence and the hyoid bone
   (d) Superior to the level of the hyoid bone
64. A lesion of the most superficial nerve in the posterior triangle of the neck would logically result in:
   (a) Difficulty swallowing
   (b) Difficulty breathing
   (c) Difficulty turning the head to the same side
   (d) Difficulty elevating (hunching) the shoulder
65. The pleural cavities:
   (a) Contain the lungs
   (b) Communicate across the midline
   (c) Are composed of inner parietal and outer visceral layers
   (d) Surround the lungs
66. A penetrating wound that enters the right fourth intercostal space in the midclavicular line would initially enter the:
   (a) Superior lobe of the right lung
   (b) Right lung below the oblique fissure
   (c) Inferior lobe of the right lung
   (d) Middle lobe of the right lung
67. *Not* participating in the formation of Hasselbach's triangle is the:
   (a) Falx inguinals (conjoined tendon)
   (b) Lateral border of the rectus abdominis
   (c) Inguinal ligament
   (d) Inferior epigastric vessels
68. The inguinal ligament extends between the:
   (a) Pubic tubercele and the anterior superior iliac spine
   (b) Anterior superior and inferior iliac spines
   (c) Greater trochanter of the femur and the pubic tubercle
   (d) Ischial spine and pubic tubercle
69. The neck of an indirect hernia is found:
   (a) Medial to the pubic tubercle
   (b) Medial to the inferior epigastric vessels
   (c) Lateral to the deep inguinal ring
   (d) Lateral to the inferior epigastric vessels
70. The renal pelvis is directed:
   (a) Anteromedially
   (b) Posteromedially

(c) Anterolaterally
(d) Posterolaterally

71. The pelvic diaphragm slopes inferiorly from:
(a) Anterior to posterior
(b) Medial to lateral
(c) Posterior to anterior
(d) The pubic symphysis to the sacral promontory

72. The superficial perineal space (pouch) is continuous with the:
(a) Subcutaneous area of the thigh
(b) Peritoneal cavity
(c) Ischiorectal fossa
(d) Fascial plane in the abdominal wall between the external abdominal oblique fascia and the membraneous layer of superficial fascia

73. All of the following are true for the plasma membrane *except:*
(a) Possesses transmembrane proteins that help to transport specific molecules into the cell
(b) Contains glycolipids and glycoproteins
(c) Possesses a double layer of phospholipid molecules whose fatty acid components make up an intermediate hydrophobic zone
(d) Is coated by a glycocalyx on both its outer and inner surfaces

74. In the mitochondria:
(a) The electron transport system of enzymes is on the inner membrane of the cristae
(b) Pyruvate is converted to acetyl-CoA between the outer and inner membranes
(c) Of pancreatic cells are found a preponderance of tubular cristae
(d) The energy that is produced is used in forming ADP

75. All of the following are true statements for cytoplasmic organelles *except:*
(a) Coated vesicles are coated with clathrin and are involved in receptor-mediated endocytosis
(b) Free ribosomes are mostly involved in the production of secretory proteins
(c) Centrioles are similar in structure to basal bodies
(d) Intermediate filaments are plentiful in epidermal cells

76. The Golgi apparatus is involved in which of the following?
(a) Concentrating secretory products
(b) Packaging secretory products in membrane-bound vesicles
(c) Producing thyroglobulin
(d) All of the above

77. Which of the following cells characteristically contain much smooth endoplasmic reticulum?
(a) Cells of the zona fasciculata of the suprarenal gland
(b) Basophilic erythroblasts
(c) Pancreatic acinar cells
(d) Neurons

78. Which of the following cells is considered to be quite phagocytic?
(a) Oligodendroglia
(b) Fibroblasts
(c) Macrophages
(d) Plasma cells

79. Which of the following statements regarding epithelia is correct?
(a) Stratified squamous epithelium comprises most glands.
(b) Transitional epithelium is well adapted for absorptive functions.
(c) All cells of pseudostratified columnar epithelium reach the basement membrane, but not all of them reach the luminal surface.
(d) Epithelial cells usually receive nutritive substances from capillaries located in the intercellular spaces of the epithelium.

80. The basement membrane consists of:
(a) Large collagen bundles
(b) Reticular fibers and a basal lamina
(c) The plasma membrane of basal epithelial cells
(d) A basal lamina only

81. Which of the following is found within the intercellular spaces between epidermal cells?
(a) Tonofilaments
(b) Microvilli
(c) Meissner's tactile corpuscles
(d) Melanocyte processes

82. Osteons (haversian systems) contain all of the following *except:*
(a) Collagen fibers that, in adjacent lamellae, run perpendicular to each other
(b) Interstitial lamellae
(c) Trabeculae of bone
(d) Canaliculi through which blood is transported to osteocytes

83. Which of the following is characteristic of both hyaline cartilage and bone?
(a) Avascular tissue
(b) Cells occurring in isogenous groups
(c) Both appositional and interstitial growth
(d) Intercellular matrix that contains numerous collagenous fibers and a mucoidal ground substance

84. Cardiac muscle differs from adult skeletal muscle in that cardiac muscle possesses:
(a) Intercalated discs
(b) Branching fibers

(c) Centrally located nuclei
(d) All of the above

85. During excitation-contraction coupling in skeletal muscle:
(a) Calcium is released from the cisterna of the sarcoplasmic reticulum
(b) The interaction of actin and myosin is regulated, at least in part, by troponin and tropomyosin
(c) A wave of membrane depolarization is carried into the depths of the muscle fiber by the T tubules
(d) All of the above

86. Glial (neuroglial) cells are components of which of the following?
(a) Pars intermedia of the hypophysis
(b) Pars distalis of the hypophysis
(c) Pineal gland
(d) Adrenal (suprarenal) medulla

87. A drug that interferes with mitosis would be likely to directly affect the division of:
(a) Metamyelocytes
(b) Reticulocytes
(c) Normoblasts
(d) Polychromatophilic erythroblasts

88. Lymphatic nodules are found in the:
(a) Spleen
(b) Lymph nodes
(c) Ileum
(d) All of the above

89. Which of the following statements about the respiratory system is true?
(a) Great alveolar (giant septal, pneumonocyte II) cells produce surfactant.
(b) Bronchioles possess elastic cartilage, which allows for expansion of bronchioles at inspiration.
(c) Alveolar ducts possess smooth muscle and alveoli.
(d) The true vocal cords (folds) and rest of the larynx are lined by pseudostratified columnar epithelium.

90. Which of the following organs possesses submucosal glands?
(a) Duodenum
(b) Fundus of the stomach
(c) Jejunum
(d) Colon

91. In which cell is there normally only 23 chromosomes (although there may be a normal diploid amount of DNA)?
(a) Parietal cell of the stomach
(b) An oocyte just after it is discharged from the ovary at ovulation
(c) Zygote
(d) Spermatid

92. Which of the following statements about the liver is correct?
(a) Discontinuities in the sinusoidal epithelium permit passage of some substances between the lumen of the sinusoid and the perisinusoidal space of Disse.
(b) In the classical liver lobule, bile as well as arterial and venous blood flows toward the center of the lobule.
(c) Hepatocytes constitute the walls of the bile canaliculi and the arterioles.
(d) All of the above

93. Following the administration of radioactive glucose, which of the following structures or substances would be labeled?
(a) The fuzz (glycocalyx) covering the free surface of the intestinal lining cell
(b) Colloid in the thyroid follicle
(c) Hyaline cartilage matrix
(d) All of the above

94. Which one of the endocrine tissues listed below is *incorrectly* matched with a mechanism that is involved in the regulation of the production and/or release of the hormone produced by that tissue?
(a) Parathyroid—increased levels of TSH
(b) Adrenal medulla—stimulation of preganglionic sympathetic neurons
(c) Pars distalis of hypophysis—releasing hormones that reach the pars distalis from hypothalamic neurons by way of the hypophyseal portal system
(d) Corpus luteum—placenta formation

95. Which of the following ''cell-secretory product'' combination is *incorrect?*
Plasma cell—circulating antibodies
(b) Mast cell—acid phosphatase
(c) Fibroblast—collagen precursor
(d) Enteroendocrine cell—serotonin

96. Which of the following ''cell-secretory product'' combinations is correct?
(a) Chief cell of the stomach—pepsinogen
(b) Acidophil of the pars distalis—growth hormone
(c) Zona glomerulosal cell of the adrenal gland—mineralocorticoids
(d) All of the above

97. A simple cuboidal or columnar epithelium with extensive basal infoldings of plasma membrane is characteristically found in:
(a) Collecting tubules of the kidney
(b) The lining epithelium of the small intestine
(c) Striated ducts of the parotid gland
(d) The lining epithelium of the oral cavity

98. Which of the following statements about the kidney is correct?
    (a) The macula densa is a region of the distal tubule that is closely associated with an afferent glomerular arteriole.
    (b) Collecting tubules are located in both the medulla and cortex.
    (c) Proximal convoluted tubules have an extensive microvillous (brush) border.
    (d) All of the above
99. Which of the following cells is correctly paired with its secretory product?
    (a) Acidophils of hypophysis—FSH (follicle-stimulating hormone)
    (b) Oxyphil cells—parathyroid hormone
    (c) Acidophils of hypophysis—prolactin (luteotrophic hormone)
    (d) Chromaffin cells of adrenal—aldosterone
100. Which of the following is neither the target cell nor organ for the hormone indicated?
    (a) Seminal vesicle—luteinizing hormone (LH)
    (b) Prostate gland—follicle-stimulating hormone (FSH)
    (c) Leydig cells—testosterone
    (d) Sertoli cells—follicle-stimulating hormone (FSH)
101. Which of the following statements regarding the testis is correct?
    (a) Some spermatogonia proliferate and remain as stem cells, while others differentiate into primary spermatocytes.
    (b) The smooth endoplasmic reticulum of Leydig cells is essential for testosterone production.
    (c) Sertoli cells help control passage of macromolecules to haploid cells.
    (d) All of the above
102. The luteal (secretory) phase of the menstrual cycle is characterized by all of the following *except:*
    (a) A coiling or sacculation of endometrial glands
    (b) Decreased amounts of progesterone in the blood plasma
    (c) The presence of a functional corpus luteum
    (d) Atresia of some ovarian follicles
103. In the membranous labyrinth of the ear:
    (a) The organ of Corti has receptors for position sense
    (b) Otoconia are components of the cristae
    (c) Efferent nerves end on some of the hair cells
    (d) Perilymph flow during head rotation produces forces on sensory hairs that cause them to fire nerve impulses
104. Which of the following statements regarding the eye is correct?
    (a) The inner nuclear layer of the retina contains the nuclei of bipolar cells, horizontal cells, and amacrine cells.
    (b) Aqueous humor passes, in sequence, through the posterior chamber, anterior chamber, trabecular meshwork (spaces of Fontana), canal of Schlemm, and veins.
    (c) Light striking the retina (excluding the fovea centralis and the optic papilla) encounters in order: ganglion cells, bipolar cells, and rods and cones.
    (d) All of the above
105. Loss of which one of the following would least likely result from bilateral destruction of the posterior white columns at spinal cord segment C5?
    (a) Fine discrimination of pain in both hands
    (b) Vibratory sense in both hands
    (c) Ability to identify objects placed in a patient's hands when the patient's hand are out of sight
    (d) Appreciation of passive limb movements in the hands and feet
106. One month after ipsilateral destruction of the C3 through T3 dorsal root ganglia, there would be ipsilateral:
    (a) Anesthesia of the upper extremity
    (b) Slight increase in deep tendon reflexes of the upper extremity
    (c) Nerve fiber degeneration in the medulla, pons, and midbrain
    (d) A complete dermatomal loss of sensation in only segments C6 to T1.
107. Two months after complete destruction of the lateral funiculus in spinal cord segments C5 and C6 there would probably be:
    (a) Ipsilateral hemiplegia
    (b) Ipsilateral hypertonus at lower levels
    (c) Absence of ipsilateral superficial (cutaneous) abdominal reflexes
    (d) All of the above
108. Two months after complete ipsilateral destruction of the ventral roots of the C5 through T1 spinal nerves, one would expect to find:
    (a) Exaggerated myotatic (stretch) reflexes in the ipsilateral upper limb
    (b) Spastic paralysis of muscles in the ipsilateral upper limb
    (c) Loss of superficial (cutaneous) abdominal reflexes
    (d) Muscle atrophy in the ipsilateral upper limb
109. When an axon is damaged there is dispersal of Nissel material in the cell body (perikaryon) of the damaged neuron, which is called chromatolysis. If the facial nerve was sectioned at its emergence

from the brain stem, in which of the following would chromatolysis be present?
(a) Nucleus solitaris
(b) Geniculate ganglion
(c) Pterygopalatine ganglion
(d) Submandibular ganglion

110. A high medullary lesion involving the spinal tract and nucleus of the trigeminal nerve on one side could:
(a) Produce some loss of sensation from the ipsilateral external auditory canal
(b) Cause contralateral and ipsilateral loss of crude touch on the face
(c) Produce no ipsilateral loss of pain on the anterior two thirds of the tongue
(d) Cause a diminished jaw-jerk reflex

111. A tumor obliterating the right striate cortex above the calcarine fissure would result in all of the above *except:*
(a) Damage to cells that receive impulses from both retinae by way of the lateral geniculate nucleus
(b) Left lower quadratic anopsia
(c) Chromatolysis of ganglion cells in the temporal half of the retina of the right eye
(d) An homonymous type of visual defect

112. All of the following structures are components of the hearing pathway *except* the:
(a) Superior olivary nucleus
(b) Inferior colliculus
(c) Lateral geniculate body (nucleus)
(d) Lateral lemniscus

113. Destruction of the entire right tegmentum at the level of the facial colliculus would result in:
(a) Contralateral loss of pain and temperature in the trunk, extremities, and part of the face
(b) Complete contralateral loss of two-point touch in the trunk, extremities, and face
(c) Paralysis of conjugate lateral gaze to both sides
(d) Babinski reflex on the left

114. A lesion of the mesencephalic tegmentum, which destroys the left oculomotor nerve, left medial lemniscus, and left red nucleus and adjacent cerebellar efferents, would *not* result in:
(a) Loss of the consensual response in the pupillary light reflex when light is shone in the left eye
(b) Intention tremor in the right upper extremity
(c) Ptosis of the left eye
(d) Loss of touch on the right side of the body

115. Destruction of which of the following structures is most likely to cause apraxia?
(a) Subthalamic nucleus
(b) Post central gyrus
(c) Left inferior parietal gyrus (area 39, angular gyrus)
(d) Supraoptic nucleus

116. Which of the following lesions would *not* produce the signs and symptoms indicated?
(a) A hemisection of the cord produces a contralateral loss of pain and temperature and ipsilateral loss of two-point touch below the level of the lesion.
(b) A lesion of the vagus nerve near its emergence from the brain stem produces chromatolysis in the dorsal motor nucleus of the vagus and the nucleus ambiguus.
(c) A lesion of the right hypoglossal nerve results in deviation of the tongue, upon protrusion, to the left side.
(d) A lesion of the inferior cerebellar peduncle causes chromatolysis in the ipsilateral nucleus dorsalis (Clarke's nucleus).

117. Which of the following statements regarding the location of the spinal nerve in the intervertebral foramen is *incorrect?*
(a) It is at the level of the intervertebral disc in the cervical region.
(b) It is above the level of the intervertebral disc in the lumbar region.
(c) It is at the level of Luschka's joint in the lower cervical region.
(d) It is at the level of the intervertebral disc in the lumbar region.

118. With respect of the support provided by the ligaments of the vertebral column:
(a) The anterior longitudinal ligament resists flexion of the vertebral column
(b) The posterior longitudinal ligament resists extension of the vertebral column
(c) The interspinous ligaments resist extension of the vertebral column
(d) The ligamenta flava resist flexion of the vertebral column

119. With respect to the location of the ligaments of the vertebral column:
(a) The ligamenta flava interconnect the lamina of adjacent vertebrae
(b) The anterior longitudinal ligament lines the anterior aspect of the vertebral canal
(c) The posterior longitudinal ligament attaches to the posterior aspects of the neural arches
(d) The anterior longitudinal ligament attaches to the pedicles of adjacent vertebrae

120. The radial nerve:
(a) Passes posteriorly around the surgical neck of the humerus

(b) Passes ventral to the medial aspect of the elbow
(c) Passes medial to the biceps tendon in the cubital fossa
(d) Passes around the neck of the radius

121. Which of the following is palpable in the anatomic snuff box?
(a) Scaphoid bone
(b) Median nerve
(c) Ulnar artery
(d) Pisiform bone

122. The function of which of the following nerves can be checked by testing the motions of the thumb?
(a) Median
(b) Ulnar
(c) Radial
(d) All of the above

123. The superficial palmar arterial arch:
(a) Is deep to the long flexor tendons
(b) Is superficial to the palmar aponeurosis
(c) Is proximal to the deep part of the flexor retinaculum
(d) Is at the same level (depth) as the common digital branches of the median nerve

124. MP flexion and IP extension of the index, middle, ring, and little fingers are produced by:
(a) The dorsal interossei muscles
(b) The lumbrical muscles
(c) The ventral interossei muscles
(d) All of the above

125. Which of the following locations of the ulnar nerve is *incorrect?*
(a) Passes posterior to the medial epicondyle of the humerus
(b) Passes medial to the pisiform
(c) Is deep to the flexor carpi ulnaris muscle in the forearm
(d) Passes superficial to the deep part of the flexor retinaculum

126. The median nerve:
(a) Is formed from both the medial and posterior cords of the brachial plexus
(b) Is deep to the flexor digitorum profundus in the forearm
(c) Is medial to the brachial artery in the cubital fossa
(d) Is lateral to the tendon of the flexor carpi radialis muscle at the wrist

127. The musculocutaneous nerve:
(a) Passes deep to the brachialis muscle
(b) Passes through the coracobrachialis muscle
(c) Is the continuation of the medial cord of the brachial plexus
(d) Passes between the two heads of the biceps brachii muscle

128. The capsule of the hip joint:
(a) Encloses the entire femoral neck
(b) Is reinforced by the iliofemoral, ischiofemoral, and pubofemoral ligaments
(c) Encloses the proximal two thirds of the femoral neck anteriorly
(d) Tightens as the femur is flexed

129. The medial part of the transverse tarsal (midtarsal) joint is formed by the:
(a) Talus and navicular
(b) Talus and calcaneus
(c) Cuboid and calcaneus
(d) Navicular and cuboid

130. The lateral collateral ligament of the ankle extends between the lateral malleolus and the:
(a) Calcaneus and talus
(b) Navicular and talus
(c) Talus and cuboid
(d) Cuboid and calcaneus

131. The femoral nerve:
(a) Is the most medial structure that passes deep to the inguinal ligament
(b) Contains fibers from spinal cord segments L1 through L5
(c) Innervates muscles that extend the knee and hip
(d) Is formed within the substance of the psoas major muscle

132. The common peroneal nerve:
(a) Is the deepest structure in the popliteal fossa
(b) Passes around the neck of the fibula
(c) Innervates the major plantar flexors of the foot
(d) Is the most medial nerve in the popliteal fossa

133. The tibial nerve:
(a) Innervates all of the intrinsic muscles of the plantar foot
(b) Enters the foot by passing behind the medial malleolus
(c) Passes through the median (middle) area of the popliteal fossa
(d) Does all of the above

134. The anterior cranial fossa is *not* related to the:
(a) Orbit
(b) Nasal cavity
(c) Maxillary sinus
(d) Ethmoid air cells

135. The lateral portion of the middle cranial fossa is related anterior to the:
(a) Infratemporal fossa
(b) Middle ear cavity
(c) Cavernous sinus
(d) Orbit

136. The phrenic nerve:
   (a) Contains fibers from spinal cord segments C3, C4, and C5
   (b) Passes posterior to the root of the lung
   (c) Passes through the scalene triangle (groove)
   (d) Contributes fibers to the cardiac plexus
137. The pterygopalatine fossa communicates with the:
   (a) Middle cranial fossa by way of the foramen ovale
   (b) Nasal cavity by way of the pterygomaxillary fissure
   (c) Oral cavity by way of the pterygopalatine canal
   (d) Orbit by way of the superior orbital fissure
138. Regarding the openings of the paranasal sinuses:
   (a) The anterior ethmoid air cells drain into the superior meatus of the nasal cavity
   (b) The maxillary sinus drains into the inferior meatus of the nasal cavity
   (c) The frontal sinus drains into the inferior meatus of the nasal cavity
   (d) The sphenoid sinus drains into the sphenoethmoidal recess of the nasal cavity
139. With respect to the areas or parts of the larynx:
   (a) The glottis includes the true and false vocal folds
   (b) The ventricle is the area between the false folds
   (c) The vestibule and supraglottic portions are the same
   (d) The additis is the connection between the larynx and trachea
140. Which of the following muscle-function pairs is correct?
   (a) Cricothyroid—relaxation of the vocal cords
   (b) Posterior cricoarytenoid—abduction of the vocal cords
   (c) Lateral cricoarytenoid—abduction of the vocal cords
   (d) Transverse arytenoid—abduction of the vocal cords
141. Relative to the heart:
   (a) Its diaphragmatic surface is formed primarily by the right and left ventricles
   (b) Its posterior surface is formed predominantly by the right atrium
   (c) Its apex projects to the left at the level of the fourth rib
   (d) Its right border is formed by the right ventricle
142. With respect to the relationships of the duodenum:
   (a) Its first part is related anteriorly to the portal vein and common bile duct
   (b) Its second part is related laterally to the head of the pancreas
   (c) Its third part is crossed anteriorly by the superior mesenteric vessels
   (d) Its third part is related posteriorly to the transverse colon
143. The stomach is related:
   (a) Posteriorly to the caudate lobe of the liver
   (b) Anteriorly to the lesser omental bursa
   (c) Anteriorly to the splenic artery
   (d) Posteriorly to the pancreas
144. The vermiform appendix:
   (a) Usually arises from the large intestine just superior to the entrance of the ileum
   (b) Arises from the cecum at the termination of the taeniae coli
   (c) Typically hangs into the (true) pelvic cavity
   (d) Is seldom retrocecal in position
145. The spleen:
   (a) Is deep to ribs 9, 10, and 11
   (b) Is related to the head of the pancreas
   (c) Is related posteriorly to the stomach
   (d) Is related to the right colic flexure
146. Pelvic splanchnic nerves:
   (a) Contain preganglionic parasympathetic nerve fibers
   (b) Contain fibers that innervate the gastrointestinal tract from the cecum to the splenic flexure
   (c) Are pelvic branches of the sympathetic trunk
   (d) Contain the same type of efferent fibers as the lumbar splanchnic nerves
147. The portal vein is formed:
   (a) Between the pancreas and the stomach
   (b) By the union of the splenic and superior mesenteric veins
   (c) By the junction of the superior and inferior mesenteric veins
   (d) Anterior to the pancreas
148. Which of the following statements regarding the pudendal nerve is *incorrect?*
   (a) It arises from spinal cord segments S2, S3, and S4.
   (b) It passes through the pudendal canal.
   (c) It passes superficial to the sacrotuberous ligament.
   (d) It passes through the greater sciatic foramen.
149. The urogenital diaphragm:
   (a) Is found both anterior and posterior to the ischial tuberosities
   (b) Is oriented parallel to the sagittal plane
   (c) Is perforated by the urethra and anal canal
   (d) Extends between the ischiopubic rami
150. Which of the following statements regarding the processes leading to protein synthesis is *incorrect?*

(a) The genetic code is found in the nitrogenous base sequence of DNA.
(b) Messenger RNA molecules are transcribed from exposed nitrogenous bases of DNA.
(c) Both rRNA and tRNA are involved in translating the mRNA message.
(d) The tRNA places an amino acid directly into the rough endoplasmic reticulum.

ONE BEST ANSWER

For each of the following groups of items you will be given a series of lettered options. Select the *one* lettered option that is most closely associated with each item. Each lettered option may be selected once, more than once, or not at all.

For each numbered structure, select the embryologic structure that most likely gives rise to it.

(a) Primitive node (Hensen)
(b) Primitive streak
(c) Yolk sac entoderm
(d) Neural crest
(e) Third pharyngeal pouch

1. Sarcomere
2. Primordial sex cell
3. Notochord
4. Cardiac muscle

For each cell function, select the most likely organelle.

(a) Smooth endoplasmic reticulum
(b) Rough endoplasmic reticulum
(c) Coated vesicle
(d) Mitochondria
(e) Lysosome

5. Endocytosis
6. Phagocytosis
7. Steroid production
8. Generation of ATP

For each product, select the cell that produces it.

(a) Growth hormone
(b) Cortisol
(c) Follicle-stimulating hormone
(d) Sodium and bicarbonate rich fluid
(e) Glucagon

9. Adrenal zona fasciculata cell
10. Acidophil of the adenohypophysis
11. Alpha cell of pancreas
12. Intercalated duct

For each lesion site, select the most likely sign or symptom that would result from this lesioned area.

(a) Upper quadrantic anopsia
(b) Lower quadrantic anopsia
(c) Bitemporal heteronymous hemianopsia
(d) Loss of smooth pursuit movements ipsilaterally
(e) Loss of pupillary light reflex

13. Rostral portion of the temporal lobe
14. Lingual gyrus
15. Optic chiasm
16. Pretectal area

For each nucleus, select the tract, pathway, or fiber bundle whose axons come from each nucleus.

(a) Contralateral medial lemniscus representing cervical levels
(b) Contralateral medial lemniscus representing sacral levels
(c) Ipsilateral posterior spinocerebellar tract
(d) Inferior cerebellar peduncle
(e) Posterior limb of the internal capsule

17. Nucleus dorsalis (Clarke)
18. Nucleus cuneatus
19. Ventral posteromedial (VPM) and ventral posterolateral nuclei (VPL)
20. Accessory cuneate nucleus

For each location, select the structure that occupies that position.

(a) Tendon of the tibialis posterior muscle
(b) Tendon of the flexor digitorum longus muscle
(c) Posterior tibial artery
(d) Tendon of the flexor hallucis longus

21. Between the tendons of the flexor digitorum longus and flexor hallucis longus muscles
22. Most posterior structure passing posterior to the medial malleolus
23. Most anterior structure passing posterior to the medial malleolus
24. Deepest structure passing posterior to the medial malleolus

For each organ, select the artery that provides the majority of its blood supply.

(a) Splenic artery
(b) Superior mesenteric artery
(c) Inferior mesenteric artery
(d) Internal iliac artery

25. Bladder
26. Pancreas
27. Descending colon
28. Jejunum

For each opening, select the structure that passes through that opening.

(a) Middle meningeal artery
(b) Cranial nerve X (vagus)
(c) Cranial nerve VII (facial)
(d) Maxillary division of cranial nerve V (trigeminal)

29. Jugular foramen
30. Foramen spinosum
31. Internal auditory (acoustic) meatus
32. Foramen rotundum

For each position, select the correct structure.

(a) Prostate
(b) Rectum
(c) Small intestine
(d) Pubic symphysis

33. Anterior to the bladder in the male
34. Inferior to the bladder in the male
35. Superior to the bladder in the male
36. Posterior to the bladder in the male

For each structure, select its proper location.

(a) Central compartment of the hand
(b) Thenar compartment of the hand
(c) Hypothenar compartment of the hand
(d) Adductor interosseous compartment of the hand

37. Superficial palmar arterial arch
38. Radial bursa
39. Opponens digiti minimi muscle
40. Lumbrical muscles

ANSWERS TO MULTIPLE-CHOICE QUESTIONS

Multiple Choice: One-Answer Type

1. b	**9.** b	**17.** a	**25.** d
2. d	**10.** c	**18.** a	**26.** c
3. c	**11.** a	**19.** c	**27.** c
4. d	**12.** c	**20.** b	**28.** b
5. b	**13.** b	**21.** c	**29.** a
6. d	**14.** c	**22.** c	**30.** a
7. d	**15.** d	**23.** a	**31.** b
8. d	**16.** a	**24.** a	**32.** c

33. d	**63.** c	**93.** d	**123.** d
34. b	**64.** d	**94.** a	**124.** d
35. b	**65.** d	**95.** b	**125.** b
36. c	**66.** d	**96.** d	**126.** c
37. c	**67.** a	**97.** c	**127.** b
38. a	**68.** a	**98.** d	**128.** b
39. c	**69.** d	**99.** c	**129.** a
40. d	**70.** a	**100.** b	**130.** a
41. a	**71.** c	**101.** d	**131.** d
42. d	**72.** d	**102.** b	**132.** b
43. c	**73.** d	**103.** c	**133.** d
44. b	**74.** a	**104.** d	**134.** c
45. c	**75.** b	**105.** a	**135.** d
46. c	**76.** d	**106.** a	**136.** a
47. c	**77.** a	**107.** d	**137.** c
48. b	**78.** c	**108.** d	**138.** d
49. b	**79.** c	**109.** b	**139.** c
50. d	**80.** b	**110.** a	**140.** b
51. a	**81.** d	**111.** c	**141.** a
52. d	**82.** c	**112.** c	**142.** c
53. b	**83.** d	**113.** a	**143.** d
54. d	**84.** d	**114.** a	**144.** b
55. a	**85.** d	**115.** c	**145.** a
56. b	**86.** c	**116.** c	**146.** a
57. c	**87.** d	**117.** d	**147.** b
58. a	**88.** d	**118.** d	**148.** c
59. d	**89.** a	**119.** a	**149.** d
60. b	**90.** a	**120.** d	**150.** d
61. c	**91.** b	**121.** a	
62. c	**92.** a	**122.** d	

Multiple Choice: One Best Answer

1. b	**11.** e	**21.** c	**31.** c
2. c	**12.** d	**22.** d	**32.** d
3. a	**13.** a	**23.** a	**33.** d
4. b	**14.** a	**24.** d	**34.** a
5. c	**15.** c	**25.** d	**35.** c
6. e	**16.** e	**26.** a	**36.** b
7. a	**17.** c	**27.** c	**37.** a
8. d	**18.** a	**28.** b	**38.** b
9. b	**19.** e	**29.** b	**39.** c
10. a	**20.** d	**30.** a	**40.** a

Rypins' Basic Sciences Review, 17th Edition,
edited by Edward D. Frohlich. Lippincott–Raven Publishers,
Philadelphia © 1997.

3

Physiology

John E. Hall, Ph.D.
Arthur C. Guyton Professor and Chairman
Department of Physiology and Biophysics
University of Mississippi Medical Center
Jackson, Mississippi

Thomas H. Adair, Ph.D.
Professor
Department of Physiology and Biophysics
University of Mississippi Medical Center
Jackson, Mississippi

Physiology is the study of function of living organisms and their parts. In human physiology, we are concerned with characteristics of the human body that allow us to sense our environment, to move about, to think and communicate, to reproduce, and to perform all of the functions that enable us to survive and thrive as living beings.

Human physiology is a very broad subject, including the functions of molecules and subcellular components of the organism, functions of organs, such as the heart, organ systems, such as the cardiovascular system, as well as interaction and communication between the various organ systems. A distinguishing feature of this scientific discipline is that it seeks to integrate the large number of individual physical and chemical events occurring at all levels of organization to understand the function of the whole organism.

Cells are the basic living units of the body. Each organism is an aggregate of many different cells held together by intercellular supporting structures. The entire body contains about 75 to 100 trillion cells, each of which is adapted to perform special functions. Although the many cells of the body differ from each other in their special functions, all of them have certain basic characteristics. They are all bathed in extracellular fluid, the constituents of which are exactly controlled. A large part of our discussion of physiology focuses on the mechanisms that regulate the constituents of the extracellular fluid; this is called ***homeostasis,*** which means simply the maintenance of constant conditions in the internal environment of the body.

This chapter is based on an earlier version written by Dr. Arthur C. Guyton, whom the authors gratefully acknowledge for his excellent contributions.

FUNCTIONAL SYSTEMS OF THE BODY

The body can be divided into several major functional systems, each of which performs a particular task in maintaining homeostasis.

The ***cardiovascular system*** transports fluid and solutes, including nutrients and waste products, through all parts of the body. It keeps the fluids of the internal environment continually mixed by pumping blood through the vascular system. As the blood passes through the capillaries, a large portion of its fluid diffuses back and forth into the interstitial fluid that lies between the cells, allowing continuous exchange of substances between the cells and interstitial fluid and between the interstitial fluid and the blood.

The ***respiratory system*** provides oxygen for the body and removes carbon dioxide.

The ***gastrointestinal system*** digests food and absorbs different nutrients, including carbohydrates, fatty acids, and amino acids into the extracellular fluid.

The ***kidneys*** regulate the extracellular fluid composition by controlling excretion of salts, water, and waste products of the chemical reactions of the cells. By controlling body fluid volumes and composition, the kidneys also regulate blood volume and blood pressure.

The ***nervous system*** directs the activity of the muscular system, thereby providing locomotion. It also controls the function of many internal organs through the autonomic nervous system, and it allows us to sense our external and internal environments and to be intelligent beings so that we can attain the most advantageous conditions for survival.

The ***endocrine glands*** provide another regulatory system. Hormones secreted by these glands control many of the metabolic functions of the cells, such as growth, rate of metabolism, and special activities associated with reproduction.

The ***musculoskeletal system*** consists of skeletal muscle, bones, tendons, joints, cartilage, and ligaments. This system provides protection of internal organs, as well as support and movement of the body.

The ***integumentary system,*** composed mainly of skin, provides protection against injury and defense against foreign invaders as well as dehydration of underlying tissue. In addition, the skin also acts as an important means of maintaining a constant temperature in the body.

The ***immune system*** also acts as one of the body's chief defense mechanisms, providing protection against foreign invaders, such as bacteria and viruses, to which the body is exposed daily.

The ***reproductive system*** provides for formation of new beings like ourselves; even this can be considered a homeostatic function, for it generates new bodies in which trillions of more cells can exist in a well-regulated internal environment.

THE CELL AND ITS FUNCTION

Cell Structure. The cell is not merely a bag of fluid and chemicals; it also contains highly organized physical structures called ***organelles*** and is surrounded by a ***cell membrane*** (Fig. 3-1). Inside the cell, there are two major structures: the ***nucleus*** and the ***cytoplasm.*** Surrounding the nucleus is a ***nuclear membrane,*** which is highly permeable, and surrounding the cytoplasm is the cell membrane, which is also permeable but much less so than the nuclear membrane. Both the nucleus and cytoplasm are filled with highly viscous fluid containing salt and

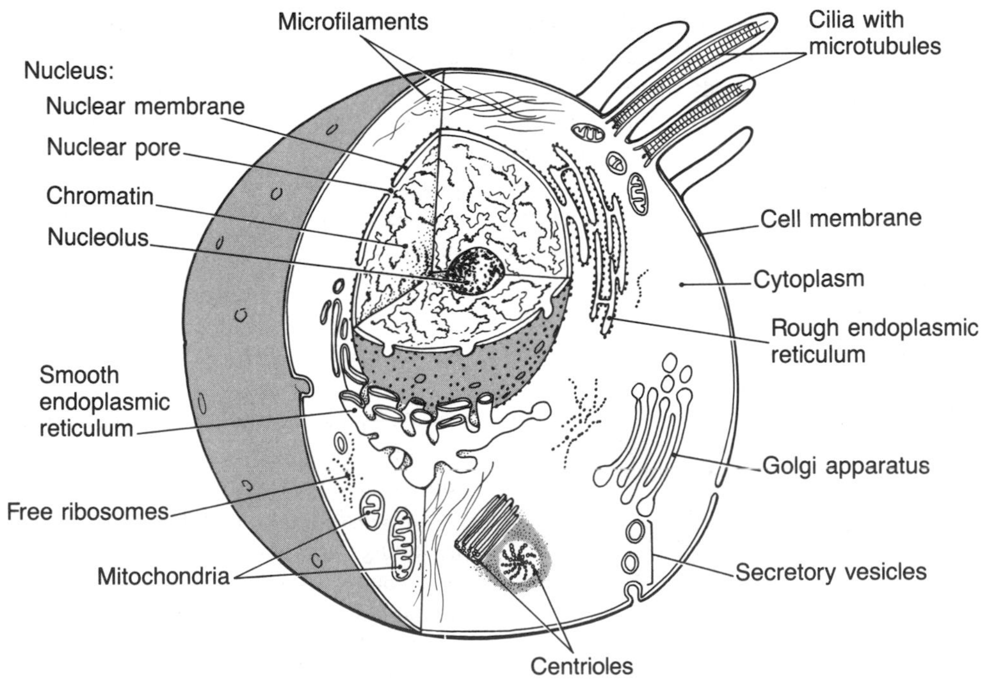

Fig. 3-1. Schematic reconstruction of a typical cell, showing the internal organelles in the cytoplasm and the cell nucleus. (Bullock BL: Pathophysiology: Adaptations and Alterations in Function, 4th ed. Philadelphia: Lippincott–Raven Publishers, 1996)

proteins, glucose, electrolytes, and many other substances. In addition to these two major organelles, there are many other structures (discussed in the following paragraphs). The nucleus contains 23 pairs of ***chromosomes,*** each of which contains several thousand sequences of ***deoxyribose nucleic acid (DNA)*** molecules that are the ***genes*** that regulate reproduction and the characteristics of the protein enzymes of the cytoplasm.

The cytoplasm contains several organelles, including the ***mitochondria,*** which are often called the powerhouses of the cell. The mitochondria contain large quantities of oxidative and other enzymes that are responsible for supplying energy to the cells, as will be discussed below. A second important structure of the cytoplasm is the ***endoplasmic reticulum,*** which is a system of tubes and vesicles that connects with the nucleus through the nuclear membrane and spreads throughout the cytoplasm.

Mitochondrial Energy Release in the Cell. An adequate supply of energy must always be available to energize the chemical reactions of the cells. This is provided principally by the chemical reaction of oxygen with any one of the three different types of foods: glucose derived from carbohydrates, fatty acids derived from fats, and amino acids derived from proteins. After entering the cell, the foods are split into smaller molecules that in turn enter the mitochondria where other enzymes remove carbon dioxide and hydrogen ions in the process called the ***citric acid cycle.*** Then an oxidative enzyme system, also in the mitochondria, causes progressive oxidation of the hydrogen atoms. The end products of the reactions of the mitochondria are water and carbon dioxide, and the energy liberated is used by the mitochondria to synthesize still another substance, ***adenosine triphosphate (ATP),*** a highly reactive chemical that can diffuse through the cell to release its energy whenever it is needed for performing cellular functions. These energy processes will be discussed in more detail later in the chapter.

Endoplasmic Reticulum—Synthesis of Multiple Substances in the Cell. The large network of tubules and vesicles, called the endoplasmic reticulum, penetrates almost all parts of the cytoplasm. The membrane of the endoplasmic reticulum provides an extensive surface area for manufacturing multiple substances that are used inside the cells and excreted from some cells. These substances include proteins, carbohydrates, lipids, and structures such as lysosomes, peroxisomes, and secretory granules.

The membranes of the endoplasmic reticulum perform many synthetic processes, and many of the substances that are formed are transported in the tubules and vesicles of the endoplasmic reticulum to other parts of the cell. Lipids are made in the structure of the endoplasmic reticulum wall. For the synthesis of proteins, ribosomes attach to the outer surface of the endoplasmic reticulum; these function in association with ***messenger RNA*** to synthesize many protein molecules that then enter the endoplasmic reticulum where the molecules are further modified before release for use in the cell. The details of protein synthesis will be discussed later.

Lysosomes. An organelle found in great numbers in cells is the lysosome. This is a small spherical vesicle surrounded by a membrane that contains digestive enzymes, which allow lysosomes to digest intracellular substances and structures, especially damaged cell structures, food particles that have been ingested by the cell, and unwanted materials such as bacteria. Ordinarily, the membranes surrounding the lysosome prevent the enclosed enzymes from coming into contact with other substances in the cell, and therefore prevent their digestive action. However, damage to these membranes releases the enzymes, which then split the organic substances with which they come into contact into highly diffusible substances such as amino acids and glucose.

Control of Protein Synthesis by Cell Genes. Proteins play a key role in almost all functions of the cell for two reasons: (1) all of the enzymes that catalyze the chemical reactions of the cells are proteins, and (2) most of the important physical structures of the cell contain structural proteins.

The genes control protein synthesis in the cell and in this way control cell function. Each gene is a double-stranded helical molecule of deoxyribose nucleic acid, called DNA, and it is composed of multiple units of (a) the sugar ***deoxyribose,*** (b) ***phosphoric acid,*** and (c) four ***nitrogenous bases,*** including two purines, ***adenine*** and ***guanine,*** and two pyrimidines, ***thymine*** and ***cytosine.*** The first stage in the formation of DNA is the combination of one molecule of phosphoric acid, one molecule of deoxyribose, and one of the four bases to form a ***nucleotide.*** Four separate nucleotides can be formed, corresponding to four different nitrogenous bases. Multiple nucleotides combine to form DNA in such a way that phosphoric acid and deoxyribose alternate with each other in the two separate strands, and these strands are held together by loose bonds between the purine and pyrimidine bases. The purine base adenine always bonds with the pyrimidine base thymine, and the purine base guanine always bonds with the pyrimidine base cytosine. The sequence of bases is different for each type of gene, and it is the specific sequence of bases in one of the two strands of DNA molecules that controls the type of protein synthesized.

The Genetic Code—Triplets of Bases. Three successive bases in the DNA strand are each called a ***code word*** and these code words control the sequence of amino acids in the protein to be formed in the cytoplasm. One code word might be composed of a sequence of adenine, thymine, and guanine, while the next code word might have a sequence of cytosine, guanine, and thymine. These two code words have entirely different meanings because their bases are different. The sequence of successive code words on the DNA strand is known as the ***genetic code.***

The Process of Transcription—Transfer of DNA Code to Ribose Nucleic Acid. Because DNA is located in the nucleus of the cell and many of the functions of the cell are carried out in the cytoplasm, there must be some means for the genes of the nucleus to control the chemical reactions of the cytoplasm. This is achieved through the intermediary of another type of nucleic acid, RNA, the formation of which is controlled by the DNA of the nucleus, a process called ***transcription.*** The RNA diffuses from the nucleus through the nuclear pores into the cytoplasm where it controls protein synthesis.

Each RNA molecule is composed of (a) the sugar ribose, (b) phosphoric acid, and (c) one of the four different pyrimidine and purine bases (the same bases as those found in DNA, except that thymine is replaced by uracil). Thus, the RNA strand is similar to the DNA strand. When the DNA strand of the gene causes formation of the RNA strand, it transfers its code to the RNA strand by controlling the sequence of bases in the RNA strand. This control is called transcription because the code of the RNA is "transcribed" onto the RNA.

During the transcription process, the two strands of DNA that make up the chromosome pull apart from each other. One of these strands then serves as the gene and attracts to it the necessary chemicals that form the RNA strand. The four separate bases that are part of the building blocks of the DNA strand are mutually attracted to four complementary bases that subsequently become part of the RNA strand (guanine attracts cytosine; cytosine attracts guanine; adenine attracts uracil; thymine attracts adenine). Thus, the code formed in the RNA strand is a complementary code to that of the gene DNA strand. Once the RNA is formed in the nucleus, it diffuses outward into the cytoplasm where it functions in the synthesis of a specific cell protein.

Three different types of RNA strands are formed: (1) ***messenger RNA (mRNA),*** which carries the genetic code to the cytoplasm for controlling the formation of the proteins; (2) ***transfer RNA (tRNA),*** which transports activated amino acids to the ribosomes to be used in assembling the proteins; and (3) ***ribosomal RNA,*** which along with other proteins forms the ***ribosomes,*** the structures in which protein molecules are actually assembled.

Ribosomal RNA becomes a major constituent of the small particles called ***ribosomes.*** Protein molecules are then manufactured by these ribosomes.

There are 20 separate types of ***transfer RNA,*** each of which combines specifically with one of the 20 different amino acids and conducts this amino acid to the ribosome, where it is combined into the protein molecule.

Translation—Polypeptide Synthesis on Ribosomes from the Genetic Code Contained in mRNA. There are many thousands of different mRNAs, each of which carries the genetic code that determines the sequence in which successive amino acids will be arranged in one specific type of protein molecule. Messenger RNA is a single-stranded, long molecule, having a succession of ***codons*** along its axis. These codons are mirror images of the code words in the gene DNA, and they also consist of three successive bases. To manufacture proteins, one end of the RNA strand enters the ribosome, and the entire strand then threads its way to the ribosome in just over a minute. As it passes through, the ribosome "reads" the genetic code and causes the proper succession of amino acids to bind together by chemical bonds called ***peptide linkages,*** which will be discussed later in the chapter. Actually, the mRNA does not recognize the different types of amino acids but instead recognizes the different transfer RNA molecules. However, each type of transfer RNA molecule carries only one specific type of amino acid that will be incorporated into the protein.

To recapitulate, as the strand of mRNA passes through the ribosome, each of its codons draws to it a specific transfer RNA that in turn delivers a specific amino acid. This amino acid then combines with the preceding amino acids by forming a peptide linkage, and the sequence continues to build until an entire protein molecule is formed. At this point, a special codon appears that indicates completion of the process, and the protein is released into the cytoplasm or through the membrane of the endoplasmic reticulum into the interior of this reticulum. This control of amino acid sequence by the RNA code during protein formation is called ***translation.***

It is estimated that there are about 100,000 different types of genes in the nucleus; therefore, one can understand that a large number of different types of proteins can also be formed in each cell. The character of each cell depends on the relative proportion of different types of proteins that are formed. Thus, the genes control the structure of the cell through the types of structural proteins formed, and the genes control the function of the cell mainly through the types of protein enzymes that are formed.

Cell Differentiation. Cell differentiation allows different cells of the body to perform different functions. As a human being develops from a fertilized ovum, the ovum divides repeatedly until trillions of cells are formed. Gradually, however, the new cells differentiate from each other, with certain cells having different genetic characteristics from other cells. This differentiation process occurs as a result of inactivation of certain genes and activation of others during successive stages of cell division.

This process of differentiation leads to the ability of different cells in the body to perform different functions.

Cellular Reproduction—The Process of Mitosis. Most cells of the body, with the exception of mature red blood cells, striated muscle cells, and neurons in the nervous system, are capable of reproducing other cells of their own type. Ordinarily, if sufficient nutrients are available, each cell grows larger and larger until it automatically divides by the process of ***mitosis*** to form two new cells. Before mitosis occurs, all the genes in the nucleus, as well as the chromosomes carrying the genes, are themselves reproduced to create a complete new set of genes. During mitosis, one set of genes enters one of the daughter cells while the other set enters the second daughter cell. Thus, not only are the physical characteristics of the two new cells alike, but they are still controlled by the same types of genes so that their functions will be very similar. If, during the process of reproduction, one or more of the genes fail to be reproduced or become suppressed, then the two new cells will not be exactly alike, and the cells will become slightly differentiated from each other.

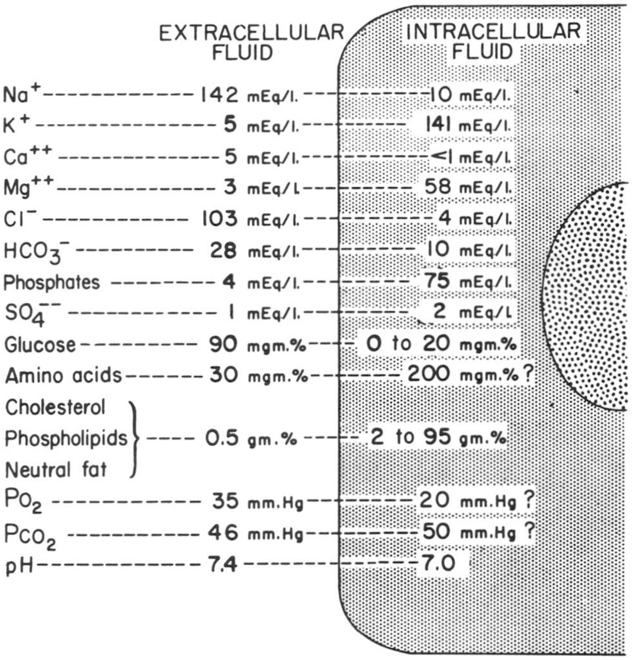

Fig. 3-2. Chemical compositions of extracellular and intracellular fluids. (Guyton AC: Textbook of Medical Physiology, 8th ed. Philadelphia: WB Saunders, 1991)

THE BODY FLUIDS

Total Body Water—Extracellular and Intracellular Fluid. In a normal 70-kg adult human, the total body water averages 60% of the body weight, or about 42 liters. This can be divided into two major compartments: the ***extracellular fluid,*** which is about 20% of total body weight (14 liters), and ***intracellular fluid,*** which is 40% of total body weight (28 liters).

The extracellular fluid can be subdivided into two main subcompartments: *the* ***plasma,*** which makes up almost one fourth of the extracellular fluid (3 liters), and the ***interstitial fluid,*** which lies between the tissue cells and amounts to more than three fourths of the extracellular fluid (11 liters). Because the plasma and interstitial fluids are separated only by highly permeable capillary membranes, their ionic compositions are similar and they are often considered together as one large compartment of homogeneous fluid. The most important difference between plasma and interstitial fluid is the higher concentration of protein in the plasma, which exists because the capillaries have a low permeability to the plasma proteins.

Comparison of Extracellular and Intracellular Fluid. Figure 3-2 shows the concentrations of the most important substances in extracellular and intracellular fluids. Both of these fluids contain nutrients that are needed by the cells, including glucose, amino acids, oxygen, and others not shown in the figure. The intracellular fluid is separated from the extracellular fluid by a cell membrane that is highly permeable to water but not to many of the electrolytes in the body, causing important differences between extracellular and intracellular fluids in electrolyte concentrations. Extracellular fluid contains large quantities of sodium and chloride ions but only small amounts of potassium, magnesium, and phosphate ions. In contrast, intracellular fluid contains large amounts of potassium and phosphate ions, moderate amounts of magnesium ions, and exceedingly few calcium ions. These differences in the ionic composition of the fluids cause a membrane potential to develop across the two sides of the cell membrane—negative on the inside and positive outside. Later in the chapter we shall see how this potential develops and the manner in which it changes during the transmission of nerve and muscle impulses. Because the cell membrane is highly permeable to water, the osmolarity (the concentration of osmotically active solute particles) of the intra- and extracellular compartments is normally the same, about 285 mosm/liter.

Measurement of Volumes in Different Body Fluid Compartments—The Indicator-Dilution Principle. The volume of a fluid compartment in the body can be measured by placing a substance in the compartment, allowing it to disperse throughout the compartment's fluid, and then analyzing the extent to which it has become diluted in the compartment. Thus, the unknown volume of the compartment (V) can be calculated by knowing the total amount of substance injected into the compartment (Q), divided by the concentration of the substance (C) after dilution in the compartment: $V = Q/C$. For this method to be used properly, the substance must be uniformly distributed in the compartment, and only in the compartment that is being measured.

Total body water is measured using substances that disperse throughout the body fluids, such as radioactive water (^3H_2O) or heavy water (deuterium, ^2H_2O). ***Extracellular fluid*** is measured using several substances that disperse in the plasma and interstitial fluid but do not permeate the cell membrane, such as radioactive sodium, insulin, and thiosulfate. ***Intracellular volume*** cannot be measured directly, but can be calculated as the difference between total body water and extracellular volume. ***Plasma volume*** is measured by injecting substances such as radioactive albumin, which do not penetrate capillary membranes and therefore remain in the vascular system. ***Interstitial fluid volume*** cannot be measured directly but can be calculated as the difference between extracellular fluid volume and plasma volume.

EXCHANGE OF FLUID AND ELECTROLYTES ACROSS THE CELL MEMBRANE

The Cell Membrane—Lipid Bilayer and Protein Channels. A thin film of lipids only two molecules thick, composed mainly of phospholipids, cholesterol, and triglycerides, covers the entire cell surface. Interspersed in this lipid film are large globular protein molecules that protrude through the membrane. Channels through the structures of the protein molecules serve as minute pores in the membrane.

The lipid bilayer part of the membrane is impermeable to the usual water-soluble substances, such as ions, glucose, urea, and others. On the other hand, fat-soluble substances such as oxygen, carbon dioxide, and alcohol move with ease through this part of the membrane. However, the lipid membrane also contains large glycoprotein molecules that penetrate the membrane. Channels through the structures of these protein molecules serve as minute pores in the membrane through which water and water-soluble substances, especially the ions, move through the membrane.

Diffusion—Net Movement of Molecules Through the Cell Membrane Along Chemical or Electrical Gradients. Substances pass through the cell membrane, back and forth between the extracellular and intracellular fluids, by the process of ***diffusion,*** which occurs because molecules migrate from a region of high concentration to one of lower concentration as a result of random motion. The rate of diffusion across the cell membrane is *directly* related to (1) the electrical potential and chemical concentration differences across the membrane, (2) the permeability of the membrane for the solute, and (3) the surface area of the membrane. Diffusion rate is *inversely* related to (1) thickness of the cell membrane and (2) the size of the solute.

Substances that are highly soluble in lipids can diffuse directly through the lipid matrix of the cell membrane. The various ions, large molecules such as glucose, and water enter and leave the cells through the membrane channels formed by glycoprotein molecules that extend all the way through the membrane. These channel proteins allow rapid passage of water and other small molecules. However, they are often highly selectively permeable to certain substances, such as the ions; depending on various conditions of the cells some of these channels are open and allow rapid diffusion of specific substances, whereas at other times the channels are closed and diffusion is greatly decreased. Thus, opening and closing these channels is a means by which movement of many substances through the cell membrane can be controlled, as we shall discuss more fully later in this chapter.

Facilitated Diffusion—Carrier-Mediated Diffusion. Many substances are transported through the cell membrane by combining chemically with a carrier, which is a protein that penetrates through the cell membrane. The carrier combines chemically with the substance and "facilitates" its diffusion through the cell membrane to the opposite side, where the substance is released. Facilitated diffusion differs from simple diffusion in the following important way: although the rate of diffusion increases proportionally with the concentration of the diffusing substance, as occurs with diffusion through an open channel, there is a ***transport maximum,*** called V_{max}, with facilitated diffusion. Among the most important substances that cross cell membranes by facilitated diffusion are ***glucose*** and ***amino acids.***

Active Transport Through the Cell Membrane Against an Electrochemical Gradient. Active transport is similar to facilitated diffusion in that the substance to be transported combines with a carrier protein and is released from the carrier on the opposite side of the membrane. However, active transport differs from facilitated diffusion in that it can transport the substance even in the absence of an electrochemical gradient, or even against an electrochemical gradient. To achieve "uphill" transport against a concentration or electrical gradient, energy is required. This energy is supplied by the high-energy compound ***adenosine triphosphate (ATP)*** or by some other high-energy phosphate compound inside the cell.

One of the most important active transport systems in the body is that for transport of sodium out of the cells and potassium into the cells, which is called the ***sodium–potassium pump*** (Fig. 3-3). The protein structure of the pump serves both as the carrier and as the energy-transferring mechanism for moving the sodium out of the

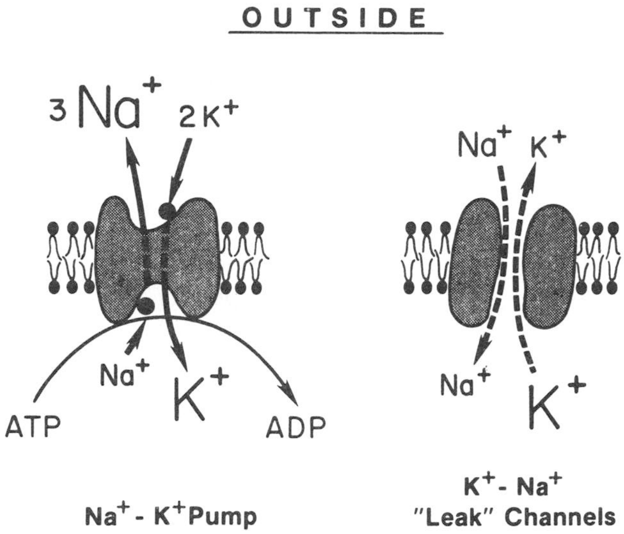

Fig. 3-3. Postulated mechanism of the sodium–potassium pump. (Guyton AC: Textbook of Medical Physiology, 8th ed. Philadelphia: WB Saunders, 1991)

cell and potassium into the cell. The pump causes the concentration of sodium inside the cell to become very low, and at the same time causes the intracellular potassium concentration to build up to a very high level. This sodium–potassium pump maintains much of the ionic concentration difference between intracellular and extracellular fluids and therefore is extremely important in controlling the volume of cells, as well as the function of excitable nerve and muscle fibers, as will be described later in the chapter. Other important primary active transport systems include (1) the ***calcium pump,*** which transports calcium to the outside of the cell membrane as well as into the internal organelles of the cell (this calcium pump maintains a very low intracellular calcium concentration); and (2) ***hydrogen pumps,*** which are especially important for secreting hydrochloric acid in the stomach and for secreting hydrogen ions into the renal tubules.

Secondary Active Transport—Co-transport and Countertransport. When sodium ions are transported out of the cells by the sodium–potassium pump, a large concentration gradient for sodium develops, with very high concentration outside the cell and low concentration inside. This gradient represents a storehouse of energy, and under appropriate conditions this diffusion energy of sodium can pull other substances along with sodium into the cell. This phenomenon is called ***co-transport*** and is one form of active transport. Examples of substances co-transported with sodium include glucose and amino acids, especially in the epithelial cells of the intestine and renal tubules.

Another form of secondary active transport is ***countertransport,*** in which the substance is transported in the *opposite direction* as sodium, again by means of a carrier protein that binds both sodium and the substance to be transported. Two very important countertransport mechanisms are ***sodium–calcium countertransport*** and ***sodium–hydrogen countertransport.***

OSMOTIC PRESSURE AND OSMOTIC EQUILIBRIA AT THE CELL MEMBRANE

Osmosis. Osmosis is the diffusion of water across a membrane. Cell membranes in the body are highly permeable to water, and whenever there is a higher concentration of solute on one side of the membrane, water rapidly diffuses across the membrane toward the region of higher solute concentration. The reason for this is that the higher the concentration of dissolved substances in a water solution, the lower the concentration of water molecules in the fluid. Therefore, if a solution with a low solute concentration (high water concentration) is placed on one side of the cell membrane, water will diffuse from the side of the membrane with the low solute concentration to the side that has the high solute concentration (low water concentration) until the water concentration on both sides becomes equal; this is osmosis.

Relationship Between Osmoles and Moles. The total number of solute particles in a solution is measured in terms of ***osmoles.*** One osmole (osm) is equal to one mole (mol; 6.02×10^{23}) of solute particles. Therefore, a solution containing one mole of glucose in each liter has a concentration of 1 osm/liter. If a molecule dissociates into two ions (giving two particles), such as sodium chloride ionizing to give chloride and sodium ions, then the solution containing 1.0 mol/liter will have an osmotic concentration of 2.0 osm/liter. For body fluids, the osmotic activity of solutes is usually expressed in terms of ***milliosmoles*** (mosm), which equals 1/1,000 osmoles.

Osmotic Pressure. If sufficient pressure is applied across the membrane through which osmosis is occurring, but the pressure is applied in the direction opposite the osmotic flow, the osmosis can be stopped. The amount of pressure that is required to stop osmosis is called the ***osmotic pressure.*** Osmotic pressure, therefore, is an indirect measurement of the water and solute concentration of a solution. The higher the osmotic pressure of a solution, the higher the solute concentration of the solution.

The osmotic pressure of a solution is directly proportional to the concentration of osmotically active particles, regardless of whether the solute is a large molecule or small molecule. Expressed mathematically, osmotic pressure (π) can be calculated as: $\pi = \mathbf{CRT}$, where C is the concentration of solute in osmoles per liter, R is the ideal gas constant, and T is the absolute temperature. For biological solutions, π calculates to be about 19,300 mmHg for a solution having a concentration of 1.0 osm/liter. This means that for a concentration of 1.0 mosm/liter, π is equal to 19.3 mmHg. Thus, for each milliosmole concentration gradient across the cell membrane, 19.3 mmHg osmotic force is exerted. This means that only small differences in solute concentration across the cell membrane can cause rapid osmosis of water.

Isotonic, Hypotonic, and Hypertonic Fluids. A solution is said to be ***isotonic*** if no osmotic force develops across the cell membrane when a normal cell is placed in the solution. This means that an isotonic solution has the same osmolarity as the cell and that the cells will not shrink or swell if placed in the solution. Examples of isotonic solutions are a 0.9% sodium chloride solution or a 5% glucose solution.

A solution is said to be ***hypertonic*** when it contains a higher osmotic concentration of substances than does the cell. In this case, osmotic force develops that causes water to flow out of the cell into the solution, thereby greatly concentrating intracellular fluid and shrinking the cell.

The solution is said to be ***hypotonic*** if the osmotic concentration of substances in the solution is less than their concentration in the cell. An osmotic force develops immediately when the cell is exposed to the solution, causing water to flow by osmosis into the cell until the intracellular fluid has about the same concentration as the extracellular fluid, or until the cell bursts from excessive swelling.

Fluid Therapy. When fluid is administered into a patient, it is usually injected into the bloodstream or is absorbed into the blood from the gastrointestinal tract, and it immediately becomes part of the extracellular fluid. If the fluid is isotonic, and if the cell membrane is relatively impermeable to the solute, as is true for sodium chloride, most of the injected fluid stays in the extracellular compartment and there is very little change in the concentration of intracellular or extracellular fluids. If the fluid is very hypotonic, large portions of the water in the fluid will diffuse into the cells by osmosis, causing expansion of the extracellular fluid volume and a decrease in osmolarity of both intracellular and extracellular fluids. On the other hand, if the fluid is hypertonic, it will draw large amounts of intracellular water out of the cells, thereby shrinking the cells and raising both intracellular and extracellular fluid osmolarity.

Dehydration means loss of water from the body. If pure water is lost, by evaporation from the respiratory tract or from the surface of the skin, this will concentrate both the extracellular and intracellular fluids. However, if pure extracellular fluid, or fluid very similar to extracellular fluid, is lost in the body, as occasionally occurs in different types of kidney disease or when a person sweats profusely, the fluid lost at first will be mainly from the extracellular compartment without affecting the intracellular fluid.

EXCHANGE OF FLUIDS AND SOLUTES THROUGH CAPILLARY MEMBRANES

Capillary Permeability. Most capillaries are very porous, with several million slits or pores between the cells that make up their walls (the widths of the pores are about 8 nm) to each square centimeter of capillary surface. Because of the high permeability of the capillaries for most solutes, as blood flows through the capillaries, very large amounts of dissolved substances diffuse in both directions through these "pores." In this way, sodium, chloride, potassium, glucose, and almost all other dissolved substances in the plasma, except the plasma proteins, continually mix with the interstitial fluid. The rate of diffusion for most solutes is so great that even cells as far as 50 microns away from the capillaries can still receive adequate quantities of nutrients. In capillaries, the most important means of moving solutes from the blood to the interstitium is by simple diffusion across the capillary wall.

Bulk Flow (Ultrafiltration) of Fluid Across the Capillary Wall. Although exchange of nutrients, oxygen, and metabolic end products across the capillaries occurs almost entirely by diffusion, the distribution of fluid across the capillary is determined by another process: the bulk flow, or ultrafiltration, of protein-free plasma. As discussed above, the capillary wall is highly permeable to water and to most plasma solutes, except for the plasma proteins. Therefore, a hydrostatic pressure difference across the capillary wall pushes a protein-free plasma (ultrafiltrate) through the capillary wall into the interstitium. The rate at which this ultrafiltration occurs depends on the difference in hydrostatic and colloid osmotic pressures of the capillary and interstitial fluid.

The ***capillary hydrostatic pressure,*** which normally averages about 17 mmHg, tends to push fluid out of the pores of the capillaries into the interstitial fluid. However, the proteins in the plasma are relatively impermeable to the capillary wall and therefore exert an osmotic force that tends to draw fluid back into the capillaries. This osmotic force is often called the ***oncotic pressure*** or ***colloid osmotic pressure,*** which averages about 28 mmHg in most capillaries. The ***interstitial fluid hydrostatic pressure*** tends to oppose fluid filtration, but in many tissues the normal interstitial fluid hydrostatic pressure averages −3 mmHg, a negative rather than a positive value. Proteins in the interstitial fluid also exert an ***interstitial fluid colloid osmotic pressure*** of approximately 8 mmHg, which tends to draw fluid out of the capillaries. Thus, there are opposing forces acting to move fluid across the capillary wall: (1) the difference between capillary hydrostatic pressure and interstitial fluid hydrostatic pressure, which tends to cause filtration out of the capillary; and (2) the difference in colloid osmotic pressure between the plasma and interstitial fluid, which favors movement of fluid into the capillary. Under normal conditions, these forces are nearly balanced so that there is very little net movement of fluid out of the capillaries. This balance between inward and outward forces is called ***Starlings' equilibrium of the capillaries,*** and it can be stated mathematically as follows: Capillary hydrostatic pressure − interstitial fluid hydrostatic pressure = plasma colloid osmotic pressure − interstitial fluid colloid osmotic pressure.

The normal values for these different pressures are as follows: capillary pressure, 17 mmHg; interstitial fluid hydrostatic pressure, −3 mmHg; plasma colloid osmotic pressure, 28 mmHg; and tissue fluid colloid osmotic pressure, 8 mmHg. Thus, the sum of forces that tend to move fluid into or out of the capillary wall are normally almost exactly balanced (Fig. 3-4). (Actually there is usually a fraction of a millimeter of mercury greater pressure tending to move fluid outward, which is what causes the formation of tissue fluid and lymph, as will be discussed later.)

Edema. ***Intracellular edema*** can occur when the cell membrane is damaged or when there is inadequate nutrition to the cells. When this happens, sodium ions are no longer pumped out of the cells, and the excess sodium ions inside the cells cause osmosis of water into the cells.

In most instances, edema occurs mainly in the ***extracellular fluid*** compartment when there is accumulation of fluid in the interstitial spaces. There are two general causes of extracellular edema: (1) abnormal leakage of fluid from the plasma to the interstitial spaces across the capillaries and (2) failure of the lymphatics to return fluid from the interstitium back to the blood.

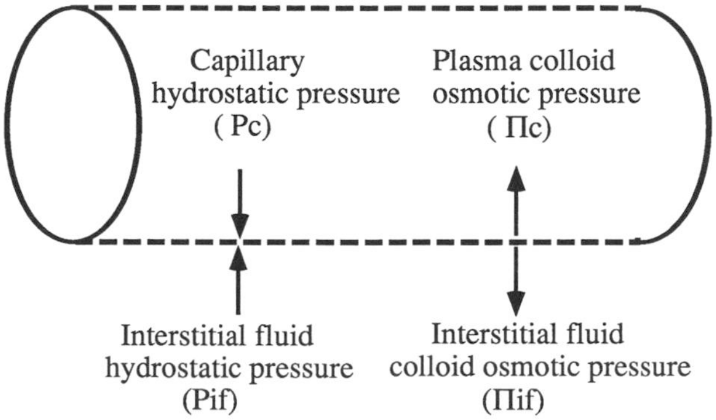

Fig. 3-4. Forces operative at the capillary membrane tending to move fluid either outward or inward through the membrane pores.

Factors That Can Increase Capillary Filtration and Cause Interstitial Fluid Edema. To understand the cause of excess capillary filtration, it is useful to state the mathematical determinants of capillary filtration:

$$\text{Filtration} = K_f \times (P_C - P_{IF} - \pi_C + \pi_{IF})$$

where K_f is the capillary filtration coefficient (the product of the permeability and surface area of the capillaries), P_{IF} is the interstitial fluid hydrostatic pressure, π_C is the capillary plasma colloid osmotic pressure, and π_{IF} is the interstitial fluid colloid osmotic pressure. From this equation, one can see that any of the following changes can increase the capillary filtration rate: (1) ***increased capillary filtration coefficient,*** which allows leakage of fluids and plasma proteins through the capillary membranes—this can occur as a result of allergic reactions, bacterial infections, and toxic substances, which injure the capillary membranes; (2) ***increased capillary hydrostatic pressure,*** which can result from obstruction of a vein, excess flow of blood from the arteries into the capillaries, or failure of the heart to pump blood rapidly out of the veins (heart failure); (3) ***decreased plasma colloid osmotic pressure,*** which can occur as a result of failure of the liver to produce sufficient quantities of plasma proteins, loss of large amounts of proteins into the urine in certain kidney diseases, or loss of large quantities of proteins through burned areas of the skin or other denuding lesions; and (4) ***increased interstitial fluid colloid osmotic pressure,*** which will draw fluid out of the plasma into the tissue spaces—this results most frequently from lymphatic blockage, which prevents the return of proteins from the interstitial spaces to the blood, as will be discussed in the following sections.

LYMPHATIC SYSTEM

The lymphatics are a system of accessory vessels that accompany blood vessels to almost all parts of the body. Minute ***lymphatic capillaries,*** like the blood capillaries, are found in almost all tissues; these lead into progressively larger lymphatic channels that finally converge mainly in the ***thoracic duct,*** which passes upward through the chest and empties into the venous system at the juncture of the left internal jugular and subclavian veins. The lymphatic capillaries are highly permeable so that bacteria, various types of debris in the interstitial fluids, and large proteins can enter the lymph from the interstitial fluid with great ease.

Because of their large molecular size, most proteins that move out of the blood capillaries into the interstitial fluids cannot pass back into the blood capillaries. After these collect in the interstitial fluid and become progressively more and more concentrated, they finally flow into the lymphatic system, and are returned to the bloodstream in this way. Approximately half of all the protein in the blood leaks into the interstitial spaces each day, and were it not for its return by the lymph to the blood, a person would lose most of the plasma colloid osmotic pressure within a few hours and would therefore no longer be able to maintain normal blood volume. Return of protein from the interstitial spaces to the blood is therefore probably the single most important function of the lymphatic system.

Lymph Formation from Interstitial Fluid. Lymph is formed from the fluid that flows out of the interstitial spaces into the lymphatic capillaries. Therefore, its constituents are almost identical to those of the interstitial fluid. Most lymph from the peripheral tissues has a protein concentration between 2 and 3 g/100 ml, while liver has a concentration of about 6 g/100 ml, and that of the intestines about 3 to 4 g/100 ml. Since the liver produces much more lymph in proportion to its weight than any other tissue in the body, the thoracic lymph has a protein concentration of about 4 g/100ml.

Control of Lymph Flow. The two main factors that control the rate of lymph flow are (1) the interstitial fluid hydrostatic pressure and (2) the pumping activity of the lymphatics. The greater the volume of fluid in the tissue spaces, the greater the interstitial fluid hydrostatic pressure. This in turn promotes increased flow of fluid into the lymphatic capillaries through their large openings. Once in the lymphatic capillaries, the lymph is pumped by intermittent compression of the lymphatic vessels. Compression results either from repetitive contraction of the lymphatic walls or from external compression of the lymph vessels by contracting muscles, joint movement, or other effects that cause tissue compression. The lymphatics contain valves that allow flow to occur only away from the tissues and toward the bloodstream. Therefore, during each compression cycle of a lymph vessel, fluid is pumped progressively along the vessel toward the circulation.

Removal of Bacteria and Debris from Tissues by the Lymphatic System at Lymph Nodes. Because of the very high degree of permeability of the lymphatic capillaries, bacteria and other small particulate matter in the tissues can pass into the lymph. However, the lymph passes through a series of nodes on its way to the blood. In these nodes, bacteria and other debris are filtered out, then phagocytized by macrophages in the nodes, and finally digested into amino acids, glucose fatty acids, and other small molecular substances before being released into the blood.

KIDNEYS

The kidneys serve multiple functions to maintain homeostasis, including (1) regulation of water and electrolyte balances in the body, (2) regulation of body fluid osmolarity and electrolyte concentrations, (3) regulation of acid-base balance, (4) excretion of metabolic waste products and foreign chemicals, (5) regulation of arterial pressure, (6) secretion of hormones (*e.g.*, erythropoietin, renin), and (7) synthesis of glucose from amino acids (gluconeogenesis).

URINE FORMATION

The kidneys perform their most important functions by ''clearing'' unwanted substance from the blood and excreting them in the urine while returning substances that are needed back to the blood. Excretion of urine begins with the filtration of fluid from the glomerular capillaries into the renal tubules, a process called ***glomerular filtration.*** As glomerular filtrate flows along the renal tubules, the volume of the filtrate is reduced, and its composition is altered by ***tubular reabsorption*** (the movement of water and solutes from the tubules back into the blood) and by ***tubular secretion*** (the net movement of water and solutes into the tubules). For each substance excreted in the urine, a particular combination of filtration, reabsorptions and secretion occurs:

$$\begin{array}{l}\text{urinary}\\ \text{excretion}\\ \text{rate}\end{array} = \begin{array}{c}\text{filtration}\\ \text{rate}\end{array} - \begin{array}{c}\text{reabsorption}\\ \text{rate}\end{array} + \begin{array}{c}\text{secretion}\\ \text{rate}\end{array}$$

As we shall discuss later, changes in urinary excretion rate of different substances that are needed to maintain body fluid and electrolyte homeostasis can occur as a result of changes in glomerular filtration, tubular reabsorption, or in some cases, tubular secretion.

Nephron—The Functional Unit of the Kidney. Each kidney in the human is made up of about 1 million nephrons, each capable of forming urine. The functional parts of the nephron are shown in Figure 3-5. Each nephron is composed of a tuft of ***glomerular capillaries*** called the ***glomerulus,*** through which large amounts of fluid are filtered from the blood; a capsule around the glomerulus called ***Bowman's capsule;*** and a long tubule in which the filtered fluid is converted into urine on its way to the ***renal pelvis,*** which receives urine from all of the nephrons. Urine passes from the renal pelvis to the ***bladder,*** where it is stored until it is eventually expelled from the body by the process of ***micturition,*** or urination.

Renal Blood Flow. Blood flows to the kidney at a rate of about 1,200 ml/min (21% of cardiac output) through the renal artery, which branches progressively to form the ***interlobar arteries, arcuate arteries, interlobular arteries,*** and ***afferent arterioles,*** which lead to the glomerular capillaries. Blood leaves the glomerular capillaries through an ***efferent arteriole,*** which empties into a second capillary network, the ***peritubular capillaries.***

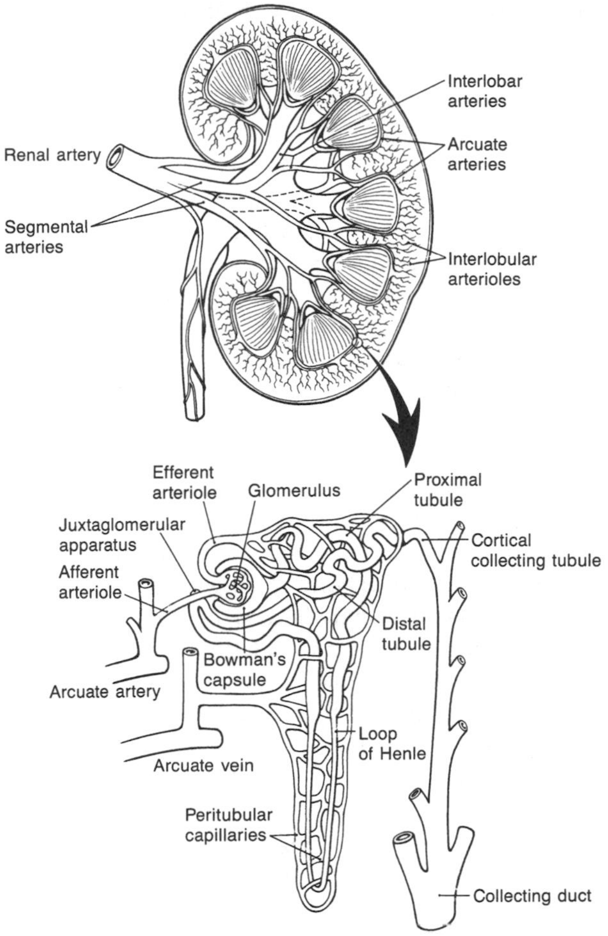

Fig. 3-5. Section of the human kidney showing the major vessels that supply blood to the kidney and schematic of the nephrons, including vascular and tubular elements. (Guyton AC, Hall JE: Textbook of Medical Physiology, 9th ed. Philadelphia: WB Saunders, 1995)

The peritubular capillaries surround the renal tubules and empty into the venous system, which leaves the kidney via the renal vein.

Glomerular Filtration—The First Step in Urine Formation. The glomerular filtrate is an ultrafiltrate of plasma that has a composition almost identical to that of plasma, except that it has almost no protein (only 0.03%). The glomerular filtration rate (GFR) is normally about 125 ml/min, or about 20% of the renal plasma flow; thus, the fraction of renal plasma flow that is filtered ***(filtration fraction)*** averages about 0.2.

As in other capillaries, the GFR is determined by the balance of hydrostatic and colloid osmotic forces across the capillary membrane and by the glomerular ***capillary filtration coefficient*** (K_f), which is the product of the permeability and surface area of the capillaries:

$$GFR = \text{net filtration pressure} \times K_f$$

The ***net filtration pressure*** represents the sum of hydrostatic and colloid osmotic forces that either favor or oppose filtration across the glomerular capillaries. These forces include (1) the hydrostatic pressure inside the glomerular capillaries (P_G), which is normally about 60 mmHg and promotes filtration; (2) the hydrostatic pressure in Bowman's capsule outside the capillaries (P_B), which is normally 18 mmHg and opposes filtration; (3) the colloid osmotic pressure of the glomerular capillary plasma proteins (π_G), which averages 32 mmHg and opposes filtration; and (4) the colloid osmotic pressure of the proteins in Bowman's capsule (π_B), which is normally near zero and therefore has little effect on filtration. Therefore,

$$\text{Net filtration pressure} = P_G - P_B - \pi_G \cong 10 \text{ mmHg}$$

This net filtration pressure can be decreased in several ways: (1) by decreasing the arterial pressure, which decreases the glomerular hydrostatic pressure; in normal kidneys, glomerular hydrostatic pressure changes only 1 to 2 mmHg occur over a wide range of arterial pressure (from 80–160 mmHg) due to ***autoregulation,*** which causes adjustments of renal arteriolar resistance; (2) by increasing the resistance of the afferent arterioles, which decreases glomerular hydrostatic pressure; (3) by decreasing resistance of the efferent arterioles, which decreases glomerular hydrostatic pressure; and (4) by increasing the glomerular plasma colloid osmotic pressure.

The GFR can also be reduced by decreasing K_f. Table 3-1 summarizes the physical determinants of GFR and physiological factors that can influence these determinants.

Tubular Secretion—Net Movement of Solutes from the Peritubular Capillaries into Tubules. Some substances are not only filtered by the glomerular capillaries but are also secreted from the peritubular capillaries into the tubules. The first step of tubular secretion is simple diffusion of the substance from the peritubular capillaries into the interstitium. The next step is movement of the substance into the tubular cell or between the tubular cells into the lumen of the tubule by active or passive transport. Substances that are actively secreted into the tubules include potassium and hydrogen ions. Certain organic acids and bases are also highly secreted into the renal tubules, leading to rapid removal of these substances from the blood and excretion in the urine.

Reabsorption of Solutes and Water from Tubules to Peritubular Capillaries. As the glomerular filtrate enters the renal tubules, it flows sequentially through four major sections of the tubule: (1) ***proximal tubules,*** (2) ***loops of Henle,*** (3) ***distal tubules,*** and (4) ***collecting tubules and ducts.*** From the 125 ml/min of glomerular filtrate, approximately 124 ml/min are normally reabsorbed by the tubules into the peritubular capil-

TABLE 3-1. Summary of Factors That Can Decrease GFR*

PHYSICAL DETERMINANTS	PHYSIOLOGICAL/PATHOPHYSIOLOGICAL CAUSES
$\downarrow K_f \rightarrow \downarrow$ GFR	↑ Sympathetic activity; renal disease; hypertension
$\uparrow P_B \rightarrow \downarrow$ GFR	Urinary tract obstruction (*e.g.*, kidney stones)
$\uparrow \pi_G \rightarrow \downarrow$ GFR $\downarrow P_G \rightarrow \downarrow$ GFR	↓ Renal blood flow; increased plasma proteins
• $\downarrow A_P \rightarrow \downarrow P_G$	↓ Arterial pressure (has only small effect due to autoregulation)
• $\downarrow R_E \rightarrow \downarrow P_G$	↓ Angiotensin II
• $\uparrow R_A \rightarrow \downarrow P_G$	↑ Sympathetic activity; ↑ vasoconstrictor hormones (*e.g.*, norepinephrine, endothelin)

* Opposite changes in the above determinants/factors usually increase GFR.

K_f = glomerular filtration coefficient
P_B = Bowman's capsule hydrostatic pressure
π_G = glomerular capillary colloid osmotic pressure
P_G = glomerular capillary hydrostatic pressure
A_P = systemic arterial pressure
R_A = afferent arteriolar resistance
R_E = efferent arteriolar resistance

lary blood, leaving only 1 ml/min to pass into the urine. Approximately 65% is reabsorbed in the proximal tubules, 15% in the loop of Henle, 10% in the distal tubule, and 9.3% in the collecting tubules and ducts. Thus, most of the reabsorption occurs in the early part of the renal tubular system.

Some substances that are filtered, such as glucose and amino acids, are almost completely reabsorbed by the tubules so that urinary excretion rate is essentially zero. Most of the ions in the plasma, such as sodium, chloride, and bicarbonate, are also highly reabsorbed, but their rates of reabsorption and urinary excretion are variable depending upon the needs of the body. Certain waste products, such as urea and creatinine, are poorly reabsorbed and excreted in relatively large amounts. Therefore, tubular reabsorption is highly selective, allowing the kidneys to regulate excretion of solutes independently of one another. This allows precise control of the composition of the body fluids.

Reabsorption in Proximal Tubules. Approximately two thirds of the water and solutes filtered are reabsorbed in the proximal tubules. Thus, one important function of the proximal tubules is to conserve substances that are needed by the body, including glucose, amino acids, proteins, as well as water and electrolytes such as sodium, potassium, and chloride. On the other hand, the proximal tubules are relatively impermeable to the waste products of the body.

Reabsorption in Loop of Henle. The loop of Henle consists of three functionally distinct segments: the descending thin segment, the ascending thin segment, and ascending thick segment. These parts of the loop of Henle dip into the inner part of the kidney, the ***renal medulla,*** and play an important role in allowing the kidney to form a concentrated urine. Normally, there is a graded increase in the osmolarity of the renal medullary interstitium, with the inner renal medulla being about 1,200 mosm/liter, more than four times as great as that of the plasma.

The descending loop of Henle is highly permeable to water, and therefore water is rapidly reabsorbed from the tubular fluid into the hyperosmotic interstitium; approximately 20% of the glomerular filtrate volume is reabsorbed in the thin descending loop of Henle, causing the tubular fluid to become hyperosmotic as it moves toward the inner part of the renal medulla.

In the thin and thick segments of the ascending loop of Henle, water permeability is virtually zero, but large amounts of sodium, chloride, and potassium are reabsorbed, causing the tubular fluid to become dilute (hypotonic) as it flows back up toward the cortex. At the same time, active transport of sodium chloride out of the ascending loop of Henle into the interstitium causes a very high concentration of these ions in the interstitial fluid of the renal medulla. This mechanism for trapping sodium chloride and building up a high osmolality of the renal medullary interstitium is called the ***countercurrent multiplier,*** which is essential for forming a highly concentrated urine, as will be discussed later.

Reabsorption in Distal and Collecting Tubules. In the later parts of the nephron, fluid and solute reabsorption can vary greatly depending on the body's needs. If the concentration of sodium is high in the body fluids, very little sodium is reabsorbed in these sections of the tubules so that large amounts of sodium are lost in the urine. It is in these parts of the renal tubule, where final processing of the urine takes place, that several hormones influence reabsorption. For example, ***aldosterone*** stimulates sodium reabsorption in these segments and ***antidiuretic hormone*** increases water reabsorption. Normally, about 5% of the glomerular filtrate is reabsorbed in the distal tubules and less than 10% in the collecting tubules and ducts.

Active and Passive Reabsorption by Renal Tubules. Reabsorption of some electrolytes, such as sodium, occurs by ***active transport,*** especially by the ***sodium–potassium ATPase pump*** (Fig. 3-6). Many of the nutrients, such as glucose and amino acids, are reabsorbed by ***co-transport*** with sodium. In most instances, reabsorption of these substances displays a ***transport maximum,*** which refers to the maximum rate of reabsorption. When the filtered load of these substances exceeds the transport maximum, the excess amount is excreted. The ***threshold***

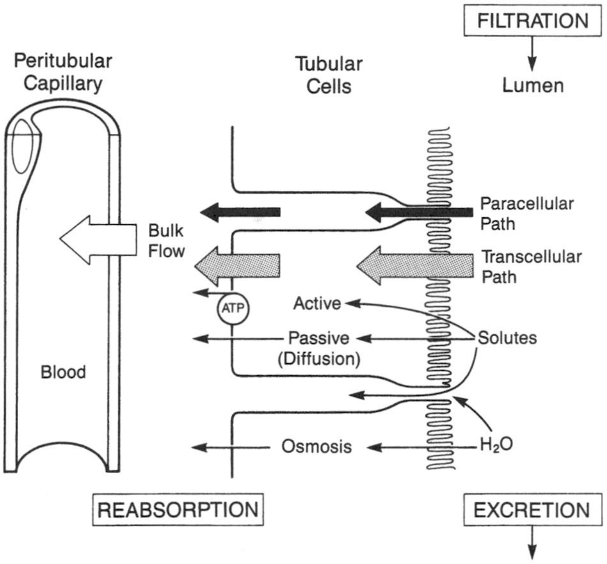

Fig. 3-6. Reabsorption of filtered water and solutes from the tubular lumen across the tubular epithelial cells, through the renal interstitium, and back into the blood. Solutes are transported through the cells (transcellular route) by passive diffusion or active transport, or between the cells (paracellular route) by diffusion. Water is transported through the cells and between the cells by osmosis. Transport of water and solutes from the interstitial fluid into the peritubular capillaries occurs by ultrafiltration (bulk flow). (Guyton AC, Hall JE: Textbook of Medical Physiology, 9th ed. Philadelphia: WB Saunders, 1995)

is the tubular load at which the transport maximum is exceeded in one or more nephrons, resulting in the appearance of that solute in the urine. Some substances, such as water and urea, are absorbed through the tubular membrane by passive diffusion and osmosis, which is called ***passive reabsorption.***

Regulation of Tubular Reabsorption. Because it is essential to maintain precise balance between tubular reabsorption and glomerular filtration, multiple nervous, hormonal, and local control mechanisms regulate the rate of tubular reabsorption as well as the rate of glomerular filtration. An important feature of tubular reabsorption is that some solutes and water can be independently regulated. Some of the mechanisms that control reabsorption are the following:

1. ***Glomerulotubular balance*** refers to the ability of the tubules to increase reabsorption rate in response to increased tubular load (increased tubular inflow of water and electrolytes).
2. Increased ***arterial pressure*** reduces tubular reabsorption and increases renal excretion of sodium and water, which are called ***pressure natriuresis*** and ***pressure diuresis,*** respectively.
3. ***Aldosterone,*** secreted by the adrenal cortex, increases sodium reabsorption and potassium secretion by the tubules; therefore, aldosterone reduces sodium excretion and increases potassium excretion.
4. ***Angiotensin II*** increases sodium reabsorption directly and indirectly by stimulating aldosterone secretion.
5. ***Antidiuretic hormone,*** secreted by the posterior pituitary gland, increases water reabsorption in the distal and collecting tubules.
6. ***Parathyroid hormone,*** increases calcium reabsorption and decreases phosphate reabsorption, leading to decreased calcium excretion and increased phosphate excretion.
7. ***Sympathetic nervous activity*** increases sodium reabsorption.

Renal Clearance. The concept of renal clearance is useful in quantitating the efficiency of the kidneys in removing a substance from the plasma. For a given substance X, renal clearance is defined as the ratio of the excretion rate of substance X to its concentration in the plasma:

$$\mathbf{C_X = (U_X * V)/P_X}$$

where C_X is renal clearance of the substance in milliliters per minute, $U_X * V$ is the excretion rate of substance X (U_X is the concentration of X in urine and V is urine flow rate in milliliters per minute), and P_X is plasma concentration of X.

Renal clearances can be used to quantitate several aspects of kidney function, including the rate of glomerular filtration, tubular reabsorption, and tubular secretion of different substances. For example, creatinine is filtered at the glomerulus but is not reabsorbed by the tubule; therefore, the entire 125 ml of plasma that filters into the tubules each minute (GFR) is cleared of creatinine (*e.g.*, creatinine clearance is 125 ml/min, which is equal to the GFR). For substances that are completely reabsorbed from the tubules (*e.g.*, amino acids, glucose), the clearance rate is zero because the urinary excretion rate is zero. For substances that are highly reabsorbed (*e.g.*, sodium), the clearance rate is usually less than 1% of the GFR, or less than 1 ml/min. In general, waste products of metabolism, such as urea, are poorly reabsorbed and have relatively high clearance rates. Some substances, such as para-aminohippuric (PAH) acid, are filtered and not reabsorbed by the tubules, but are secreted into the tubules. Therefore, the renal clearance of these substances is greater than GFR. In fact, about 90% of the plasma flowing through the kidney is completely cleared of PAH, and the renal clearance of PAH (C_{PAH}) can be used to estimate the renal plasma flow

$$C_{PAH} = (U_{PAH*}\ V)/P_{PAH} \cong \text{Renal Plasma Flow}$$

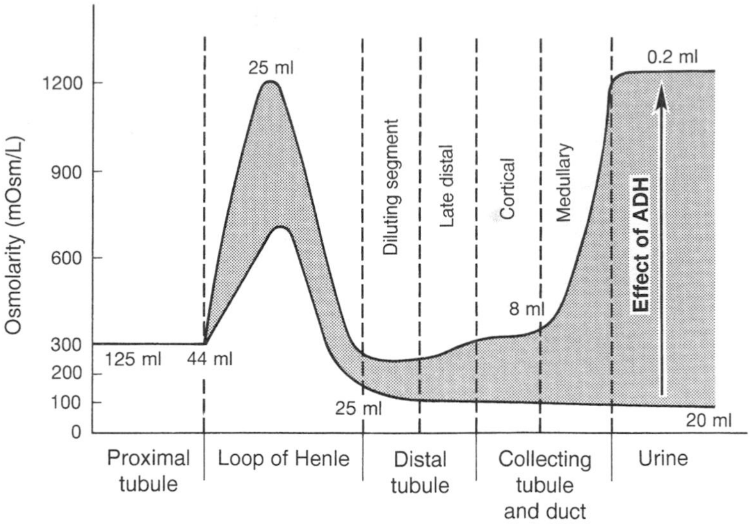

Fig. 3-7. Changes in osmolarity of the tubular fluid as it passes through the different tubular segments in the presence of high levels of ADH and in the absence of ADH. (Numerical values indicate the approximate volumes in milliliters per minute or osmolarities in milliosmoles per liter of fluid flowing along the different tubular segments.) (Guyton AC, Hall JE: Textbook of Medical Physiology, 9th ed. Philadelphia: WB Saunders, 1995)

where U_{PAH} and P_{PAH} are urine and plasma concentrations of PAH, respectively, and V is urine flow rate.

Urine Concentration. Urine can be more dilute or more concentrated than plasma. The kidneys can produce urine with a range of osmolarity from 50 to 1,400 mosm/liter. The ability to dilute the urine depends on decreased ***antidiuretic hormone*** (ADH) secretion, which reduces the permeability of the distal and collecting tubules to water and therefore prevents water from being reabsorbed in these parts of the nephron. In the absence of ADH, solutes continue to be reabsorbed from the tubules, but water cannot be effectively reabsorbed in the distal and collecting tubules, making very dilute urine (Fig. 3-7).

The formation of a concentrated urine depends on (1) high ADH levels, which increase permeability of the distal and collecting tubules to water; and (2) a high osmolarity of the renal medulla. Tubular fluid flowing out of the loop of Henle is dilute, with an osmolarity of only about 50 to 100 mosm/liter. As fluid flows into the distal and collecting tubules, it can equilibrate with the surrounding interstitium when high levels of ADH are present and the tubules are permeable to water. The medullary interstitium outside the collecting tubules is normally very concentrated with sodium and urea due to the operation of the ***countercurrent multiplier,*** which depends on the special permeability characteristics of the loop of Henle discussed previously. Thus, as fluid flows into the distal tubules and finally into the collecting tubules and ducts, water is reabsorbed until the tubule osmolarity equilibrates with medullary interstitial fluid osmolarity. This leads to a highly concentrated urine with an osmolarity of 1,200 to 1,400 mosm/liter when high levels of ADH are present.

The ***vasa recta*** are specialized peritubular capillaries that act as a countercurrent exchange system to preserve solute concentration in the renal medulla. However, excessively high blood flow in the vasa recta can "wash out" the medullary interstitium and reduce urine concentrating ability.

The inability to form a highly concentrated urine can also be caused by (1) decreased secretion of ADH ***("central" diabetes insipidus);*** (2) a lack of responsiveness of the renal tubules to ADH ***(nephrogenic diabetes insipidus);*** or (3) drugs that interfere with the operation of the countercurrent multiplier (*e.g.*, certain diuretics).

Osmoreceptor–ADH System Regulation of Extracellular Sodium Concentration and Osmolarity. There are two primary mechanisms for controlling the concentration of osmotically active substances in the body fluids: (1) the ***hypothalamic-pituitary antidiuretic hormone feedback system*** and (2) **the *thirst mechanism.*** When extracellular fluid osmolarity is increased above normal, both of these systems are activated, causing increased thirst, and therefore increased intake of water, and stimulation of ADH secretion, which increases water reabsorption in the renal tubules and decreases water excretion. Therefore, the quantity of water in the body increases, diluting the concentration of solutes. The opposite effect occurs with low plasma osmolarity, which reduces both ADH secretion and thirst.

Regulation of Sodium Balance and Extracellular Fluid Volume. Sodium and chloride are the most abundant ions in the extracellular fluid. Consequently, changes in sodium chloride content of the extracellular fluid usually cause parallel changes in extracellular fluid volume, provided the ADH-thirst mechanisms are operative. When the ADH-thirst mechanisms are functioning normally, a change in the amount of sodium chloride in the extracellular fluid is matched by a similar change in the amount of extracellular water, so that osmolarity and sodium concentration are maintained relatively constant.

The total amount of sodium in the extracellular fluid is determined by the balance between sodium intake and sodium excretion by the kidneys. Although sodium intake and excretion must be precisely balanced under steady-state conditions, temporary imbalances can lead to changes in extracellular fluid sodium content and consequently extracellular fluid volume. Because sodium intake is usually governed more by one's eating and drinking habits than by physiological control mechanisms, the regulation of extracellular fluid volume is vested largely in the control of renal sodium excretion. The two variables that control renal sodium excretion ($U_{Na}V$) are (1) the rate of sodium filtration ($GFR * P_{Na}$) and (2) the rate of tubular sodium reabsorption:

$$U_{Na}V = (GFR * P_{Na}) - (\text{tubular sodium reabsorption})$$

As discussed previously, glomerular filtration and tubular reabsorption are regulated by multiple factors, including hormones, sympathetic activity, and arterial pressure.

Perhaps the most powerful mechanism for control of blood volume and extracellular fluid volume, as well as for the maintenance of sodium balance, is the effect of blood pressure on sodium excretion, called ***pressure natriuresis,*** as discussed previously. When extracellular fluid volume and blood volume increase, this also increases arterial pressure. The increased pressure in turn has a potent effect to increase the rate of sodium excretion by the kidneys, thereby reducing extracellular fluid volume back toward the normal level. This mechanism for control of extracellular fluid volume and blood volume is called the ***renal-body fluid feedback mechanism.***

One important aspect of the renal-body fluid feedback is that nervous and hormonal factors act in concert with pressure natriuresis to make this mechanism more effective in minimizing changes in blood volume, extracellular fluid volume, and blood pressure in response to day-to-day challenges. For example, with increased sodium intake there are reductions in angiotensin II and aldosterone formation that decrease sodium reabsorption and add to the direct effect of blood pressure to raise sodium excretion. Increased extracellular fluid volume also reduces sympathetic nervous system activity and increases secretion of ***atrial natriuretic factor (ANF)*** (a hormone secreted by the cardiac atria), which both decrease sodium reabsorption, causing the kidneys to excrete increased amounts of sodium and water and reducing extracellular fluid volume and blood volume back toward normal. Thus, combined activation of natriuretic systems and suppression of sodium and water retaining systems leads to increased sodium excretion when sodium intake and extracellular fluid volume are increased. The opposite changes take place when sodium intake and extracellular fluid volume are reduced below normal.

Regulation of Potassium Excretion. Extracellular potassium concentration normally is regulated precisely at about 4.2 mEq/liter. A special difficulty in regulating extracellular potassium concentration is the fact that over 98% of the total body potassium is contained in the cells and only about 2% in the extracellular fluid. Therefore, it is extremely important to maintain a precise balance between potassium intake and potassium excretion, which occurs mainly via the kidneys. Renal potassium excretion in turn is determined by the sum of three processes: (1) potassium filtration at the glomerulus, (2) potassium reabsorption by the tubules, and (3) potassium secretion by the tubules.

Normally, most of the daily variation in potassium excretion occurs by changes in potassium secretion in the distal and collecting tubules, rather than by changes in glomerular filtration or tubular reabsorption of potassium. The cells in the late distal tubules and cortical collecting tubules that secrete potassium are called ***principal cells.*** Secretion of potassium from the peritubular capillary blood into the tubular lumen is a three-step process, beginning with passive diffusion of potassium from the blood to the interstitium, active transport of potassium from the interstitium into the cell by the sodium–potassium–ATPase pump at the basolateral membrane, and finally passive diffusion of potassium from the cell interior into the tubular fluid. The primary factors that *increase potassium secretion* by the principal cells include (1) increased extracellular potassium concentration, (2) increased aldosterone concentration, and (3) increased tubular flow rate. One factor that *decreases* potassium secretion is increased hydrogen ion concentration (acidosis).

Increased extracellular potassium concentration stimulates potassium excretion directly as well as indirectly by stimulating aldosterone secretion. ***Aldosterone***, a hormone secreted by the adrenal cortex, increases sodium reabsorption and increases potassium secretion by the distal and collecting tubules, which reduces urine excretion of sodium and increases potassium excretion. Aldosterone is the primary hormonal mechanism for regulating potassium ion concentration because there is a direct feedback by which aldosterone and potassium ion concentration are linked. This feedback mechanism operates as follows: Whenever extracellular fluid potassium concentration rises above normal, this stimulates secretion of aldosterone, which then increases renal excretion of potassium, returning extracellular fluid potassium concentration toward normal. The opposite changes take place when potassium concentration is too low.

Regulation of Other Extracellular Fluid Electrolytes. Other extracellular fluid electrolytes that are also closely regulated include calcium, magnesium, chloride, and bicarbonate. For example, a decrease in calcium ion concentration stimulates ***parathyroid hormone*** secretion, which in turn increases calcium reabsorption by the renal tubules and decreases loss of calcium in the urine. Hydrogen and bicarbonate ion concentrations are adjusted by the renal and respiratory mechanisms for control of acid–base balance, as explained in the following paragraphs.

Regulation of Acid–Base Balance (Hydrogen Ion Concentration). Hydrogen ion concentration $[H^+]$ in the extracellular fluid is precisely regulated, averaging only 0.00004 mEq/liter (40 nm/liter). Normally, hydrogen ion concentration is expressed in terms of *p*H, which is the logarithm of the reciprocal of the hydrogen ion concentration:

$$pH = \log(1/[H^+]).$$

Arterial blood has a normal *p*H of 7.4. A *p*H of 7.8 is considered to be highly alkaline, while a *p*H of 7.0 is considered to be highly acidic.

The body has three primary lines of defense against changes in hydrogen ion concentration: (1) ***acid–base buffer systems,*** which react within seconds to prevent changes in concentration; (2) the ***lungs,*** which eliminate carbon dioxide and therefore carbonic acid (H_2CO_3; sometimes called volatile acid)—this mechanism operates within seconds to minutes and acts as a second defense; (3) the ***kidneys,*** which can excrete hydrogen ions, reabsorb bicarbonate (HCO_3^-), and produce new bicarbonate ions, this mechanism is a third line of defense that operates slowly but very powerfully in regulating acid balance.

Acid–Base Buffer Systems. One of the most important buffer systems of the body fluids is the ***proteins*** of the cells, and to a lesser extent, the proteins of the plasma and interstitial fluids. The ***phosphate buffer system*** ($HPO_4^{2-}/H_2PO_4^-$) is not a major buffer in extracellular fluid but is important as an intracellular buffer and as a buffer in renal tubular fluid. The most important extracellular fluid buffer is the ***bicarbonate buffer system*** (HCO_3^-/P_{CO_2}) primarily because the components of this system, carbon dioxide and bicarbonate, are closely regulated by the lungs and the kidneys, respectively.

The *p*H of extracellular fluid can be expressed as a function of the concentration of the components of the bicarbonate buffer system according to the ***Henderson–Hasselbalch equation:***

$$pH = 6.1 + \log \frac{HCO_3^-}{0.03 * P_{CO_2}}$$

In this equation, bicarbonate is expressed in millimoles per liter, and P_{CO_2} is expressed as millimeters of mercury. The greater the P_{CO_2}, the lower the *p*H; the greater the bicarbonate the higher the *p*H.

Respiratory Regulation of Hydrogen Ion Concentration. Because the lungs expel carbon dioxide from the body, rapid ventilation by the lungs decreases the concentration of carbon dioxide in the blood, which in turn reduces carbonic acid (H_2CO_3) and hydrogen ion concentration in the blood. Conversely, decreasing pulmonary ventilation increases the concentration of carbon dioxide and hydrogen ions in the blood.

Because increased hydrogen ion concentration stimulates respiration and alveolar ventilation, which in turn decreases hydrogen ion concentration, the respiratory system acts as a negative feedback controller of hydrogen ion concentration. Thus, when hydrogen ion concentration increases above normal, the respiratory system is stimulated and alveolar ventilation increases, thereby reducing P_{CO_2} and hydrogen ion concentration back toward normal. Conversely, if the hydrogen ion concentration falls below normal, the respiratory center becomes depressed, and alveolar ventilation decreases and increases back toward normal. The respiratory system can return $[H^+]$ and pH about two-thirds of the way back toward normal within a few minutes after a sudden disturbance of acid–base regulation.

Regulation of Acid–Base Balance by the Kidneys. When the respiratory system fails to completely restore hydrogen ion concentration to normal, the kidneys are capable of bringing it back toward normal within 12 to 24 hours in most cases. If the kidneys have sufficient time to function, they are many times as effective as either the buffers or the respiratory mechanism in adjusting the *p*H of the body fluids.

The kidneys readjust the hydrogen ion concentration by excreting either an acidic or basic urine. Excreting an acidic urine reduces the amount of acid in the extracellular fluid, whereas excreting a basic urine removes base from the extracellular fluid, which is the same as adding hydrogen ions.

The overall mechanism by which the kidneys excrete acid or basic urine is as follows: large amounts of bicarbonate ions are filtered continuously into the tubules, and if they are excreted in the urine, this removes base from the blood. On the other hand, large numbers of hydrogen ions are also secreted into the tubular lumen by the epithelial cells, thus removing acid from the blood. If more hydrogen ions are secreted than bicarbonate ions are filtered, there will be a net loss of acid from the extracellular fluids. Conversely, if more bicarbonate ions are filtered than hydrogen ions are secreted, there will be a net loss of base.

When there is a reduction in extracellular fluid hydrogen ion concentration ***(alkalosis),*** the kidneys fail to reabsorb all of the filtered bicarbonate, thereby increasing excretion of bicarbonate. Because bicarbonate ions normally buffer hydrogen ions in the extracellular fluid, the loss of bicarbonate ions is the same as adding hydrogen ions to the extracellular fluid. Thus, in alkalosis the removal of bicarbonate ions raises the extracellular fluid $[H^+]$ and decreases *p*H back toward normal.

When hydrogen ion concentration in the extracellular fluid increases ***(acidosis),*** the kidneys do not excrete bicarbonate in the urine, but reabsorb all of the filtered bicarbonate and actually produce new bicarbonate, which is added back to the extracellular fluid. This reduces extracellular fluid $[H^+]$ toward normal. Bicarbonate is not reabsorbed directly by the tubules but occurs as a result of the combination of secreted hydrogen ions, with filtered bicarbonate ions in the tubular fluid under the influence of carbonic anhydrase in the tubular epithelium. Secreted hydrogen ions are consumed by reaction with bicarbonate, forming carbonic acid, which dissociates to carbon dioxide and water. The carbon dioxide diffuses into the cell and is used to reform HCO_3^- which is reabsorbed. The hydrogen ions remaining in excess of that which reacts with bicarbonate can react with other urinary buffers, especially ammonia and phosphate, and is then excreted as buffer salts. For each hydrogen ion secreted that combines with a non-bicarbonate buffer, a new bicarbonate ion is formed within the renal tubular cells and added to the body fluids.

Acid–Base Disturbances. The condition of ***acidosis*** occurs when arterial *p*H is below 7.4, whereas ***alkalosis*** occurs when arterial *p*H is above 7.40. An abnormality of *p*H that results primarily from a change in bicarbonate concentration is called ***metabolic*** acidosis or alkalosis, whereas a disturbance that results primarily from a change in Pco_2 is called ***respiratory*** acidosis or alkalosis.

Respiratory acidosis results from high Pco_2 due to the failure of the lungs to eliminate carbon dioxide adequately. As a compensation, increased Pco_2 stimulates hydrogen ion secretion by the renal tubular cells, causing increased bicarbonate reabsorption; the excess hydrogen ions remaining in the renal tubular cells combines with buffers, especially ammonia in chronic acidosis, which leads to generation of new bicarbonate ions, which are added back to the blood. These changes return plasma *p*H toward normal.

In ***respiratory alkalosis,*** Pco_2 is reduced due to excessive ventilation. Renal compensation for this includes a reduction in hydrogen ion secretion, which results in incomplete bicarbonate reabsorption and a loss of bicarbonate in the urine, thereby restoring plasma *p*H toward normal.

Metabolic acidosis results from a loss of buffer, such as bicarbonate, or too much acid in the body fluids. The compensatory responses include stimulation of the respiratory centers that eliminate carbon dioxide and return *p*H toward normal. At the same time, renal compensation increases reabsorption of bicarbonate and excretion of buffer salts, which leads to new bicarbonate formation and a return of hydrogen ion and bicarbonate ion concentrations toward normal.

Metabolic alkalosis results from excessive loss of hydrogen ions (*e.g.*, loss of HCl) or excessive intake or retention of bases. This raises bicarbonate ion concentration, thereby decreasing hydrogen ion concentration and increasing *p*H. The compensatory responses include a reduction in respiration rate, causing retention of carbon dioxide and an increased renal excretion of bicarbonate, which both help return plasma *p*H toward normal. Table 3-2 shows the different types of acid–base disturbances and the characteristic changes in plasma *p*H, hydrogen ion concentration, Pco_2 and hydrogen ion concentration.

TABLE 3-2. Characteristics of Primary Acid–Base Disturbances

	*p*H	H^+	Pco_2	HCO_3^-
Respiratory acidosis	↓	↑	⇑	↑*
Respiratory alkalosis	↑	↓	⇓	↓*
Metabolic acidosis	↓	↑	↓**	⇓
Metabolic alkalosis	↑	↓	↑**	⇑

The primary event is indicated by the double arrows (⇑ or ⇓). Note that respiratory acid–base disorders are initiated by an increase or a decrease in Pco_2, whereas metabolic disorders are initiated by an increase or decrease in HCO_3^-.

* Denotes compensatory changes in HCO_3^- caused by the kidneys.

** Denotes the compensatory changes in Pco_2 by the lungs.

Micturition—The Process of Urination. The urinary bladder empties when it becomes filled through two main steps: The bladder fills progressively until the tension in its walls rises above a threshold level, which elicits the second step; (2) a nervous reflex called the ***micturition reflex*** occurs and empties the bladder or, if this fails, at least causes a conscious desire to urinate. Although the micturition reflex is a spinal cord reflex, it can also be inhibited or facilitated by centers in the cerebral cortex of the brain stem.

BLOOD, HEMOSTASIS, AND IMMUNITY

BLOOD COMPONENTS

Red Blood Cells. Red blood cells (erythrocytes) are anuclear, biconcave disks. They average 7 μm in diameter, but their extreme pliability allows them to squeeze through capillaries of less than 5 μm in diameter. The body contains about 25 trillion red blood cells in an average concentration of about 5 million per mm^3 of blood. The percentage of the total blood volume comprised of red blood cells is called the ***hematocrit,*** and this is normally about 40% in females and about 45% in males.

Red Blood Cell Function. The main function of red blood cells is to transport hemoglobin. In turn, hemoglobin transports oxygen from the lungs to the tissues and transports carbon dioxide from the tissues back to the lungs. Also, hemoglobin is an excellent ***acid–base buffer*** (as is true of most proteins), providing most of the buffering power of whole blood.

Red Blood Cell Formation. The mass of red blood cells in the circulation is regulated within narrow limits to provide adequate oxygenation of the tissues, but not so concentrated as to impede blood flow to the tissues. The general mechanism of this is the following: Tissue hypoxia causes the kidneys to release a hormone called ***erythropoietin,*** which then flows in the blood to the bone marrow where it stimulates ***erythropoiesis.*** Once formed, the average life span of the red blood cells is 120 days in the circulatory system.

Factors that decrease tissue oxygenation and stimulate red blood cell production include low blood volume, anemia, low hemoglobin, poor blood flow, and pulmonary disease. In persons residing at very high altitudes where oxygen concentration is low, the number of red blood cells sometimes becomes as much as 50% greater than normal. The condition is called ***polycythemia.***

Role of Vitamin B_{12} and Folic Acid in Maturation of Red Blood Cells. The process of red blood cell formation can be divided into two principal processes: (1) formation of the cell structure itself and (2) formation of hemoglobin. The red cell is formed in the bone marrow by a series of divisions from the ***hemocytoblast.*** Two vitamins, vitamin B_{12} and folic acid, are essential for the synthesis of DNA. Lack of either vitamin leads to decreased DNA and thus failure of nuclear maturation and division. The erythroblastic cells of the bone marrow become larger than normal and are called ***megaloblasts.*** The adult red blood cell has a flimsy membrane and is often large, with an ovoid shape rather than the usual biconcave disk shape. Therefore, vitamin B_{12} or folic acid deficiency causes ***maturation failure*** in the process of erythropoiesis.

Lack of Iron and Hypochromic Anemia. A primary nutritive factor necessary for formation of hemoglobin is iron. Iron is present in the diet in only very small quantities, and even then is rather poorly absorbed from the gastrointestinal tract; therefore, many persons fail to form sufficient quantities of hemoglobin to fill the red blood cells as they are being produced. This causes ***hypochromic anemia,*** in which the number of cells may be normal but the amount of hemoglobin in each cell is far below normal.

White Blood Cells. The number of white cells (leukocytes) in the blood is normally only 1/600 the number of red blood cells, about 8,000 per mm^3 of blood. They perform the very important function of protecting or helping to protect the body from invasion by infectious agents. The white cells consist of neutrophils, eosinophils, basophils, monocytes, and platelets, all formed in the bone marrow, and lymphocytes formed in the lymph nodes.

Neutrophils. The neutrophils are the most numerous of the white blood cells. They represent about 60% of the total white cells in the blood. They are highly motile, highly phagocytic, and are attracted out of the blood into tissue areas where tissue destruction is occurring by a process called ***chemotaxis,*** which means attraction by the destruction products from the damaged tissues. Once in the tissue area, the neutrophils phagocytize bacteria and small amounts of dead tissue debris.

The Monocyte-Macrophage System. The ***monocytes*** are much larger cells than the neutrophils, and large numbers of them normally wander through the capillary membranes and into the tissues all of the time. Many of them become attached to tissue cells, and they become very large and are called ***macrophages.*** They can phagocytize five to ten times as many bacteria and much larger particles of tissue debris than can the neutrophils. Almost all tissues of the body contain macrophages, but they are especially abundant in those tissues that are routinely exposed to bacteria, such as the lung alveoli, the sinusoids of the liver, the sinusoids of the bone marrow, the sinusoids of the lymph nodes, and the subcutaneous tissue. This extensive ***monocyte-macrophage system*** is frequently also called the ***reticuloendothelial system.***

Macrophage and Neutrophil Response to Inflammation. The macrophages already present in a tissue provide the ***first line of defense*** against infection. Within a few hours, neutrophils present in the blood invade the inflamed area, providing the ***second line of defense.*** At the same time, the number of neutrophils in the blood can increase several fold, resulting in ***neutrophilia.*** Neutrophilia is caused by products from the infected or inflamed tissues that enter the blood stream and are transported to the bone marrow where they mobilize stored neutrophils. Several days later, the concentration of macrophages in the inflamed tissue becomes very high, the macrophages replacing most of the neutrophils. This is the ***third line of defense.*** The ***fourth line of defense*** consists of increased production of white blood cells by the bone marrow, which is stimulated by products released from the infected or inflamed tissues.

Eosinophils and Parasitic Infections. Eosinophils constitute about 2% of all blood leukocytes and are similar to the neutrophils, except that they are less chemotactic and less phagocytic. Eosinophils are produced in large numbers in persons with parasitic infections. The parasites are usually too large to be phagocytized, but the eosinophils attach themselves to the surface and release lethal substances that can kill many of the parasites. Large numbers of eosinophils also appear in the blood in allergic conditions and may help to detoxify toxins that are released by allergic reactions.

Mast Cells and Basophils. The type of antibody, the IgE type, that causes allergic reactions binds to mast cells and basophils, causing them to release various inflammatory products that in turn cause many of the manifestations of allergic reactions. Also, basophils and mast cells liberate heparin into the blood, a substance that can prevent blood coagulation.

Platelets. Platelets are fragments of megakaryocytes. Like heparin, they, too, are important in the blood coagulation process, but instead cause coagulation, as will be discussed below.

BLOOD COAGULATION

Blood Clot. When a blood vessel ruptures, a blood clot develops within a few minutes to fill the gap and stop the bleeding—if the rupture is not too large. This process is caused by polymerization of plasma ***fibrinogen*** molecules into long ***fibrin threads*** that entrap large numbers of red blood cells, white blood cells, platelets, and plasma to form a soft gelatinous mass, the blood clot. The fibrin threads gradually contract, expressing most of the plasma from the clot, which leaves a reasonably solid barrier in the opening of the blood vessel.

Initiation of Blood Clotting. Prothrombin is a plasma protein continually formed by the liver that can be split into two smaller molecules, one of which is thrombin. Thrombin is an enzyme that then enzymatically causes polymerization of the plasma fibrinogen molecules into the fibrin threads that lead to blood clotting. In the normal circulation, very little prothrombin is converted into thrombin, and blood clotting does not occur. Two principal conditions that can lead to blood clotting are (1) damage to the vessel wall and (2) damage to the blood itself.

Extrinsic Pathway for Prothrombin Activation. The damaged tissues in the wall of the vessel release a substance called ***tissue thromboplastin.*** This is mainly composed of phospholipids from the damaged tissues. The thromboplastin in turn catalyzes a series of enzymatic reactions among multiple blood plasma proteins called ***blood coagulation factors.*** These reactions eventually form ***prothrombin activator,*** which causes the prothrombin to change into thrombin and thereby initiate blood coagulation.

Intrinsic Pathway for Prothrombin Activation. Damage to the blood causes direct activation of special protein blood coagulation factors. Also, damage to the platelets of the blood causes release of ***platelet thromboplastin,*** which has effects similar to those of tissue thromboplastin released by torn blood vessels. The combined activation of the protein coagulation factors and release of the platelet thromboplastin lead eventually to the formation of prothrombin activator. Then, the prothrombin activator converts prothrombin to thrombin, which subsequently causes blood clotting.

Hemophilia. Hemophilia occurs exclusively in males, usually because of a deficiency in Factor VIII, or ***antihemophilic factor,*** which is required for function of the intrinsic pathway of blood coagulation. Excessive bleeding will usually not occur without trauma, but the amount of trauma required to cause severe and prolonged bleeding is hardly noticeable.

Liver Disease and Vitamin K Deficiency. Most of the coagulation factors are formed in the liver. Therefore, hepatitis, cirrhosis, and other diseases of the liver can depress the normal coagulation system, causing a person to bleed excessively. Another cause of decreased coagulation factor production by the liver is vitamin K deficiency. Vitamin K is necessary for formation of prothrombin, Factor VII, Factor IX, and Factor X.

Thrombocytopenia and Petechial Hemorrhages. Thrombocytopenia means that the number of platelets in the blood is greatly reduced. Platelets, aside from their capability to induce blood clotting, also have the ability to attach themselves to very minute rupture points in blood vessels and thereby close these holes, even without causing actual blood coagulation. In thrombocytopenia this function is lost, and as a result the person develops many minute bleeding spots, called petechial hemorrhages, throughout all of the organs and beneath the skin.

IMMUNITY

Immunity means resistance of the body to invasion by bacteria, viruses, or other infectious agents or toxins.

Innate Immunity. Each person is born with a certain amount of innate immunity that results from several special mechanisms: (1) the reticuloendothelial system and the white blood cells, which have already been discussed; (2) resistance of the intact skin to invasion by microorganisms; (3) destruction of bacterial organisms by the digestive enzymes in the stomach; and (4) substances circulating in the blood.

Acquired Immunity. In addition to the natural immunity that normally exists in all persons, a person can develop acquired immunity to many destructive agents to which he is not naturally immune. Most destructive agents, such as bacteria, viruses, or toxins, are mostly composed of protein molecules. On entering the body, these proteins act as antigens and cause two types of immunity: one is called ***humoral immunity*** and the other ***cell-mediated immunity.***

Humoral Immunity. Foreign antigens first enter the lymphoid tissue, especially the lymph nodes. There they cause plasma cells, which are derived from lymphocytes, to produce large quantities of antibodies that are specifically reactive for the type of protein (or other chemical) that initiated their production. Once these antibodies have been formed and released into the body fluids, which usually requires a week to several weeks, they then destroy the specific invader that had caused their formation and can also destroy any future invader of this same type.

Antibodies. Antibodies are large protein molecules, usually gamma globulins, that attach to the surfaces of bacteria or viruses, or they combine directly with toxins. They either destroy the invading agent or make it more susceptible to phagocytosis by the tissue macrophages or by white blood cells. Or, in the case of toxins, the antibodies can simply neutralize these by combining chemically with them.

Lymphocytes. In early fetal development of the lymph nodes, no lymphocytes are present in the nodes. Instead, the early lymphocytes are formed and processed in the liver and the thymus gland. After processing, the lymphocytes are released into the circulating blood and eventually become entrapped in the lymph nodes. Once in these nodes, those lymphocytes processed in the liver eventually are converted into plasma cells that become part of the humoral immune process to form antibodies.

Cell-Mediated Immunity. The lymphocytes that are processed in the thymus gland also end up in the lymph nodes and other lymphoid tissues of the body. However, instead of forming antibodies when the lymph node is exposed to antigens, these cells form so-called ***sensitized lymphocytes,*** also called ***T cells*** because of their earlier processing in the thymus. The T cells form chemical substances that are similar to antibodies, but these remain attached to the cell membranes of the lymphocytes. Large numbers of T cells are then released into the circulating blood, and they spread throughout the body.

Major Types of Sensitized T Cells. ***Cytotoxic T cells*** combine directly with antigens on the surfaces of invading organisms and can therefore destroy the organisms. ***Helper T cells*** function mainly in association with the plasma cells in the lymph nodes; they multiply manyfold the capability of the plasma cells to produce humoral antibodies in response to antigens. ***Suppressor T cells*** suppress some of the immune reactions, in this way preventing the immune system from running wild and being destructive to normal tissues.

Immune Tolerance. The immune process of the normal human body does not develop antibodies or sensitized lymphocytes that can destroy the body's own tissues, despite the fact that the body tissues are to a great extent like bacteria in their chemical composition. This phenomenon is called ***tolerance*** to the body's own proteins and tissues. This results mainly from destruction during fetal life of those primordial lymphocytes in the thymus and liver capable of forming antibodies or sensitized lymphocytes against the body's own proteins and tissues. It is likely that special suppressor T cells also develop to help cause tolerance.

Failure of Immune Tolerance. Autoimmunity occurs particularly in older age or after some disease causes destruction of large amounts of body tissue with release of tissue antigens into the circulating body fluids. Once the immune process has caused production of antibodies or sensitized lymphocytes that can attack the body's own tissues, these will then react against specific tissues and cause serious debility. Examples of autoimmune disease include rheumatic heart disease, rheumatoid arthritis, thyroiditis, acute glomerulonephritis, myasthenia gravis, and lupus erythematosus.

ALLERGY

There are multiple different types of allergy, some of which can occur under appropriate conditions in normal persons and some only in persons who have a specific allergic tendency.

Allergy in Normal Persons. Delayed-reaction allergy can occur in the normal person. It is caused by sensitized lymphocytes and not by antibodies. A typical example is the reaction to poison ivy. The toxin of poison ivy becomes deposited in the skin, and a small portion of it finds its way to the lymph nodes, which, over a period of several days to a week or so, form sensitized lymphocytes. These then are carried by the blood back to the original site of entry of the poison ivy toxin. Reaction of the lymphocytes with the toxin in direct association with the cells produces severe local tissue damage, which is the well-known rash and blisters associated with poison ivy.

Allergy in Allergic Persons. Allergy in allergic persons is characterized by excess IgE antibodies. These IgE antibodies are called ***reagins.*** They have a protein structure different from that of normal IgG antibodies. Also, the reagins tend to attach themselves to basophils and mast cells throughout the tissues. When the specific antigen (called the ***allergen***) that reacts with the reagin enters the tissue, it combines with the reagin. This combination, occurring on the cell surface of the basophils and mast cells, causes cellular damage with release of histamine and proteolytic enzymes from the affected cells. Severe local tissue damage can result. Types of allergies of this type are hay fever, asthma, urticaria (called also hives), and some types of anaphylaxis.

BLOOD GROUPS AND TRANSFUSION

Successful transfusion of blood from the donor to the recipient is mainly a problem of immunity; the recipient may already be immune to the transfused blood, or she may develop immunity, which then causes damage or death to the red blood cells in the transfusion.

Transfusion Reaction. A transfusion reaction is likely to occur if the host is already immune to the transfused blood or becomes immune soon after the transfusion. The antibodies, called ***agglutinins,*** attach themselves to the surfaces of the red blood cells and make them ***agglutinate*** with each other, which means that the cells stick together in clumps. Occasionally the antibodies are powerful enough to cause the cells to rupture. However, even if the cells do not rupture from this cause, the clumped cells become caught in the capillaries of the circulatory system and during the next few hours become ruptured because of progressive trauma or attack by white blood cells or by tissue macrophages. Thus, the final result in all transfusion reactions is rupture of the red cells, which is called ***hemolysis,*** with release of hemoglobin and other intracellular substances into the blood.

Acute Renal Shutdown. Much of the free hemoglobin in the blood resulting from a transfusion reaction filters through the glomerular membrane into the renal tubules; then water is reabsorbed from the tubules, allowing the hemoglobin to become so concentrated that it precipitates. If large amounts of blood are hemolyzed, this process can block many or most of the tubules of the kidneys, causing either oliguria or anuria. As a result, a person occasionally dies a week or so later of uremia rather than as the immediate result of the transfusion reaction.

A-B-O Blood Groups. The membranes of the red blood cells in about 60% of all human beings contain one or both of two very important antigens, called ***group A*** or ***group B agglutinogens,*** that frequently cause transfusion reactions. The bloods of different persons are generally ***typed,*** as illustrated in Table 3-3, on the basis of the presence or the absence of these agglutinogens in the blood cells. Thus, the four major blood groups of humans are ***group A,*** which contains type A agglutinogen; ***group B,*** which contains type B agglutinogen; ***group AB,*** which contains both A and B agglutinogens; and ***group O,*** which contains neither.

Agglutinins and Agglutinogens. The agglutinins, like other antibodies, are gamma globulins that develop in response to small numbers of group A and B antigens that enter the body in food, bacteria, and in other ways. Antibodies that agglutinate the A agglutinogen are called ***anti-A agglutinins,*** while those that agglutinate the B agglutinogen are called ***anti-B agglutinins.*** Thus, type A blood contains ***anti-B agglutinins,*** type B blood contains ***anti-A agglutinins;*** type AB blood contains neither of the agglutinins; and type O blood, both anti-A and anti-B agglutinins. Therefore, mixing bloods of different types will often cause agglutination of at least some of the cells and can result in a transfusion reaction.

TABLE 3-3. The Blood Groups Showing Their Genotypes and Their Agglutinogens and Agglutinins

GENOTYPES	BLOOD GROUPS	AGGLUTINOGENS (CELL ANTIGENS)	AGGLUTININ (SERUM ANTIBODIES)
OO	O	—	Anti-A and anti-B
OA or AA	A	A	Anti-B
OB or BB	B	B	Anti-A
AB	AB	A and B	—

Rh Antigen. The blood cells of about 85% of all white persons, 95% of North American blacks, and virtually 100% of African blacks contain another antigen, called the ***Rh antigen,*** which exists in several different forms. Those persons who have the Rh antigen are said to be Rh positive while those who do not have any Rh antigen are said to be Rh negative.

Rh Transfusion Reaction. A transfusion reaction can occur when Rh-positive blood is transfused into an Rh-negative person. However, a reaction will not occur unless the Rh-negative person has been exposed previously to Rh-positive blood because, contrary to the anti-A and anti-B agglutinins, anti-Rh antibodies do not occur spontaneously in the blood. Yet, if the Rh-negative person has been exposed previously to Rh-positive blood, he or she will have developed anti-Rh antibodies against the Rh factor, and a subsequent transfusion with Rh-positive blood can cause an equally severe transfusion reaction as one that occurs with the A-B-O blood groups.

Erythroblastosis Fetalis. If the mother is Rh negative, and the baby inherits the Rh-positive trait from the father, some of the Rh-positive antigens from the baby can sometimes cause the mother to develop anti-Rh antibodies; these antibodies then diffuse through the placenta into the baby and cause agglutination of the baby's circulating red cells. This effect rarely occurs with the first Rh-positive baby, but occurs much more frequently during subsequent pregnancies. The reason is that immunity develops in the mother after birth of the baby in response to antigens entering her blood from degenerating products of the placental tissues. If the mother is given antiserum against the Rh factor immediately after each delivery, most instances of immunization can be prevented. But without such preventive measures, death will occur in large numbers of newborn or unborn children. The clinical condition, when present, is called ***erythroblastosis fetalis*** because the fetus responds with an erythroblastic reaction to form more blood cells.

NERVE AND MUSCLE

FUNCTION OF THE NERVE FIBER

Negative Membrane Potential. A membrane potential exists across the membranes of all cells. In large nerve and muscle cells this potential amounts to about 90 millivolts during resting conditions, with the inside of the cell negatively charged with respect to the outside. The development of this ***resting membrane potential*** occurs as follows: All cell membranes contain sodium–potassium pumps that transport sodium to the outside of the cell and potassium to the inside. Because more sodium is transported outward than potassium inward, the net effect of these pumps is principally to transport sodium outward. This active transport of sodium, which is a positively charged ion, to the outside of the membrane causes loss of positive charges from inside the membrane and gain of positive charges on the outside, thus creating negativity inside the membrane and positivity outside. Also, the membrane is relatively permeable to potassium, so potassium can leak out of the cell with ease. This leakage of positively charged potassium ions out of the cell contributes greatly to the development of negativity inside the cell. The resulting membrane potential is the basis of conduction of all impulses by nerve and muscle fibers.

Depolarization of Action Potential. The action potential is a sequence of changes in the membrane potential that occurs within a small fraction of a second when a nerve or muscle membrane impulse spreads over its surface. Any factor that makes the cell membrane suddenly excessively permeable to sodium ions can elicit an action potential. Such factors include passing an electrical current through the membrane, pinching the nerve fiber, pricking it with a pin, crushing it, or applying a drug such as acetylcholine. When the membrane becomes very permeable to sodium, the positive sodium ions on the outside of the membrane now flow rapidly to the inside. Therefore, the negative potential inside the membrane suddenly becomes greatly reduced or even reversed, with positivity on the inside and negativity on the outside. This process is called ***depolarization*** because the polarity across the cell membrane decreases.

Repolarization of Action Potential. When depolarization has occurred, and the negative potential on the inside of the membrane has been lost, the movement of sodium ions to the interior of the cell decreases, and the permeability to sodium returns to its resting state. At the same time, the permeability to potassium increases greatly. This low permeability to sodium and high permeability to potassium permit only a few sodium ions to pass to the inside, but large numbers of potassium ions to pass to the outside, since these are present inside the cell in high concentration. Because potassium ions are also positively charged, this once again causes loss of positive charges from the inside of the membrane, reestablishing the normal negative membrane potential. This process is called ***repolarization,*** and the total sequence of depolarization and repolarization is called the ***action potential.***

Bi-directional Propagation of Action Potentials. An action potential elicited at one point on an excitable membrane can excite adjacent portions of the membrane, thus causing the action potential to spread in both directions. The mechanism of this is the following: Each time an action potential begins at any given point on the membrane, the normal negative charge on the inside of the membrane is lost, which causes an electrical current to flow to adjacent and as yet unexcited regions, where an ***electrotonic potential*** is generated. This potential reaches the ***threshold value*** and serves as the stimulus for exciting these adjacent regions of the membrane. As a result, an action potential then occurs at each of these points, and the process is repeated again and again until the action potential has spread to both ends of the fiber.

Conduction Velocity. The velocity of conduction in very large myelinated nerve fibers can be as great as 100 meters per second and as little as only 0.5 meters per second in very small unmyelinated fibers.

Refractory Period. The refractory period of the action potential is the duration of time between the beginning of depolarization and the end of repolarization. In large nerve fibers, the repolarization process follows about 1/2,500 second after the depolarization process. Therefore, as many as 2,500 nerve impulses (action potentials) can be transmitted along a large nerve fiber per second. On the other hand, the process of repolarization is so slow in some smooth muscle fibers that not over one impulse in every few seconds can be transmitted.

The All-or-Nothing Law. A very important aspect of nerve function is that a stimulus usually causes a nerve fiber either to transmit a complete impulse (action potential) or, if the stimulus is too weak, none at all. This is called the all-or-nothing law of excitation. Furthermore, once an impulse begins, it normally travels in all directions over the fiber—either backward or forward and into all branches of the fiber—until each portion of the neuronal membrane has become depolarized.

Energy Requirement of Action Potential. The energy required to reestablish the sodium and potassium concentrations across the membrane following a large number of action potentials is derived from the metabolic processes of the cell. However, the number of sodium and potassium ions that move across the cell membrane with each action potential is so infinitesimal that tens of thousands of action potentials can be transmitted by a nerve fiber after the metabolic machinery of the cell has been poisoned. Therefore, nerve metabolism can be blocked for as long as several hours at a time without greatly affecting transmission of the impulse, for, once the differences in ion concentration across the cell membrane have been built up, impulse transmission is purely a physical phenomenon without involving the enzymatic metabolic processes of the cells.

THE NEUROMUSCULAR JUNCTION

Skeletal muscles are innervated by large, myelinated nerve fibers called motor neurons, or ***motoneurons.*** The neuromuscular junction is the point of connection between a motor nerve fiber and a skeletal muscle fiber. The nerve ending, where it lies on the skeletal muscle fiber, branches to form a complex of 50 or more nerve terminals, and the entire structure is called the ***motor endplate.*** The nerve terminals in this motor endplate synthesize and store a chemical transmitter substance called acetylcholine.

Release of Acetylcholine at Neuromuscular Junction. When a nerve impulse reaches the motor endplate, portions of acetylcholine stored in small vesicles are released into the ***synaptic cleft*** between the nerve terminals and the muscle membrane. The acetylcholine binds to receptors on the muscle membrane, increasing its permeability to sodium and thus depolarizing the muscle fiber. Within another 1/500 second a protein enzyme called cholinesterase destroys the acetylcholine. Thus, the net result of a nerve impulse reaching the motor endplate is the release of a small pulse of acetylcholine that lasts only a few milliseconds at most but still long enough to stimulate the muscle fiber.

Acetylcholine Initiation of the Endplate Potential. When the short pulse of acetylcholine increases the permeability of the muscle membrane, sodium ions immediately begin to pour to the inside of the fiber, causing a depolarization in the immediate vicinity of the endplate. This change in potential is called the endplate potential. The endplate potential is nearly always above the ***threshold value*** of the membrane, and the action potential that follows spreads over the entire muscle fiber as described above for nerve fibers.

Myasthenia Gravis and Muscle Paralysis. Myasthenia gravis is an autoimmune disease in which the immune system has produced antibodies against acetylcholine receptors on the muscle membrane. The endplate potentials are often too small to stimulate the muscle fibers, and the result is muscle weakness. In severe cases, the patient dies following paralysis of the respiratory muscles. When treated with a drug, such as neostigmine, that can inactivate the enzyme that normally inactivates acetylcholine, the levels of acetylcholine build and thereby enhance neuromuscular transmission.

FUNCTION OF SKELETAL MUSCLE

Physiologic Anatomy. Skeletal muscle is composed of muscle fibers that run the entire length of the muscle. The cytoplasm of the muscle fiber contains myofibrils that consist of ***actin filaments*** and ***myosin filaments*** arranged linearly in the muscle fiber so that the myosin filaments alternate with the actin filaments. The portion of a myofibril that lies between two successive ***Z discs*** is called the ***sarcomere,*** which is the basic functional unit of skeletal muscle. The resting length of the typical sarcomere is about 2 micrometers. The interdigitating actin and myosin filaments within a sarcomere cause myofibrils to have alternate light and dark bands, which give skeletal and cardiac muscle their striated appearance. The light bands contain only actin filaments and are called ***I bands,*** and the dark bands contain both actin and myosin filaments and are called ***A bands.***

Molecular Characteristics of Contractile Filaments. Although the myosin filaments are composed entirely of myosin molecules, the actin filament is composed of long threads of ***actin*** and ***tropomyosin*** wrapped around each other in a helical manner. Also, attached periodically to the tropomyosin is a protein complex called ***troponin.*** The troponin and tropomyosin control muscle contraction.

Sliding Filament Theory of Contraction. When an action potential passes over the muscle fiber membrane, the actin and myosin filaments interact with each other so that they slide past each other, thus shortening the fiber. Figure 3-8 shows the relaxed and contracted state of four successive sarcomeres. During the relaxed state, the actin filaments connected to the Z discs barely overlap each other but overlap the myosin filaments completely. In the contracted state, the actin filaments have been pulled inward among the myosin filaments, and the two successive Z discs are now much closer together. As soon as the action potential is over, the interaction between the actin and myosin filaments disappears so that the alternating sets of filaments then slide away from each other.

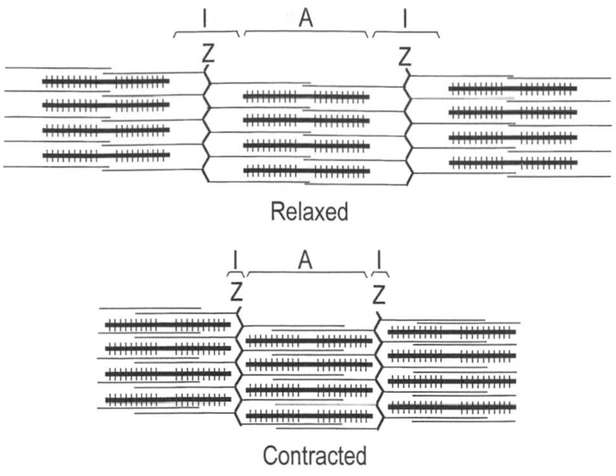

Fig. 3-8. Relaxed and contracted states of a myofibril showing sliding of the actin filaments into spaces between myosin filaments. Note that actin filaments are connected to Z discs and that myosin filaments have crossbridges (Adapted from Guyton AC, Hall JE: Textbook of Medical Physiology, 9th ed. Philadelphia: WB Saunders, 1995:76)

Connection of Actin Filaments with Myosin Crossbridges. The nature of the forces that cause the actin and myosin filaments to slide along each other during the contractile process is not entirely understood. One theory is that myosin filaments have arms, called ***crossbridges,*** that extend outward from the main filament. The end of each crossbridge has a head that connects with an active site on the actin filament. Molecular forces between the heads of the crossbridges and the actin filament cause the heads to bend and the actin filament to be pulled inward along the myosin filament in a ratcheting motion. This so-called walk along theory of contraction applies to skeletal and cardiac muscle.

Length–Tension Relationship. Figure 3-9 illustrates the effect of sarcomere length (actin and myosin overlap) on tension development in contracting muscle. The degree of actin and myosin overlap at different points along the curve is shown to the right. Note at points B and C that maximum tension develops in association with maximum overlap of actin and myosin filaments at this ideal sarcomere length. Any increase or decrease in sarcomere length from this ideal position decreases overlap of actin and myosin filaments and thus decreases the development of tension. Point D indicates that zero tension is developed when zero overlap occurs. This diagram indicates that maximum contraction occurs with maximum overlap of actin and myosin filaments and supports the idea that the number of myosin crossbridges pulling on actin filaments controls the strength of a muscle contraction.

INITIATION OF CONTRACTION: EXCITATION-CONTRACTION COUPLING

Transmission of an action potential over the muscle fiber membrane causes the fiber to contract a few milliseconds later, which is called ***excitation-contraction coupling.*** The mechanism by which this occurs is described in the following sections.

Transverse Tubule Conduction of Action Potential to Interior of Muscle Fiber. Minute tubules, called transverse tubules, or T tubules, pass transversely all the way through the muscle fiber from one side of the fiber membrane to the other side. The action potential, on reaching one of these tubules, travels to the interior of the muscle fiber along the membranes of the tubules. Thus, electrical current from the action potential is distributed to the inner substance of the muscle fiber as well as along its surface. The T tubules make physical contact inside the muscle fiber with many additional very fine tubules called ***longitudinal tubules.*** These are part of the endoplasmic reticulum and are collectively called the ***sarcoplasmic reticulum;*** they lie parallel to the myofibrils that cause muscle contraction. Also, they contain large amounts of highly concentrated calcium ions.

Calcium Release from Longitudinal Tubules. When the action potential travels along the T tubules, electrical currents spread from these to the longitudinal tubules and cause a pulse of calcium ions to be released from the longitudinal tubules into the fluid surrounding the actin and myosin filaments of the myofibrils. The calcium ions then combine with the troponin complex, and in some way not yet understood, this changes the physical relationship of the tropomyosin and actin molecules; the net result is exposure of active electrical sites on the actin filament that attract the heads of the myosin

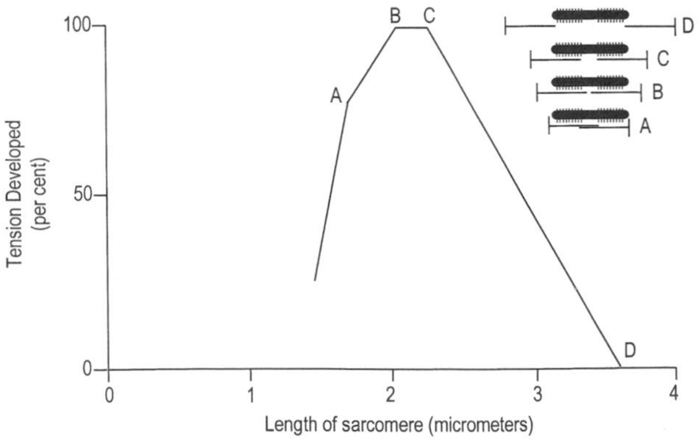

Fig. 3-9. Length-tension diagram for single sarcomere, illustrating maximum strength of contraction when sarcomere is 2.0 to 2.2 μm in length. The degree of actin and myosin overlap at different points along the curve is shown on the upper right. (Adapted from Guyton AC, Hall JE: Textbook of Medical Physiology, 9th ed. Philadelphia: WB Saunders, 1995:79)

filament, causing contraction of the muscle. Within another small fraction of a second the calcium ions are actively transported back into the longitudinal tubules, which decreases the calcium ion concentration back to a very low value and thereby inactivates the myosin, allowing relaxation of the muscle.

Adenosine Triphosphate and the Myosin Crossbridge. Contraction of the muscle requires energy. Each time a muscle fiber contracts, a certain amount of adenosine triphosphate, the energy-rich compound that is synthesized during the metabolism of food, is destroyed. It is believed that one molecule of adenosine triphosphate is degraded each time the head of a crossbridge bends to cause movement of the actin filament. The energy derived from this adenosine triphosphate is used to return the head back to its original ''cocked'' position. In this way the energy is stored in the cocked head, and it is the release of this energy that provides the force exerted by the head to pull the actin filament forward.

The more times a muscle fiber contracts and the greater the load against which the muscle contracts, the greater is the quantity of adenosine triphosphate that is degraded. During extreme muscle activity, the rate of metabolism in individual muscles sometimes rises to more than 50 times the metabolic rate of the resting muscle.

Regulation of Strength of Muscle Contraction. A skeletal muscle is composed of many muscle fibers connected in parallel with each other. The strength of contraction of the entire muscle can be increased by (1) multiple motor unit summation, in which many parallel muscle fibers contract simultaneously; and (2) frequency summation, in which successive contractions of each muscle fiber occur so close together that they actually fuse into one long continuous contraction rather than many individual twitches. This latter effect is called ***tetanization.***

FUNCTION OF CARDIAC AND SMOOTH MUSCLE

Calcium Initiation of Contraction. The basic contractile mechanism of both cardiac and smooth muscle is similar to that of skeletal muscle. An exception is that in smooth muscle the actin and myosin filaments are not arranged in distinct alternate segments as is true in both skeletal and cardiac muscle. Nevertheless, an action potential traveling over the membrane causes contraction as a result of the release of calcium ions that makes the actin and myosin filaments attract each other.

Rhythmic Contractions in Cardiac and Smooth Muscle. A distinguishing characteristic of both cardiac and smooth muscle is that they can exhibit repetitive rhythmic contractions. These rhythmic contractions are caused by spontaneously occurring action potentials in the muscle fibers. Each time the membrane potential returns to the resting state, a new action potential begins because the membranes of these types of muscle are naturally very permeable to sodium ions. The sodium ions leak into the muscle fiber, cause a decrease in the local membrane potential as well as an increase in membrane permeability, and these effects initiate an action potential.

The action potential of cardiac muscle lasts about 0.3 second and of smooth muscle from as little as 0.01 second in some types of smooth muscle to more than a second in others. Also, these two types of muscle contract for more prolonged periods than the very short period that occurs in skeletal muscle, from 0.3 second to several seconds.

Smooth Muscle Tone. Another important distinguishing characteristic of smooth muscle is that it can contract continuously in addition to the rhythmic contractions. The continuous contraction is called ***tone.*** The degree of tone can change from time to time, becoming almost none or increasing to a truly strong contraction. The intermittent rhythmic contractions are then superimposed on the basic tone. Thus, in the gastrointestinal tract, tonic contraction maintains a basal amount of pressure in the lumen of the gut, while rhythmic contractions superimposed on this cause propulsion of food along the gastrointestinal tract.

HEART

FUNCTIONAL ANATOMY OF THE HEART

The heart is actually two separate pumps, a ***right heart*** that pumps blood through the lungs and a ***left heart*** that pumps blood through the peripheral organs. Each of these two pumps is in turn comprised of two chambers, an ***atrium*** and a ***ventricle.*** Located between the atria and ventricles on both sides of the heart are the ***atrioventricular (A-V)*** valves, which normally allow blood to flow from the atrium to the ventricle but prevent backward flow from the ventricles to the atria. The right A-V valve is called the ***tricuspid valve,*** and the left is called the ***mitral valve.*** Blood exits from the right ventricle through the ***pulmonary valve*** into the pulmonary artery, and from the left ventricle through the ***aortic valve*** into the aorta. The pulmonary and aortic valves allow blood to flow into the arteries during ventricular contraction ***(systole)*** but prevent blood from moving in the opposite direction during ventricular relaxation ***(diastole).***

The walls of the heart (called the ***myocardium***) are composed primarily of cardiac muscle cells ***(myocytes).*** The inner surface of the myocardium, which comes in contact with the blood within the cardiac chambers, is lined with a layer of cells called ***endothelial cells,*** which provide a smooth surface throughout the cardiovascular system, including the blood vessels, and help to prevent blood clotting.

The cardiac muscle cells are arranged in layers that completely encircle the chambers of the heart. When the walls of the chambers contract, this exerts pressure on the blood that the chambers enclose and propels the blood forward. Cardiac muscle cells are striated and have typical myofibrils containing ***actin*** and ***myosin*** filaments, similar to those found in skeletal muscle, which slide along each other during the process of contraction. Adjacent cardiac muscle cells are joined end to end at structures called ***intercalated discs,*** which are actually cell membranes that have very low electrical resistance. This permits ions, and therefore action potentials, to move with ease from one cardiac muscle cell to another. Therefore, cardiac muscle is a ***syncytium*** of many myocytes that are interconnected; when one of these cells becomes excited, the action potential spreads rapidly throughout the interconnections.

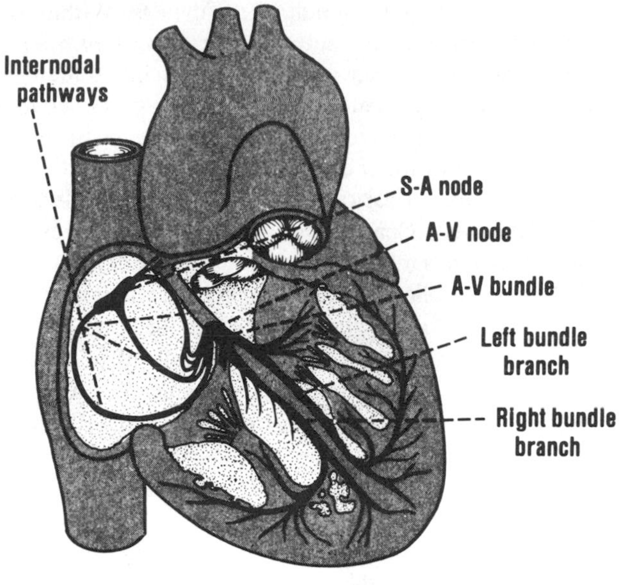

Fig. 3-10. The excitation system of the heart—the Purkinje system. (Guyton AC: Textbook of Medical Physiology, 8th ed. Philadelphia: WB Saunders, 1991)

RHYTHMICAL EXCITATION OF THE HEART

Action Potentials in Cardiac Muscle. Contraction of cardiac muscle, similar to contraction of other muscles, is triggered by depolarization of the cell membranes and development of action potentials, which spread from one cell to another. The resting membrane potential of normal ventricular muscle is approximately −90 mV. As in skeletal muscle, depolarization and development of action potentials in cardiac muscle are due mainly to a sudden increase in sodium permeability caused by opening of voltage-sensitive ***fast sodium channels*** that allow large numbers of sodium ions to enter the muscle fibers. However, in cardiac muscle, unlike skeletal muscle, the action potential has a plateau and is prolonged because of opening of ***slow calcium channels,*** which remain open for several tenths of a second, allowing large amounts of calcium and sodium ions through these channels to the interior of the cardiac cell; this maintains a prolonged period of depolarization, causing a plateau in the action potential. Eventually repolarization occurs when the permeabilities of calcium and potassium return to their original state and the slow calcium channels close.

The action potentials of atrial cells have similar shape, except that the duration of their plateau phase is shorter. In contrast, the action potentials in the conducting system of the heart (described later) differ considerably from that of the ventricular cells just described. In some parts of the conducting system of the heart there is a gradual, progressive depolarization, resulting in a rhythmic cell excitation of the cardiac tissue.

Pacemaker Function of Sinoatrial Node. The heart is also endowed with a specialized system that initiates rhythmic contraction of the heart and rapidly conducts signals throughout the heart, thus controlling the heart contraction (Fig. 3-10). Although many cardiac fibers have the capability of self-excitation, initial depolarization normally arises in a small group of specialized cardiac cells, called the ***sinoatrial (S-A) node,*** located in the wall of the right atrium near the opening of the superior vena cava. The S-A node has a natural rate of rhythmicity of about 72 times per minute, whereas the natural rate of rhythmicity of atrial muscle, if separated from the S-A node, is only 40 to 60 times per minute, and that of the ventricular muscle is about 15 to 30 times per minute. Thus, the more rapid basic rhythmicity of the S-A node usually initiates the heartbeat, and for this reason, the S-A node normally serves as the ***pacemaker*** of the heart.

The pacemaker function of the S-A node is accomplished as follows: Every time the muscle fibers of the S-A node contract, an impulse is transmitted to the rest of the atrial muscle and from there to the ventricular muscle. Thus, contraction of the S-A node causes contraction of the entire heart. Then, long before the atria or the ventricles can recover enough to contract again spontaneously, another excitatory impulse arrives from the S-A node. Therefore, the more slowly contracting parts of the heart are never allowed to contract at their natural rates of rhythm under normal conditions.

Purkinje System and Conduction of Impulses. The Purkinje fibers are modified cardiac muscle cells that allow a single impulse to rapidly spread over the entire heart muscle mass. In the ventricles, the Purkinje fibers conduct impulses at a velocity of approximately 2 m per second, which is four to six times the velocity in normal cardiac muscle. This rapid conduction allows all portions of the ventricular muscle to contract almost at the same time, rather than one part contracting ahead of another part; this in turn allows effective and forceful pumping by the heart.

The Purkinje system begins in the S-A node and from here passes through the atria by way of the ***internodal pathways*** to the ***A-V node,*** which lies in the posterior wall of the right atrium near the tricuspid valve. From the A-V node, a large bundle of Purkinje fibers called the ***A-V bundle*** (also called the ***bundle of His***) passes into the ventricular wall. Then the bundle divides into the ***left and right bundle branches,*** which spread, respectively, around the endocardial surfaces of the left and right ventricles. The atria and the ventricles are separated from each other by fibrous tissue everywhere, except where the A-V bundle passes into the ventricles. Therefore, in the normal heart the only pathway by which the impulse can travel from the atria to the ventricles is through the A-V bundle.

Another very important feature of the Purkinje system is the ***junctional fibers*** that occur in the A-V node. These fibers are very small and have extremely slow velocity of impulse transmission, only about one tenth the velocity of transmission in normal cardiac muscles. This slow velocity allows the prolonged delay of the impulse so that the atria contract 0.1 to 0.2 second ahead of the ventricles. This allows the atria to pump blood into the ventricles before the ventricles begin their pumping cycle.

Conduction Disorders Caused by Damage to A-V Node or A-V Bundle. Occasionally, pathologic conditions destroy or damage the A-V bundle or A-V node so that impulses no longer pass from the atria to the ventricles. When this occurs, the atria continue to beat at the normal rate of the S-A node, while the ventricles establish their own rate of rhythm. This condition is called ***heart block.*** Usually the Purkinje fibers in the A-V bundle or one of the bundle branches of the ventricles become the ***ventricular pacemaker,*** because these fibers have a higher rate of rhythm than the muscle fibers of the ventricles. The natural rate of rhythm in the ventricles after heart block can be as slow as 15 beats per minute or as rapid as 60 beats per minute. In heart block, the atrial contractions are not coordinated with ventricular contractions, which prevents the ventricles from becoming as well filled before contraction as in the normal heart. Loss of this coordinated atrial function impairs maximal heart pumping about 30%; however, a person with heart block can live for many years because the normal heart has tremendous reserve capacity for pumping blood.

Cardiac Flutter and Fibrillation—The Circus Movement. Occasionally an impulse in the heart continues all the way around the heart, and when arriving back at the starting point, reexcites the heart muscle to cause still another impulse that goes around the heart, continuing indefinitely. This is called circus movement. This does not occur in the normal heart for two reasons: First, normal cardiac muscle has a long refractory period, usually about 0.25 second, which means the muscle fiber cannot be reexcited during this time. Second, the impulse of the normal heart travels so rapidly that it will normally pass over the entire atrial or ventricular muscle mass in about 0.06 second, and therefore disappears before the heart muscle becomes reexcitable.

In the abnormal heart, however, the circus movement can occur in the following conditions: (1) when the refractory period of cardiac muscle becomes much less than 0.25 second; (2) when the Purkinje system is destroyed so that impulses take a far longer time to travel through the ventricles because of the slow conduction in the muscle fibers; (3) when the atria or the ventricles become dilated so that the length of the pathway around the heart is greatly increased, thereby increasing the time required for the impulse to travel around the heart; and (4) when the impulse does not travel directly around the heart, but instead travels in a zigzag direction, which lengthens the pathway to as much as ten times the direct distance around the heart; this obviously prolongs the time for transmission of the impulse and can result in reexcitation of the cardiac muscle.

In the atria, a regular circus movement around and around the atria causes ***atrial flutter,*** whereas zigzag impulses cause ***atrial fibrillation.*** The zigzag impulses in fibrillation also divide into multiple impulses so that there may be as many as five to ten impulses traveling in different directions at the same time. As a result, the atria remain partially contracted all the time, but they never contract rhythmically to provide any pumping action.

Flutter only very rarely occurs in the ventricles, but ***ventricular fibrillation,*** with many zigzag impulses spreading in all directions at once, is a major cause of cardiac failure and death. Either an electric shock to the ventricles or ischemia of the ventricular muscle as a result of coronary thrombosis can initiate ventricular fibrillation.

THE ELECTROCARDIOGRAM—INDIRECT RECORDING OF ELECTRICAL POTENTIALS OF THE HEART

The principles and clinical uses of electrocardiography obviously cannot be presented in this chapter, but the normal electrocardiogram (ECG), illustrated in Figure 3-11, can be related to the rhythmic excitation of the heart.

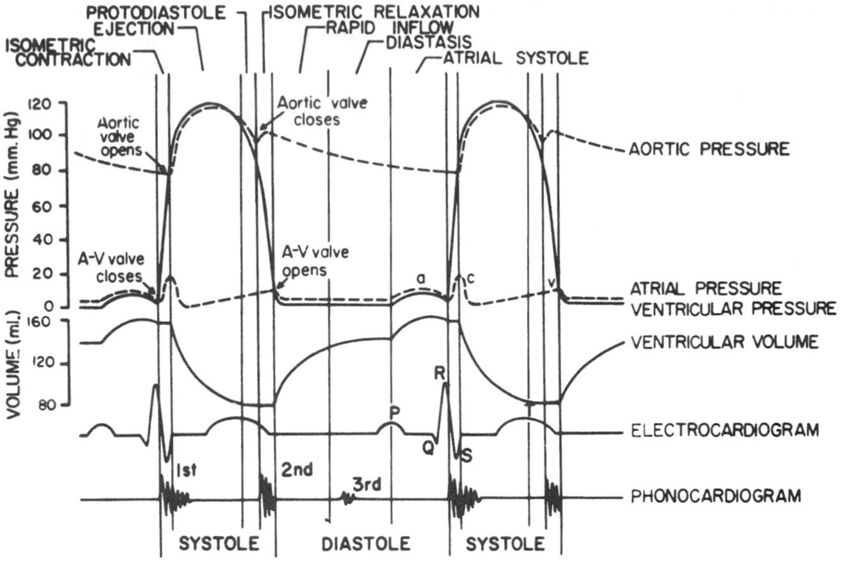

Fig. 3-11. The changes in cardiovascular pressures and ventricular volume during the cardiac cycle, and the relationship of the ECG and phonocardiogram to other events of the cycle. (Guyton AC: Textbook of Medical Physiology, 8th ed. Philadelphia: WB Saunders, 1991)

The normal ECG consists of a ***P wave,*** which is caused by the depolarization process in the atria; a ***QRS complex*** of waves, which is caused by the depolarization process of the ventricles; and the ***T wave,*** which is caused by repolarization of the ventricles.

The PQ Interval—The Time Between Atrial and Ventricular Depolarization. Normally, depolarization begins in the atria approximately 0.16 second before it begins in the ventricles. Therefore, the length of time between the beginning of the P wave and the Q wave, called the PQ interval (or PR interval when the Q wave is absent), is normally 0.16 second. Abnormally slow conduction of the impulse through the A-V bundle, as occurs when the bundle becomes ischemic following coronary thrombosis or when it becomes inflamed in the acute phase of rheumatic fever, prolongs the PQ interval to as much as 0.25 to 0.4 second. The process of rheumatic inflammation of the heart can be assessed by following the changes in the PQ interval. As the disease becomes worse, the PQ interval often increases, and as it becomes better the PQ interval decreases toward normal. When the PQ interval becomes very long, conduction to the A-V bundle will eventually cease, causing heart block, as explained earlier.

Abnormal QRS Waves. Since the QRS wave represents passage of the depolarization process through the ventricles, any condition that causes abnormal impulse transmission will alter the shape, the voltage, or the duration of the QRS complex. For example, hypertrophy of one ventricle will cause increased voltage and is likely to increase predominantly the R or the S wave, depending on the electrocardiographic lead and the ventricle affected. Also, damage to any portion of the Purkinje system will delay transmission of the impulse through the heart and therefore cause an abnormal shape of the QRS complex as well as prolongation of the complex.

Abnormal T Wave. Some diseases damage the ventricular muscle just enough that it becomes difficult for the muscle to reestablish normal membrane potentials after each heartbeat. As a result, some of the ventricular fibers may continue to emit electrical current longer than usual, which causes a bizarre pattern to the T wave, such as a biphasic pattern, or sometimes inversion of the T wave. Thus, an abnormal T wave ordinarily means mild to severe damage to at least a portion of the ventricular muscle.

Elevated or Depressed S-T Segment—Current of Injury. Occasionally the ECG segment between the S and T waves is displaced either above or below the major level of the ECG. This is caused by failure of some of the cardiac muscle fibers to repolarize between each two heartbeats. As a result, between heartbeats these fibers continue to emit large quantities of electrical current, called ***current of injury,*** which causes an elevated or depressed S-T segment. Therefore, when an elevated or depressed S-T segment is observed, one can be certain that at least some portion of the ventricular muscle is severely damaged, as occurs after acute heart attacks.

Abnormal Rhythms. The ECG can also be used to diagnose abnormal cardiac rhythms. For example, in heart block the P waves are completely dissociated from the QRS and T waves because of blocked conduction from the atria to the ventricles through the A-V bundle. In atrial fibrillation, no true P wave can be discerned, but many very fine waves continue indefinitely in the ECG. Finally, in extrasystoles of the heart, occasional QRST waves appear in the record points completely out of rhythm with the remaining portions of the ECG.

It should be emphasized that the ECG does not record changes in membrane potential across the individual cardiac muscle cells, but is a measure of electrical activity of many cells. In some cases, changes in mechanical and pumping ability of the heart can occur without measured changes in electrical activity, and therefore no major changes in the ECG. However, despite this limitation, the ECG can be a powerful tool for diagnosing many types of heart disease.

MECHANICS AND REGULATION OF HEART PUMPING

Cardiac Cycle. The two major phases of the cardiac cycle are both named for events occurring in the ventricles: (1) a period of ventricular relaxation, called ***diastole,*** lasting for about 0.5 second, in which the ventricles fill with blood; and (2) a period of ventricular contraction and blood ejection, called ***systole,*** lasting about 0.3 second. Thus, at a normal heart rate of about 72 beats/min, the entire cardiac cycle lasts about 0.8 second. As the heart rate increases, the fraction of the cardiac cycle in diastole decreases, which means that the heart beating very fast may not remain relaxed long enough to allow complete filling of the ventricles before the next contraction.

Figure 3-11 shows the pressure changes in the heart during the cardiac cycle and the relationship to the ECG, the heart sounds, and ventricular volume changes. Important events during the transition from diastole to systole include closure of the A-V (mitral and tricuspid) valves, which causes the first heart sound, a brief period of isovolumic contraction, and opening of the aortic and pulmonary valves. This transition period begins with the heart at the largest volume seen during the cardiac cycle—the ***end-diastolic volume.*** At the end of ventricular contraction, the heart has its smallest volume during the cardiac cycle—the ***end-systolic volume.*** During this period, the aortic and pulmonary valves close, causing the second heart sound and preventing backflow from the aorta into the ventricles; other events occurring during this transition from systole to diastole include isovolumic relaxation and opening of the A-V (mitral and tricuspid) valves. Because the aorta and large arteries are distensible, the blood pumped into the arterial system during systole is stored in these vessels and continues to flow through the systemic circulation, even during diastole. At the end of diastole, the cycle begins again.

Note that the P wave of the ECG occurs slightly before atrial contraction, the QRS waves occur at the onset of ventricular contraction, and the T wave occurs at the time of ventricular relaxation.

Cardiac Function Curve. When increased amounts of blood flow into the heart from the veins and distend its chambers, the stretched cardiac muscle automatically contracts with increased force. This increased force, in turn, pumps the extra blood through the heart into the arterial system. This is called the ***Frank-Starling law of the heart,*** and it allows the heart to adjust its pumping capacity automatically to the amount of blood that needs to be pumped. This mechanism also permits the heart to pump as much as two times the normal amount of blood even without increasing the heart rate, although there is a plateau in cardiac output at very high filling pressure. This plateau can be increased by sympathetic stimulation or decreased by heart failure. The ***ejection fraction*** is the ratio of stroke volume to end-diastolic volume. Normally, this is about 0.6, but the ejection fraction can increase with sympathetic stimulation and decrease during heart failure.

Autonomic Nervous Control of the Heart. There are two types of nerve fibers that supply the heart: ***parasympathetic fibers,*** which are carried in the vagus nerve; and ***sympathetic fibers,*** which are carried in the sympathetic nervous system. Stimulation of the sympathetic nerves releases ***norepinephrine*** at the nerve endings, causing increased heart rate and an increased force of contraction. Conversely, stimulation of the parasympathetics releases ***acetylcholine,*** which decreases heart rate. In certain conditions, such as exercise, there is a simultaneous increase in sympathetic stimulation and an inhibition of parasympathetic stimulation, causing marked increases in heart rate and overall pumping ability. Conversely, during rest, the sympathetics are inhibited and the parasympathetics again transmit a moderate amount of impulses to the heart so that the degree of activity of the heart lessens.

CIRCULATION AND ITS REGULATION

DYNAMICS OF BLOOD FLOW THROUGH THE CIRCULATION

Circulation as a Complete Circuit. Contraction of the left heart propels blood into the systemic circulation through the aorta, which empties into smaller arteries, arterioles, and eventually the capillaries where exchange of nutrients and waste products between the blood and the tissues occurs. Because blood vessels are distensible, each contraction of the heart distends the vessels; during relaxation the heart and vessels recoil, thereby continuing flow to the tissues even between heartbeats. Multiple regulatory mechanisms normally keep the average systemic arterial pressure within a range that is adequate for perfusion of the tissues. Pulsatile pressure in the aorta is dampened in the smaller arterioles so that pressure and flows in the capillary feeding the tissues are relatively steady.

The thin walls of the capillaries allow exchange of the nutrients and waste products between the blood and the tissues. Blood leaving the capillaries enters the venules and larger veins, which carry the blood to the right heart, which then pumps the blood through the pulmonary artery, smaller arteries, arterioles, and capillaries, where oxygen and carbon dioxide are exchanged between the blood and the tissues. From the pulmonary capillaries, blood flows into venules and large veins and empties into the left atrium and left ventricle before it is pumped again to the systemic circulation (Fig. 3-12).

Because blood flows around and around through the same vessels, any change in flow in a single part of the circuit alters flow in other parts. For example, strong constriction of the arteries in the systemic circulation can reduce the total cardiac output, in which case, blood flow through the lungs will be decreased equally as much as flow through the systemic circulation. Another important aspect of the circulation is that sudden constriction of a blood vessel must always be accompanied by opposite dilation of another part of the circulation, because blood volume cannot change rapidly and blood itself is incompressible. For instance, strong constriction of the veins in the systemic circulation displaces blood into the heart, dilating the heart and causing it to pump with increased force. This is one of the mechanisms by which cardiac output is regulated. With sustained constriction, changes in total blood volume can occur through exchange with the interstitial fluid or because of changes in fluid excretion by the kidneys.

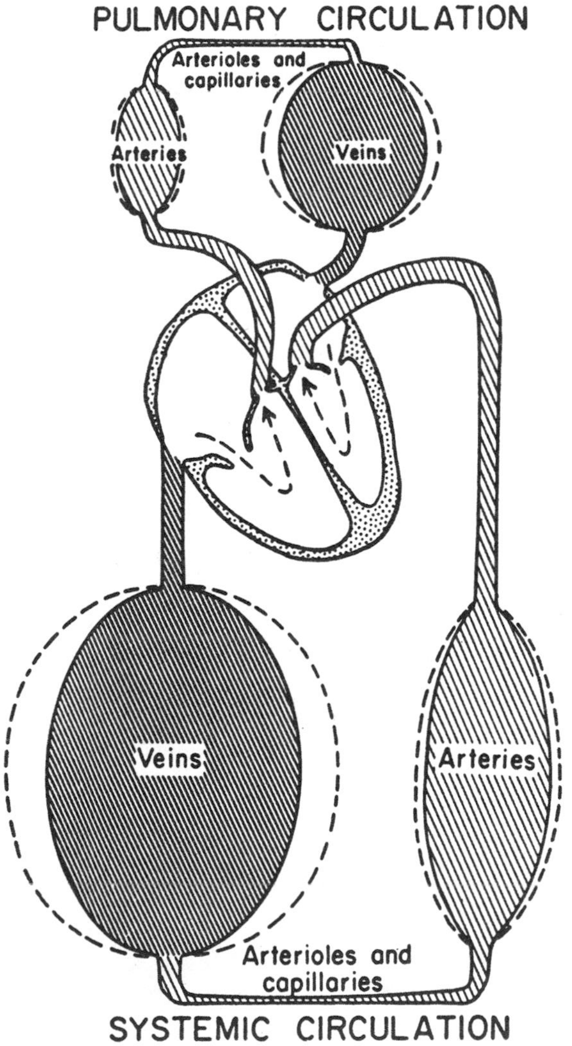

Fig. 3-12. Schematic of the circulatory system showing the flow of blood through the circulation and the distribution of blood volume in the different parts of the circulatory system. (Guyton AC: Textbook of Medical Physiology, 8th ed. Philadelphia: WB Saunders, 1991)

Blood Volume Distribution. About 84% of the total blood volume is in the systemic circulation, 9% is in the pulmonary circulation, and 7% is in the heart. Within each of these circulations, about three fourths of the blood is in the veins, about one sixth in the arteries, and one twelfth in the arterioles and capillaries. Thus, although the capillary blood exchanges nutrients and waste products in peripheral tissues and gases in the lungs, only a small part of the total blood volume is in the capillaries at any given time.

Blood Flow. When a blood vessel has a high pressure at one end and a lower pressure at the other, the rate of blood flow through the vessel is directly proportional to the difference in pressure between the two ends of the vessel and inversely proportional to the resistance to blood flow along the vessel. This relationship can be expressed as

$$\text{Blood Flow (Q)} = \frac{\text{Pressure Difference } (\Delta P)}{\text{Resistance}}$$

Blood pressure is usually expressed in millimeters of mercury and blood flow in milliliters per minute. Therefore, vascular resistance is expressed as millimeters of mercury per milliliter per minute. According to the ***theory of Poiseuille,*** vascular resistance is directly proportional to the viscosity of the blood and the length of the blood vessel, and inversely proportional to the radius of the vessel raised to the fourth power:

$$\frac{\text{Resistance } \alpha \text{ (Constant} \times \text{Viscosity} \times \text{Length)}}{\text{Radius}^4}$$

Thus, increased viscosity, which is determined principally by the concentration of red cells in the blood, raises vascular resistance. Decreased radius of the blood vessels also increases vascular resistance. Because vascular resistance is inversely related to the fourth power of the radius, even a small change in radius can cause a very large change in resistance. Thus, small vessels in the circulation have the largest amount of resistance, while large vessels have very little resistance to blood flow.

Vascular Compliance (Capacitance). The total quantity of blood that can be stored in a given part of the circulation for each millimeter of mercury of pressure is called the ***compliance*** (also called ***capacitance***) of the vascular bed:

$$\text{Vascular Compliance} = \frac{\Delta\ \text{Volume}}{\Delta\ \text{Pressure}}$$

The greater the compliance of the vessel, the more easily it can be distended by pressure. Compliance is related to ***distensibility*** of the vessel as follows:

$$\text{Compliance} = \text{Distensibility} \times \text{Volume}$$

The compliance of a vein is about 24 times as great as its corresponding artery because it is about eight times as distensible and has a volume three times as great ($8 \times 3 = 24$).

SYSTEMIC CIRCULATION

Systemic Arterial Pressure. The left ventricle normally pumps about 5 liters of blood into the aorta each minute. Each heartbeat ejects approximately 70 ml of blood into the aorta; this is called the ***stroke volume output.*** As a result, the arteries become greatly distended during cardiac systole, and during diastole the recoil of the arteries causes blood stored in the arterial tree to ''run off'' through the systemic vessels to the veins. Thus, the aortic pressure rises to its highest point, the ***systolic pressure,*** during systole and falls to its lowest point, the ***diastolic pressure,*** at the end of diastole. In the normal adult, the systolic pressure is approximately 120 mmHg and diastolic pressure is 80 mmHg. This is usually written 120/80.

The difference between systolic and diastolic pressure ($120 - 80 = 40$ mmHg) is called the ***pulse pressure.*** The two most important factors that can *increase* pulse pressure are (1) increased stroke volume and (2) decreased arterial compliance. Decreased arterial compliance can result from ''hardening'' of the arteries that occurs with aging or arteriosclerosis.

Arterial pressure changes throughout the cardiac cycle. The ***mean arterial pressure,*** however, is not simply the value halfway between systolic and diastolic pressure, because diastole usually lasts longer than systole. True mean arterial pressure can be measured with a catheter placed in the arteries, but a fairly accurate estimate of mean arterial pressure can also be obtained from the systolic and diastolic pressure as follows:

$$\begin{matrix}\text{Mean Arterial} \\ \text{Pressure}\end{matrix} = \begin{matrix}\text{Diastolic} \\ \text{Pressure}\end{matrix} + \begin{matrix}\text{1/3 Pulse} \\ \text{Pressure}\end{matrix}$$

From the example given above, mean arterial pressure equals 80 plus 1/3 ($120 - 80$) $= 93.3$ mmHg.

Because resistance to blood flow through the major arteries is so slight, the mean arterial pressure does not change markedly until the arteries become very small. In the arterioles, the major site of resistance to blood flow along the vasculature, there is a large drop in pressure to about 30 mmHg at the juncture of the arterioles and capillaries. The capillaries also contribute a moderate amount of resistance, causing the mean arterial pressure to fall to about 10 mmHg at the juncture of the capillaries and the veins. Resistance in the venous system is relatively slight, and pressure falls only 10 mmHg in the entire system; the pressure in the right atrium is approximately 0 mmHg.

Blood Flow Velocity. The total cross-sectional area of the systemic circulation increases from about 2.5 cm^2 in the central aorta to 2,500 cm^2 in the capillaries. The gathering of venules and veins decreases cross-sectional area to about 8 cm^2 at the level of the right atrium. Because the velocity of blood flow is inversely related to the cross-sectional area of the vessels, the blood flow velocity is greatest in the central aorta, reaches its lowest value in the capillary beds (about 1/100 as great as velocity in the aorta), then progressively increases in the venules and veins as the cross-sectional area decreases. The low velocity of blood flow in the capillaries is important in allowing efficient exchange of nutrients and waste products between the capillary blood and the tissues.

Regulation of Blood Flow by Arterioles. The arterioles not only have a high basal level of vascular resistance, but also have the capacity to change resistance by increasing or decreasing their diameters. Arteriolar walls are very muscular and respond to nervous, hormonal, and local control mechanisms that can constrict so intensely as to almost completely block blood flow, or dilate the vessels to increase blood flow as much as 7 to 20 times normal.

Local Tissue Autoregulation of Blood Flow. In most tissues, blood flow is autoregulated, which means that the tissue itself regulates its own blood flow. This is beneficial to the tissue because it allows the rate of tissue delivery of oxygen and nutrients and removal of waste products to parallel the rate of tissue activity; also, autoregulation permits blood flow to one tissue to be regulated independently of flow to another tissue.

The precise means by which tissues autoregulate their blood flow is still unknown. In many tissues, autoregulation appears to be linked to oxygen delivery or release from the tissues of metabolic waste products, such as adenosine and carbon dioxide, that cause vasodilation. For example, in metabolically active tissues, rapid utilization of oxygen tends to reduce oxygen tension in vascular smooth muscle. This, in turn, dilates the arterioles, increases blood flow, and delivers more oxygen to the active tissues. At the same time, a high rate of metabolism causes increased formation of vasodilatory metabolites, which also increase blood flow; the higher rate of blood flow removes the waste products of metabolism, restoring their tissues levels toward normal. As discussed in other sections of this chapter, some tissues, such as the kidneys, have special means of autoregulation that are not directly linked to metabolism.

Sympathetic Nervous System Reduction of Tissue Blood Flow. In almost all areas of the body, the arterioles are innervated by sympathetic nerve fibers that release ***norepinephrine,*** which then acts on ***α-adrenergic receptors*** in the vascular smooth muscle to cause vasoconstriction and decreased blood flow. Conversely, decreased sympathetic stimulation relaxes the arterioles and increases tissue blood flow.

In general, activation of the sympathetic nervous system reduces blood flow in many parts of the body at the same time. For example, when a person stands up, many of the blood vessels of the body, especially the veins, are reflexly constricted. This offsets the tendency of blood to ''pool'' in the lower part of the body and therefore allows plenty of blood to flow back to the heart, and keeps the cardiac output near normal, instead of falling as would otherwise occur. The sympathetic nervous system also causes vasoconstriction in many regions of the circulation when there is a tendency for blood pressure or blood volume to decrease, as occurs with hemorrhage; this vasoconstriction helps to minimize the fall in blood pressure that would otherwise occur with hemorrhage.

Endothelial Cell Release of Vasodilator (Endothelial-Derived Relaxing Factor) and Vasoconstrictor (Endothelin) Substances. Endothelial cells of blood vessels, especially large blood vessels, release several substances that then diffuse to the adjacent vascular smooth muscle and induce either relaxation or vasoconstriction. One of these substances, ***endothelial-derived relaxing factor (EDRF),*** is believed to be ***nitric oxide*** and normally dilates only the local blood vessels near its release because it is rapidly destroyed in the blood. One of the factors that stimulates EDRF release is distortion of the endothelial cells caused by the shear stress of blood flowing along the vessel. With increased amounts of blood flowing into the vessel, increased shear stress on the endothelial cells releases EDRF, causing the vessel to dilates so that the increased quantity of blood can flow with greater ease at a lower velocity.

Endothelin is a powerful vasoconstrictor that is released by endothelial cells in response to damage to the endothelium. For example, after severe blood vessel damage caused by crushing of the tissues, endothelin release and subsequent vasoconstriction may help to prevent excessive bleeding from the vasculature.

SPECIAL AREAS OF THE SYSTEMIC CIRCULATION

Muscle Circulation. During strenuous exercise, blood flow through a muscle can increase as much as 25-fold. This increase is caused mainly by local regulatory mechanisms that cause vasodilation secondary to increased muscle metabolic activity. In most cases, skeletal muscle blood flow is proportional to the workload of the muscle, ranging from a low of 4 ml/min per 100 g of tissue at rest to nearly 100 ml/min per 100 g of tissue during strenuous exercise. Because a trained athlete's body often contains more than 20 kg of skeletal muscle, total muscle blood flow can be as high as 20 liters/min in these individuals during strenuous exercise.

Skin Circulation. The skin plays a major role in regulating heat loss from the body. Skin blood flow in turn is controlled by the central nervous system via sympathetic nerves. When body temperature rises above normal, sympathetic activity is reduced, causing the skin blood vessels to dilate and allowing rapid flow of warm blood into the skin and loss of heat. Conversely, when the internal temperature of the body is too low, the skin vessels constrict, the skin becomes cold, and very little heat is lost.

Heart Blood Flow. Blood flow through cardiac tissue is nearly proportional to myocardial metabolic activity, which in turn depends on the myocardial workload. Because the rate of coronary blood flow parallels very closely the rate of oxygen consumption of heart muscle, many physiologists believe that low oxygen concentration in the heart tissue is in some way involved in the autoregulatory process, either through the direct effect of low oxygen to cause arteriolar vasodilation or indirectly by causing the tissues to release ***adenosine,*** which also dilates the blood vessels.

Coronary blood flow is normally about 4% of the resting cardiac output, but with increased myocardial workload, the coronary blood flow can increase as much as three- to fivefold.

Cerebral Circulation. Blood flow through the brain is normally almost constant due to autoregulation. When blood flow to the brain is threatened, as occurs with low blood pressure, this causes a buildup of carbon dioxide to the brain tissue, which in turn dilates cerebral arterioles and helps to restore blood flow toward normal. This interrelationship between brain tissue carbon dioxide and blood flow provides a stable environment for neuronal function, which is highly dependent on changes in carbon dioxide and tissue *p*H.

Decreased blood *p*H or decreased oxygen concentration will also increase brain blood flow when either of

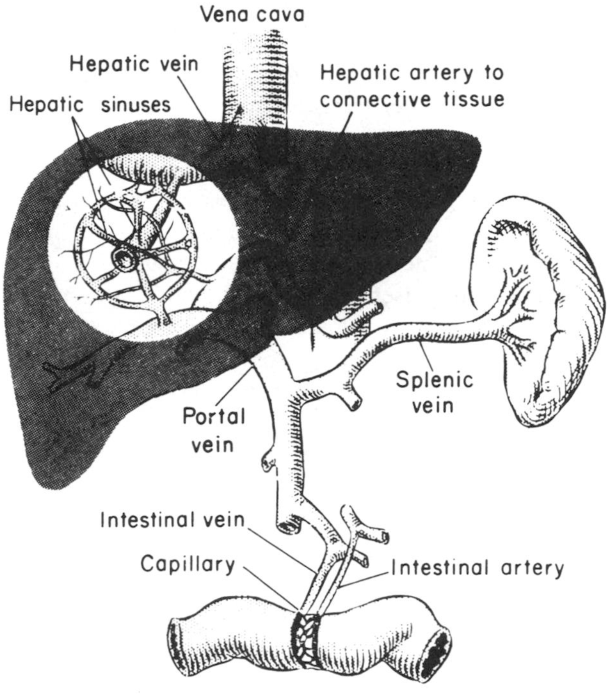

Fig. 3-13. The splanchnic circulation. (Guyton AC: Textbook of Medical Physiology, 8th ed. Philadelphia: WB Saunders, 1991)

these effects is severe. However, the normal blood flow to the brain is relatively constant at about 700 to 800 ml per minute, or about 15% of the cardiac output.

Splanchnic Circulation. The circulation of several abdominal organs, including the gastrointestinal tract, spleen, pancreas, and liver, are collectively referred to as the splanchnic circulation. Figure 3-13 shows the special arrangement of the venous circulation from the gastrointestinal tract, which is called the ***portal circulation.*** Note that blood flows from the gastrointestinal tract and from the spleen into the portal vein and then through the liver before emptying into the systemic veins. Normally the liver vessels offer reasonable amounts of resistance to blood flow, and portal venous pressure is about 8 mmHg. However, in liver disease, such as ***liver cirrhosis,*** this resistance can increase so greatly that portal venous pressure may rise to as high as 20 mmHg or more. This causes the portal capillary pressure also to rise to a very high value, which in turn causes large amounts of fluid to leak out of the capillaries into the peritoneal cavity.

Together, the splanchnic organs receive about 25% of the cardiac output at rest. However, increased metabolic activity of the gastrointestinal organs, such as occurs after eating a large meal, can raise tissue blood flow as much as 50% to 100%. In emergency circumstances, such as acute hemorrhage, activation of sympathetic nerves can markedly reduce splanchnic blood flow.

PULMONARY CIRCULATION

Relationship of Pulmonary Blood Flow to Cardiac Output. Because the circulatory system is a circuit, the same amount of blood flowing through the entire systemic circulation must also flow through the lungs. However, resistance to blood flow in the lungs is only about one eighth of that in the systemic circulation, and the pressures are correspondingly smaller. The pulmonary arterial systolic pressure averages 25 mmHg, and diastolic pressure averages 8 mmHg. The mean pulmonary artery pressure is about 15 mmHg, and left atrial pressure is 2 mmHg, giving a total pressure drop through the pulmonary circulation of only 13 mmHg. The pulmonary capillary pressure is about 7 mmHg, which is only a few millimeters greater than the left atrial pressure. This low capillary pressure is important in keeping the alveoli of the lungs dry, which will be discussed later in this chapter.

Effect of Blood Flow on Pulmonary Vascular Resistance. During strenuous exercise and in other states of physiologic stress, cardiac output sometimes increases as much as four- to fivefold, and blood flow through the lungs also increases by the same amount. However, pulmonary arterial pressure rises only a moderate amount for two reasons: (1) As flow increases, many pulmonary capillaries that are normally closed open up, and those that are already open dilate even more; and (2) the pulmonary vessels are highly distensible and therefore stretch as blood flow increases, decreasing pulmonary vascular resistance. As a result, the pulmonary vascular resistance decreases markedly as cardiac output increases, and mean pulmonary pressures usually rise only a few millimeters.

Blood Shifts Between Systemic and Pulmonary Circulations. Normally, only about 10% of the blood in the circulatory system is in the lungs, and about 80% is in the systemic circulation, the remainder being in the heart. However, the amounts of blood in the two circulations can change when one side of the heart fails. If the right heart fails, the pressure in the right atrium increases, and some of the blood normally pumped by the right heart builds up in the systemic circulation. Conversely, if the left heart fails, a portion of the systemic blood fails to be pumped into the systemic circulation and is displaced into the lungs, sometimes increasing pulmonary blood volume as much as two times normal. This can lead to pulmonary edema, as discussed below.

Relationship of Low Pulmonary Capillary Pressure to Alveoli. Normal pulmonary capillary pressure is only about 7 mmHg, while normal colloid osmotic pressure of the plasma is 28 mmHg. Thus, the pressure tending to force fluid out of the pores of the capillary (capillary pressure) is less than the force tending to cause absorption of fluid in the capillaries (plasma colloid osmotic pressure). Consequently, there is a large excess of "absorption pressure" at the pulmonary capillary membrane, which causes any fluid that enters the alveoli to be absorbed, thus keeping the alveoli dry.

Pulmonary Edema. Whenever excess blood shifts into the lungs, as a result of failure of the left heart to pump adequately, all of the pressures throughout the lungs, including the capillary pressure, rise. As long as the capillary pressure remains less than about 30 mmHg, the alveoli of the lungs will remain dry, but as soon as capillary pressure rises above the plasma colloid osmotic pressure, large amounts of fluid immediately begin to filter out of the capillaries into the interstitial fluid, and usually also through the alveolar membranes into the alveoli. This condition is called ***pulmonary edema,*** and it greatly impairs gas exchange between the alveoli and the blood capillaries.

Normally, there are safety factors that prevent pulmonary edema with moderate increases in pulmonary capillary pressure. However, if pulmonary capillary pressure rises acutely to about 50 mmHg, sufficient pulmonary edema can develop in 20 minutes to cause death; if pulmonary capillary pressure rises acutely to only 30 mmHg, sufficient pulmonary edema can still develop in 3 to 6 hours to cause death. However, in chronic conditions such as mitral valve stenosis, pulmonary capillary pressure can remain as high as 40 mmHg for long periods of time without causing severe pulmonary edema, probably because very large lymphatic vessels develop in the lungs and provide extra drainage of fluid from the tissues.

REGULATION OF SYSTEMIC ARTERIAL PRESSURE

Because systemic arterial pressure is the driving force for blood flow through the tissues of the body, it is not surprising that it is carefully regulated. Under resting conditions, the mean arterial pressure is approximately 100 mmHg, but for short periods of time, such as during strenuous exercise, mean arterial pressure may rise to as high as 150 mmHg in the normal person. In chronic hypertension, the pressure remains elevated indefinitely, or until treatment is instituted to lower pressure.

Blood pressure regulation is so important for homeostasis that the body is endowed with multiple short-term and long-term control mechanisms that keep mean arterial pressure relatively constant. The short-term control mechanisms, especially the nervous reflexes, operate within seconds to minimize changes in arterial pressure during acute disturbances, such as sudden blood loss or changes in body posture. Other mechanisms act very slowly, but powerfully, to keep mean arterial pressure relatively constant over a period of days, weeks, and months.

Cardiovascular Autonomic Reflexes as Pressure Control Mechanisms. The ***baroreceptor reflexes*** are initiated by changes in mechanical stretch of receptors, called ***baroreceptors,*** located in the walls of the internal carotid arteries, the aorta, and in other regions of the circulation. When the arterial pressure becomes excessively high in these vessels, these receptors are stimulated and impulses are transmitted to the brain to inhibit the sympathetic nervous system. As a result, the normal sympathetic impulses throughout the body are reduced, causing decreased heart rate, decreased strength of heart contraction, and decreased peripheral vascular resistance, which together help to reduce the blood pressure back toward normal. Conversely, a fall in blood pressure decreases the number of impulses transmitted by the baroreceptors; these impulses then no longer inhibit the sympathetic nervous system so that it becomes very active, causing the blood pressure to increase back toward normal.

There are also stretch receptors located in other regions of the circulation, such as the atria, the ventricles, and the pulmonary artery. These receptors, called ***cardiopulmonary baroreceptors,*** also function in a manner similar to the arterial baroreceptors to keep the cardiovascular control centers informed about pressures in the venous side of the systemic circulation as well as in the pulmonary circulation. Increased pressure in these regions inhibits sympathetic activity, whereas decreased pressure stimulates sympathetic activity.

Chemoreceptors also exist in the brain and in the peripheral circulation. For example, an increase in carbon dioxide concentration excites the neurons of the vasomotor centers of the brain stem, resulting in strong sympathetic stimulation throughout the body and an increase in blood pressure. This mechanism helps to ensure adequate pressure during stressful conditions, since physical stress to the body often increases the basal level of metabolism and the production of carbon dioxide. There are also small structures known as ***carotid and aortic bodies,*** located in the arch of the aorta, that respond to changes in arterial blood oxygen. When blood oxygen tension decreases, these chemoreceptors cause reflex activation of the sympathetic nervous system, thereby raising blood pressure. The increased blood pressure in turn helps to maintain adequate delivery of oxygen to vital organs, especially the brain, in which sympathetic stimulation does not markedly increase vascular resistance. However, these receptors are much more important for control of respiration than for blood pressure regulation.

Cerebral ischemia, a lack of adequate blood flow to the brain, is also a potent stimulus for activation of the sympathetic nervous system and increased blood pressure. In brain ischemia, the vasomotor center of the brain automatically becomes highly excited, probably because of the failure of the blood to carry carbon dioxide out of the vasomotor center rapidly enough. As a result, ***central nervous system ischemic reflexes*** initiate strong sympathetic stimulation throughout the body, immediately elevating the arterial pressure; this in turn increases cerebral blood flow back toward normal and helps to relieve the effects of ischemia.

Hormonal Control of Arterial Pressure. Several hormonal mechanisms also provide moderately rapid control of arterial blood pressure. Sympathetic stimulation to the adrenal medulla causes release of ***norepinephrine*** and ***epinephrine,*** which add to the vasoconstrictor effect of increased sympathetic stimulation. A second hormonal system, involved in both short-term and long-term blood pressure regulation, is the ***renin-angiotensin system.*** This system acts in the following manner for acute blood pressure control: (1) A decrease in blood pressure stimulates the juxtaglomerular cells of the kidney to secrete ***renin*** into the blood, (2) renin catalyzes the conversion of ***renin substrate (angiotensinogen)*** into the peptide ***angiotensin I,*** and (3) angiotensin I is converted into ***angiotensin II*** by the action of ***converting enzyme,*** present in the lungs and many of the blood vessels. Angiotensin II, the primary active component of this system, is a potent vasoconstrictor and raises arterial pressure. As described previously in this chapter, angiotensin II directly causes the kidneys to retain sodium and water and stimulates ***aldosterone*** secretion, which also decreases renal sodium and water excretion and helps to expand blood volume, actions that are especially important in long-term blood pressure regulation.

Another hormone that is released when blood pressure falls too low is ***vasopressin*** (also called ***antidiuretic hormone*** or ***ADH***). Vasopressin has a direct vasoconstrictor effect on peripheral blood vessels and also decreases renal excretion of water, thereby increasing blood volume. The various hormonal mechanisms, together with the cardiovascular reflexes, provide a powerful means of resisting changes in blood pressure under acute conditions, such as when a person stands after having been in a lying position or when a person bleeds severely. However, the cardiovascular reflex mechanisms are probably not of great importance in long-term blood pressure regulation because most of them eventually adapt (or ''reset'') to the prevailing pressure level.

Role of Kidneys in Long-Term Regulation of Arterial Pressure and Circulatory Volume. The most important mechanism for long-term control of arterial pressure is linked to control of circulatory volume by the kidneys, a mechanism known as the ***renal-body fluid feedback mechanism.*** When arterial pressure rises too high, the kidneys excrete increased quantities of sodium and water. As a result, the extracellular fluid volume and blood volume both decrease, and continue to decrease until arterial pressure returns back to normal and the kidneys excrete normal amounts of sodium and water. Conversely, when arterial pressure falls too low, the kidneys reduce their rate of sodium and water excretion and over a period of hours to days, if the person drinks enough water and eats enough salt to increase blood volume, arterial pressure will return to its previous level. This mechanism for blood pressure control is very slow to act, sometimes requiring several days or perhaps as long as a week or more to come to equilibrium. Therefore, it is not of major importance in acute control of arterial pressure. On the other hand, it is by far the most potent of all long-term arterial pressure controllers.

This basic mechanism for long-term control of blood volume and arterial pressure is enhanced by some of the hormonal mechanisms discussed above, especially the renin-angiotensin and aldosterone systems. For example, increasing intake of salt tends to raise blood volume and arterial pressure, which in turn increases renal salt and water excretion through ***pressure natriuresis,*** as discussed previously in this chapter. The increased renal excretion eliminates the extra salt, with relatively small changes in blood volume and arterial pressure, as long as the renin-angiotensin and aldosterone systems are functioning normally. Most persons can easily eliminate extra salt intake, with very small increases in arterial pressure and blood volume, because increased salt intake also reduces the formation of angiotensin II and aldosterone, which helps to eliminate the additional sodium. As long as the renin-angiotensin-aldosterone systems are fully operative, salt intake can be as low as one-tenth normal or as high as 10 times normal with only a few millimeters of change in blood pressure. However, when the renin-angiotensin-aldosterone systems are not functioning, changes in salt intake have a much greater effect on blood volume and arterial pressure.

HYPERTENSION

Hypertension is a syndrome characterized by elevated systemic arterial pressure; a person is usually considered to be clinically hypertensive if the arterial pressure is greater than 140/90. Approximately 25% to 30% of the population in westernized societies is hypertensive, although the incidence of hypertension is much higher in elderly subjects. Hypertension is one of the principal risk factors for the development of stroke, myocardial infarction, and kidney disease. Yet despite the great incidence of hypertension in the population and its important consequences, its precise cause in most people is still unknown. This type of hypertension is called ***essential hypertension.*** In the remaining cases, the cause is usually renal disease or nervous or hormonal disorders that affect the kidney pressure regulatory system.

Renal Hypertension. Any condition that reduces the ability of the kidney to excrete water and salt will usually cause hypertension. Such conditions include pyelonephritis, glomerulonephritis, polycystic kidney disease, arteriosclerosis, renal artery stenosis, and many other types of renal disease. One type of renal dysfunction that reduces water and salt excretion is renal vascular damage, such as stenosis of the arteries of the kidneys, constriction of the afferent arterioles, or increased resistance to fluid filtration through the glomerular membrane. Each of these factors reduces the ability of the kidneys to form glomerular filtrate, which in turn causes fluid and electrolyte retention, as well as increased blood volume and increased blood pressure. The rise in blood pressure then helps to return glomerular filtration rate toward normal and reduces tubular reabsorption, permitting renal excretory function to return to normal in the face of the vascular disorders.

The amount of long-term increase in blood volume required to cause hypertension is only a few percent and is much less than that required to cause acute increases in blood pressure. The reason for this is that acute increases in blood volume activate rapid blood pressure control mechanisms, especially the baroreceptor mechanisms, that oppose increased arterial blood pressure. Therefore, an increase in volume will not immediately raise blood pressure, but instead will cause pressure to rise slowly over days to weeks. Even when hypertension is associated with marked increases in blood volume, the cardiac output normally rises significantly above normal only during the first day or two of hypertension, because the increased output also causes excess blood flow to the body's tissues, which automatically causes constriction of the arterioles of the tissues; this process, called autoregulation, helps to return tissue blood flow toward normal. Therefore, the cardiac output returns to normal while peripheral vascular resistance becomes elevated, even though the initiating cause of the hypertension was increased blood volume and a rise in cardiac output.

Ischemia of the kidneys can also increase the arterial pressure by causing excess formation of renin and therefore angiotensin II, which constricts the arterioles throughout the body, thereby rapidly increasing arterial pressure. This effect occurs especially in malignant hypertension and in hypertension caused by unilateral renal artery disease when the renal ischemia fails to be relieved by the high blood pressure. However, increased angiotensin II levels are not elevated in most essential hypertensive patients.

Hormonal Hypertension. Oversecretion of certain hormones, especially the adrenal medullary hormones and the adrenocortical hormones, can cause hypertension. For example, a tumor of the adrenal gland called ***pheochromocytoma*** occasionally secretes large amounts of norepinephrine and epinephrine. These two substances have almost exactly the same effect on the circulatory system as stimulation of the sympathetic nervous system, thereby elevating the mean arterial pressure. Occasionally a tumor of the adrenal cortex or hyperplastic adrenal cortices (called ***primary aldosteronism***) secrete excessive quantities of adrenal cortical hormones, such as aldosterone or cortisone. These hormones can cause the kidneys to reabsorb large amounts of sodium and water from the tubules, and this in turn leads to an elevated blood volume and high blood pressure.

Possible Mechanisms of Essential Hypertension. Patients who develop essential hypertension slowly over many years almost always have significant changes in kidney function. Most important, the kidneys cannot excrete adequate quantities of water and salt at normal arterial pressures, but instead require a high arterial pressure to maintain normal balance between intake and output of water and salt. In theory, abnormal renal excretory capability could be caused either by renal vascular disorders that reduce glomerular filtration or by tubular disorders that increase reabsorption of salt and water. Because patients with essential hypertension are very heterogeneous with respect to the characteristics of their hypertension, it seems likely that both types of disorders contribute to increased blood pressure in hypertensive subjects.

Recent studies indicate that excessive weight gain and advanced age contribute to increased blood pressure in a high percentage of essential hypertensive patients. The precise mechanisms by which aging and weight gain raise blood pressure are still not known, but some studies suggest that weight gain may activate the sympathetic nervous system and cause changes in the kidneys that lead to increased tubular reabsorption of salt and water. With advancing age, the development of atherosclerosis may also contribute to increased renal vascular resistance and further impairment of kidney function.

A widely held belief is that genetic abnormalities may contribute to increased blood pressure in 20% to 30% of hypertensive patients. For example, some investigators believe that hypertensive persons may have genetic abnormalities of vascular smooth muscle, perhaps of the smooth muscle cell membranes, that cause excessive constriction of the small arterioles throughout the body, including the renal arterioles, which leads to hypertension.

REGULATION OF CARDIAC OUTPUT

Cardiac output is the amount of blood pumped by the left or right ventricle each minute. ***Venous return*** is the amount of blood flowing into the left or right atrium each minute. Although transient differences between cardiac output and venous return can occur, these two variables are equal in the steady state.

The normal cardiac output (and venous return) in the adult is approximately 5 liters per minute, but may increase to four to five times this value during strenuous exercise. Because the cardiac output is the sum of flow to all of the tissues of the body, it is regulated in proportion to the need for blood flow through the body tissues. That is, each tissue controls its own blood flow mainly by autoregulation, which matches the blood flows through the tissues to their metabolic needs, and the cardiac output is then regulated to supply the required blood flows. For example, cardiac output may reach over 25 liters per minute in a young athlete performing vigorous exercise, or it may be greatly reduced in a very inactive person with muscle atrophy. Loss of a limb by amputation or an organ because of injury or surgery likewise reduces the cardiac output by an amount equal to the flow to the lost limb or organ.

Changes in cardiac output can be effected in two different ways: (1) by ***changing the pumping ability of the heart*** and (2) by ***changing the venous return*** of blood into the heart from the systemic vessels.

Regulation of Pumping Ability of the Heart. One of the two primary mechanisms that controls the pumping action of the heart is the ***Frank-Starling mechanism,*** which refers to the ability of the heart to modify its stroke volume in response to variations in the amount of diastolic filling; within limits, the more the heart is filled during diastole, the greater the initial length of cardiac muscle fibers and the more forceful the ventricular contraction, causing a greater stroke volume. Figure 3-14 shows the ventricular function curve, in which cardiac output is plotted as a function of left ventricular end-diastolic pressure. The greater the left ventricular end-diastolic pressure, the greater the stretch of cardiac muscle fibers just before contraction begins. This is frequently referred to as ***ventricular preload;*** within certain limits, the greater the ventricular preload, the greater the force of contraction of cardiac muscle. This mechanism has two important characteristics: (1) It occurs on a beat-by-beat basis to match cardiac pumping with venous return, and (2) it is a property of cardiac muscle fibers that is independent of innervation.

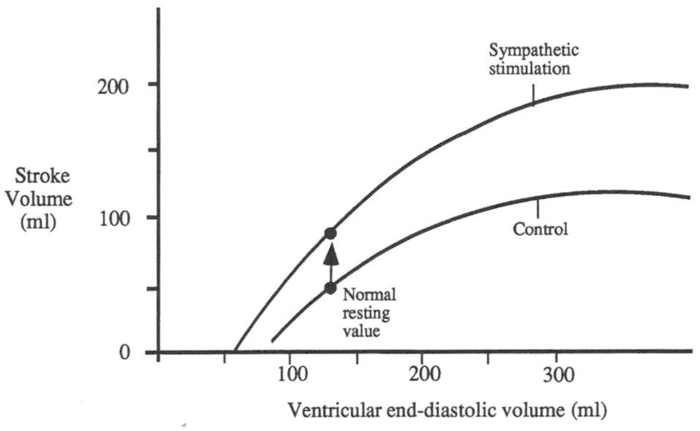

Fig. 3-14. Relationship between left ventricular end-diastolic volume and stroke volume, illustrating the basic Frank-Starling mechanism, as well as the effects of sympathetic stimulation to increase the pumping ability of the heart.

A second factor that influences cardiac pumping ability is ***contractility*** of cardiac muscle. This refers to the ability of cardiac muscles to contract independent of changes in the initial length of the muscle fibers. Increased contractility shifts the relationship between left ventricular end-diastolic pressure and cardiac output to higher levels. As discussed earlier, increased sympathetic stimulation to the heart increases the cardiac contractility as well as the heart rate. Decreased cardiac contractility shifts the ventricular function curve downward and to the right. This can occur, for example, with myocardial infarction, which causes ischemia and impaired contraction of the cardiac muscle.

Regulation of Venous Return. Venous return is regulated by three primary factors: (1) the average pressure of the blood in the systemic circulation, called the mean systemic filling pressure; (2) the right atrial pressure; and (3) the resistance to flow of blood through the systemic vessels.

In the normal circulatory system, the right atrial pressure is not a primary factor regulating venous return, because as discussed previously, the heart normally pumps all the blood that comes into it and therefore maintains the right atrial pressure near zero. For this reason, thc two other factors, the mean systemic filling pressure and the resistance to blood flow through the vessels, are the major controllers of venous return.

The ***mean systemic filling pressure*** is the average of all the pressures in the systemic circulation, which is usually about 7 mmHg in the normal animal. It is this low because most of the blood is in the veins where the pressure is low rather than in the arteries where the pressure is high. Factors that can increase the mean systemic filling pressure and therefore return of blood to the heart include (1) increased blood volume or (2) constriction of the blood vessels. Symphathetic constriction of the veins is especially important because most of the blood is stored in the veins. When the veins constrict, large amounts of blood are forced into the heart, thus distending the heart chambers and transiently increasing the cardiac output.

Reducing the ***resistance to blood flow*** also increases flow from the systemic vessels toward the heart, thereby increasing venous return. This is a primary means by which venous return is controlled; when the tissues become metabolically active, their blood vessels dilate, causing blood to flow more rapidly from the arteries into the veins and increasing venous return and cardiac output. Thus, an adequate amount of blood flow is automatically made available to the active tissues while non-active tissues maintain their same resting blood flow. Thus, increased cardiac output during strenuous exercise is caused mainly by increased flow to the actively exercising muscles. After eating a large meal, there is a reduction in resistance to blood flow in the gastrointestinal tract, allowing increased blood flow necessary for the increased activity of these tissues associated with digestion.

Regulation of Venous Pressure. Venous pressure is regulated mainly by the same two factors that regulate cardiac output—the ability of the heart to pump blood and the venous return to the heart. The normal heart is capable of pumping all of the blood that returns to it and therefore keeps the right atrial pressure at near 0 mmHg. However, if the heart is weakened by injury or disease, or if the venous return to the heart becomes so much greater than normal that the heart cannot pump it all, blood begins to dam up in the right atrium, and the right atrial pressure rises. Thus, the balance between pumping of the heart and venous return determines the right atrial pressure. The right atrial pressure in turn is an important determinant of peripheral venous pressure; the greater the right atrial pressure, the higher the peripheral venous pressure must be to keep blood flowing toward the heart. In most cases, the right atrial pressure must rise about 5 to 6 mmHg before significant distention of the peripheral veins occurs.

The Venous Pump. In the standing position blood does not flow with ease uphill through the veins. However, the veins are provided with valves, and when the surrounding muscles intermittently contract and compress the veins, this acts as a pump to keep blood flowing toward the heart. If a person stands completely still and the veins are not intermittently compressed, or if the valves of the veins have been destroyed, as occurs in varicose veins, then the venous pump is no longer effective. Under these conditions, the weight of the blood in the veins makes the venous pressure in the foot of a standing person as high as 75 to 90 mmHg.

PHYSIOLOGY OF HEART FAILURE

Coronary Atherosclerosis and Thrombosis. The most frequent cause of heart failure is insufficient coronary blood flow to the heart muscle, which causes ischemia and weakness and, in some cases, destruction of the cardiac muscle. The most frequent cause of insufficiency of coronary blood flow is ***atherosclerosis,*** which means fatty-fibrotic lesions of the coronary vessels that cause progressive, usually localized blockage of blood flow. This occurs, to some extent, in most older individuals. In some persons, another condition, ***coronary thrombosis,*** occurs acutely as a result of a blood clot in the coronary artery, leading to the well-known "heart attack." Both coronary atherosclerosis and coronary thrombosis normally occur from ***atheromata,*** which means infiltration of the coronary wall with cholesterol and other fatty substances. The deposits of cholesterol attract the growth of fibrous tissue and thereby cause the sclerosis, or occasionally the cholesterol protrudes to the intima into the lumina of the vessel and causes a blood clot to form, thereby occluding the vessel rapidly and producing a heart attack.

Heart Failure and Cardiac Output. One of the immediate effects of heart failure is the diminished pumping ability of the heart, which in turn reduces cardiac output and causes blood to dam up in one or both atria. If cardiac output remains low, and if the rise in atrial pressures are severe, edema can occur in peripheral tissues and in the lungs, which can rapidly cause death.

Heart Failure and the Sympathetic Nervous System. The fall in cardiac output that occurs immediately after an acute heart attack also decreases systemic arterial pressure and initiates intense cardiovascular reflexes that activate the sympathetic nervous system. The sympathetic nervous activation in turn helps to compensate for decreased pumping ability of the heart in two ways: (1) Sympathetic stimulation increases the strength of contraction of the nondamaged portion of the heart, and (2) sympathetic stimulation increases vasomotor tone throughout the systemic circulation, which results in increased venous return of blood to the heart and maintains arterial pressure sufficiently high to perfuse vital organs, including the brain. In severe heart attacks the nervous compensations are unable to return the cardiac output to normal, but nevertheless do help maintain perfusion of the brain and thereby help prevent death of the patient.

Heart Failure and Renal Fluid Retention. With a reduction in blood pressure immediately after an acute heart attack, the urine output by the kidneys is reduced for three reasons: (1) Sympathetic reflexes cause intense afferent arteriolar constriction of the kidney and reduced glomerular filtration rate, as well as increased tubular reabsorption of sodium and water; (2) the low cardiac output and reduced arterial pressure also contribute to decreased glomerular filtration rate; and (3) the low cardiac output and reduced arterial pressure stimulate the kidneys to secrete large amounts of renin, causing increased angiotensin II formation. The increased angiotensin II levels directly stimulate sodium reabsorption by the kidneys and indirectly increase sodium reabsorption by stimulating aldosterone secretion. Consequently in severe, acute cardiac failure, a person may become completely ***anuric*** (which means complete cessation of urine formation), or in milder degrees of cardiac failure, the person may become ***oliguric*** (which means a state of reduced urine formation).

The fluid retention by the kidneys increases the extracellular fluid volume, but much of this leaks out of the capillaries into the interstitial spaces and causes edema. However, some of the volume remains in the blood and increases the blood volume. Moderate degrees of fluid retention are beneficial because the increased blood volume promotes return of blood to the heart, which allows increased cardiac pumping. Beyond a certain degree of venous return, the heart muscles can become overstretched, and further retention of fluid then becomes detrimental to heart function. Also, excessive fluid retention can promote pulmonary edema and death.

Effects of Left Heart Failure Versus Right Heart Failure. Since the heart is actually two separate pumps, one side of the heart can fail independently of the other. More often, the left heart fails because most coronary thromboses affect principally the left ventricle. However, right heart failure occurs in patients who have pulmonary hypertension or in patients with certain types of congenital heart defects.

Some of the differences between left and right heart failure are obvious. Left heart failure causes a shift of fluid into the lungs with resulting pulmonary edema, while right heart failure causes shift of fluid into the systemic circulation.

In right heart failure, only a small amount of venous congestion occurs immediately in the systemic circulation, since only small amounts of extra blood are available in the lungs to shift into the systemic circulation. Therefore, peripheral edema does not occur to any significant extent immediately after *acute* right heart failure, but instead must await retention of fluid by the kidneys.

On the other hand, in acute left heart failure, a shift of blood into the lungs from the very voluminous systemic circulation can result in severe pulmonary edema and death within a matter of minutes. Sometimes pulmonary capillary pressure rises only a moderate amount immediately after the failure, not enough to cause significant edema. During the next few days, however, as the kidneys retain fluid, pulmonary capillary pressure may rise still higher, causing more severe pulmonary edema and respiratory death.

PATHOPHYSIOLOGY OF CIRCULATORY SHOCK

Circulatory shock occurs when the cardiac output is so greatly reduced that tissues throughout the body begin to deteriorate for lack of adequate nutrition. Any circulatory abnormality that greatly reduces cardiac output can cause circulatory shock. There are four major classifications of shock: (1) cardiogenic, (2) hypovolemic, (3) septic, and (4) neurogenic.

Cardiogenic Shock. This occurs most frequently in acute heart failure, in which the cardiac output falls because of impaired pumping ability of the heart itself.

Hypovolemic Shock. This type of shock results from reduced blood volume caused by (1) blood loss, (2) plasma loss, and (3) dehydration. Hypovolemic shock decreases the venous return to the heart, thereby reducing cardiac output.

Septic Shock. This condition, formally known as "blood poisoning," refers to widely disseminated infection to many areas of the body, with the infection being borne through the blood from one tissue to another, causing extensive damage. Some of the typical causes of septic shock include (1) peritonitis caused by spread of infection in the gastrointestinal tract; (2) generalized infection resulting from spread of simple skin infection, such as streptococcal infection; (3) generalized gangrenous infection; (4) infection spreading into the blood from the kidney or urinary tract; and (5) endotoxin shock, which occurs when a large segment of the gut loses much of its blood supply and results in proliferation of bacteria in the gut that release a toxin called ***endotoxin.***

In septic shock, once the bacteria or endotoxin enter the bloodstream, this results in severe dilation of the blood vessels of the body, resulting in reduced blood pressure. Also, further compounding circulatory depression is a direct effect of endotoxins on the heart to decrease myocardial contractility.

Neurogenic Shock. This is a circulatory shock that results from sudden inhibition of the sympathetic nervous system throughout the body. This allows all the systemic vessels to dilate and the blood to "pool" in the lower part of the body rather than returning to the heart. If a person with loss of sympathetic tone is kept in the standing position, this can actually cause death, but if the person is placed in a horizontal or head down position, sufficient blood will usually still flow back to the heart to allow survival.

Cyclical Nature of Circulatory Shock. One of the key features of circulatory shock is that it creates a vicious cycle and tends to make the shock itself worse. That is, the shock causes poor blood flow to the tissues of the body, including the tissues to the heart and the vascular system; this causes deterioration of the heart and blood vessels, causing still further decreases in cardiac output and further tissue deterioration. This vicious cycle continues unless the cardiovascular reflexes and other compensatory mechanisms overcome the progressive tendency of shock or unless therapy is instituted; if not, the vicious cycle continues until death.

Irreversible Circulatory Shock. Another distinguishing characteristic of shock is that, beyond a certain stage of progressive deterioration, any amount of therapy becomes ineffective in preventing death of the patient.

This is called the irreversible stage of shock. Often, different types of therapy, such as blood transfusion, will return the arterial pressure to normal and above normal. Yet, after a brief period, the blood pressure begins to fall again because the cardiovascular tissues have already been damaged too much, and further therapy fails to keep this cycle from proceeding on to death.

RESPIRATORY SYSTEM

The respiratory system supplies oxygen to the tissues and removes carbon dioxide. Major functional events of respiration include (1) ventilation, which is how air moves in and out of the alveoli; (2) diffusion of oxygen and carbon dioxide between the blood and alveoli; (3) transport of oxygen and carbon dioxide to and from the peripheral tissues; and (4) regulation of respiration.

VENTILATION OF THE LUNGS

Lung Volume and the Thoracic Cavity. The lungs float freely in the thoracic cavity, and anytime the length or thickness of the thoracic cavity increases or decreases, simultaneous changes in lung volume must also occur. The space between the visceral pleura of the lungs and the parietal pleura of the thoracic cage is called the ***intrapleural space.*** Continuous absorption of fluid by lymphatic channels keeps the space nearly empty except for a few milliliters of pleural fluid that provides lubrication for the moving lungs.

Diaphragm. Contraction of the diaphragm elongates the thoracic cavity, causing the lungs to expand. Other muscles of inspiration include the ***external intercostals*** and neck muscles, which pull the rib cage upward and forward in a ''bucket handle'' motion, increasing the thickness of the chest cavity.

Expiration. The lungs and chest wall are elastic and tend to return to their resting positions following inspiration. Expiration becomes an active process during exercise and other strenuous activities in which breathing increases greatly. The major muscles of expiration are the ***abdominal muscles;*** contraction of these forces the abdominal viscera upward against the bottom of the diaphragm. The ***internal intercostals*** help with expiration by pulling the chest cage downward, which decreases the thickness of the chest cavity.

Surfactant in the Alveoli. If the alveoli were lined with pure water, the surface tension would be so great that they would likely remain collapsed all the time. Fortunately, surfactant is secreted into the alveoli by type II epithelial cells, which line the alveoli. This substance acts to decrease the surface tension of the fluid lining the alveoli, which allows normal expansion of the lungs. Surfactant is formed relatively late in fetal life, and some newborn babies without adequate quantities may develop respiratory distress and die.

Pneumothorax. When a hole is made in the chest wall, the elastic lungs immediately collapse, and the chest wall springs outward, sucking air into chest cavity. This is called a pneumothorax. When the person tries to breathe, air moves in and out of the hole in the chest, and death can occur by suffocation.

Pulmonary Volumes and Capacities. Figure 3-15 shows a recording for successive breath cycles at different depths of inspiration and expiration. The recording was made using an apparatus called a ***spirometer,*** which is a drum inverted in water, with a tube extending

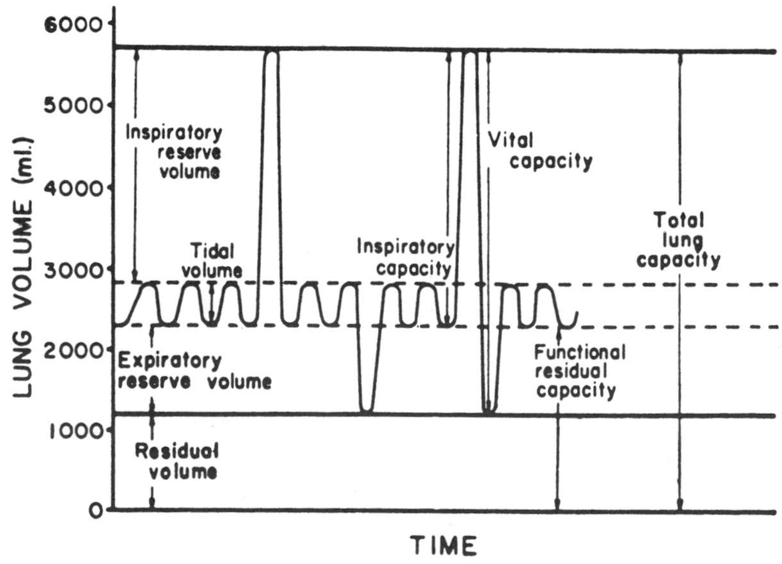

Fig. 3-15. Changes in lung volume during normal breathing and during maximal inspiration and expiration. (Guyton AC: Textbook of Medical Physiology, 8th ed. Philadelphia: WB Saunders, 1991)

from the air space in the drum to the mouth of the person being tested. As the person breathes in and out, the drum moves up and down, and a recording of the movement is made. In the illustration, note that neither the functional residual capacity nor the residual volume can be measured with a spirometer. The four volumes and four capacities shown are described below.

Tidal volume (~500 ml): the amount of air inspired and expired with each normal breath

Inspiratory reserve volume (~3,000 ml): the amount of air that can be inspired beyond the tidal volume

Expiratory reserve volume (~1,100 ml): the amount of air that can be expired by forceful expiration at the end of a normal tidal expiration

Residual volume (~1,200 ml): the amount of air in the lungs after a maximal expiration

Vital capacity (~4,600 ml): the range in lung volume from maximum inspiration to maximum expiration

Functional residual capacity (~2,300 ml): the volume of air in the lungs after a normal expiration

Inspiratory capacity (~3,500 ml): the maximum volume of air a person can inspire beginning from the end of a normal expiration

Total lung capacity (~5,800 ml): the maximum volume of air that the lungs can hold after the greatest possible inspiration.

Total Ventilation. The total ventilation, also called minute respiratory volume, is the sum of all the tidal air breathed during a minute. Since the normal respiratory rate is about 12 breaths per minute, and the normal tidal volume is 500 ml, the normal total ventilation is about 6,000 ml per minute.

Alveolar Ventilation. Each time a person inspires, part of the new air must be used to fill the passageways between the nose and the alveoli. Since this portion of the inspired air does not reach the alveoli, it is called the ***anatomic dead space volume*** and is normally about 150 ml. Thus, with each normal tidal volume of air, 150 ml of the 500 ml fails to reach the alveoli and therefore is not available to aerate the blood. That portion of the air that does reach the alveoli is called the alveolar ventilatory air, and it normally amounts to about 350 ml with each breath. With a normal respiratory rate of 12 per minute, this amounts to an alveolar ventilation of 4,200 ml per minute.

PARTIAL PRESSURES OF RESPIRATORY GASES

Movement of Respiratory Gases. In essentially all respiratory studies gas concentration is expressed not in terms of percentage but in ***partial pressures.*** The partial pressure of a gas is the amount of pressure exerted by that gas alone. Partial pressures (Table 3-4) are used to express the concentrations of gases because it is pressure that causes the gases to move by diffusion from one part of the body to another.

Calculation of Partial Pressure. The partial pressure of a gas is calculated by multiplying its concentration by the total pressure. For example, dry atmospheric air is 20.93% oxygen. The partial pressure of oxygen PO_2 at sea level is equal to 760 mmHg (atmospheric pressure) $\times$ 20.93/100 = 159.1 mmHg. Air becomes humidified in the warm, moist respiratory airways, and its vapor pressure is 47 mmHg. When water vapor pressure is subtracted from the total pressure (760 − 47), the total pressure is 713 mmHg. Therefore, the oxygen tension of moist tracheal air is 713 $\times$ 20.93/100 = 149.2 mmHg.

TRANSPORT OF OXYGEN AND CARBON DIOXIDE BETWEEN ALVEOLI AND TISSUES

Partial Pressures of Oxygen and Carbon Dioxide in Arterial Blood. Oxygen diffuses from the alveoli into the mixed venous blood entering the pulmonary capillaries along a partial pressure gradient of 64 mmHg, as shown in Table 3-4. Carbon dioxide diffuses in the opposite direction along a gradient of 6 mmHg. The partial pressure of oxygen (100 mmHg) and carbon dioxide (40 mmHg) in the arterial blood leaving the lungs is nearly equal to the alveolar values.

Rate of Gas Diffusion Across Pulmonary Membrane. The rate of gas diffusion across the pulmonary membrane is proportional to the membrane area and partial pressure gradient, and inversely proportional to membrane thickness. The total surface area of the pulmonary

TABLE 3-4. Values of Total and Partial Pressures for Respiratory Gases (in mmHg)

	DRY AIR	MOIST TRACHEAL AIR	ALVEOLAR GAS	ARTERIAL BLOOD	MIXED VENOUS BLOOD
PO_2	159.1	149.2	104	100	40
PCO_2	0.3	0.3	40	40	46
PH_2O	0.0	47.0	47	47	47
PN_2	600.6	563.5	569	573	573
P total	760.0	760.0	760	760	706

membrane is 50 to 100 square meters, and its thickness averages about 0.5 micrometer. The rate of diffusion is also proportional to the diffusion constant for the gas, which is proportional to the solubility of the gas and inversely proportional to the molecular weight of the gas. Since carbon dioxide has a much greater solubility, compared to oxygen, but a similar molecular weight, carbon dioxide diffuses through the pulmonary membrane far more easily than does oxygen.

Diffusing Capacity of the Lungs. The rate at which a gas will diffuse from the alveoli into the blood for each millimeter of mercury pressure difference is called the diffusing capacity of the lungs for that particular gas. The diffusing capacity of the lungs for oxygen when a person is at rest is approximately 22 ml/mmHg/min. The diffusing capacity for carbon dioxide is about 20 times this value, or approximately 440 ml/mmHg/min.

Oxygen Transport by Hemoglobin. About 97% of the oxygen is carried to the tissues in chemical combination with hemoglobin. The remaining 3% is carried to the tissues in the dissolved state in the water of the plasma and cells. Hemoglobin combines with large quantities of oxygen when the Po_2 is high, and then releases the oxygen when the Po_2 falls. Therefore, when blood passes through the lungs, where the blood Po_2 rises to 100 mmHg, hemoglobin picks up large quantities of oxygen. Then as it passes through the tissue capillaries, where the Po_2 falls to about 40 mmHg, large quantities of oxygen are released from the hemoglobin. The free oxygen then diffuses to the tissue cells.

Hemoglobin Release of Oxygen to Tissues. Hemoglobin is normally about 97% saturated, with oxygen at a normal alveolar Po_2 of 104 mmHg. If the oxygen in the alveolar air rises even as high as 1,000 mmHg, the hemoglobin can only become 100% saturated with oxygen, so that even with large increases in atmospheric oxygen, essentially the same amount of oxygen is carried by the hemoglobin to the tissues. As the blood passes through the capillaries, its Po_2 normally falls to about 40 mmHg before it enters the veins. During high metabolic activity of the tissues, this value may fall to as low as 15 to 20 mmHg.

Maximum Oxygen Transport by Hemoglobin. In a normal person, each 100 ml of blood contains about 15 of hemoglobin, and each gram of hemoglobin can bind with about 1.34 ml of oxygen when it is 100% saturated ($15 \times 1.34 = 20$ ml O_2/100 ml blood). The hemoglobin in venous blood leaving the peripheral tissues is about 75% saturated with oxygen, so the amount of oxygen transported by hemoglobin in venous blood is about 15 ml O_2/100 ml blood. Therefore, about 5 ml of oxygen is normally transported to the tissues in each 100 ml of blood.

Effects of Carbon Monoxide on Oxygen Transport. Carbon monoxide interferes with oxygen transport because it has about 250 times the affinity of oxygen for hemoglobin. For this reason, relatively small amounts of carbon monoxide can tie up a large portion of the hemoglobin, making it unavailable for oxygen transport. A patient with severe carbon monoxide poisoning can be helped by administration of pure oxygen, because oxygen at high alveolar pressures displaces carbon monoxide from its combination with hemoglobin more effectively than oxygen at low atmospheric pressures.

Carbon Dioxide Transport. About 70% of the carbon dioxide is transported to the lungs in the form of bicarbonate ions. Dissolved carbon dioxide reacts with water inside red blood cells to form ***carbonic acid.*** This reaction is catalyzed by a protein enzyme in the red cells called ***carbonic anhydrase.*** Most of the carbonic acid immediately dissociates into bicarbonate ions and hydrogen ions, the hydrogen ions in turn combining with hemoglobin. Approximately 23% of the carbon dioxide produced in the tissues combines directly with hemoglobin to form ***carbaminohemoglobin,*** and an additional 7% is transported in the dissolved state in the water of the plasma and cells. When the blood arrives in the lungs, the carbon dioxide diffuses from the blood into the alveoli, causing rapid reversal of these chemical reactions.

REGULATION OF RESPIRATION

Respiratory Rhythm. The respiratory center is located in the brain stem in the reticular substance of the medulla and the pons. This center has a basic oscillating mechanism that causes it to emit rhythmic impulses to the respiratory muscles. However, the intensity of this rhythmic excitation of respiration can be increased or decreased by changes in the chemical composition of the blood and also by sensory signals from the lungs.

Hering-Breuer Reflex. This reflex is initiated by nerve receptors that detect the degree of stretch of the lungs. When the lungs become overly inflated, the receptors send signals through the vagi into the respiratory center to inhibit inspiration and to excite expiration, thus preventing overinflation of the lungs.

Carbon Dioxide. Carbon dioxide is the most powerful blood stimulus for increasing the rate and depth of alveolar ventilation. When increased quantities of carbon dioxide are formed in the body cells and carried in the blood to the respiratory center in the brain stem, the ventilation sometimes increases to as high as ten times normal. This in turn blows off the extra quantity of carbon dioxide from the lungs.

Hydrogen Ions. Increased blood hydrogen ion concentration (*i.e.,* decreased *p*H) increases alveolar ventilation. This increase in alveolar ventilation can be as much as four times normal. The effects of blood hydrogen ion concentration on ventilation are thought to be mediated by way of peripheral chemoreceptors (discussed below) in addition to direct effects on the respiratory center.

Indirect Effect of Carbon Dioxide on Alveolar Ventilation. Carbon dioxide itself has little direct effect in stimulating the respiratory center. However, carbon dioxide reacts with water to form carbonic acid, which in turn dissociates into hydrogen and bicarbonate ions. The increase in ventilation causes increased quantities of carbon dioxide to be blown off from the blood, which in turn decreases the amount of blood carbonic acid. Since carbonic acid is in constant equilibrium with hydrogen ions of the blood, the hydrogen ion concentration also decreases back toward normal.

Effect of Carbon Dioxide on Respiratory Center. Why is it that blood carbon dioxide has a more potent effect in stimulating the respiratory center than do blood hydrogen ions? The blood-brain barrier is almost totally impermeable to hydrogen ions, so that increases in the blood hydrogen ion concentration have relatively little effect on the hydrogen ion concentration in the vicinity of the respiratory center. Carbon dioxide on the other hand permeates the blood brain barrier with ease and immediately reacts with water to form hydrogen ions. Thus, more hydrogen ions are released in the respiratory center when the blood carbon dioxide concentration increases than when the blood hydrogen ion concentration increases.

Lack of Oxygen and Rate of Alveolar Ventilation. Lack of oxygen in the blood can also increase the rate of alveolar ventilation. However, unlike the effects of carbon dioxide and hydrogen ion concentration, oxygen lack does not directly stimulate the respiratory center. Instead, it excites special nerve receptors called ***chemoreceptors*** located in minute ***carotid*** and ***aortic bodies*** that lie, respectively, in the carotid bifurcations and along the aorta. Each of these bodies has a special artery that supplies abundant amounts of arterial blood to the chemoreceptors. When the arterial oxygen concentration falls, signals from the chemoreceptors are transmitted to the respiratory center where they cause an increase in alveolar ventilation.

Relative Importance of Carbon Dioxide, Hydrogen Ions, and Oxygen Lack on Alveolar Ventilation. Stimulation of alveolar ventilation by excess carbon dioxide and low *p*H is great compared to the oxygen lack stimulus. Maximal increase in carbon dioxide can increase alveolar ventilation about tenfold; maximal increase in hydrogen ion concentration can increase it about fourfold; but maximal oxygen lack (under acute conditions) can increase alveolar ventilation only by about one and two thirds.

Why is oxygen lack a relatively poor stimulus for alveolar ventilation? One often wonders why the evolutionary processes have made oxygen lack such a poor stimulus of respiration in comparison with carbon dioxide and hydrogen ions. However, oxygen concentration in the tissues is regulated principally by the manner in which it is released from hemoglobin as discussed above, while carbon dioxide and hydrogen ion concentration is regulated almost entirely by alveolar ventilation. Therefore, there usually is less need for oxygen to control respiration than for carbon dioxide and hydrogen ion concentration to control it.

Exercise and Alveolar Ventilation. Exercise can cause alveolar ventilation to increase as much as 30-fold. This increase in alveolar ventilation is even more than the increase that occurs as a result of maximal carbon dioxide or maximal hydrogen ion stimulation. The precise cause of the greatly increased respiration during exercise has not been determined, but it is believed to result from nerve signals transmitted during exercise from other centers of the brain that provide the nervous drive for the exercise itself, and possibly from sensory signals originating in the active muscles.

PHYSIOLOGY OF RESPIRATORY DISORDERS

Hypoxia signifies insufficient availability of oxygen to support normal tissue metabolism. If the hypoxia is severe enough, it can depress mental activity, sometimes causing coma, and reduce the work capacity of the muscles. The different possible causes of hypoxia are listed in Table 3-5.

Oxygen Therapy for Hypoxia. Oxygen therapy can relieve certain types of hypoxia. This is particularly true of atmospheric hypoxia, hypoventilation hypoxia, and hypoxia caused by impaired alveolar membrane diffusion. In each of these instances, an increase in the oxy-

TABLE 3-5. Causes of Hypoxia

Inadequate Oxygenation of Normal Lung
Deficiency of oxygen in atmosphere
Hypoventilation (neuromuscular disorders)
Pulmonary Disease
Hypoventilation (airway obstruction or decreased pulmonary compliance)
Uneven alveolar ventilation/pulmonary capillary blood flow
Decreased respiratory membrane diffusion
Venous-to-Arterial Shunts ("right-to-left" cardiac shunts)
Inadequate Transport of Oxygen by Blood to Tissues
Anemia or abnormal hemoglobin
General or local circulatory deficiency
Tissue edema
Inadequate Tissue Capacity to Use Oxygen
Poisoning of cellular enzymes
Diminished cellular metabolic capacity caused by toxicity, vitamin deficiency, or other factors

gen concentration increases the P_{O_2} in the alveoli and thereby promotes increased oxygen diffusion into the blood. In other types of hypoxia, the problem is mainly diminished transport of oxygen to the tissues or diminished use of oxygen by the tissues. In these types of hypoxia, oxygen therapy may be of some benefit, but not nearly so much as in the types mentioned above.

AVIATION AND HIGH-ALTITUDE PHYSIOLOGY

Hypoxia at High Altitudes. A major problem in aviation physiology is a progressive decrease in P_{O_2} at higher and higher altitudes. A normal person often becomes lethargic and loses much mental alertness at about 12,000 to 15,000 feet. At 18,000 feet, a person can become so disoriented that judgment is lost; pilots may actually fly still higher rather than returning to a lower level to correct the hypoxic condition. And at about 23,000 feet, an unacclimatized aviator will become comatose in 20 to 30 minutes.

Breathing pure oxygen can improve tolerance to high altitude. If pure oxygen is used rather than normal air, a pilot can ascend to an altitude of about 45,000 feet before becoming hypoxic, because the oxygen replaces the nitrogen that normally fills the major amount of space in the alveoli.

Acclimatization to Hypoxia. Though an aviator almost never remains at a high altitude long enough to become adjusted to the altitude, mountain climbers often become acclimatized sufficiently that they can live and work at altitudes many thousand feet higher than normal persons. Acclimatization results from three major physiologic changes:

1. **Increased pulmonary ventilation.** The oxygen lack mechanism for control of pulmonary ventilation normally increases ventilation only about 65%, but after a person remains at high altitudes for several days, this mechanism becomes progressively more effective and increases ventilation about 400% instead of the normal 65%, thus providing much greater amounts of oxygen for the alveoli.
2. **Increase in red blood cells and hemoglobin.** When one stays at a high altitude for several weeks, the hypoxia causes greatly increased production of red blood cells by the mechanism explained earlier in the chapter, sometimes increasing the total red cell mass to as much as 80% above normal and the hematocrit to 50% above normal. This obviously increases the ability of the blood to transport oxygen to the tissues.
3. **Increased capillarity in the tissues.** Associated with the increased blood cell mass is a slight increase in the number of blood vessels in the tissues or in their sizes so that increased quantities of blood can flow through the tissues, thus again increasing the available oxygen in the tissues.

Acceleratory Forces in Aviation. Another major problem in aviation is ***centrifugal acceleration,*** which means that a person tends to be pushed in one direction or another when the airplane turns to one side or up or down. Centrifugal acceleration is of special importance when one comes out of a dive or when one goes through a tight turn. Sometimes the aviator is pressed downward against the seat of the airplane with a force many times the weight of his or her body. The normal weight of the body is said to be 1 gravity *(g),* but if the total force against the seat is two times body weight, the acceleration is 2 *g*. A person can withstand up to about 4 *g* without harm, but 5 *g* or more for only 10 seconds usually causes blackout because of ''centrifuging'' the blood out of the head and into the vessels of the legs and abdomen.

SPACE PHYSIOLOGY

Linear Acceleration and Deceleration. The problem of ***linear acceleration*** exists principally when the spaceship leaves the earth, for the ship must be accelerated to the velocity required to escape the pull of earth's gravity. Approximately the highest degree of linear acceleration developed is about 9 *g*—that is, the body is pushed backward against the seat with a force about nine times its own weight. The human body can stand 9 *g* in a horizontal or reclining position though not in the upright position. Therefore, takeoff has to be accomplished with the body horizontal to the line of takeoff. Linear ***deceleration*** occurs during reentry, and the problems are the same.

Weightlessness. The sensation of weightlessness that occurs in an orbiting spaceship is not caused by lack of gravity because gravity from earth is still active. However, the gravity pulls on the person and spaceship at the same time, and since there is no resistance to movement in space, both are pulled at exactly the same acceleratory forces, so they essentially fall together at the same speed. For this reason, the person is not attracted to the top, bottom, or sides of the spacecraft and thus simply floats in the ship.

Physiologic Problems of Weightlessness. Most of the problems are related to (1) motion sickness for the first few days of spaceflight, (2) transfer of fluid from the tissues of the lower body because the usual hydrostatic pressure gradients are absent, and (3) decreased use of skeletal muscles because the body is weightless. The effects of prolonged exposure to weightlessness include the following: decreased blood volume and red cell mass, decreased muscle strength and work capacity, decreased maximum cardiac output, and loss of calcium and phosphate from the bones with actual bone loss.

DEEP-SEA DIVING PHYSIOLOGY

Gaseous Pressures. When a person descends deep under the sea, air must be pumped into the lungs with progressively more and more pressure so that the chest can withstand the pressure of the water on the outside; otherwise, the chest would collapse. At a depth of 33 feet, the pressure must be two times normal atmospheric pressure; at 66 feet, 3 atmospheres; at 100 feet, 4 atmospheres; and so forth.

High Oxygen Pressures. High pressures of oxygen cause mental disorientation followed by irritability and possibly convulsions and coma. Other symptoms include nausea, muscle twitchings, dizziness, and visual disturbances. The cause of nervous system oxygen toxicity is thought to be increased concentrations of oxidizing free radicals, such as the superoxide free radical (O_2^-). The oxidizing free radicals cause destruction of many essential elements of the cells and thereby hamper normal metabolic processes.

High Nitrogen Pressures. Sufficient exposure to high nitrogen pressures first causes mild narcosis characterized by joviality and loss of inhibitions. This is followed by lethargy, a somnolent state, and finally total anesthesia. The mechanism of nitrogen narcosis is thought to be the same as that of other gaseous anesthetics—that is, alteration of electrical conductance of the membranes, which reduces their excitability.

Helium Replacement. The deepest sea depth that a person can survive while breathing pure air for more than an hour is about 300 feet, at which depth the pressure is 10 atmospheres. At this pressure the nitrogen narcosis effect approaches the somnolent level, and the oxygen effect approaches the convulsion level. For safety's sake, a person rarely works below 250 feet even for short periods of time when breathing compressed air. For deeper levels, the nitrogen and part of the oxygen are replaced by helium, which causes far less of the narcotic or convulsive effects of nitrogen or oxygen.

Bubble Formation on Rapid Ascent. Another major problem in deep-sea diving physiology is the tendency for divers to develop bubbles in their body fluids as they ascend from the depths. When the body is exposed to high pressure, the inert gases of the breathing mixture, such as nitrogen or helium, become dissolved in high concentrations in all of the body fluids. Then, when the person is again exposed to low pressure, these gases must diffuse out of the tissue spaces into the blood and then through the lungs into the expired air. This ''degassing'' process sometimes requires as much as 6 or more hours, and, if the pressure around the body is decreased rapidly rather than slowly, these gases will simply form bubbles in the body fluids rather than diffusing out through the lungs. Therefore, it is essential that the diver ascend from depths slowly or be decompressed slowly over a long period in a decompression chamber.

Decompression Sickness. The development of bubbles in the body fluids can cause serious damage in the tissues or can cause gas emboli in the circulating blood. Two of the most distressing effects are (1) air emboli in the pulmonary vessels, which causes the ''chokes''; and (2) disruption of nerve pathways in the nervous system, which causes serious pain or even paralysis. This condition is generally called decompression sickness, the bends, caisson disease, or diver's paralysis.

CENTRAL NERVOUS SYSTEM

BASIC ORGANIZATION OF THE CENTRAL NERVOUS SYSTEM

The nervous and endocrine systems provide most of the control systems of the body. The nervous system generally controls rapid functions of the body, such as muscle contractions, and the endocrine system mainly controls metabolic functions of the body. Three main parts of the nervous system important for controlling bodily functions include (1) the sensory system, (2) the motor system, and (3) the integrative system.

Sensory Receptors. The sensory receptors include any type of nerve ending in the body that can be stimulated by some physical or chemical stimulus originating either outside or within the body. Examples include visual receptors, auditory receptors, tactile receptors, taste receptors, and so forth. The sensory experience can produce an immediate reaction, or information can be stored for many weeks, months, or years before a final reaction takes place.

Motor System. Some of the most important motor functions include contraction of skeletal muscle, contraction of smooth muscle in the internal organs, and secretion by endocrine or exocrine glands. The muscles and glands that perform the ***motor functions*** are called ***effectors*** because they perform the motor functions dictated by the nerve signals.

Reflex Arc. A reflex arc is a complete neuronal network extending from the peripheral receptor through the central nervous system and then to the peripheral effector. Reflex arcs can be as simple as withdrawing the hand from a hot object or blinking when the cornea is touched, or they can involve more complicated actions such as coughing, sucking, sneezing, and protecting the body from the environment. Other reflexes include circulatory reflexes, digestive reflexes, sexual reflexes, and respiratory reflexes.

Integrative Centers of Nervous System. Those parts of the nervous system that put many different types of sensory signals together before causing a reaction or that first store the information and later cause a reaction are called the integrative centers of the nervous system. The brain stem is the integrative center for most respiratory control, for most nervous control of arterial pressure, and for control of swallowing; the motor area of the cerebral cortex, the cerebellum, the basal ganglia, and large parts of the reticular substance of the brain stem are major parts of the integrative centers for control of muscular movement.

FUNCTION OF THE SINGLE NEURON

The nervous system contains between 100 and 200 billion neurons, one of which is illustrated in Figure 3-16. The sum of all the actions of the single neurons determines the overall function of the brain. Therefore, it is necessary to understand the functional abilities of single neurons in order to comprehend the manner in which these operate together to give the integrative functions of the nervous system.

The Synapse. The neurons of the nervous system are arranged so that each neuron stimulates other neurons,

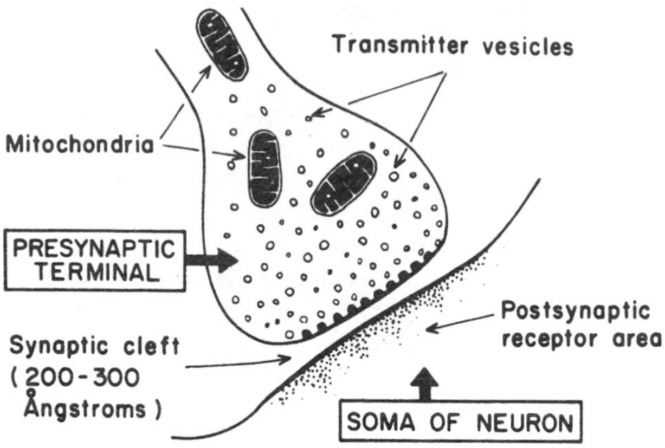

Fig. 3-17. Physiologic anatomy of the synapse. (Guyton AC: Textbook of Medical Physiology, 8th ed. Philadelphia: WB Saunders, 1991)

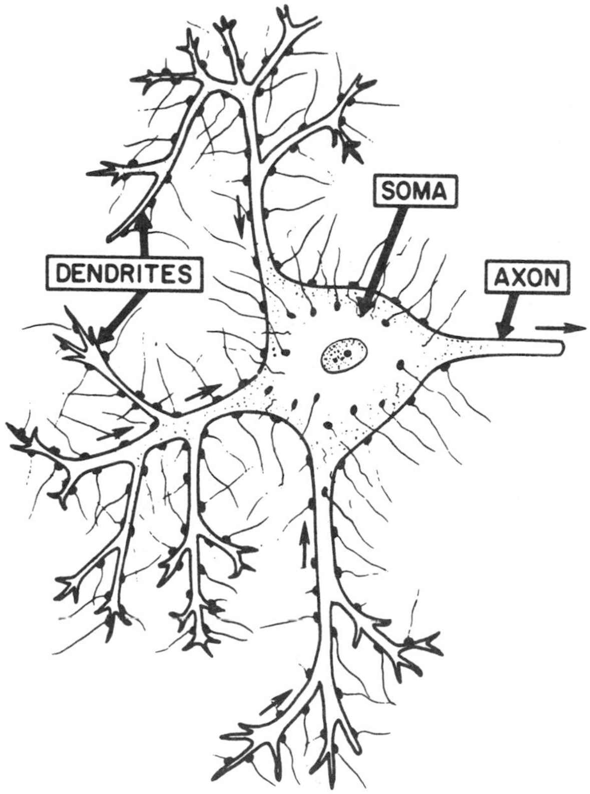

Fig. 3-16. Typical motor neuron, showing presynaptic terminals on the neuronal soma and dendrites. Note also the single axon. (Guyton AC, Hall JE: Textbook of Medical Physiology, 9th ed. Philadelphia: WB Saunders, 1995)

and these in turn stimulate still others until the functions of the nervous system are performed. The point of contact between successive neurons, illustrated in Figure 3-17, is called a synapse, and the terminal endings of the nerve filaments that synapse with the next neuron are called ***presynaptic terminals, synaptic knobs, boutons,*** or simply ***end feet.*** Usually, there are many thousand presynaptic terminals on each neuron, these having originated from preceding neurons. Each terminal secretes a particular transmitter substance that may either excite the next neuron or inhibit it. These substances are called ***excitatory*** or ***inhibitory transmitters.***

Transmitter Substances. More than 40 different types of chemical substances have been postulated to act as synaptic transmitters. Each presynaptic terminal generally secretes one characteristic transmitter substance, but often more than one. Each transmitter is synthesized within the terminal and stored in thousands of small vesicles. When an action potential spreads over the end of the nerve fiber, the depolarization of the terminal causes migration of a few of the vesicles to the membrane surface of the terminal, and these vesicles then extrude their contents of transmitter substance into the synaptic cleft between the terminal and the membrane of the succeeding neuron. The transmitter then combines with a receptor (a protein molecule) that is an integral part of the subsequent neuronal membrane. This opens a channel through the receptor in the membrane and allows ions to move through the channel.

Excitatory and Inhibitory Receptors. If the receptor is ***excitatory,*** it opens sodium channels, allowing sodium ions to move selectively to the inside of the membrane, which partially depolarizes the neuron and therefore stimulates it. In the case of the ***inhibitory receptor,*** the channels become permeable to chloride and potassium ions. Movement of these ions through the membrane ***hy-***

perpolarizes the neuron (makes the inside of the membrane more negative), and this inhibits the neuron rather than exciting it. Whether a given transmitter substance will be excitatory or inhibitory depends on both the transmitter and the nature of the receptor. Some transmitters can be either excitatory or inhibitory, depending on the type of receptor with which they bind. However, other transmitters are almost always either inhibitory or excitatory.

Acetylcholine as Classical Excitatory Transmitter. Acetylcholine is released by a large number of presynaptic terminals in the central nervous system. Acetylcholine stimulates the successive neuron in exactly the same way that it stimulates a muscle fiber at the neuromuscular junction, that is, by increasing the permeability of the neuronal membrane to sodium. Sodium leaks rapidly to the interior of the cell, causing a sudden loss of electrical potential across the membrane (*i.e.,* causing depolarization). Other transmitter substances that often function as excitatory transmitters include norepinephrine, epinephrine, glutamic acid, enkephalin, and substance P. However, some of these also function as inhibitory transmitters in the presence of inhibitory receptor types.

Gamma Aminobutyric Acid (GABA) and Glycine as Classical Inhibitory Transmitters. Other transmitters that sometimes but not always serve as inhibitory transmitters (in the presence of inhibitory receptors) include norepinephrine, epinephrine, serotonin, and dopamine. Synapses terminating on the presynaptic neuron, called presynaptic terminals, secrete inhibitory transmitters rather than excitatory transmitters. In fact, there are many more inhibitory synapses in the central nervous system than most individuals might imagine, for the function of large parts of the brain, including the cerebral cortex, the basal ganglia, the thalamus, and the cerebellum, depend almost as much on inhibition of neurons as upon excitation. It is probable that as many as a third or even more of the synapses are of the inhibitory type rather than of the excitatory type.

FUNCTIONS OF "POOLS" OF NEURONS

Each part of the brain usually contains large numbers of similar types of neurons that lie close to each other and are interconnected by means of many fine nerve filaments. Each such group of neurons is called a ***neuronal pool.*** Different patterns of nerve filament interconnections exist in different pools, and the type of pattern in turn determines the manner in which the pool operates in the overall function of the brain. In general, three basic types of circuits occur in neuronal pools: (1) the diverging circuit, (2) the converging circuit, and (3) repetitive firing circuits.

Diverging Circuit. This circuit is the simplest of all that occur in the neuronal pools. The nerve fibers entering the pool divide many times so that a few nerve fibers entering the pool branch many times and excite many different new neurons, causing a large number of impulses to leave the pool.

The diverging circuit is typified by the nervous control of muscular activity. Stimulation of a single large neuron in the motor cortex can stimulate many interneurons in the spinal cord, and these in turn might then stimulate as many as 50 to 100 anterior motor neurons, which in turn stimulate thousands of muscle fibers.

Converging Circuit. A converging circuit is one that, after receiving incoming signals from several sources, determines the level of reaction that will occur. That is, impulses "converge" into the pool, some from inhibitory nerves, some from excitatory nerves, some from peripheral nerves, and some from parts of the brain.

The overall response of a converging circuit depends on multiple factors. These are (1) the basic excitability of the neurons in the pool, (2) the number of excitatory impulses entering the pool, (3) the number of inhibitory impulses entering the pool, (4) whether there might be some diverging circuits also in the pool, (5) the distribution of excitatory and inhibitory impulses to the different neurons, and so forth. From this list of possible factors that can affect the output from the neuronal pool, one can readily understand that basic differences in the anatomic organization of different neuronal pools can give thousands of different responses to incoming signals.

Thresholds of Neuronal Pools. A pool may have a high threshold into which many excitatory impulses must arrive before an effect will occur. It might be a low threshold pool into which only a few impulses must arrive before an effect will occur. The low-threshold circuit is typified by the neuronal response that causes withdrawal of a limb when only a few pain receptors are stimulated, while the high-threshold circuit is typified by withdrawal of a hand only when tremendous numbers of touch receptors are stimulated.

Repetitive Firing Circuit. In a repetitive firing circuit the neuronal pool emits a series of impulses lasting long after the incoming signal is over. This is among the most important types of circuits in the nervous system. Three types of circuits can cause this: The first is a pool of neurons consisting of very excitable neurons, each one of which has a natural tendency to fire repetitively. The second is a ***long chain of neurons*** arranged one after another so that an incoming stimulus activates each one in succession. From each neuron of the chain a nerve fiber extends to some outlying neuron. Thus, this outlying neuron receives repetitive impulses from the successive neurons of the chain, but after all these have fired, the repetitive firing from the output neuron ceases. The third is the reverberating circuit discussed below.

Reverberating Circuit. In a reverberating circuit an incoming impulse is passed along a succession of neurons until one of the neurons restimulates an earlier neuron in the succession. This is probably the most important type of repetitive firing circuit. The impulse goes around the reverberating circuit again and again. Every time around the circuit, collateral impulses are emitted into outgoing nerve fibers that spread to other parts of the nervous system. Theoretically, this type of circuit might continue to oscillate indefinitely, but more usually the oscillation ceases when some of the neurons in the circuit become too fatigued to continue. The continual respiratory rhythm represents a continually reverberating circuit, while the thought processes of the cerebral cortex probably represent circuits that reverberate for short periods until neurons in the circuit fatigue or are inhibited so that the thought ceases.

To summarize, the nervous system is actually made up of many neuronal pools, each of which has specific circuit characteristics that allow it to emit a certain pattern of output impulses in response to incoming signals. By combining the functional characteristics of the many different pools in the nervous system, one can achieve almost any type of integrative function in one portion of the nervous system or another.

THE PROCESS OF CEREBRATION

Thoughts. The bases of cerebration are the individual thoughts, many of which occur directly as a result of incoming sensory impulses. For instance, the impulses from the eyes when a person is looking at a beautiful scene, certainly generate a number of different thoughts. The precise mechanisms of thoughts in the brain are not understood, but one of the suggestions is that a thought represents a pattern of impulses passing through particular neurons in multiple simultaneous areas of the conscious brain.

Memory. Memory is believed to result from permanent facilitation of synapses. This means simply that excitation of a synapse repetitively over a time will cause that synapse to become more and more effective in stimulating the neuron. In other words, the fact that an impulse passes through a synapse once makes it easier for successive impulses to pass through the same synapse. Therefore, if a thought pattern is evoked over and over by incoming sensory stimuli, eventually the pathway for transmission of impulses through that particular thought channel becomes facilitated so that even the slightest stimulus entering this pathway at a later time can elicit the entire thought. For instance, such a facilitated thought pathway might develop in response to seeing the beautiful scene referred to above. Then a year later, some stray impulse from another part of the brain might enter this particular thought pathway and allow the person to see the scene again in his or her mind. This is believed to be the basis of memory.

Cerebral Cortex and Memory. The cerebral cortex is the portion of the brain most concerned with memory. All through the cerebral cortex are located neuronal pools that can be facilitated by sensory impulses so that subsequent signals entering these pools will evoke specific reactions. The storage of information in the brain is mostly lost when the cortex is gone.

Experiments in lower animals have demonstrated one possible type of memory circuit. When repetitive signals are passed through the synapses of the brain's memory system, the surface areas of the activated presynaptic terminals grow larger; also, increased numbers of synaptic vesicles appear adjacent to the new presynaptic membrane area. Therefore, at any later time when still newer signals enter the same neuronal pathway, far greater quantities of synaptic transmitter are secreted into the synaptic cleft. Obviously, this enhances the sensitivity of the memory pathway and allows one to reactivate the memory circuit with ease.

Programming of Thoughts. Everyone is familiar with the fact that different thoughts usually occur in rapid succession, and that each succeeding thought usually has some association with the preceeding thought. Many sequences of thoughts are initiated by incoming sensory signals, whether these originate from the skin, from the eyes, from the ears, and so forth. For instance, a sudden knife cut on the leg would elicit first a thought of pain, then another thought that localizes the cut on the body, this followed by integrative processes that make the person turn the eyes and head to look at the pained area, followed by visual input impulses that combine with the previous thoughts to determine the nature of the stimulus causing the pain, and, finally, a series of integrations that cause motor movements to remove the painful object from the body. In this sequence of cerebration, the person must call forth memories from past experiences in order to understand why and how the leg is being pained, for, if he or she has never seen a knife before and is not familiar with its cutting capabilities, simply looking at the leg and seeing a knife against the skin will not explain the cause of the pain. In short, for cerebration to occur, the thoughts must be programmed.

Some part of the brain must determine where the attention of the mind will be directed. That is, whether the mind will be directed to the incoming sensory signals from the leg, to the movement of the head and the eyes, or to one of the memory circuits to call forth information. The nature of this programming system of the brain is still unclear. However, the anatomic locations of the thalamus and the reticular substance of the mesencephalon have made many neurophysiologists point to these two areas as possible programming centers. Also, stimulation of specific points in these two areas causes highly specific patterns of reaction to occur in other parts of the brain and cord.

THE SOMATIC SENSORY SYSTEM

The general plan for transmission of sensory signals from all parts of the body into the central nervous system is illustrated in Figure 3-18. The five basic types of sensory receptors are listed below.

Mechanoreceptors detect various mechanical stimuli, with some receptors responding to high-frequency vibrations and others to constant pressure.

Thermoreceptors can be subdivided into warm receptors and cold receptors that respond to a respective rise or fall in temperature.

Nociceptors (pain receptors) detect physical or chemical damage occurring in the tissues.

Electromagnetic receptors detect light on the retina of the eye.

Chemoreceptors detect taste, smell, oxygen level, carbon dioxide level, osmolarity in body fluids, and other chemical substances.

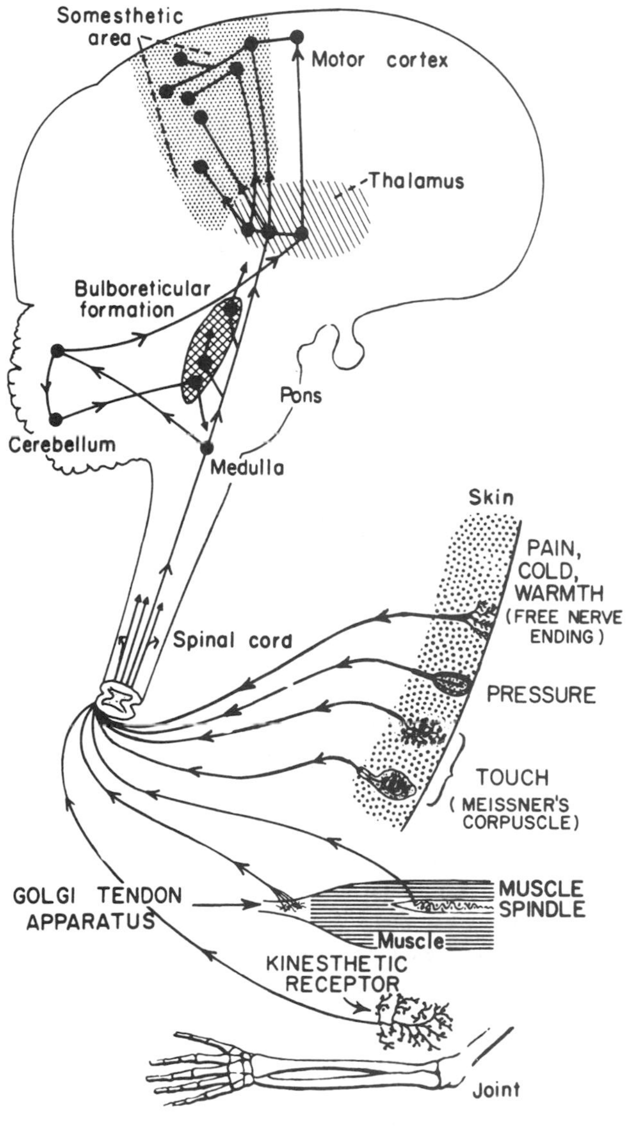

Fig. 3-18. The somatic sensory system. (Guyton AC: Textbook of Medical Physiology, 8th ed. Philadelphia: WB Saunders, 1991)

The Free Nerve Ending. The most common type of sensory receptor is the free nerve ending. The free nerve ending, illustrated in Figure 3-18, is nothing more than a filamentous end of a nerve usually interwoven with other filamentous nerve endings. Different types of free nerve endings can transmit relatively crude sensations such as pain, crude touch, tickle, heavy pressure, and temperature. In addition to the free nerve endings, the skin contains a number of specialized endings that are adapted to respond to some specific type of physical stimulus. For instance, one of these endings, called a ***Meissner's corpuscle,*** is most numerous in the skin over the fingertips and responds specifically to light touch.

Proprioceptive Sensations. Proprioceptive sensations are detected by specialized sensory receptors. These include ***joint receptors,*** which detect the degree of angulation of the joints; ***pacinian corpuscles,*** which detect high-frequency vibration and very rapid changes in pressure; ***Golgi tendon apparatuses,*** which detect the degree of tension in the tendons; and ***muscle spindles,*** which detect the degree of elongation of the muscle fibers. In general, the proprioceptive impulses are transmitted by ***large type A nerve fibers*** that can transmit at velocities as high as 100 m per second. This rapid velocity is especially important when a person is moving rapidly, for the nervous system needs to know during each split second the positions of all parts of the body.

The Labeled-Line Law. Each type of sensory nerve fiber transmits only one modality of sensation—the Labeled-Line Law. ''Modality'' of sensation means the particular type of sensation felt, such as pain, touch, temperature, pressure, and so forth. If a sensory nerve fiber is stimulated by an electrical stimulus, a person will perceive only one particular modality of sensation. For instance, excitation of a pain fiber will cause pain, and excitation of a warmth fiber will cause the sensation of warmth.

Modalities of Sensation. It is not the type of receptor that determines the modality of sensation transmitted, but, instead, it is the point in the central nervous system to which the fiber from the receptor connects that determines the modality. For instance, pain fibers end in a slightly different point in the thalamus from the warmth fibers, and in a different point from the cold fibers.

Transmission of Somatic Sensory Signals. The impulses generated in the sensory receptors are transmitted first into the spinal nerves and then through the dorsal roots of the spinal nerves into the spinal cord. The nervous signals are then carried up the spinal cord by way of the ***dorsal column–medial lemniscal system*** or the ***anterolateral system,*** depending on the origin of the sensory signal.

The dorsal column–medial lemniscal system is composed of large, myelinated nerve fibers that transmit signals to the brain at velocities ranging from 30 to 110 m/sec. The anterolateral system is composed of much smaller myelinated fibers and can only transmit signals at lower velocities. The dorsal column–medial lemniscal system also has a much higher degree of spatial orientation with respect to the origin of the nerve signals on the surface of the body. A special feature of the anterolateral system is the capability to transmit a broad spectrum of sensory modalities, such as pain, warmth, cold, crude tactile sensations, tickle and itch, and sexual sensations. The dorsal column–medial lemniscal system transmits position sensations and more refined pressure and touch sensations.

Localization of Somatic Sensory Signals. Since some modalities of sensation, such as pain and temperature sensations, can still be perceived even when the sensory portions of the cerebral cortex are removed, it is believed that sensory centers in the brain stem and the thalamus can determine at least some of the different sensory modalities. On the other hand, a person cannot localize sensations in different parts of his or her body accurately when the sensory portions of the cerebral cortex have been destroyed. Therefore, discrete localization is principally a function of the somatic sensory cortex, though the thalamus by itself is capable of crude localization to general areas of the body.

PAIN

Stimulation of Pain Fibers. Pain fibers are stimulated any time a tissue is being damaged or being overstressed. However, once the damage is complete, the pain sensation generally disappears in a few minutes or sometimes even in a few seconds. Pain nerve endings can be stimulated by mechanical trauma to the tissues; excess heat; excess cold; chemical damage; certain types of radiation damage, such as the pain associated with sunburn; and even lack of adequate blood flow to a tissue area, which causes ischemic pain.

Control of Pain Pathways. The brain controls the sensitivity of pain pathways by sending centrifugal inhibitory signals from the brain to the brain stem and spinal cord to control pain signal transmission. The analgesia system consists of three main components. Neurons from the ***periaqueductal gray area*** surrounding the aqueduct of Sylvius in the mesencephalon and upper pons send signals to the ***raphe magnus nucleus*** located in the lower pons and upper medulla. The signals are then transmitted to a ***pain inhibitory complex*** located in the dorsal horns of the spinal cord where the analgesia signals can block pain before it is relayed to the brain.

Enkephalin and Serotonin. Enkephalin and serotonin are transmitter substances involved in the analgesia system. Nerve fibers derived from the periaqueductal gray area secrete enkephalin at their terminations in the raphe magnus nucleus. Fibers originating in the raphe magnus nucleus secrete serotonin at their endings in the dorsal horns of the spinal cord, which in turn excite other dorsal horn neurons to secrete enkephalin; the enkephalin then acts on the pain-conducting neurons to block the pain signals.

Visceral Pain. Visceral pain usually occurs only on stimulation of pain endings over a wide area. Internal organs of the body have a sparse supply of pain endings compared to the skin and are relatively insensitive to a sharp knife cut since there are insufficient pain endings in any minute area to cause pain. Therefore, in general, sharp pain is much less likely to occur from the viscera than is the generalized aching or burning type of pain, and the pain usually occurs only on stimulation of pain endings over a wide area. However, this is not true in the periosteum of the bones, in the walls of the arteries, in the parietal pleura, and in the parietal peritoneum; these areas are almost equally as susceptible to pain as the skin.

Visceral pain can be caused by many types of stimuli. The different types of stimuli that are particularly prone to cause visceral pain are (1) overdistension of a hollow organ, (2) spasm of the smooth muscle of an organ, (3) too little blood flow to an organ, and (4) chemical damage such as that produced by spillage of acid gastric juice into the peritoneal cavity through a ruptured peptic ulcer.

Referred Pain. Pain in a visceral organ is not always felt directly over the organ itself, but may be referred to a distant area of the body. For instance, pain originating in the heart is often felt mainly in the left arm or shoulder. This is called referred pain. Referred pain usually results from collateral neuronal connections between the visceral pain fibers and the somatic pain pathways in the cord, the visceral impulses exciting the somatic pathways and the person localizing the pain in some nonvisceral part of the body.

SPINAL CORD REFLEXES

Many central nervous system functions occur locally in the spinal cord without the aid of the brain. The cord especially integrates many specific reflexes that help to control muscle movements.

Stretch Reflex. The stretch reflex utilizes the muscle spindle to prevent the length of a muscle from changing rapidly. The stretch reflex is elicited by stretching the muscle. In its simplest form, the stretch reflex involves only two neurons, the sensory neuron from the muscle spindle to the anterior motor neuron and the anterior motor neuron back to the muscle. Stretch of the muscle spindle increases the number of impulses transmitted by the spindle, and this increases the number of impulses transmitted by the anterior motor neuron back to the muscle. Therefore, muscle stretch enhances the contractile tension in the muscle. This tension in turn tends to shorten the muscle back to its initial length. Thus, the stretch reflex opposes changes in muscle length.

The stretch reflex has both a dynamic and a static component. These are called respectively the ***dynamic stretch reflex*** and the ***static stretch reflex.*** The dynamic effect occurs only when the muscle is stretched rapidly because the spindles are very strongly stimulated during the actual instant of stretching; the strong signal from the spindle causes extreme feedback contraction of the muscle to oppose the sudden stretch. The static stretch reflex is much weaker than the dynamic reflex, but it maintains muscle contraction for minutes or hours when the muscle remains stretched beyond its normal length.

Signals from the brain stem can alter the overall reactivity of the muscles. The muscle spindles themselves are provided with excitatory nerve fibers from the spinal cord called ***gamma efferent fibers,*** and these in turn are controlled by signals from the reticular formation of the brain stem. Impulses transmitted through the gamma fibers can increase the degree of activity of the muscle spindle and therefore can also increase the intensity of either the dynamic stretch reflex or the static reflex.

Muscle spindles continually send impulses into the spinal cord to excite the anterior motor neurons; these in turn transmit impulses back to the respective muscle. This continual flow of impulses helps to maintain muscle tone.

Withdrawal Reflexes. Withdrawal reflexes function to move any pained part of the body away from the object causing the pain. For instance, if the hand is placed on a hot stove, impulses are transmitted from the pain receptors to the cord and immediately back to the flexor muscles of the arm to withdraw the hand. Because the flexor muscles are involved in this instance, this particular withdrawal reflex is called a ***flexor reflex.*** Part of the withdrawal response involves impulses transmitted to the opposite side of the body to extend the opposite limb, thereby pushing the whole body away from the vicinity of the painful object. This extensor effect is called the ***crossed extensor reflex.***

Positive Supportive Reflex. Pressure on the bottoms of the feet causes the extensor muscles of the legs to tighten, which helps the legs to support the weight of the body against gravity. This reflex is integrated entirely in the few segments of the spinal cord that control the activity of each respective limb.

Walking Movements. In an opossum with a transection in the thorax, the hind limbs can "walk" but without coordination with the movements of the forelimbs. If the cord is transected in the neck, rhythmic to-and-fro coordinated walking movements among all four limbs can occur. Occasionally, trotting movements also occur and, very rarely, galloping movements. However, with a neck transection, equilibrium cannot be maintained, so that the animal cannot actually make forward progression.

The basic patterns for walking and other movements of locomotion are integrated in the spinal cord. The nerve fiber tracts that coordinate the functions of the superior and the inferior segments of the cord are the ***propriospinal fiber pathways*** that lie near the cord gray matter and account for approximately one half of all the fiber tracts in the cord.

FUNCTIONS OF THE BRAIN STEM

Support Against Gravity. Even though the spinal cord is capable of providing the positive supportive reflex that helps to support the body against gravity and also of supplying walking reflexes, the human body still cannot stand and certainly cannot walk without the aid of higher central nervous system centers. With progression from lower phylogenetic types to the higher types of animals, more and more of the control systems have gradually shifted from the cord toward the brain. As stated above, a lower animal, such as an opossum, can still walk quite well with its hind limbs, even when its spinal cord is transected in the thorax. In the dog, basic walking movements can occur in the hind limbs with the thoracic cord transected, but these cannot be coordinated sufficiently to provide functional walking. In the human being, even these walking reflexes are crude when the cord is cut.

Vestibular and Reticular Nuclei of Brain Stem. The vestibular and reticular nuclei transmit impulses especially to the extensor muscles, tightening the muscles of the trunk, the buttocks, the thighs, and the lower legs to allow the body to stand in an upright position. Therefore, it is frequently said that the brain stem supplies the nervous energy required for supporting the body against gravity.

The Vestibular Apparatus. Closely associated with the support of the body against gravity is the maintenance of equilibrium. The vestibular and reticular nuclei of the brain stem can vary the degree of tension in the different extensor muscles in proportion to the need for maintenance of equilibrium. To do this, these nuclei in turn are controlled by the vestibular apparatuses located on the two sides of the head in close association with the ears.

Vestibular Receptor Systems. One of the receptor systems of the vestibular apparatus is the maculae of the utricle and saccule. The maculae contain large numbers of small calcified crystals called ***otoliths,*** which lie on "hairs" projecting from sensory receptor cells called ***hair cells.*** Leaning of the head to one side or forward or backward causes these otoliths to fall toward the direction of leaning, thus bending the hairs. Because the different hair cells are oriented in all of the different directions, this bending of the hairs causes signals to be transmitted into the brain informing the brain of the position of the head in relation to the direction of gravitational pull.

Another receptor system of the vestibular apparatus is the semicircular ducts. This system consists of three circular ducts on each side of the head. Each of the ducts is oriented in one of the three planes of space. The ducts are filled with fluid so that any time the head rotates in any plane, inertia of the fluid causes it to move through one or more of the ducts and thereby to stimulate hair cells located in the ***ampullae*** of the semicircular ducts. Thus, rotating movements of the head are also made known to the nervous system.

INTEGRATION OF SENSORY AND MOTOR FUNCTIONS IN THE CEREBRAL CORTEX

Signals from each type of sensory receptor are transmitted to a specific area of the cerebral cortex.

Somatic sensations are relayed by the thalamus directly to the somatic sensory cortex located anteriorly in the parietal lobes.

Visual sensations are relayed from the optic tract by the lateral geniculate bodies of the thalamus directly to the visual cortex in the calcarine fissure area of the occipital lobes.

Auditory impulses from the auditory nerves are relayed by the medial geniculate bodies of the thalamus to the auditory cortex in the central portion of the superior temporal gyri.

Taste impulses are relayed through the nuclei of the tractus solitarius and the thalamus to a small area of the cerebral cortex deep in the fissure of Sylvius.

Olfactory sensations are relayed to the amygdala (a subcortical mass of neurons in the anterior temporal lobe) and the pyriform area of the cortex.

Spatial Orientation of Sensory Information. Spatial orientation of sensory information is maintained in the cerebral cortex. In the visual system each minute area of the retina is connected directly to a minute area of the visual cortex. In the somatic sensory system each point on the surface of the body connects with a specific point in the somatic sensory cortex, as illustrated in Figure 3-19, so that stimulation of a finger, for instance, will excite only a minute area of the cortex. In the auditory cortex certain sound frequencies stimulate one portion of the auditory cortex, while others stimulate other portions.

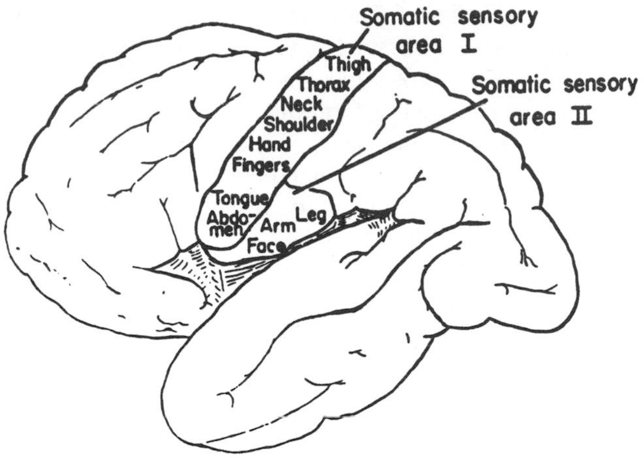

Fig. 3-19. Localization of sensory perception in the cerebral cortex. (Guyton AC: Textbook of Medical Physiology, 8th ed. Philadelphia: WB Saunders, 1991)

Memories of Past Sensory Associations. Located immediately adjacent to the primary sensory areas are the sensory association areas, which receive direct communications from the primary sensory areas. In the sensory association areas many memories of past sensory associations are stored, and here the new information arriving from the primary sensory areas is compared with information that has been stored from the past. In this way the significance of the new sensory signals is determined. For instance, when a person hears a word, he or she will not know that it is a word unless memory of that word has been stored in the auditory association areas. Likewise, when a person sees an airplane, the primary visual cortex is unable to determine the nature of the object, but, on transmission of appropriate information into the visual association areas, the person becomes aware that she is seeing an object that she has seen before and classifies it as an airplane. Similar functions are performed by somatic, taste, and smell association areas.

Wernicke's Area. Brain surgeons have found that destruction of the posterior part of the superior gyrus of the temporal lobe, called ***Wernicke's area,*** in the left hemisphere of the right-handed person will destroy the ability to put together information from the different sensory association areas and thereby determine the overall meaning. For this reason, this region of the brain has been called the ***gnostic center,*** which means simply the "knowing center." This area is well located for this purpose because it lies at the juncture of the temporal, the parietal, and the occipital lobes in very close association with most of the sensory association areas of the cortex.

Wernicke's area is necessary for ideomotor function of the brain. Once all the information from the different sensory association areas has been integrated into a distinct conscious meaning, the brain then decides what type of physical reaction should occur—from no reaction at all to very violent reaction. This is called the ideomotor function of the brain. Again, in neurosurgical patients it has been found that damage to Wernicke's area will cause a person to lose ideomotor ability. After all sensory information is put together, appropriate signals are then sent to the motor portion of the brain, which in turn causes muscular movements.

THE MOTOR PATHWAYS

The motor axis of the nervous system for controlling skeletal muscle contraction is shown in Figure 3-20. Muscle contraction can be controlled at many different levels in the central nervous system. These include the spinal cord, the reticular substance of the brain stem, the basal ganglia, the cerebellum, and the motor cortex.

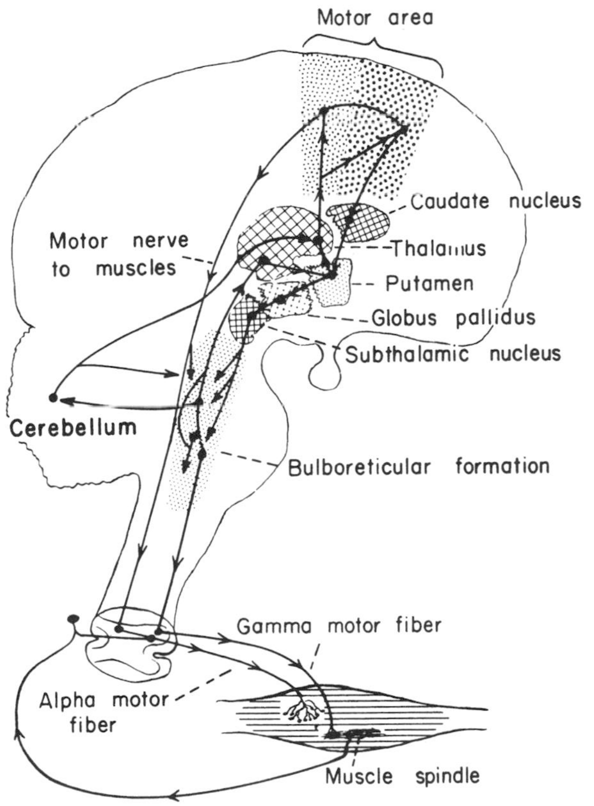

Fig. 3-20. The motor nervous system. (Guyton AC: Textbook of Medical Physiology, 8th ed. Philadelphia: WB Saunders, 1991)

Somatotopic Organization of Motor Cortex. The motor cortex is somatotopically organized. In other words, there is point-to-point communication between the primary motor cortex and specific muscles everywhere in the body. The primary motor cortex is a strip of the cortex averaging about 2 cm in width and lying horizontally all the way across the cortex, located immediately in front of the central sulcus of the brain. Stimulation of discrete points in the primary motor cortex will cause contraction of discrete muscles in the body. For instance, stimulation of the primary motor cortex at a point on top of the brain where it dips into the longitudinal fissure will cause contraction of a leg muscle on the opposite side of the body, while stimulation of the primary motor cortex where it begins to dip into the fissure of Sylvius will contract a muscle somewhere on the opposite side of the face.

The thumb, finger, mouth, and throat muscles are represented to the greatest extent in the motor cortex. Stimulation of a small area of the motor cortex might cause a large group of muscles in the trunk to contract, whereas stimulation of the same amount of cortical tissue in the mouth area might cause only one small muscle to contract. The degree of representation of the mouth and throat and also of the thumb and fingers is as much as 100 times that of the trunk muscles. This high level of representation allows the cerebral cortex to control with extreme fidelity the movement of the hands, and the special representation of the mouth and throat accounts for the ability of the human being to talk.

Pyramidal Tract. The ***pyramidal tract*** (corticospinal tract) is the most important output pathway from the motor cortex. In the primary motor cortex of each hemisphere are some 30,000 large neuronal cells called ***pyramidal*** or ***Betz cells.*** Fibers from these cells pass downward through the ***pyramidal tracts*** all the way into the spinal cord. This means that in human beings some of the axons must be over 1 m long. The majority of pyramidal axons cross in the brain stem to the contralateral side and end on ***interneurons*** located in the posterolateral gray matter of the cord.

Extrapyramidal Pathways. Unlike the pyramidal pathways, the ***extrapyramidal pathways*** do not cross to the contralateral side and have one or more synapses along their route to the spinal cord. Another important difference is that the extrapyramidal motor pathways originate not only in the motor cortex but also in other brain structures such as the cerebellum and the vestibular nuclei. Extrapyramidal pathways are thought to transmit many of the stereotyped and subconscious movements of the body.

Premotor Cortex. Located anterior to the motor cortex is still another strip averaging about 2.5 cm in width called the premotor cortex. Stimulation of a discrete point in the premotor cortex usually does not cause contraction of a discrete muscle but, instead, causes a "pattern" of muscle contraction. That is, it might cause the whole arm to rise upward, or it might cause the whole hand to flex forward, or stimulation of still another point might cause the thumb and the forefinger to move toward each other as if cutting with scissors.

Perhaps not more than a few hundred different patterns of movement are stored in the normal premotor cortex. However, considering the thousands to millions of different combinations into which these patterns of movement can be organized, even this small number of movements could allow almost any type of activity. It is believed that the ideomotor function of the cortex from Wernicke's area controls the sequence of patterns of movement.

FUNCTION OF THE BASAL GANGLIA

The basal ganglia are an accessory motor system that function in close association with the cerebral cortex and pyramidal system. Major portions of the basal ganglia include the caudate nucleus, the putamen, and the globus pallidus; physiologically related structures include the subthalamus and substantia nigra. The basal ganglia have very extensive neuronal connections with the premotor and primary motor portions of the cortex, with the somatic sensory cortex, with the thalamus, and with some nuclei of the brain stem. They have four clinical functions.

Patterns of Movements. The basal ganglia in association with the premotor and the motor cortex operate to help control most of the patterns of movements. Damage to certain areas of the basal ganglia will cause abnormal and often continuous movements such as choreiform movements, writhing movements, and so forth.

Degree of Activity. The basal ganglia help to control the basal degree of activity of the entire motor system. Damage to certain areas of the basal ganglia can cause portions of the motor system to become greatly overexcitable, resulting in intense tonic contraction of either localized portions of the body or of the whole body. This results in a state of rigidity.

Movements of Postural Muscles. The basal ganglia operate in conjunction with the nuclei of the brain stem to damp the antagonistic movements of the postural muscles. For instance, if an extensor muscle should attempt to extend a limb, this would immediately elicit certain proprioceptive reflexes that would make flexor muscles tend to contract. This in turn would tend to make the extensor muscles contract again, and, as a result, a continuous state of oscillation would develop. However, this effect is normally damped by some of the lower basal ganglia so that antagonistic movements throughout the body are normally very smooth rather than tremorous. But in patients who have ***Parkinson's disease,*** which results from damage to the ***substantia nigra,*** one of the brain stem nuclei connected with the basal ganglia, a continuous tremor exists between the antagonistic pairs of muscles either in the entire body or in certain affected areas.

Voluntary Muscle Activity. The basal ganglia become activated before the primary motor cortex when a person performs voluntary muscle activity. Other studies have shown that, before the onset of muscle activity, portions of the sensory cortex also become activated, even before the basal ganglia. Therefore, a suggested scheme to explain voluntary motor activity is: First, the nature of the motor act is probably conceived in the sensory cortex. Then signals are sent to the middle regions of the brain's motor system such as the basal ganglia, the reticular formation in the brain stem, and even the cerebellum to initiate the more gross aspects of the motor act. Finally, the primary motor cortex is called into play to control the more discrete actions of the peripheral parts of the body, such as the hands, fingers, and feet.

FUNCTION OF THE CEREBELLUM

The cerebellum helps the motor system to stop when the mission has been accomplished. The cerebellum receives collateral signals from the pyramidal and extrapyramidal fibers whenever they are stimulated by the primary motor cortex, by the premotor cortex, and by the basal ganglia, and it also receives impulses from proprioceptor nerves originating in all peripheral parts of the body. Thus, every time a motor movement is instituted by the brain, the cerebellum receives direct information of the projected movement from the cerebrum and receives information from the peripheral parts of the body telling it whether the movement has been accomplished and how much so. Putting these different types of information together, the cerebellum helps the motor system to stop the movements when the mission has been accomplished. To do this, the cerebellum performs two basic functions.

1. **Predictive function.** From the proprioceptor impulses the cerebellum can tell how rapidly a part of the body is moving and from this can predict when the part will get to a desired position. As it approaches the appropriate point, impulses are transmitted from the cerebellum through the thalamus to the motor cortex and basal ganglia, there initiating the motor signals that stop the movement.
2. **Damping function.** The damping function of the cerebellum is closely associated with the predictive function. By starting to stop the movement of a limb before it gets to the desired point, the momentum of the limb will not carry it beyond its intended position. However, if the cerebellum has been destroyed,

the momentum will carry the limb beyond the position. Then the other areas of the brain attempt to bring it back again to the desired position, but again the limb overshoots, and this continues several times until the intended movement is finally accomplished.

Intention Tremor. Cerebellar damage can cause tremors very similar to those resulting from basal ganglia damage. However, there is one particular difference: The basal ganglia tremor continues almost all the time when the person is awake, while the cerebellar tremor occurs only during movements associated with specific voluntary motor acts such as intentional movement of the hand from one point to another. In other words, cerebellar damage produces an ***intention tremor.***

Control of Rapid Motor Movements. Failure of the predictive and the damping functions of the cerebellum causes a person to walk with ataxic movements, causes hand movements to be jerky if they are performed rapidly, and even causes speech to become dysarthric, which means that some sounds are overemphasized or held too long while other sounds are underemphasized to such an extent that the words are frequently unintelligible. It should be emphasized, though, that a person without a cerebellum can still perform most functions, even with precision, if he or she performs them very, very slowly. Therefore, the cerebellum is a system for helping to control rapid motor movements while they are actually occurring, keeping them precise despite rapidity of movement.

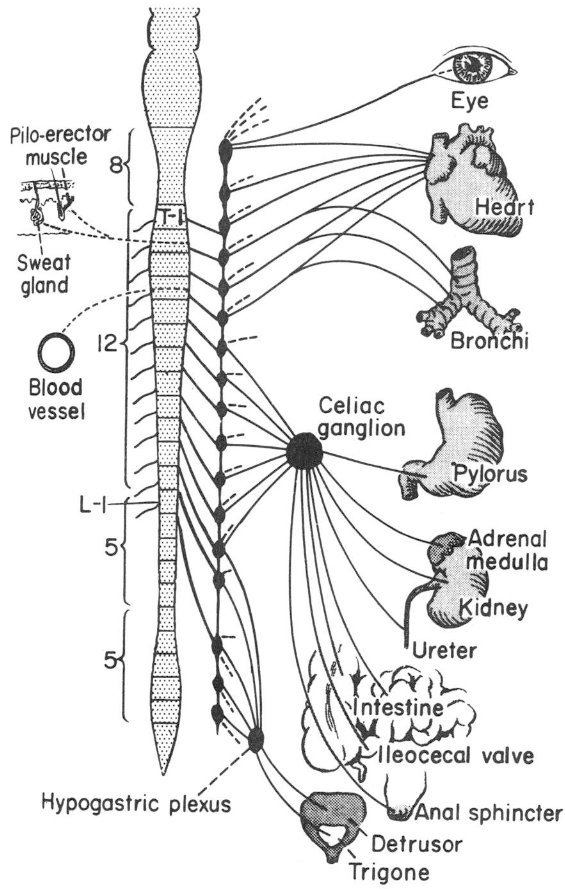

Fig. 3-21. The sympathetic nervous system. (Guyton AC: Textbook of Medical Physiology, 8th ed. Philadelphia: WB Saunders, 1991)

AUTONOMIC NERVOUS SYSTEM

The motor impulses from the central nervous system to the visceral portions of the body are transmitted differently from those to the skeletal muscles. These pass through two different divisions of the autonomic nervous system called the sympathetic and the parasympathetic systems, which are illustrated in Figures 3-21 and 3-22.

Sympathetic System. The sympathetic nervous system originates in neurons located in the lateral horns of the gray matter in the spinal cord between the first thoracic cord segment and the second lumbar segment. Nerve fibers pass by way of the anterior spinal roots first into the spinal nerves and then branch immediately into the sympathetic chain. From here, fiber pathways are transmitted to all portions of the body, especially to the different visceral organs and to the blood vessels.

Most sympathetic nerve endings secrete norepinephrine. Norepinephrine excites most of the visceral structures but inhibits a few. In general, it excites the heart and most of the blood vessels of the body, causing increased force of cardiac contraction and increased total peripheral resistance, with a resultant rise in arterial pressure. It inhibits the activity of the gastrointestinal tract, thereby slowing peristalsis, and it inhibits the urinary bladder, dilates the pupil of the eye, excites the liver to cause release of glucose, and increases the rate of metabolism of essentially all cells of the body.

Secretion of Epinephrine and Norepinephrine by Adrenal Medullae. Sympathetic nerves also control the rate of secretion of both epinephrine and norepinephrine by the adrenal medullae, the central portions of the two adrenal glands. These hormones are carried by the blood and cause essentially the same effects in most parts of the body as those caused by direct sympathetic stimulation in each respective part. Furthermore, these hormones reach some cells that have no sympathetic nerve supply. They especially increase the rate of metabolism in all cells of the body, an effect that is much more potent for epinephrine than norepinephrine.

The adrenal medullae represent a second means by which the central nervous system can cause sympathetic effects throughout the body. When sympathetic nerves to some organs have been destroyed, the sympathetic hor-

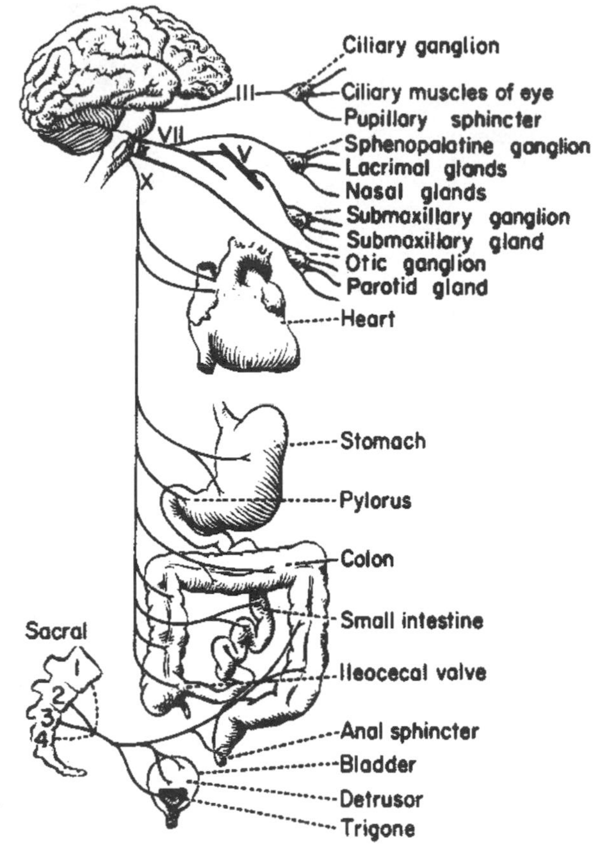

Fig. 3-22. The parasympathetic nervous system. (Guyton AC: Textbook of Medical Physiology, 8th ed. Philadelphia: WB Saunders, 1991)

mones can still elicit the usual sympathetic functions when the overall sympathetic nervous system is excited.

Parasympathetic System. Parasympathetic fibers pass mainly through the vagus nerves. A few fibers pass through several of the other cranial nerves and through the anterior roots of the sacral segments of the spinal cord. Parasympathetic fibers do not spread as extensively through the body as do sympathetic fibers, but they do innervate some of the thoracic and abdominal organs, as well as the pupillary sphincter and ciliary muscles of the eye and the salivary glands.

Parasympathetic nerve endings secrete acetylcholine. Like norepinephrine, acetylcholine stimulates some organs and inhibits others. In general, it inhibits the heart and those very few blood vessels that have parasympathetic innervation, but it excites the ciliary and the pupillary sphincter muscles of the eye, the glandular and motor functions of the gastrointestinal tract, the urinary bladder, and the gallbladder.

Control of Autonomic Nerves by Central Nervous System. The activities of the sympathetic and the parasympathetic nerves are controlled in four different levels in the central nervous system:

1. **Spinal cord.** Autonomic cord reflexes have to do principally with local reactions in discrete parts of the body. For instance, excess filling of the rectum causes a parasympathetic reflex from the sacral cord that promotes emptying of the rectum. Visceral pain from the small intestine causes reflex sympathetic inhibition of the gastrointestinal tract, and excess heat to a skin area causes reflex sympathetic vasodilatation and sweating, which help to reduce the local skin temperature.
2. **Brain stem.** The brain stem controls such factors as blood pressure, swallowing, vomiting, salivary secretion, stomach and pancreatic secretion, and, to a certain extent, emptying of the urinary bladder.
3. **Hypothalamus.** The autonomic centers of the hypothalamus control such functions as body temperature, degree of overall excitability of the body, and various responses of the viscera to emotions. To perform these functions, the hypothalamus transmits signals into the lower brain stem and thence either into the vagus nerves or down into the spinal cord to stimulate the spinal autonomic centers.
4. **Cerebral cortex.** Centers in the cerebral cortex can elicit almost any type of autonomic response. These responses are often of an emotional nature, such as fainting caused by widespread vasodilation through the body. Also, some are associated with muscular exercise, such as a rise in blood pressure and vasodilation in the muscles. The responses caused by the cerebral cortex are transmitted mainly through the autonomic centers in the hypothalamus and the lower brain stem.

EYE

OPTICS OF THE EYE

The eye is constructed very much like a camera, as illustrated in Figure 3-23. The ***retina*** is analogous to the film

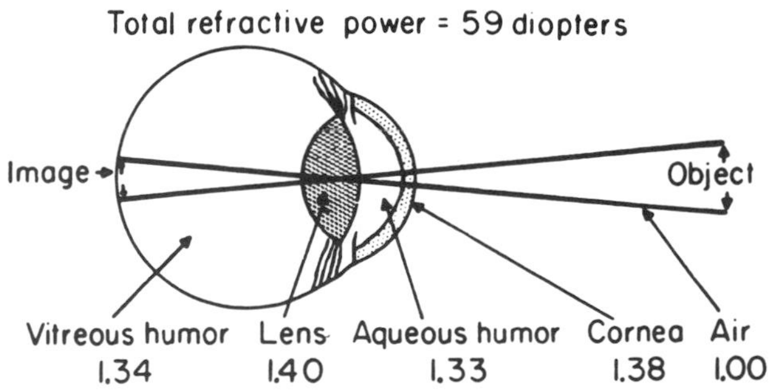

Fig. 3-23. The eye as a camera. The numbers are the refractive indices, which are the reciprocals of the light velocities. (Guyton AC: Textbook of Medical Physiology, 8th ed. Philadelphia: WB Saunders, 1991)

in a camera, the ***cornea*** and the ***lens*** of the eye are analogous to the lens system of a camera, and the ***pupil*** is analogous to the diaphragm of a camera.

The Retinal Image. Because light rays travel at different velocities in the eye fluids, the cornea, and the lens, the rays are refracted; that is, they are bent. Refraction occurs at four different corneal and lens surfaces: (1) the anterior surface of the cornea, (2) the posterior surface of the cornea, (3) the anterior surface of the lens, and (4) the posterior surface of the lens. This bending of the light rays allows an image of the scene in front of the eyes to be focused on the retina in exactly the same way that an image is focused by the lens system of a camera on the film. The image is upside down and reversed to the opposite side from the orientation of the object in front of the eyes.

Mechanism of Focusing. For a clear image to be formed on the retina, the surfaces of the cornea and of the lens of the eye must have the appropriate curvatures in relation to the distance of the retina behind the lens system. That is, the image must be focused on the retina. The eye can change the curvature of the lens in the following way: Attached around the periphery of the lens are approximately 70 ligaments that pull continually to the side, keeping the lens normally in a flattened, ovoid shape. The lens itself is a very elastic structure so that when these ligaments are loosened, it assumes a round, globular shape. When an object comes close to the eye, the more rounded shape of the lens is required to focus a clear image on the retina.

The shape of the lens is controlled by the ***ciliary muscle.*** This muscle is a circular sphincter extending all the way around the peripheral attachments of the ligaments, and on contraction the circle of the sphincter becomes smaller so that the ligaments are loosened. This automatically allows the lens to change from its normal ovoid shape to a more rounded shape, thereby assuming far greater curvature and allowing adequate focusing of the images of nearby objects.

The tension on the lens ligaments must be controlled very exactly, or the lens might become too round for adequate focusing. This is controlled by the cerebral cortex. If the image is in poor focus, the visual image in the brain is indistinct, and appropriate impulses are transmitted back through the visceral nucleus of the third nerve and finally through the third cranial nerve to the ciliary muscle to adjust the degree of contraction.

Function of the Pupil. The diameter of the pupil of the eye is controlled by a nervous reflex originating in the retina called the ***light reflex.*** Signals caused by strong light on the retina are transmitted along the optic nerve and optic tract into the pretectal nuclei of the midbrain, from there to the visceral nucleus of the third nerve, and then back to the pupillary constrictor to decrease the pupillary aperture, thus decreasing light intensity on the retina. Conversely, in darkness, lack of light signals from the retina reverses the reflex and causes the diameter of the pupil to increase.

The pupil alters the ***depth of focus*** of the eye. When the image on the retina is not in exact focus, the light rays passing through the peripheral edges of the lens will be much more out of focus than those passing through the very center of the lens. However, as the pupillary diameter becomes smaller, the light rays entering the peripheral edges of the eye are blocked and do not reach the retina. Therefore, by constricting the size of the pupil, which occurs in bright light, a person whose lens is not in exact focus will still have fairly clear vision; that is, he or she has increased "depth of focus."

FUNCTION OF THE RETINA

Rods and Cones. Rods and cones are the photoreceptor cells of the retina. The rods outnumber the cones in a ratio of about 125 million to 4 million. The rods distinguish only the white and the black aspects of an image while the cones are capable of distinguishing its colors as well. In general, one or more cones plus 50 to 400 rods are connected to a single optic nerve fiber. However, in the very central portion of the retina a single cone is connected to a single optic nerve fiber. As a result, minute points of light on the retina can be localized to very discrete positions by the cones but can be localized far less acutely by the rods. Thus, very acute and clear vision of objects is mediated by the cones, while only a more diffuse type of vision is mediated by the rods.

The foveal region of the retina is capable of very sharp vision. A person normally has very acute vision only in the central portion of the visual field. The reason is that a small area in the center of the retina having a diameter of only 0.4 mm is especially capable of detailed vision. This special area, called the ***fovea,*** has only cones, the cones are smaller in diameter, and the ratio of cones to optic nerve fibers is close to one. Also, the blood vessels and nerves are pulled to one side, so that light can pass with ease directly to the deep layers of the retina where the cones are located. The peripheral areas, which contain progressively more and more rods, have progressively more diffuse vision.

Rhodopsin Utilization by Rods. For a person to see an image, the light energy entering the eye must be changed into nerve impulses. In the rods this is accomplished by means of a chemical system called the rhodopsin-retinal cycle. Large quantities of the light-sensitive substance ***rhodopsin,*** also known as ***visual purple,*** are present in the rods. When light impinges on the rods, a small portion of the rhodopsin is transformed immediately into another substance called ***lumi-rhodopsin,*** which is a very unstable compound that lasts for only a minute fraction of a second. It degenerates through a series of chemical steps to form two substances called ***retinal*** and ***scotopsin*** (a protein). But, during the split second while the rhodopsin is being degraded, the rod becomes excited, sending nerve impulses from the retina into the optic nerve.

The retinal and scotopsin are gradually recombined by the metabolic processes of the rod to reform rhodopsin, thereby continually supplying the rod with new rhodopsin.

Night Blindness. Night blindness occurs in severe vitamin A deficiency. Retinal is derived from vitamin A. Therefore, when a person has a very serious deficiency of vitamin A in the diet, the retina is not able to form adequate quantities of retinal and thus becomes relatively insensitive to light.

Light and Dark Adaptation. The retina is capable of adapting its sensitivity so that the eye can see almost equally as well in both very bright light and in dim light. This adaptation is a far more powerful mechanism than the pupillary adaptation discussed above, though it requires several minutes to several hours to develop fully each time the person changes to a new level of light intensity. The mechanism of dark and light adaptation is the following:

Light adaptation. When a person remains in very bright light for a long time, extremely large quantities of rhodopsin are split into retinal and scotopsin; this reduces the quantity of rhodopsin in the rods and therefore makes them become insensitive to light.

Dark adaptation. When a person spends a long time in darkness, only very small amounts of rhodopsin are split while the metabolic systems of the rods are continually building more and more rhodopsin. Consequently, rhodopsin collects in very high concentration after a while and greatly increases the sensitivity of the retina.

Color Vision. The cones of the eye function in very much the same way as the rods except that the light-sensitive chemicals are slightly different from rhodopsin. These chemicals still utilize retinal as the basis for light sensitivity, but the retinal combines with a different ***photopsin*** for each of the three primary colors rather than with scotopsin. Each photopsin, like scotopsin, is a protein, but slightly different from other photopsins. The nature of this protein determines the color sensitivity of the light-sensitive chemical. There are three major groups of cones that respond especially intensely to certain colors of light. These cones are classified as ***blue cones, green cones,*** and ***red cones.***

The eye determines the color of an object by the relative intensities of stimulation of the different types of cones. For instance, yellow is a color with a wavelength midway between green and red. Therefore, it stimulates the green and the red cones about equally, which gives one the sensation of seeing the color yellow. Orange has a wavelength somewhat closer to that of red light than of green light. Therefore, it stimulates the red cones about twice as much as it does the green cones, giving the sensation of orange. Finally, pure red light stimulates the red cones very strongly while stimulating the green and blue cones only weakly. This gives the sensation of red. The same principles hold true for the different shades of color between green, blue, and yellow.

Analysis of Visual Image in the Retina. In the retina are several other types of neuronal cells in addition to the rods and cones. These are the bipolar cells, the horizontal cells, the amacrine cells, and the ganglion cells. Some of these are inhibitory while others are excitatory. By combining excitatory and inhibitory signals from the excited rods and cones, the signals that finally reach the ganglion cells of the retina are initiated almost entirely by three types of visual effects: (1) spots or borders in the retinal image where there is a sudden change from light to dark or dark to light (*i.e.,* sudden change in contrast in the image), (2) sudden increases or decreases in light intensity from one instant to another, and (3) changes in color from one area to another. In other words, those portions of the visual image that do not have any contrast in intensity or color in them do not stimulate the ganglion cells to a great extent. It is mainly where contrast borders occur that the ganglion cells are strongly stimulated. Also, some ganglion cells are stimulated strongly when there is a sudden change in light intensity. Thus, these contrast borders and the changes in light intensity send most of the signals to the primary visual cortex.

Transmission of Signals from Retina to Cerebral Cortex. Each point of the retina connects with a discrete point in the ***visual cortex*** of the brain located in the calcarine fissure area of the occipital cortex. Therefore, every time a single point on the retina is stimulated, a corresponding point is stimulated in the visual cortex. From here, other signals pass to the visual association areas and then to Wernicke's area for analysis of the visual images, as described earlier in the chapter.

EAR

Transmission of Sound from Tympanic Membrane to Cochlea. Figure 3-24 illustrates the functional parts of the ear. Sound is caused by compression waves that travel through the air at a velocity of about 1/5 mile per second. As each compression wave strikes the ***tympanic membrane*** (or "eardrum"), the membrane is forced inward, and between compressions it moves outward. The center of the tympanic membrane is connected to the ***ossicular system,*** which consists of three bony le-

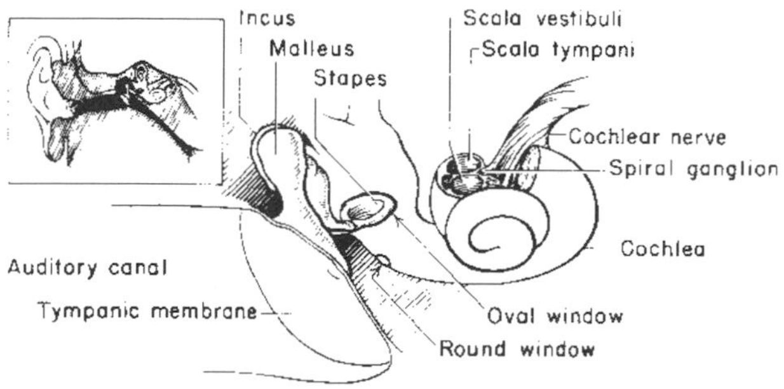

Fig. 3-24. The tympanic membrane, the ossicular system of the middle ear, and the inner ear. (Guyton AC: Textbook of Medical Physiology, 8th ed. Philadelphia: WB Saunders, 1991)

vers (the malleus, incus, and stapes) that transmit the sound vibrations into the cochlea at the oval window.

The tympanic membrane and the ossicular system function as a sound "transformer." The tympanic membrane has a surface area some 20 times the surface area of the oval window. Therefore, the force of sound vibrations reaching the oval window has been increased by 20-fold.

Function of the Cochlea. Figure 3-25 illustrates the fluid system in the cochlea. The cochlea is composed of two major fluid-filled tubes, the scala vestibuli and the scala tympani, which lie side by side in a coil and are separated by the basilar membrane. Inward movement of the stapes against the oval window, which is at the end of the scala vestibuli, pushes the fluid deeper into the scala vestibuli, and this in turn causes the basilar membrane to bulge and push the fluid in the scala tympani. Finally, the fluid in the scala tympani pushes outward against the round window, which is at the end of this scala. Thus, every time the stapes moves inward, the round window bulges outward into the middle ear.

Low-frequency sound causes the stapes to move back and forth very slowly, which allows the pressure waves to travel far up into the scala vestibuli before maximum bulging of the basilar membrane into the scala tympani occurs. On the other hand, high-frequency sound waves cause very rapid vibration of the stapes, and the waves have enough time between waves to travel only a short distance into the scala vestibuli before maximum bulging occurs. In this way a form of resonance occurs in the cochlea, with low-frequency waves causing maximum back-and-forth vibration of the basilar membrane near the far tip of the cochlea and high-frequency sound causing vibration of the basilar membrane near the base of the cochlea, that is, close to the oval and round windows. The brain determines the pitch of the sound mainly from the portion of the basilar membrane that vibrates; high pitch is near the base of the cochlea and low pitch is near the apex.

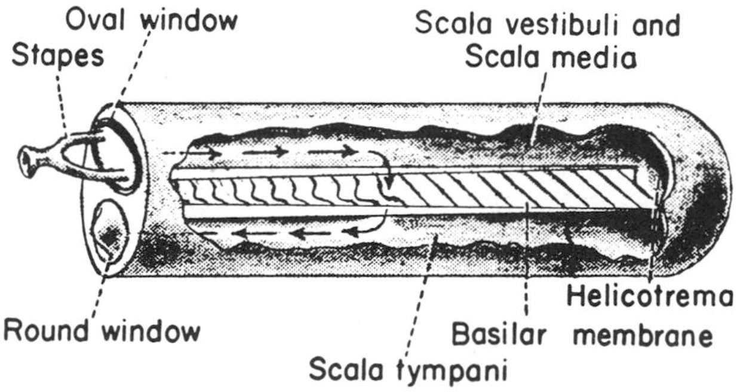

Fig. 3-25. Vibration of the basilar membrane in response to sound. (Guyton AC: Textbook of Medical Physiology, 8th ed. Philadelphia: WB Saunders, 1991)

Organ of Corti. The organ of Corti is the receptor organ that generates nerve impulses in response to vibration of the basilar membrane. The actual sensory receptors of the organ of Corti are hair cells that synapse with a network of cochlear nerve endings. Bending of the hair cells in one direction depolarizes the hair cells, and bending them in the opposite direction hyperpolarizes them. The more forceful the vibration and subsequent bending of the hair cells, the greater the rate of nerve impulses. The loudness of the sound is determined by the rate of impulse transmission from the hair cells into the brain by way of the cochlear nerve.

Spatial Orientation of Auditory Impulses. Approximately 25,000 nerve fibers are attached to the hair cells of the cochlear apparatus. The auditory signals in the auditory nerves go first to the cochlear nuclei located in the brain stem; from here they pass upward to the inferior colliculus, then to the medial geniculate body, and finally to the ***primary auditory cortex*** in the middle of the superior temporal gyrus of the temporal lobe. The spatial orientation of the nerve fibers is maintained all the way from the basilar membrane to the auditory cortex so that one sound frequency excites specific areas of the auditory cortex while another sound frequency excites other areas. The meanings of the auditory signals are then interpreted in the auditory association areas immediately adjacent to the primary auditory cortex.

CHEMICAL SENSES

TASTE

Taste Buds. Located on the surfaces of the tongue, especially on the papillae and most importantly on the circumvallate papillae, which lie in a V line on the posterior part of the tongue, and also in small numbers on the lateral walls of the pharynx, are many small taste receptor organs called taste buds. One of these is illustrated in

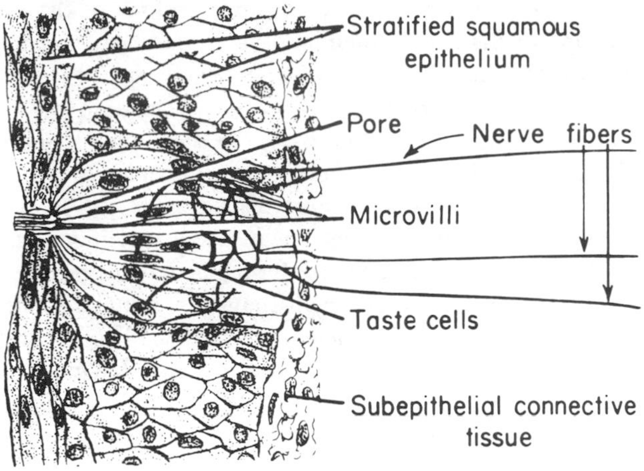

Fig. 3-26. The taste bud. (Guyton AC: Textbook of Medical Physiology, 8th ed. Philadelphia: WB Saunders, 1991)

Figure 3-26. Each taste bud has a hollow cavity that communicates through a small ***taste pore*** with the mouth. Lining the cavity are sensory taste receptor cells, and cilia called taste ''hairs'' protrude from the ends of these cells into the pore. Certain types of chemicals diffuse into the taste pores and excite the hairs of the taste cells.

The four types of taste buds respond to saltiness, sweetness, sourness, and bitterness. The first three of these taste sensations help the person to select the quality of food that he eats and in some instances even makes him desire certain substances such as salt that may be deficient in his body. The last of the taste sensations, bitterness, is principally for protection, because most of the naturally occurring poisons among plant foods elicit a bitter taste that normally will cause an animal to reject the food.

Transmission of Taste Signals to Primary Taste Cortex. Most of the taste signals are transmitted by way of the ***chorda tympani*** into the ***seventh nerve*** and then into the brain stem; the remainder are transmitted through the ninth and tenth nerves into the brain stem. The signals pass first to the ***nucleus of the tractus solitarius,*** then to the ***thalamus*** and finally to the ***primary taste cortex,*** which lies far laterally in the parietal cortex immediately posterior to the central sulcus of the brain and deep in the fissure of Sylvius (also called the lateral fissure).

SMELL

The Olfactory Epithelium. Located in the superiormost part of each nostril is a small area having a surface of about 2.5 cm^2 called the olfactory epithelium. This contains large numbers of nervous receptors called ***olfactory cells*** that send long cilia (''olfactory hairs'') into the mucus on the surface of the epithelium. Almost any chemical substance that can diffuse through the mucus and then into these cilia will stimulate one or more of the olfactory cells. Since the cilia themselves have lipid membranes, lipid-soluble substances stimulate the cells much more readily than nonlipid-soluble substances. The precise types of chemicals that stimulate different types of olfactory cells are not known, for it has been very difficult to study by either subjective or objective means the olfactory stimulus from a single olfactory cell. It is believed that there might be 7 to 50 primary sensations of smell and that the many thousands of different smells to which we are accustomed are actually combinations of these primary sensations.

TRANSMISSION OF OLFACTORY SIGNALS INTO THE BRAIN

From the olfactory cells signals are transmitted first to thc olfactory bulb of the first cranial nerve and then through the olfactory tract into several midline nuclei of the brain that lie superior and anterior to the hypothalamus, and also into the pyriform cortex, the amygdala, and the thalamus. The midline nuclei are associated with the crude functions of smell, such as eliciting salivation or licking the lips. The pyriform cortex, amygdala, and thalamus deal with olfactory conditioned reflexes that determine appetite and the social responses to food.

GASTROINTESTINAL TRACT

The alimentary tract provides water, electrolytes, and nutrients for the body. This requires (1) propulsion and mixing of gastrointestinal contents, (2) secretion of digestive juices, (3) digestion of food, and (4) absorption of digestion products, water, and electrolytes. The entire alimentary tract is shown in Figure 3-27.

MOTOR MOVEMENTS OF THE GASTROINTESTINAL TRACT

The intestinal wall has an outer longitudinal muscle layer and an inner circular muscle layer required for the two basic types of movements in the gastrointestinal tract: ***propulsive movements*** that propel food forward along the tract and ***mixing movements*** that mix food with the gastrointestinal secretions.

Propulsive Movements. ***Peristalsis*** is a wave of contraction passing along the gastrointestinal tract. The intensity and frequency of peristalsis vary greatly from one part of the tract to another. In the stomach, the intensity of peristalsis is usually sufficient to cause movement of the food through the stomach within 1 to 3 hours after a meal. The peristaltic waves are less intense in the small

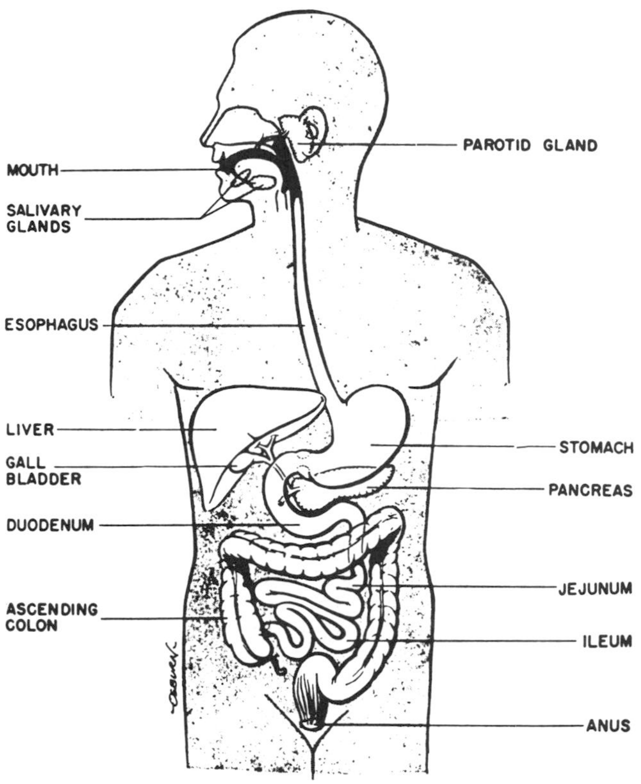

Fig. 3-27. The alimentary tract. (Guyton AC: Textbook of Medical Physiology, 8th ed. Philadelphia: WB Saunders, 1991)

intestine and they spread along only 10 to 15 cm at a time so that about 3 to 10 hours is required to move the food through the small intestine. In the large intestine, the propulsive movements are a modified type of peristalsis, called ***mass movements,*** that are often very strong but last only a fraction of an hour out of each day.

Distention is the usual stimulus for peristalsis. If food collects at any point in the gut and stretches the gut wall, a constrictive ring moves forward along the gut, pushing any material in the gut ahead of the constriction. This is known as the ***law of the intestines.*** Peristalsis is caused by nerve impulses that move along a nerve plexus, called the ***myenteric plexus,*** in the wall of the gut. Stimulation at any point of the plexus causes nerve impulses to travel around the gut and also in both directions along the gut. Impulses traveling around the gut cause it to constrict, and impulses traveling lengthwise along the gut cause the constriction to move in the analward direction.

Peristalsis is regulated by the autonomic nervous system. Peristalsis is far more intense when the parasympathetic nerves are stimulated, and less intense when the sympathetic nerves are stimulated. Strong stimulation of the sympathetic nervous system can totally block movement of food through the gastrointestinal tract.

Intestinal motility is regulated by neural reflexes. The ***intestinointestinal reflex*** inhibits contraction of the remaining bowel when a portion of the bowel is severely distended. The ***gastroileal reflex*** results in the movement of ileal contents into the large intestine following a meal.

Swallowing (deglutination) is a special type of propulsive movement. When food is pushed into the back of the mouth by the tongue, nerve receptors in the pharynx elicit an automatic swallowing process that occurs entirely in less than 2 seconds. Signals are transmitted from these receptors to the brain stem, integrated there, and a sequence of swallowing signals is then transmitted back through the pharyngeal and vagus nerves to the pharynx and upper esophagus. A peristaltic wave begins in the pharyngeal constrictors, the glottis closes so that food cannot pass into the trachea, and the upper esophageal constrictor muscle at the opening of the esophagus relaxes so that the food will enter the esophagus. Then, after this swallowing process is over, the peristaltic wave proceeds downward along the upper esophagus. All of this is controlled directly by nerve impulses from the brain stem. On reaching the lower half of the esophagus, the natural peristaltic process of the myenteric plexus in the gastrointestinal tract takes over and propels the food the rest of the way to the stomach.

The stomach smooth muscle has three functions: (1) The muscle relaxes to accommodate a meal, (2) the ingested meal is mixed with gastric juices to facilitate digestion, and (3) smooth muscle contractions propel the stomach contents into the duodenum at an optimal rate.

Mixing Movements. Peristaltic waves of constriction pass over the ***antrum*** at the lower end of the stomach toward the pylorus, yet the opening of the pylorus is too small to allow the antral contents to be expelled into the duodenum. Therefore, most of the contents are squirted backward through the peristaltic ring toward the body of the stomach, providing an intense type of mixing called "retropulsion." The mixture of food and secretions that results is called ***chyme.***

Intermittent constrictive rings occur several times a minute, dividing the small intestine into segments. Then the first constrictions relax and others occur at other points. In this way the chyme is chopped again and again into small portions. These movements are called ***segmenting contractions.*** In the large intestine similar but much slower contractions called ***haustrations*** occur; these slowly roll the fecal matter over and over, allowing almost complete absorption of the water and electrolytes.

SECRETIONS IN THE GASTROINTESTINAL TRACT

Secretion of Saliva. Saliva is secreted principally by the parotid, submaxillary, and sublingual glands. It is composed of a mucus secretion containing ***mucin*** and a serous secretion containing the enzyme ***ptyalin,*** which is an ***α-amylase.*** The mucus functions to provide lubrication for swallowing, and the ptyalin functions to begin digestion of starches and other carbohydrates in the food. Saliva is also important for oral hygiene by virtue of its washing and bactericidal actions.

Salivary secretions are controlled by parasympathetic nervous signals from the salivatory nuclei. Salivatory nuclei in the brain can be stimulated by taste and tactile stimuli from the tongue and mouth. Salivation can also be stimulated from higher centers in the central nervous system, for example, when favorite foods are smelled or eaten. Drugs like atropine and scopolamine block the acetylcholine receptors and abolish salivary secretions, whereas drugs such as neostigmine that inhibit acetylcholinesterase increase salivation.

Gastric Secretion. The three phases of gastric secretion are shown in Figure 3-28. The ***cephalic phase*** accounts for 30% of the response to a meal and is initiated by the anticipation of eating and the smell and taste of food. It is mediated entirely by the vagus nerve. The ***gastric phase*** accounts for 60% of the acid response to a meal. It is initiated by distention of the stomach, which leads to nervous stimulation of gastric secretion. In addition, partial digestion products of proteins in the stomach cause ***gastrin*** to be released from the antral mucosa. The gastrin then passes by way of the bloodstream to the ***gastric glands*** located in the upper three quarters of the stomach, called the ***fundus*** and ***body,*** to cause secretion of a highly acidic gastric juice. The ***intestinal phase*** (10% of the response) is initiated by nervous stimuli associated with distention of the small intestine. The presence of digestion products of proteins in the small intestine can also stimulate gastric secretion by a humoral mechanism.

Pancreatic Secretion. The chyme, on entering the small intestine, causes the release of two different hormones from the intestinal mucosa, ***secretin*** and ***cholecystokinin,*** and these are carried in the blood to the pancreatic secretory cells. Secretin causes the pancreatic ducts to secrete large amounts of a highly alkaline, watery solution, and cholecystokinin causes the pancreatic acinar cells to release larger quantities of digestive enzymes into this solution. Secretin is released from the intestinal mucosa mainly in response to acid emptied from the stomach into the duodenum; the alkaline pancreatic secretion in turn neutralizes the acid. Cholecystokinin is released mainly in response to the presence of fats and proteins in the chyme, and the secreted enzymes in turn help to digest the proteins and fats.

Intestinal Secretion. Intestinal fluid is secreted by epithelial cells in the crypts of Lieberkühn. Intestinal secretion normally results from either mechanical stimulation of the mucosa by the chyme or distention of the gut, and is mediated by intramural nervous reflexes in the submucosal and myenteric plexuses. Intestinal fluid is almost pure extracellular fluid, providing a watery vehicle for absorption of substances from the chyme.

Secretion of Mucus. Mucus protects the mucosa of the gastrointestinal tract. Mucus is secreted in all parts of the gastrointestinal tract, from the salivary glands all the way to the mucosal glands of the large intestine. Mucus is an excellent lubricant and is also very resistant to chemical destruction, either by the gastric and intestinal juices or by different types of foods.

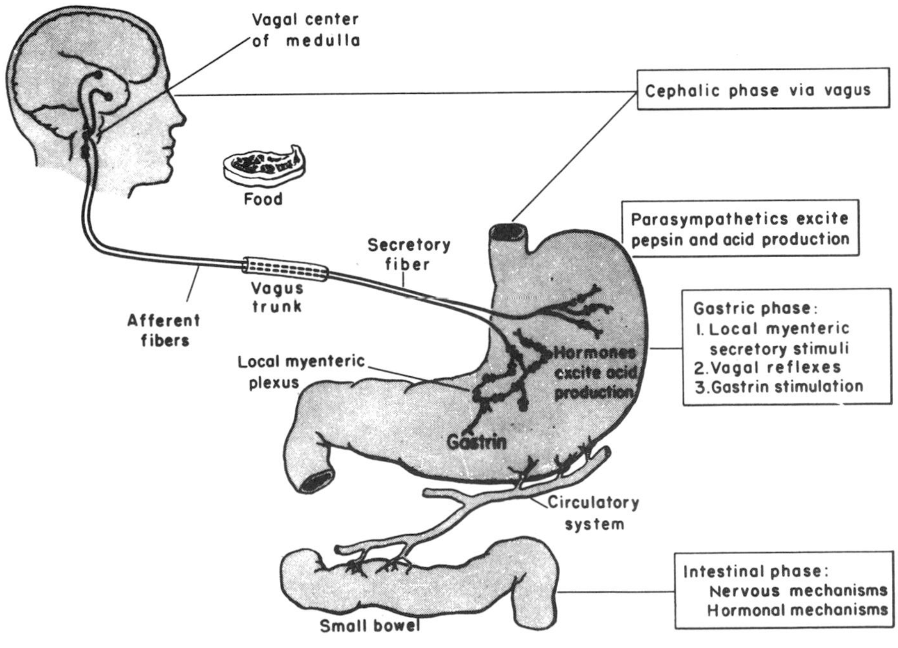

Fig. 3-28. The phases of gastric secretion and their regulation. (Guyton AC: Textbook of Medical Physiology, 8th ed. Philadelphia: WB Saunders, 1991)

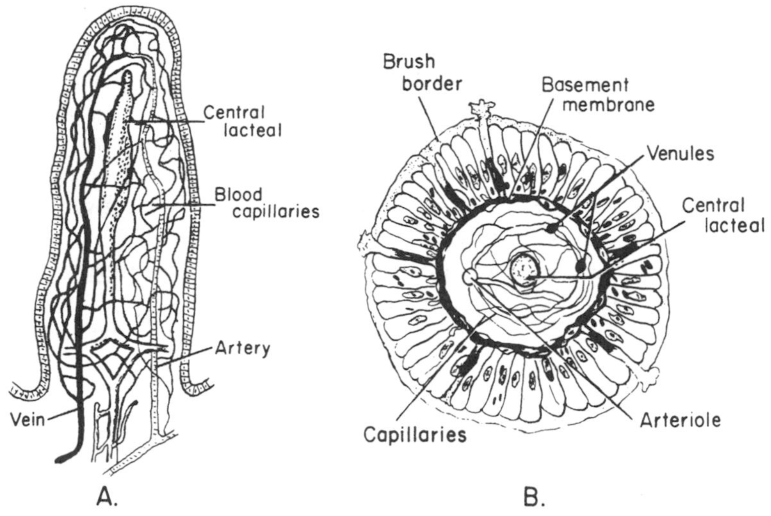

Fig. 3-29. Structure of the intestinal villus. A, Longitudinal section. B, Cross-section. (Guyton AC: Textbook of Medical Physiology, 8th ed. Philadelphia: WB Saunders, 1991)

DIGESTION IN THE INTESTINAL TRACT

Hydrolysis is the basic chemical process of digestion. This means that the food molecule splits into two smaller molecules, and at the same time a hydrogen atom from a water molecule combines with one of the food products at the point of splitting while the remaining hydroxyl radical from the water combines with the other food product. The carbohydrates are hydrolyzed into monosaccharides, the fats into glycerol and fatty acids, and the proteins into amino acids.

Hydrolysis is catalyzed by digestive enzymes. Digestion of carbohydrates is begun by ***salivary amylase*** secreted in the saliva, and their digestion is carried still further by ***pancreatic amylase*** secreted in the pancreatic juice. After the action of these two, the carbohydrates will have been split principally into disaccharides. Then four enzymes in the epithelial cells of the small intestinal mucosa, ***sucrase, maltase, isomaltase,*** and ***lactase,*** split the disaccharides into monosaccharides, principally ***glucose, fructose,*** and ***galactose.***

The fats are split into ***glycerol*** and ***fatty acid*** molecules by ***lipases*** secreted mainly in the pancreatic juice but to a very slight extent in other digestive secretions.

Protein digestion begins in the stomach under the influence of ***pepsin*** and ***hydrochloric acid.*** Then it continues in the upper small intestine under the influence of ***trypsin*** and ***chymotrypsin*** secreted by the pancreas. At this point, the proteins will have been digested into large polypeptides. Then several different ***peptidases*** secreted in the pancreatic juice or located in or on the surfaces of the intestinal epithelial cells split the polypeptides into amino acids.

ABSORPTION FROM THE GASTROINTESTINAL TRACT

Role of Intestinal Villi. Located on the mucosal surface of the small intestine are millions of small intestinal villi, each of which projects about 1 mm into the intestinal lumen, as shown to the left in Figure 3-29. These villi increase the surface area of the small intestine about tenfold. The end products of digestion are absorbed through the epithelial cells lining these villi into sublying villar blood vessels and lymphatics.

Microvilli increase the intestinal surface area by 20-fold. In addition to the increased surface area caused by the presence of the villi, each epithelial cell has approximately 600 microvilli, each 1 micron in length. In all, the total area for absorption is about 250 m^2 for the entire small intestine.

Active Absorption. This active absorption is very similar to that which occurs in the kidney tubules, which was explained earlier in the chapter. Substances that can be actively absorbed are most monosaccharides (especially glucose, fructose, and galactose), the amino acids, and several ions including sodium, calcium, iron, potassium, and others.

Passive Absorption. Water, chloride ions, and some fats are passively absorbed. Passive absorption means absorption of substances simply by diffusion through the membrane. When substances in the chyme are actively absorbed, such as glucose, the amount of osmotically active substances increases in the fluids on the outer side of the intestinal membrane while the amount decreases in the chyme. As a result, tremendous quantities of water are osmotically absorbed from the gut. Also, when positively charged ions such as sodium ions are actively absorbed, a positive charge builds up on the other side of the membrane, and this pulls negatively charged substances such as chloride ions through the membrane.

Portal and Lymphatic Routes. Almost all of the water-soluble substances are absorbed directly into the blood capillaries of the villi, and then pass with the portal blood through the liver sinusoids and into the general circulatory system. This is called the portal route of absorption, and the substances absorbed in this way are (1) most of the water and electrolytes, (2) the carbohydrates, and (3) the amino acids.

Fatty acids are not absorbed into the blood of the villi but, instead, while passing through the epithelium of the villus, recombine with glycerol to form triglycerides (neutral fat). This then passes into the lymphatics and is transmitted upward along the thoracic duct in the form of minute fatty globules called ***chylomicrons*** to be emptied into the veins of the neck.

GASTROINTESTINAL DISORDERS

Peptic Ulcer. ***Peptic ulcers*** form when the damaging effects of acid and pepsin overcome the protective actions of bicarbonate secretion, mucus, and normal renewal of the cells. Because gastric and duodenal ulcers result from mucosal digestion by acid and pepsin, they are both categorized as peptic ulcers. However, their etiologies are quite different. ***Duodenal ulcers*** result from excessive secretion of acid and pepsin. Duodenal ulcer patients have higher than normal serum gastrin levels in response to a meal. Also, patients with ***gastrinoma,*** a gastrin-secreting tumor, always develop duodenal ulcers, never gastric ulcers. ***Gastric ulcers*** appear to result from a defect in the mucosa itself. Factors that can damage the so-called ***gastric mucosal barrier*** and thus promote gastric ulcer formation include abnormalities in mucosal blood flow, decreased mucus secretion, bacterial infection, and irritants such as alcohol and aspirin.

Diarrhea. Irritation is the most common cause of diarrhea. Almost any irritation of the gastrointestinal mucosa greatly increases the local rate of secretion of intestinal juices and also the intensity of peristalsis. This causes a ''washout'' phenomenon, the material in the irritated area following rapidly toward the anus. In addition to irritation and bacterial toxins, diarrhea can also result from excessive activity of the parasympathetic nervous system, because parasympathetic stimulation increases the secretory and propulsive activites of the entire gastrointestinal tract but especially to the latter half of the large intestine.

Cholera toxin causes severe diarrhea. The rate of fluid secretion from intestinal epithelial cells can increase severalfold causing as much as 5 to 10 liters of diarrhea fluid to be lost during the first day of infection. Circulatory shock by dehydration will occur within a few hours if the body fluids are not replaced.

Pernicious Anemia. Gastric atrophy can cause pernicious anemia. Normal gastric secretions contain a glycoprotein called intrinsic factor that is required for absorption of vitamine B_{12} by the ileum. In the absence of intrinsic factor, ***maturation failure*** occurs in the production of red blood cells, resulting in pernicious anemia.

Achalasia. ***Achalasia*** is characterized by failure of the lower esophageal sphincter to relax. This results in accumulation of food in the esophagus, sometimes causing an extreme enlargement of the esophagus called ***megaesophagus.*** It is caused by dysfunction of the myenteric plexus in the lower half of the esophagus. The musculature at the lower end of the esophagus remains tonically contracted, and the myenteric plexus has lost its ability to transmit signals necessary for relaxation of the gastroesophageal sphincter.

METABOLISM AND ENERGY

METABOLISM OF CARBOHYDRATES AND SYNTHESIS OF ADENOSINE TRIPHOSPHATE

Glucose. The digestive products of essentially all carbohydrates are glucose, fructose, and galactose. Much of the fructose is converted to glucose as it is absorbed by the intestinal epithelium, and the remaining fructose and the galactose, after being absorbed, are transmitted by the portal blood mainly to the liver, where they are almost all also converted into glucose. This glucose eventually passes back out of the liver cells into the blood to join the glucose that is absorbed directly from the gastrointestinal tract.

Liver Glycogen. Large quantities of glucose, either that converted from fructose and galactose or that directly absorbed from the gastrointestinal tract, can be stored in the liver cells in the form of glycogen granules, glycogen being a polymer of glucose. Special enzymes in the liver cells cause the polymerization of glucose into glycogen. When the glucose level in the blood falls too low, the glycogen is split by still other enzymes back into glucose, which then passes into the blood to be utilized elsewhere in the body. In this way extra glucose is removed from the blood when the blood glucose concentration is too high, and then is returned when the blood glucose falls too low.

Insulin. Glucose is transported through the cell membrane by a facilitated diffusion mechanism, as was discussed in the early part of this chapter. The activity of this mechanism for glucose transport is controlled by the amount of insulin secreted by the pancreas. Large amounts of insulin increase the rate of glucose transport to about 15 times the rate when no insulin is available. When the pancreas fails to secrete insulin, very little glucose can enter most cells, but when excess insulin is secreted, glucose enters the cells so rapidly that the blood glucose falls to a very low level.

Glycolysis. After entry into the cells, glucose can be polymerized into glycogen and stored temporarily as glycogen granules, or it can be used immediately to provide energy for cellular functions. The initial process for providing energy is principally glycolysis. Each molecule of glucose is split to form pyruvic acid by a series of chemical reactions involving several stages of phosphorylation and several transformations, all catalyzed by protein enzymes in the cells.

Glycolysis provides a net yield of two molecules of adenosine triphosphate (ATP) for every molecule of glucose converted into pyruvic acid. In this way a small portion (about 3%) of the energy stored in the glucose molecule is transferred to ATP molecules. The ATP in turn is very highly reactive and can provide immediate energy to other functional systems of the cells as needed.

Citric Acid Cycle. The two molecules of pyruvic acid formed from glucose in the glycolysis process still contain about nine tenths of the energy originally in the glucose molecule. To make this available to the cell, each molecule of pyruvic acid is first split into carbon dioxide and hydrogen. This occurs principally by means of a series of chemical reactions called by various names: the ***Krebs cycle,*** the ***tricarboxylic acid cycle,*** or the ***citric acid cycle.***

Chemical reactions in the citric acid cycle are catalyzed by decarboxylases (which remove carbon dioxide) and dehydrogenases (which remove hydrogen). The pyruvic acid is first decarboxylated to form ***acetyl coenzyme A,*** and this immediately combines with oxaloacetic acid to form citric acid. The citric acid is then progressively decomposed, liberating carbon dioxide and hydrogen atoms. The carbon dioxide diffuses out of the cells and is blown off by the lungs into the expired air. However, the hydrogen atoms are made available to react with oxygen, a process that provides tremendous amounts of energy to the cell, as will be discussed below. After the carbon dioxide and hydrogen atoms have been removed, the residue of the citric acid molecule is a new molecule of oxaloacetic acid that can be used over and over again in the citric acid cycle.

Oxidative Phosphorylation. Most of the hydrogen that is released during the breakdown of pyruvic acid combines with nicotinamide adenine dinucleotide (NAD) and is then rapidly passed to another substance, a flavoprotein. The hydrogen then leaves the flavoprotein to become hydrogen ions, each hydrogen losing one electron in the process. The electrons removed from the hydrogen atoms are passed through a series of electron carriers, including cytochrome B, cytochrome C, cytochrome A, and cytochrome oxidase, and finally are combined with water and the dissolved oxygen in the fluids of the cell to convert these into hydroxyl ions. The presence of both hydrogen and hydroxyl ions in the same fluid allows immediate combination of the two to form water. The important features about this oxidation of hydrogen is not the formation of water but, instead, the use of energy from the hydrogen and oxygen atoms for synthesis of ATP.

Hydrogen atoms are utilized to cause the formation of ATP. The first step is ionization of the hydrogen atoms and passage of the electrons removed during the ionization process through the electron carrier system. The electron carriers are large protein molecules that are integral parts of the inner wall of the mitochondrion. As the electrons pass from one carrier to the next, they give up energy, and the energy is used to pump the hydrogen ions from the central cavity of the mitochondrion into the outer chamber between the two mitochondrial walls. This creates a high concentration of hydrogen ions in this outer chamber.

The Chemiosmotic Mechanism. The entire process of oxidative phosphorylation occurs inside the mitochondria. The large hydrogen ion gradient across the inner wall of the mitochondrion causes the hydrogen ions to leak back through the inner wall toward the central cavity. This flow of hydrogen ions through the inner wall of the mitochondria from the outer mitochondrial chamber to the central cavity occurs through very large protein molecules called APT synthetase. Each of these molecules is an ATPase enzyme capable of using the energy derived from the flow of hydrogen ions through its molecular matrix to convert adenosine diphosphate (ADP) plus a phosphate radical into ATP, that is, to cause synthesis of ATP. Thus, in this roundabout way, the tremendous energy that had been present in the glucose molecule is finally used to form ATP, which itself stores a large portion of this energy and uses it later to energize almost all intracellular reactions.

Oxidative phosphorylation accounts for more than 90% of ATP production. Thirty-six molecules of ATP are produced for each molecule of glucose oxidized, 18 times as many molecules as are formed by the process of glycolysis alone.

ATP is a highly labile compound, the formula for which is shown in Figure 3-30. The point where the last two phosphate radicals attach (indicated by the curving bonds) are called high-energy phosphate bonds. These bonds provide from 7,000 to 12,000 calories of energy for each mole of ATP, the exact amount depending on concentrations and other conditions of the reactants. The two phosphate radicals on the end of the molecule can split away with great ease and can transfer this energy to other chemical processes in the cells. Thus, ATP is almost an explosive compound that is ready to act immediately. After it begins to be consumed, more ATP is formed by the processes described above.

ATP is needed for almost all chemical reactions. Some of the specific functions of ATP are (1) to provide the immediate energy needed for contraction of muscle cells, (2) to provide the energy needed to pump sodium out of

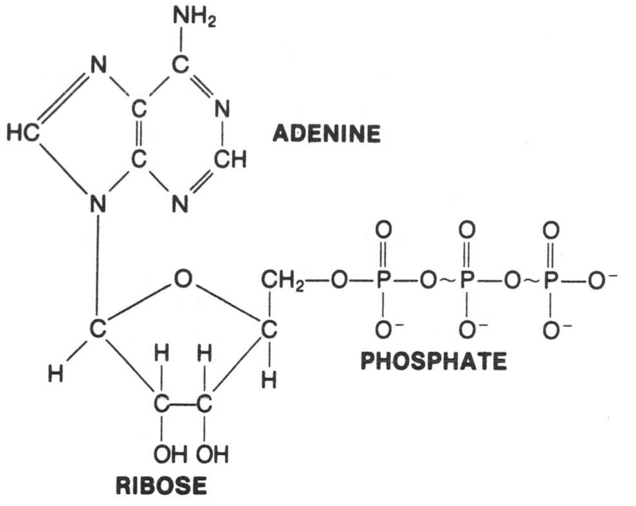

Fig. 3-30. Structure of adenosine triphosphate. (Guyton AC: Textbook of Medical Physiology, 8th ed. Philadelphia: WB Saunders, 1991)

nerve and muscle cells so that action potentials can be transmitted along the membranes, (3) to provide the energy needed to synthesize new proteins by the ribosomes in the cytoplasm, and (4) to provide the energy needed for synthesis and secretion of almost all substances formed by the glands. These are only a few of the functions of ATP.

METABOLISM OF FATS

Chylomicrons. Fatty acids absorbed from the small intestine immediately recombine in the intestinal epithelial cells with glycerol to form minute particles of triglycerides (neutral fat). The triglycerides then aggregate with small amounts of protein to form fat globules called ***chylomicrons,*** which have an average size of 0.4 micron. These pass into the intestinal lymphatics and along the thoracic duct, eventually to empty into the blood. Within an hour or so after a meal has been completely absorbed, most of the chylomicrons will have been removed from the circulating blood, some of them being absorbed by the liver cells and a very large portion being split by an enzyme, lipoprotein lipase, into fatty acids that are either metabolized for energy or are resynthesized into fat by the fat cells and stored.

Lipoproteins. Most fatty substances are not soluble in the body fluids. Therefore, lipids (95%) are transported in the blood in the form of minute suspended particles, called ***lipoproteins.*** Lipoproteins are composed of triglycerides, phospholipids, cholesterol, and protein. The fatty substances in the lipoproteins are loosely bound with varying amounts of protein. The proteins in turn, being miscible with water, increase the suspension stability of the lipoproteins in the plasma and prevent excessive adherence of them to each other or to the endothelium.

Free Fatty Acids. A very small amount of fatty acids, about 15 mg per 100 ml, is present in the plasma in combination with the albumin of the plasma proteins. These are called ***free fatty acids.*** Despite this very small concentration, this free fatty acid is transferred extremely rapidly back and forth with the tissue fats, as much as one half of it transferring every 2 to 3 minutes. Such rapid mobility makes this the principal means of transport of most of the fat from one area of the body to another.

Fat Depots. All of the fat in the fat cells of the body is known collectively as ***fat depots.*** When the amount of circulating fatty acid falls very low in the blood during the interdigestive period between meals, the stored ***triglycerides*** are split by tissue lipoprotein lipase to release free fatty acids, which are then transported in the blood to other cells of the body where they may be needed.

Fats as a source of energy. Fats provide energy in nearly the same manner as carbohydrates. The chemical processes for deriving energy from fats include the following stages: (1) The triglycerides are split inside the fat cells into glycerol and fatty acids. The glycerol, having a chemical composition very similar to that of certain glucose breakdown products, can easily be oxidized to energize the formation of ATP molecules. (2) The fatty acid molecules are partially oxidized, mainly in the liver cells, by a process called ***beta carbon oxidation,*** which causes the fatty acid to split and form many ***acetyl coenzyme A*** molecules. These in turn enter the mitochondria where they are decomposed by the citric acid cycle and then completely oxidized by the oxidative phosphorylation process to synthesize large numbers of ATP molecules in exactly the same way that the acetyl coenzyme A derived from pyruvic acid is used for the same purpose. Thus, fats provide energy in nearly the same manner as carbohydrates except that the initial stage for spliting carbohydrates is mainly the glycolysis mechanism while the initial stage for splitting fats is principally the beta carbon oxidation mechanism.

A large share of all fatty acid degradation begins in the liver, but only a small portion of the acetyl coenzyme A formed in the liver cells is used for energy in the liver itself. Instead, it is transported away from the liver by the blood in the form of ***acetoacetic acid,*** a condensation product of two molecules of acetyl coenzyme A. This in turn is absorbed by the other cells of the body where it is split again into two molecules of acetyl coenzyme A, then enters the citric acid cycle, and is used for energy.

Phospholipids. Phospholipids are chemical substances derived mainly from fat and have certain of the physical and chemical characteristics of fats. All cells of the body synthesize phospholipids, but most of these are synthesized in the liver or intestinal epithelial cells. The phospholipids are used by the cells to form the most significant part of the cellular membrane, different intracellular membranes, and other intracellular structures.

Cholesterol. Cholesterol absorbed from the intestinal tract is called ***exogenous cholesterol,*** but an even greater quantity of cholesterol, called ***endogenous cholesterol,*** is formed in the cells of the body. Cholesterol is used along with phospholipids and small amounts of triglycerides in composing the different membranous structures of cells. An especially large amount of cholesterol is formed by the liver, and about 80% of this is then used by the liver to synthesize bile acids that are secreted in the bile into the small intestine. These in turn promote emulsification of fats in the gastrointestinal tract so that they can be digested, and they also promote fat absorption. Cholesterol is also a precursor for a number of steroid hormones.

Atherosclerosis. Unfortunately, large quantities of cholesterol are occasionally either synthesized by the walls of the arteries or are deposited there from the blood. As a result, large plaques of cholesterol frequently develop in the arterial walls and protrude through the intima into the flowing arterial blood. This disease is called ***arteriosclerosis.*** Blood clots often develop on the protruding cholesterol plaques, at times becoming large enough to occlude completely the lumen of the vessel. This is the cause of most acute coronary occlusions that bring about heart attacks. Thrombosis or hemorrhage of arteries in the brain can lead to stroke and cause other problems in other organs, such as kidney, liver, gastrointestinal tract, limbs, and so forth.

Ingestion of saturated fats increases the severity of arteriosclerosis. The rate at which cholesterol is deposited in the walls of the arteries is directly proportional to the intake of calories in the diet, especially when this is above the daily requirements for energy and also when the diet contains a high percentage of cholesterol and fat. Atherosclerosis also seems to be more severe when most of the intake of calories is in the form of highly saturated fats rather than in the form of unsaturated fats, proteins, and carbohydrates. Certain persons with a hereditary disease called ***familial hypercholesterolemia*** are inclined to very severe arteriosclerosis.

METABOLISM OF PROTEINS

Amino Acids. The ***amino acids,*** which are the end products of protein digestion in the gastrointestinal tract, are absorbed into the portal blood and then are disseminated into all parts of the body. Some of the amino acids are transported into the liver cells and are temporarily stored there, though this is of minor importance in comparison with the storage of glucose and fat by the liver. Most of the amino acids are rapidly absorbed directly into all the cells of the body by active transport or facilitated diffusion mechanisms.

Most amino acids are synthesized into proteins. This process is controlled by messenger ribonucleic acid molecules that act as templates for the formation of the protein molecules in the ribosomes. Some of these proteins include fibrous proteins such as collagen, elastins, keratins, and actin and myosin; plasma proteins such as albumin, globulin, and fibrinogen; and, various enzymes, hormones, and growth factors. Amino acids can also be used to produce energy, as discussed below.

Essential Amino Acids. Essential amino acids cannot be synthesized in the cells. The usual proteins of the body contain 20 different amino acids, and these are available in almost all protein foods that are eaten. However, an occasional dietary protein has a deficiency of one or more of the usual amino acids. Often one of the available amino acids can be converted into the missing one, but 10 of the 20 amino acids cannot be formed this way and must be present in the diet in order for the cells to synthesize their normal complements of proteins. These 10 amino acids are called ***essential amino acids.*** The other 10 ***non-essential amino acids*** are *essential* for the formation of proteins but it is not *essential* that they be present in the diet.

Catabolism of Proteins. A small concentration of amino acids, about 30 mg per 100 ml, is always maintained in the plasma and interstitial fluid. When this amount decreases, amino acids are transported out of the cells, and this causes the proteins of the cells to begin to be catabolized into amino acids. This catabolism is catalyzed by intracellular enzymes called ***cathepsins,*** which are digestive enzymes released from lysosomes in the cells. In this way a small concentration of amino acids is always maintained in the body fluids. Then, if a particular cell becomes damaged or for some other reason needs an immediate source of amino acids to repair its structural and enzyme systems, the amino acids are available. Amino acid mobilization is greatly accelerated by glucocorticoid hormones.

Deamination of Amino Acids. If a person eats more protein than the amount needed to maintain adequate protein stores in the cells, all the excess amino acids are degraded and then used for energy as carbohydrates and fats are used. The first stage in this process is ***deamination,*** which means removal of the amino radical from the amino acid. This is accomplished by a specific enzyme system in the liver cells. The amino radical is then synthesized into urea, which is excreted through the kidneys into the urine.

Many of the deaminated amino acids are similar to pyruvic acid and can enter the citric acid cycle either directly or after a few stages of minor alterations. In this way, the amino acids become oxidized in very much the same way as carbohydrates and fats, and large quantities of ATP are formed to be used as an energy source everywhere in the cells.

NUTRITION

The Calorie. Energy is generally expressed in terms of Calories (spelled with a capital C), which are equivalent to kilocalories. A calorie (spelled with a lower case c) is the amount of heat required to heat one gram of water 1°C. The different types of food are not equal in their capabilities for supplying energy. One gram of carbohydrate or 1 g of protein supplies 4.1 Calories of energy to the body, while 1 g of fat supplies 9.3 Calories of energy. Therefore, it is evident that over twice as much carbohydrate or protein must be eaten to provide the same amount of energy as a specified quantity of fat.

A normal adult burns about 1,600 Calories each day simply to exist. To provide the energy needed for sitting, another 200 to 400 Calories is required; and for walking and working moderate amounts, still another 500 Calories. The total daily energy requirement for the average person adds up to about 2,500 Calories. This is called the metabolic rate of the body. For performing very heavy physical labor, this can occasionally be as great as 6,000 to 7,000 Calories per day.

Basal Metabolic Rate. The basal metabolic rate is the metabolic rate of an awake person whose body is as inactive as possible. To attain the basal state a person must have had essentially no exercise for the past 8 to 10 hours, no food for the past 12 hours, and he or she must have quiet conditions and normal room temperature. The normal basal metabolic rate of the young male adult is about 40 Calories per square meter of body surface area per hour or a total of about 70 Calories per hour for the whole body.

Proteins. The body continues to degrade proteins into amino acids, even when proteins are absent from the diet. This *obligatory loss* of proteins amounts to about 20 to 30 g of protein each day. Because not all proteins contain amino acids in the same proportions as the bodily proteins and because not all proteins are used completely by the body, it is usually necessary to ingest 60 to 75 g of protein each day to avoid significant protein loss.

Short-Term Food Intake. Whenever the gastrointestinal system becomes overly filled, nervous signals passing from the intestinal tract to the brain diminish one's desire for food and therefore diminish the intake of food. The degree of distention of the stomach and upper portions of the small intestine is particularly important. Since about 20 minutes or so is required for the nervous signals from a full stomach to make a person begin to lose his or her appetite for food, eating a meal very slowly can be an effective means of reducing caloric intake.

Long-Term Food Intake. Located in the lateral nucleus of the hypothalamus is a feeding center, which, when stimulated, increases the food intake. Located in the ventromedial nucleus of the hypothalamus is a center that makes a person feel satisfied and therefore inhibits food intake; therefore, this center is called the satiety center. The degree of activity of the feeding center of the hypothalamus is determined by the metabolic status of the body. When a person becomes overweight, the activity of the feeding center diminishes. On the other hand, in starvation, the feeding center becomes greatly activated. The exact feedback signals to the feeding center that activate or inactivate it are not well understood, but it is known that increased levels of glucose and amino acids in the blood will inhibit feeding, while diminished quantities of these excite feeding. It is probable that the level of fatty acids in the circulating blood also is an important factor in controlling the activity of the feeding center.

Obesity. When more foods are ingested than are utilized each day, the extra amount is stored in the form of fat. Even excess carbohydrates and proteins are converted into fat and then stored. Thus, obesity actually develops from an excess intake of energy each day over utilization of energy. A common ***psychological factor*** that contributes to obesity is the notion that three meals are required every day and that each meal should result in complete satiation. This false notion often develops during childhood from overzealous parents. ***Genetic factors*** contributing to obesity can involve abnormalities of the feeding centers or psychic abnormalities that cause a person to eat as a release mechanism. ***Childhood overnutrition*** can increase the proliferation of fat cells in the first few years of life and thereby promote the development of obesity throughout the life of the individual.

Metabolic Processes During Starvation. Sufficient glycogen is stored in the liver and muscle cells to provide significant amounts of energy for about one half to one day. Beyond that, almost all the energy made available to the body at first comes from the stored fat, this sometimes lasting for as long as 3 to 8 weeks. However, during the entire process of starvation, a small amount of body protein is continually degraded and used for energy as well, and when the fat stores begin to run out, tremendous amounts of protein then begin to be used for energy. When this happens, the functional state of the cells quickly deteriorates, and death soon follows. However, it is fortunate that most of the proteins are spared until the last.

Vitamins. The functions of some of the important vitamins are the following:

Vitamin A is used to synthesize rhodopsin, which is a chemical necessary for vision. It also important for the normal growth of most cells, especially epithelial cells.

Thiamine (vitamin B_1) functions as a cocarboxylase, mainly for decarboxylation of pyruvic acid. Thus, thiamine is necessary for normal metabolism of carbohydrates and many amino acids.

Niacin (nicotinic acid) functions in the body as coenzymes in the forms of nicotinamide adenine dinucleotide (NAD) and nicotinamide adenine dinucleotide phosphate (NADP). These act as hydrogen acceptors when hydrogen is removed from the foods; therefore, they are important in the oxidation of food.

Riboflavin (vitamin B_2) is used to form flavoprotein, which is also a hydrogen carrier in the oxidation of foodstuffs.

Vitamin B_{12} and ***folic acid*** were discussed earlier in the chapter as substances needed for the maturation of red blood cells in the bone marrow.

Pantothenic acid is a precursor of coenzyme A, which is needed for acetylation of many substances in the body. It is especially needed for the formation of acetyl coenzyme A prior to oxidation of both glucose and fatty acids.

Pyridoxine is used as a coenzyme in many reactions involving amino acid metabolism, one of which acts to transfer amino radicals from one substance to another, and another of which causes deamination.

Ascorbic acid (vitamin C) is a strong reducing compound that acts in several metabolic processes in which electrons are exchanged with oxidative chemicals. Though the precise nature of all these specific chemical reactions is not known, the major physiologic function of ascorbic acid is to maintain normal intercellular substances, including normal collagen fibers and normal intercellular cement substance between the cells.

Vitamin D increases absorption of calcium from the gastrointestinal tract and also helps to control calcium deposition in the bone.

Vitamin K is needed in the synthetic processes of the liver for formation of prothrombin, Factor VII, and several other factors that are utilized in blood coagulation. Therefore, vitamin K deficiency retards blood clotting.

REGULATION OF BODY TEMPERATURE

The temperature of the body is determined by the balance between the rate of heat production and the rate of heat loss. If the rate of heat production exceeds the rate of heat loss, the body temperature will rise. If the rate of loss is greater, then the body temperature will fall.

Heat Production. All the metabolic processes of the body produce heat as a byproduct, for almost all the energy in the food eventually becomes heat after it performs its other functions. Thus, in the average person about 2,500 Calories of heat are formed each day.

Under basal conditions it is mainly the internal organs—the brain, the heart, the kidneys, the gastrointestinal tract, and especially the liver—that produce most of the heat. However, when a person uses muscles for various activities, these produce tremendous amounts of heat. During extreme muscular activity, the total heat production of the body can increase temporarily to as much as 15 to 20 times normal, over 90% of the heat then coming from the muscles.

Heat Loss. Normally, about 60% of the heat loss from a nude person sitting in a room at 70°F (21°C) is by ***radiation.*** Heat loss in this manner results from heat waves, a type of electromagnetic radiation, that are transmitted from the surface of the body to surrounding objects. Approximately 18% of the heat that is lost by the nude person is by ***conduction*** to objects touching the body or to the surrounding air and then by ***convection*** of the heated air away from the body. Finally, a small amount of water continually diffuses through the skin, and evaporation of each gram of water removes about one-half calorie of heat from the body. ***Evaporation*** of water accounts for about 22% of the heat loss from the nude person.

Heat loss is controlled by blood flow to the skin. The skin is supplied with an abundant vasculature, but the amount of blood that flows through the skin vessels is controlled very exactly by the sympathetic nervous system so that when the body becomes overly heated, skin blood flow will be tremendous, and when the body is underheated, skin blood flow will be negligible. Rapid flow of blood heats the skin, allowing large amounts of heat to be lost to the surroundings. Also, sympathetic stimuli to the sweat glands increase sweat production and consequently greatly increase the evaporative loss of heat. Slow blood flow prevents heat loss because the internal heat of the body cannot be carried to the skin, and the skin temperature falls rapidly to approach that of the surroundings.

The Hypothalamic Thermostat. The preoptic area of the anterior hypothalamus contains heat-sensitive neurons as well as cold-sensitive neurons. These neurons are thought to function as temperature sensors for controlling body temperature. The ***heat-sensitive neurons*** increase their rate of firing when the body becomes too hot, and the ***cold-sensitive neurons*** increase their firing rate when the body becomes too cold. The temperature sensory signals from the anterior hypothalamus are transmitted to the posterior hypothalamus where they are integrated with signals from periphery to make appropriate adjustments in heat production and heat loss.

Temperature-Increasing Mechanisms. Constriction of the skin blood vessels reduces the rate of heat loss because the skin temperature approaches the temperature of the surrounding air. Heat production is increased by (1) shivering, which increases the muscle metabolic rate; and (2) sympathetic release of epinephrine, which effects an increase in the metabolic rate of all cells in the body. The result of these effects is an increase in the body temperature back toward normal.

Temperature-Decreasing Mechanisms. When the preoptic area becomes too hot, the temperature control system decreases heat production by reducing the tone of the skeletal muscles throughout the body and reducing the sympathetic release of epinephrine. More important, however, it increases the rate of heat loss in two ways: (1) Lack of sympathetic vasoconstriction allows the blood vessels of the skin to become greatly dilated—the skin temperature rises, and increased amounts of heat are lost to the surroundings; and (2) stimulation of a sweat center, also located in the heat center of the hypothalamus, causes sweating over the entire body, with resultant evaporative loss of heat.

Summary of Hypothalamic Control of Body Temperature. If the preoptic area of the anterior hypothalamus becomes too hot, heat production is decreased while heat loss is increased, and the body temperature falls back toward normal. Conversely, if the preoptic area becomes too cold, heat production is increased, while heat loss is decreased so that the body temperature now rises toward normal.

Temperature Signals from Skin. When the skin becomes too warm, nerve impulses are transmitted from the skin warm receptors all the way to the preoptic area of the hypothalamus to increase sweating, and this obviously increases body heat loss. Conversely, when the skin becomes too cold, signals from the skin cold receptors are transmitted to the posterior hypothalamus where they activate shivering, which in turn helps to increase the body temperature back toward normal. Therefore, body temperature control is vested in an integrated mechanism in which the hypothalamus is the central integrator, but reacts to signals both from the preoptic area and from the skin.

ENDOCRINE CONTROL SYSTEMS

The endocrine glands secrete ***hormones*** that control many of the body's functions. Hormones are chemical messengers that are carried by the blood from endocrine glands to the cells in which they act, often referred to as ***target cells*** for that hormone. In general, the hormone systems function to (1) control transport of substances through cell membranes; (2) control the activity of specific cellular genes, which in turn determine the formation of specific enzymes and other cell factors; (3) control directly some metabolic systems of the cells.

Hormone Structure, Synthesis, and Secretion. There are three general classes of hormones: (1) steroids, such as cortisol and estrogen; (2) proteins and polypeptides, such as adrenocorticotropic hormone (ACTH) and growth hormone; and (3) amino acid derivatives, such as epinephrine and thyroxine. Most hormones are water soluble and there are no hormones known that are polysaccharides or nucleic acids.

Steroid hormones are synthesized from cholesterol and are lipid-soluble substances consisting of three cyclohexyl rings and one cyclopentyl ring combined into a single structure. Steroids are synthesized and secreted by the adrenal cortex and the gonads (including the testes and ovaries) as well as the placenta during pregnancy. Because the steroids are highly lipid soluble, once they are synthesized they simply diffuse across the cell membrane of the steroid-producing cell and enter the interstitial fluid and then the blood. The circulatory half-life of most steroids is between 60 and 100 minutes.

Protein and polypeptide hormones comprise the majority of hormones in the body and range in size from small peptides of a few amino acids to small proteins. In many cases, they are synthesized first as larger proteins that are cleaved to form ***prohormones,*** which in turn must be modified by the secretory cells to produce biologically active hormones. Protein and polypeptide hormones are usually stored in subcellular membrane-bound secretory granules within the cytoplasm of the different endocrine cells. The hormones are released into the blood by ***exocytosis,*** which occurs when the secretory granule is fused with the cell membrane and the granular contents are then extruded into the interstitial fluid or directly into the bloodstream. In many cases, the stimulus for exocytosis is an increase in cytosolic calcium concentration caused by depolarization of the plasma membrane. The circulatory half-life of protein and peptide hormones is relatively short, lasting for as little as 2 to 3 minutes to as long as 60 minutes for some hormones.

Amine hormones are derived from the amino acid tyrosine and are sometimes called phenolic derivatives; these hormones include ***epinephrine, norepinephrine, triiodothyronine*** (T_3) and ***thyroxine*** (T_4). The thyroid hormones T_4 and T_3 are synthesized and stored in the thyroid gland and incorporated into molecules of the protein ***thyroglobulin.*** Hormone secretion occurs when T_4 and T_3 are split from the thyroglobulin, and the free hormones are then released into the bloodstream. After entering the blood, most of the T_4 and T_3 combine with plasma proteins, especially thyroxin-binding globulin, which slowly releases the hormones to the tissue cells.

The hormones epinephrine and norepinephrine are formed in the adrenal medulla, which normally secretes about four times more epinephrine than norepinephrine. Both of these catecholamines exist in the plasma in free form or in conjugation with other substances; most of the circulating epinephrine is bound to plasma proteins, especially albumin, whereas norepinephrine does not significantly bind to plasma proteins. The circulatory half-life of norepinephrine and epinephrine is about 1 to 3 minutes.

Mechanisms of Hormone Action. The first step of a hormone's action is to bind to a specific ***receptor*** in the target cell; cells that lack specific receptors for the hormone do not respond. For some hormones (*e.g.*, peptide hormones), receptors are located on the target cell membrane. In other instances, the cell receptors are located in the cytoplasm (*e.g.*, steroids) or at the nucleus (*e.g.*, thyroid hormones). Lipid-soluble hormones can cross the cell membrane, interact with specific intracellular receptors, and increase or decrease protein synthesis by stimulating or inhibiting the production of mRNA. These either bind to specific receptors in the cytoplasm or diffuse through the nuclear membrane and bind to specific receptors in the nucleus. Activation of these intracellular receptors then elicits a sequence of events that produces the hormone effects by regulating expression of specific genes in the cell nucleus.

Peptide hormones and catecholamines cannot penetrate cell membranes and therefore must interact with receptors on the exterior surface of the cell. Coupling of the receptor to the intracellular enzymes that control cell function results from generation of intracellular ***signal transduction mechanisms*** and ***second messengers.*** In some cases, the hormone receptor itself contains an ion channel, and activation of the receptor causes the channel to open, resulting in increased diffusion across the plasma membrane of ions specific for the channel. The altered ion concentration of the cell then elicits the cell responses to the hormone.

Figure 3-31 shows the ***adenylate cyclase/cyclic AMP second messenger system*** for many hormones, including most polypeptides and catecholamines. Binding of the hormone to its receptor allows coupling of the receptor to a ***G protein*** (called a ***G_s protein,*** denoting a stimulatory G protein). This stimulates adenylate cyclase, a membrane-bound enzyme, which then catalyzes the formation of cyclic AMP (cAMP) inside the cell. This then activates ***cAMP-dependent protein kinase,*** which phosphorylates specific proteins in the cell, triggering the various biochemical reactions that ultimately lead to the cell's response to the hormone.

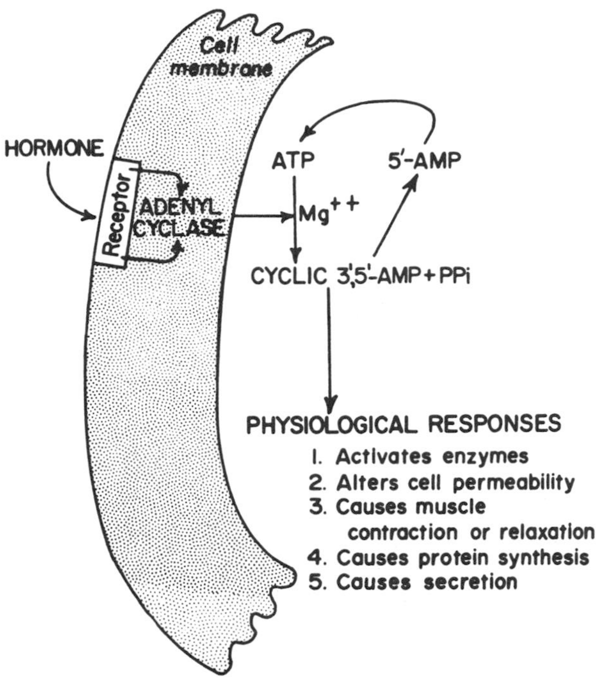

Fig. 3-31. Cyclic AMP second messenger system. (Guyton AC: Textbook of Medical Physiology, 8th ed. Philadelphia: WB Saunders, 1991)

THE HYPOTHALAMUS–PITUITARY HORMONE SYSTEM

The ***pituitary gland,*** located at the base of the brain just below the brain area called the ***hypothalamus,*** secretes a large number of peptide hormones that regulate many body functions. The pituitary is connected to the hypothalamus by a stalk that contains nerve fibers and blood vessels and is divided into two major parts: the ***anterior pituitary*** and the ***posterior pituitary*** glands. Six well-known hormones are secreted by the anterior pituitary gland, including (1) growth hormone, (2) thyroid-stimulating hormone, (3) adrenocorticotropic hormone (ACTH), (4) prolactin, (5) luteinizing hormone, and (6) follicle-stimulating hormone. The posterior pituitary gland secretes two primary hormones: antidiuretic hormone (ADH) and oxytocin.

Control of Anterior Pituitary Hormone Secretion. If the anterior pituitary gland is separated from the hypothalamus, secretion of most of its hormones, with the exception of prolactin, decreases to very small amounts. This occurs because secretion of the anterior pituitary gland is controlled mainly by additional hormones formed in the hypothalamus, which are then conducted to the pituitary through the ***hypothalamic-hypophyseal venous portal system,*** shown in Figure 3-32. The system consists of small veins that carry blood (and therefore hormones) from capillaries in the lower hypothalamus to the venous sinuses of the anterior pituitary gland. Here, the hormones from the hypothalamus act directly on the anterior pituitary cells to control secretion of the pituitary hormones. Most of the hormones from the hypothalamus stimulate hormone secretion from anterior pituitary cells, but some of them inhibit release of hormones.

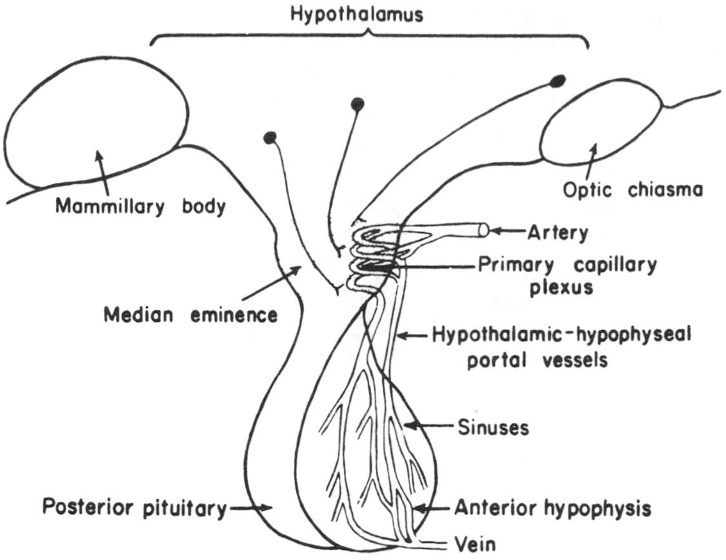

Fig. 3-32. The hypothalamic-hypophyseal portal system. (Guyton AC: Textbook of Medical Physiology, 8th ed. Philadelphia: WB Saunders, 1991)

Some of the most important hormones that control the function of the anterior pituitary gland are the following:

Growth hormone–releasing hormone (GHRH), which causes release of growth hormone

Corticotropin-releasing hormone (CRH), which causes release of adrenocorticotropic hormone

Thyrotropin-releasing hormone (TRH), which causes release of thyroid-stimulating hormone

Gonadotropin-releasing hormone (GnRH), which causes release of two gonadotropins, luteinizing hormone (LH) and follicle-stimulating hormone (FSH)

Prolactin inhibitory hormone, believed to be ***dopamine,*** which inhibits the release of prolactin; in the absence of this hormone, the rate of prolactin secretion increases to about 3 times normal

Somatostatin or ***somatropin-releasing inhibiting factor*** (SRIF), which inhibits the secretion of growth hormone, thyroid-stimulating hormone, and possibly other hormones.

Adrenocorticotropic Hormone. Adrenocorticotropic hormone (ACTH) strongly stimulates ***cortisol*** production of the adrenal cortex and to a lesser extent the production of other adrenocortical hormones. Cortisol in turn has many different metabolic effects on the body, including degradation of proteins in the tissues, release of amino acids into the circulating blood, conversion of many of these amino acids into glucose (the process of gluconeogenesis), and decreased utilization of glucose by the tissues. These effects will be discussed later in relation to the adrenal hormones.

Figure 3-33 shows that the secretion of ACTH by the anterior pituitary is controlled mainly by CRH released by the hypothalamus. The rate of secretion of CRH in turn is strongly stimulated by stressful states such as disease, trauma to the body, and even emotional excitement. When excess quantities of cortisol are present in the blood, these feed back on the hypothalamus and anterior pituitary cells to decrease the rate of secretion of ACTH, thus providing a negative feedback mechanism for controlling cortisol concentration in the blood.

Thyroid-Stimulating Hormone. Thyroid stimulating hormone (TSH) stimulates the thyroid gland follicles in several ways: (1) It increases the rate of synthesis

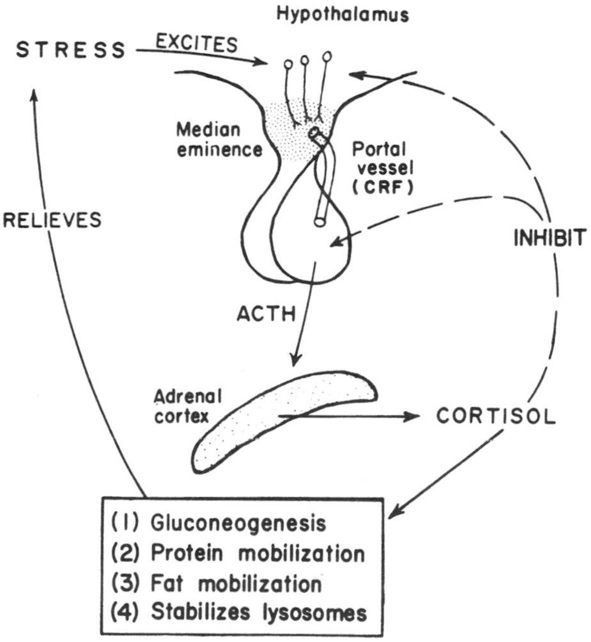

Fig. 3-33. Regulation of ACTH and cortisol secretion, and multiple actions of cortisol. (Guyton AC: Textbook of Medical Physiology, 8th ed. Philadelphia: WB Saunders, 1991)

of thyroglobulin, (2) it increases the uptake of iodide ions from the blood by the glandular cells, and (3) it activates all of the chemical processes that cause thyroxine production and release by the thyroid gland. Therefore, TSH indirectly increases the overall rate of metabolism of the body through increased formation and release of thyroxine.

The rate of TSH secretion by the anterior pituitary is controlled mainly by the negative feedback effect of thyroxine on the hypothalamus. When thyroxine concentrations are high, this decreases the rate of secretion of TSH by the hypothalamus and production of thyroxine by the anterior pituitary.

Growth Hormone. The anterior pituitary gland secretes growth hormone throughout life, not only while a person is growing. However, growth hormone does not markedly influence fetal growth and is not a major growth factor during the first few months after birth. On the other hand, growth hormone is essential for normal body growth during childhood and adolescence. It causes enlargement and proliferation of cells in all parts of the body, resulting in progressive growth of the body stature until adolescence. At this time, the epiphyses of the long bones unite with the shafts of the bones so that further increase in height of the body cannot occur. However, certain of the "membranous" bones such as the bones of the nose and certain bones of the skull, as well as the solid tissues of some of the internal organs, can continue to grow under the influence of excess growth hormone.

In addition to its growth promoting action, growth hormone also has effects on lipid, carbohydrate, and protein metabolism. For example, growth hormone is believed to modulate some of the actions of insulin on the liver and peripheral tissues, inhibiting glucose used by muscle and fat and increasing glucose production by the liver. In addition, growth hormone also stimulates mobilization of triglycerides from fat depots in the body. For this reason, excess secretion of growth hormone can produce metabolic disturbances much like those in individuals with non-insulin–dependent diabetes mellitus.

The precise mechanism by which growth hormone exerts its effect on cells is not clear. However, it is known to act on the liver to cause formation of several small protein substances called ***somatomedins,*** one of which is called ***insulin-like growth factor I (IGF-1).*** IGF-1 is produced by many cells of the body and released in the bloodstream, but the liver is the primary source of IGF-1 in the blood. IGF-1 in turn has a negative feedback effect to decrease the secretion of growth hormone.

Growth hormone specifically promotes transport of some amino acids through cell membranes, thereby making more of these available to the cells. In addition, (1) it activates the RNA translation process to stimulate formation of proteins by the ribosomes; (2) it increases the rate of DNA transcription to increase the amount of mRNA; (3) it increases the replication of DNA, which causes increased production of the cells themselves; (4) it decreases the rate of breakdown of proteins in the cells. Thus, growth hormone has a potent effect to enhance all aspects of protein synthesis and storage in the cells of the body.

After adolescence, growth hormone continues to be secreted at about two thirds the pre-adolescent rate. Although most of the growth of the body stops at this time, primarily because the growth potential of the long bone ceases when the epiphyses unite with the shafts, the other metabolic effects of the growth hormone continue.

Growth hormone secretion is controlled by GHRH that is secreted in the hypothalamus and transported to the anterior pituitary through the hypothalamic-hypophyseal portal system. When nutritional debility causes protracted hypoglycemia or reduces the body's protein storage, the secretion of GHRH and therefore the rate of growth hormone secretion are increased. Also, other types of physical or mental stress often greatly increase the rate of growth hormone secretion.

Gonadotropic Hormones. The anterior pituitary secretes two hormones that regulate many male and female sexual functions. These are FSH and LH, which influence virtually every aspect of the reproductive process. The rates of secretion of these hormones are controlled mainly by LH-releasing hormone from the hypothalamus, but feedback from the sex hormones also helps to control their rates of secretion. The gonadotropic hormones will be discussed in more detail later in relation to reproduction.

Prolactin. Prolactin is important in the development of the breast during pregnancy and in promoting milk secretion by the breast after birth of the baby. These functions will also be discussed in more detail in relation to milk production.

The secretion of prolactin is controlled mainly by ***prolactin inhibitory hormone*** in the hypothalamus, which reduces the secretion of prolactin. There are also ***prolactin releasing factors(s)*** released by the hypothalamus, but these have not been fully characterized. Prolactin secretion increases about tenfold during pregnancy. This rate of secretion is also increased by suckling of the nipples by the baby, which in turn causes production of more milk.

Posterior Pituitary Hormones. The posterior pituitary is, to a large extent, a neural extension of the hypothalamus. The hormones of the posterior pituitary are synthesized in the cell bodies of the hypothalamus whose axons pass through the ***median eminence*** and enter the posterior pituitary. These hormones move down the neural axons to accumulate at the axon terminals in the posterior pituitary. When the hypothalamus neurons receive input signals for ADH or oxytocin secretion, action potentials are generated in these cells and travel down the axons to trigger the release of ADH or oxytocin from the axon terminal. These substances then diffuse into the capillaries and enter the systemic circulation.

Secretion of ***ADH,*** discussed earlier in relation to water reabsorption by the renal tubules, is stimulated when the body fluids become excessively concentrated. Neuronal cells in or near the ***supraoptic nucleus*** of the hypothalamus, called ***osmoreceptors,*** are stimulated by increased osmolality or cell shrinkage and cause the release of ADH from the posterior pituitary gland. On reaching the kidney, ADH increases the rate of water reabsorption from the renal tubules and tends to correct the overconcentration of the body fluids.

ADH secretion is also stimulated by decreased blood pressure or decreased blood volume, through baroreceptor and cardiopulmonary reflexes, which send signals to the hypothalamus. ADH, in addition to causing water retention, also constricts the arterioles and causes the arterial pressure to rise the primary reason it is also called ***vasopressin.***

Oxytocin causes contraction especially of the uterus and to a lesser extent other smooth muscles of the body. Oxytocin is released by the posterior pituitary gland in increased amounts during parturition and may play a significant role in initiating birth of the baby. Oxytocin also plays a role in lactation in the following ways: Sucking on the breast initiates nerve impulses that pass all the way from the nipple to the hypothalamus, which then sends signals to the posterior pituitary gland to stimulate release of oxytocin. The oxytocin in turn stimulates ***myoepithelial cells*** in the breast that constrict the alveoli of the breast in a manner that makes the milk flow into the ducts. This is called ***milk ejection*** or ***milk let down.***

ADRENOCORTICAL HORMONES

The adrenal cortex secretes three different types of steroid hormones that are chemically similar but physiologically very different. These are (1) ***mineralocorticoids,*** represented principally by aldosterone; (2) ***glucocorticoids,*** represented mainly by cortisol; and (3) several ***androgens,*** which have masculine sexual effects.

The adrenal cortex of the adult human consists of three distinct layers: (1) the ***zona glomerulosa,*** the outer zone, which produces aldosterone; (2) the ***zona fasciculata,*** the middle layer, which produce glucocorticoids and androgens; and (3) the ***zona reticularis,*** the inner layer of the cortex, which also produces glucocorticoids and androgens.

Mineralocorticoid Control of Electrolyte Balance. Although several mineralocorticoid hormones are secreted by the adrenal cortex, about 95% of the total mineralocorticoid activity is due to ***aldosterone.*** As discussed earlier in this chapter, aldosterone enhances sodium reabsorption from the renal tubules into the blood and at the same time increases potassium transport from the blood into the tubules. Therefore, aldosterone causes the body to conserve sodium while increasing the excretion of potassium in the urine.

Aldosterone also increases reabsorption of chloride ions and water from the tubules in parallel with increased sodium reabsorption, as explained previously. As a result, increased aldosterone secretion causes the kidneys to retain water and sodium and to increase extracellular fluid volume.

The main factors that control aldosterone secretion are as follows: (1) An increased ***potassium ion*** concentration stimulates aldosterone secretion by the adrenal gland. This provides an important negative feedback control system for extracellular fluid potassium ion concentration because aldosterone then promotes excretion of excess potassium from the extracellular fluid into the urine. (2) ***Angiotensin II*** also stimulates secretion of aldosterone, an effect that provides important feedback control of extracellular fluid volume. When extracellular fluid volume or blood pressure decreases, this stimulates the kidney to release renin, which in turn stimulates angiotensin II formation and aldosterone secretion. The increased aldosterone concentration causes the renal tubules to reabsorb more sodium, chloride, and water, thus returning extracellular fluid volume and blood pressure toward normal. (3) Decreased ***sodium ion*** concentration in the extracellular fluid also stimulates aldosterone secretion. (4) ***ACTH*** transiently increases aldosterone secretion and also plays a permissive role in allowing other stimuli, such as potassium and angiotensin II, to exert their long-term effects on aldosterone secretion.

A deficiency of aldosterone secretion, such as occurs in ***Addison's disease,*** is associated with a tendency toward decreased extracellular fluid volume and accumulation of potassium. Excess secretion of aldosterone, as occurs in ***primary aldosteronism (Conn's syndrome),*** causes sodium and water retention, mild expansion of extracellular fluid volume, and hypokalemia (decreased plasma potassium concentration).

Glucocorticoid Effects on Metabolism and Inflammation. Several different glucocorticoids are secreted by the adrenal cortex, but most of the glucocorticoid activity is caused by ***cortisol,*** also called ***hydrocortisone.*** Cortisol reduces glucose uptake into cells and also reduces the rate of utilization of glucose by the cells. It also increases the rate of gluconeogenesis in liver cells, which convert amino acids into glucose. Thus, several different effects of glucocortisol cause the blood concentration of glucose to increase.

Cortisol also causes degradation of proteins and decreases protein synthesis in most tissues of the body. This causes amino acids to be released from the cells and therefore increases their concentration in the blood. In the liver, however, cortisol has the opposite effect—it increases amino acid uptake. These amino acids are used to synthesize large quantities of plasma proteins, to provide metabolic energy for the liver, and to be converted into glucose by the process of gluconeogenesis as discussed previously.

Cortisol also increases the use of fat for energy. This results mainly from an effect of cortisol to activate ***hormone-sensitive lipase*** in fat cells, which causes splitting of the fat and release of amino acids into the circulating blood.

Cortisol can also suppress inflammation by stabilizing cellular lysosomes, preventing them from rupturing and releasing their digestive enzymes as well as histamine, bradykinin, and other factors that promote inflammation. Cortisol also reduces the permeability of capillary membranes, which minimizes leakage of fluid into the tissues during inflammation. Because of the antiinflammatory effect of cortisol, it is often administered clinically to reduce inflammation in certain allergic reactions, to treat bursitis and arthritis, and in some types of infection.

One of the primary controls for glucocorticoid secretion is ACTH, which increases cortisol secretion. Secretion of both cortisol and ACTH usually follows a circadian pattern, dependent on the sleep/wake cycle, with levels of both hormones increasing during waking hours. Other important stimuli for ACTH secretion, and there fore cortisol secretion, include emotional and physical stress, trauma, shock, infection, and hypoglycemia. There is also feedback inhibition of ACTH secretion by glucocorticoids acting at the pituitary as well as the hypothalamus to inhibit CRH.

Deficiency of glucocorticoid production (as occurs in Addison's disease) reduces the ability to cope with stress, to form glucose during fasting, and to mobilize lipids for use by peripheral tissues. Conversely, excess glucocorticoid production, as occurs in ***Cushing's disease,*** is associated with increased production and decreased utilization of glucose and therefore a tendency toward hyperglycemia. In addition, prolonged exposure of the body to large amounts of glucocorticoids causes breakdown of peripheral tissue proteins, increased mobilization of lipid from fat stores, and a redistribution of fat on the abdomen, shoulders, and face. Although Cushing's syndrome can be caused by primary hypersecretion of cortisol by the adrenal gland, it usually occurs in response to hypersecretion of ACTH by the pituitary.

Although the most important androgen in the body is testosterone, secreted by the testes, the adrenal cortex also secretes several androgenic hormones. These are normally of minor importance, but when an adrenal tumor develops or when adrenal glands become hyperplastic and secrete excess quantities of hormones, the amounts of androgens then secreted occasionally become great enough to cause even a child or an adult female to take on adult masculine characteristics.

THYROID HORMONES

The thyroid gland, located immediately below the larynx on either side and to the front of the trachea, secretes two hormones, ***thyroxine*** and ***triiodothyronine,*** that have marked effects on the metabolic rate of the body. The thyroid gland also secretes ***calcitonin,*** a hormone that is important for calcium metabolism and will be considered later.

Synthesis and Secretion of Thyroxine and Triiodothyronine. The thyroid gland is composed of follicles lined with thyroid glandular cells, shown in Figure 3-34. These cells secrete a very large glycoprotein called ***thyroglobulin*** to the inside of the follicles. They also absorb iodide ions from the circulating blood and secrete these in an oxidized form into the follicles along with the thyroglobulin. This oxidized iodine combines with tyrosine amino acid molecules that are integral parts of the thyroglobulin molecule. In this manner, large quantities of thyroxine and smaller amounts of triiodothyronine are formed within the thyroglobulin molecule, and the thyroglobulin then remains stored in the thyroid follicles for an average of about 6 weeks.

As thyroid hormones are needed in the circulating blood, some of the thyroglobulin is reabsorbed back into the glandular cells by the process of pinocytosis. Then the thyroglobulin is digested by proteases formed by lyso-

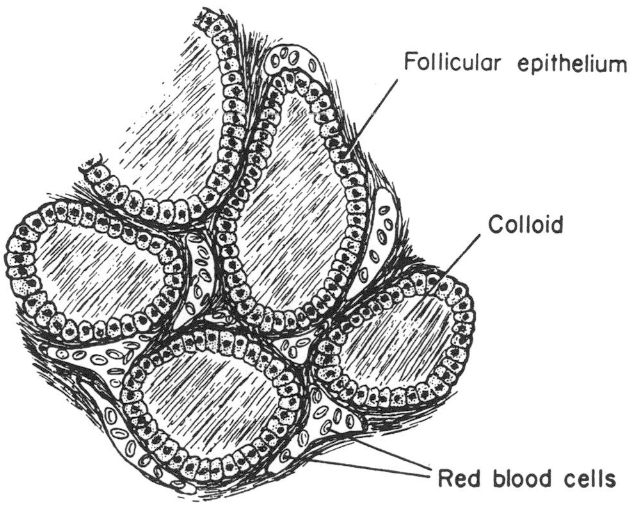

Fig. 3-34. Microscopic appearance of the thyroid gland. (Guyton AC: Textbook of Medical Physiology, 8th ed. Philadelphia: WB Saunders, 1991)

somes in the cells, thus releasing thyroxine and triiodothyronine into the blood.

The rate of formation of the thyroid hormones, and especially their rate of release from thyroglobulin, is controlled to a large extent by TSH released from the anterior pituitary gland, as discussed earlier. The thyroid hormones in turn regulate their own secretion by exerting an inhibitory effect on TSH secretion. Consequently, when circulating concentrations of thyroid hormones are too high, the rate of TSH secretion is reduced and the secretion of thyroid hormones returns toward normal.

Once the thyroid hormones have been released into the blood, they combine with several different plasma proteins. Then during the next week they are slowly released from the blood into the tissue cells.

Effect of Thyroxine and Triiodothyronine on Metabolic Activity of Cells. The overall action of the thyroid hormones is to increase the metabolic activity in almost all cells of the body. They also increase the breakdown of cell foodstuffs and the rate of release from the cells. Thyroxine (T_4) is the major circulating form of thyroid hormone, although triiodothyronine has the same effects as thyroxine, except that it acts more rapidly.

A second important effect of thyroid hormones is to influence growth and differentiation. Fetal or neonatal thyroid deficiency leads to ***cretinism,*** a condition associated with abnormal structure of the face, reduced neuronal development, and delayed skeletal maturation. Unfortunately, the exact mechanisms by which the thyroid hormones perform their functions in the cells are still unknown. However, they increase the rate of synthesis of proteins in almost all cells, and especially the rate of synthesis of the different intracellular enzymes that are the basis for increased metabolic activities of the cells. They also increase the sizes and numbers of mitochondria in the cells and these in turn increase the rate of production of ATP, which also promotes enhanced cellular metabolism.

Metabolic and Nervous Disorders Caused by Hyperthroidism. One of the most common causes of excess thyroid hormone production in the human is ***Graves's disease,*** an autoimmune disease believed to be caused by antibodies formed against certain components of follicular cell membranes, causing enlargement of the thyroid gland and oversecretion of the thyroid hormones. The main effects caused by excess thyroid activity include (1) greatly increased rate of metabolism throughout the body; (2) increased heart rate and increased cardiac output; (3) increased gastrointestinal secretion and motility; (4) increased activity of the nervous system, sometimes causing a fine tremor of the muscles; (5) increased respiratory rate; (6) frequent abnormal glandular secretion by the endocrine systems; and (7) severe loss of weight in extreme cases. In general, hyperthyroid individuals are nervous and irritable and experience physical weakness and fatigue, gradual destruction of body tissue, and weight loss despite increased food intake.

Decreased Metabolic Activity Caused by Hypothroidism. A deficiency of thyroid hormone greatly inhibits activity of almost all functional systems, causing (1) a decrease in metabolic rate to as low as 40% below normal, (2) lethargy so that a person may sleep 14 to 16 hours a day and have difficulty cerebrating even when awake, and (3) collection of mucinous fluid in the tissue spaces between the cells, creating an edematous state called ***myxedema.***

THE PANCREATIC HORMONES: INSULIN AND GLUCAGON

The pancreas has thousands of small clusters of cells, called ***islets of Langerhans,*** one of which is illustrated in Figure 3-35. These islets are composed of four main cell types, including (1) ***alpha cells,*** which secrete ***glucagon;*** (2) ***beta cells,*** which secrete ***insulin;*** (3) ***delta cells,*** which secrete ***somatostatin;*** and (4) ***F cells,*** which secrete ***pancreatic polypeptide***. The precise roles of pancreatic somatostatin and pancreatic polypeptide have not been elucidated, but both insulin and glucagon are known to be important in the storage and use of the fuels and in regulating metabolism.

Insulin is a small protein with a molecular weight of about 6,000 and is often referred to as the storage hormone because its secretion is greatly increased immediately after a meal and because it causes cellular storage of all the different food stuffs, including carbohydrate, fat, and protein. Glucagon, on the other hand, has effects

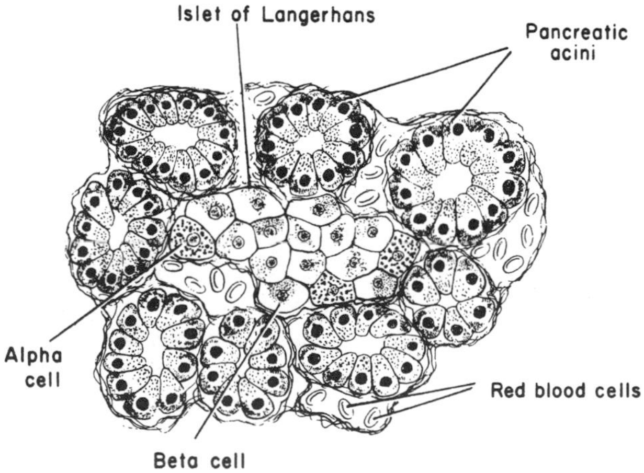

Fig. 3-35. Anatomy of an islet of Langerhans in the pancreas. (Guyton AC: Textbook of Medical Physiology, 8th ed. Philadelphia: WB Saunders, 1991)

that are in many ways opposite those of insulin, as will be discussed later.

Insulin Regulation of Blood Glucose Concentration. Insulin is perhaps the most important hormone in maintaining normal blood glucose concentration. After a large meal, increased secretion of insulin prevents the glucose concentration from rising too high by causing storage of approximately 60% of the absorbed glucose in the liver and 15% in the skeletal muscle, with the remaining glucose used for energy. Then, between meals the secretion of insulin is markedly decreased, and most of the glucose returns to the blood because of continual breakdown of glycogen in the liver when insulin is not present. This maintains a relatively constant blood glucose concentration in the fed and fasting states, which assures a relatively constant rate of delivery of glucose to the brain. Because the brain cells utilize fats and proteins very poorly for energy, the precise regulation of blood glucose concentration helps to maintain a steady rate of neuronal activity.

The mechanisms by which insulin promotes glucose storage in the liver are quite different from the storage mechanism in muscle. In the liver, glucose can rapidly diffuse across the cell membrane without the action of insulin; once glucose diffuses across the cell membrane, it is trapped in the hepatic cells by being converted first into glucose-6-phosphate and then into glycogen. Insulin promotes this effect by greatly increasing the activity of two liver enzymes, ***glucokinase*** and ***glycogen synthetase***. Insulin also reduces hepatic glucose output by inhibiting ***glycogenolysis*** (breakdown of glycogen) through rapidly decreasing glycogen phosphorylase activity and gradually by decreasing glucose-6-phosphatase levels. In addition, insulin also inhibits ***gluconeogenesis*** by decreasing hepatic uptake of precursor amino acids, which are used to synthase glucose.

In skeletal muscle and in most other cells of the body besides the liver and the brain, insulin greatly stimulates glucose transport across the cell membrane. In the presence of large amounts of insulin, the cell membrane of resting skeletal muscle is about 15 times as permeable to glucose as it is when there is no insulin. Insulin also activates glycogen synthetase and ***phosphofructokinase,*** which cause glycogen synthesis and glucose utilization, respectively, in skeletal muscle. And finally, insulin also increases muscle blood flow due to its metabolic effects, which in turn causes more delivery of glucose to the skeletal muscle.

In adipose tissue, as in skeletal muscle, insulin stimulates the transport of glucose into the cells. This glucose is then used for esterification of fatty acids and permits their storage as triglycerides. In the brain, insulin has little or no effect on transport of glucose across the cell membrane. Instead, the rate of glucose diffusion to these cells is directly proportional the blood glucose concentration.

Insulin Reduction of Lipolysis and Stimulation of Storage of Triglycerides. Insulin has both direct and indirect effects on fat metabolism. The direct effect is to reduce the rate of fatty acid release (lipolysis) from fat tissues in the body fluids. The mechanism of this is mainly intense depression of ***hormone-sensitive lipase*** by insulin; this prevents the hydrolysis of triglycerides in the fat tissue and therefore prevents fatty acid release. When there is very little insulin, this enzyme becomes active and causes large quantities of fatty acids to be released into the tissue fluids. In this way, fatty acids become mobilized and are utilized for energy in place of glucose that cannot be effectively utilized in most tissues of the body without insulin.

The indirect effect of insulin on fat metabolism occurs secondarily to insulin-induced changes in carbohydrate metabolism. As discussed above, insulin has the same effect on fat cells that it has on muscle cells to cause increased glucose transport into the cells. This causes some increase in formation of fatty acids in these cells and then storage of these in the form of triglycerides. However, the most important effect is that the glucose inside the fat cells is used to form the glycerol portion of the stored triglycerides.

In the liver, fatty acids are also synthesized from glucose under the influence of insulin. These fatty acids are then transported to the fat cells where they combine with the glycerol to form still more triglycerides that are stored. In the absence of insulin, large amounts of fatty acids are released from the fat cells, and many of these are transported to the liver where they form excessive quantities of (1) stored fat in the liver; (2) cholesterol, phospholipids, and triglycerides, which are released into the blood; and (3) acetoacetic acid, which is also released into the blood. In prolonged periods of low insulin secretion (*e.g.*, diabetes mellitus), the acetoacetic acid can become so great that it causes severe acidosis.

Effect of Insulin on Normal Growth and Protein Metabolism. Even growth hormone will not cause significant growth in an animal in the absence of insulin. Insulin probably has this effect because it increases the formation of protein in cells. It does this by promoting active transport of some of the amino acids through the cell membranes to the interior of the cell, by increasing the number of functional ribosomes for forming proteins, and by increasing the activity of the DNA-RNA system that controls protein formation. *Thus, insulin is an anabolic hormone.*

Stimulation of Insulin Secretion by Increased Blood Glucose. The rate of secretion of insulin by the pancreas is controlled mainly by the concentration of glucose in the circulating blood, but also by the concentration of amino acids. When glucose concentration increases, large quantities of insulin are secreted, and the insulin in turn promotes the storage of glucose in the body cells, especially in the liver. When blood glucose concentration decreases, the rate of insulin secretion also decreases, and glucose is then transported out of the liver back into the blood, helping to prevent excessive decreases in plasma glucose concentration.

Glucagon. In almost all respects, the actions of glucagon are exactly opposite those of insulin. Glucagon promotes mobilization rather than storage of fuels, especially glucose. The most important site of action of glucagon is in the liver, where it has a hyperglycemic action resulting mainly from stimulation of hepatic glycogenolysis. Over a longer period of time, glucagon also causes marked increases in liver gluconeogenesis, which is the process by which amino acids are converted into glucose. The mechanism by which glucagon causes glucose release in the liver cells is the following: glucagon activates adenylate cyclase in the liver cell membranes. This in turn causes formation of cAMP in the cells, which then activates phosphorylase, the enzyme that causes glycogen to split into glucose molecules.

When the blood concentration of glucose falls below normal, the pancreas secretes large amounts of glucagon. The blood glucose–raising effect of glucagon then helps to correct the hypoglycemia. Therefore, glucagon, like insulin, is also important for control of blood glucose concentration.

Diabetes Mellitus. There are two types of diabetes mellitus, caused by either insufficient secretion of insulin, referred to as ***insulin-dependent diabetes mellitus (IDDM, or type I),*** or resistance to the metabolic effects of insulin on the target tissue, referred to as ***non-insulin-dependent diabetes mellitus (NIDDM, or type II).*** In both of these types of diabetes mellitus, metabolism of all the basic foodstuffs is altered. The basic effect on glucose metabolism is to prevent the efficient uptake and utilization of glucose by most of the cells of the body, except those of the brain. As a result, blood glucose concentration increases, cell utilization of glucose falls lower and lower, and fat utilization increases.

Insulin-Dependent Diabetes Mellitus. Any disease or injury to the beta cells that impairs insulin production can lead to IDDM. Most often, beta cell injury is caused by an autoimmune disorder in which the beta cells are destroyed by the immune system, or in some cases by viral infections that destroy the beta cells. The usual age of onset is at about 12 years of age, and for this reason IDDM is often called ***juvenile diabetes mellitus.*** There is considerable evidence that IDDM has a genetic basis, but environmental factors, especially viral infections, also may be involved.

The lack of insulin secretion results in four principal sequelae. First, the blood glucose concentration rises to very high levels because the efficiency of peripheral glucose utilization is reduced and glucose production is augmented. Increased plasma glucose then causes multiple effects throughout the body, especially injury to the blood vessels and the kidneys; diabetes is one of the leading causes of end-stage kidney disease and an important contributor to the mortality and morbidity associated with cardiovascular diseases. The high blood glucose also causes more glucose to filter into the renal tubules than can be reabsorbed. This creates an osmotic pressure in the tubules that prevents reabsorption of much of the tubular water, thereby promoting very rapid diuresis and requiring the person to drink large amounts of water to maintain fluid balance. Thus, one of the classic symptoms of diabetes mellitus is polyuria (excessive urine excretion) and increased thirst.

A second effect of diabetes mellitus is increased utilization of fats for energy. This causes the liver to release acetoacetic acid into the plasma more rapidly then it can be taken up and oxidized by the tissue cells. As a result, the patient develops severe acidosis from the excessive acetoacetic acid, which, in association with dehydration due to the excessive urine formation, can cause diabetic coma. This leads rapidly to death unless the condition is treated immediately with large amounts of insulin.

A third effect is to cause, over a prolonged period of time, depletion of the body's proteins. Also, failure to utilize glucose for energy leads to decreased storage of fat as well. Therefore, a person with severe untreated diabetes mellitus suffers rapid weight loss and often death within a few weeks.

Fourth, over a long period of time, the excess fat utilization in the liver causes large amounts of cholesterol in the circulating blood and increased deposition of cholesterol in the arterial walls. This leads to severe arteriosclerosis and other vascular lesions.

NON-INSULIN-DEPENDENT DIABETES MELLITUS

NIDDM is far more common than IDDM, accounting for about 80% to 90% of all diabetics. This syndrome is characterized by impaired ability of target tissues to respond to the metabolic effects of insulin, a condition referred to as ***insulin resistance.*** There are multiple causes of insulin resistance, but the most common is ***obesity***. In most cases, the onset of IDDM is gradual, with relatively mild hyperglycemia occurring after ingestion of carbohydrates. However, higher rates of insulin secretion by the pancreas are required to maintain normal blood levels of glucose because of the insulin resistance. Because the average age of onset of NIDDM is 50 to 60 years, this syndrome has often been referred to as ***adult-onset diabetes.*** In many instances, NIDDM can be effectively treated, at least in the early stages, with caloric restriction and weight reduction, and no exogenous insulin administration is required. However in the later stages, when the pancreatic beta cells can no longer secrete enough insulin to prevent hyperglycemia, insulin administration is required.

PARATHYROID HORMONE AND PHYSIOLOGY OF BONE

Formation of Bone by Osteoblasts. Before explaining the function of parathyroid hormone (PTH), the basic physiology of bone and its relation to calcium and phosphates in the extracellular fluids must be discussed. Bone is formed by ***osteoblasts,*** which line the outer surfaces of all bones and are also present inside most of the bone cavities. The osteoblasts secrete a very strong ***protein bone matrix,*** compromised mainly of collagen fibers, which gives the bone its toughness. This matrix has the special property of causing phosphate ions to combine with calcium ions, precipitating a complicated salt of calcium and phosphate called ***hydroxyapatite*** in the protein matrix to make it extremely hard. The strength of the collagen fibers gives the bone tremendous tensile strength, while the hardness of bone gives it compressive strength.

When calcium is not available in large quantities in the body fluids, bone is poorly formed. Calcium is not well absorbed from the gastrointestinal tract, and when it fails to be absorbed, phosphate is also poorly absorbed because the two substances form insoluble compounds in the gut. However, ***vitamin D*** greatly increases calcium absorption, which in turn allows increased phosphate absorption. Therefore, lack of vitamin D reduces the amount of available calcium and phosphate for bone formation and can result in poor mineralization of the bones, so that they no longer resist compressive forces. This is the disease known as ***rickets.***

Before vitamin D can increase calcium absorption by the gastrointestinal tract, it must be converted from its natural form into the substance ***1,25-dihydroxycholecalciferol.*** The first stage of this conversion occurs in the liver and the second stage in the kidney; the second stage requires the presence of PTH. Therefore, severe liver disease, kidney disease, or lack of PTH can lead to diminished calcium absorption by the intestinal tract.

Resorption of Bone by Osteoclasts. Bone is continually being broken down (resorbed) by large numbers of ***osteoclasts*** present in the bone cavities. Osteoclasts are large multinucleated cells that secrete hydrogen ions (which dissolve the crystals) and hydrolytic enzymes, which digest the collagen matrix. This resorption of bone has two major functions: (1) In all bones the protein matrix becomes aged and loses its toughness, thereby allowing the bones to become brittle. The osteoclastic resorptive process removes the aging bone, which is then continuously replaced by new bone formation by the osteoblasts. (2) Resorption of bone provides a means by which calcium ions can rapidly be made available to the extracellular fluids.

Parathyroid Hormone Regulation of Plasma Calcium Concentration. PTH is secreted by the ***parathyroid glands,*** which are embedded in the surface of the thyroid gland, but are distinct from it. PTH secretion is controlled primarily by changes in plasma calcium concentration; decreased plasma calcium concentration stimulates PTH secretion, whereas increased calcium concentration reduces PTH secretion.

PTH in turn has several actions that tend to increase plasma calcium concentration: (1) PTH increases the activity of osteoclasts and therefore causes resorption of bone; this results in movement of calcium and phosphate from bone into the extracellular fluid. (2) PTH stimulates the activation of vitamin D, which increases intestinal calcium reabsorption. (3) PTH increases renal tubular calcium reabsorption, thereby reducing urinary excretion of calcium; and (4) PTH reduces phosphate reabsorption by the kidney, thereby increasing excretion of phosphate and lowering extracellular phosphate concentration. Although PTH releases phosphate from the bones, it does not increase the plasma phosphate concentration because of the increased loss of phosphate by the kidneys.

The regulation of calcium ion concentration by PTH is very important, because all of the excitable tissues in the body, including nerves, skeletal muscles, the heart, and smooth muscles, depend on well-regulated calcium ion concentration for normal function. For instance, low calcium ion concentration causes an extreme increase in irritability of the peripheral nerves so that they begin to emit impulses spontaneously, causing a state of continual muscle contraction called ***tetany.*** Also, a greatly decreased calcium ion concentration reduces the contractility of cardiac muscle. PTH secretion is the principal method by which normal calcium ion concentration is maintained in the body fluids, and the bones act as a large reservoir of calcium to be used for this purpose.

Calcitonin. The hormone calcitonin, when injected into an animal, causes rapid deposition of calcium into the bones and therefore rapid decrease in calcium ion concentration of the body fluids. This hormone is secreted by special cells, called ***parafollicular cells,*** located between the follicles and the thyroid gland in the human. Its rate of secretion increases when the calcium ion concentration rises above normal. Therefore, it functions in exactly the opposite manner of PTH, returning calcium ion concentration back toward normal when this concentration rises too high. Further, it responds more rapidly than does PTH. However, the quantitative role of calcitonin in calcium ion regulation is far less than that of parathyroid hormone. Also, its effect usually does not continue for more than a few hours to a few days.

MALE REPRODUCTIVE FUNCTIONS

Spermatogenesis. The basic reproductive function of the male is the formation of sperm by the testes. The seminiferous tubules of the testes contain a basal layer of ***germinal epithelium,*** the cells of which divide through several stages and gradually form the sperm. During sperm formation, essentially all of the cytoplasm is lost from the cell, and the cell membrane elongates in one direction to form a tail. Also, at one stage of division, the 23 chromosome pairs (46 chromosomes) split into two unpaired sets of 23 chromosomes, one of these sets going to one sperm and the other to the second sperm. One pair of chromosomes, called the ***XY pair,*** is known as the sex pair. After separation of this chromosome pair in the process of sperm formation, half of the sperm carry an X chromosome and the other half a Y chromosome. The X chromosome causes a female child to be formed, while the Y chromosome causes a male child to be formed. Thus, the sex of the offspring is determined by the type of sperm that fertilizes the ovum. Furthermore, this division of chromosomes allows half of the genes of the father to be inherited by the child, while the other half come from the mother.

In addition to the germinal cells, the seminiferous tubules contain large ***Sertoli cells,*** from which the developing sperm obtain nutrient substances.

Transport, Storage, and Ejaculation of Sperm. After sperm are formed in the seminiferous tubules, they pass into the ***epididymis*** where they remain for approximately one day while they mature within this new environment. From there, they pass into the ***vas deferens*** and the ***ampulla*** where they are stored. During coitus, sexual stimulation transmits impulses to the spinal cord that cause reflex erection of the penis mediated by parasympathetic impulses. Then at the height of sexual stimulation, rhythmic peristalsis, which is mediated by the sympathetic nervous system, begins in the epididymis and spreads up the vas deferens, into the ampulla and seminal vesicles, and finally through the prostrate gland. This expels the semen into the posterior urethra, a process called ***emission.*** Then, rhythmical contractions of the bulbocavernosus muscle cause rhythmic compression of the urethra, and about 3 ml of semen is expelled. This process is called ***ejaculation.***

The ejaculate is composed of a mixture of (1) sperm from the testes, (2) a highly mucid fluid from the seminal vesicles, and (3) a highly alkaline fluid from the prostate gland. The alkalinity of the prostate fluid causes the sperm to become immediately motile by activating movement of the sperm tail, permitting the sperm to travel at a velocity as much as 1 to 4 mm/min, and to pass through the uterus and the fallopian tubes to fertilize the ovum.

Failure of the male to expel more than 60 to 80 million sperm in each ejaculate usually results in sterility. This is probably caused by the lack of sufficient hyaluronidase and various proteolytic enzymes that are secreted by the sperm. These enzymes dissolve the mucus plug of the female cervix and possibly also help to break granulosa cells away from the surface of the ovum to allow the sperm to penetrate the ovum.

Testosterone Formation. Large amounts of testosterone are formed by the interstitial cells of the testes located between the seminiferous tubules. This testosterone has a local effect in the testes to promote sperm production by the seminiferous tubules, and without it spermatogenesis cannot occur. However, testosterone is also secreted into the blood and causes development of the sexual and secondary sexual characteristics of the male, including (1) formation of the penis when the fetus is developing; (2) descent of the testes into the scrotum; and in the adult life of the male, (3) development of the enlarged musculature, (4) increase in the thickness of the skin, (5) deepening of the voice, resulting from growth of the larynx, (6) growth of the beard and hair in many areas of the body, and (7) baldness in those individuals who are genetically predisposed.

Regulation of Testicular Function by Anterior Pituitary Gland. At least two gonadotropic hormones, FSH and LH, are secreted by the pituitary gland and help to control spermatogenesis and testosterone secretion by the testes. During childhood, almost no gonadotropic hormones are secreted by the anterior pituitary gland, but at puberty both FSH and LH begin to be secreted; the FSH hormone promotes division of the germinal cells to initiate spermatogenesis, while LH stimulates the interstitial cells to produce testosterone. Testosterone in turn is required for proper development and maturation of the sperm. The testes continue to produce both sperm and testosterone from puberty until death, although beyond approximately the fortieth year of life, the rates of production gradually decline.

Luteinizing Hormone–Releasing Hormone Control of Gonadotropic Hormone Secretion. The rate of secretion of gonadotropic hormones by the anterior pituitary is controlled mainly by LH-releasing hormone, as discussed previously. This hormone causes both LH and FSH to be released from the anterior pituitary gland.

Testosterone secreted by the testes inhibits the formation of LH-releasing hormone by the hypothalamus, thus providing a negative feedback mechanism for control of testosterone secretion. In addition, a substance called ***inhibin*** is secreted by the Sertoli cells and suppresses FSH secretion by the anterior pituitary, thus providing a feedback mechanism for controlling sperm formation.

During childhood the rate of secretion of LH-releasing hormone is very low because the hypothalamus is extremely sensitive to the inhibitory effects of even small amounts of circulating testosterone. However, at approximately 12 years of age, the hypothalamus loses most of this inhibitory sensitivity and large amounts of LH-releasing hormone then begin to be secreted, and the sex life of the male begins. This initiates the period of ***puberty.***

FEMALE REPRODUCTIVE FUNCTIONS

Ovarian Cycle and Oogenesis. The newborn female has about two million ***primordial ova*** in her two ovaries. Many of these degenerate during childhood, and only about 70,000 to 400,000 remain at puberty. At that time, under the stimulation of gonadotropic hormones from the anterior pituitary, the rhythmic monthly sexual cycle begins. At the beginning of each month, the cells surrounding a few of the ova, the ***granulosal*** and the ***thecal cells,*** begin to proliferate, and these secrete large quantities of ***estrogens,*** one of the female sex hormones. Fluid is secreted by the granulosa and thecal cells, forming cavities around these few ova, called ***follicles.*** After approximately 14 days of growth, one of the growing follicles breaks open and expels its ovum into the abdominal cavity. Then, all of the other growing follicles begin to degenerate within a few hours, a process called ***atresia.*** Presumably, this results from an inhibitory hormone action on the ovaries after ovulation from the first follicle occurs. The result is normally the release of one single ovum each month at approximately the fourteenth day of the sexual cycle.

Immediately after the ovum has been expelled, the granulosal and thecal cells undergo rapid fatty changes and considerable swelling, a process called ***luteinization,*** and they begin to secrete large amounts of progesterone in addition to estrogens. This modified mass of cells, now called a ***corpus luteum,*** persists for another 14 days, after which time it degenerates. Then a new set of follicles begins to develop, and at the end of another 14 days another ovum is expelled into the abdominal cavity, with the cycle continuing on and on.

At about the same time the ovum is expelled from the follicle, the nucleus of the ovum divides two times in rapid succession. During one of these divisions, the pairs of chromosomes separate and half of them are expelled from the ovum, leaving 23 unpaired chromosomes in the final mature ovum, which is then ready for fertilization.

Effect of Estrogens and Progesterone on the Uterine Endometrium. The estrogens and progesterone secreted by the ovaries prepare the uterine endometrium for implantation of the fertilized ovum. The estrogen secreted during the first half of the monthly ovarian cycle causes very rapid proliferation of the endometrial stroma and glandular cells. Then during the second half of the monthly cycle, progesterone causes the stromal and glandular cells to begin secreting a serous fluid, while the stromal cells store large quantities of protein and glycogen in preparation for supplying nutrition to the developing ovum.

Menstruation. When the corpus luteum degenerates at the end of the monthly cycle, very little estrogen or progesterone is secreted by the ovaries for the next few days. Lack of the normal stimulatory effect of these hormones causes the endometrial cells to lose their stimulus for increased activity. This results in rapid necrosis of the superficial two thirds of the endometrium, with the dead tissue sloughing away and being expelled through the vagina along with about 40 ml of blood and at least this much additional serous exudate. This process, called ***menstruation,*** normally lasts about 4 days. By the end of menstruation, new follicles have begun to develop, and the ovaries are beginning to secrete estrogens once again. Under the influence of these estrogens, the endometrium begins a new cycle of development.

Effects of Estrogens and Progesterone on Other Tissues. Estrogens and progesterone, in addition to their effects on the endometrium, produce other effects throughout the body. Estrogens cause proliferation and enlargement of the smooth muscle cells in the uterus, increasing the uterine size after puberty to about double the childhood size. Estrogens also cause proliferation of the glandular cells of the breast and deposition of fat in the breast tissue, the hips, and other points that give the characteristics of the adult female. They cause very rapid growth of bones immediately after puberty but also promote early uniting of the epiphyses with the shafts of the long bones so that the final height of the woman, despite her rapid growth immediately after puberty, is less than it otherwise would have been. Finally, estrogens cause enlargement of the external genitalia.

Progesterone has very much the same effect on the breast that it has on the uterine endometrium, causing the glandular cells to increase in size and to develop secretory granules in their cells. In addition, progesterone causes accumulation of fluid and electrolytes in the breast tissue, making them swell during the latter half of each monthly sexual cycle.

Regulation of Female Sexual Cycle by the Hypothalamus and Anterior Pituitary Gland. Until the child is about 12 years of age, the anterior pituitary secretes no gonadotropic hormones, as is also true in the male. This is thought to be caused by a very high sensitivity of the hypothalamus to the inhibitory effect of even small amounts of estrogen and progesterone secreted by the ovaries. However, at puberty, the hypothalamus loses

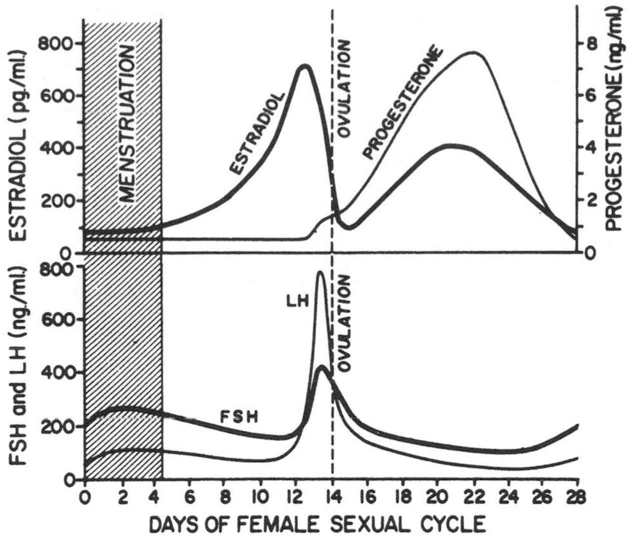

Fig. 3-36. Approximate plasma concentrations of the gonadotropins and ovarian hormones during the normal female sexual cycle. (Guyton AC: Textbook of Medical Physiology, 8th ed. Philadelphia: WB Saunders, 1991)

this inhibitory sensitivity and begins to secrete LH-releasing hormone in the same manner that this occurs in the male. This hormone in turn stimulates the secretion of both LH and FSH in the monthly cycles by the anterior pituitary gland, as shown in the lower curve of Figure 3-36. The FSH causes initial growth of the ovarian follicles during the first few days of the monthly cycle. Then this hormone, aided by LH as well, causes the thecal cells and possibly also the granulosal cells to secrete estrogen (the ''estradiol'' curve in the upper part of the figure) plus large quantities of fluid into the developing follicles.

At about the thirteenth day of the ovarian cycle, a very large amount of LH is secreted by the anterior pituitary, which is called the ***LH surge.*** The excess LH, in some way not completely understood, causes ovulation about 24 hours later. The LH also causes the granulosal and thecal cells to change into ***lutein cells,*** which in the aggregate become the corpus luteum. LH then stimulates the corpus luteum to produce large amounts of both progesterone and estrogen during the latter half of the sexual cycle. Finally, when the corpus luteum degenerates at the end of the cycle, the resulting lack of progesterone and estrogen leads to menstruation, as described above.

The exact mechanisms that control secretion of FSH, LH, estrogen, and progesterone during the sexual cycle are not completely understood. However, it is known that estrogen and progesterone normally cause feedback inhibition of LH-releasing hormone secretion by the hypothalamus. Therefore, during the latter part of the ovarian cycle, when large amounts of progesterone and estrogen are secreted by the corpus luteum, secretion of both FSH and LH by the anterior pituitary decreases markedly. This in turn leads to degeneration of the corpus luteum and greatly decreased production of progesterone and estrogen. Next, lacking the feedback inhibition of these two hormones, the hypothalamus and pituitary gland become active once again during the next few days, and the rates of secretion of FSH and LH rise again, thus beginning a new cycle.

Menopause. At 40 to 50 years of age, essentially all of the ova in the ovaries have been used up, a few expelled into the abdominal cavity by ovulation and large numbers degenerated *in situ* in the ovaries. Therefore, no follicles or any corpus luteum can develop in the ovaries to secrete either estrogens or progesterone. The anterior pituitary gland continues to secrete large amounts of gonadotropic hormones, but since no estrogen or progesterone can be secreted to inhibit the hypothalamus or the pituitary, no monthly sexual cycle occurs thereafter.

PHYSIOLOGY OF PREGNANCY

Ovum Fertilization and Implantation in Endometrium. After coitus, millions of motile sperm make their way up to the uterus and fallopian tubes. The sperm are capable of living in the genital tract of the female for as long as 72 hours but are very fertile for only about 24 hours. If during this time an ovum is expelled from the ovary, or if an ovum has been expelled up to 24 hours prior to coitus, then a sperm can cause fertilization. In the process of fertilization, the head of the sperm combines with the nucleus of the ovum. Since each of these contains 23 unpaired chromosomes, the combination restores the normal cellular complement of 23 pairs of chromosomes. The fertilized ovum then contains 44 autosomal chromosomes and either two X chromosomes, which causes a female child to develop, or an X and a Y chromosome, which causes a male child to develop. After fertilization, the process of division begins, the first division occurring approximately 30 hours after fertilization. Subsequent divisions occur at a rate of about once every 18 to 24 hours.

The ovum usually passes, shortly before fertilization, to one of the two fallopian tubes, the fimbriated ends of which lie in approximation to the ovaries. The cilia that line the fallopian tube beat toward the uterus and slowly move the dividing ovum downward along the tube to reach the uterus in about 3 days.

The dividing ovum develops an outer layer of ***trophoblast cells;*** these are capable of phagocytizing nutrient materials from the secretions of the fallopian tube and uterus, thus making nutrients available to the developing mass of cells. The trophoblast cells also secrete proteolytic enzymes that allow the developing cell mass to eat its way into the endometrium and thereby implant itself. Once implantation occurs, the trophoblastic and underlying cells proliferate rapidly.

Secretion of Chorionic Gonadotropin by Trophoblast Cells. When the corpus luteum degenerates at the end of the normal monthly menstrual cycle, the endometrium of the uterus sloughs away and menstruation occurs. However, when the ovum becomes fertilized it is important that the endometrium remain intact for the early developing fetus to implant and grow. Fortunately, the trophoblast cells secrete a hormone, called ***human chorionic gonadotropin (HCG),*** that has the same effects on the corpus luteum as LH secreted by the pituitary gland. Therefore, this hormone keeps the corpus luteum from degenerating and keeps it secreting large quantities of estrogens and progesterone; as a result, menstruation does not occur. Instead the endometrium actually grows thicker and the large endometrial cells, called ***decidual cells,*** are gradually phagocytized by the growing fetal tissues, providing the major portion of the nutrition for the fetus during the first 8 to 12 weeks of pregnancy.

After the first 2 to 4 months of pregnancy, the placenta begins to secrete large amounts of estrogen and progesterone. From then on, the hormones from the corpus luteum are not needed and it degenerates.

Placenta as Organ of Exchange. During the early weeks of pregnancy, the trophoblast cells and other fetal tissues gradually develop the ***placenta.*** This organ contains multiple large chambers filled with the mother's blood, and into these chambers project millions of small villi containing blood capillaries from the fetus. Trophoblast cells cover the surfaces of the villi, and these actively reabsorb many nutrients from the mother's blood and transport them into the fetal blood during the early weeks of pregnancy. However, after 4 to 8 weeks most of the necessary nutrients are absorbed passively from the mother's blood into the fetal blood. This occurs because the concentrations of the nutrients are greater in the mother's blood than in the fetal blood, and as a result they can diffuse through the placental membrane into the fetal blood. Conversely, waste products of metabolism, such as urea, uric acid, and creatinine accumulate in higher concentrations in the fetal blood and diffuse through the placental membrane into the mother's blood, and then are excreted by the mother's kidneys.

Placental Secretion of HCG, Estrogen, and Progesterone. In addition to secreting HCG, the placenta also secretes other important hormones, especially estrogens and progesterone. After approximately the third month of pregnancy, the secretion of HCG becomes greatly reduced, and the corpus luteum begins to degenerate. From that time onward, the estrogens and progesterone from the placenta are essential for the maintenance of pregnancy. Toward the end of pregnancy, the rate of secretion of active estrogens is about 30 times that during the normal ovarian cycle, and the rate of secretion of progesterones is about 10 times as great. Estrogens and progesterone are essential for the growth and development of the fetus.

The progesterone secreted by the placenta is formed from cholesterol derived from the mother's blood. However, secretion of estrogens by the placenta requires a two-stage process. The first stage is the formation of large quantities of androgens by greatly enlarged adrenal cortices in the fetus. These androgens are then carried into the blood to the placenta where they are converted into several different types of estrogens, including ***estradiol,*** the most potent of all of the estrogens.

The placenta also produces large amounts of another hormone, called ***human chorionic somatomammotropin.*** This hormone has several important effects: (1) It promotes growth of the fetus. (2) It causes increased use of fatty acids by the mother for energy and decreased use of glucose; this makes the excess glucose of the mother available for use by the fetus. (3) It aids in the growth and development of the breasts during pregnancy, thus preparing the breast for lactation following birth of the baby.

Growth of Fetus. During the first few weeks of pregnancy, the fetus hardly grows at all, though the surrounding fetal membranes, especially the placenta, develop very rapidly. After 4 to 5 weeks, however, the length of the fetus increases approximately in proportion to the time of gestation, and the weight increases with the cube of the time. Thus, at 6 months, the length is approximately six ninths the final length, but the weight is still only about one fourth the final weight. Thus, the greatest growth in weight of the fetus occurs in the last 3 months, and during this time pregnancy makes many demands on the mother for nutritive substances needed by the baby, including especially proteins, vitamins, large amounts of calcium for the bones, and iron for the red blood cells.

Parturition. When the fetus is fully formed, approximately 9 months after fertilization, the uterus becomes more excitable than usual, labor begins, and the baby is expelled. This is called ***parturition.*** The precise factors that initiate parturition are uncertain, but a combination of several different factors progressively increase the excitability of the uterine musculature: (1) Near term, the placenta begins to secrete a progressively higher ratio of estrogens to progesterone. Since estrogens normally excite uterine activity while progesterone inhibits it, this change in ratio increases the excitability of the uterine musculature. (2) The fetus itself increases in size, which stretches the uterus, thus increasing its excitability. (3) The head of the fetus presses downward against the cervical opening of the uterus and begins to stretch the cervix; this also increases the excitability of the uterus. (4) The posterior pituitary gland begins to secrete additional amounts of oxytocin, and at the same time the sensitivity of the uterus to oxytocin increases greatly, both of which increase the excitability of the uterine musculature.

As a result of all of these factors, the rhythmic contractions of the uterus become stronger and stronger. Finally, they become strong enough to begin pushing the baby into the birth canal. This stretches the cervix very rapidly, causing still greater increase in the excitability of the uterus and making it contract even harder. Also, sensory signals from the cervix to the hypothalamus cause progressively increasing secretion of oxytocin, which excites the uterus even more. Thus, a positive feedback cycle is set up as follows: strong uterine contraction stretches the cervix, which stimulates even stronger uterine contraction, causing still more stretch of the cervix, and so forth, until the baby is expelled.

Changes in the Baby Immediately After Birth. Prior to birth, the baby receives its nutrition and oxygen through the placenta. Normally, the first function performed by the newborn baby is rapid expansion of its lungs and onset of respiration to oxygenate its own blood. A baby can usually go as long as 4 to 6 minutes without breathing before neuronal cells in the brain are damaged.

In the fetus, blood bypasses the lungs by two routes: (1) Some of it flows directly from the right atrium through the ***foramen ovalae*** directly into the left atrium. (2) Most of the remaining blood that does not take this route is pumped by the right ventricle into the pulmonary artery and then through the ***ductus arteriosus*** directly into the aorta rather than through the lungs. Growth of the baby changes these directions of blood flow in the following ways: (1) Loss of blood flow through the placenta after birth greatly increases the total peripheral resistance in the baby's systemic circulation. (2) Expansion of the lungs expands the pulmonary blood vessels, and this greatly reduces the resistance to blood flow through the pulmonary circulation. As a result, the ratio of resistance in the systemic circulation to resistance in the pulmonary circulation increases severalfold, allowing much easier flow of blood through the lungs but considerably more difficult flow through the systemic circulation. Because of this, the pulmonary artery pressure falls, while the systemic arterial pressure rises, so that blood now begins to flow backward from the aorta through the ductus arteriosus rather than forward. This brings arterialized blood, containing a high oxygen concentration, into contact with the ductus, and the oxygen constricts the ductus, causing functional closure within a few hours. Then fibrous tissue grows into the ductus and causes permanent closure in 1 to 2 months (except in one baby in several thousand).

Also, immediately after birth, the increased resistance in the systemic circulation raises the load on the left heart and therefore increases the left atrial pressure. At the same time, the decreased resistance in the lungs reduces the right atrial pressure. This higher pressure in the left atrium than the right atrium closes a valve-like structure over the foramina ovalae, preventing backflow through this route. Thus, these two changes in the circulatory system provide normal blood flow through the lungs.

LACTATION

During pregnancy, large amounts of estrogens and progesterone are secreted by either the corpus luteum or the placenta. Estrogens cause proliferation of the glandular tissues of the breasts, and progesterone causes development of the alveoli and storage of nutrient materials in the glandular cells. Other hormones that help to promote breast development during pregnancy include ***prolactin*** and ***growth hormone*** from the mother's anterior pituitary gland, ***insulin*** from her pancreas, ***glucocorticoids*** from her adrenal glands, and ***human chorionic somatomammotropin*** from the placenta. However, progesterone and estrogens also inhibit milk production despite their effects on breast proliferation. Therefore, before birth of the baby, the mother does not secrete milk. Loss of the placenta from the mother's body when the baby is born removes the source of progesterone and estrogen so that the breasts are no longer inhibited, and within 24 to 48 hours, milk begins to flow.

During pregnancy, the mother's anterior pituitary gland produces increased amounts of prolactin, increasing to about 10 times the normal rate of secretion. This hormone is required to cause final development of the breasts and to cause them to secrete milk. After the birth of the baby, continued suckling of the breast stimulates the anterior pituitary gland to continue secreting large quantities of prolactin, and this in turn causes the breasts to continue producing milk. When milk is no longer needed by the child and is no longer removed from the breast, the anterior pituitary gland stops producing prolactin, and milk production ceases within a few days.

Oxytocin secreted by the posterior pituitary gland during the suckling process is also important for lactation, causing milk ejection from the alveoli of the breasts.

QUESTIONS IN PHYSIOLOGY

Essay Questions

FUNCTIONAL SYSTEMS OF THE BODY

What is meant by homeostasis?

What is meant by the internal environment of the body?

What are the functional systems of the body, and how does each one help to provide homeostasis?

THE CELL AND ITS FUNCTION

Describe the major parts of the cell, including the different organelles and their overall functions.

What are the principal mechanisms by which energy is released in the cell and the role of mitochondria in energy release?

What is the function of the endoplasmic reticulum?

How do the genes regulate protein synthesis in the cell?

What are the functions of mRNA, transfer RNA, and ribosomal RNA?

What is the process of mitosis, and how does cellular reproduction occur?

THE BODY FLUIDS

How are the body fluids distributed between the extracellular and intracellular compartments?

What are the differences between the ionic compositions of extracellular and intracellular fluids?

Describe the basic structure of the cell membrane.

Explain the differences between active and passive transport, between primary and secondary active transport, and between simple and facilitated diffusion.

Describe the mechanisms for co-transport of glucose and amino acids with sodium, and countertransport of sodium and hydrogen ion in the cell membrane.

Explain the mechanism of osmosis through cell membrane and how osmotic pressure develops across a semipermeable membrane.

What is meant by isotonic, hypertonic, and hypotonic fluids? What are the changes in intracellular and extracellular fluid volumes and osmolarity after intravenous administration of isotonic, hypertonic, and hypotonic fluids?

What are the functional differences between the capillary membrane and the cell membrane?

What are the forces that determine fluid movement across the capillary membrane?

What are the different factors that can cause interstitial fluid edema?

What is the major function of the lymphatics? What are the two main factors that control the rate of lymph flow?

KIDNEYS

List seven major functions of the kidney in maintaining homeostasis.

What is the overall relationship between glomerular filtration, tubular reabsorption, and tubular secretion in urine formation?

Describe the basic anatomy of the nephron, including vascular and tubular elements.

What are the effects of the following changes on glomerular filtration rate: (1) decreased glomerular capillary filtration coefficient, (2) decreased glomerular hydrostatic pressure, (3) increased afferent arteriolar resistance, and (4) decreased efferent arteriolar resistance.

Explain how solutes are secreted from the peritubular capillaries into the tubules.

Explain how water and solutes are reabsorbed from the tubules into the peritubular capillaries.

Explain the differences between the functions of the following tubular segments: (1) the proximal tubules, (2) the descending and ascending segments of the loop of Henle, and (3) the distal and collecting tubules.

Explain the different tubular effects of the following hormones: aldosterone, angiotensin II, antidiuretic hormone, and atrial natriuretic peptide.

What is meant by renal clearance? How is renal clearance used to calculate glomerular filtration, renal plasma flow, and tubular reabsorption?

What are the factors that determine whether the kidneys form a concentrated or a dilute urine?

Explain the role of the osmoreceptor-ADH-thirst systems in controlling extracellular sodium concentration and osmolarity.

What is meant by pressure natriuresis, and how does this mechanism regulate extracellular fluid volume?

Explain the mechanisms that cause potassium secretion in the distal and collecting tubules; what are the factors that regulate potassium secretion in these tubular segments?

What are the three primary lines of defense against changes in body fluid hydrogen ion concentration?

Why is the bicarbonate buffer system so important as an extracellular fluid acid–base buffer?

How is the bicarbonate buffer system regulated?

How does the respiratory system regulate hydrogen ion concentration?

What are the mechanisms by which the kidneys secrete hydrogen ion, reabsorb bicarbonate, and generate new bicarbonate?

What are the characteristic changes in plasma *p*H, hydrogen ion concentration, P_{CO_2}, and plasma bicarbonate concentration in the following acid–base disturbances: respiratory acidosis, respiratory alkalosis, metabolic acidosis, and metabolic alkalosis?

BLOOD, HEMOSTASIS, AND IMMUNITY

What is meant by the hematocrit?

About many red blood cells does the body contain?

What are three important functions of hemoglobin?

What are the normal concentrations of red and white cells in the blood?

How is the concentration of the red cells in the blood regulated?

What are the roles of vitamin B_{12} and folic acid in red blood cell production?

Lack of iron causes which type of anemia?

Give the basic functions of the different types of white blood cells.

Describe the four lines of defense against infection.

Describe how initiation of coagulation differs between the extrinsic and intrinsic pathways.

Why does liver disease often lead to blood-clotting abnormalities?

Explain the cause of bleeding in hemophilia, in thrombocytopenia, and in prothrombin deficiency.

Define the concept of immunity, indicating the difference between acquired and passive immunity and between cellular and humoral immunity.

Describe how antibodies destroy an invading agent.

Identify the differences between T lymphocytes and B lymphocytes.

Explain the difference in function between antibodies and T cells in the process of immunity.

What are the three major types of sensitized T cells?

What is meant by immunologic tolerance?

What is the basic cause of autoimmune disease?

What is the significance of IgE antibodies in allergy?

How does histamine enter into allergic reactions?

Describe the possible effects of a transfusion of mismatched blood.

What is meant by the A-B-O blood groups, and how can mismatching of these groups cause transfusion reactions?

How do the Rh blood types differ from the A-B-O blood groups in causing transfusion reactions?

Describe the cause of erythroblastosis fetalis.

NERVE AND MUSCLE

What causes the membrane potential to be negative?

Explain the mechanism of the action potential.

How does an action potential spread along a nerve membrane?

What is meant by the all-or-nothing law?

If oxidative metabolism in the nerve suddenly stops, can the nerve continue to transmit nerve impulses?

Describe the mechanism by which an impulse is transmitted through a neuromuscular junction.

How is contraction initiated in a skeletal muscle fiber?

What determines the amount tension that can be developed by a contracting muscle?

Explain the mechanism of muscle tetanization.

What is the importance of the transverse tubules of a muscle fiber?

Describe the involvement of adenosine triphosphate in the contractile process.

Describe the role of calcium in the contractile process.

What factors control the strength of a muscle contraction?

How does smooth muscle differ from skeletal and cardiac muscle?

How does cardiac muscle differ from smooth and skeletal muscle?

Describe the disease myasthenia gravis, its cause, and its treatment.

HEART

Explain the differences in the action potential of cardiac muscle, compared with skeletal muscle.

Explain the basic mechanisms for control of rhythmicity in the heart, including the pacemaker function of the S-A node.

Trace the conduction of the cardiac impulse through the heart.

What is the significance of the junctional fibers in the Purkinje system?

What is meant by heart block, and how does it occur?

Explain circus movement of electrical impulses in the heart, and describe the mechanisms of flutter and fibrillation.

What does the P-Q interval in the electrocardiogram represent?

What conditions cause abnormal QRS waves in the electrocardiogram?

What conditions cause abnormal T waves in the electrocardiogram?

Describe the pressure changes in the heart during the cardiac cycle and the relationship to the electrocardiogram, the heart sounds, and ventricular volume changes.

Explain the Frank-Starling law of the heart.

What are the types of autonomic nerve fibers that supply the heart, and what is the function of each type?

CIRCULATION AND ITS REGULATION

Trace the flow of blood from the left ventricle until it returns to the left atrium; explain the ''circuit'' concept of the circulation.

Give the approximate percentage of the total blood volume distributed in the systemic circulation, the pulmonary circulation, and the heart. Within these circulations, what fraction of blood is in the veins compared to the arteries, and the arterioles and capillaries?

What are the determinants of blood flow through a blood vessel? Give the formula relating blood flow to blood pressure and vascular resistance.

What are the factors that determine the resistance to blood flow in a blood vessel?

What is vascular compliance, and how is it related to distensibility of the vasculature?

Define the following terms: stroke volume, diastolic pressure, systolic pressure, and pulse pressure.

What is the relationship between blood flow velocity and total cross-sectional area of blood vessels? What part of the vasculature has the lowest blood flow velocity?

How is blood flow regulated in local tissues by the arterioles?

What is meant by autoregulation of blood flow?

What effect does activation of the sympathetic nervous system have on blood flow in most tissues?

Explain the special mechanisms for blood flow regulation in the following tissues: skeletal muscle, skin, heart, and the brain.

Explain the special arrangement of the venous circulation from the gastrointestinal tract, called the portal circulation.

Compare the pressures in the pulmonary circulation with the pressures in the systemic circulation.

What effect does increased blood flow have on pulmonary vascular resistance?

Under what conditions can significant quantities of blood shift from the pulmonary circulation to the systemic circulation, and vice versa?

Under what conditions can pulmonary edema develop?

Describe the cardiovascular autonomic reflexes and their role in short-term blood pressure regulation. Why does cerebral ischemia elevate blood pressure?

What are the effects of each of the following hormones on blood pressure: angiotensin II, norepinephrine, aldosterone, vasopressin?

Describe the renal–body fluid feedback mechanism for long-term regulation of mean arterial pressure.

What type of renal abnormalities can lead to chronic hypertension?

Discuss the possible basic causes of essential hypertension.

What are the two primary mechanisms that regulate pumping action of the heart?

What are the three main factors that regulate venous return?

What is meant by systemic filling pressure?

What are the two main factors that regulate venous pressure?

Why does activation of the sympathetic nervous system help to compensate for mild heart failure?

How does renal fluid retention help to compensate for mild heart failure? Under what conditions can excessive fluid retention be of harm in heart failure?

What are the main differences that occur in the circulation in left heart failure, compared with right heart failure?

What are the four major classifications of circulatory shock, and what are the main causes of each type of shock? What is meant by irreversible circulatory shock, and how does this occur?

Respiratory System

What are the muscles of inspiration, and which is most important?

Describe the different mechanisms of expiration, comparing quiet breathing to heavy breathing.

What is a major function of surfactant?

Define and give the values for tidal air, minute respiratory volume, vital capacity, maximum rate of pulmonary ventilation, alveolar ventilation per minute, dead space, and functional residual capacity.

List the concentrations and the partial pressures of the different gases in the alveoli.

Why is it important that gases utilized by the respiratory system be expressed in terms of partial pressure?

Which factors determine the rate of diffusion of a gas across the pulmonary membrane?

What is the diffusing capacity of a gas?

Why does carbon dioxide diffuse through the pulmonary membrane far more rapidly than does oxygen?

Explain the mechanism by which hemoglobin transports oxygen in the blood.

How much oxygen in normally carried in each 100 ml of blood?

Give the different mechanisms by which carbon dioxide is transported in the blood.

What causes the continual respiratory rhythm?

How do carbon dioxide, blood *p*H, and oxygen lack increase pulmonary ventilation?

List the different causes of hypoxia.

Oxygen therapy is beneficial to which causes of hypoxia?

How high can an aviator ascend without developing coma from hypoxia?

What are the mechanisms by which a person becomes acclimatized to hypoxia?

What is meant by an acceleratory force of 5 *g*, and approximately how much centrifugal acceleratory force can an aviator stand?

What are the particular physiologic problems involved in space travel?

What are the toxic effects of high oxygen pressure and high nitrogen pressure on the body?

What is decompression sickness, and what is its cause in deep-sea diving?

Why does helium replacement allow deeper diving?

CENTRAL NERVOUS SYSTEM

What are the three parts of the nervous system for controlling body functions?

Describe the basic mechanism of the reflex arc.

What is meant by the integrative centers of the nervous system?

Describe the synapse and its functions.

What is meant by an excitatory transmitter, and under what conditions will it excite a neuron?

What is meant by an inhibitory transmitter, and how does it function at the synapse?

Give examples of classical excitatory and inhibitory transmitters.

Describe the basis of the diverging circuit, and give an example of a system that utilizes it.

Explain the mechanism and the significance of a converging or an integrative circuit in a neuronal pool.

Give the types of repetitive firing circuits in a neuronal pool, and describe their specific characteristics.

Describe a possible mechanism by which thoughts occur in the central nervous system.

Describe a possible mechanism of memory.

Which portion of the brain is most concerned with memory?

What is meant by programming of thoughts?

List the five basic types of sensory receptors.

List the different modalities of sensation.

What determines the modality of sensation that will be felt when a nerve fiber is electrically stimulated?

What is meant by the ''labeled-line'' law?

Describe the ''purpose'' of pain, and the stimuli that cause it.

What is the basic stimulus necessary to cause pain?

How does the brain control the sensitivity of the pain pathways?

What types of stimuli can cause visceral pain?

Why are the internal organs relatively insensitive to the feel of a sharp knife cut?

What is referred pain? Explain the mechanism by which it occurs.

Describe the stretch reflex, and give its functions.

Describe the withdrawal response, and explain its relationship to the flexor reflex and the crossed extensor reflex.

Describe the positive supportive reflex, and explain its importance.

How are walking reflexes integrated in the spinal cord?

Explain the function of the brain stem in the support of the body against gravity.

What is the difference between the functions of the macula of the utricle and the semicircular canals in equilibrium?

List the locations of the primary sensory areas of the cerebral cortex.

What is meant by sensory association areas, and what are the functions of the somatic, the auditory, and the visual sensory association areas?

What is meant by the gnostic function of the brain?

What is the ideomotor function of the brain?

Explain the functions of Wernicke's area.

Trace the pyramidal system from the motor cortex to the spinal cord.

Describe some basic differences between the pyramidal pathways and extrapyramidal pathways.

Which portions of the musculature are represented to the greatest extent in the cerebral cortex?

What is the function of the premotor cortex in the control of muscular movements?

List the functions of the basal ganglia in the control of muscular movements.

How does the cerebellum damp the movements of the body?

Why does cerebellar dysfunction frequently cause ataxic movements?

What are the hormones secreted by the sympathetic and the parasympathetic nerve endings?

Describe how the central nervous system controls function of the autonomic nervous system.

EYE

Describe how the lens system of the eye functions as a camera.

What are the four refractive surfaces of the eye?

Explain the mechanism by which the eye focuses images on the retina.

What is the relationship of the pupil to the depth of focus of the eye?

What controls the shape of the lens and what is the involvement of the cerebral cortex?

Give the mechanism of the pupillary light reflex.

Distinguish between the functions of the rods and the cones.

Explain how the rhodopsin-retinal cycle of the rods operates.

Explain the mechanism of dark and light adaptation.

Explain the method by which the eye distinguishes different colors.

Trace the transmission of nerve impulses from the retina to the cerebral cortex.

EAR

Explain the mechanics of sound transmission from the tympanic membrane to the cochlea.

How does resonance occur in the cochlea?

Explain how the frequency of sound is determined by the cochlea.

Explain how the cochlea determines the loudness of a sound.

Trace the transmission of auditory impulses into the brain.

CHEMICAL SENSES

Trace the transmission of taste impulses into the brain.

What types of substances can stimulate the olfactory cells?

Describe the taste bud, and identify the four primary taste sensations.

GASTROINTESTINAL TRACT

List the major types of movements in the gastrointestinal tract.

Explain the mechanism of peristalsis and its control.

Explain how mixing occurs in the stomach, small intestine, and large intestine.

Describe three major functions of the stomach.

Describe the mechanism of swallowing.

Describe the functions of saliva and the manner in which salivary secretion is controlled.

Describe the three phases of gastric secretion and the quantitative importance of each phase.

Explain how pancreatic secretion is controlled.

What is the major mechanism by which small-intestine secretion is controlled?

What is the purpose of mucus secretion in the gastrointestinal tract?

Explain the mechanisms of digestion of carbohydrates, fats, and proteins in the gastrointestinal tract.

What substances are absorbed into the portal blood?

What substances are absorbed into the lymphatic system of the gastrointestinal tract?

What substances are absorbed by diffusion?

What substances are actively absorbed from the gastrointestinal tract?

What causes peptic ulcers to develop in the stomach or duodenum?

What is the basic cause of megaesophagus?

METABOLISM AND ENERGY

Explain how liver glycogen provides a blood glucose–buffering function.

How does insulin affect the transport of glucose into cells?

Describe the basic process of glycolysis.

What is the citric acid cycle, and what are its final products?

Describe the mechanisms by which adenosine triphosphate can be formed in the cells.

Describe the mechanism of adenosine triphosphate production by oxidative phosphorylation.

What is the chemiosmotic mechanism?

How are fats transported in the plasma?

What is the composition of chylomicrons?

What are fat depots?

How can fat be utilized to synthesize adenosine triphosphate?

In what form are fats transported in the plasma?

What are the functions of phospholipids and cholesterol in the body?

Discuss what is known about the cause of atherosclerosis.

How are amino acids transported, and how are they stored in the body?

What is meant by an essential amino acid?

What is the fate of most amino acids?

Under what conditions does catabolism of proteins occur in the cells?

Why must deamination of amino acids occur before these can be used for energy?

Define the calorie and the Calorie.

Explain the energy equivalent of foods, and give the energy equivalents for carbohydrates, fats, and proteins.

What are some of the causes of obesity?

What are the daily energy requirements of the body under different physiologic conditions?

Define the basal metabolic rate, and describe its measurement.

What types of stored foods are utilized by the body in starvation?

Discuss the mechanisms that regulate food intake.

List the vitamins, and give the principal function(s) of each vitamin.

Explain why blood flow through the skin is so variable and why it is controlled almost entirely by the nervous system in contrast to most other tissues in which blood flow is controlled mainly by local regulatory factors.

What are the mechanisms by which heat is produced in the body?

What are the mechanisms by which heat is lost from the body?

Explain the hypothalamic mechanism for automatic control of body temperature.

ENDOCRINE CONTROL SYSTEMS

What are the three general classes of hormones? Give examples of each class and the differences in their chemical structures.

Describe the general mechanisms of action for hormones that have receptors located on the cell membrane compared to hormones that interact with specific intracellular receptors.

Explain how cyclic AMP acts as an intracellular hormonal ''second messenger.''

List six hormones released by the hypothalamus that control function of the anterior pituitary gland, as well as their actions.

List six major hormones secreted by the anterior pituitary gland.

List the functions of adrenocorticotropic hormone (ACTH).

What are the major functions of thyroid-stimulating hormone?

How does growth hormone promote tissue growth?

What are the two principal gonadotrophic hormones, and what are their major actions?

What are the two principal hormones secreted by the posterior pituitary gland, and what are their major actions?

What are the three major types of steroid hormones secreted by the adrenal cortex, and what are their principal actions?

What are the major effects of excess secretion of mineralocorticoids (e.g., primary aldosteronism)?

What is the function of cortisol, and how is its secretion regulated?

What are the basic effects of thyroxine and triiodothyronine on cell function?

What are the pathophysiological effects of hyperthyroidism?

What specific cell types of the pancreas secrete glucagon and insulin?

Describe the basic effects of insulin on carbohydrate metabolism in skeletal muscle compared to liver.

How does insulin affect fat metabolism?

What are the most important effects of glucagon?

What are the two types of diabetes mellitus and their primary causes?

Outline the principal steps in the formation of bone.

Which cells resorb bone, and what is the function of bone resorption?

What are the mechanisms by which parathyroid hormone regulates plasma calcium concentration?

How does calcitonin affect calcium ion concentration?

Describe the formation of sperm by the testes.

What are the physiologic functions of testosterone?

How is testicular function controlled by the anterior pituitary gland?

Explain the events associated with formation of ova.

What are the principal effects of estrogens and progesterone on the uterine endometrium?

Describe the events of the ovarian cycle during the female sexual month.

What are the effects of estrogens and progesterone on the tissues of the body other than the sex organs?

What are the roles of the hypothalamus and anterior pituitary in regulating the female sexual cycle?

How does the ovum become fertilized and implanted in the endometrium?

Why is human chorionic gonadotropin necessary for the continuation of pregnancy?

Describe the nutritive functions of the placenta.

Outline the schedule of growth of the fetus during gestation.

Explain the mechanisms of parturition.

Describe specifically the changes that occur in the baby's respiration and circulation immediately after birth.

What are the factors that cause growth of the mother's breasts and then milk secretion following birth of the baby?

What is the function of oxytocin in lactation?

Multiple Choice Questions

Choose the *best* answer. Answers are at the end of this chapter.

1. What is the probable structure of pores in the cell membrane?
   (a) A cylindrical hole through the membrane
   (b) A protein molecule in the membrane with a channel through it
   (c) A phospholipid molecule entrapped in the membrane
   (d) A large polysaccharide molecule entrapped in the membrane
   (e) A slit in the membrane
2. All of the following have an important role in protein synthesis *except*:
   (a) Ribosomal RNA
   (b) Transfer RNA
   (c) Messenger RNA
   (d) Lysosomes
   (e) Ribosomes
3. The formation of proteins on the ribosomes is a process called:
   (a) Transcription
   (b) Translation
   (c) Transduction
   (d) Replication
4. Oxidative phosphorylation occurs in which of the following organelles?
   (a) Lysosome
   (b) Nucleus
   (c) Ribosome

(d) Mitochondria
(e) Golgi apparatus

5. The cell membrane is least permeable to which of the following?
(a) Water
(b) Sodium
(c) Oxygen
(d) Ethanol
(e) Carbon dioxide

6. Transport pathways through cell membranes are highly selective for specific substances *except*:
(a) Simple diffusion through lipid bilayer
(b) Simple diffusion through protein channels
(c) Facilitated diffusion via carrier proteins
(d) Active transport via carrier proteins

7. Intracellular and interstitial body fluids have similar
(a) Potassium ion concentrations
(b) Colloid osmotic pressures
(c) Sodium ion concentrations
(d) Chloride ion concentrations
(e) Total osmolarity

8. Infusion of hypertonic NaCl solution will
(a) Increase both intracellular and extracellular fluid volumes
(b) Increase intracellular osmolarity only
(c) Increase extracellular osmolarity only
(d) Decrease both intracellular and extracellular fluid volumes
(e) Increase extracellular volume and decrease intracellular volume

9. A man drinks 2 liters of water to replenish the fluids lost by sweating during a period of exercise. Compared with the situation prior to the period of sweating:
(a) His intracellular fluid will be hypertonic
(b) His extracellular fluid will be hypertonic
(c) His intracellular fluid volume will be greater
(d) His extracellular fluid volume will be greater
(e) His intracellular and extracellular fluid volumes will be unchanged

10. Calculate the *net* pressure difference across the capillary wall given the following conditions:
Interstitial fluid hydrostatic pressure = −3 mmHg
Plasma colloid osmotic pressure = 28 mmHg
Capillary hydrostatic pressure = 17 mmHg
Interstitial fluid colloid osmotic pressure = 8 mmHg
(a) −2 mmHg
(b) −1 mmHg
(c) 0 mmHg
(d) 1 mmHg
(e) 2 mmHg

11. Extracellular edema may result from all of the following *except*:
(a) Increased plasma colloid osmotic pressure
(b) Lymphatic blockage
(c) Increased capillary permeability
(d) Increased capillary pressure
(e) Increased interstitial fluid colloid osmotic pressure

12. The most important physiologic function of the lymphatic system is to:
(a) Transport fluid and proteins away from the interstitium
(b) Concentrate proteins in the lymph
(c) Remove particulate materials from the interstitium
(d) Transport antigenic materials to lymph nodes
(e) Create negative pressure in the free interstitial fluid

Questions 13 and 14. The following test results were obtained on specimens from a person during a 24-hour period:

Urine flow rate: 2.0 ml/min
Urine inulin: 1.0 mg/ml
Plasma inulin: 0.01 mg/ml
Urine urea: 220 mmol/liter
Plasma urea: 5 mmol/liter

13. What is the glomerular filtration rate?
(a) 100 ml/min
(b) 125 ml/min
(c) 150 ml/min
(d) 175 ml/min
(e) 200 ml/min

14. What is the urea clearance?
(a) 4.4 ml/min
(b) 22 ml/min
(c) 44 ml/min
(d) 88 ml/min
(e) 440 ml/min

15. All of the following statements concerning the determinants of glomerular filtration rate (GFR) and renal blood flow (RBF) are correct *except*:
(a) Constriction of the afferent arteriole decreases both RBF and GFR.
(b) An increase in RBF, even with little change in glomerular pressure, increases GFR.
(c) In a normal kidney, an increase in systemic arterial pressure from 100 to 150 mmHg increases GFR severalfold.
(d) Constriction of the efferent arteriole decreases RBF and slightly increases GFR.

Questions 16–18: Below are four hormones (letter choices a through d). Below these choices are three numbered descriptions. Match each number with the appropriate letter choice. Letter choices may be used once, more than once, or not at all.

(a) Angiotensin II
(b) Aldosterone
(c) Antidiuretic hormone
(d) Atrial natriuretic peptide

16. Increases urea and water permeability in the collecting duct
17. Is produced by the adrenal glands
18. Increases urinary excretion of sodium
19. Which of the following changes would tend to *decrease* glomerular filtration rate?
(a) Increased afferent arteriolar resistance
(b) Increased glomerular capillary filtration coefficient
(c) Decreased hydrostatic pressure in Bowman's capsule
(d) Decreased plasma colloid osmotic pressure
20. All of the following statements are correct *except*:
(a) Countercurrent flow in the vasa recta minimizes solute loss from the medulla of the kidney.
(b) There is net movement of water out of the descending limb of the loop of Henle.
(c) The thick ascending limb of the loop of Henle is highly permeable to water.
(d) Blood flow through the vasa recta is very slow, compared to blood flow through peritubular capillaries of cortical nephrons.
21. Vasodilation of the *efferent* arterioles of the kidney causes all of the following *except*:
(a) Increased renal blood flow
(b) Decreased glomerular filtration rate
(c) Decreased peritubular capillary hydrostatic pressure
(d) Decreased glomerular capillary hydrostatic pressure
22. For which of the following substances would you expect the renal clearance to be the *lowest*, under normal conditions?
(a) Urea
(b) Creatinine
(c) Sodium
(d) Glucose
(e) Water
23. Which of the following changes would *not* occur as a result of dehydration (loss of water, but not solute)?
(a) Increased secretion of antidiuretic hormone
(b) Increased plasma sodium concentration
(c) Decreased permeability of the collecting ducts to water
(d) Increased solute concentration in the renal medulla
24. During chronic respiratory acidosis, all the following will occur in a person with normal kidneys *except*:
(a) Almost all of the filtered HCO_3^- will be reabsorbed by the kidney.
(b) The production of ammonia by the kidney will increase.
(c) H^+ secretion in the distal nephron will be enhanced.
(d) Glutamine uptake by the kidney will be enhanced.
(e) The urinary *p*H will be increased.
25. When a person is dehydrated, hypotonic fluid will be found in the:
(a) Glomerular filtrate
(b) Proximal tubule
(c) Distal end of the ascending loop of Henle
(d) Late distal convoluted tubule
(e) Collecting duct
26. Destruction of the supraoptic nuclei of the brain will produce which of the following changes in urinary volume and concentration? (Assume that fluid intake equals fluid loss.)
(a) Increased urinary volume and a very dilute urine
(b) Increased urinary volume and a concentrated urine
(c) Decreased urinary volume and a very dilute urine
(d) Decreased urinary volume and a concentrated urine
(e) None of the above
27. A normal individual on a diet high in K^+ exhibits increased K^+ excretion. The major cause of this increased renal excretion of K^+ is:
(a) Increased secretion of K^+ by the distal and collecting tubules
(b) Decreased reabsorption of K^+ by the proximal tubule
(c) Decreased reabsorption of K^+ by the loop of Henle
(d) Decreased aldosterone secretion
(e) Increased glomerular filtration rate

Questions 28–32. The following table shows the arterial blood acid–base data for five individuals who are designated by the letters a–e. For each of the following descriptions of acid–base status, choose the individual with the appropriate acid–base data.

	P_{CO_2} (mmHg)	$[HCO_3^-]$ (mmol/L)	*p*H
(a)	29	22.0	7.50
(b)	33	32.0	7.61
(c)	35	17.5	7.32
(d)	40	25.0	7.41
(e)	60	37.5	7.42

28. Normal
29. Partially compensated metabolic acidosis
30. Fully compensated respiratory acidosis
31. Uncompensated respiratory alkalosis
32. Combined respiratory and metabolic alkalosis
33. Macrophages are the mature form of:
    (a) Neutrophils
    (b) Eosinophils
    (c) Basophils
    (d) Monocytes
    (e) Lymphocytes
34. Hemophilia is most commonly caused by deficiency of which of the following clotting factors?
    (a) Platelet Factor III
    (b) Factor V
    (c) Thromboplastin
    (d) Factor VIII
    (e) Factor XII
35. When infection occurs in a tissue, what type of white blood cell is first attracted from the blood into the tissue by the process of chemotaxis?
    (a) Neutrophils
    (b) Monocytes
    (c) Eosinophils
    (d) Basophils
    (e) Plasma cells
36. What is the first important event in hemostasis following severe tissue injury?
    (a) Blood coagulation
    (b) Formation of a platelet plug
    (c) Vascular spasm
    (d) Formation of thromboplastin
    (e) Formation of prothrombin activator
37. Vitamin B_{12} is essential for what aspect of blood cell reproduction?
    (a) Formation of hemoglobin
    (b) Extrusion of the nucleus from the normoblasts
    (c) Formation of DNA
    (d) Activation of erythropoietin
    (e) Promotion of iron absorption from the intestinal tract
38. What cells found in lymph nodes phagocytize unwanted particles in the lymph?
    (a) Neutrophils
    (b) Lymphocytes
    (c) Plasma cells
    (d) Microphages
    (e) Macrophages
39. Which of the following types of agglutinins are found in the plasma of a person with type O blood?
    (a) None
    (b) Anti-A
    (c) Anti-B
    (d) Anti-A and anti-B
40. In most instances of erythroblastosis fetalis:
    (a) The mother is Rh-positive, the father Rh-negative, and the baby Rh-negative
    (b) The mother is Rh-negative, the father Rh-positive, and the baby Rh-negative
    (c) The mother is Rh-negative, the father Rh-negative, and the baby Rh-negative
    (d) The mother is Rh-positive, the father Rh-positive, and the baby Rh-positive
    (e) The mother is Rh-negative, the father Rh-positive, and the baby Rh-positive
41. The repolarization phase of a nerve action potential is mainly caused by which of the following?
    (a) Increased potassium permeability
    (b) Decreased potassium permeability
    (c) Increased sodium permeability
    (d) The sodium–potassium pump
42. Tension development in skeletal muscle is proportional to the:
    (a) Magnitude of muscle action potentials
    (b) Length of muscle action potentials
    (c) Frequency of muscle action potentials
    (d) Duration of muscle action potentials
43. Troponin is believed to play what role in the muscle contractile process?
    (a) It provides the major amount of elastic tension during the contractile process.
    (b) It is believed that in the resting state it covers the active sites on the actin strands of the actin helix.
    (c) Combination of this complex with myosin excites the activity of the "power stroke."
    (d) Combination of calcium with the troponin is believed to trigger muscle contraction.
44. If the membrane of a large nerve fiber is not able to pump sodium and potassium ions through the membrane, but otherwise it is in the normal resting state, approximately how many nerve impulses can be transmitted by the nerve fiber before it cannot transmit any more impulses?
    (a) 1
    (b) About 10
    (c) About 5,000
    (d) Usually 50,000 or more
45. Skeletal muscle contraction is excited when the intracellular concentration of which ion rises

above a critical level in the sarcoplasm of the muscle cells?
(a) Sodium
(b) Calcium
(c) Magnesium
(d) Potassium
(e) Chloride

46. Which ions are probably most important in causing release of transmitter vesicles at nerve endings?
(a) Calcium ions
(b) Potassium ions
(c) Magnesium ions
(d) Sodium ions
(e) Chloride ions

47. The conduction velocity of an action potential is greatest in:
(a) Small, myelinated axons
(b) Small, unmyelinated axons
(c) Large, myelinated axons
(d) Large, unmyelinated axons

48. Which of the following heart murmurs can be heard only during systole?
(a) Interventricular septal defect
(b) Aortic regurgitation
(c) Mitral stenosis
(d) Patent ductus arteriosus
(e) Pulmonary valve regurgitation

49. The first heart sound is associated with:
(a) Inrushing of blood into the ventricles due to atrial contraction
(b) Closing of the A-V valves
(c) Closing of the semilunar valves
(d) Opening of the A-V valves
(e) Inrushing of blood into the ventricles in the early to middle part of diastole

50. The T wave of the normal electrocardiogram is caused by:
(a) Ventricular depolarization
(b) Ventricular repolarization
(c) Atrial repolarization
(d) Atrial depolarization

51. A heart murmur that is present during systole suggests:
(a) Aortic stenosis
(b) Mitral stenosis
(c) Aortic insufficiency

52. In the cardiac cycle, the period of isometric contraction occurs:
(a) During the second heart sound
(b) During the P wave of the electrocardiogram
(c) During the maximum ventricular ejection
(d) With the aortic valve closed

53. The natural rate of rhythmic discharge is greatest in which part of the heart?
(a) Ventricular myocardium
(b) Atria
(c) Sinoatrial node
(d) Purkinje fibers
(e) A-V node

54. The velocity of impulse transmission is slowest in the:
(a) A-V node
(b) Ventricular myocardium
(c) Atria
(d) Purkinje system
(e) Sinoatrial node

55. Cardiac muscle:
(a) Has a velocity of conduction of action potentials of 0.3 to 0.5 m per second
(b) Never contracts for more than 0.12 second
(c) Is not influenced by norepinephrine
(d) Has a longer duration of contraction during tachycardia
(e) All of the above

56. During the middle of diastole:
(a) The second heart sound is heard
(b) The mitral valve is closed
(c) Aortic pressure is falling
(d) The A-V valve is closing

57. During the middle of systole:
(a) The pulmonic valve is open
(b) The QRS complex is occurring
(c) Ventricular volume is increasing
(d) The aortic valve is closing

58. The delay between the P wave and the Q wave in the normal electrocardiogram is primarily caused by:
(a) A slow transmission through the A-V node and junctional fibers
(b) Delay at the internodal pathways
(c) Circus movement
(d) The slow rate of conduction in atrial heart muscle

59. Autoregulation of tissue blood flow in response to an increase in arterial pressure occurs as a result of:
(a) A decrease in vascular resistance
(b) An initial decrease in vascular wall tension
(c) Excess delivery of nutrients such as oxygen to the tissues
(d) A decrease in tissue metabolism

60. All of the following statements are correct *except*:
(a) Blood flow velocity in the capillaries is greater than in the large veins.
(b) Total surface area of the capillaries is much greater than of the large veins.

(c) Reduced oxygen tension in the tissues tends to relax precapillary sphincters.
(d) Increased sympathetic nerve stimulation tends to constrict the small arterioles.

61. The blood vessels of the systemic circulation responsible for most of the resistance to blood flow in the circulation are the:
(a) Aorta and large arteries
(b) Arterioles
(c) Capillaries
(d) Venules
(e) Venae cavae and large veins

62. Moderate fluid retention:
(a) Is detrimental in mild heart failure
(b) Is beneficial in mild heart failure
(c) Has no effect in mild heart failure

63. The renal–body fluid volume mechanism for regulating arterial pressure is important for:
(a) Raising the pressure when a person stands suddenly after having been in a lying position
(b) Minimizing a decrease in arterial pressure immediately following severe hemorrhage
(c) Increasing arterial pressure during strenuous physical exercise
(d) Maintaining arterial pressure at a normal level over a period of weeks, months, or years

64. Which type of heart failure is most likely to be associated with pulmonary edema?
(a) Heart failure resulting from an arteriovenous fistula
(b) High cardiac-output heart failure
(c) Left heart failure without right heart failure
(d) Left heart failure with right heart failure
(e) Right heart failure without left heart failure

65. Which of the following factors probably affects myocardial blood flow to the greatest extent under normal conditions?
(a) Degree of parasympathetic stimulation of coronary vessels
(b) Rate of release of adenosine from the myocardium
(c) Degree of sympathetic stimulation of coronary vessels
(d) Myocardial carbon dioxide concentration
(e) Rate of release of potassium from the myocardium

66. The most important factor for regulating cerebral blood flow under normal conditions is the:
(a) Rate of cerebral carbon dioxide formation
(b) Rate of cerebral oxygen consumption
(c) Degree of sympathetic stimulation of cerebral vasculature
(d) Rate of release of adenosine from the cerebrum
(e) Rate of release of potassium from the cerebrum

67. The pressure at one end of an artery is 60 mmHg, the pressure at the other end of the artery is 20 mmHg, and the flow through the artery is 200 ml/min. What is the resistance of the artery expressed in the above units?
(a) 0.05
(b) 0.1
(c) 0.2
(d) 0.4
(e) 0.6

68. The resistance of a blood vessel is 16 peripheral resistance units (PRU). Doubling the vessel diameter would change the resistance to:
(a) 10 PRU
(b) 8 PRU
(c) 4 PRU
(d) 2 PRU
(e) 1 PRU

69. Sympathetic stimulation of which vessels causes the greatest increase in total peripheral resistance?
(a) Veins
(b) Venules
(c) Capillaries
(d) Arterioles
(e) Arteries

70. Which of the following would not be expected to occur during strenuous physical exercise?
(a) Large increase in pulmonary blood flow
(b) Large increase in pulmonary arterial pressure
(c) Large decrease in pulmonary vascular resistance
(d) Pulmonary capillary distension
(e) Pulmonary capillary recruitment

71. Which one of the following would result in an increase in tissue blood flow?
(a) An increase in tissue oxygen concentration
(b) A decrease in tissue carbon dioxide concentration
(c) An increase in tissue adenosine concentration
(d) A decrease in tissue lactic acid concentration
(e) None of the above

72. A decrease in blood pressure at the level of the internal carotid artery would result in:
(a) A decrease in nerve impulses from carotid sinus nerves
(b) An increase in heart rate
(c) An increase in total peripheral resistance
(d) An increase in the strength of heart muscle contraction
(e) All of the above

73. Arteriosclerosis is associated with an increase in pulse pressure because:

(a) Stroke volume is decreased
(b) Compliance of the arterial tree is decreased
(c) Vascular conductance is increased
(d) Total peripheral resistance is decreased
(e) None of the above

74. If the baroreceptor reflexes are fully functional when upright posture is assumed:
(a) The blood vessels of the arms will become vasodilated
(b) Arterial pressure in the foot will decrease markedly
(c) Bradycardia will occur
(d) Cerebral blood flow will not change appreciably

75. The most important factor that tends to collapse the lungs (the recoil tendency) is the:
(a) Elastic fibers in the lungs
(b) Intrapleural fluid pressure
(c) Total intrapleural pressure
(d) Tension in the intercostal muscles
(e) Surface tension of the alveolar fluid

76. Oxygen therapy has significant value in all the following types of hypoxia *except:*
(a) Atmospheric hypoxia
(b) Hypoventilation hypoxia
(c) Hypoxia due to pulmonary edema
(d) Hypoxia due to decreased hemoglobin in the blood
(e) Histotoxic hypoxia due to cyanide poisoning

77. Contraction of which of the following muscles is most important for causing forceful expiration?
(a) Internal intercostals
(b) Diaphragm
(c) Abdominals
(d) Sternocleidomastoids
(e) External intercostals

78. Which of the following factors has no direct stimulatory effect on the medullary respiratory center?
(a) Changes in arterial Pco_2
(b) Changes in arterial *p*H
(c) Chances in arterial Po_2

79. In which of the following diseases would you expect to find an increase in thickness of the respiratory membrane?
(a) Asthma
(b) Emphysema
(c) Pulmonary edema
(d) Pulmonary artery thrombosis
(e) Skeletal abnormalities of the chest

80. Which of the following would not be expected to cause hypoxia?
(a) Hyperpnea
(b) Hypoventilation
(c) Reduced ventilation-to-perfusion ratio
(d) Diminished diffusing capacity for oxygen
(e) Excessive blood flow through venous to arterial shunts

81. If a person has a tidal volume of 411 ml, a physiologic dead space volume of 100 ml, and a respiratory minute ventilation of 3,600 ml/min, what is his or her approximate alveolar ventilation?
(a) 3,600 ml/min
(b) 3,000 ml/min
(c) 2,700 ml/min
(d) 1,500 ml/min
(e) 900 ml/min

82. The major factor regulating alveolar ventilation during rest is:
(a) Arterial Po_2
(b) Arterial Pco_2
(c) Arterial *p*H
(d) Nervous output from the joint proprioceptors

83. Sudden exposure of an unacclimatized subject to 25,000 feet would produce which of the following after 10 minutes?
(a) Improved night vision
(b) Falling *p*H
(c) Helium bubbles in the blood
(d) Coma

84. If a neurotransmitter is considered to be excitatory in nature, its effect on the postsynaptic membrane would most likely be:
(a) A decrease in sodium permeability
(b) A decrease in calcium permeability
(c) An increase in sodium permeability
(d) A decrease in potassium permeability

85. Damage to which area of the cerebral cortex is likely to cause the greatest degree of loss of intellectual capabilities in a right-handed person?
(a) The frontal lobes
(b) The left posterior superior temporal gyrus
(c) The right somesthetic sensory and sensory association areas
(d) The left somesthetic sensory and sensory association areas
(e) The right posterior temporal and angular gyrus regions

86. Which of the following types of stimuli may excite a nociceptor?
(a) Mechanical stimuli
(b) Chemical stimuli
(c) Thermal stimuli
(d) Tissue damage
(e) All of the above

87. The additive effect of a number of rapidly occurring postsynaptic potentials that result in the firing of an action potential by the postsynaptic neuron is an example of:

(a) Spatial summation
(b) Facilitation
(c) Temporal summation
(d) Reverberation
(e) Electrotonic summation

88. What provides most of the energy used to maintain a normal resting membrane potential of about 70 millivolts inside the neuronal soma?
(a) The chloride pump
(b) The bicarbonate pump
(c) The sodium–potassium pump
(d) The calcium pump
(e) Diffusion of chloride ions

89. Which theory probably best explains long-term memory?
(a) That actual physical or chemical changes occur at the synapses
(b) That there is change in RNA inside the soma of the neuron
(c) That the glial cells around the neuron change
(d) That the ionic composition of the neurons changes
(e) That the electrical potential of the neuron changes

90. The phenomena of referred pain:
(a) Explains why pains from the heart may be localized to the arm and neck
(b) Results from the extensive branching of the peripheral process (axon) of nociceptors
(c) Is useful in diagnosis, as the pain is always referred to the immediate overlying area
(d) Explains why headaches are so common
(e) Feels real, but is psychosomatic

91. What part of the lower regions of the brain probably plays the most significant role in directing one's attention to one particular type of brain activity?
(a) The thalamus
(b) The hypothalamus
(c) The mesencephalon
(d) The pons
(e) The septal region of the limbic system

92. The transmission of pain, thermal, tickle, itch, and sexual sensations is provided by the:
(a) Pyramidal tract
(b) Anterolateral pathway
(c) Spinocerebellar pathway
(d) Dorsal column medial lemniscal pathway

93. In the autonomic nervous system, preganglionic transmission is exclusively:
(a) Cholinergic
(b) Adrenergic
(c) Sympathetic
(d) Parasympathetic

94. Which of the following statements is true?
(a) The transmitter secreted at the endings of the sympathetic preganglionic neurons is norepinephrine.
(b) The transmitter secreted at the endings of the preganglionic neurons of the parasympathetic neurons is epinephrine.
(c) The transmitter secreted at the postganglionic neuron endings of the parasympathetic neurons is atropine.
(d) The transmitter secreted at most postganglionic neuron endings of the sympathetic nervous system is norepinephrine.

95. Almost all of the cerebral cortex has direct two-way communication with which one of the following subcortical structures?
(a) Cerebellum
(b) Thalamus
(c) Hypothalamus
(d) Bulboreticular facilitory area
(e) Putamen

96. In what part of the central nervous system do the signals probably originate to provide most of the support of the body against gravity?
(a) Brain stem
(b) Basal ganglia
(c) Motor cortex
(d) Cerebellum
(e) Spinal cord

97. Where are the centers located for causing such gross stereotype body movements as rotational movements of the head, raising movements of the head and body, flexing movements of the head and body, and turning movements of the body?
(a) Motor cortex
(b) Cerebellum
(c) Amygdala
(d) Mesencephalon

98. The portion of the vestibular system that is most important for preventing a person from suddenly falling if he or she makes a sudden turn while moving forward is the:
(a) Saccule
(b) Utricle
(c) Cochlea
(d) Otoconia
(e) Semicircular canals

99. Where is motor activity probably initiated in the brain?
(a) Motor cortex
(b) Premotor cortex
(c) Basal ganglia
(d) Cerebellum
(e) Somatic sensory cortex

100. To what part of the brain do most of the signals from the Golgi tendon apparati and muscle spindles go?
   (a) Somatic sensory cortex
   (b) Thalamus
   (c) Basal ganglia
   (d) Motor cortex
   (e) Cerebellum
101. What probably causes stimulation of the thermal receptors?
   (a) Change in the membrane permeability caused by heat or cold
   (b) Change in the number of protein receptors in the nerve ending
   (c) Change in the vicosity of the fluid surrounding the neuron
   (d) Change in the concentration of sodium ions outside the neuron caused by changes in temperature
102. Kinesthetic sensations are detected mainly by what type of receptors?
   (a) Muscle spindles
   (b) Golgi tendon apparati
   (c) Skin receptors
   (d) Joint receptors
103. Which primary cortical sensory area is located in the middle of the superior temporal gyrus?
   (a) Vision
   (b) Hearing
   (c) Somatic sensation
   (d) Taste
   (e) Smell
104. When a person wishes to speak a certain thought, where does the thought originate?
   (a) Broca's area
   (b) Wernicke's area of the temporal cortex
   (c) Supramarginal gyrus
   (d) Facial region of the motor cortex
   (e) Prefrontal cortex
105. What determines whether norepinephrine circulating in the body fluids will be excitatory or inhibitory in a particular organ?
   (a) The nature of the receptor in the cells of the organ
   (b) The intensity of nerve stimulation of the organ
   (c) The chemical changes that occur in the norepinephrine before it excites the cells
   (d) The position on the cells where norepinephrine is secreted by the nerve endings
106. The fovea is especially adapted for high acuity vision because:
   (a) The fovea has a very large surface area
   (b) The fovea contains a high density of rods
   (c) The fovea is covered by numerous blood vessels
   (d) The ratio of cones to optic nerve fibers in the fovea is close to 1
   (e) Cones of the fovea have a larger diameter than those of the peripheral retina
107. Going from bright sunlight to a dark room will result in:
   (a) Improved color vision
   (b) Depletion of the stores in rhodopsin
   (c) Twofold increase in retinal sensitivity
   (d) Net accumulation of rhodopsin in the rods
   (e) Hundredfold increase in retinal sensitivity
108. The red cones and the green cones are stimulated approximately equally. What color will the person see?
   (a) Red
   (b) Yellow
   (c) Green
   (d) Purple
   (e) Blue
109. The sensory receptor responsible for the perception of sound is the:
   (a) Golgi apparatus
   (b) Organ of Corti
   (c) Organ of Ruffini
   (d) Corpus geniculatum
   (e) Krause's corpuscle
110. The type of taste that provides protection against ingesting poisonous plant products is the:
   (a) Sour taste
   (b) Salty taste
   (c) Sweet taste
   (d) Bitter taste
111. The most frequent stimulus of peristalsis is:
   (a) Distention
   (b) Sympathetic stimulation
   (c) Acid chyme
   (d) Alkaline chyme
112. Hydrochloric acid is secreted by the:
   (a) Paneth cells
   (b) Goblet cells
   (c) Chief cells
   (d) Parictal cells
113. The three phases of gastric secretion are:
   (a) First, second, and third
   (b) Cephalic, gastric, and intestinal
   (c) Ptyalin, gastrin, secretin
   (d) Gastric, intestinal, colonic
114. Which of the following hormones stimulate the rate of stomach emptying:
   (a) Gastrin
   (b) Cholecystokinin
   (c) Secretin

(d) Somatostatin
(e) Epinephrine

115. Which of the following chemical processes is the basis of food digestion?
(a) Oxidation
(b) Reduction
(c) Hydration
(d) Hydrolysis
(e) Nucleophilic substitution

116. Pepsinogen is secreted by the:
(a) Paneth cells
(b) Goblet cells
(c) Chief cells
(d) Parietal cells

117. The hormone generally considered to be the major stimulus for enzyme secretion by the pancreas is:
(a) Cholecystokinin
(b) Secretin
(c) Trypsin
(d) Gastrin

118. Which of the following enzymes requires an acid *p*H of approximately 2.0 to function optimally?
(a) Trypsin
(b) Chymotrypsin
(c) Pepsin
(d) Pancreatic lipase
(e) Parotid amylase

119. Amino acids are transported in the blood mainly:
(a) In the form of plasma proteins
(b) In the form of lipoproteins
(c) In combination with a carbohydrate carrier
(d) In combination with a phospholipid carrier
(e) In the form of amino acids themselves

120. Which ionic gradient across the inner mitochondrial membrane provides the electromotive force for the production of adenosine triphosphate?
(a) Sodium gradient
(b) Calcium gradient
(c) Chloride gradient
(d) Potassium gradient
(e) Hydrogen ion gradient

121. When the temperature of the surroundings is greater than the body temperature, heat loss is possible only through which of the following?
(a) Radiation
(b) Convection
(c) Conduction
(d) Evaporation
(e) Forced convection

122. If a person whose normal core body temperature is 98.6°F is placed in air that is 98°F, and the person is breathing air that is 98°F and 100% humidified:
(a) The person's core temperature will rise
(b) The person's core temperature will fall to 98°F
(c) Shivering is likely
(d) Sweating will occur and maintain constant body temperature

123. At normal room temperature most body heat loss is by:
(a) Convection
(b) Direct conduction
(c) Radiation
(d) Sweating

124. Integration of temperature information by the nervous system occurs mainly in the:
(a) Spinal cord
(b) Hypothalamus
(c) Amygdala
(d) Peripheral receptors

125. Menstruation is caused by the:
(a) Surge of LH just prior to midcycle
(b) Failure of the corpus luteum to involute
(c) Sudden reduction of progesterone and estrogen at the end of the ovarian cycle
(d) Excessive secretion of estrogen and progesterone at the end of the ovarian cycle

126. The secretion of parathyroid hormone is controlled by the concentration of:
(a) Extracellular ionized calcium
(b) Calcium bound to citrate anions
(c) Calcium bound to plasma proteins
(d) Calcium inside of the bone matrix

127. Important effects of testosterone include all of the following *except:*
(a) Formation of the fetal penis
(b) Descent of the testes into the scrotum
(c) Increased muscle development
(d) Initiation of ejaculation
(e) Increased thickness of the skin

128. Penile erection is caused primarily by:
(a) Reflex-sympathetic constriction of the arterioles
(b) Parasympathetically induced dilation of the arterioles
(c) Contraction of the bulbocavernosus muscle
(d) Reflex-parasympathetic constriction of the venules
(e) Sympathetic-induced constriction of the veins

129. During a normal menstrual cycle a large surge of FSH and LH occurs:
(a) During menstruation
(b) One or two days before ovulation
(c) One or two days before menstruation
(d) During the days following ovulation

130. In Graves' disease, one would least likely expect:
(a) Goiter
(b) Weight loss

(c) Increased sweating
(d) Increased metabolic rate
(e) Increased TSH secretion

131. Which of the following hormones impairs hydrolysis of triglycerides to fatty acids?
(a) Insulin
(b) Glucagon
(c) Cortisol
(d) Growth hormone

132. Increased plasma parathyroid hormone concentration tends to increase all of the following *except:*
(a) Number of active osteoclasts
(b) Extracellular phosphate concentration
(c) Absorption of calcium from the gastrointestinal tract
(d) Absorption of calcium from the renal tubules
(e) Absorption of phosphate from bone

133. The active form of vitamin D is:
(a) Calcitonin
(b) 1,25-dihydroxycholecalciferol
(c) Parathyroid hormone
(d) Cholecalciferol

134. High plasma levels of thyroxine can lead to all of the following *except:*
(a) Increased cardiac output
(b) Increased plasma triglyceride concentration
(c) Increased heart rate
(d) Decreased body weight
(e) Increased metabolic rate

135. Cortisol can cause all of the following *except:*
(a) Inflammation to be suppressed
(b) Fat to be used for energy
(c) Lysosomal membranes to become unstable
(d) Blood glucose concentration to increase
(e) Proteins to be degraded in many tissues

136. Growth hormone increases all of the following *except:*
(a) Blood glucose concentration
(b) Blood free fatty acid concentration
(c) Protein synthesis
(d) Storage of protein in cells
(e) Metabolism of carbohydrates

137. Glucagon:
(a) Is secreted by beta cells of the islets of Langerhans
(b) Helps correct hyperglycemia
(c) Is secreted by alpha cells of the islets of Langerhans
(d) Promotes glycogen storage by the liver
(e) Decreases gluconeogenesis

138. All of the following hormones mediate their major effects without actually entering the target cell *except:*
(a) Cortisol
(b) Insulin
(c) Growth hormone
(d) Glucagon
(e) Parathyroid hormone

139. Blockage of the hypothalamic-hypophyseal venous portal system would be expected to cause increased secretion of:
(a) Growth hormone
(b) Adrenocorticotropic hormone
(c) Thyroid-stimulating hormone
(d) Prolactin
(e) Follicle-stimulating hormone

140. The basic effects of growth hormone on body metabolism include:
(a) Decreasing the rate of protein synthesis
(b) Increasing the rate of use of carbohydrates
(c) Decreasing the mobilization of fats
(d) Increasing the use of fats for energy
(e) None of the above

141. Almost all of the active thyroid hormone entering the circulation is in the form of:
(a) Triiodothyronine
(b) Thyroxine
(c) Thyroglobulin
(d) Thyrotropin
(e) Long-acting thyroid stimulator

142. Which of the following produces human chorionic gonadotropin?
(a) The follicle
(b) The corpus luteum
(c) The trophoblasts
(d) The anterior pituitary gland

143. Which of the following stimulates milk production by breasts?
(a) Oxytocin
(b) Prolactin
(c) Estrogen
(d) Dopamine

144. Which of the following will lead to release of calcium from bone?
(a) Stimulation of the activity of osteoblasts
(b) Stimulation of activity of the osteocytes
(c) Stimulation of the activity of the osteoclasts
(d) Elevation of extracellular calcium ion activity

145. How many chromosomes are present in a normal mature sperm cell?
(a) 21
(b) 23
(c) 46
(d) 92

146. When is the rate of estrogen secretion highest?
(a) During menstruation
(b) Three days before ovulation
(c) One day after ovulation
(d) One day before menstruation

ANSWERS TO MULTIPLE-CHOICE QUESTIONS

1. b
2. d
3. b
4. d
5. b
6. a
7. e
8. e
9. c
10. c
11. a
12. a
13. e
14. d
15. c
16. c
17. b
18. d
19. a
20. c
21. c
22. d
23. c
24. e
25. c
26. a
27. a
28. d
29. c
30. e
31. a
32. b
33. d
34. d
35. a
36. c
37. c
38. e
39. d
40. e
41. a
42. c
43. d
44. d
45. b
46. a
47. c
48. a
49. b
50. b
51. a
52. d
53. c
54. a
55. a
56. c
57. a
58. a
59. c
60. a
61. b
62. b
63. d
64. c
65. b
66. a
67. c
68. e
69. d
70. b
71. c
72. e
73. b
74. d
75. e
76. e
77. b
78. c
79. c
80. a
81. c
82. b
83. d
84. c
85. b
86. e
87. c
88. c
89. a
90. a
91. a
92. b
93. a
94. d
95. b
96. a
97. d
98. e
99. e
100. e
101. a
102. d
103. b
104. b
105. a
106. d
107. d
108. b
109. b
110. d
111. a
112. d
113. b
114. a
115. d
116. c
117. a
118. c
119. e
120. e
121. d
122. a
123. c
124. b
125. c
126. a
127. d
128. b
129. b
130. e
131. a
132. b
133. b
134. b
135. c
136. e
137. c
138. a
139. d
140. d
141. b
142. c
143. b
144. c
145. b
146. b

Rypins' Basic Sciences Review, 17th Edition,
edited by Edward D. Frohlich. Lippincott–Raven Publishers,
Philadelphia © 1997.

4

Biochemistry

Robert Roskoski, Jr., M.D., Ph.D.
Fred G. Brazda Professor and Head
Department of Biochemistry
and Molecular Biology
Louisiana State University Medical Center
New Orleans, Louisiana

INTRODUCTION TO BIOCHEMISTRY AND MOLECULAR BIOLOGY

Biochemistry is the study of life at the molecular level. Biochemistry includes a study of the molecular composition of living systems and the chemical reactions that living systems undergo. Biochemistry is also concerned with the production and use of fuel molecules that provide living organisms with the chemical energy required to maintain their highly organized state. In addition to the chemical energy required for biosynthesis, biochemistry considers the mechanisms responsible for the work of transport, intracellular movement, and muscle contraction. Biochemistry and molecular biology also entail a consideration of replication, differentiation, development, maintenance, healing or repair, and aging.

Besides addressing physiological processes, biochemistry plays an important role in understanding the pathogenesis of diseases. A complete understanding of pathological processes occurs only after the biochemical mechanisms have been discovered. The frequent reference to protein factors and the elucidation of the structure of a gene associated with a disease in the current health science literature conveys the importance of biochemistry.

The complexity of living systems and attempts to understand the biochemistry of humans and human pathogens can be daunting and bewildering. The large number of components involved adds to the difficulty. However, recognizing that all forms of life are made up of about 50 fundamental building blocks and their derivatives constitutes a major step in simplifying the science of biochemistry. A list of additional unifying principles is given in Table 4-1, and these principles can be reviewed during the study of subsequent sections in this chapter.

The Cell

Humans, other animals, plants, and microorganisms are composed of fundamental units called ***cells*** (Table 4-1). All cells are surrounded by a ***plasma membrane,*** the boundary between the cell interior and the surrounding environment. The plasma membrane regulates and limits the influx and efflux of fuel molecules, such as glucose, and ions, such as sodium and potassium. Intracellular metabolites such as glucose 6-phosphate and citrate bear electrical charges and pass through the plasma membrane with difficulty, if at all. Those charged molecules that cross the plasma membrane are transported by specific proteins called ***translocases.***

Cells arise from other cells by the process of cell division. Organisms are divided into two major classes based on the presence or absence of a discrete cell nucleus. Humans and other organisms whose cells contain a nucleus are called ***eukaryotes;*** cell division occurs by mitosis. The four stages of the cell cycle include G_1, S, G_2, and M. G_1 and G_2 are *g*rowth phases. S refers to the DNA *s*ynthesis phase, and M refers to *m*itosis. Microorganisms that lack a well-defined nucleus are called ***prokaryotes.*** *Escherichia coli* and *Streptococcus pneumoniae* are examples. Prokaryotes divide by binary fission.

A diagram of a prototypic animal cell is shown in Fig-

TABLE 4-1. Fundamental Principles of Biochemistry and Molecular Biology

1. All forms of life are constructed from fundamental units called cells (the cell theory of Schleiden and Schwann).
2. Cells obey the laws of chemistry and physics.
3. Biochemical reactions are catalyzed by enzymes.
4. Enzymes are protein catalysts (Sumner's law). Ribozymes are RNA catalysts (Cech's law).
5. The sun is the ultimate source of energy for life on earth.
6. Biochemical processes proceed with the liberation of free energy.
7. ATP is the common currency of energy exchange in all forms of life (Lipmann's law).
8. The final common pathway in oxidative metabolism of aerobic organisms is the Krebs citric acid cycle.
9. A proton motive force furnishes the energy for ATP synthesis in (1) oxidative phosphorylation in aerobes and (2) photophosphorylation in photosynthetic organisms (Mitchell's chemiosmotic theory).
10. ATP hydrolysis provides energy for establishing ion gradients. Ion gradients provide energy for metabolite transport.
11. NADH is the hydrogen carrier in most catabolic processes; NADPH is the hydrogen carrier or reductant in most anabolic processes.
12. Activated monomers are the precursors for condensation and polymerization reactions.
13. The generation of inorganic pyrophosphate and its subsequent hydrolysis catalyzed by pyrophosphatase serves to pull biochemical reactions toward completion. This explains why ATP with its two high-energy bonds and not ADP with its single high-energy bond is the common currency of energy exchange.
14. The primary structure of a protein governs its secondary and tertiary structure (Anfinsen's law).
15. Biomolecules that interact have complementary structures (Fischer's lock and key hypothesis).
16. Enzymes may be regulated by noncovalent or allosteric agents (theory of Monod, Wyman, and Changeux) and by covalent modification such as that of phosphorylation.
17. Metabolic regulation and molecules with regulatory activities (allosteric effectors) follow a pattern that makes physiological sense (the molecular logic of the cell).
18. Various forms of life are continually giving rise to slightly different forms, some of which are adapted to multiply more effectively (Darwin's theories of evolution and natural selection).
19. A single gene codes for one enzyme or polypeptide (the one gene–one enzyme hypothesis of Beadle and Tatum).
20. DNA is the molecule of heredity (law of Avery, MacLeod, and McCarty). In some viruses RNA performs this function (law of Gierer and Schramm).
21. DNA forms an antiparallel double helix with Watson-Crick base pairing (A with T; G with C in DNA; A with U in RNA).
22. DNA biosynthesis is semiconservative (law of Messelson and Stahl).
23. The flow of information in biological systems is from DNA to DNA and from DNA to RNA to protein (Crick's law of molecular biology). In some cases, information flows from RNA to DNA (Temin's law).
24. The genetic code is triplet in nature (a sequence of three nucleotides encodes one amino acid) and mRNA is read in the 5′- to 3′-direction.
25. The genetic code is (almost) universal.
26. Complementary nucleotide base pairing is antiparallel in nature.
27. Nucleic acid elongation reactions proceed in the 5′ to 3′ direction; amino acid elongation reactions in protein synthesis proceed from the amino to carboxyl terminus.
28. Eukaryotes possess interrupted genes. Intervening sequences in RNA are removed by splicing reactions.

ure 4-1. The constituent parts and the biochemical reactions associated with each part are listed in Table 4-2. This table can be used as a reference for other sections of this chapter. The ***nucleus*** is the repository of genetic information that is composed of DNA. ***Chromatin*** refers to a combination of DNA, histone and nonhistone proteins, and nascent RNA. The nucleus is surrounded by a double membrane that contains nuclear pores (Fig. 4-1).

The mitochondrion is the powerhouse of the cell and is responsible for most of the cell's adenosine triphosphate (ATP) production. The mitochondria contain an ***outer membrane*** that is freely permeable to small organic molecules and some larger proteins. The ***inner mitochondrial membrane,*** in contrast, exhibits restricted permeability. Except for a few uncharged substances such as oxygen, carbon dioxide, and urea, the passage of metabolites through the mitochondrial inner membrane is mediated by specific translocases. For example, a specific protein

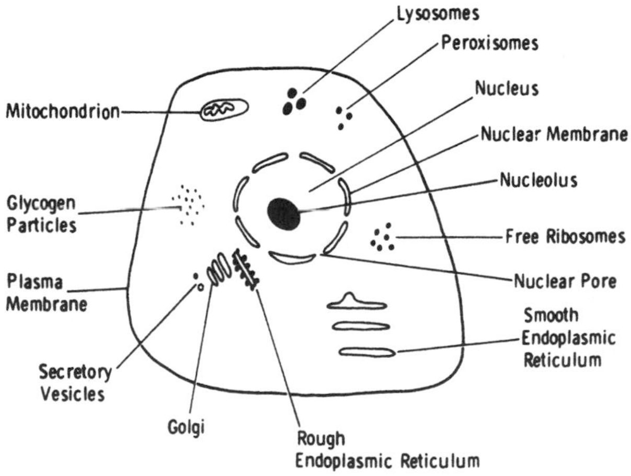

Fig. 4-1. Diagram of a prototypical human cell and its subcellular components.

TABLE 4-2. Properties of Eukaryotic Cell Components

COMPONENT	GENERAL PROPERTIES	ASSOCIATED BIOCHEMICAL PROCESSES	PERCENT VOLUME	NUMBER PER CELL
Cytosol	Nonsedimentable	Glycolysis, glycogenesis; glycogenolysis, pentose phosphate pathway, gluconeogenesis, fatty acid synthesis, steroid synthesis, purine and pyrimidine formation, carbamoyl-phosphate synthetase II, protein synthesis (free ribosomes)	54	1
Nucleus	Repository and expression of genes	DNA replication, RNA synthesis and processing; contains chromatin, histones, and nonhistones	6	1
Mitochondrion	Powerhouse of the cell; major site of ATP formation	Citric acid cycle; β-oxidation of fatty acids; oxidative phosphorylation and ATP synthesis; pyruvate dehydrogenase, citrate synthase, carbamoyl-phosphate synthetase I (liver); some DNA, RNA, and protein synthesis; metabolic water formed here	22	1,700
Lysosome	Waste basket of the cell	Acid phosphatase, cathepsins (degrade several classes of proteins), DNAse, RNAse, hexosaminidase, and many other hydrolytic activities	1	300
Peroxisome	Hydrogen peroxide metabolism	Catalase, peroxidase	1	400
Rough endoplasmic reticulum and Golgi	Synthesis of membrane proteins and proteins for export	Membrane-bound ribosomes, protein processing, and glycosylation	9	1
Smooth endoplasmic reticulum	Complex lipid biosynthesis	Cytochrome P-450 electron transport, steroid hydroxylation, fatty acid desaturation, phospholipid biosynthesis	6	1
Plasma membrane	Boundary between cell exterior and interior	Na^+/K^+ ATPase, adenylyl cyclase, many receptors (*e.g.*, insulin, β-adrenergic, HDL receptor), ion channels, glucose, and amino acid transport proteins		1

carrier translocates ATP from the mitochondrion in exchange for adenosine diphosphate (ADP). This is an example of ***antiport:*** one substance moves in one direction and the other moves in the opposite direction. In a ***symport*** process, both substances move in the same direction. The transport of glucose across the intestinal epithelium, for example, is accompanied and driven by the cotransport of sodium. The impermeability of the inner mitochondrial membrane to protons is important for the biosynthesis of ATP. The infoldings of the inner mitochondrial membrane are ***cristae.*** The infoldings represent a way for increasing membrane surface area. The compartment within the inner mitochondrial membrane is called the mitochondrial ***matrix.***

Membranes are composed of phospholipid ***bilayers*** with a hydrophilic exterior and hydrophobic interior. ***Integral membrane proteins*** are imbedded in or course through the membrane. Lipids and proteins readily move laterally in the two-dimensional plane of the membrane; lateral movement is termed ***fluidity.*** The existence of proteins within the lipid scaffold or sheet is termed a ***mosaic.*** Both properties (fluidity and mosaicism) are important and have given rise to the ***fluid–mosaic model*** of membranes.

Lysosomes are membrane-bound organelles that participate in the hydrolytic degradation of several types of compounds. The interior of lysosomes is acidic (pH ≈5) relative to the cytosol (*p*H ≈7). The degradative enzymes found in lysosomes exhibit an acid pH optimum. The hereditary absence of specific enzymes is associated with several lysosomal diseases, including Gaucher and Tay-Sachs disease.

The ***endoplasmic*** (inside the cell) ***reticulum*** (network) is a membranous structure that participates in a wide variety of activities (Table 4-2). When associated with ribosomes ***(rough endoplasmic reticulum),*** the endoplasmic reticulum plays a role in protein synthesis. The ribosomes attached to the endoplasmic reticulum exhibit a studded or roughened appearance as observed by electron microscopy. Many reactions of lipid synthesis occur in the ***smooth endoplasmic reticulum*** because of the solubility of lipids in membranes.

The dimensions of cells vary considerably. A cuboidal liver cell is about 20 μm × 20 μm × 20 μm. The circular mature human erythrocyte is about 7 μm in diameter and 2 μm thick. Erythrocytes (7 μm diameter) serve as an important relative standard when viewing tissues by microscopy. An *E. coli* cell and a liver mitochondrion are about 1 μm in diameter and 2 μm in length.

The mammalian ***erythrocyte*** lacks a nucleus, mito-

TABLE 4-3. Elements of the Human Body

ELEMENT	MASS IN 70-Kg HUMAN		COMMENTS
Organic matter and water			
Carbon	12.6	kg	Organic chemicals
Hydrogen	7.0	kg	Organic chemicals and water
Oxygen	45.5	kg	Organic chemicals and water
Nitrogen	2.1	kg	Nucleic acids and amino acids
Phosphorous	0.7	kg	Nucleic acids and many metabolites; constituent of bones and teeth
Sulfur	0.175	kg	Connective tissue and proteins
Bulk minerals			
Sodium	105	g	Principal extracellular cation
Potassium	245	g	Principal intracellular cation; diffusion through cell membrane generates, in part, the negative intracellular electromotive force; obligatory loss of 40 mEq/day in urine
Magnesium	35	g	Cofactor for ATP and other nucleotide reactants; a calcium antagonist; $MgSO_4$ used in treatment of ecclampsia to decrease nerve excitability
Calcium	1,050	g	Constituent of teeth and bones; intracellular second messenger; triggers muscle contraction and exocytosis
Chloride	105	g	Major extracellular anion; activates amylase
Fluoride	8	g	Increases hardness of bones and teeth; excess produces dental fluorosis
Trace minerals			
Manganese	20	mg	Mitochondrial superoxide dismutase
Iron	3,000	mg	Found in hemoglobin, myoglobin, cytochromes, iron-sulfur proteins; transported as transferrin and stored as ferritin; deficiency leads to a microcytic anemia
Cobalt	5	mg	Constituent of vitamin B_{12}
Copper	100	mg	Component of cytochrome a,a_3 and tyrosinase (in melanin formation); transported in blood by ceruloplasmin; bound to erythrocuprein of the red blood cell; Wilson's disease (hepatolenticular degeneration) is a rare hereditary disorder involving brain and liver with abnormal copper metabolism; cytosolic superoxide dismutase
Zinc	2,300	mg	Cofactor for carbonic anhydrase, carboxypeptidase, and cytosolic superoxide dismutase
Molybdenum	Trace		Xanthine dehydrogenase of purine metabolism and aldehyde oxidase in catecholamine metabolism
Iodine	Trace		Required for production of thyroid hormones T_4 and T_3 (formed from thyroglobulin); deficiency of thyroid hormone produces cretinism in children and myxedema in adults; hyperthyroidism with thyroid hyperplasia is treated with radioiodine
Selenium	Trace		Glutathione peroxidase

chondria, endoplasmic reticulum, and other membranous organelles. Erythrocytes obtain their energy by anaerobic glycolysis. Mature erythrocytes cannot participate in DNA, RNA, or protein synthesis. Erythrocytes contain hemoglobin and 2,3-bisphosphoglycerate at a concentration of about 5 mM each. Hemoglobin accounts for about 90% of the red blood cell protein. Erythrocytes function in both oxygen and carbon dioxide transport.

The Structural Chemistry of Biomolecules

ELEMENTS

The components of matter that constitute humans can be classified as (1) elements of organic matter and water, (2) abundant minerals, and (3) trace minerals. The identity of these elements and their approximate mass in a 70-kg human are given in Table 4-3. Oxygen is the most abundant element in the body (in terms of mass, not number of atoms). The average adult is composed of 55% water, 19% protein, 19% fat, 7% inorganic matter, and less than 1% carbohydrate and nucleic acid. The preponderance of water accounts for the large mass of oxygen in humans. Although calcium is predominantly extracellular (as solid hydroxyapatite in bones and teeth and as a 2-mM solution in the extracellular space), calcium plays an important regulatory role within cells. Changes in intracellular concentration from 10^{-8} M to 10^{-7} M or more trigger muscle contraction, exocytosis, and other cellular processes. Hydroxyapatite is a calcium phosphate–calcium hydroxide complex with the following formula: $Ca_{10}(PO_4)_6(OH)_2$.

The other elements are mentioned as appropriate in the text and are addressed again under nutrition.

CHEMICAL BONDS

Four types of chemical bonds are important in the formation of molecules in biological systems: (1) covalent bonds, (2) ionic bonds (salt bridges), (3) hydrogen bonds, and (4) hydrophobic bonds. ***Covalent bonds*** are composed of a pair of electrons. Covalent bonds are strong (400 kJ/mol) and account for the stability of carbohydrates, fats, proteins, and nucleic acids. In aqueous solution ***salt bridges,*** or ***ionic bonds,*** between positively and negatively charged species are weaker (20 kJ/mol) than covalent bonds. ***Hydrogen bonds*** refer to the sharing of a hydrogen atom between electronegative oxygen atoms, nitrogen atoms, or a combination of the two. The hydrogen atom is covalently linked to one atom of the pair and interacts electrostatically with the second. The strength of hydrogen bonds is dependent on direction. Although these bonds are individually weak (10–30 kJ/mol), formation of a large number promotes stability. ***Hydrophobic*** (water-fearing) ***bonds*** are apolar bonds between hydrocarbon-containing compounds. It is energetically favorable to sequester hydrocarbons in hydrophobic domains and minimize their contact with polar water molecules in solution. Although hydrophobic bonds are individually weak (1 kJ/mol), formation of a large number results in a stable structure.

FUNCTIONAL GROUPS IN BIOCHEMICALS

In considering the reactions of metabolism, it is important to understand the chemistry of the participating functional groups. Examining the precise bonds that are made and broken during a chemical transformation aids in understanding and analysis of a biochemical process. The main functional groups are listed in Table 4-4. Most of these compounds are familiar from organic chemistry. Organic chemistry is often described as the chemistry of carbon. Bond making and breaking usually involve a carbon atom. In biochemistry, however, reactions often involve processes at phosphorus, oxygen, and nitrogen as well as carbon.

Most biomolecules contain more than one functional group. ***Carbohydrates,*** for example, contain an aldehyde or ketone and two or more alcohol groups. ***Amino acids,*** as their name indicates, contain both amino and carboxylic acid groups. Although there is incredible diversity among all forms of life, only about 50 fundamental compounds constitute the major mass of living organisms. This unity in nature makes our task easier. Besides the fundamental building blocks, there are a few hundred other metabolites that constitute the vast majority of com-

TABLE 4-4. Functional Groups in Biochemicals

GROUP		EXAMPLE WITH GROUP
Hydrocarbons		
Alkyl groups	$CH_3(CH_2)_n{}^-$	
		Leucine
Alkenes	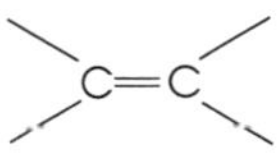	Fumarate
Aromatic	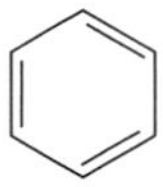	Phenylalanine
Alcohol	R—OH	Ethanol
Amines	R—NH_2	Glycine
Sulfur Derivatives		
Sulfhydryl group (mercaptan)	R—SH	Cysteine
Disulfide	R—S—S—R[1]	Cystine
Thioethor	R—S—R[1]	Methionine
Sulfate	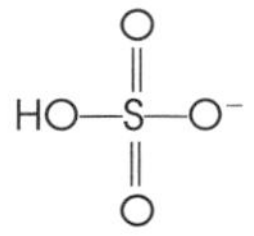	

(continued)

TABLE 4-4. Functional Groups in Biochemicals (*continued*)

GROUP		EXAMPLE WITH GROUP
Sulfur Derivatives		
Sulfate ester	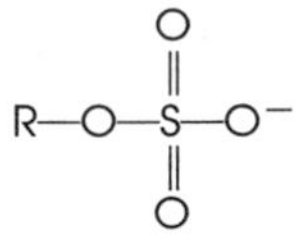	Chondroltin sulfate
Carbonyl groups	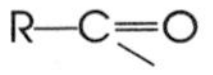	
Aldehyde	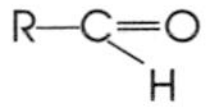	Glyceraldehyde-3-phosphate
Ketone	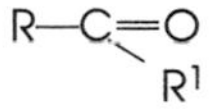	Dihydroxyacetonephosphate
Carboxylic acid	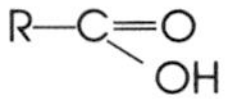	Palmitic acid
Ester	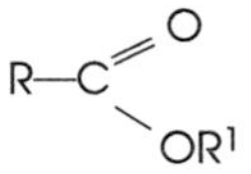	Triglyceride
Amide	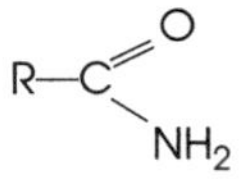	Glutamine
Thioester	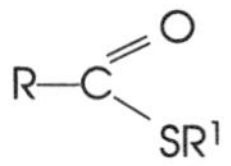	Acetyl-CoA
Combinations		
Hemiacetal	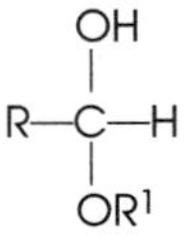	Glycopyranose
Acetal	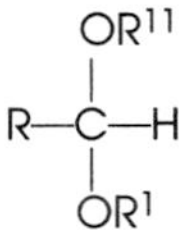	Glycogen
Hydroxyacid	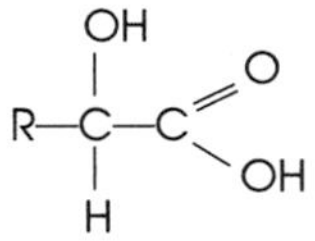	Lactate
Ketoacid	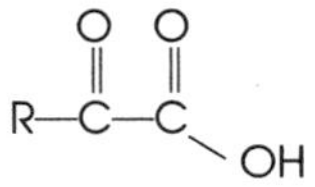	Pyruvate
Combinations		
Dicarboxylate	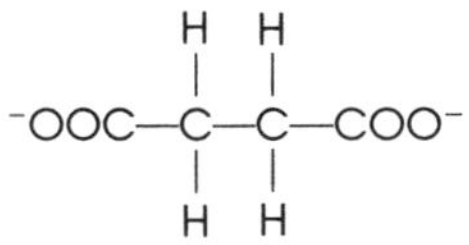	Succinate

TABLE 4-4. Functional Groups in Biochemicals (*continued*)

GROUP		EXAMPLE WITH GROUP
Phosphates		
Phosphoric acid (P_i)	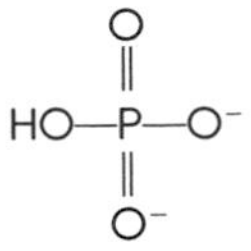	
Pyrophosphate (PP_i)	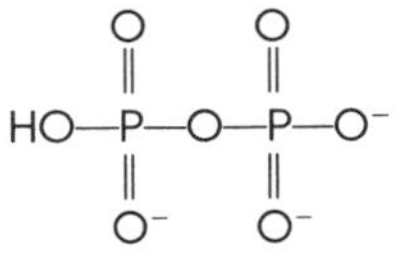	
Phosphomonoester	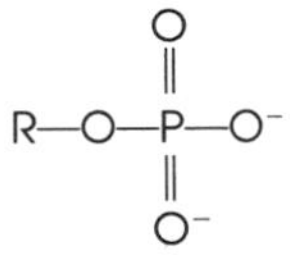	Glucose 6-phosphate
Phosphodiester	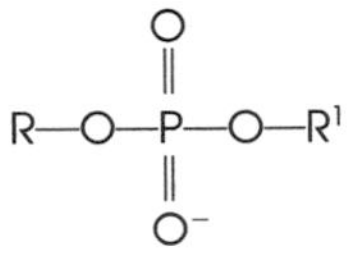	Cyclic AMP, DNA, RNA
Bisphosphate	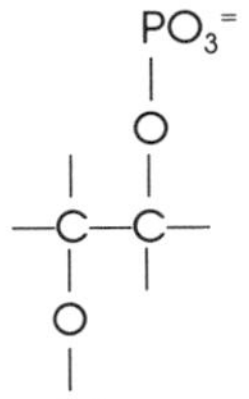	2,3-Bisphosphoglycerate
Trisphosphate	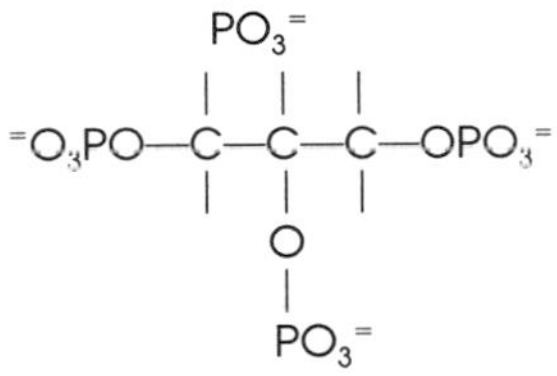	Inositol trisphosphate
Diphosphate	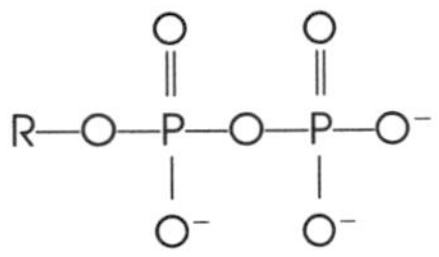	Adenosine diphosphate (ADP)
Triphosphate	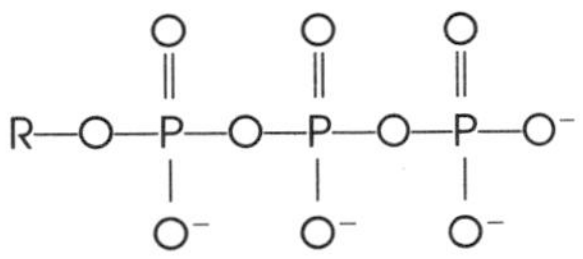	Adenosine triphosphate (ATP)
Phosphoenol group	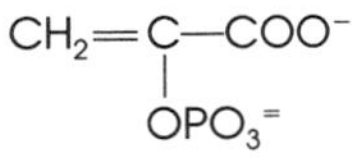	Phosphoenol pyruvate
Phosphoramidate	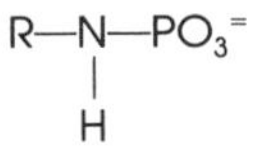	Creatine phosphate
Acylphosphate	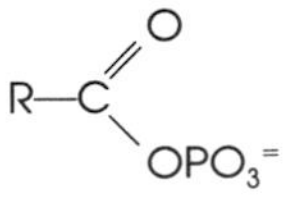	1,3-Bisphosphoglycerate

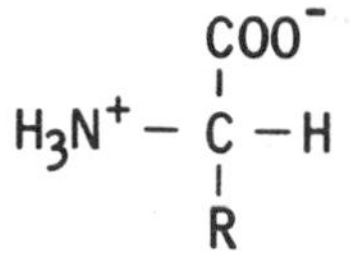

Fig. 4-2. Structure of an α-amino acid.

pounds with which biochemists are concerned. The number and diversity of protein molecules in humans, for example, greatly exceed those of the low–molecular mass compounds, or metabolites.

Protein Structure

Proteins perform a number of essential functions in all forms of life. The name, moreover, is derived from Greek *protos* meaning "first" or "primary." Proteins serve a structural role within the cell (cytoskeleton) and within the connective tissue and skeleton of the whole organism. Proteins also function, *inter alia,* as catalysts, receptors, translocases, antibodies, and hormones. About 19% of the human body is protein in nature. It is noteworthy (for examination purposes) that ***collagen,*** a connective tissue protein, is the most abundant protein in humans. ***Proteins*** are polymers of α-amino acids. There are 20 amino acids that are genetically encoded and serve as precursors for protein biosynthesis on ribosomes. Some of these amino acid residues are modified or derivatized after biosynthesis (posttranslational modification). Specific protein serines, for example, are phosphorylated to produce a phosphoseryl residue. Phosphoserine per se is not incorporated into the nascent or growing polypeptide chain. Other posttranslational modifications include hydroxylation, carboxylation, methylation, glycosylation, myristoylation, farnesylation, and acetylation.

AMINO ACIDS

Let us now consider the identity and structures of the 20 genetically encoded, or standard, amino acids. The amino acids found in proteins are α-amino acids (Fig. 4-2). With the exception of glycine, which lacks a chiral carbon atom (a carbon atom with four different substituents), the amino acids found in proteins possess the ***L-configuration*** (the absolute configuration corresponds to the standard L-glyceraldehyde).

The amino acids with hydrocarbon side chains are shown in Figure 4-3. Glycine is the simplest and is so named because of its sweet taste (*gly,* sugar). The side chains of valine, leucine, and isoleucine are hydrophobic. Four amino acids are dicarboxylic acids (aspartate and glutamate) or their derivatives (asparagine and glutamine) and are polar (Fig. 4-4). Asparagine was first isolated from asparagus. Three amino acids contain basic, nitrogen-containing, polar side chains. These are lysine, arginine, and histidine (Fig. 4-5). Three amino acids are aromatic (phenylalanine, tyrosine, and tryptophan), and these are hydrophobic (Fig. 4-6). Two amino acids contain sulfur: cysteine and methionine (Fig. 4-7). And two amino acids contain a polar alcohol side chain: serine and threonine (Fig. 4-8). The remaining genetically encoded amino acid, proline, is cyclic (Fig. 4-9). Note that the nitrogen atom of proline is linked to two carbon atoms. There are a large number of amino acids in nature that are not found in proteins. Examples include ornithine and citrulline, which are important intermediates in urea biosynthesis.

Glycine lacks a chiral carbon atom. Two amino acids, isoleucine and threonine, contain two asymmetric carbon atoms. The β-carbon atom in each case constitutes the second asymmetric center. The amino acids are designated by a three-letter or single-letter abbreviation (Table 4-5).

PROTEINS

The reaction of an α-amino group of one amino acid with the carboxyl group of a second amino acid with the elimination of water results in the formation of a ***peptide bond.*** The resulting compound is a ***dipeptide.*** A ***tripeptide***

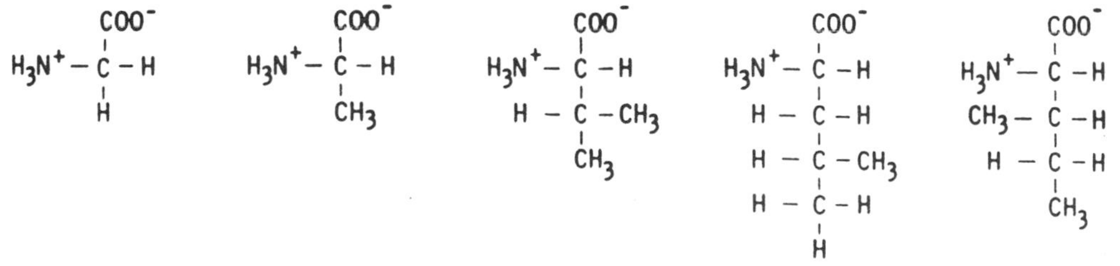

Glycine Alanine Valine Leucine Isoleucine

Fig. 4-3. Aliphatic amino acids.

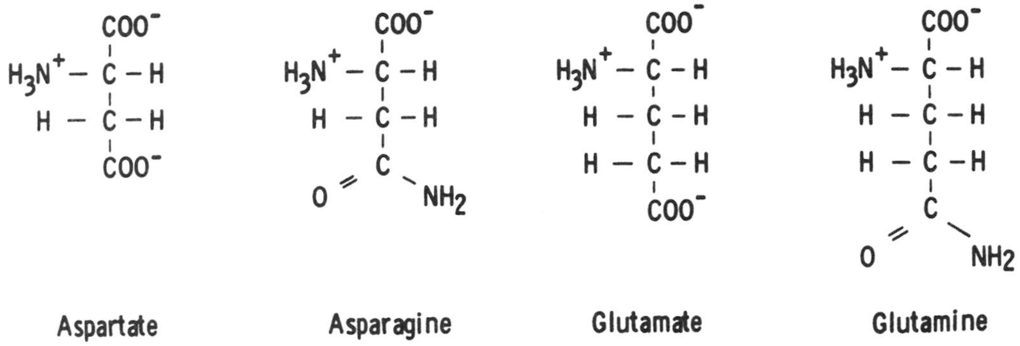

Fig. 4-4. Acidic amino acids and their amides.

contains three amino acid residues, an ***oligopeptide*** contains a few, and a ***polypeptide*** contains many amino acid residues. The peptide bond is planar. The carbonyl group and substituted amide occur in a plane, and rotation about the C–N bond is prohibited. This limits the conformations that a polypeptide chain may assume.

Proteins are polypeptides consisting of amino acid residues. The hormone insulin contains 51 amino acids (30 in the A chain and 21 in the B chain). Many biochemists consider this molecule as a protein, and others regard it as a polypeptide. The reader should thus be aware that the distinction between polypeptide and protein is not absolute. All proteins are polypeptides and not vice versa. An average polypeptide chain in a protein contains about 500 amino acid residues; a few contain more than 2,000 amino acid residues. The range of molecular masses of single polypeptide chains ranges from about 5,000 to 300,000. To determine the approximate number of amino acids in a protein, divide the molecular mass by 110. This value (110) approximates the average molecular mass of an amino acid residue in an average protein.

Proteins consist of one or more polypeptide chains. ***Myoglobin,*** an intracellular oxygen storage protein containing heme, consists of a single polypeptide chain and is a monomer. Hemoglobin, the oxygen-transport protein found in erythrocytes, consists of two pairs of identical subunits, which form a tetramer. ***Hemoglobin*** contains two α-chains and two β-chains, and the tetramer is denoted as $\alpha_2\beta_2$.

The structure of proteins is considered in a hierarchical fashion comprising four levels: primary, secondary, tertiary, and quaternary. The ***primary structure*** refers to the sequence of amino acids and the nature and position of any covalently attached derivatives. Peptides have a directionality with an amino group (not in peptide linkage) at one end and a carboxyl group (not in peptide linkage) at the other. The terminal amino or carboxyl groups may be free or they may be derivatized. By convention, structures are written with the amino terminus on the left and carboxyl terminus on the right. The dipeptide Gly-Ala differs from Ala-Gly.

The ***secondary structure*** of a protein refers to the pattern of hydrogen bonding. Two major classes of hydrogen-bonded structures are associated with secondary structure. The first to be described, the ***α-helix,*** refers to a helix stabilized by hydrogen bonding between a carbonyl group of one peptide bond and the N–H group on the peptide bond on the chain four residues away (*i.e.*, the residues are close together). The second form of second-

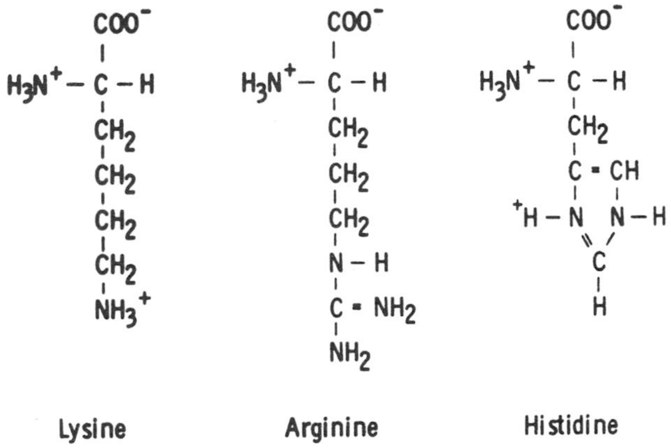

Fig. 4-5. Basic amino acids.

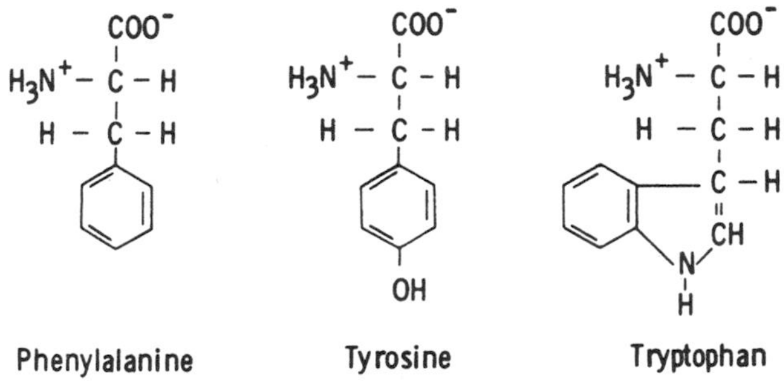

Fig. 4-6. Aromatic amino acids.

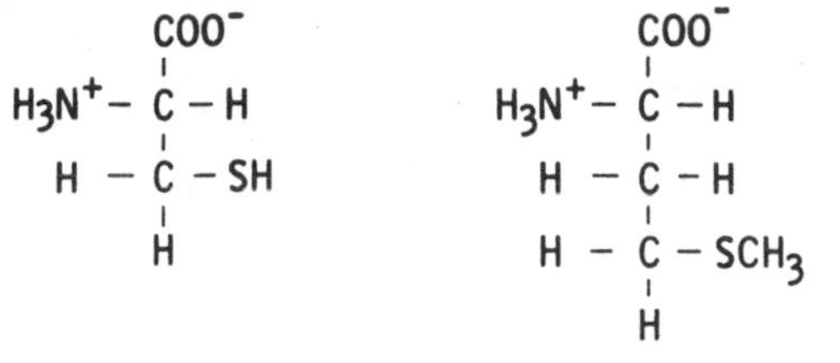

Cysteine   Methionine

Fig. 4-7. Sulfur-containing amino acids.

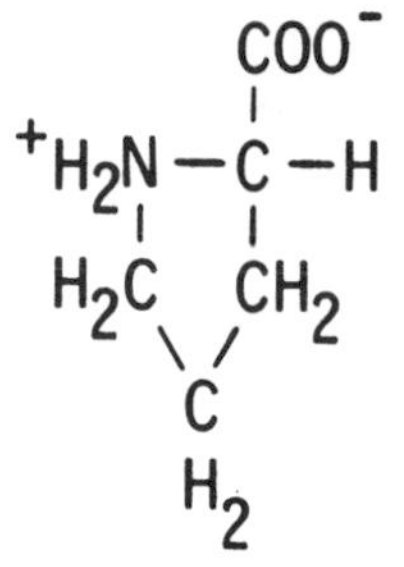

Proline

Fig. 4-9. Proline, an Imino acid.

ary structure to be described is the ***β-pleated sheet.*** Here >N–H and >C=O (carbonyl) groups from residues very far apart on the polypeptide chain or even residues on a different polypeptide chain form hydrogen bonds. Two varieties of β-pleated sheet are recognized depending on the polarity of the participating polypeptide chains. When the chains course in the same direction from the amino to carboxyl end of the molecule, the structure is a ***parallel β-pleated sheet.*** When the participating chains course in opposite directions with respect to the amino and carboxyl termini, the structure is an ***antiparallel β-pleated sheet.*** Reversal in the direction of the polypeptide chain occurs with the formation of a ***β-bend.*** This configuration involves the formation of a loop in which a residue's carbonyl group forms a hydrogen bond with the amide NH group of the residue three positions farther along the polypeptide chain.

The ***tertiary structure*** of a protein refers to the three-dimensional arrangement of the atoms of the molecule in space. For a monomeric protein such as myoglobin, the tertiary structure is the highest order of structure. The ***quaternary structure*** refers to the manner in which subunits of a multimeric protein interact. During the oxygenation of hemoglobin, a tetrameric protein, the subunits move relative to each other. This aspect of structure is the quaternary structure.

The physiologically active conformation of a protein is called the ***native*** structure. The forces responsible for maintaining the active conformation include covalent bonds, salt bridges, hydrogen bonds, and hydrophobic bonds. The contributions of the latter three in maintaining the active conformation probably vary among proteins. When these forces are disturbed as a result of exposure to extremes of *p*H (acid or alkali), high temperature (50° C or greater), 6 M urea (an unphysiological concentration), or treatment with charged detergents such as sodium dodecylsulfate, the native conformation is destroyed and a ***denatured*** structure results. The native state corresponds to one or a few active conformations, but the denatured state may be associated with multiple but inactive conformations.

The sequence of amino acids in a polypeptide chain determines the structure and properties of the protein. Secondary, tertiary, and quaternary structures are determined by the primary structure. This is a statement of Anfinsen's law (Table 4-1). The substitution of an amino acid by a similar one, for example, the replacement of leucine by valine, usually is not of great consequence. However, substitution by unlike residues can result in a protein with greatly different properties. For example, substitution of valine for glutamate at position 6 (from the amino terminus) in the β-chain of human hemoglobin produces ***hemoglobin S*** (sickle cell hemoglobin). Deoxygenated sickle cell hemoglobin assumes an abnormal conformation and is poorly soluble under physiological conditions. This leads to hemolysis and the circulatory abnormalities in the disease of ***sickle cell anemia.***

Serine   Threonine

Fig. 4-8. Hydroxyl-containing amino acids.

pH and the Henderson-Hasselbalch Equation

The properties of water are important in the maintenance of life's processes. Water constitutes about 70% of the lean body mass of humans, and water is an essential nutrient. Water dissociates into a proton and a hydroxyl group:

$$H_2O \rightleftharpoons H^+ + OH^-$$

TABLE 4-5. Genetically Encoded Amino Acids

NAME	ABBREVIATION	NUMBER OF CODONS	pK_a OF SIDE CHAIN	COMMENTS
Aliphatic				
Glycine	Gly G	4		Every third residue of collagen
Alanine	Ala A	4		
Valine	Val V	4		Hydrophobic
Leucine	Leu L	6		Hydrophobic
Isoleucine	Ile I	3		Hydrophobic
Carboxylate-Related				
Aspartate	Asp D	2	4	Anionic
Glutamate	Glu E	2	4	Anionic
Asparagine	Asn N	2		
Glutamine	Gln Q	2		
Basic				
Lysine	Lys K	2	10.5	Cationic
Arginine	Arg R	6	12.5	Cationic
Histidine	His H	2	7	
Aromatic				
Phenylalaine	Phe F	2		Hydrophobic
Tyrosine	Tyr Y	2	10.1	Rarely phosphorylated
Tryptophan	Trp W	1		Hydrophobic; single codon
Sulfur-Containing				
Methionine	Met M	1		Initiator of protein synthesis
Cysteine	Cys C	2	8.3	Oxidized to cystine
Hydroxyl-Containing				
Serine	Ser S	6		Chief phosphorylated residue of proteins
Threonine	Thr T	4		Occasionally phosphorylated
Imino				
Proline	Pro P	4		Occurs at bends in protein chain

In pure water $[H_2O] = 55.6$ M (1,000 g/L / 18 g/mol).

$$[H^+] = 10^{-7}M$$

$$[OH^-] = 10^{-7}M$$

The concentrations of $[OH^-]$ and $[H^+]$ are in reciprocal relationship to each other. When $[H^+]$ increases, $[OH^-]$ decreases and vice versa. Their product is 10^{-14} M^2.

$$[H^+] \times [OH^-] = 10^{-14}$$

When $[H^+] = 10^{-4}$ M, for example, then $[OH^-] = 10^{-10}$ M.

The pH is defined by the following equation:

$$pH = -\log [H^+]$$

At neutrality (when $[H^+] = [OH^-]$):

$$pH = -\log [10^{-7}]$$

$$= -(-7) = +7$$

The pH of blood and physiological fluids is 7.4.

$$7.4 = -\log [H^+]$$

$$3.98 \times 10^{-8}M = [H^+]$$

The pH of blood is maintained at 7.4 ± 0.05. ***Buffers*** are substances that diminish the change in pH when acid or alkali is added to a solution. Buffers are composed of weak acids and their conjugate bases or weak bases and their conjugate acids. The physiologically important buffers in blood and saliva are (1) H_2CO_3–HCO_3^-, (2) $H_2PO_4^-$–HPO_4^{2-}, and (3) protein–protein$^-$.

The ***Henderson-Hasselbalch equation*** provides a convenient way to describe and think about buffers and *p*H:

$$pH = pKa + \log \frac{[\text{unprotonated species}]}{[\text{protonated species}]}$$

or equivalently

$$pH = pKa + \log \frac{[\text{salt}]}{[\text{acid}]}$$

For the phosphate system,

$$H_2PO_4^- \rightleftharpoons H^+ + HPO_4^{2-}$$

$$pH = pKa + \log \frac{[HPO_4^{2-}]}{[H_2PO_4^-]}$$

When $[HPO_4^{2-}] = [H_2PO_4^-]$, the concentration of the protonated form equals that of the unprotonated form, and their ratio is 1.

$$pH = pKa + \log 1$$

$$pH = pKa$$

For phosphate at physiological ionic strength, the pK_a = 6.8. The pK_a is the pH at which the concentration of salt and acid is identical. Having this value, we can calculate the pH when the concentrations of $[HPO_4^{2-}]$ and $[H_2PO_4^-]$ are known. At a given pH we can calculate the ratios of the two forms. When $[HPO_4^{2-}]/[H_2PO_4^-] = 10$, then

$$\begin{aligned} pH &= 6.8 + \log 10 \\ &= 6.8 + 1 \\ &= 7.8 \end{aligned}$$

When $[HPO_4^{2-}]/[H_2PO_4^-] = 0.1$, then

$$\begin{aligned} pH &= 6.8 + \log 0.1 \\ &= 6.8 - 1.0 \\ &= 5.8 \end{aligned}$$

The CO_2 system can be expressed as follows:

$$CO_2 + H_2O \rightleftharpoons H_2CO_3$$

$$H_2CO_3 \rightleftharpoons H^+ + HCO_3^-$$

$$pH = 6.1 + \log \frac{[HCO_3^-]}{[CO_2 + H_2CO_3]}$$

The pK_a of the CO_2 system is 6.1. At pH 7.4, the ratio of $[HCO_3^-]/[CO_2 + H_2CO_3]$ is about 20.

The pK_a values of various R groups of proteins have been determined. If the pK_a of an aspartate of a polypeptide is 4.1, this means that at pH 4.1, at any instant half of these residues in a solution containing this protein are protonated and half are unprotonated. When the pH is increased to 7.4, protons are liberated and these aspartyl groups bear a net negative charge. If the pK_a of a lysine is 8.3, this means that at pH 8.3, at any instant the concentration of $R{-}NH_2$ and $R{-}NH_3^+$ in a solution containing this protein are the same. When we lower the pH to 7.4, more of these lysyl residues become protonated (because the solution is more acidic) and these lysine residues bear a net positive charge.

The imidazole of histidine is the only side chain with a pK_a in the physiological range near 7 (Table 4-5). If the pK_a of a protein–histidine is 6.9, then at pH 6.9, at any instant half of these residues in a solution containing these molecules are protonated (bearing a positive charge) and half are unprotonated (uncharged). At pH 7.4, about a third of the imidazoles of this protein–histidine in a solution are positively charged. The pK_a of the side chain of amino acids varies with the protein and the specific residue in the protein. The pK_a generally differs from that of the free amino acid. For this reason, the pK_a values given in Table 4-5 are representative or approximate.

Enzymes

GENERAL PROPERTIES

One important function of proteins is that of a catalyst. Almost all reactions of a biochemical nature occur under physiological conditions of temperature and pH because of the existence of ***enzymes,*** or protein catalysts (Table 4-1). The definition of a protein was considered in the previous section and denotes a polypeptide made up of α-amino acids. A ***catalyst*** is a substance that alters the rate of a chemical reaction without itself being permanently changed into another compound. A catalyst increases the rate at which a thermodynamically feasible reaction attains its equilibrium without altering the position of the equilibrium. The rate of a catalyzed reaction ranges from 10^3- to 10^{11}-fold greater than that of an uncatalyzed reaction. A catalyst accelerates a reaction by decreasing the free energy of activation denoted by $\Delta G\ddagger$ (Fig. 4-10). An enzyme provides an alternative and more speedy reaction route. The development of the science of biochemistry has proceeded concurrently with the development of the science of enzymology.

Enzymes are divided into two general classes. Some are ***simple proteins*** that contain only amino acids. Examples include the digestive enzymes ribonuclease, trypsin, and chymotrypsin. Others are ***complex proteins*** that contain amino acids and a non–amino acid cofactor. The complete enzyme is called a ***holoenzyme*** and is composed of a protein portion (apoenzyme) and cofactor.

$$\text{holoenzyme} = \text{apoenzyme} + \text{cofactor}$$

A metal ion may serve as a cofactor for an enzyme. Zinc, for example, is a cofactor for the enzymes carbonic anhydrase, carboxypeptidase, and cytosolic superoxide dismutase. An organic molecule such as pyridoxal phosphate or biotin may serve as a cofactor. Cofactors such as biotin, which are covalently linked or tightly bound to the enzyme, are called ***prosthetic groups*** (compare, *prosthesis*).

Besides their enormous ***catalytic power,*** which accelerates reaction rates, enzymes exhibit exquisite ***specificity*** in the types of reactions that each catalyzes as well as specificity for the substrates upon which they act. Phosphofructokinase catalyzes a reaction between ATP and fructose 6-phosphate. The enzyme does not catalyze a reaction between other nucleoside triphosphates and other sugars to a physiologically meaningful extent. Hexokinase catalyzes a reaction between ATP (but not other

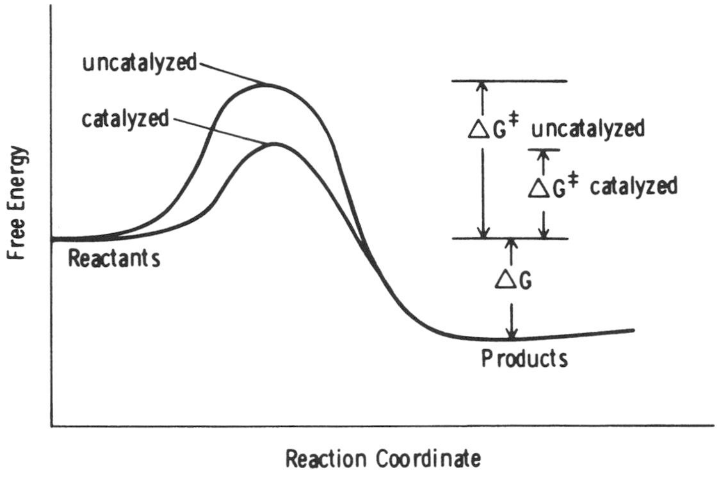

Fig. 4-10. A catalyst lowers the free energy of activation of a reaction.

nucleoside triphosphates) and glucose, fructose, or mannose (but not galactose). It is noteworthy that ***trypsin*** catalyzes the hydrolysis of peptides and proteins only on the carboxyl side of polypeptidic lysines or arginines (positively charged, basic residues). ***Chymotrypsin*** catalyzes the hydrolysis of peptides and proteins on the carboxyl side of polypeptidic phenylalanine, tyrosine, and tryptophan (aromatic residues), as well as other hydrophobic amino acids. Many enzymes exhibit trypsinlike specificity. These include blood-clotting factors and enzymes that process hormonal peptides.

TABLE 4-6. Enzyme Classification

CLASS	REACTION
Major Classes	
Oxidoreductases	Transfer hydrogen atom or hydride ion ($H:^-$); act on H_2O_2; act on O_2
Transferases	Transfer carbon, phosphoryl, glycosyl, acyl, and amino groups
Hydrolases	Cleave wide variety of substrates by adding water across bond
Lyases	Cleave carbon bound to carbon, nitrogen, or oxygen
Isomerases	Racemases, epimerases, intramolecular oxidoreductases, intramolecular transferases
Ligases	ATP- or nucleoside triphosphate–dependent condensation reaction
Selected Subclasses	
Kinases	Transfer phosphoryl group from ATP and other nucleotides; transferases
Mutases	Move phosphoryl or other group intramolecularly; isomerases
Phosphorylases	Cleave by adding phosphate across bond; transferases
Decarboxylases	Carboxylate liberated as CO_2; lyases
Hydratases	Add water to double bond and the reverse; lyases
Synthetases	ATP (or equivalent nucleotide)–dependent synthesis; ligases
Synthases	ATP-independent synthesis (*e.g.*, UDPG + glycogen → $glycogen_{n+1}$ + UDP); transferases

Enzymes are divided into six classes based on the type of reaction that they catalyze (Table 4-6). Oxidation–reduction reactions are important in energy metabolism. Kinases are a class of transferase, and kinases catalyze the transfer of the terminal phosphoryl group of ATP to acceptor substrates. Transfer of acyl groups and amino groups is prevalent in biochemistry. ***Hydrolases*** catalyze the hydrolysis (lysis, or cleavage, by water) of proteins, nucleic acids, and a variety of other compounds; hydrolase reactions are unidirectional. ***Lyases*** catalyze the nonhydrolytic cleavage of molecules and result in the formation of one more double bond in the products when compared with the reactants (lyases also catalyze the reverse reunification reaction). Lyase reactions, except for decarboxylation reactions, are bidirectional. Aldolase, an enzyme of the glycolytic pathway, is an example of a lyase. ***Isomerases*** catalyze the conversion of aldehydes to ketones and of L-compounds to D-compounds; isomerase reactions are generally bidirectional. ***Ligases*** (compare, *ligature*) catalyze the ATP-dependent condensation of one molecule with another; ligase reactions are generally bidirectional. The combination of an amino acid with its corresponding transfer RNA (tRNA), catalyzed by an aminoacyl–tRNA synthetase, is one example of a ligase reaction.

KINETICS AND INHIBITORS

In an enzyme-catalyzed reaction, there is an increase in reaction velocity with an increase in substrate concentration. Often a plot of the velocity as a function of substrate concentration yields a ***rectangular hyperbola*** (Fig. 4-11).

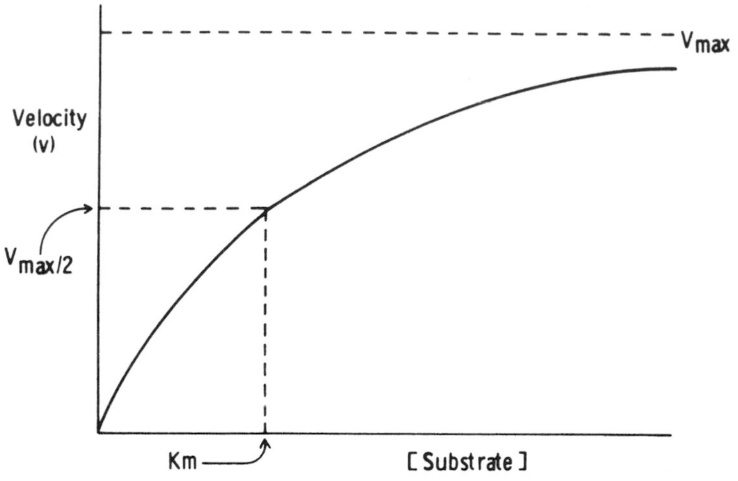

Fig. 4-11. A rectangular hyperbola illustrating saturation kinetics.

As substrate concentrations increase, the increase in activity is progressively smaller. Such data demonstrate that enzymes exhibit saturation. This is consistent with the notion that substrates interact with a finite number of catalytic molecules and are converted into products. In an uncatalyzed process, the reaction increases indefinitely as reactant concentration increases. Under defined conditions and with specific amounts of protein, an enzyme exhibits a ***maximum velocity*** (V_{max}), which approaches a limit as the substrate concentration approaches infinity. The K_m ***(Michaelis constant)*** is the substrate concentration at half the maximal velocity ($V_{max}/2$) as illustrated in Figure 4-11. The ***Michaelis-Menten equation*** is an expression for the reaction velocity (v) as a function of substrate concentration ([S]) and the kinetic constants (V_{max} and K_m) as follows:

$$v = \frac{V_{max} \times [S]}{K_m + [S]}$$

When $v = V_{max}/2$, the reader can verify the result that $K_m = [S]$. It is difficult to determine the K_m and V_{max} values from a rectangular hyperbola. Several methods are available for obtaining accurate values for these parameters, including the use of computer programs. A traditional way for determining the kinetic constants is through the use of a double reciprocal plot. When the reciprocal of the substrate concentration (1/S) is plotted versus the reciprocal of the velocity (1/v), results similar to those demonstrated in Figure 4-12 are obtained. The value of $1/V_{max}$ is obtained by extrapolation, and it corresponds to the velocity at an infinite substrate concentration. The plot also yields $-1/K_m$. Because this is a reciprocal plot, note that a larger V_{max} corresponds to a smaller value of the ordinate (*y*-axis). Similarly, a larger K_m corresponds to a less negative value of the abscissa (along the *x*-axis).

Double reciprocal plots are helpful in studying enzyme inhibition. Enzyme inhibitors are classified as reversible and irreversible. ***Irreversible inhibitors*** usually react covalently with an enzymic amino acid residue and render the enzyme inactive. The rate constant for the reaction of the inhibitor with the enzyme can be measured. ***Reversible inhibitors*** generally interact noncovalently and virtually instantaneously with an enzyme; the interactions of this class of inhibitor with enzyme can be studied by steady-state enzyme kinetics. There are two major classes of reversible inhibitor: competitive and noncompetitive. ***Competitive inhibitors*** are structural analogues of the substrate whose concentration is being varied. Consider the following hypothetical enzyme-catalyzed reaction:

Fig. 4-12. A double reciprocal or Lineweaver-Burk plot.

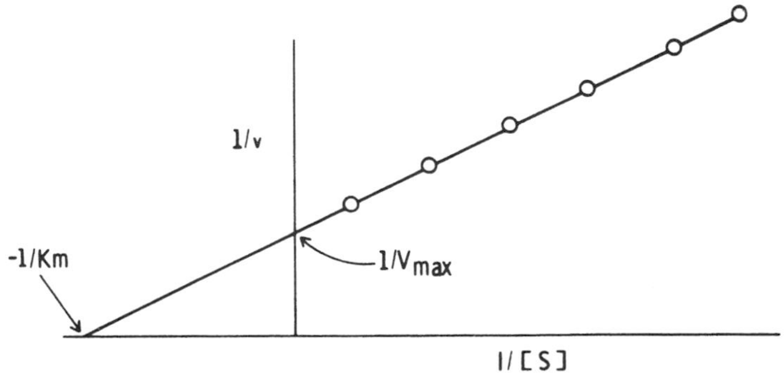

$$A + B \rightleftharpoons X + Y$$

Let us assume that B′ is a substrate analogue of B, and B′ interacts with the enzyme but fails to undergo a reaction. If we measure the velocity as a function of the concentration of B at a few fixed concentrations of B′ and in its absence, we find that at a higher concentration of B (fixed B′) the magnitude of inhibition is decreased. In fact at infinite concentrations of B (determined by extrapolation), inhibition is overcome. The location on an enzyme where catalysis occurs is named the ***active site.*** In this example, a portion of the active site corresponds to A and another portion corresponds to B. B′ inhibits the enzyme by interacting with the enzyme at the site corresponding to B, and it thereby prevents catalysis. By increasing the concentration of B, its effect overrides that of B′, and inhibition is overcome. This is illustrated by the unchanged V_{max} for competitive inhibition shown in Figure 4-13.

Let us now consider the effects of varying the concentration of A while keeping B constant. Increasing B′ increases the degree of inhibition. However, increasing concentrations of A cannot completely override the effects of B′, and the V_{max} at infinite A is decreased (noncompetitive, Fig. 4-13). This is because A and B′ do not bind to the same site. No matter how large the concentration of A, B′ may still bind to and inhibit the enzyme. This type of inhibition cannot be overcome by increasing the concentration of substrate that is not homologous to the reversible inhibitor. Moreover, B′ does not alter the K_m for A. In the case of competitive inhibition, B′ increases the apparent K_m of B (Fig. 4-13).

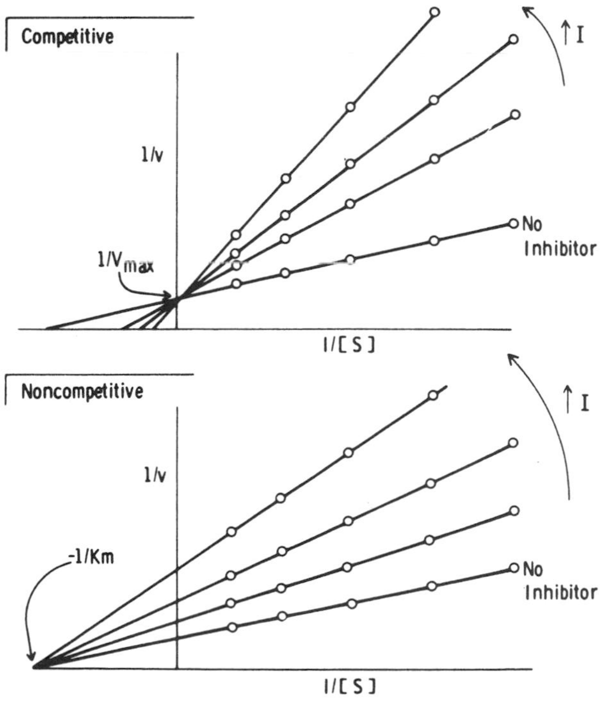

Fig. 4-13. Double reciprocal plots illustrating the effects of competitive and noncompetitive inhibitors.

In examining double reciprocal plots to determine the type of inhibition (Fig. 4-13), examine the V_{max}. If the V_{max} is unchanged, the inhibition is competitive. If the V_{max} is decreased and the K_m is unchanged, inhibition is noncompetitive. If similar experiments are conducted with an irreversible inhibitor, a pattern similar to that of noncompetitive inhibition is seen. The irreversible inhibitor inactivates some of the enzyme. The underivatized enzyme is normal (no change in K_m), but there is less active enzyme, and this is reflected by a decrease in V_{max}. As noted above, the chief utility of steady-state enzyme kinetics is in the study of instantaneous, reversible inhibitors and not in the study of irreversible inhibitors.

One of the concepts to emerge from a theoretical consideration of steady-state enzyme kinetics is that the enzyme binds with a substrate to form an enzyme–substrate complex. The enzyme is said to contain an ***active,*** or ***catalytic, site.*** After binding of the substrate(s), the enzyme promotes a reaction and the products dissociate. The active site contains residues that participate in the reaction. Amino acids that have been shown to participate in enzymic catalysis include the serine hydroxyl, the cysteine sulfhydryl, the γ-carboxyl of aspartate, the imidazole of histidine, and the ϵ-amino group of lysine as well as others. Only one, two, or three residues usually participate in reactions in a particular enzyme-active site; additional residues may participate in binding the substrate to the enzyme.

REGULATION OF ENZYME ACTIVITY

The activity of enzymes in the cell is subject to a variety of regulatory mechanisms. The amount of enzyme can be altered by increasing or decreasing its synthesis or degradation. Enzyme ***induction*** refers to an enhancement of enzyme biosynthesis. Enzyme ***repression*** refers to a decrease in enzyme biosynthesis. Enzyme activity also can be altered by ***covalent modification*** (Table 4-1). Phosphorylation of specific serine residues by protein kinases increases or decreases catalytic activity, depending on the enzyme. Proteolytic cleavage of proenzymes (chymotrypsinogen, trypsinogen, proelastase, clotting factors) converts an inactive form into an active form.

Enzyme activity also can be regulated by ***noncovalent*** or ***allosteric mechanisms*** (Table 4-1). Isocitrate dehydrogenase is an enzyme in the Krebs cycle that is activated by ADP. ADP is neither a substrate nor a substrate analogue. ADP binds to the enzyme at a site distinct from the active site called the ***allosteric site.*** Allosteric regulation is common, and the changes in activity in response to allosteric effectors make a kind of physiological sense that is called the molecular logic of the cell (Table 4-1). When it is realized that a primary function of the Krebs cycle is to provide reducing equivalents for ATP biosynthesis, then we can rationalize Krebs cycle regulation by ADP. When the concentration of ATP decreases, the concentration of ADP increases and serves as a signal to active ATP formation. ADP regulates one of the early reactions of the Krebs cycle (isocitrate dehydrogenase) and promotes greater activity. Besides activation, some enzymes are subject to ***allosteric inhibition.*** In *E. coli,* for example, threonine deaminase catalyzes the first step in the reaction pathway for isoleucine biosynthesis. When isoleucine is plentiful, it produces ***feedback inhibition*** of the first enzymatic reaction and the committed step of the pathway. This inhibition decreases the synthesis of an already abundant compound.

Some enzymes fail to conform to simple saturation kinetics and do not exhibit a rectangular hyperbola when velocity is measured as a function of substrate concentration. In the most common case, a sigmoidal curve is observed (Fig. 4-14). A sigmoidal curve is the *sine qua non* for ***positive cooperativity.*** Positive cooperativity is the condition under which the binding of one substrate (or ligand) makes it easier for the second to bind. In the case of four binding sites per protein, binding of the second molecule facilitates binding of a third molecule, and such binding facilitates the binding of the fourth molecule. This finding is reflected by the increasing slope on the initial portion of the sigmoidal curve. The sigmoidal curve indicates only positive cooperativity. Oxygen binding to hemoglobin is cooperative. Allosteric enzymes often but not invariably exhibit positive cooperativity. A sigmoidal binding curve does not indicate that an enzyme has an allosteric site distinct from an active site. The phenomena of cooperativity and allosterism are distinct.

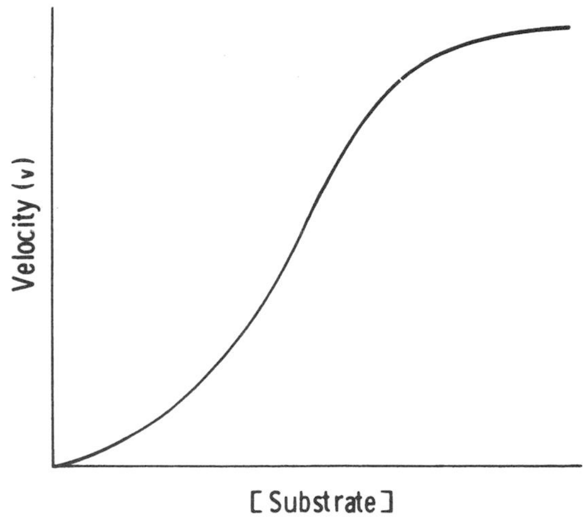

Fig. 4-14. A sigmoidal curve illustrating positive cooperativity.

Bioenergetics

FREE ENERGY CHANGES

Bioenergetics is the study of energy changes that accompany biochemical reactions. A ***chemical reaction*** is the process whereby one or more substances are converted into other substances. For example, dihydroxyacetone phosphate (one biochemical compound) is converted into glyceraldehyde 3-phosphate (another compound) in the cell. The reaction is catalyzed by triose phosphate isomerase. The most important thermodynamic parameter in bioenergetics is the ***free energy change,*** denoted by ΔG (G is named for J. Willard Gibbs, who made fundamental contributions to the study of thermodynamics). This is an energy change occurring at constant temperature and pressure (the usual condition for biochemical reactions). The expression corresponding to this reaction is

$$\Delta G = \Delta G^\circ + RT \ln [\text{G 3-P}]/[\text{DHAP}]$$

ΔG = free energy change
ΔG° = standard free energy change
R = gas constant (8.314 J K^{-1} M^{-1}) where K is the absolute temperature (273 + °C, × 2 corresponds to degrees Celsius)
T = absolute temperature
[G 3-P] = concentration of glyceraldehyde 3-phosphate (the product)
[DHAP] = concentration of dihydroxyacetone phosphate (the reactant)

For a reaction $A + B \rightleftharpoons C + D$:

$$\Delta G = \Delta G^\circ + RT \ln \frac{[C][D]}{[A][B]}$$

ΔG° corresponds to the free energy change when a mole of each reactant is converted to a mole of each product and all are present at 1 M concentration. Because biochemical reactions occur in aqueous solution and the concentration of water is constant, the effective concentration of water is given a value of 1. It would be impractical, moreover, to perform biochemical reactions in 1 M water. When $[H^+]$ is a reactant or product, it is also given a value of 1 because its concentration under physiological conditions (10^{-7} M) is also constant. The constant pH is usually designated by including a prime (′) with ΔG and ΔG° ($\Delta G'$ and $\Delta G^{\circ\prime}$).

Thermodynamically favorable reactions proceed with the liberation of free energy and are exergonic (Table 4-1). The free energy of the products is less than that of the reactants; that is, ΔG is negative.

TABLE 4-7. Free Energy Changes and Reaction Directionality

ΔG	DIRECTION OF REACTION FAVORED	CATEGORY
Negative	Toward products	Exergonic
Zero	Equilibrium	Isoergonic
Positive	Toward reactants	Endergonic

$$\Delta G = \text{free energy of products} - \text{free energy of reactants}$$

At equilibrium $\Delta G = 0$ and the reaction is isoergonic. When the free energy of the products is greater than that of the reactants, the reaction is thermodynamically unfavorable (endergonic), and ΔG is positive (Table 4-7).

At equilibrium no free energy is obtainable, and ΔG is zero. The following important result can then be derived:

$$\Delta G = \Delta G^\circ + RT \ln \frac{[C][D]}{[A][B]}$$

$$0 = \Delta G^\circ + RT \ln \frac{[C][D]}{[A][B]}$$

$$\Delta G^\circ = -RT \ln \frac{[C][D]}{[A][B]}$$

Because the reaction is at equilibrium, the values of A, B, C, and D are the concentrations at equilibrium to reflect this situation.

$$\Delta G^\circ = -RT \ln K_{eq}$$

From the equilibrium constant (K_{eq}), one can calculate the standard free energy change (ΔG°) and vice versa. The free energy change (ΔG) can be larger or smaller than the standard free energy change (ΔG°). Increasing the concentrations of reactants or decreasing the concentration of products produces a larger decrease in free energy or ΔG (the reaction is more exergonic). Decreasing the concentration of reactants or increasing the concentration of products produces a smaller decrease in free energy (the reaction is less exergonic).

A note of caution is appropriate here. The free energy changes indicate whether or not a reaction under specified conditions is thermodynamically feasible. It fails to provide any information about the rate or kinetics of a reaction. Many thermodynamically feasible reactions are unimportant or irrelevant in biochemistry because of the absence of an enzyme to mediate the reaction in a reasonable time. For example, although the oxidation of cholesterol to carbon dioxide and water is thermodynamically feasible, humans lack the enzymes that might catalyze such a reaction, and this process does not occur in human cells.

A nonbiological example may help clarify the distinction between thermodynamics and kinetics. The reaction of oxygen with gasoline to form CO_2 and H_2O is exergonic and proceeds with the liberation of considerable free energy. Gasoline, however, is stable in the presence of oxygen. The reaction occurs only under appropriate conditions, such as encountered in an internal combustion engine with an electrical spark initiating the process. The system (gasoline and oxygen) is said to be kinetically stable (unreactive) but thermodynamically unstable (exhibiting the potential for reacting).

ENERGY–RICH COMPOUNDS

The complete oxidation of glucose to carbon dioxide and water is associated with the liberation of 2,870 kJ free energy ($\Delta G^\circ = -2{,}870$ kJ). These changes in living systems occur in a graded and not an explosive fashion. Energy is released in a stepwise fashion and is coupled to the biosynthesis of ATP from ADP and inorganic phosphate (P_i). The ATP–ADP couple receives and distributes chemical energy in all living systems. This is a statement of ***Lipmann's law*** and is a cornerstone of biochemistry (Table 4-1). ATP serves as the common currency of energy exchange in living systems.

ATP is an energy-rich compound and serves as a donor of chemical energy for muscle contraction, ion transport, and biosynthetic reactions. The structure of ATP is shown in Figure 4-15. ATP is composed of a nitrogen-containing base (adenine), a five-carbon sugar (ribose), and three phosphates. The three phosphates are designated α, β, and γ from ribose to the terminus. The β- and γ-linkages are ***acid anhydrides*** (water removed from phosphoric acid). These bonds are ***energy rich*** in nature and are associated with the following reactions: (1) ATP + $H_2O \rightarrow$ ADP + P_i, and (2) ADP + $H_2O \rightarrow$ AMP + P_i. The $\Delta G^{\circ\prime}$ for these reactions is about -30 kJ/mol. Compounds with a standard free energy of hydrolysis of -30 kJ/mole or more negative are classified as energy-rich compounds.

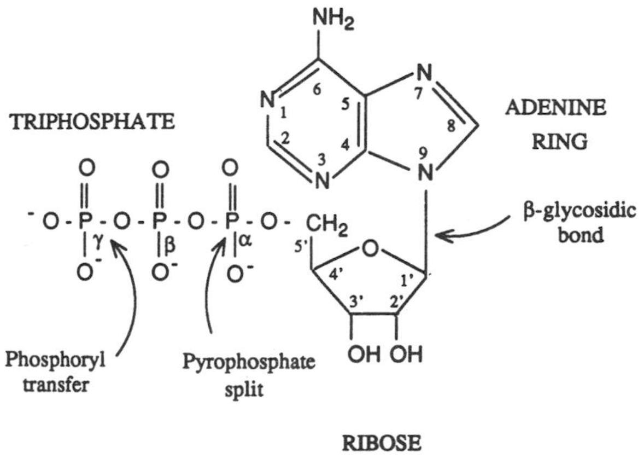

Fig. 4-15. Structure of adenosine triphosphate (ATP).

The reaction ATP + H_2O → AMP + PP_i (inorganic pyrophosphate) is also associated with the liberation of considerable free energy (about −30 kJ/mol). The α-phosphate bond (AMP + H_2O → adenosine + P_i) is low energy (−12 kJ/mol) and is a phosphate ester (phosphoric acid + alcohol − H_2O) and not an acid anhydride. The pyrophosphate (1), ADP (1), ATP (2), phosphoenolpyruvate (1), acylphosphate as found in 1,3-bisphosphoglycerate (1), and phosphoramidate as found in creatine phosphate (1) are high-energy compounds, where the number in parentheses denotes the quantity of high-energy bonds per molecule. Thioesters, such as acetyl coenzyme A (acetyl-CoA), also contain a high-energy bond.

The following examples illustrate the utility of energy-rich and energy-poor compounds in understanding whether a reaction is favorable (exergonic) or unfavorable (endergonic). Functionally isoergonic reactions are equipoised and may proceed in either direction depending upon the circumstances. The following is a prominent reaction in biochemistry:

$$\text{ATP (2)} + \text{glucose (0)} \rightarrow \text{ADP (1)} + \text{glucose 6-phosphate (0)}$$

The number of high-energy bonds on the left side is 2 and on the right side is 1 as indicated. The reaction proceeds with the loss of a high-energy bond; the reaction is exergonic and proceeds to the right. The reaction from right to left in endergonic and does not proceed to a physiologically significant extent. Another example involves the interconversion of two low-energy compounds:

$$\text{glucose 6-phosphate (0)} \rightleftharpoons \text{fructose 6-phosphate (0)}$$

The structures and energy richness of the two compounds are similar, and the reaction is isoergonic.

A similar analysis obtains for the case where the number of high-energy bonds is the same:

$$\text{ADP (1)} + \text{1,3-bisphosphoglycerate (1)} \rightleftharpoons \text{ATP (2)} + \text{3-phosphoglycerate (0)}$$

This reaction is approximately isoergonic, and the reaction proceeds without providing or using much free energy.

The hydrolysis of both energy-rich and energy-poor compounds is exergonic, and the equilibrium constant is much greater than 1. The reverse reaction is endergonic and is thermodynamically unfavored. Decarboxylations are exergonic; carboxylation reactions usually require the input of energy in the form of ATP. Simple dehydrogenation reactions (not associated with decarboxylation) are generally reversible in nature. Reactions with molecular oxygen are exergonic, and the reverse reaction fails to occur to a meaningful extent. Reactions in which an uncharged aldehyde is oxidized to a carboxylate are exergonic because of the ionization of the carboxylic acid to form a carboxylate ion and a proton. Lyase reactions are bidirectional with the exception of decarboxylation reactions.

METABOLISM

Metabolism refers to all the chemical reactions undergone by an organism. The term metabolism is derived from a Greek word meaning change. Nearly all reactions in living systems are catalyzed by enzymes (Table 4-1). The chemical reactions or metabolism of living organisms are not random; rather, they are directed along specific sequences called ***metabolic pathways.*** A metabolic pathway may be composed of from two to 20 enzyme-catalyzed steps necessary for the conversion of a molecule into a product. Each of the participant compounds is a ***metabolite.***

The process of ***catabolism*** refers to the conversion of large, complex molecules to simpler, smaller molecules. Some of these reactions release chemical energy; a portion of this chemical energy is conserved during the metabolic conversion of ADP to ATP. ***Anabolism*** refers to the conversion of small molecules to larger ones in the process of biosynthesis. These reactions require chemical energy, which is ultimately derived from ATP.

In general, the pathway for biosynthesis of a compound is not the simple reversal of its pathway for catabolism. The pathways may be completely independent, or they may share common intermediates. The conversion of glucose to pyruvate involves 12 specific enzyme-catalyzed reactions. The conversion of pyruvate to glucose requires 13 reactions. Of these reactions, nine are common to both synthesis and degradation and the others are unique. The different or unique steps occur in such a fashion that the reactions of the entire pathway are bioenergetically favorable and exergonic.

A consequence of this biochemical strategy of independent pathways for synthesis and degradation is that it permits independent regulation of the flux of metabolites through the pathway. For example, the biosynthetic rates can be increased and degradative rates can be decreased because of the occurrence of reactions unique to biosynthesis and degradation. If all the steps were common, alteration of an enzyme activity would increase or decrease both pathways simultaneously. Regulatory enzymes are generally unique to the synthetic or degradative pathway. Moreover, metabolic regulation generally occurs at the first or early step in a pathway. The regulated reaction is often physiologically irreversible and usually constitutes a committed step in metabolism.

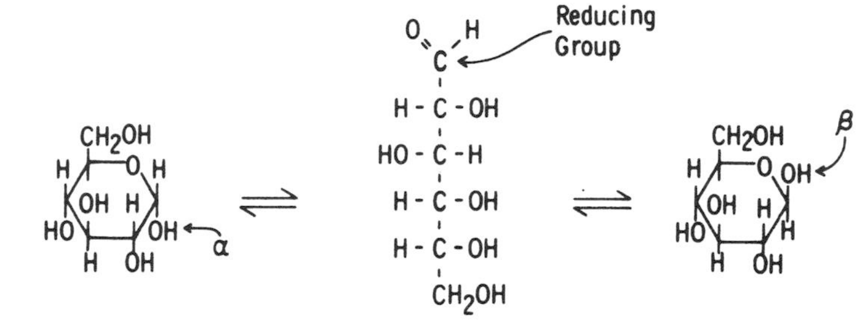

Fig. 4-16. Forms of glucose in aqueous solution.

Intermediary metabolism is addressed later in this chapter. This topic traditionally includes glycolysis and the conversion of pyruvate and fatty acids to acetyl-CoA, the oxidation of acetyl-CoA in the Krebs cycle, and the reactions of electron transport phosphorylation yielding ATP. Amino acids are also degraded to pyruvate, acetyl-CoA, or intermediates of the Krebs cycle and then oxidized. In oxidative phosphorylation, reducing equivalents are transported sequentially and stepwise in an electron transport chain to oxygen. Electron transport is exergonic. Some of the energy conserved as a proton gradient is established across a membrane in a process energized by electron transport. Protons then move down the established electrochemical gradient to drive ATP formation from ADP and P_i. ATP formation is an endergonic process energized by the proton-motive force.

Carbohydrate Chemistry

Carbohydrates are polyhydroxy aldehydes or ketones. Formulas representing D-glucose, the most common sugar in nature, are shown in Figure 4-16. The structure in the middle of the figure represents the open-chain form, and it shows the positions of the hydroxyl group on each of the chiral carbon atoms in the Fischer projection formula. The hydroxyl group on C5 forms a hemiacetal adduct with the carbonyl group on C1 and a stable six-membered ring results. This generates a new chiral carbon atom at position one. The hydroxyl group on C1 occurs with the α- or β-configuration as shown. It is noteworthy that glucose with the β-configuration is one of the most stable sugar structures in nature. First, the six-membered ring is itself stable. Second, the hydroxyl groups occupy equatorial positions and are as far apart from one another as possible.

The ring structures of sugars are shown in the Haworth projection format. If one recognizes and can draw the structure of the β-enantiomer of D-glucose, then the other common hexoses can be deduced from it. If one draws the six-membered ring (five carbons and one oxygen) and places C6 with its hydroxyl group above the ring, then the other hydroxyl groups alternate from top to bottom in regular fashion on C4 (bottom), C3 (top), C2 (bottom), and C1 (top, as the β-anomer) as shown. If the configuration of the hydroxyl on C1 is below, then the α-anomer results. Mannose differs from glucose by the hydroxyl configuration about C2; galactose differs at C4 (Fig. 4-17). These three compounds (glucose, mannose, and galactose) are epimers. The term ***anomer*** refers to differences of configuration at the hemiacetal (*e.g.*, α-D-glucose and β-D-glucose) or hemiketal (*e.g.*, α-D-fructose and β-D-fructose) carbon; the term ***epimer*** refer to differences of configuration at the other carbons (exclusive of the hemiacetal or hemiketal linkage).

The aldehyde group of glucose, mannose, and galactose constitutes a reducing component in alkaline copper solutions, and these substances are reducing sugars. The disaccharide lactose contains a hemiacetal group, which also makes it a reducing sugar (Fig. 4-18). In the disaccharide sucrose, the hemiacetal linkage of glucose and hemiketal linkage of fructose are further derivatized to form a glycoside bond. The absence of a simple hemiacetal or hemiketal bond makes sucrose a nonreducing sugar in alkaline copper solution, and this is a noteworthy property.

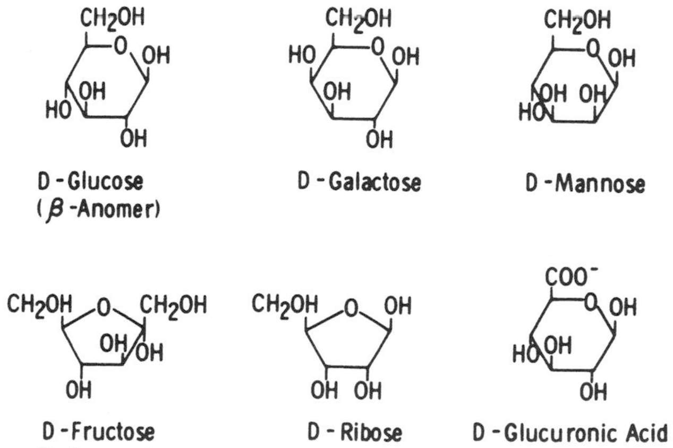

Fig. 4-17. Structure of some physiologically important sugars.

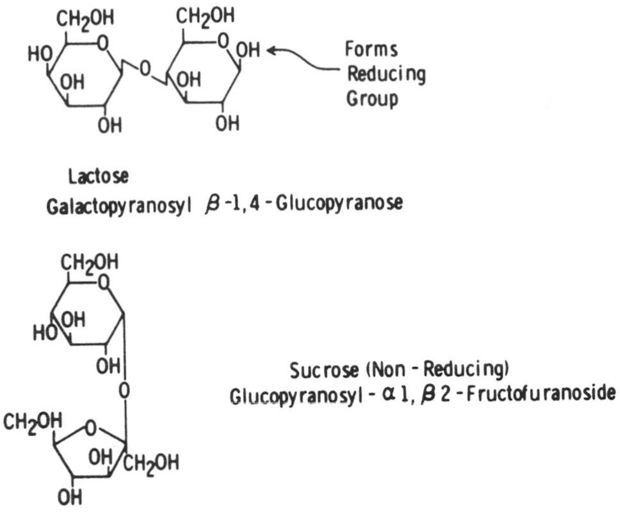

Fig. 4-18. Structures of lactose and sucrose.

Carbohydrate Metabolism

GLYCOLYSIS

The initial steps in the catabolism of glucose constitute the ***Embden-Meyerhof glycolytic pathway.*** This pathway and its enzymes are present in all human cells and are located in the cytosol (Table 4-1). The overall reaction is abbreviated as follows:

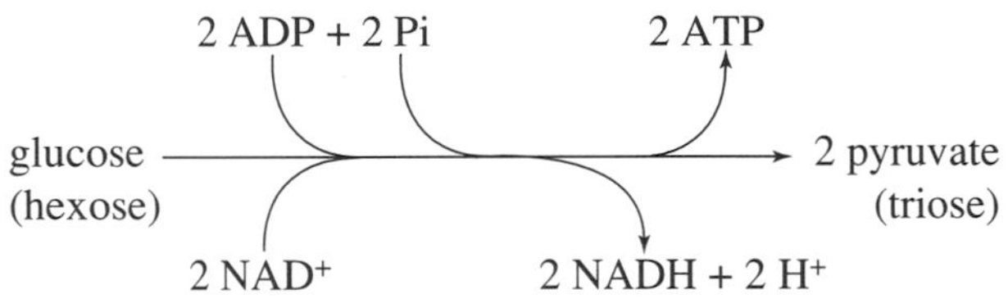

During the stepwise conversion of glucose to pyruvate, two molecules of nicotinamide-adenine dinucleotide phosphate (NADH) are formed, and there is a net production of two ATP molecules. In the first stage of glycolysis, two ATP molecules are consumed in priming reactions to produce fructose 1,6-bisphosphate. This substance is cleaved into two triose phosphates. Two molecules of glyceraldehyde 3-phosphate undergo oxidation to yield two molecules of NADH and two molecules of 1,3-bisphosphoglycerate. Two molecules of 1,3-bisphosphoglycerate, each of which contains an energy-rich acylphosphate linkage, donate their activated phosphoryl group to two molecules of ADP to yield two molecules of ATP. Subsequently, two molecules of phosphoenolpyruvate are formed, which donate their energy-rich phosphoryl group to two molecules of ADP to yield two additional molecules of ATP. Two net ATP molecules result ($-2 + 4 = 2$) per molecule of glucose. Let us now consider the reactions in this process.

The first step in glycolysis involves the phosphorylation of glucose by ATP (Fig. 4-19). The enzyme that catalyzes this exergonic and unidirectional reaction is ***hexokinase,*** and hexokinase is found in all cells. Hexokinase also catalyzes the phosphorylation of mannose and fructose to yield the respective hexose 6-phosphate. Liver contains a second enzyme that catalyzes glucose phosphorylation named ***glucokinase.*** Glucokinase does not catalyze the phosphorylation of mannose or fructose. Glucokinase exhibits a higher K_m for glucose than does hexokinase (10 mM vs. 30 μM) and is thus not saturated by the high glucose concentrations delivered to the liver by the portal vein postprandially. Glucokinase is not inhibited by glucose 6-phosphate as is hexokinase. However, glucokinase is inhibited by a complex of a regulatory protein and fructose 6-phosphate. The β-cell of the islets of Langerhans in the pancreas, which synthesize and release insulin, also contains glucokinase.

Phosphohexose isomerase catalyzes the conversion of glucose 6-phosphate to fructose 6-phosphate. The interconversion of these two energy-poor compounds is functionally isoergonic. ***Phosphofructokinase*** (PFK) catalyzes the second phosphorylation. This reaction is exergonic and unidirectional. PFK catalyzes the rate-limiting or pacemaker reaction of glycolysis. Aldolase then catalyzes the cleavage of fructose 1,6-bisphosphate to glyceraldehyde 3-phosphate and dihydroxyacetone phosphate, a bidirectional lyase reaction. ***Triose phosphate isomerase*** catalyzes the interconversion of these two compounds. ***Glyceraldehyde 3-phosphate dehydrogenase*** mediates a reaction between the designated compound, NAD^+, and P_i to yield 1,3-bisphosphoglycerate. Next, ***phosphoglycerate kinase*** catalyzes the reaction of the latter, an energy-rich compound, with ADP to yield ATP and phosphoglycerate. ***Phosphoglycerate mutase*** catalyzes the transfer of the phosphoryl group from C3 to C2 to yield 2-phosphoglycerate. This compound contains an energy-poor phosphate ester linkage. ***Enolase*** catalyzes an isoergonic dehydration (a lyase reaction) to yield PEP. This compound contains a very energy-rich phosphate bond. Its standard free energy of hydrolysis is -60 kJ/mol. PEP then donates its phosphoryl group to ADP to yield ATP and pyruvate in a reaction catalyzed by ***pyruvate kinase.*** Although the number of high-energy bonds is the same in the reactants and products (two), the reaction is highly exergonic and is physiologically irreversible.

To recapitulate, the three irreversible steps of glycolysis include the reactions catalyzed by hexokinase, PFK, and pyruvate kinase; the other reactions in glycolysis are bidirectional. PFK is the rate-limiting enzyme of the pathway. PFK is also the main regulatory enzyme. PFK is activated by ***adenosine monophosphate*** (AMP), and ***fructose 2,6-bisphosphate*** and inhibited by ATP and cit-

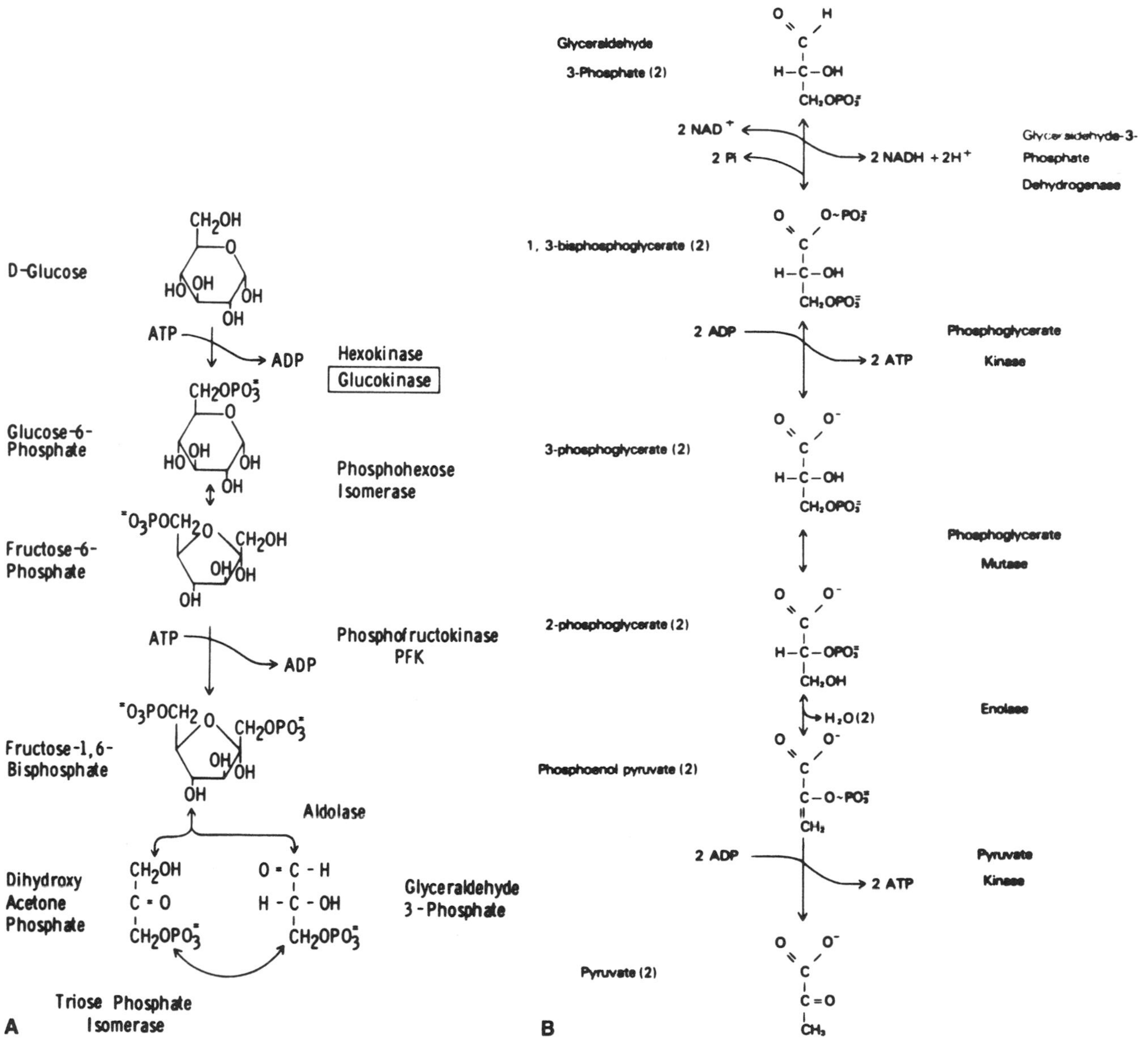

Fig. 4-19. Embden-Meyerhof glycolytic pathway.

rate. Note that ATP is both a substrate and an allosteric modulator. One function of glycolysis is to generate chemical energy as ATP. When the cellular concentrations of ATP are high, glycolysis is inhibited. When ATP levels decrease, ADP and AMP are formed and AMP activates phosphofructokinase. Under conditions whereby fatty acids serve as a fuel, citrate levels increase and glycolysis decreases. The regulatory role of fructose 2,6-bisphosphate is addressed under gluconeogenesis. High concentrations of ***fluoride*** inhibit the enolase reaction. The ATP formed in glycolysis results from ***substrate level phosphorylation.*** An energy-rich metabolite is produced, and it leads to ATP formation. This is in contrast to ***oxidative phosphorylation,*** in which ATP is produced by reactions involving electron transport, a proton-motive force, and an ATP synthase.

A note regarding nomenclature is appropriate here. When phosphates are linked together as in ADP and ATP, the appropriate prefix is *di* or *tri,* respectively. When the phosphates are not attached to one another, as in fructose 1,6-bisphosphate or inositol trisphosphate, the prefix *bis* or *tris* is appropriate (Table 4-4).

HEXOSE METABOLISM

We now consider the metabolism of fructose (from fruit) and galactose (from milk). In addition to hexokinase, the liver contains a specific ***fructokinase,*** which catalyzes the phosphorylation of fructose by ATP to yield ***fructose 1-phosphate*** in an exergonic and unidirectional process. The product is cleaved in a reaction catalyzed by aldolase to form glyceraldehyde and dihydroxyacetone phosphate. ***Glyceraldehyde kinase*** mediates the phosphorylation of glyceraldehyde by ATP to yield glyceraldehyde 3-phosphate.

The catabolism of galactose is more complex than that of the sugars covered to this point. Galactose (Fig. 4-17) is derived from the disaccharide lactose (Fig. 4-18) found in milk. Lactose is hydrolyzed by a digestive enzyme (lactase), absorbed by the gut, and transported to the liver. In the liver it is phosphorylated by ATP in a unidirectional reaction catalyzed by ***galactokinase*** to yield ADP and galactose 1-phosphate. Galactose is the only common aldohexose that is not a substrate for hexokinase. The reaction is also unusual in that the hydroxyl group of a hemiacetal linkage is derivatized (the hydroxyl of fructose on carbon one is not in hemiacetal or hemiketal linkage). Galactose 1-phosphate reacts with uridine diphosphoglucose (UDP-glucose) to yield UDP-galactose and glucose 1-phosphate. The reaction is catalyzed by ***galactose-1-phosphate uridyltransferase*** (Fig. 4-20). Glucose 1-phosphate is converted to glucose 6-phosphate by ***phosphoglucomutase*** in an isoergonic reaction. Glucose 6-phosphate is metabolized by the reactions of the Embden-Meyerhof pathway as previously considered.

UDP-galactose must be converted to UDP-glucose to

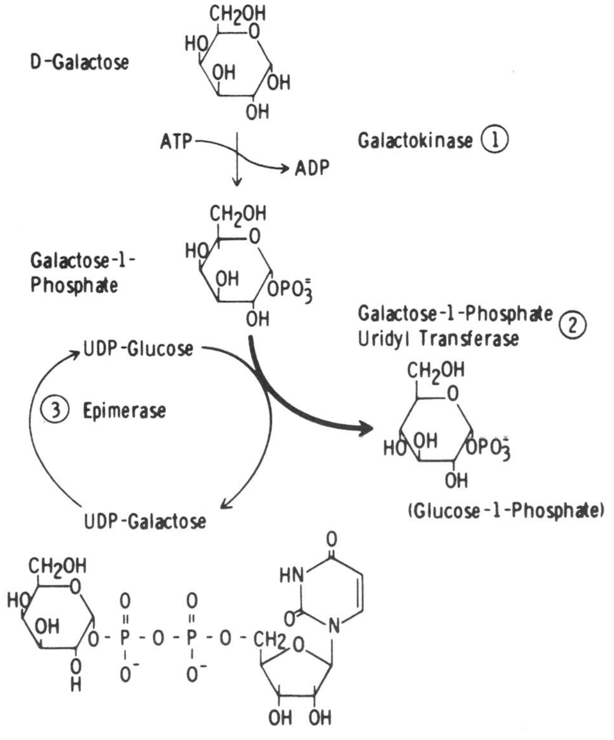

Fig. 4-20. Galactose catabolism.

regenerate the initial reactant. This reaction is catalyzed by an epimerase that converts the hydroxyl on C4 of UDP-galactose to a ketone and then reduces it to give the hydroxyl of the alternative configuration found in UDP-glucose. The epimerase contains tightly bound NAD^+ as cofactor. UDP-glucose can now react with a second molecule of galactose 1-phosphate to yield glucose 1-phosphate and UDP-galactose. The UDP moiety is thus used repeatedly in a cyclic fashion to mediate the conversion of appreciable galactose 1-phosphate to glucose 1-phosphate. UDP-glucose is said to function in a catalytic fashion; UDP-glucose is regenerated after every reaction.

The disease called ***galactosemia*** is due to a deficiency of ***galactose 1-phosphate*** uridyltransferase. Excessive galactose 1-phosphate accumulates in cells with consequent deleterious effects. A diet lacking milk and milk products (specifically lactose) constitutes treatment. Galactose forms an essential component of many carbohydrate-containing glycoproteins. Withholding galactose is not harmful because the epimerase can catalyze the formation of UDP-galactose from UDP-glucose as necessary. A milder form of galactosemia is due to a hereditary deficiency of galactokinase. The second type of galactosemia is less severe than classical galactosemia because there is not accumulation of charged intracellular metabolites.

For continued glycolysis, it is necessary to regenerate ADP and NAD^+. ATP is used in many of the cell's reactions as the common currency of energy exchange resulting in the formation of ADP. We briefly address the metabolism of NADH.

In erythrocytes, which lack mitochondria, and in other cells where NADH production exceeds the capacity for electron transport, NAD^+ is regenerated by the ***lactate dehydrogenase*** reaction. Pyruvate and NADH + H^+ react to yield lactate and NAD^+. The regenerated NAD^+ can participate again in glycolysis. The lactate is released from the erythrocyte or exercising skeletal muscle and is carried to the liver by the circulation. Under opportune conditions, lactate reacts with NAD^+ to yield NADH and pyruvate. Pyruvate may be reconverted to glucose by the process of gluconeogenesis. The glucose can be released from the liver and return to other tissues. The conversion of glucose to lactate in extrahepatic tissues, the resynthesis of glucose from lactate in liver, and subsequent transport to extrahepatic tissues is called the ***Cori cycle.*** The reoxidation of NADH to NAD^+ under aerobic conditions involving the ***malate–aspartate shuttle*** system or the ***glycerol phosphate shuttle*** is addressed in a later section.

Pyruvate Metabolism

The complete oxidation of pyruvate occurs within mitochondria. Pyruvate is transported through the inner mito-

TABLE 4-8. The Pyruvate Dehydrogenase Multienzyme Complex

ENZYME	COFACTOR	VITAMIN
E1 Pyruvate decarboxylase	Thiamine pyrophosphate	Thiamine
E2 Dihydrolipoyltransacetylase	Lipoate	
	Coenzyme A	Pantothenate
E3 Dihydrolipoyldehydrogenase	Flavine adenine dinucleotide (FAD)	Riboflavin
	Nicotinamide adenine dinucleotide (NAD^+)	Niacin

chondrial membrane by a specific translocase. Pyruvate is oxidized to acetyl-CoA and CO_2 by the ***pyruvate dehydrogenase*** multienzyme complex found in the mitochondrial matrix (Table 4-2). A ***multienzyme complex*** is an aggregate of enzymes that catalyze a series of reactions. The intermediates in the sequence may be covalently bound to the complex (as in the case of pyruvate dehydrogenase) and are not free to diffuse throughout the surrounding solution. The pyruvate dehydrogenase complex contains three enzyme activities and five cofactors (Table 4-8).

Pyruvate is converted to CO_2 and a two-carbon hydroxyethyl moiety covalently linked to the thiamine pyrophosphate of E1. The hydroxyethyl group is transferred to lipoate on E2. In the process, it becomes the more oxidized acetyl group and it is covalently linked to sulfur (as an energy-rich thioester). E2 transfers the acetyl group to CoA, yielding acetyl-CoA. E3 catalyzes the oxidation of reduced lipoate as flavin adenine dinucleotide (FAD) is converted to reduced FAD ($FADH_2$). $FADH_2$ is then oxidized to FAD; NADH + H^+ result. After this reaction, the enzyme complex is now in its original form. Pyruvate dehydrogenase catalyze the net reaction:

$$\begin{array}{ccc} \text{pyruvate}^{-1} & & CO_2 \\ + & & + \\ \text{coenzyme A} & \rightarrow & \text{acetyl-CoA} \\ + & & + \\ NAD^+ & & NADH \end{array}$$

The reaction is highly exergonic and unidirectional.

Pyruvate dehydrogenase is activated by NAD^+ and coenzyme A and inhibited by NADH and acetyl-CoA. However, the mechanism is indirect. ***Pyruvate dehydrogenase kinase*** is a protein kinase associated with the dehydrogenase in mitochondria. After phosphorylation by ATP as catalyzed by the kinase, pyruvate dehydrogenase exhibits less activity. Acetyl-CoA and NADH activate pyruvate dehydrogenase kinase; coenzyme A and NAD^+ inhibit it. A phosphoprotein phosphatase catalyzes the hydrolytic removal of phosphate from pyruvate dehydrogenase to generate the initial enzyme form.

The Krebs Cycle

The Krebs citric acid cycle, or tricarboxylic acid cycle, is often called the final common pathway of metabolism. The catabolism of glucose and fatty acids yields acetyl-CoA; metabolism of amino acids yields acetyl-CoA or actual intermediates of the cycle. The Krebs cycle provides a pathway for the oxidation of acetyl-CoA. The reactions occur in the mitochondria (Table 4-2). The pathway includes eight discrete steps. Seven of the enzyme activities are found in the mitochondrial matrix; the eighth (succinate dehydrogenase) is associated with the electron-transport chain within the inner mitochondrial membrane.

The net reaction catalyzed during each revolution of the Krebs cycle can be depicted as follows:

$$\begin{array}{ccc} \text{acetyl-CoA} & & 2\ CO_2 \\ + & & + \\ 2\ H_2O & & \text{CoA} \\ + & & + \\ 3\ NAD^+ & \rightarrow & 3\ NADH + 3\ H^+ \\ + & & + \\ FAD & & FADH_2 \\ + & & + \\ GDP + Pi & & GTP \end{array}$$

CO_2 is an end product of metabolism. CoA can be reused for a variety of reactions. The reduced cofactors donate their reducing equivalents to the electron-transport chain and oxygen to yield H_2O and the oxidized cofactors. Guanosine triphosphate (GTP) is formed by substrate-level phosphorylation. GTP is bioenergetically equivalent to ATP and serves a variety of functions. Note that acetyl-CoA is the substrate of the cycle, and any metabolite must be converted to acetyl-CoA in order to be oxidized by this pathway. An overview of the cyclic pathway depicts the location of CO_2 production and NADH and $FADH_2$ formation (Fig. 4-21). The production of 9 ATP equivalents by oxidative phosphorylation and 1 GTP by substrate-level phosphorylation is also noted.

The reactions of the cycle are shown in Figure 4-22. ***Citrate synthase*** catalyzes a reaction between acetyl-CoA, oxaloacetate, and water to yield citrate (a tricarboxylic acid) and CoA. This reaction is associated with the hydrolytic removal of CoA, which is a highly exergonic process and renders the reaction unidirectional. A note about nomenclature is appropriate here. The distinction between ***synthases*** and ***synthetases*** is that synthetases require ATP or an equivalent nucleoside triphosphate as

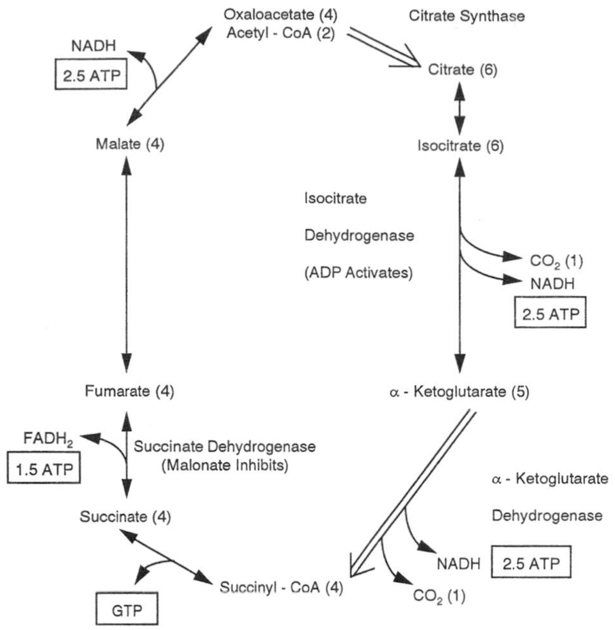

Fig. 4-21. Overview of the Krebs citric acid cycle.

an energy source (Table 4-6). Citrate synthase, in contrast, is a biosynthetic enzyme that does not use a nucleoside triphosphate such as ATP as a reactant. ***Aconitase*** catalyzes an isoergonic isomerization to yield isocitrate. Although citrate lacks an asymmetric carbon, it is prochiral and the hydroxyl is moved away from the two-carbon end just derived from the acetyl group. Isocitrate undergoes an oxidative decarboxylation reaction involving NAD^+ that is catalyzed by ***isocitrate dehydrogenase;*** the products include α-ketoglutarate, CO_2, NADH, and H^+. The reaction is modestly exergonic. The high ratio of NAD^+/NADH in mitochondria pulls the reaction in the forward direction. Isocitrate dehydrogenase is a main regulatory enzyme in the Krebs cycle. ADP serves as a positive allosteric effector. High ADP levels serve as a signal to enhance the flux of substrates through the cycle.

α-Ketoglutarate dehydrogenase catalyzes the reaction between substrate, NAD^+, and CoA to yield succinyl-CoA, CO_2, NADH, and H^+. The protein is a multienzyme complex that is analogous to the pyruvate dehydrogenase complex considered in the previous section (three enzyme activities and five cofactors). The reaction is physiologically irreversible, and the α-ketoglutarate dehydrogenase reaction ensures that the Krebs cycle is unidirectional. The next reaction is catalyzed by ***succinate thiokinase.*** This reaction is an example of substrate level phosphorylation conserving the energy-rich thioester bond of succinyl-CoA as the terminal phosphoanhydride bond of GTP. Succinyl-CoA, P_i, and guanosine diphosphate (GDP) form succinate and GTP. (Because GDP + $P_i \rightarrow$ GTP + H_2O, this reaction serves indirectly as a source of water. This property is used in calculating the stoichiometry of the cycle.)

Succinate dehydrogenase has three notable properties. First, it is the only enzyme of the Krebs cycle found within the inner mitochondrial membrane. Succinate dehydrogenase is thus localized contiguous to the electron-transport chain, where it passes its reducing equivalents. Second, only 1.5 moles of ATP is produced by electron transport (in contrast to 2.5 moles of ATP from 1 mole of NADH) from the enzyme's flavin adenine nucleotide (FAD) prosthetic group. Third, succinate dehydrogenase is inhibited competitively by malonate ($^-OOCCH_2$-COO^-). This inhibition was an important property that helped Hans Krebs elucidate the nature of the cycle. Succinate dehydrogenase mediates the conversion of substrate to fumarate (note that fumarate has the *trans* configuration at the double bond). ***Fumarase*** catalyzes the addition of water to fumarate (a hydration), yielding malate, a bidirectional lyase reaction. ***Malate dehydrogenase*** catalyzes the regeneration of oxaloacetate by the reduction of NAD^+ to NADH and H^+. Although the malate dehydrogenase reaction is bidirectional, it is endergonic.

The Krebs cycle is catalytic in nature. A *catalyst* is an agent that mediates a process and that is unchanged at its completion. In the Krebs cycle, one molecule of oxaloacetate mediates the oxidation of many molecules of acetyl-CoA because oxaloacetate is regenerated at the end of each oxidative sequence. Because it starts and ends with oxaloacetate, in this sense the Krebs cycle functions catalytically. In contrast to oxaloacetate, the acetyl group is formally consumed during each reaction cycle. Acetyl-CoA is called the ***stoichiometric substrate,*** and oxaloacetate is called the ***regenerating substrate.***

To recapitulate, the citrate synthase and α-ketoglutarate dehydrogenase reactions are unidirectional. Isocitrate dehydrogenase is the pacemaker reaction of the pathway and is allosterically activated by ADP. Succinate thiokinase catalyzes a substrate-level phosphorylation. The two molecules of CO_2 given off during a single turn of the cycle are not those immediately derived from the acetyl group. Moreover, three molecules of NADH and one molecule of $FADH_2$ are generated during each turn of the cycle.

Besides its role in catabolism, metabolites of the Krebs cycle serve as precursors for the biosynthesis of amino acids and heme. A process playing a role in both catabolism and anabolism is called ***amphibolic.*** The following reaction, catalyzed by ***pyruvate carboxylase,*** plays the important role of replenishing intermediates that are used for biosynthesis. The reaction involves ATP, HCO_3^-, and pyruvate; oxaloacetate, ADP, and P_i are products. The cofactor for the enzyme is ***biotin.*** Biotin is covalently linked to the enzyme and serves as a prosthetic group. Pyruvate carboxylase is allosterically activated by acetyl-

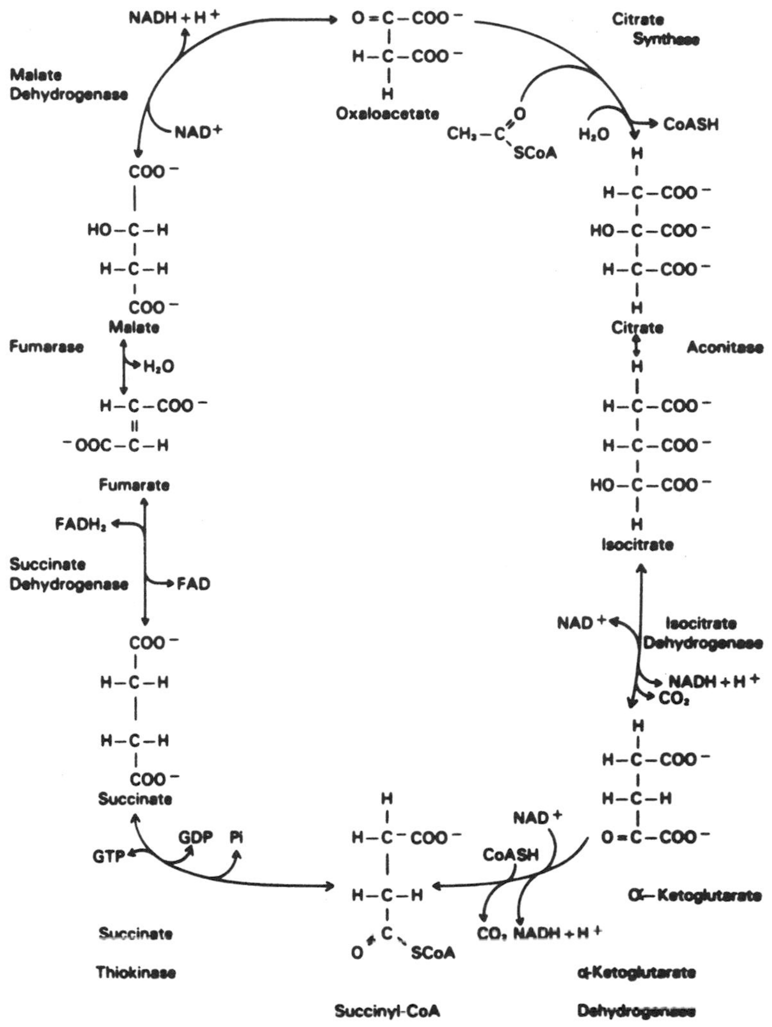

Fig. 4-22. Krebs citric acid cycle.

CoA and requires acetyl-CoA for the expression of its activity. The overall reaction is depicted by the following chemical equation:

$$\text{pyruvate}^{-} + \text{ATP} + HCO_3^{-} \rightleftarrows \text{oxaloacetate}^{-2} + \text{ADP} + \text{Pi}$$

Oxidative Phosphorylation

The term ***oxidative phosphorylation*** refers to reactions associated with oxygen consumption and the phosphorylation of ADP to yield ATP. Oxidative phosphorylation is associated with an ***electron-transport chain*** or ***respiratory chain,*** which is found in the inner mitochondrial membrane of eukaryotes (Table 4-2). A similar process occurs within the plasma membrane of prokaryotes such as *E. coli*. The importance of oxidative phosphorylation at this juncture is that it accounts for the reoxidation of reducing equivalents generated in the reactions of the Krebs cycle as well as in glycolysis. Oxidative phosphorylation accounts for the preponderance (95% or more) of ATP production in humans. The electron-transport chain transfers electrons from reductants to oxygen in a series of exergonic reactions. According to ***Mitchell's chemiosmotic theory,*** a portion of the liberated free energy energizes the transport of protons from inside to outside of the inner mitochondrial membrane (or the plasma membrane of prokaryotes). Such reactions result in energy conservation or storage of chemical energy in the form of a proton gradient. The ***proton-motive force*** exhibits a voltage component (inside negative) and a concentration component (external pH $<$ internal pH). The protons move down their electrochemical gradient (from outside to inside of the mitochondrion or the bacterial cell) in an exergonic process and drive the conversion of ADP + P_i $\rightarrow$ ATP + H_2O in a reaction catalyzed by ***ATP synthase*** (Table 4-1). The enzyme is located on the inner face of the inner mitochondrial membrane; ATP synthase catalyzes a reversible reaction and can synthesize or hydrolyze substrate (ATPase) depending on the experimental conditions. Its function in humans *in vivo* is ATP synthesis.

THE ELECTRON–TRANSPORT CHAIN

The components of the electron-transport chain include iron-sulfur proteins; cytochromes c_1, c, b, and aa_3, and coenzyme Q, or ubiquinone. The pathway of electrons along the chain is shown in Figure 4-23. Reducing equivalents can enter the chain at two locations. Electrons from NADH are transferred to NADH dehydrogenase. In reactions involving FMN and iron-sulfur proteins, electrons are transferred to coenzyme Q; protons are translocated from the interior to exterior of the mitochondrion during this process. Electrons entering from succinate dehydrogenase ($FADH_2$) are donated to coenzyme Q. This transfer is not associated with proton translocation. Electrons are transported from reduced coenzyme Q to cytochrome b and then to cytochrome c_1. This step is associated with the translocation of protons. Electrons are then carried by cytochrome c to cytochrome aa_3. Cytochrome aa_3 is also known as ***cytochrome oxidase,*** which catalyzes a reaction of electrons and protons with molecular oxygen to produce water. Cytochrome oxidase actively translocates protons across the inner mitochondrial membrane.

The three positions for active proton translocation by the electron transport chain are called sites 1, 2, and 3. Site 1 occurs between NADH dehydrogenase and coenzyme Q, site 2 occurs between coenzyme Q and cytochrome *c*, and site 3 occurs between cytochrome *c* and molecular oxygen. The sites were named on the basis of the effects of inhibitors of electron transport and before the notion of discrete proton translocating locations. The site-specific inhibitors are given in Table 4-9. Rotenone is commonly used as a rat poison. Cyanide is a powerful inhibitor of cytochrome oxidase in humans and other animals, and this accounts for cyanide's toxic and lethal effects. Carbon monoxide also binds tightly to cytochrome oxidase. However, its major toxicity is related to the formation of a complex with hemoglobin, which abolishes its oxygen-binding and transport capacity.

TABLE 4-9. Inhibitors of the Electron-Transport or Respiratory Chain

SITE	INHIBITOR
I	Rotenone
II	Antimycin A
III	Cyanide (CN^-)
	Azide (N_3^-)
	Carbon monoxide (CO)

Cytochrome *c* is a small (molecular mass = 10,000), water-soluble, heme protein. All the other proteins of the electron transport chain are water insoluble and are found embedded in the inner mitochondrial membrane as integral membrane proteins. Coenzyme Q is a lipid-soluble organic compound. It is noteworthy that coenzyme Q and cytochrome *c* are mobile electron carriers; the other components of the electron transport chain are less mobile. NAD^+, FAD, and coenzyme Q are two-electron carriers; the cytochromes (with their iron-heme) and iron-sulfur proteins are one-electron carriers. Cytochrome oxidase contains two iron atoms and two copper atoms, each of which is thought to function in one-electron transfers in series. The reduction of oxygen to water, which is catalyzed by cytochrome oxidase, is a four-electron reaction.

Note that more than 95% of oxygen consumed by humans involves a reaction catalyzed by cytochrome oxidase. When oxygen transport to tissues is blocked as the result of an arterial occlusion, serious disease or death ensues. The occlusion produced by coronary artery disease resulting in a myocardial infarction (heart attack), or cerebrovascular disease resulting in a stroke, cogently illustrates the importance of the cytochrome oxidase reaction. The product of oxygen reduction is water. In humans, reduction of oxygen accounts for the production of about 300 ml of metabolic water per day.

The precise mechanism of proton translocation at each of the three sites is unknown. An important aspect of the chemiosmotic theory is that a membrane is required, and the membrane must be relatively impermeable to protons. Protons are transported by specific transport proteins and do not simply diffuse through the membrane. Next we address the issue of how the proton-motive force drives ATP synthesis.

ATP SYNTHESIS

An intricate enzyme called ***ATP synthase*** is associated with the inner aspect of the inner mitochondrial membrane. As protons move down their electrochemical gradient in an exergonic fashion, they provide the energy for the reaction of ADP and P_i to give ATP and H_2O (Table 4-1). The synthase is made up of two domains. The F_o domain (o stands for *o*ligomycin, an inhibitor of the overall synthase reaction) is embedded in the inner membrane. The F_1 complex forms a knoblike structure in association with F_o. In the intact structure, the membrane is proton impermeable. When F_1 is removed from F_o, the membrane transmits protons. This observation provides evidence that protons course directly through the ATP synthase. The F_1 complex contains binding sites for ATP, ADP, and P_i. Movement of protons down their thermodynamic gradient provides the energy to drive the endergonic portion of the reaction (ADP + $P_i \rightarrow$ ATP

+ H_2O). The number of protons that move down their gradient to drive the synthesis of one ATP is three. An additional proton is required to translocate P_i from the cytosol to the interior of the mitochondrion. Thus, a total of four protons is required to sustain the synthesis of each molecule of ATP.

One of the triumphs of the chemiosmotic theory is the explanation of the necessity of a membrane in oxidative phosphorylation. The theory also explains the effects of uncouplers of oxidative phosphorylation. ***2,4-Dinitrophenol*** is the prototype of an uncoupler. An uncoupler does not inhibit electron transport from reductant to oxygen; uncouplers actually enhance the rates of oxygen uptake. 2,4-Dinitrophenol, however, abolishes phosphorylation or ATP formation. This explains the term "uncoupler," because oxidation occurs but phosphorylation does not. 2,4-Dinitrophenol and other uncouplers dissipate the proton gradient. Uncouplers ferry protons across the membrane and abolish the proton-motive force. In the presence of an uncoupler, proton translocation by the electron transport system is not opposed by an existing proton gradient, and electron transport to oxygen is increased. Parenthetically, 2,4-dinitrophenol was used in the treatment of human obesity in the 1930s. Because of its low therapeutic index, several deaths ensued and the practice was abolished.

Experiments show that the P:O ratio (number of ATPs formed from ADP + P_i per gram atom of oxygen consumed) using NADH as substrate is 2.5, and the P:O ratio with succinate is substrate is 1.5. Sites 1 and 3 are associated with the generation of a proton gradient sufficient for the formation of 1 ATP, and site 2 with 0.5 ATP. Succinate circumvents site 1 and results in the production of only 1.5 ATP molecules (Fig. 4-23).

To recapitulate, we note four properties of oxidative phosphorylation. First, transport of electrons from reductant to oxygen along the respiratory chain is a very exergonic process. Second, part of the chemical energy is conserved as protons are translocated from the inside to the outside of the inner mitochondrial membrane to establish a proton gradient. Third, the membrane is not freely permeable to protons. Fourth, protons then move down their electrochemical gradient (an exergonic process) and drive ATP formation in a process involving the ATP synthase of the inner mitochondrial membrane. A total of four protons are required for the synthesis of each ATP: one for the translocation of phosphate and three for ATP synthase.

METABOLITE TRANSPORT ACROSS THE INNER MITOCHONDRIAL MEMBRANE

The lipid portion of the inner mitochondrial membrane is relatively impermeable to ionic metabolites, phosphate, hydroxide, and especially protons. It is important in metabolism to transport compounds generated in one cellular compartment into another. Specific proteins, sometimes called translocases, mediate transport across membranes. The identification of a number of such translocases and their physiological role are considered in this section.

ATP is generated within the mitochondrion and functions predominantly in the cytosol, where it is converted to ADP and P_i. Two different translocases are necessary for transporting these substances. ATP is transported out of the mitochondrion in exchange for ADP (an antiport system). Both ATP and ADP are transported down a concentration gradient. Under physiological conditions, ADP is transported down its gradient into the mitochondrial matrix. These processes are inhibited by a plant-derived toxin called ***atractyloside.*** Phosphate is transported into the mitochondrion in exchange for intramitochondrial hydroxide (the export of mitochondrial hydroxide is formally equivalent to the translocation of a proton into the mitochondrion). Translocases also exist for the exchange

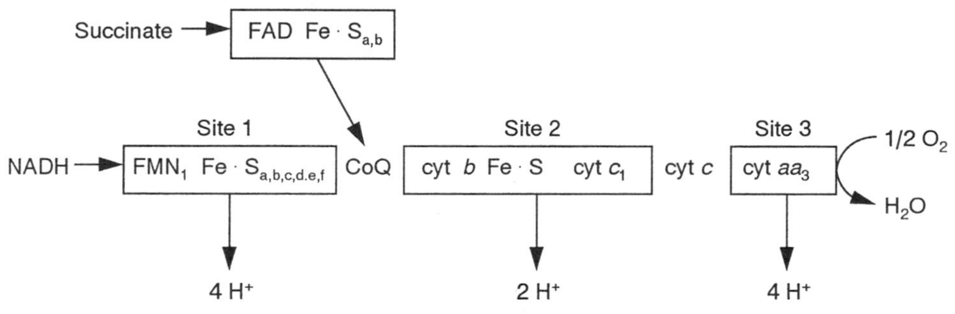

CoQ, coenzyme Q; cyt, cytochrome; FAD, flavin adenine dinucleotide; FMN, flavin mononucleotide; Fe · S, iron sulfur

Fig. 4-23. Mitochondrial electron-transport chain.

of α-ketoglutarate for malate, citrate for malate, phosphate for malate, and aspartate for glutamate. Transport proteins do not exist for the following substances, and the biochemical ramifications are discussed in appropriate sections: NAD^+, NADH, $NADP^+$, NADPH, CoA, acyl-CoA, and oxaloacetate.

We now address the transport of reducing equivalents into the mitochondrion. One important source of cytosolic reductant includes the NADH (two per mole of glucose metabolized) generated during glycolysis. Only a small proportion of NAD^+ is regenerated by the lactate dehydrogenase reaction in most cells (except mature erythrocytes) under aerobic conditions. Because a mitochondrial translocase for NADH is nonexistent, the cell uses indirect methods called the ***malate–aspartate shuttle*** or the ***glycerol phosphate shuttle*** for moving reducing equivalents from the cytosol into the mitochondrion.

Let us first consider the malate–aspartate shuttle. Two membrane translocases are required: one is specific for malate and α-ketoglutarate, and the second exchanges the amino acids aspartate and glutamate. Two sets of two enzymes also are required: mitochondrial and cytosolic malate dehydrogenase and mitochondrial and cytosolic aspartate aminotransferase. Let us begin with NADH in the cytosol, shown on the upper left of Figure 4-24. Malate dehydrogenase catalyzes a reaction between oxaloacetate and NADH + H^+ to yield NAD^+ and malate. The NAD^+ can now participate in the glyceraldehyde 3-phosphate dehydrogenase reaction of glycolysis. Malate is translocated into the mitochondrial matrix, and α-ketoglutarate is transported outward. Inside the mitochondrion, malate dehydrogenase catalyzes a reaction of substrate with NAD^+ to yield oxaloacetate and NADH + H^+. The latter serves as a reductant for the respiratory chain and leads to the formation of 2.5 moles of ATP per mole of NADH. Two NADH equivalents in the cytosol generated from a mole of glucose (two moles of triose phosphate) yields five moles of ATP. If a malate–oxaloacetate exchange protein were to occur, the shuttle would be much less complex. However, such a system does not exist, and additional processes are necessary to reestablish the initial conditions. Oxaloacetate (a C_4 compound derived from malate) reacts with glutamate to yield aspartate (C_4) and α-ketoglutarate. Aspartate is transported in exchange for glutamate. To resume the initial conditions, external aspartate (C_4) reacts with α-ketoglutarate to yield oxaloacetate (C_4) and glutamate. The biochemical machinery for the malate–aspartate shuttle exists in the liver and heart.

Brain and muscle contain a different shuttle, the ***glycerol phosphate shuttle,*** for transporting reducing equivalents into the mitochondrion. The components include a cytosolic glycerol phosphate dehydrogenase and an inner mitochondrial membrane glycerol phosphate dehydrogenase (Fig. 4-24). NADH converts dihydroxyacetone phosphate to glycerol phosphate in the cytosol. Glycerol

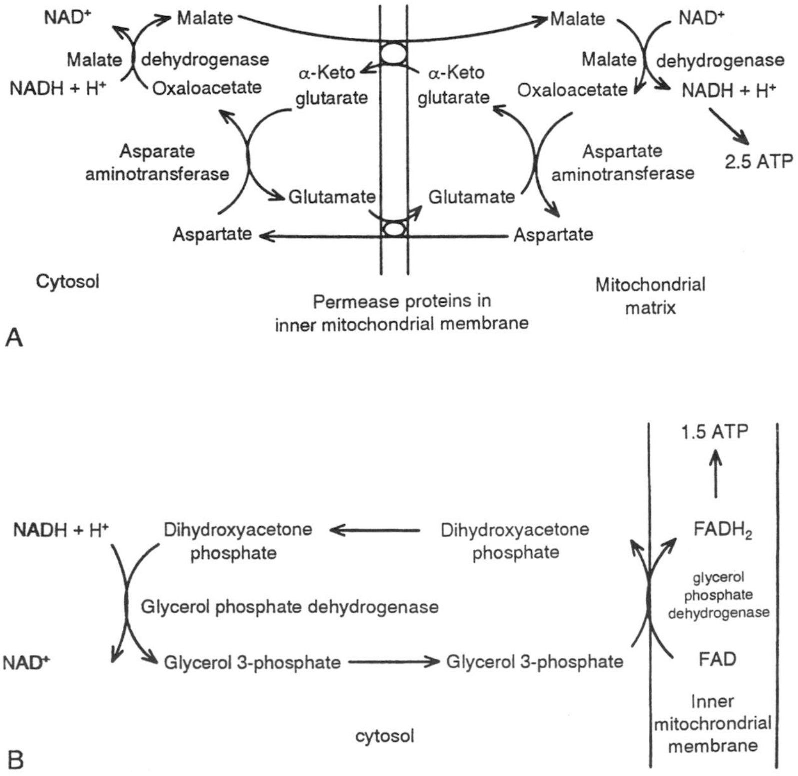

Fig. 4-24. Malate-aspartate shuttle (A) and glycerol phosphate shuttle (B) for transporting reducing equivalents into the mitochondrion.

phosphate flows through the outer mitochondrial membrane and donates electrons to the glycerol phosphate dehydrogenase imbedded within the inner mitochondrial membrane with the attendant formation of dihydroxyacetone phosphate. The electrons are passed from the dehydrogenase to coenzyme Q, and 1.5 moles of ATP is formed via oxidative phosphorylation from each mole of glycerol phosphate. Dihydroxyacetone phosphate is able to recycle, or it is metabolized by its usual reactions.

ATP YIELD

We have seen that the conversion of 1 mole of glucose to 2 moles of pyruvate during glycolysis results in the net formation of 2 ATP equivalents. Let us now consider the energy yield after the complete oxidation of glucose by the Krebs cycle and oxidative phosphorylation. We can also determine the yield of ATP from selected intermediates. We noted that 1 mole of intramitochondrial NADH yields 2.5 moles of ATP. FAD-containing enzymes such as succinate dehydrogenase, which donate reducing equivalents into the respiratory chain at the level of coenzyme Q, yield 1.5 moles of ATP per mole of coenzyme QH_2. Table 4-10 summarizes the various reactions in the catabolism of glucose. A net yield of 32 ATP equivalents is associated with the use of the malate–aspartate shuttle. A net yield of 30 ATP equivalents is associated with the use of the glycerol phosphate shuttle. We also can deduce that a mole of pyruvate yields 12.5 moles of ATP, and 1 mole of acetyl-CoA yields 10 moles of ATP. The reader should verify the correctness of these values.

TABLE 4-10. ATP Molecules Generated During the Complete Oxidation of One Molecule of Glucose by Glycolysis with the Malate–Aspartate Shuttle (Glycerol Phosphate Shuttle), Citric Acid Cycle Reactions, and Oxidative Phosphorylation

PROCESS OR REACTION	ATP YIELD
Glycolysis (glucose → 2 pyruvate)	2
2 NADH from glyceraldehyde-3-phosphate dehydrogenase and malate (glycerol phosphate) shuttle	5 (3)
Pyruvate dehydrogenase (2 NADH)	5
Isocitrate dehydrogenase (2 NADH)	5
α-Ketoglutarate dehydrogenase (2 NADH)	5
Succinate thiokinase (2 substrate level)	2
Succinate dehydrogenase	3
Malate dehydrogenase (2 NADH)	5
Total	32 (30) ATP yield per hexose
NADH (1)	2.5
$FADH_2$ (1)	1.5
Acetyl-CoA (1)	10
Pyruvate (1)	12.5

Glycogen Metabolism

Before studying the catabolism of lipids and amino acids, we address here some additional aspects of carbohydrate metabolism. We first cover the pathways for glycogen formation (glycogenesis) and glycogen degradation (glycogenolysis). In the next sections we discuss the pentose phosphate pathway and gluconeogenesis. Gluconeogenesis refers to the pathway for glucose biosynthesis from pyruvate, lactate, citric acid cycle intermediates, amino acids, and glycerol.

GLYCOGENESIS

Glycogen serves as a reservoir or storage form of carbohydrate. Glycogen is a polymer of glucose residues and is found in all cells except mature erythrocytes. The major glycogen stores in humans occur in liver and muscle. Muscle glycogen is a source of fuel for muscle contraction. Glycogen is a branched, treelike molecule with a high molecular mass (it can be more than one million daltons). The straight-chain portions are composed of α-1,4-glycosidic bonds, and the branch points occur at α-1,6 bonds. Branches occur about every 10th residue (Fig. 4-25).

Glycogen biosynthesis begins with glucose 6-phosphate. Phosphoglucomutase (PGM) catalyzes the isoergonic conversion of glucose 6-phosphate to glucose 1-phosphate. The next reaction is designed to produce an activated high-energy form of glucose for biosynthesis, which is UDP-glucose. UDP-glucose pyrophosphorylase catalyzes a reaction between uridine triphosphate (UTP) and glucose 1-phosphate to produce UDP-glucose and PP_i. This reaction is endergonic but bidirectional (the reactants contain two high-energy bonds, and the products contain three high-energy bonds). We see for the

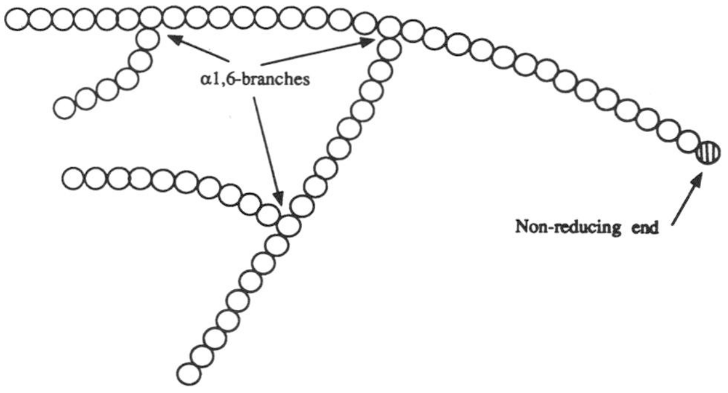

Fig. 4-25. Branched structure of glycogen.

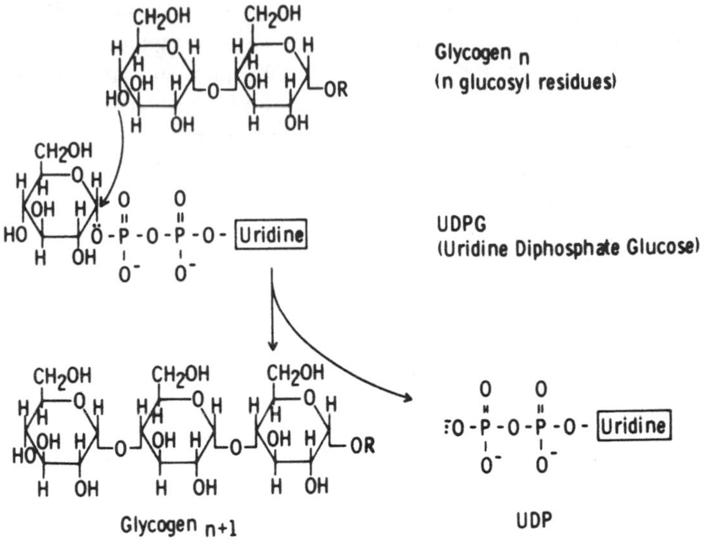

Fig. 4-26. Glycogen synthesis.

first time a reaction in which PP_i is a product. Its only known metabolic fate in humans is a hydrolysis to yield two P_i molecules; the reaction is catalyzed by a ubiquitous and separate inorganic pyrophosphatase. Hydrolysis of PP_i is exergonic and physiologically irreversible. The formation of PP_i and its hydrolysis represents one mechanism for pulling reactions forward. This is a rather general and noteworthy principle of metabolism (Table 4-1). Many reactions are associated with the so-called pyrophosphate split, and invariably the bioenergetics and principles are those stated here. The glycosidic bond between a sugar and pyrophosphate as found in UDP-glucose is energy rich with a standard free energy of hydrolysis of −30 kJ/mol.

Two enzyme activities are required for glycogen biosynthesis. The first (glycogen synthase) is responsible for the formation of linear chains, and the second (branching enzyme) is responsible for the formation of branch points. ***Glycogen synthase*** catalyzes the reaction between glycogen$_n$ (containing n glycosyl residues) and UDP-glucose to yield glycogen$_{n+1}$ and UDP. The high-energy bond of UDP-glucose is converted into a low-energy glycosidic bond, and the reaction is exergonic and unidirectional (Fig. 4-26). After 12 to 16 glucosyl residues are added distal to a branch point, then ***branching enzyme*** transfers a block of six or so residues to yield a new branch. Both ends of the branch can now be elongated in reactions catalyzed by glycogen synthase.

GLYCOGENOLYSIS

Two enzymes are necessary for glycogenolysis (the degradation or lysis of glycogen). ***Glycogen phosphorylase*** (usually called phosphorylase) catalyzes a reaction between P_i and glycogen to yield glucose 1-phosphate and glycogen$_{n-1}$(Fig. 4-27). This phosphorolysis (lysis by phosphate) reaction occurs at α-1,4-glycosidic bonds and is modestly exergonic under physiological conditions. Note that this is not a hydrolysis reaction. An additional noteworthy property of phosphorylase is that it contains pyridoxal phosphate as a cofactor. Phosphorylase reactions occur until a glucose residue about four residues from a branch point is reached. Then a single protein with two enzymatic activities, called a ***debranching enzyme,*** mediates the elimination of the branch. A glucosyltransferase activity moves three glucosyl residues as a block, leaving a single glucose in α-1,6 linkage at a branch point. The glycosyl group is added elsewhere to extend a straight chain with the α-1,4 bond (Fig. 4-28). Then the

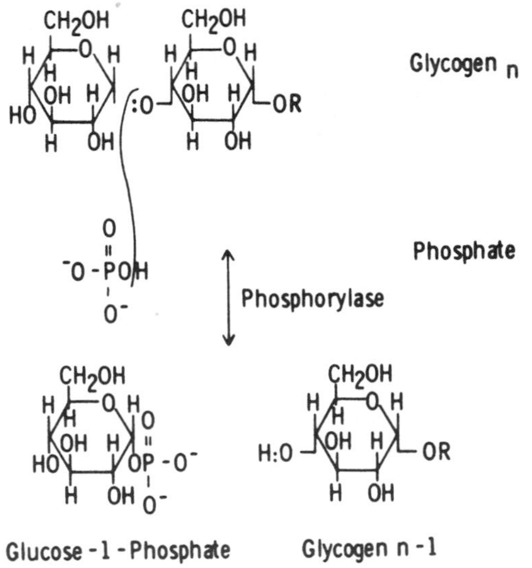

Fig. 4-27. Glycogen phosphorylase catalyzes a phosphorylytic cleavage of glycogen to yield glucose-1-phosphate.

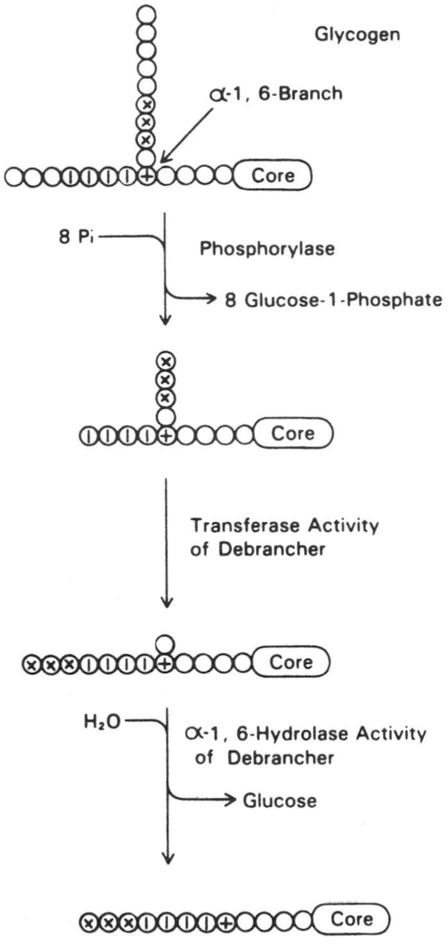

Fig. 4-28. Glycogenolysis requires phosphorylase and debrancher activities.

debrancher catalyzes the hydrolytic removal of glucose at the branch point to yield free glucose and the remainder of the glycogen molecule (Fig. 4-29).

Most of the glucosyl residues from glycogen are released as phosphate esters by the phosphorylase reaction. The resulting glucose 1-phosphate is converted to glucose 6-phosphate by phosphoglucomutase. About 10% of the residues are hydrolytically released as free glucose by the debranching reaction. For metabolism, free glucose must be phosphorylated by ATP to form glucose 6-phosphate in a reaction catalyzed by hexokinase or glucokinase. Several inborn errors of metabolism, called glycogen storage diseases, have been described. Their names and associated enzyme deficiencies are given in Table 4-11.

REGULATION OF GLYCOGENESIS AND GLYCOGENOLYSIS

The biosynthesis and degradation of glycogen are the result of distinct enzyme-catalyzed reactions. This allows

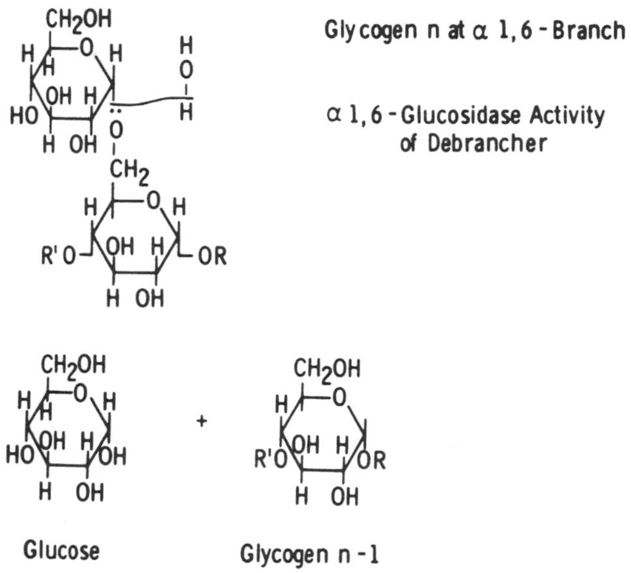

Fig. 4-29. Debranching enzyme catalyzes a hydrolysis reaction, yielding free glucose.

for enhancement of the activity of one process with concomitant inhibition of the other. It was through the study of the regulation of these processes that the metabolic regulation by the cyclic AMP second messenger system was first described. We address here the mechanism of hyperglycemia after the secretion of glucagon. Glucagon activates its receptor found in the liver cell membrane. The activated receptor interacts with a G_S protein (guanine nucleotide–binding protein, stimulatory). G_S is composed of three subunits (α, β, and γ). The α-subunit exchanges GTP for GDP and $G_S\alpha$/GTP dissociates from the β/γ complex, and $G_S\alpha$/GTP interacts with adenylyl cyclase and activates it. Adenylyl cyclase catalyzes the formation of cyclic AMP and PP_i from ATP. Cyclic AMP then activates a cognate protein kinase (cyclic AMP–dependent protein kinase, or protein kinase A [PKA]). The following equation describes this activation:

$$R_2C_2 + 4 \text{ cyclic AMP} \rightleftharpoons 2\text{ C} + R_2 - \text{cyclic AMP}_4$$
(less active) (more active)

R designates a regulatory subunit, and C designates a catalytic subunit.

Let us first consider how protein kinase A activates glycogenolysis, and then we will consider how this enzyme inhibits glycogenesis. The catalytic subunit of protein kinase A catalyzes the phosphorylation of a second protein kinase called ***phosphorylase kinase.*** The activity of phosphorylase kinase is thereby increased. Phosphorylase kinase enzyme now catalyzes the phosphorylation of the enzyme (glycogen) phosphorylase. The phosphorylated enzyme, called ***phosphorylase a,*** is the more active form. The unphosphorylated enzyme is called ***phospho-***

TABLE 4-11. Glycogen-Storage Diseases

TYPE	NAME	DEFICIENCY	COMMENTS
I	von Gierke*	Glucose-6-phosphatase	Liver and kidney have increased glycogen of normal structure
II	Pompe*	α-1 → 4 Glucosidase	Lysosomal disease
III	Cori	Debrancher	Highly branched glycogen
IV	Andersen	Brancher	Sparsely branched glycogen
V	Mcardle*	Muscle phosphorylase	Proved role of glycogen synthase in glycogenesis
VI	—	Liver phosphorylase	—

* Noteworthy.

rylase b and is less active. Phosphorylase *a* then catalyzes the degradation of glycogen. Consider the role of glycogenolysis *in vivo*. The major metabolite, glucose 1-phosphate, is converted into glucose 6-phosphate, which can in turn be hydrolyzed to glucose and released into the blood stream. The enzyme catalyzing this reaction is glucose 6-phosphatase, which is present in the liver and kidney. All other tissues lack glucose 6-phosphatase. The liver is the most important organ in releasing carbohydrate into the blood stream as glucose, but the kidney assumes an important role after fasting for 2 or more days. Other organs are unable to do so because they lack glucose 6-phosphatase.

An enhancement of the activity of the degradative enzyme represents one side of the coin. Let us now consider how glucagon decreases the rate of biosynthesis of liver glycogen. The regulatory scheme parallels that described above in that an activation of protein kinase A occurs. The inhibition of the chief biosynthetic enzyme, namely glycogen synthase, is produced in a direct fashion without the intermediacy of another protein kinase. The activated protein kinase A catalyzes the direct phosphorylation of glycogen synthase. After phosphorylation, glycogen synthase is less active.

Let us examine the processes that reestablish the initial state of the enzymes when the stimulus subsides. Decreasing glucagon concentration decreases receptor occupation. The α-subunit of G_S catalyzes the hydrolysis of GTP to GDP and P_i. $G_S\alpha$/GDP then recombines with the $\beta\gamma$-complex, and adenylyl cyclase activity returns to unstimulated or basal levels. A cyclic AMP phosphodiesterase catalyzes the hydrolysis and destruction of cyclic AMP by converting it to 5′-AMP. A decrease in cyclic AMP concentration favors the reassociation of the catalytic and regulatory subunits of protein kinase A, rendering the enzyme less active. Both phosphorylase kinase and glycogen synthase are regenerated from their phosphorylated forms after hydrolytic reactions catalyzed by phosphoprotein phosphatase-1. There is a family of protein phosphatase enzymes that participate in the many phosphorylation-dephosphorylation reactions in biochemistry, including phosphoprotein phosphatases-1, -2A, -2B, and -2C.

To summarize this section, two enzymes are required for glycogen biosynthesis, and two are required for its degradation. The synthetic enzymes are ***glycogen synthase*** and ***brancher;*** the catabolic enzymes are ***phosphorylase*** and ***debrancher.*** Glucose 1-phosphate is the product of phosphorylase, and free glucose results from the action of debrancher. Cyclic AMP and its cognate protein kinase enhance glycogenolysis by protein phosphorylation. Phosphorylase kinase is the target enzyme. Phosphorylase kinase then catalyzes the ATP-dependent phosphorylation and activation of phosphorylase. Protein kinase A catalyzes the direct phosphorylation of glycogen synthase, rendering it less active. Protein phosphorylation can change the activity of the target enzyme in the positive or negative direction; the result depends on the enzyme.

Other mechanisms come into play in the regulation of glycogen metabolism. Elevated 5′-AMP activates phosphorylase *b* allosterically. 5′-AMP serves as a signal that ATP levels are low. Furthermore, ionic calcium activates phosphorylase kinase; one of the subunits of phosphorylase kinase is calmodulin, and the formation of a calcium-calmodulin complex leads to greater enzyme activity. Glucose decreases phosphorylase activity in an allosteric fashion and thereby inhibits glycogenolysis.

Elevated blood glucose stimulates the release of insulin from the β-cells of the pancreas. Insulin promotes glucose transport from the extracellular space into muscle and adipose tissue by recruiting GLUT4 (one of seven glucose transporters) to the plasma membrane; insulin has no direct effect on glucose transport into liver cells, which contain GLUT1. Insulin also increases glycogen synthase activity in liver cells by enzyme induction. Glucagon release is enhanced at low blood glucose concentrations. Glucagon interacts with its specific receptor in the liver cell membrane, which in turn activates adenylyl cyclase and leads to glycogenolysis via the protein kinase A cascade as outlined above.

Gluconeogenesis

The supply of hepatic glycogen is limited, and other fuels must be used to maintain normal blood glucose levels after an overnight fast. ***Gluconeogenesis*** is the process responsible for converting lactate (produced by red blood cells, muscle, and other tissues), glycerol (produced from lipolysis or triglyceride catabolism), pyruvate, and intermediates of the Krebs cycle (derived from amino acid catabolism) into glucose. Lactate is also produced by muscle during anaerobic conditions and functions as part of the Cori cycle mentioned earlier. Gluconeogenesis occurs in the liver and kidney. The pathway is absent in muscle, heart, and brain tissue as well as in other organs. Although muscle and heart can use other metabolic fuels such as free fatty acids and ketone bodies (see below), the red blood cell and brain are dependent on circulating glucose, and it is for this reason that adequate blood glucose levels must be maintained. After an overnight fast, the liver produces glucose by gluconeogenesis, whereas the brain and red blood cells metabolize glucose by glycolysis; both processes occur simultaneously but in different cells.

Let us consider the general strategy of gluconeogenesis. As noted earlier, nine enzyme-catalyzed reactions are shared by glycolysis and gluconeogenesis. Three reactions of glycolysis are highly exergonic and biochemically irreversible. These are the reactions catalyzed by hexokinase, phosphofructokinase, and pyruvate kinase. The process of gluconeogenesis can be more easily understood if we consider how these three irreversible reactions are bypassed. The four enzymes involved in the bypass reactions include pyruvate carboxylase, PEP carboxykinase (both of which are required to bypass the pyruvate kinase step), fructose-1,6-bisphosphatase, and glucose-6-phosphatase.

First, we consider gluconeogenesis from lactate. Lactate is oxidized in the cytosol to form NADH and pyruvate as catalyzed by lactate dehydrogenase. The NADH is used as a reductant in the cytosol for the glyceraldehyde-3-phosphate dehydrogenase reaction of gluconeogenesis. The large negative free energy of hydrolysis of PEP (-60 kJ/mol) is an indication that PEP is energy rich, and the direct phosphorylation of pyruvate by ATP does not occur to a physiologically important extent. To overcome the thermodynamic barrier, nature uses a two-step pathway. Pyruvate is translocated into the mitochondrion, and ***pyruvate carboxylase*** catalyzes a reaction between ATP, pyruvate, and bicarbonate to yield oxaloacetate, ADP, and P_i. ***Phosphoenolpyruvate carboxykinase*** (PEP carboxykinase) then catalyzes a reaction between oxaloacetate and GTP to yield PEP, GDP, and P_i. Two high-energy bonds ($\Delta G^{\circ\prime}$ of hydrolysis of -30 kJ/mol) are expended to form the energy-rich linkage of PEP ($\Delta G^{\circ\prime} = -60$ kJ/mol). Mitochondrial phosphoenolyruvate is translocated into the cytosol in exchange for P_i.

An alternative route is operative for the conversion of pyruvate and Krebs cycle intermediates into phosphoenolpyruvate. Pyruvate, which is translocated into the mitochondrion from the cytosol, is converted to oxaloacetate by the pyruvate carboxylase reaction. As noted previously, oxaloacetate per se cannot be transported across the inner mitochondrial membrane. Oxaloacetate is converted to malate, transported outside the mitochondrion, and oxidized to yield oxaloacetate and NADH. This is the route followed by pyruvate and Krebs cycle intermediates, which, unlike lactate, do not generate cytosolic NADH. Transport of malate, however, results in the translocation of reducing equivalents to the cytosol that can be used in gluconeogenesis. Oxaloacetate is converted to PEP in a reaction catalyzed by cytosolic PEP carboxykinase. In humans, the activities of mitochondrial and cytosolic PEP carboxykinase are about equal.

Next, the enzymes of glycolysis convert phosphoenolpyruvate to fructose 1,6-bisphosphate. Circumventing the phosphofructokinase reaction, ***fructose-1,6-bisphosphatase*** catalyzes the hydrolysis of this compound to yield fructose 6-phosphate and P_i; this is an exergonic reaction and is unidirectional. After a reaction catalyzed by phosphohexose isomerase, ***glucose 6-phosphatase*** catalyzes the hydrolysis of its substrate to yield glucose and P_i; the reaction is unidirectional.

The stoichiometry for the gluconeogenesis pathway is demonstrated in the following equation:

$$\begin{array}{ccc} 2\ \text{pyruvate} & & \text{glucose} \\ + & & + \\ 2\ \text{NADH} + 2\text{H}^+ & & 2\ \text{NAD}^+ \\ + & & + \\ 2\ \text{GTP} & \rightarrow & 2\ \text{GDP} \\ + & & + \\ 2\ \text{ATP} & & 2\ \text{ADP} \\ + & & + \\ 4\ \text{H}_2\text{O} & & 4\ \text{P}_i \end{array}$$

Note that six high-energy bonds are expended and two moles of reduced NADH are required.

Let us next consider the regulation of gluconeogenesis. When glucose and insulin levels are low, there is an increase in catabolism of fatty acids in the liver. This is accompanied by an increase in the concentrations of citrate and acetyl-CoA. ***Acetyl-CoA*** is required for pyruvate carboxylase activity (the first step in gluconeogenesis). Acetyl-CoA also inhibits pyruvate dehydrogenase by activating pyruvate dehydrogenase kinase. Furthermore, citrate inhibits phosphofructokinase and decreases catabolism by glycolysis. ***Fructose 2,6-bisphosphate*** is another allosteric regulator of glycolysis and gluconeogenesis; it interacts with phosphofructokinase and fructose-1,6-bisphosphatase. Fructose 2,6-bisphosphate activates phosphofructokinase and inhibits fructose-1,6-bisphosphatase in liver. Fructose 2,6-bisphosphate promotes glycolysis. Under conditions favoring gluconeogenesis, the concentration of fructose 2,6-bisphosphate declines. This decrease removes a stimulus for phosphofructokinase and an inhibitor of fructose-1,6-bisphosphatase.

Fructose 2,6-bisphosphate is formed in a reaction involving fructose 6-phosphate and ATP; ADP is the other product. Fructose 2,6-bisphosphate is degraded by hydrolysis to form fructose 6-phosphate and P_i. A single protein contains the kinase and phosphatase activities that catalyze the formation and degradation of fructose 2,6-bisphosphate. The phosphorylation of the kinase/phosphatase by protein kinase A increases the phosphatase activity and decreases the fructose-6-phosphate 2-kinase activity. Kinase/phosphatase phosphorylation occurs under conditions of low plasma glucose and insulin, or high glucagon, levels. Agents that elevate cyclic AMP levels in the liver promote gluconeogenesis, and this observation can be used to rationalize the reciprocal effects and levels of fructose 2,6-bisphosphate.

The simultaneous operation of two opposing pathways such as glycolysis and gluconeogenesis is called a ***futile cycle.*** The net transformation of metabolites fails to occur. Futile cycles are associated with the loss of ATP, as illustrated in the following equation:

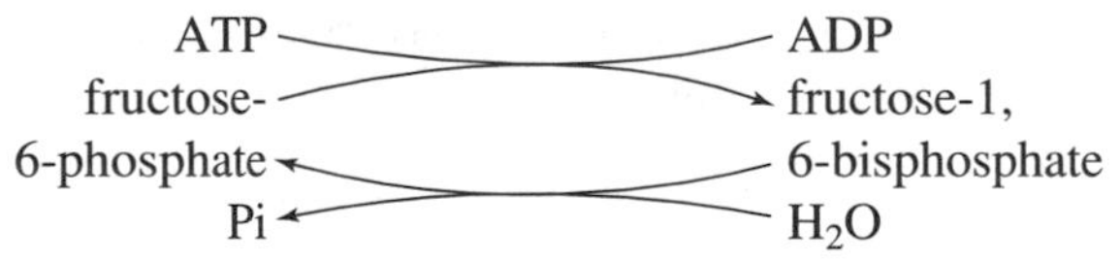

Regulatory mechanisms operate to minimize futile cycles *in vivo.*

Let us now consider the feeder pathways for other substances that serve as substrates for gluconeogenesis. Alanine is converted to pyruvate by alanine aminotransferase in one step. The resulting pyruvate is translocated into the mitochondrion and is converted to oxaloacetate and then malate, which is exported into the cytosol as a reductant and precursor of glucose. Alanine, which is mobilized from muscle, is one of the most important substrates for human gluconeogenesis. Amino acids that can be converted into Krebs cycle intermediates also serve as substrates for gluconeogenesis. They can be converted to malate in the Krebs cycle, and the subsequent reactions of gluconeogenesis follow. It appears that lactate, which produces reducing equivalents in the cytosol, eventually uses the mitochondrial PEP carboxykinase, whereas alanine and Krebs cycle intermediates are exported as malate and use the cytosolic PEP carboxykinase.

The β-oxidation of fatty acids containing an even number of carbon atoms (the most common case) yields acetyl-CoA. In humans, acetyl-CoA cannot lead to a net increase in glucose and other carbohydrates. This is because of the unidirectional nature of the Krebs cycle. After the reaction with oxaloacetate to yield citrate, two carbon atoms are eliminated during the conversion to malate (Fig. 4-21). Owing to the lack of a net increase in the number of carbon atoms in the resulting metabolite, acetyl-CoA cannot serve as a source for the net production of carbohydrate. This is the explanation for the often cited and noteworthy aphorism that fat (fatty acids) cannot be converted to carbohydrate in humans.

Pentose Phosphate Pathway

In addition to the Embden-Meyerhof glycolytic pathway, the Warburg-Dickens pentose phosphate pathway represents a scheme for the metabolism of glucose 6-phosphate. The function of the pathway is twofold. First, it is responsible for the production of biosynthetic reducing equivalents as NADPH. One of the noteworthy principles of biochemistry is that NADPH is used in biosynthetic reactions, and NADH is produced in catabolic reactions (Table 4-1). NADPH is important in fatty acid and steroid biosynthesis. The tissues and organs that exhibit high activities of the enzymes of the pentose phosphate pathway include the liver (for cholesterol and fatty acid synthesis), adrenal cortex (steroid hormone synthesis), and lactating mammary gland (lipid synthesis). The second major function of the pentose phosphate pathway is the generation of five-carbon sugars. These occur in nucleotides such as ATP, NAD^+, $NADP^+$, FAD, CoA, RNA, and DNA. We see that NADPH is produced concomitantly with pentose phosphates. However, the requirement for NADPH is generally much greater than that of the pentose phosphates. Enzymes exist that convert the pentose phosphates to triose phosphate and glucose 6-phosphate to salvage the five-carbon sugar derivatives. The pentose phosphate pathway is a flexible one and allows for the interconversion of many carbohydrate intermediates. The components of the pentose phosphate pathway and glycolysis are located in the cytosol (Table 4-2).

The pentose phosphate pathway can be divided into two portions. The first is the ***oxidative segment*** and is associated with NADPH production. The second is the ***nonoxidative segment*** and is associated with the interconversion of several pairs of sugar phosphates. These range from trioses (C_3) to heptoses (C_7). A simplified stoichiometry of the pathway is demonstrated in the following equation:

$$\text{3 glucose-6-phosphate} + 6\,NADP^+ \rightarrow \text{2 glucose-6-phosphate} + 3\,CO_2 + \text{1 glyceraldehyde-3-phosphate} + 6\,NADPH + 6\,H^+$$

Let us first consider the oxidative segment. ***Glucose 6-phosphate dehydrogenase*** catalyzes a reaction between substrate and $NADP^+$ to form 6-phosphogluconolactone and NADPH + H^+ in a reversible fashion. Next, a specific ***lactonase*** catalyzes the hydrolysis of the lactone to yield 6-phosphogluconate in a unidirectional hydrolytic reaction. ***6-Phosphogluconate dehydrogenase*** catalyzes an oxidative decarboxylation, yielding ***ribulose 5-phosphate,*** CO_2, NADPH, and H^+. Two moles of NADPH are generated per hexose phosphate. This concludes the oxidative segment.

Let us now consider the nonoxidative portion of the pathway, which involves four enzymes: two enzymes catalyze specific reactions, and two enzymes catalyze general reactions. The specific enzymes include a ***3-epimerase,*** which mediates the reversible interconversion of ribulose 5-phosphate and xylulose 5-phosphate. The second is a ***keto isomerase,*** which catalyzes the reversible interconversion of ribulose 5-phosphate (a ketopentose) and ribose 5-phosphate (an aldopentose). The two general enzymes are ***transaldolase*** and ***transketolase.*** Transaldolase contains an essential lysine residue that mediates the transfer of a three-carbon fragment from a donor to an acceptor. Transketolase contains ***thiamine pyrophosphate*** as an essential cofactor and mediates the transfer of a two-carbon ketonyl fragment to an appropriate acceptor. From the reactants and products of a reaction, one can deduce whether the enzyme is a transketolase (two-carbon transfer) or transaldolase (three-carbon transfer). The association of vitamin deficiency and alcoholism has prompted an examination of the properties of transketolase in such individuals. Initial studies suggest that the activity of transketolase is altered in alcoholism, but additional work is required to establish the significance, if any, of this finding.

Next let us consider the pathway for the transformation of 3 moles of ribulose 5-phosphate (15 carbon atoms) to 2 moles of glucose 6-phosphate (12 carbon atoms) and 1 mole of glyceraldehyde 3-phosphate (three carbon atoms). Two moles of ribulose 5-phosphate are transformed into xylulose 5-phosphate by the 3-epimerase, and 1 mole of ribulose 5-phosphate is transformed into ribose 5-phosphate by keto isomerase. Then transketolase transfers a two-carbon fragment from xylulose 5-phosphate to ribose 5-phosphate to form sedoheptulose 7-phosphate and glyceraldehyde 3-phosphate. Transaldolase then operates on these two substrates and transfers a three-carbon fragment from sedoheptulose-7-phosphate to glyceraldehyde 3-phosphate, yielding fructose 6-phosphate and erythrose 4-phosphate. Fructose 6-phosphate can be metabolized by glycolysis or converted to glucose 6-phosphate and metabolized by the pentose phosphate pathway. Transketolase then catalyzes the transfer of a two-carbon fragment from xylulose 5-phosphate and erythrose 4-phosphate to yield fructose 6-phosphate and glyceraldehyde 3-phosphate. Both compounds are intermediates for glycolysis or gluconeogenesis and will be further metabolized depending on metabolic need. Despite extensive investigation, knowledge of the mechanism of regulation of the pentose phosphate pathway is incomplete. The $NADP^+$/NADPH ratio is considered to be important. A high ratio promotes pentose phosphate cycle activity at the glucose-6-phosphate dehydrogenase step. Insulin action may also lead to induction of enzymes of the pathway.

The pentose phosphate pathway plays an important role in maintaining the mature erythrocyte. The pentose phosphate pathway provides NADPH for the reduction of oxidized glutathione. ***Glutathione*** is a tripeptide (γ-glutamylcysteinylglycine). Glutathione exists as the reduced (G–SH) and oxidized forms (G–S–S–G). ***Glutathione reductase*** converts the oxidized to the reduced form:

$$\begin{matrix} \text{GSSG} & & \text{2 GSH} \\ + & \longrightarrow & + \\ \text{NADPH} + H^+ & & NADP^+ \end{matrix}$$

Reduced glutathione is a substrate for ***glutathione peroxidase*** (selenium is a cofactor, Table 4-3):

$$2\ \text{GSH} + H_2O_2 \rightarrow \text{GSSG} + 2\ H_2O$$

Glutathione peroxidase plays an important role in destroying H_2O_2 in the erythrocyte. Recall that the mature erythrocyte lacks membranous cellular organelles, such as peroxisomes, which are found in nucleated cells. Catalase in peroxisomes mediates the conversion of H_2O_2 to water and molecular oxygen ($H_2O_2 \rightarrow H_2O + \frac{1}{2} O_2$). Glutathione peroxidase functions in the red blood cell to destroy H_2O_2, as catalase functions in other cells. A deficiency of glucose 6-phosphate dehydrogenase is associated with drug-induced hemolytic anemias produced by primaquine (an antimalarial agent) and a variety of other substances. Hemolysis may be related to deficient NADPH production for the glutathione peroxidase reaction.

Fatty Acid Metabolism

The important classes of lipids in humans include triglycerides (triacylglycerols), phospholipids, and steroids. Triglyceride serves as the main storage form of metabolic fuel in humans. Triglyceride is the most concentrated form of metabolic energy (9 kcal/g). Moreover, triglyceride, which is stored in an anhydrous state, represents an average of 19% of the total body mass (the percentage varies considerably among individuals from a minimum of about 9%). Triglyceride can subserve humans for weeks or months of starvation. In contrast, stored carbo-

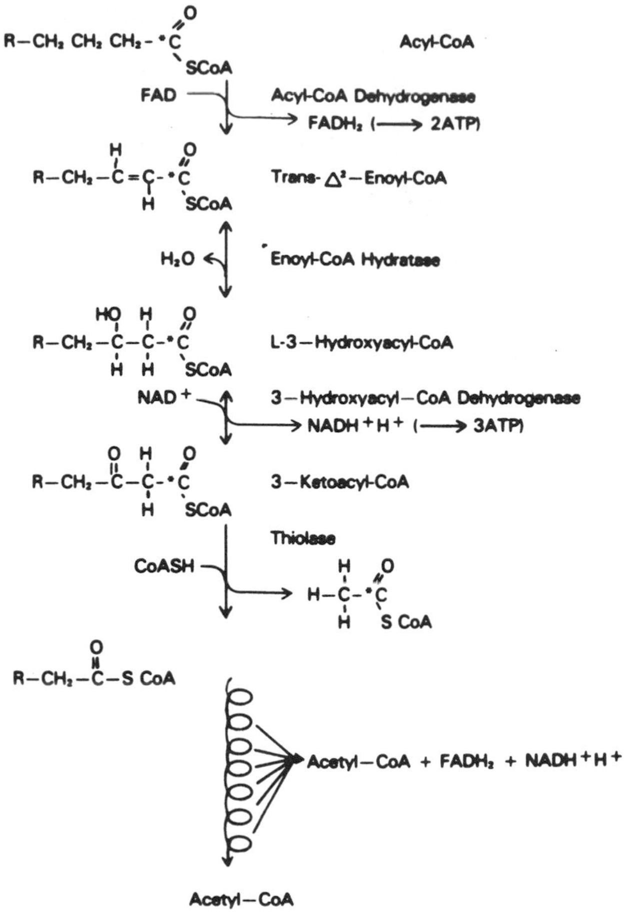

Fig. 4-30. *β*-oxidation of fatty acyl-CoA.

hydrate is depleted in a day or so and must be replenished by gluconeogenesis. Glycogen is extensively hydrated, and this increases its bulk. A gram of tissue glycogen contains an equivalent amount of bound water. Glycogen does not represent as efficient an energy storage form as triglyceride does. Amino acids and proteins are not stored to any appreciable extent in humans.

Fatty acids stored in adipose tissue are released from triglycerides by hydrolysis reactions catalyzed by triglyceride lipase. This enzyme is also called ***hormone-sensitive lipase*** because it responds to circulating epinephrine by undergoing phosphorylation by protein kinase A and concomitant activation. Hormone-sensitive lipase, moreover, is inhibited by the action of insulin. The liberated fatty acids, bound to albumin, are transported in the circulation, and the fatty acids are taken up by most organs or tissues (except the brain). After entering the cells, the fatty acids must be derivatized as thioesters with CoA before metabolism. A family of ***fatty acyl–CoA synthetases*** and a single ***pyrophosphatase*** catalyze these reactions in the cytosol.

(a) $$\text{fatty acid} + \text{ATP} + \text{coenzyme A} \rightleftharpoons \text{fatty acyl-CoA} + \text{AMP} + \text{PP}_i$$

(b) $$\text{PP}_i + H_2O \rightarrow 2\ \text{P}_i$$

The first part of the reaction involves the formation of an intermediate fatty acyladenylate and PP_i. In the second part of the reaction, CoA displaces adenylate to yield fatty acyl–CoA and AMP. The family of fatty acyl–CoA synthetases differs in chain length specificity. Long-chain (16 carbon atoms or more), intermediate-chain (six to 14 carbon atoms), and short-chain (two to four carbon atoms) specific enzymes have been described. Thioesters are energy-rich bonds. To pull the reaction forward, as mentioned in Table 4-1, pyrophosphatase (a separate enzyme) catalyzes the hydrolysis of PP_i to yield two P_i molecules in an exergonic and unidirectional reaction.

As noted previously, CoA and its derivatives do not pass through the inner mitochondrial membrane. To effect the transfer of fatty acids into the mitochondrial matrix (the site of fatty acid oxidation; Table 4-2), the formation of fatty acylcarnitine is required. This isoergonic process is catalyzed by carnitine acyltransferase I:

$$\begin{matrix} \text{fatty acyl-CoA} & & \text{fatty acylcarnitine} \\ + & \rightleftharpoons & + \\ \text{carnitine} & & \text{coenzyme A} \end{matrix}$$

The fatty acylcarnitine is transported into mitochondria in exchange for carnitine. Once inside the mitochondrion, carnitine acyltransferase II catalyzes the reverse reaction, yielding fatty acyl–CoA and free carnitine. Carnitine ($[CH_3]_3N^+CH_2CH[OH]CH_2COO^-$) forms an ester linkage through its *β*-OH group with the carboxyl group of the fatty acid.

β-OXIDATION

The conversion of fatty acyl–CoA to acetyl-CoA requires the action of four enzymes. The stoichiometry for the conversion of stearoyl-CoA (C_{18}) to 9 moles of acetyl-CoA is described as follows:

$$\begin{matrix} \text{steroyl-CoA} & & \text{9 acetyl-CoA} \\ + & & + \\ \text{8 FAD} & & \text{8 FADH}_2 \\ + & \rightarrow & + \\ \text{8 NAD}^+ & & \text{8 NADH} + \text{8 H}^+ \\ + & & \\ \text{8 coenzyme A} & & \end{matrix}$$

The cyclic pathway for *β*-oxidation is illustrated in Figure 4-30. An ***acyl–CoA dehydrogenase*** catalyzes an isoergonic oxidation to yield *trans*-enoyl-CoA and $FADH_2$. The reducing equivalents are donated to the electron transport chain at the level of coenzyme Q and provide energy for the formation of 1.5 moles of ATP per mole of $FADH_2$. Next, ***enoyl-CoA hydratase*** catalyzes an isoergonic hydration yielding an L-β-hydroxyacyl–CoA. The resulting compound is oxidized by NAD^+ in a reaction catalyzed by ***hydroxyacyl–CoA dehydrogenase*** to give β-ketoacyl–CoA, NADH, and H^+. Oxidation of 1 mole NADH by the respiratory chain yields 2.5 moles of ATP. Next, ***β-ketothiolase*** (thiolase) catalyzes an exergonic cleavage or thiolysis by CoA to yield acetyl-CoA and a fatty acyl–CoA lacking the two carbon atoms. For stearoyl-CoA, the β-oxidation spiral (Fig. 4-30) occurs eight times.

This series of reactions in β-oxidation can be more easily remembered and understood by comparison with three analogous reactions in the Krebs cycle. The pattern of the first oxidation in β-oxidation by FAD is analogous to the succinate dehydrogenase reaction. The hydration reaction in β-oxidation parallels that catalyzed by fumarase. Finally, the oxidation of an alcohol by NAD^+ to form a ketone parallels that of the malate dehydrogenase reaction.

Let us now consider the number of moles of ATP formed from ADP and P_i as a result of the β-oxidation of the 18-carbon stearic acid and reactions of the Krebs cycle and oxidative phosphorylation. The value is shown in Table 4-12. The net production of ATP takes into account the requirement that the fatty acid must be converted to a CoA derivative with the expenditure of two high-energy bonds ($ATP + H_2O \rightarrow AMP + 2\ P_i$).

A small percentage of fatty acids in the human diet contains an odd number of carbon atoms. These fatty acids undergo β-oxidation and yield propionyl-CoA (propionate = C_3) and acetyl-CoA (acetate = C_2) after the final thiolytic cleavage. Propionyl-CoA is also produced during the catabolism of several amino acids (valine, isoleucine, and methionine). The pathway for the metabolism of propionyl-CoA is quantitatively more important for amino acid metabolism than for the metabolism of the uncommon odd-chain fatty acids. Propionyl-CoA metabolism requires the participation of vitamin B_{12}, and this is a distinctive property.

TABLE 4-12. ATP Yield from the Complete Oxidation of Stearic Acid (C_{18})

PROCESS	ATP RESULTING	
8 $FADH_2$	8 × 1.5	12
8 NADH + 8 H^+	8 × 2.5	20
9 Acetyl-CoA	9 × 10	90
		122
ATP required for stearyl-CoA formation*		−2
Net ATP production		120

* $ATP \rightarrow AMP + 2\ P_i$

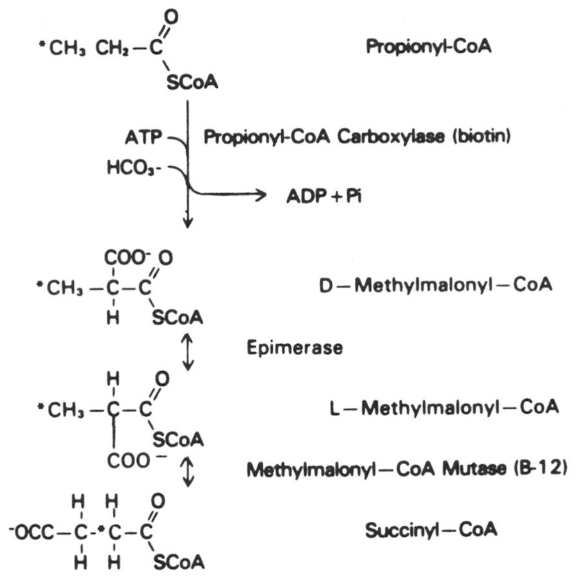

Fig. 4-31. Conversion of propionyl-CoA to succinyl-CoA.

Propionyl-CoA carboxylase catalyzes a reaction between substrate, bicarbonate, and ATP to yield D-methylmalonyl-CoA, ADP, and P_i (Fig. 4-31). This ATP-dependent carboxylation reaction, like several others, involves a biotin prosthetic group. An ***epimerase*** catalyzes an isoergonic conversion of D-methylmalonyl-CoA to the L-isomer. ***Methylmalonyl-CoA mutase*** (a vitamin B_{12}–dependent enzyme) catalyzes the conversion of L-methylmalonyl-CoA to succinyl-CoA. The carbonyl-SCoA is transferred to the carbon marked with the asterisk to yield the final product (Fig. 4-31). Succinyl-CoA is an intermediate in the Krebs cycle and is metabolized by familiar reactions. The association of ***vitamin B_{12}*** with ***methylmalonyl-CoA mutase*** is noteworthy.

The metabolism of fatty acids with double bonds beginning at even-numbered carbon atoms, such as the Δ^{12} position of linoleate, requires two additional enzyme activities not required for saturated fatty acid metabolism: ***2,4-dienoyl-CoA reductase*** and ***enoyl-CoA isomerase.*** A Δ^2-*trans*,Δ^4-*cis* double bond results from the action of acyl-CoA dehydrogenase on linoleate. 2,4-Dienoyl-CoA reductase catalyzes a reaction of the substrate with ***NADPH*** to form a Δ^3-*trans* derivative. Note that this is an unusual case where NADPH is required for catabolism. Enoyl-CoA isomerase catalyzes the conversion of the Δ^3-*trans* derivative to the Δ^2-*trans* derivative, a substrate for the hydratase of β-oxidation. The metabolism of fatty acids with double bonds beginning at odd-numbered carbon atoms, such as the Δ^9 position of linoleate, requires a third enzyme—***3,5-dienoyl-CoA isomerase.*** A Δ^2-*trans*,Δ^4-*cis* metabolite of linoleate is acted on by enoyl-CoA isomerase to form a Δ^3-*trans*,Δ^5-*cis* derivative. This substrate for 3,5-dienoyl-CoA isomerase is converted to a *Δ^2-trans,Δ^4-trans* metabolite that is in turn a substrate for 2,4-dienoyl-CoA reductase. The resulting *Δ^3-trans* compound is a substrate for enoyl-CoA isomerase, and β-oxidation can proceed.

BIOSYNTHESIS

The reactions of fatty acid biosynthesis take place on a ***fatty acid synthase multienzyme complex.*** A priming reaction using acetyl-CoA initiates the process. Then malonyl-CoA adds successive two-carbon fragments to the primer. After each addition, four reactions convert a β-ketoacyl compound to the reduced acyl derivative. NADPH serves as reductant. The fatty acid synthase contains ***acyl carrier protein*** (ACP). This is a small protein containing covalently bound ***4′-phosphopantetheine.*** The latter constitutes part of the molecular structure of CoA, and ACP can be considered to represent protein-bound CoA. ACP carries covalently linked intermediates from the various active sites necessary for biosynthesis. The −SH group of ACP is called the ***central thiol.*** An enzymic cysteine constitutes a ***peripheral thiol.*** After the 16-carbon palmitoyl group is formed, free palmitate is released by hydrolysis.

Let us now consider the pathway for palmitate biosynthesis. Acetyl-CoA initiates the process by reacting with the multienzyme complex to yield an acetyl-enzyme thioester intermediate involving the peripheral thiol group. This acetyl group contributes carbon atoms 15 and 16 of the 16-carbon palmitate. They are at the omega *(ω)* end of the fatty acid, that is, the farthest removed from the carboxyl group. The other 14-carbon atoms are contributed by malonyl-CoA. Let us consider the formation of malonyl-CoA as catalyzed by ***acetyl-CoA carboxylase:***

$$\text{ATP} + \text{HCO}_3^- + \text{acetyl-CoA} \rightleftharpoons \text{malonyl-CoA} + \text{ADP} + \text{P}_i$$

Acetyl-CoA carboxylase is the rate-limiting step in fatty acid biosynthesis and is activated by citrate. Malonyl-CoA reacts with the acetyl-fatty acid synthase complex to yield CoA and the malonyl group bound to the central thiol of ACP (Fig. 4-32).

The sequential series of reactions begins as the α-carbon of malonyl-ACP attacks the carbonyl group of acetyl-CoA in a condensation reaction catalyzed by ***3-ketoacyl***

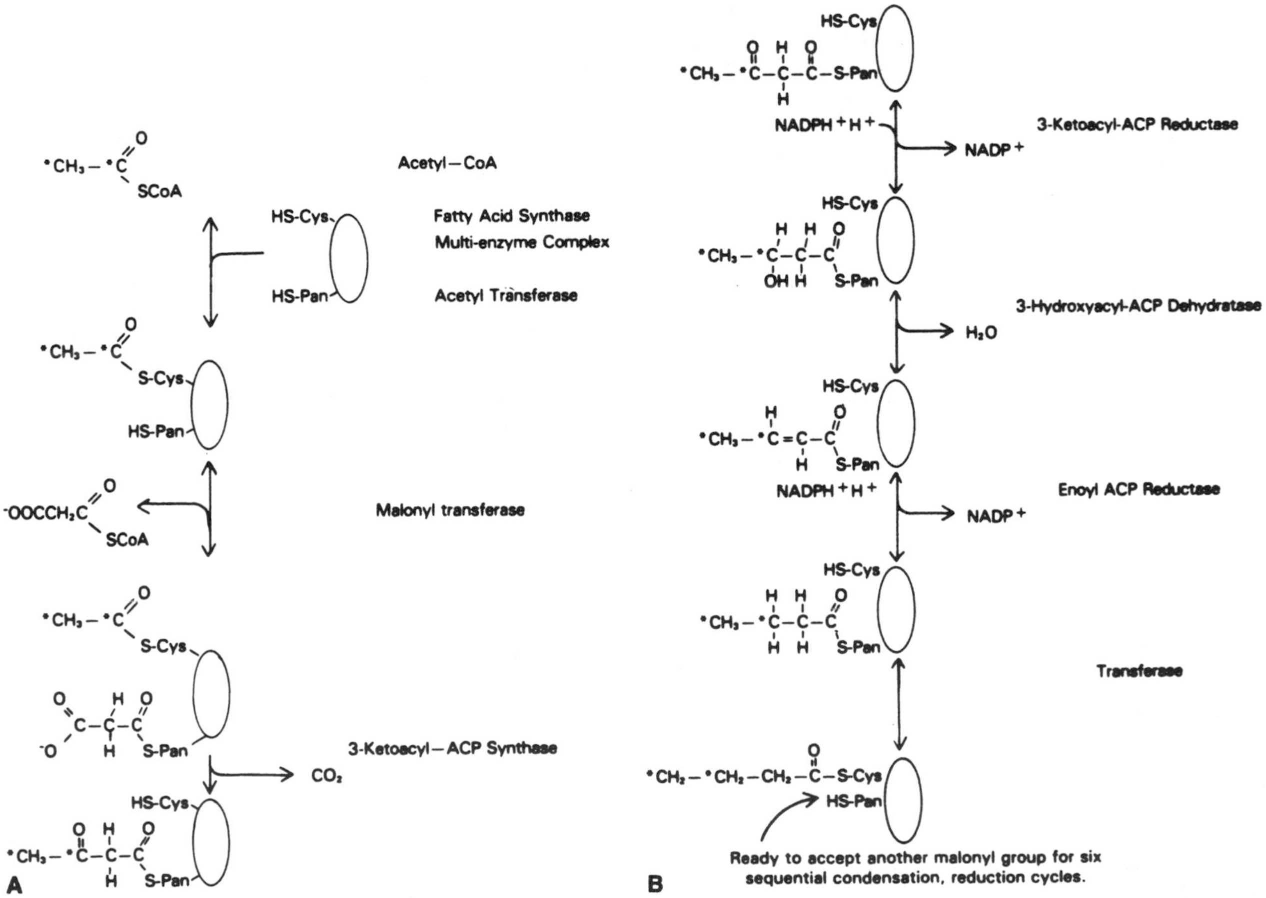

Fig. 4-32. Pathway for fatty acid biosynthesis.

synthase (Fig. 4-32). A β-ketoacyl group is attached to the central thiol as the peripheral thiol is freed, and carbon dioxide is displaced. This decarboxylation renders the process exergonic. The exergonic decarboxylation accounts for the formation and use of the malonyl group; the carboxyl group activates the tail of the acetyl group within malonyl-CoA for this condensation reaction. A ***3-ketoacyl reductase*** catalyzes a reaction with NADPH + H^+ to form D-β-hydroxyacyl–ACP and $NADP^+$. A ***dehydratase*** catalyzes the elimination of water, yielding a 2,3-unsaturated acyl-ACP. An ***enoyl reductase*** catalyzes a reaction with NADPH + H^+ to yield acyl-ACP. The acyl group, now elongated by two carbons, is parked on the peripheral thiol. Next, malonyl-CoA reacts with the acyl-enzyme, and the malonyl group is linked to the central thiol. This is followed by another condensation reaction resulting in the formation of a β-ketoacyl group elongated by two carbon atoms, and carbon dioxide is the other product. The sequence of reactions is repeated as a reduction, dehydration, and second reduction occurs. The acyl group is transferred to the peripheral thiol.

A total of seven condensation reactions is required to produce the palmitoyl-enzyme. A thioesterase catalyzes the hydrolytic cleavage and release of palmitate, and the free enzyme is regenerated. That fatty acids longer than palmitate cannot be synthesized by the complex is probably related to a limitation in the size of one of the active sites of the complex. In a figurative sense, the fatty acid synthase complex counts to 16 carbons and releases palmitate.

A comparison of fatty acid oxidation and synthesis is given in Table 4-13. The separate pathways and intracellular localization (Table 4-2) permit independent regulation of the processes. Although carbon dioxide as bicarbonate is required for malonyl-CoA formation, the added carbonyl group is released during the condensation reactions, and bicarbonate is not a direct source of the carbon atoms in fatty acids. All the carbon atoms are derived from acetyl-CoA; the two on the ω-end are derived directly from acetyl-CoA, and the others are derived from malonyl-CoA.

TABLE 4-13. Comparison of Fatty Acid Oxidation and Synthesis

	OXIDATION	SYNTHESIS *de novo*
Acetyl-CoA required	+	+
Malonyl-CoA required	−	+
NAD^-	+	−
NADPH	+	+
CoA	+	+
ACP (acyl carrier protein)	−	+
Mitochondria	+	−
Cytosol	−	+
Multienzyme complex	−	+
L-Hydroxyacyl intermediate	+	−
D-Hydroxyacyl intermediate	−	+

Let us now consider the source of NADPH and acetyl-CoA used as substrates for palmitate biosynthesis. In liver, which is the predominant triglyceride-synthesizing organ in humans, most of the NADPH is derived from the pentose phosphate pathway. In adipocytes, about half the NADPH results from the reaction catalyzed by ***malic enzyme*** (NADP-malate dehydrogenase) shown here:

$$\text{malate} + NADP^+ \rightarrow \text{pyruvate} + CO_2 + NADPH + H^+$$

The producers and consumers of NADPH occur within the cytosol, so that no barrier to effective use occurs.

The provision of cytosolic acetyl-CoA, however, requires transport across the mitochondrial membrane. Glucose serves as the source of carbon atoms for much of the fatty acid biosynthesis that occurs in the liver. Glucose is converted to pyruvate by glycolysis. Pyruvate is transported into the mitochondrion by its specific translocase and is converted to acetyl-CoA in a reaction catalyzed by pyruvate dehydrogenase. CoA and its derivatives are not directly transportable through the inner membrane. The transport of acetyl groups occurs via citrate. Citrate is formed by the usual Krebs cycle reaction involving acetyl-CoA, oxaloacetate, and water. Citrate is transported through the inner mitochondrial membrane in exchange for malate. Once in the cytosol, ***ATP-citrate lyase*** (citrate cleavage enzyme) catalyzes a reaction with substrate, CoA, and ATP to yield acetyl-CoA, oxaloacetate, ADP, and P_i. Acetyl-CoA then functions as a precursor for fatty acid formation. Oxaloacetate is reduced to malate and can be transported into the mitochondrion in exchange for citrate.

The provision of cytosolic acetyl-CoA by mitochondrial citrate provides a likely explanation for the regulation of the Krebs cycle at the isocitrate dehydrogenase reaction. This allows for the biosynthesis of citrate and still permits the regulation of the Krebs cycle by ADP at a distal step, that is, at the isocitrate dehydrogenase reaction. Also note that cytosolic citrate activates the acetyl-CoA carboxylase reaction (the rate-limiting reaction in fatty acid biosynthesis). Citrate serves both as a precursor and feed-forward activator of fatty acid biosynthesis.

Lipid Metabolism

TRIGLYCERIDE BIOSYNTHESIS

The precursors for triglyceride, or triacylglycerol, synthesis include 3 moles of fatty acyl–CoA and glycerol phosphate. The palmitate produced by synthesis *de novo* is thioesterified as palmitoyl-CoA in a reaction catalyzed by fatty acyl–CoA synthetase. Fatty acid, ATP, and CoA are reactants, and fatty acyl–CoA, AMP, and PP_i are products. Palmitoyl-CoA also may be elongated, desaturated, or both before incorporation into triglyceride. Dietary fatty acids, derived from triglyceride, are a major precursor of stored triglyceride. Glycerol phosphate can be obtained by the reduction of dihydroxyacetone phosphate catalyzed by ***glycerol phosphate dehydrogenase*** or by the ATP-dependent phosphorylation of glycerol as catalyzed by ***glycerol kinase.*** The fatty acyl–CoA groups are energy-rich and activated forms of fatty acids, which are logical donors in biosynthetic reactions. The following four reactions yield triglyceride. Glycerol phosphate acyltransferase catalyzes the first reaction between fatty acyl–CoA, which is activated like a warhead, and glycerol 3-phosphate to yield 1-acylglycerol 3-phosphate. An acyltransferase catalyzes the addition of the next acyl group from fatty acyl–CoA (usually unsaturated) to yield 1,2-diacylglycerol 3-phosphate (also called phosphatidate) as shown in Figure 4-33. Next, a phosphatidate phosphatase catalyzes a hydrolysis to yield 1,2-diacylglycerol and P_i. Finally, 1,2-diacylglycerol acyltransferase catalyzes a reaction of diacylglycerol with fatty acyl–CoA to yield triacylglycerol, or triglyceride, and CoA. Each of the four reactions is highly exergonic. The fatty acid thioesterified to CoA constitutes a high-energy and activated form of the fatty acid. Activated monomers serve as energetically favorable precursors in condensation reactions (Table 4-1).

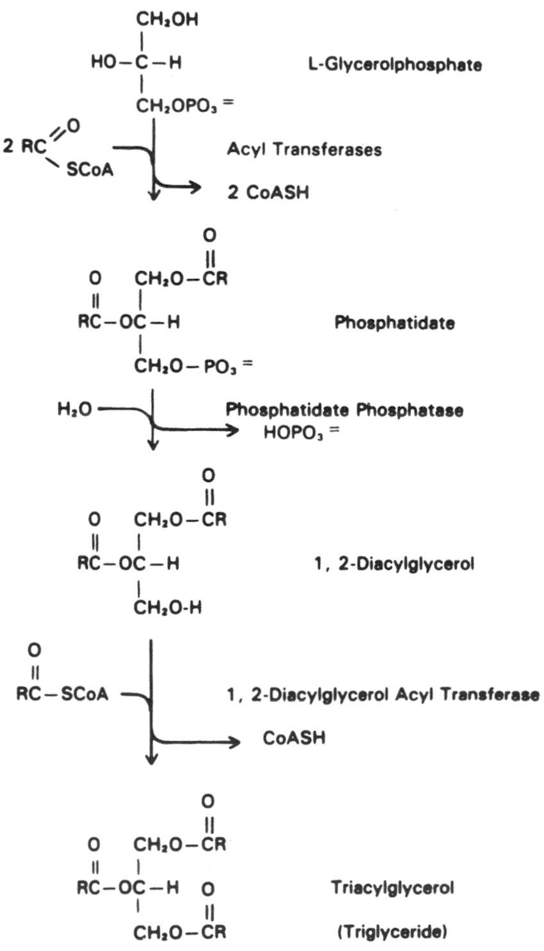

Fig. 4-33. Biosynthesis of triacylglycerol.

PHOSPHOLIPID BIOSYNTHESIS

Important phospholipids include ***phosphatidylcholine (lecithin), phosphatidylserine,*** and ***phosphatidylethanolamine.*** The latter two compounds can be converted into phosphatidylcholine. Let us consider the pathway for phosphatidylcholine formation beginning with free choline and 1,2-diacylglycerol. This is called the salvage pathway because preformed choline is salvaged or used. In contrast, in the *de novo* pathway, choline is formed from phosphatidylethanolamine.

In the first step of the salvage pathway for phosphatidylcholine biosynthesis, choline is phosphorylated by ATP to yield phosphocholine and ADP in a reaction catalyzed by choline kinase (Fig. 4-34). Phosphocholine must now be converted to an activated or energy-rich form before combining with an acceptor molecule (Table 4-1). The activated form is cytidine diphosphate–choline (CDP-choline). The diphosphate linkage is that of an acid anhydride and is energy rich with a $\Delta G^{\circ\prime}$ of hydrolysis of -30 kJ/mol. The activation process involves a reaction of cytidine triphosphate (CTP) and phosphocholine to yield CDP-choline and PP_i and is catalyzed by CTP-phosphocholine cytidyltransferase. The number of high-energy bonds is the same in the reactants and products, and this is an isoergonic reaction. The process is coupled to the hydrolysis of PP_i catalyzed by pyrophosphatase, which serves to pull the reaction forward (Table 4-1). CDP-choline reacts with 1,2-diacylglycerol to yield phosphatidylcholine and cytidine monophosphate (CMP) in a reaction catalyzed by a choline phosphotransferase.

The pathway for phosphatidylethanolamine biosynthesis is analogous to that for phosphatidylcholine biosynthesis by the salvage pathway. Ethanolamine is phosphorylated by ATP to form ethanolamine phosphate (Fig. 4-35). The latter reacts with CTP to form CDP-ethanolamine, which then reacts with 1,2-diacylglycerol to form phosphatidylethanolamine. Phosphatidylethanolamine can be converted into phosphatidylcholine by three successive transmethylation reactions involving *S*-adenosylmethionine (Fig. 4-35). Phosphatidylethanolamine and phosphatidylcholine occur in the lipid bilayer of cell membranes.

Another cytidine derivative important in lipid metabo-

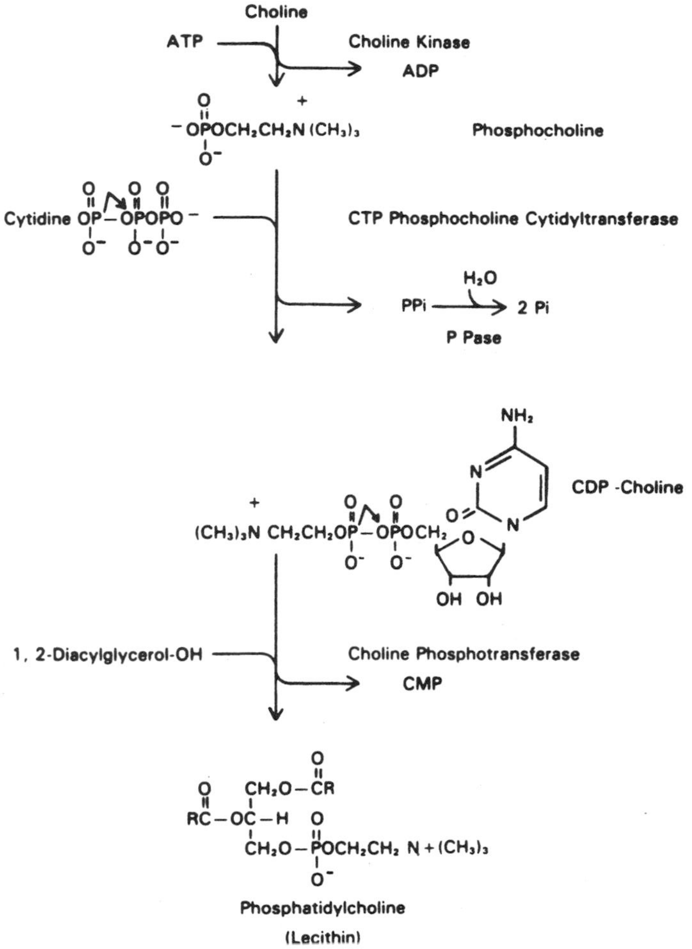

Fig. 4-34. Phosphatidylcholine biosynthesis by the salvage pathway.

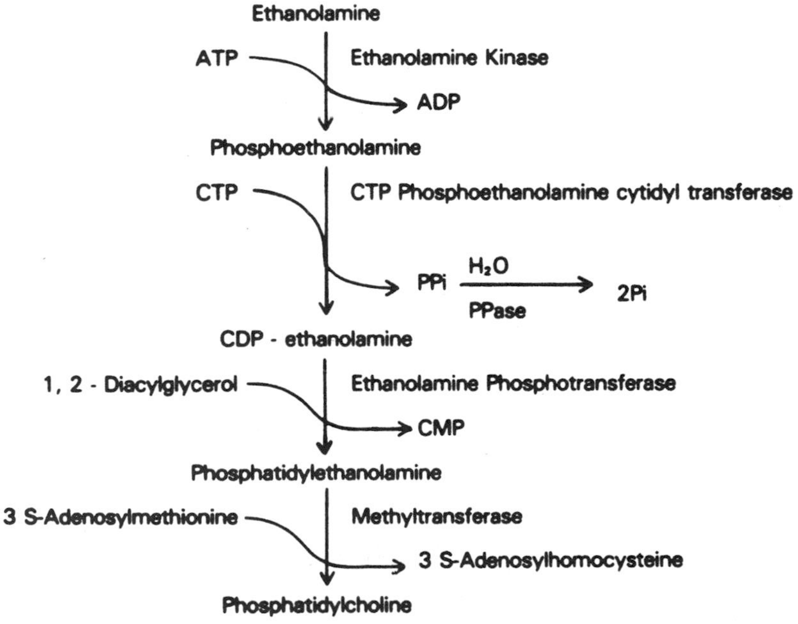

Fig. 4-35. Phosphatidylcholine biosynthesis *de novo.*

lism is CDP-diacylglycerol. CDP-diacylglycerol results from a reaction involving phosphatidate and CTP and yields CDP-diacylglycerol and PP_i. CDP-diacylglycerol reacts with inositol (a hexitol) to form phosphatidylinositol and CMP. Phosphatidylinositol is phosphorylated by ATP to form ADP and phosphatidylinositol 4-phosphate (PIP). The latter is phosphorylated by ATP to form ADP and phosphatidylinositol 4,5-bisphosphate (PIP_2). PIP_2 is an important precursor for two intracellular second messengers: inositol 1,4,5-trisphosphate (IP_3) and diacylglycerol, or diglyceride. The physiological roles of these agents are discussed later.

SPHINGOLIPID BIOSYNTHESIS

This group of phospholipids contains a complex amino alcohol named sphingosine; sphingolipids lack glycerol. ***Sphingosine*** is formed in a three-step process from palmitoyl-CoA and serine. In a reaction catalyzed by a pyridoxal phosphate–dependent enzyme, the 16-carbon palmitoyl-CoA reacts with the three-carbon serine to yield the 18-carbon dehydrosphinganine (3-ketosphinganine), carbon dioxide (from serine), and CoA (Fig. 4-36). Dihydrosphingosine reacts with acyl-CoA to form CoA and *N*-acyldihydrosphingosine. The latter is oxidized to yield *N*-acylsphingosine, or ceramide.

Ceramide (*N*-acylsphingosine) is a key intermediate in sphingolipid biosynthesis. Ceramide is converted to ***sphingomyelin*** (*O*-phosphocholine ceramide) after a reaction with CDP-choline. Ceramide is also converted to ***cerebrosides*** and ***gangliosides.*** The alcohol group of ceramide reacts with an activated UDP-sugar to yield cerebroside and UDP (Fig. 4-37). The addition of several (up to five) sugars to ceramide yields a family of gangliosides. These are glycolipids (sugars attached to lipid).

PHOSPHOLIPID DEGRADATION

The specificity of several phospholipases is indicated in Figure 4-38. Two phospholipases have been implicated in several regulatory processes. Phospholipase A_2, for example, catalyzes the hydrolysis of the fatty acid at C^2 of the derivatized glycerol. Arachidonate and other polyunsaturated fatty acids are often attached to C^2. Arachidonate is converted into biologically active eicosanoids (prostaglandins [PGs], prostacyclins [PGIs], thromboxanes [TXs], and leukotrienes [LTs]). Phospholipase A_2 is the rate-limiting enzyme in eicosanoid biosynthesis. Phospholipase C catalyzes the removal of a sugar alcohol at position 3. Important products derived from phosphatidylinositol 4,5-bisphosphate include inositol trisphosphate (IP_3) and diacylglycerol, or diglyceride.

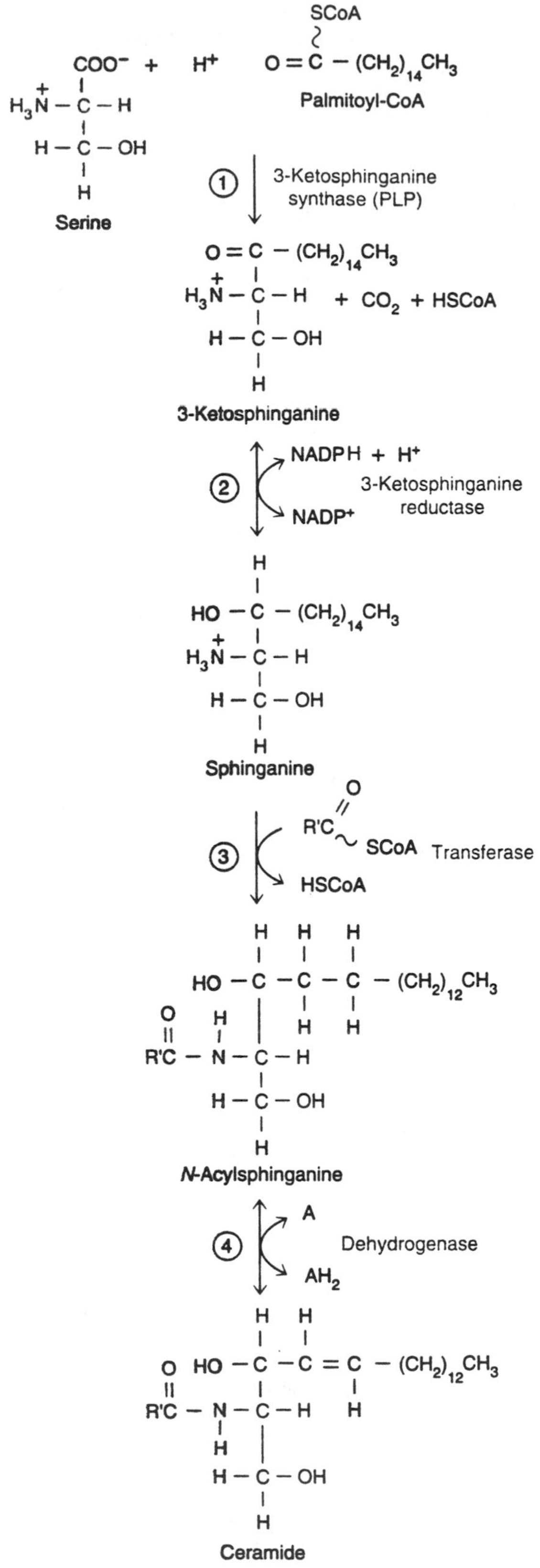

Fig. 4-36. Conversion of palmitoyl-CoA and serine to sphingosine.

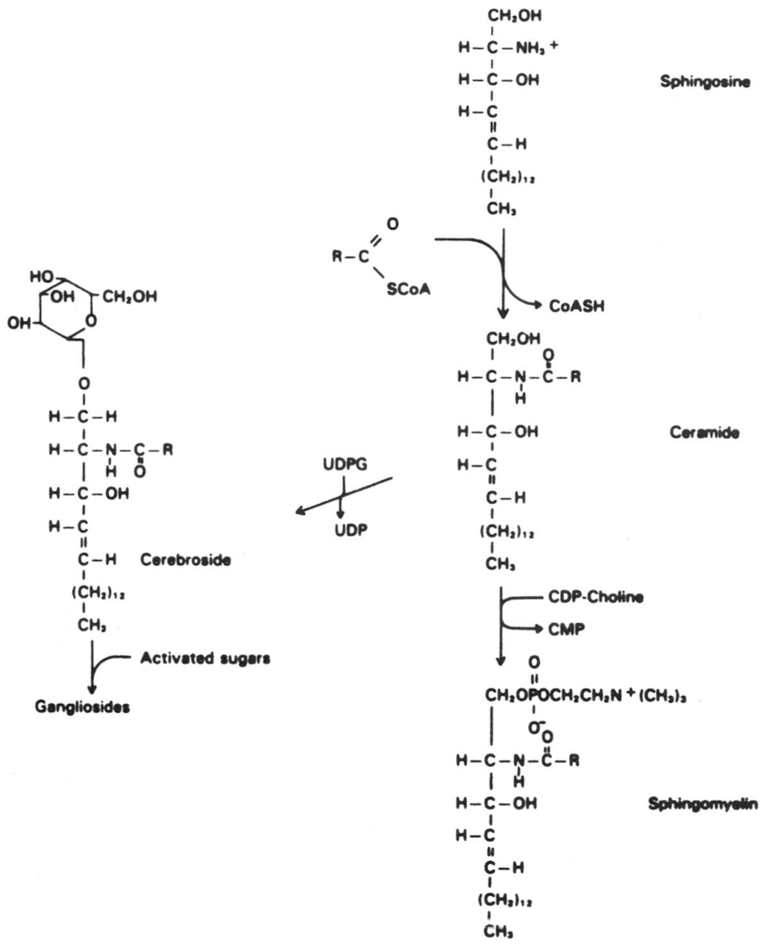

Fig. 4-37. Sphingomyelin and ganglioside biosynthesis.

SPHINGOLIPID DEGRADATION

A number of diseases, called ***sphingolipidoses,*** are caused by the deficiency of a lysosomal enzyme that catalyzes the hydrolysis of sphingolipids. Selected sphingolipidoses are listed in Table 4-14. In the absence of hydrolytic activity, the sphingolipid that cannot be degraded accumulates and produces the characteristic pathology. The diseases have been known much longer than has the existence and functions of lysosomes. Basic research has provided an intellectual and scientific framework for understanding these disorders. It is possible to diagnose affected individuals *in utero*. Diagnosis is based on enzyme activity measurements or DNA analysis. The design of curative or effective palliative treatment has yet to be developed.

Ketone Body Metabolism

Ketone bodies are a group of three related compounds including ***acetoacetate, β-hydroxybutyrate,*** and ***acetone.*** The condition of ketosis occurs during carbohydrate deprivation and starvation. A more severe form of ketosis is that of diabetic ketoacidosis. Ketosis occurs in humans during the extensive mobilization of fatty acids. Ketone bodies are synthesized, but not used by the liver. They are transported to extrahepatic tissues, where they are metabolized to provide reducing equivalents for oxidative phosphorylation. Although a paradoxical contradiction in terms, ketone bodies can be considered as water-soluble lipids.

Let us first consider the biosynthesis of ketone bodies. Like fatty acids, ketone bodies are derived from acetyl-CoA. Two moles of acetyl-CoA condense to yield acetoacetyl-CoA and CoA. This process constitutes the reversal of the ***thiolase*** reaction of β-oxidation and is endergonic. Acetoacetyl-CoA is also produced by β-oxidation per se. One might envisage the synthesis of acetoacetate by hydrolysis of its CoA thioester. However, this pathway is not prominent or is nonexistent. The absence of such a hydrolytic enzyme prevents the loss of acetoacetyl-CoA formed during the course of the β-oxidation of fatty acids. Acetyl-CoA condenses with acetoacetyl-CoA followed by hydrolysis of one thioester bond to yield CoA and 3-hydroxy-3-methylglutaryl-CoA (HMG-CoA) in a highly exergonic reaction catalyzed by ***HMG-CoA synthase.***

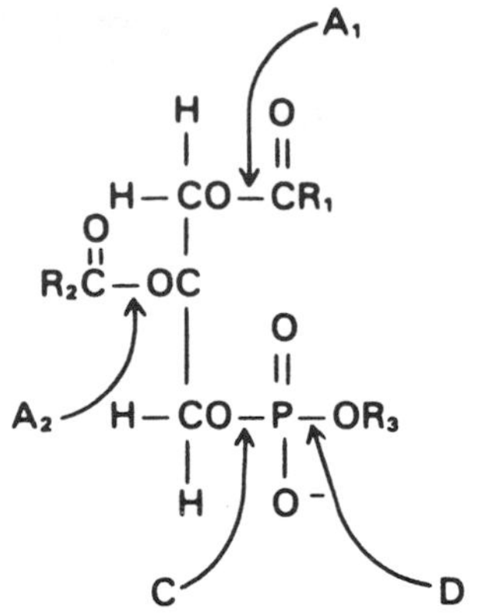

Fig. 4-38. Bonds hydrolyzed by phospholipases A_1, A_2, C, and D.

HMG-CoA is a substrate for ***HMG-CoA lyase,*** which catalyzes the nonhydrolytic conversion of substrate to acetoacetate and acetyl-CoA. HMG-CoA synthase and lyase occur in liver mitochondria. This localization accounts for the exclusive production of ketone bodies by the liver. This pathway is active under conditions that favor fatty acid oxidation.

A portion of acetoacetate is reduced to form β-hydroxybutyrate by β-hydroxybutyrate dehydrogenase. β-Hydroxybutyrate dehydrogenase is found in liver and extrahepatic tissues. The reaction is reversible and functions *in vivo* in both directions depending on metabolic need. Acetoacetate undergoes a nonenzymatic decarboxylation reaction to yield CO_2 and acetone. Acetone constitutes a metabolic dead end and is excreted in the urine or exhaled by the lungs. It does not form to a significant extent during human fasting. However, small amounts form during diabetic ketoacidosis. A suggestive diagnosis of ketoacidosis can be made by smelling acetone in the breath of a comatose patient. It is reminiscent of the odor associated with fruity chewing gums.

β-Hydroxybutyrate and acetoacetate are transported from the liver to extrahepatic organs, where they are taken up by cells. The β-hydroxybutyrate is oxidized to acetoacetate. Acetoacetate is derivatized in mitochondria in a reaction catalyzed by succinyl-CoA:acetoacetyl-CoA transferase; CoA is transferred from succinyl-CoA, yielding succinate and acetoacetyl-CoA. The latter is a substrate for thiolase and yields 2 moles of acetyl-CoA. The HMG-CoA synthase and lyase in the liver explain ketone body synthesis there. Liver tissue lacks the CoA transferase, which is present in extrahepatic tissues. The distribution of the enzymes explains why ketone bodies are not catabolized in the liver but are catabolized in other tissues.

Cholesterol Metabolism

Cholesterol is an essential constituent of human cell membranes, and depriving mammalian cells of cholesterol results in cell death. ***Cholesterol*** makes up about 40% by mass of the Golgi and plasma membranes, but it is present to a lesser extent in the endoplasmic reticulum and nuclear membranes. Cholesterol is converted by the liver into ***bile salts,*** which are important in lipid digestion and in absorption from the intestine. Cholesterol is also converted into steroid hormones, including estradiol, progesterone, testosterone, cortisol, and aldosterone. The structure and numbering system for cholesterol, a C_{27} compound, are shown in Figure 4-39. There are two sources of cholesterol in humans: (1) *de novo* synthesis in all nucleated cells and (2) animal products in the diet. About 1 g/day is synthesized *de novo,* and 0.3 g/day is absorbed from the gut.

Animals lack the ability to degrade the steroid nucleus, or ring system (Fig. 4-39), to carbon dioxide and water. Conversion of cholesterol into bile acids and excretion into the feces represents the quantitatively important routes of its elimination. Conversion to steroid hormones, although important biologically, constitutes a quantitatively minor route of metabolism.

TABLE 4-14. Enzyme Deficiencies in Selected Sphingolipidoses

DISEASE	ENZYME	SITE OF DEFICIENT REACTION (DENOTED BY /)
Gaucher*	β-Glucosidase	Cer/Glc
Krabbe	β-Galactosidase	Cer/Gal
Niemann-Pick*	Sphingomyelinase	Cer/P-Choline
Metachromatic leukodystrophy	Arylsulfatase A	Ger-Gal/OSO_3^-
Tay-Sachs*	Hexosaminidase A	Cer-Glc-Gal(NeuAc)/GalNac

* Noteworthy.
Cer = ceramide.
Glc = glucose.
Gal = galactose.
NeuAc = *N*-acetylneuraminic acid.
GalNAc = *N*-acetylgalactosamine.

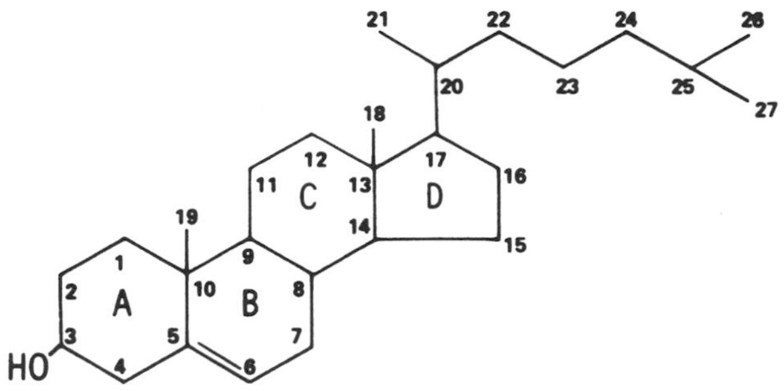

Cholesterol

Fig. 4-39. Structure of cholesterol.

Here we address in detail only a few of the steps in cholesterol biosynthesis. Cholesterol is derived entirely from acetyl-CoA. Acetyl-CoA is converted into the six-carbon HMG-CoA (Fig. 4-40) as previously described for ketone body formation, except that the reactions occur in the cytosol (Table 4-2) and not in mitochondria, as in the case of ketone bodies. The synthesis of HMG-CoA by ***HMG-CoA synthase*** is an important regulatory step. Then ***HMG-CoA reductase*** catalyzes a reaction between HMG-CoA and two molecules of NADPH to form 2 $NADP^+$ and ***mevalonate*** (Fig. 4-40). Mevalonate undergoes three successive phosphorylation reactions by ATP,

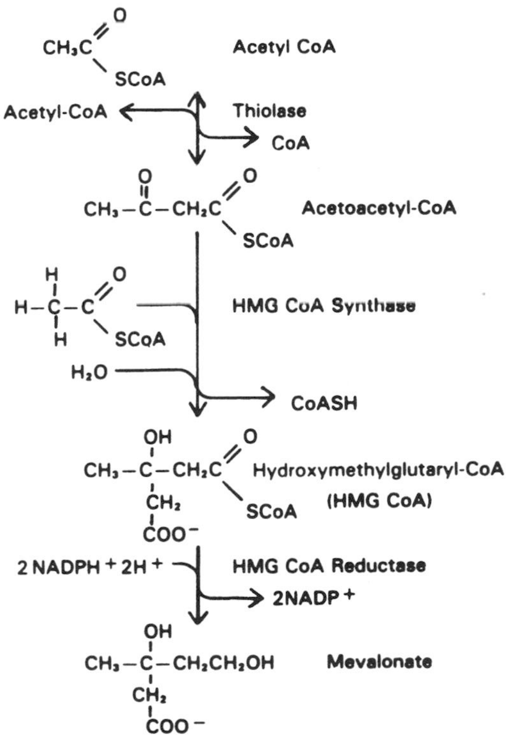

Fig. 4-40. First stage of cholesterol biosynthesis: conversion of acetyl-CoA to mevalonate.

yielding mevalonate phosphate, mevalonate pyrophosphate, and mevalonate-3-phospho-5-pyrophosphate (Fig. 4-41). The last compound undergoes decarboxylation and elimination of P_i to yield ***isopentenyl pyrophosphate*** (isopentenyl-PP_i). Isopentenyl-PP_i undergoes an isomerization reaction to form ***dimethylallyl pyrophosphate.***

The conversion of these isoprenoid compounds to cholesterol is outlined in Figure 4-41. Two five-carbon fragments (isopentenyl-PP_i and dimethylallyl-PP_i) condense to form the 10-carbon ***geranyl-PP_i***. The latter reacts with the five-carbon isopentenyl-PP_i to yield the 15-carbon ***farnesyl-PP_i***. Two of these react to form the 30-carbon ***squalene*** (first isolated from *Squalus,* a genus of shark). In a reaction involving molecular oxygen, squalene is converted into the four-membered ring system of steroids

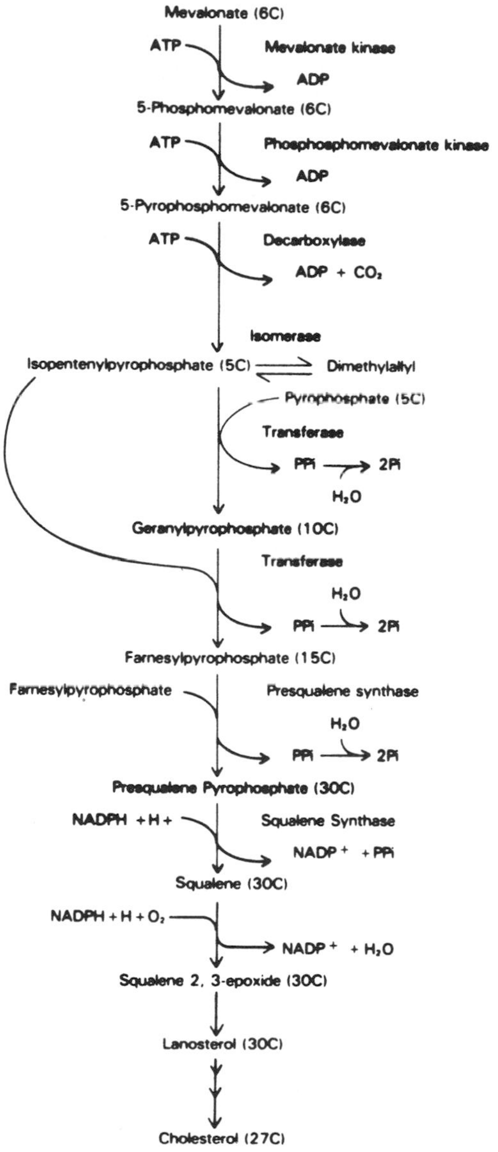

Fig. 4-41. Second stage of cholesterol biosynthesis.

in the form of the 30-carbon ***lanosterol.*** Formate is released in an oxygen-dependent reaction, and this step is followed by two decarboxylations, resulting in the 27-carbon ***zymosterol.*** Zymosterol, in turn, is converted to cholesterol, which also contains 27 carbon atoms.

Eicosanoid Metabolism

Arachidonate (5,8,11,14 eicosatetraenoate) gives rise to eicosanoids (20-carbon acids), including prostaglandins (PGs), prostacyclins (PGIs), thromboxanes (TXs), and leukotrienes (LTs). Humans cannot synthesize arachidonate *de novo.* Arachidonate is derived from linoleate. Linoleate is termed an ***essential fatty acid*** to reflect the inability of humans to synthesize this required compound. The eicosanoids have multiple and diverse effects. Thromboxanes, for example, are synthesized in platelets and produce vasoconstriction and platelet aggregation. Prostacyclins are produced by blood vessel walls and inhibit platelet aggregation. Prostaglandins increase cyclic AMP levels in platelets, the anterior pituitary, and lung but lower cyclic AMP levels in renal tubules and adipose cells. Leukotrienes are produced in leukocytes, platelets, and macrophages, and they attract and activate leukocytes. They also play a role in inflammation and hypersensitivity reactions, including asthma. Eicosanoids are synthesized on demand (they are not stored) and are released and act locally in an autocrine or paracrine fashion. These compounds have an evanescent existence. Only the general pathway for biosynthesis is considered here.

Arachidonate is derived from phospholipids in the plasma membrane by hydrolysis as catalyzed by phospholipase A_2 (Fig. 4-38). This is the rate-limiting enzyme in the pathway. Phospholipase A_2 activity is stimulated by angiotensin II, bradykinin, epinephrine, and thrombin under specific conditions. Phospholipase A_2 stimulation involves a cell surface receptor and the action of a specific G-protein. Phospholipase A_2 is inhibited by antiinflammatory corticosteroids. Arachidonate exists at a branch point in metabolism. Under the action of cyclooxygenase, it reacts with 2 moles of oxygen to form a prostanoid termed PGG_2. PGG_2 is converted to one of the prostaglandins, prostacyclins, or thromboxanes by specific enzymes (Fig. 4-42). ***Cyclooxygenase*** is inhibited by aspirin and indomethacin, and this is a noteworthy property.

Arachidonate, in a reaction catalyzed by 5-lipoxygenase, is converted to 5-hydroperoxyeicosatetraenoate (***5-HPETE;*** Fig. 4-42). This is converted to 5-hydroxyeicosatetraenoate ***(5-HETE)*** or to the leukotrienes. Leukotrienes are potent constrictors of bronchial smooth muscle. Leukotriene A_4 forms a covalent adduct via a thioether linkage with glutathione to yield leukotriene C_4. Glutamate is hydrolytically removed, yielding leukotriene D_4, and glycine is hydrolytically removed to yield leukotriene E_4. Sophisticated chemical techniques, including gas chromatography/mass spectrometry, were required to elucidate the reactions outlined in Figure 4-42, which is given for reference purposes.

Lipid Transport and Lipoproteins

Glucose, amino acids, and ketone bodies are soluble in water. In contrast, fatty acids, triglycerides, and cholesteryl esters are sparingly soluble in water. There are two general processes for mediating the transport of lipids. Free fatty acids are transported as a complex with albumin. Albumin has a low capacity for binding and transporting fatty acids and an even lower capacity for binding and transporting cholesterol. A second system with larger capacity for triglyceride and cholesterol is composed of four classes of lipoproteins. The lipoproteins are made up of a hydrophilic phospholipid monolayer exterior, specific proteins (apolipoproteins) associated with the phospholipid surface, and an apolar lipid core. Lipoproteins mediate the transport of lipids in the extracellular compartments between the intestine, liver, adipose tissue, and other peripheral organs. Lipoprotein solubility and transport are dependent on the hydrophilic nature of the particle exterior. We next consider the transport of free fatty acids.

FREE FATTY ACID TRANSPORT

Adipose tissue is a storage depot for triglyceride. A ***hormone-sensitive lipase*** catalyzes the hydrolysis of two of the three fatty acids of triglyceride. A second enzyme catalyzes the removal of the third fatty acid. The fatty acids are released into the circulation, where they are transported as a complex with albumin. Nearly all cells except the brain and erythrocytes can take up fatty acid. Fatty acids furnish between one quarter and one half of the required metabolic energy under fasting conditions. The plasma content of underivatized fatty acid (bound to albumin) is about 0.5 mM postabsorptively and 0.8 mM after an overnight fast.

TRIGLYCERIDE AND CHOLESTEROL TRANSPORT

There are four major classes of lipoproteins. They are (in order of decreasing percentage of lipid and increasing density) ***chylomicrons,*** very low density lipoprotein ***(VLDL),*** low-density lipoprotein ***(LDL),*** and high-density lipoprotein ***(HDL).*** The major function of chylomicrons is to transport triglyceride and cholesterol, derived from the diet, from the intestine to other tissues (Table 4-15). Chylomicrons are synthesized by the intestine but derive some apolipoproteins from HDL. Lipoprotein lipase in the capillary endothelium throughout the body

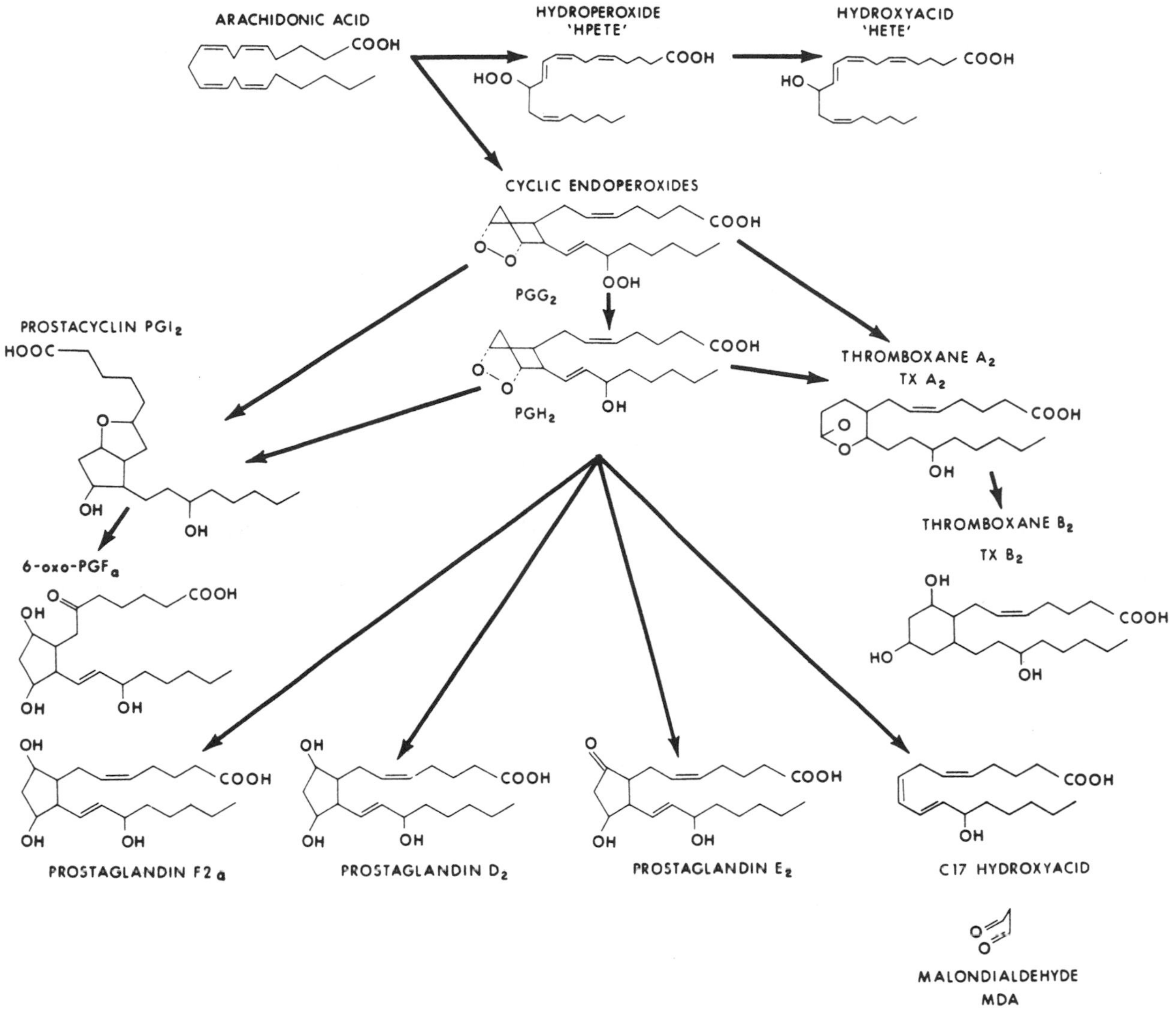

Fig. 4-42. Metabolic conversions of arachadonic acid. (Reproduced with permission from Moncada S, Vane JR: Mode of action of aspirinlike drugs. In Stollerman GH et al. (eds): Advances in Internal Medicine, Vol 24. Copyright © 1979 by Year Book Medical Publishers, Chicago)

catalyzes the hydrolysis of triglyceride to fatty acids, which are then taken up by cells of the tissues or organs. Chylomicron remnants return apoproteins to HDL, and the remnants are taken up and metabolized by the liver.

The function of VLDL is to transport triglyceride from liver to extrahepatic tissues. Lipoprotein lipase catalyzes the hydrolysis and release of fatty acids from the core triglyceride. VLDL is synthesized by the liver and also receives apoproteins from HDL. After transporting a portion of its triglyceride and after returning specific apoproteins to HDL, VLDL is converted into intermediate-density lipoprotein ***(IDL)*** and then LDL by the liver.

The main function of LDL is to transport cholesterol from the liver to extrahepatic tissues. This process has been implicated as a potential factor in atherogenesis, and sometimes LDL is called ''bad'' cholesterol. The LDL complex is recognized by specific plasma membrane receptors in most cells. LDL is taken up by the cell by receptor-mediated endocytosis and is delivered to the lysosomes. The latter degrade the apoproteins and hydrolyze cholesteryl ester to cholesterol. Cholesterol acts to decrease the synthesis of HMG-CoA synthase, HMG-CoA reductase, and the LDL receptor and thereby decreases intracellular cholesterol levels. The regulation of metabolic pathways at more than one step is called the dispersive control of metabolism. The LDL receptor is

TABLE 4-15. Composition and Function of the Major Classes of Lipoproteins

PARTICLE	FUNCTION	ORIGIN	FATE	APOLIPOPROTEINS
Chylomicron	Transports dietary triglyceride and cholesterol from gut to other tissues	Gut and HDL	Liver and HDL	Apo B-48 Apo CII, and CIII Apo E
VLDL	Transports triglyceride from liver to other tissues	Liver and HDL	Converted into LDL	Apo B-100 Apo CI, CII, CIII Apo E
LDL	Transports cholesterol from liver to other tissues (bad cholesterol)	Formed from VLDL by liver	Taken up by target cells	Apo B-100
HDL	Transports cholesterol to liver from other tissues (good cholesterol)	From chylomicrons and liver	Liver	Apo AI, AII Apo B Apo CI, CII, CIII Apo D, Apo E

nonfunctional in ***familial hypercholesterolemia,*** an autosomal-dominant disease.

The main function of HDL is to transport cholesterol from extrahepatic tissues to the liver. HDL is sometimes called ''good'' cholesterol because it removes cholesterol from peripheral tissues. HDL is synthesized in the liver and donates and receives components from chylomicrons and VLDL. VLDL is degraded by the liver. These properties are summarized in Table 4-15.

The proteins that constitute the various classes of lipoprotein particles are endowed with properties important in secretion, cell recognition, and activation of participating enzymes. Apoprotein AI, for example, is an activator of lecithin-cholesterol acyltransferase (LCAT). LCAT converts cholesterol and lecithin on the surface of HDL to cholesteryl ester and lysolecithin. The cholesteryl ester is incorporated into the interior of HDL, and lysolecithin is transferred to albumin. ***Apoprotein CII*** activates lipoprotein lipase, which catalyzes triglyceride hydrolysis. Chylomicrons and VLDL serve as substrates for this lipase. Most of the released free fatty acid is transported into the tissues that contain lipoprotein lipase. ***Apoprotein B-100*** is recognized by the LDL receptor. Apoprotein E is recognized by the LDL receptor and by the chylomicron remnant receptor.

Amino Acid Metabolism and Urea Biosynthesis

Oxidation of the carbon skeletons of amino acids accounts for about 15% of the metabolic energy of humans. The amino groups are converted to ammonia and urea. The metabolism of some amino acids involves complex pathways and will be covered in abbreviated form. Amino acids are derived from the breakdown of body proteins and of dietary protein. About 85% of the amino acids resulting from the breakdown of endogenous body proteins is used for protein synthesis. The breakdown of proteins into amino acids and their reuse for protein synthesis is called ***turnover.***

The metabolism of amino acids is divided into three categories. Amino acids are designated as ***glycogenic*** if they lead to carbohydrate formation, ***ketogenic*** if they lead to ketone body formation, and both glycogenic and ketogenic if they lead to increases in both types of compound. This classification was derived from experiments performed by administering each amino acid to animals and determining whether there was an increase in blood glucose (glycogenic amino acid), circulating ketone bodies (ketogenic amino acid), or both. Ketogenic amino acids are catabolized to acetyl-CoA, acetoacetyl-CoA, or both. The general classification of amino acids in this fashion is given in Table 4-16. Note that ***leucine*** is the sole amino acid that is ketogenic only (lysine administration leads to an elevation of both glucose and ketone bodies, but the metabolic pathway given in textbooks indicates that it is ketogenic only, indicating that our knowledge of lysine catabolism is incomplete). The aromatic amino acids, lysine, and isoleucine are both glycogenic and ketogenic, and the remainder are glycogenic only. Before examining the fate of the carbon skeletons of the amino acids, we discuss (1) transamination reactions, (2) ammonium ion production, and (3) urea biosynthesis.

TABLE 4-16. Classification of Glycogenic and Ketogenic Amino Acids

GLYCOGENIC ONLY		BOTH GLYCOGENIC AND KETOGENIC	KETOGENIC ONLY
Gly	Arg	Ile	*Leu
Ala	His	Lys	
Val	Ser	Phe	
Asp	Thr	Tyr	
Asn	Cys	Trp	
Glu	Met		
Gln	Pro		

* Noteworthy.

TRANSAMINATION REACTIONS

Transamination reactions, which are isoergonic, are pivotal for both the degradation and biosynthesis of the majority of the genetically encoded amino acids. The following equation is representative of all the reactions.

$$
\begin{array}{ccccccc}
 & COO^- & & COO^- & & COO^- & & COO^- \\
 & | & & | & & | & & | \\
H_3N^+\text{—} & C\text{—}H & + & O\text{=}C & \rightleftharpoons & O\text{=}C & + \; H_3N^+\text{—} & C\text{—}H \\
 & | & & | & & | & & | \\
 & R1 & & R2 & & R1 & & R2
\end{array}
$$

Several enzymes catalyze this reaction, and ***pyridoxal phosphate*** (a derivative of vitamin B_6) is the cofactor. Transaminases generally demonstrate a preference for one of the pairs of amino group donor and acceptor and exhibit a varying latitude for the reciprocal cognate pair. The involvement of glutamate and α-ketoglutarate as substrate is prevalent and pivotal. The ability of most amino acids to donate their amino groups to α-ketoglutarate to form glutamate is responsible in part for the central role of glutamate in nitrogen metabolism. Glutamate is also a common amino group donor in the formation of many other amino acids. The transaminase enzymes occur in the cytosol and mitochondria of all human cells. Aminotransferases also occur in human blood plasma in low but measurable amounts. An increase in serum transaminases occurs during hepatitis, in other liver diseases, and accompanying the tissue necrosis due to a myocardial infarction. Clinical chemistry laboratories routinely measure serum glutamate oxaloacetate transaminase (SGOT) serum glutamate pyruvate transaminase (SGPT) for a variety of diagnostic purposes.

Glutamate is a source of free ammonium ion. ***Glutamate dehydrogenase*** catalyzes a reversible reaction involving the following components:

$$
\begin{array}{ccc}
\text{glutamate} & & \alpha\text{-ketoglutarate} \\
+ & & + \\
NAD(P)^+ & \rightleftharpoons & NAD(P)H \\
+ & & + \\
H_2O & & NH_4^+
\end{array}
$$

Both NAD^+ and $NADP^+$ are substrates for this enzyme. The glutamate dehydrogenase reaction is amphibolic and can function in biosynthesis or degradation depending on physiologic need.

UREA FORMATION

The most important excretory product of nitrogen metabolism in humans is urea. A human consuming about 100

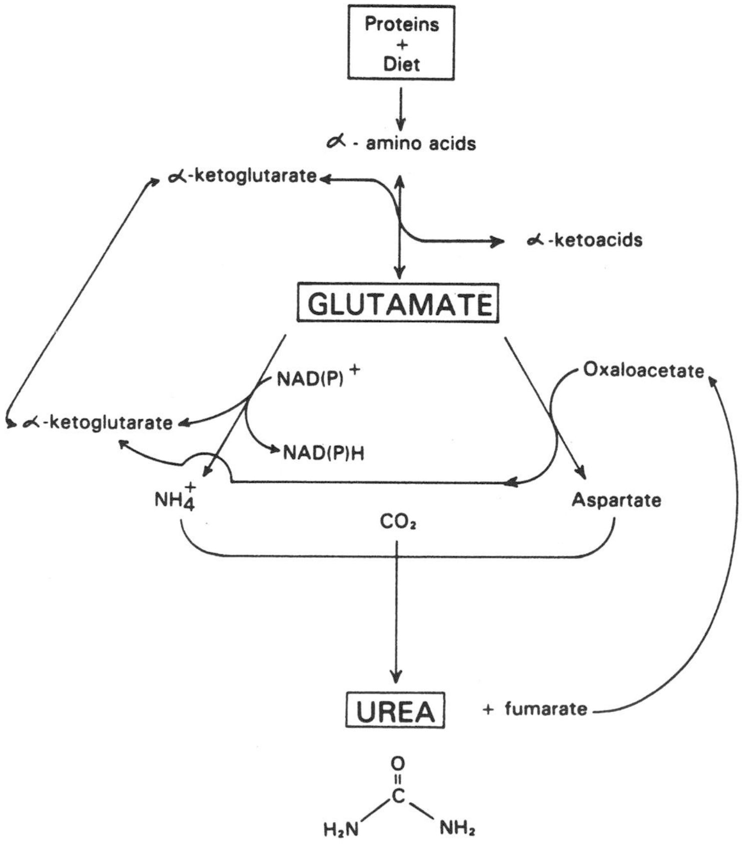

Fig. 4-43. Glutamate plays a central role in amino acid metabolism.

g of protein daily excretes about 16.5 g of nitrogen per day. About 80% to 90% of this is in the form of urinary urea. A small proportion is excreted as uric acid and free ammonium ion. About 5% of nitrogen is eliminated in organic form in the feces. Urea is synthesized in the liver (and to a lesser extent in the kidney) but not in other tissues or organs. The precursors of urea are shown in Figure 4-43. One nitrogen of urea is derived from ***ammonium ion,*** and the second is derived from ***aspartate.*** The carbonyl group is derived from carbon dioxide (as bicarbonate). Amino groups are funneled into glutamate (Fig. 4-43). Glutamate is oxidized, and one precursor (ammonia) is formed; glutamate donates its amino group to oxaloacetate to yield the second precursor (aspartate).

The pathway for urea biosynthesis was elucidated by Hans Krebs and a medical student, Kurt Henseleit, who was performing a research project. The process involves a cyclic metabolic pathway called the Krebs urea cycle, or urea cycle. This was the first cyclic pathway to be discovered, and the urea cycle represents the intellectual cornerstone for the elucidation of the citric acid cycle.

The urea cycle pathway involves a complex interplay of mitochondrial and cytosolic reactions. The stoichiometry of the overall process is given as follows:

$$\begin{array}{ccc} NH_3 & & 2\ ADP + 2\ P_i \\ + & & + \\ HCO_3^- & & AMP + PP_i \\ + & & + \\ \text{aspartate}^- & \rightarrow & \text{fumarate}^{-2} \\ + & & + \\ 3\ ATP & & \text{urea} \\ + & & \\ H_2O & & \end{array}$$

The first step in the urea cycle involves the formation of active carbamate as ***carbamoyl phosphate.*** Its formation requires the expenditure of two high-energy bonds from two ATP molecules and is catalyzed by carbamoyl-phosphate synthetase I, a mitochondrial enzyme. This enzyme requires **N-*acetylglutamate*** as an allosteric activator. Carbamoyl-phosphate synthetase I is distinct from the cytosolic enzyme that is involved in pyrimidine formation, carbamoyl-phosphate synthetase II (Fig. 4-44). Active carbamate reacts with ornithine in a reaction catalyzed by ***ornithine transcarbamoylase*** to yield citrulline. ***Citrulline*** is transported into the cytosol (in exchange for ornithine) before the subsequent reactions of urea formation (Fig. 4-45). Aspartate, ATP, and citrulline react to form AMP, PP_i, and argininosuccinate in a reaction catalyzed by ***argininosuccinate synthetase.*** PP_i is hydrolyzed by pyrophosphatase to pull the reaction forward. Next, ***argininosuccinase*** catalyzes a lyase (not hydrolase) reaction to yield arginine and fumarate. ***Arginase*** catalyzes the hydrolysis of arginine to form urea and ornithine.

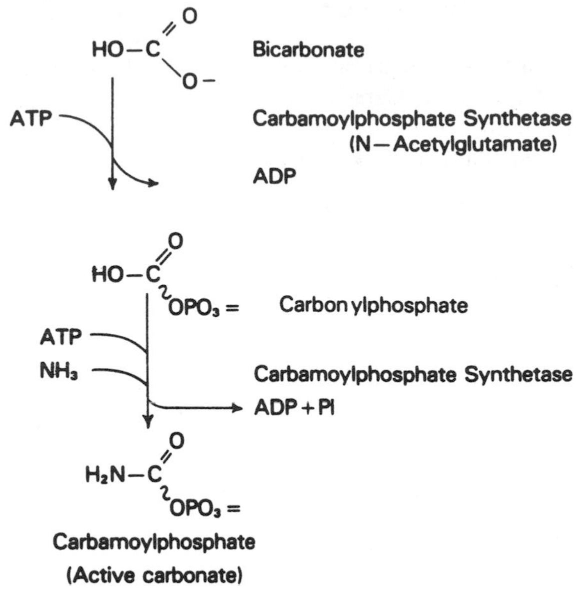

Fig. 4-44. Synthesis of carbamoyl phosphate.

Ornithine is transported into mitochondria in exchange for citrulline.

From the stoichiometry of the cycle, we see that three ATP molecules and four energy-rich bonds are expended (2 ATP → 2 ADP + 2 P_i [2], and ATP → AMP + 2P_i [2]). The overall process is exergonic. Renal disease is often associated with an elevation of the ***blood urea nitrogen*** (BUN). In severe liver disease, there is an elevation of blood ammonia. One mechanism proposed for the toxicity of ammonia involves the depletion of mitochondrial citric acid cycle intermediates by converting α-ketoglutarate to glutamate in the reaction catalyzed by glutamate dehydrogenase. Krebs citric acid cycle function and aerobic metabolism are especially important in the brain, and ammonium toxicity leads to hepatic encephalopathy with confusion, stupor, or even coma and death. Inborn errors of urea cycle metabolism have been reported that involve each of the urea cycle enzymes except for arginase (Table 4-17). Defects in the urea cycle are unusual in that these inborn errors of metabolism are not associated with metabolic acidosis.

CATABOLISM OF THE CARBON SKELETONS OF THE AMINO ACIDS

Amino acids that give rise to pyruvate and intermediates of the citric acid cycle (α-ketoglutarate, succinyl-CoA, fumarate, and oxaloacetate) are glycogenic. These compounds can furnish mitochondrial malate, a substrate for gluconeogenesis. In contrast, those amino acids that di-

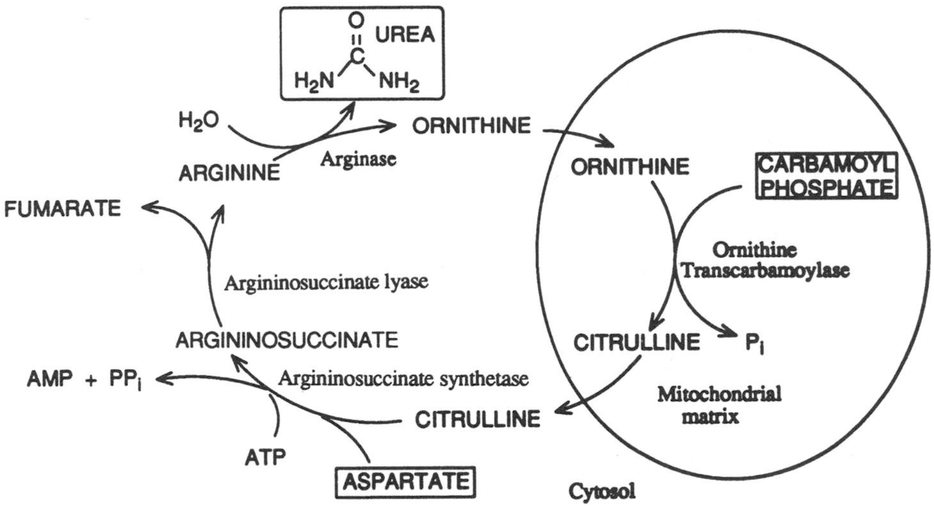

Fig. 4-45. The urea cycle.

rectly yield acetyl-CoA or acetoacetyl-CoA cannot support gluconeogenesis. These compounds yield ketone bodies. Several amino acids exhibit multiple pathways of metabolism, which are not considered here.

Four amino acids (alanine, glycine, serine, and cysteine) are converted to pyruvate. ***Alanine*** undergoes a transamination reaction and yields pyruvate directly. ***Glycine*** reacts with N^5,N^{10}-methylenetetrahydrofolate and water to yield ***serine*** and tetrahydrofolate. Serine dehydratase catalyzes the pyridoxal phosphate–dependent elimination of ammonia with a rearrangement to yield pyruvate. Note that the initial steps in the catabolism of threonine, glycine, and serine do not involve transaminations. The main pathway for ***cysteine*** metabolism in humans involves oxidation of the thiol group to sulfinate ($R{-}SO_2^-$), transamination, and then hydrolysis (releasing $HO{-}SO_2^-$), yielding pyruvate.

Five amino acids (proline, arginine, histidine, glutamine, and glutamate) are metabolized to α-ketoglutarate. ***Proline*** is dehydrogenated (NAD^+), forming a double bond in the ring between the α-carbon and nitrogen (Δ1-pyrroline-5-carboxylate), and this compound is hydrolyzed between the α-carbon and nitrogen atoms to form L-glutamate semialdehyde. A dehydrogenase (NAD^+) oxidizes the aldehyde on C^5 to yield glutamate. ***Glutamate*** is converted into α-ketoglutarate by transamination or by dehydrogenation (glutamate dehydrogenase). ***Arginine*** is hydrolyzed to urea and ornithine. Ornithine undergoes a transamination reaction to form L-glutamate semialdehyde, whose metabolism we have just considered. ***Histidine*** metabolism is too complex to consider fully. Histidine ammonia-lyase catalyzes the elimination of ammonia to form urocanate (first isolated in canine urine). Urocanate undergoes two successive hydrolysis reactions to yield *N*-formimino-L-glutamate (FIGLU). This reacts with tetrahydrofolate to form L-glutamate and N^5-formiminotetrahydrofolate. In folic acid deficiency, FIGLU is excreted in the urine and forms the basis of a

TABLE 4-17. Inborn Errors of Urea Cycle and Amino Acid Metabolism

NAME	ENZYME DEFICIENCY	METABOLISM AFFECTED
Argininosuccinaturia	Argininosuccinase	Urea cycle
Citrullinemia	Argininosuccinate synthetase	Urea cycle
Hyperammonemia I	Ornithine transcarbamoylase	Urea cycle
Hyperammonemia II	Carbamoyl-phosphate synthetase	Urea cycle
Alkaptonuria*	Homogentisate oxidase	Phe, Tyr
Argininemia	Arginase	Arg
Cystathionuria	Cystathionase	Cys, Met, Ser
Histidinemia	Histidine ammonia lyase	His
Homocystinuria	Cystathionine synthase	Cys, Met, Ser
Maple syrup urine* disease	Branched-chain ketoacid dehydrogenase	Val, Leu, Ile
Phenylketonuria*	Phenylalanine hydroxylase	Phe

* Noteworthy.

diagnostic test after a large dose of histidine. Glutaminase catalyzes the hydrolysis of the amide group of ***glutamine*** to yield glutamate and ammonia. It is noteworthy that the glutaminase reaction in the kidney is responsible for the generation of most of the ammonium ion excreted in the urine. Glutamate is converted into α-ketoglutarate in one step by transamination or dehydrogenation.

Valine, isoleucine, threonine, and methionine are metabolized to succinyl-CoA. The pathway from ***valine*** to succinyl-CoA is composed of eight steps and is not described in its entirety here. The first step is a transamination to form α-ketoisovalerate. This undergoes an oxidative decarboxylation involving NAD^+ and CoA. The reaction is catalyzed by a ***branched-chain keto acid dehydrogenase,*** discussed later. The reaction is analogous to the pyruvate dehydrogenase and α-ketoglutarate dehydrogenase reactions (three enzymes and five cofactors). Subsequent steps eventually yield methylmalonyl-CoA, which is metabolized in a vitamin B_{12}–dependent pathway that was considered in the metabolism of fatty acids with an odd number of carbon atoms (Fig. 4-31). Methylmalonyl-CoA is converted to succinyl-CoA in this process.

Isoleucine is first transaminated to form α-keto-β-methylvalerate, which undergoes an oxidative decarboxylation by the same branched-chain keto acid dehydrogenase mentioned above. After several more steps, a thiolytic cleavage produces propionyl-CoA and acetyl-CoA. Propionyl-CoA is converted to succinyl-CoA by the B_{12}–dependent pathway (Fig. 4-31). Propionyl-CoA is glycogenic and acetyl-CoA is ketogenic, accounting for isoleucine's classification in Table 4-16. ***Threonine*** undergoes a dehydration–deamination reaction catalyzed by serine/threonine dehydratase to yield α-ketobutyrate. Serine/threonine dehydratase contains pyridoxal phosphate as cofactor. α-Ketobutyrate undergoes an NAD^+–dependent oxidative decarboxylation reaction to form propionyl-CoA, CO_2, and NADH and H^+. α-Ketobutyrate dehydrogenase is made up of three different proteins and requires the same five cofactors as pyruvate dehydrogenase. Propionyl-CoA is converted into succinyl-CoA (Fig. 4-31).

The metabolism of ***methionine*** is complex. We address the reactions of its derivative, *S*-adenosylmethionine, in some detail later. **S-*Adenosylmethionine*** is an important methyl donor in several reactions. The conversion of phosphatidylethanolamine to phosphatidylcholine, for example, was considered previously (Fig. 4-35). ***Homocysteine,*** which forms after transmethylation and hydrolysis, is a four-carbon homologue of cysteine with the thiol group on the γ-carbon. Homocysteine reacts with serine to yield ***cystathionine*** ($HOOCCH[NH_2]$-$CH_2CH_2SCH_2CH[NH_2]COOH$) and water. Cystathionine is cleaved in a lyase reaction catalyzed by cystathionase to form cysteine, ammonia, and α-ketobutyrate; the latter is derived from the four carbons of methionine after hydrolysis of the amino group. α-Ketobutyrate undergoes an oxidative decarboxylation as catalyzed by its dehydrogenase (noted in the previous paragraph for threonine metabolism) to yield propionyl-CoA. The latter is converted to succinyl-CoA by the vitamin B_{12}–dependent pathway (Fig. 4-31). Valine, isoleucine, threonine, and methionine constitute the succinyl-CoA family.

Phenylalanine and tyrosine are converted to fumarate (glycogenic) and acetoacetyl-CoA (ketogenic) and are thus both glycogenic and ketogenic. ***Phenylalanine*** (essential) is converted into tyrosine (nonessential) in a reaction catalyzed by ***phenylalanine hydroxylase,*** which occurs only in the liver. ***Tetrahydrobiopterin*** is the reductant, and molecular oxygen is required. The products include tyrosine, dihydrobiopterin, and water. The hereditary deficiency of phenylalanine hydroxylase is associated with ***phenylketonuria*** (PKU), one of the more common inborn errors of metabolism. Tyrosine undergoes a transamination reaction with α-ketoglutarate to yield 4-hydroxyphenylpyruvate and glutamate; the enzyme catalyzing this reaction is ***tyrosine aminotransferase.*** In a reaction involving molecular oxygen, 4-hydroxyphenylpyruvate is decarboxylated, hydroxylated, and rearranged to produce ***homogentisate.*** Homogentisate undergoes a reaction with oxygen catalyzed by ***homogentisate oxidase,*** which opens the aromatic ring yielding ***maleylacetoacetate.*** This undergoes an isomerization to ***fumarylacetoacetate.*** A lyase then catalyzes the formation of ***fumarate*** (glycogenic) and ***acetoacetate*** (ketogenic). Acetoacetate is transported from the liver for metabolism in extrahepatic tissues as a ketone body.

Asparagine and aspartate are metabolized to oxaloacetate. Asparaginase catalyzes the hydrolytic removal of the amide group of ***asparagine*** to yield ammonia and aspartate. ***Aspartate*** undergoes transamination and yields oxaloacetate. The complete oxidation of any Krebs cycle metabolite is not as trivial as one might expect. Recall the Krebs cycle is catalytic and results in the catabolism of acetyl-CoA; the Krebs cycle intermediates are regenerated and not catabolized. The oxidation of Krebs cycle intermediates requires their conversion first to pyruvate and then acetyl-CoA. To achieve this requirement, Krebs cycle metabolites are converted to malate. A mitochondrial malic enzyme mediates the reaction of malate with $NAD(P)^+$ to pyruvate, CO_2, and NAD(P)H. Pyruvate is converted to acetyl-CoA, the stoichiometric substrate of the Krebs cycle, in a reaction catalyzed by pyruvate dehydrogenase, also a mitochondrial enzyme. The yield of ATP from the oxidation of NADPH is equivalent to that of NADH (2.5 moles of ATP per mole of NADH or NADPH).

Leucine, lysine, and tryptophan are converted to acetoacetyl-CoA. ***Leucine*** is converted to α-ketoisocaproate by transamination. This substance undergoes an oxidative decarboxylation by the branched-chain keto acid dehydrogenase and yields isovaleryl-CoA. (We see that branched-chain keto acid dehydrogenase operates on valine, isoleucine, and leucine metabolites). In three enzyme-catalyzed reactions, 3-hydroxy-3-methylglutaryl-CoA is formed from isovaleryl-CoA. HMG-CoA lyase catalyzes its conversion to acetyl-CoA and acetoacetate. It is noteworthy that leucine is the only genetically encoded amino acid that is entirely ketogenic (Table 4-16).

Lysine metabolism is complex and incompletely understood. α-Ketoadipate (a six-carbon dicarboxylic acid) is an intermediate metabolite. It is converted in several steps to acetyl-CoA (ketogenic). Studies in animals indicate that lysine is both glycogenic and ketogenic, and how lysine metabolites lead to the formation of net glucose is unknown. Because of this uncertainty, lysine is classified in some texts as ketogenic only, but this classification does not agree with metabolic studies *in vivo.*

Tryptophan metabolism is complex. Moreover, tryptophan is metabolized in humans to nicotinic acid, a vitamin, and this is a noteworthy property. The first reaction in tryptophan catabolism involves its reaction with both atoms of an oxygen molecule, which opens the five-membered ring of imidazole and yields *N*-formyl kynurenine. After the hydrolytic cleavage of formate, ***L-kynurenine*** results. This undergoes hydroxylation (O_2 and NADPH are reactants) and is followed by the elimination of alanine (glycogenic) and the formation of ***3-hydroxyanthranylate,*** which has two possible fates. The intermediate can be converted into α-ketoadipate, also a lysine metabolite. 3-Hydroxyanthranylate is also converted into quinolinate, which can be converted into ***nicotinic acid ribose phosphate.*** Nicotinic acid is a vitamin in humans because this pathway fails to provide physiologically adequate amounts of nicotinic acid. The formation of quinolinate from tryptophan decreases the requirement for niacin in humans.

There are a large number of inborn errors in the metabolism of amino acids. The most common is phenylketonuria, and its incidence is 1/10,000 live births. Classical ***phenylketonuria*** is due to a relative deficiency of phenylalanine hydroxylase (Table 4-17). Because phenylalanine cannot be degraded, alternative metabolites accumulate. These include phenylpyruvate (the phenylketone excreted in urine), phenyllactate, and phenylacetate. Although several commercial methods are available as screening tests for this disorder, the definitive diagnosis requires a determination of plasma phenylalanine levels. The treatment includes a diet deficient in phenylalanine. Variants of phenylketonuria exist. One is due to a deficiency of dihydropteridine reductase activity. This enzyme is responsible for regenerating tetrahydrobiopterin from dihydrobiopterin.

Alkaptonuria is another disorder of phenylalanine and tyrosine metabolism. Alkaptonuria is attributable to a deficiency in ***homogentisate oxidase;*** homogentisate is excreted in the urine, which turns dark due to autoxidation of the aromatic derivative. Alkaptonuria is a benign disorder in contrast to the morbidity associated with phenylketonuria. Archibald Garrod, who coined the term ''inborn error of metabolism,'' studied the biochemistry of alkaptonuria, which serves as a prototype of such genetic diseases.

Maple syrup urine disease is a rare genetic disorder associated with a deficiency of the branched-chain keto acid dehydrogenase involved in the metabolism of valine, leucine, and isoleucine (Table 4-17). There are elevated levels of each of these three amino acids and their corresponding α-keto acids in plasma. The disease is so named because of the odor of urine (and perspiration) in affected individuals, which is reminiscent of maple syrup.

AMINO ACID BIOSYNTHESIS

There are 20 genetically encoded amino acids (Table 4-5). If one of these amino acids is present in inadequate amounts, then protein synthesis is correspondingly diminished. ***Nonessential amino acids*** can be produced from endogenous metabolites. In contrast, ***essential amino acids*** cannot be derived from endogenous metabolites in required amounts, if at all, and must be obtained from the diet. A relative deficiency of an essential amino acid impairs protein synthesis and leads to a ***negative nitrogen balance*** (nitrogen excretion exceeds nitrogen intake). In healthy adults, ***nitrogen balance*** exists (intake equals excretion). In growing children in whom nitrogen intake exceeds excretion, ***positive nitrogen balance*** occurs. Negative nitrogen balance results from a variety of nonphysiological conditions, including infections, burns, and postsurgical stress. Negative nitrogen balance results in part from increased glucocorticoid secretion from the adrenal cortex.

Experiments with normal adult volunteers have yielded results indicating that eight of the 20 amino acids are essential and must be provided in the diet. Moreover, it is thought that human infants require arginine for optimal growth. When human volunteers are fed a diet lacking histidine, they do not experience negative nitrogen balance. The pathway for histidine synthesis, which is intricate in bacteria and plants, has not been demonstrated in humans. However, human muscle contains carnosine, a dipeptide made of histidine and β-alanine. During starvation, the levels of carnosine decrease. It is postulated that carnosine masks the essential nature of histidine. A mnemonic for the essential amino acids is the acronym PVT

TIM *HALL* ("private Tim Hall"). The letters correspond to *p*henylalanine, *v*aline, *t*hreonine, *t*ryptophan, *i*soleucine, *m*ethionine, *h*istidine, *a*rginine, *l*eucine, and *l*ysine. If one remembers that tyrosine is nonessential, because it is derived from phenylalanine (essential), then the mnemonic is less ambiguous. HA is italicized to signify that arginine is required in infants and that histidine is postulated to be essential.

In this section we sketch the pathways for the synthesis of the nonessential amino acids. The pathways for the biosynthesis of essential amino acids that occur in plants and microorganisms are intricate and are not discussed. Glycine is formed by multiple pathways, including the pathway from serine by way of the hydroxymethyltransferase reaction involving tetrahydrofolate. Alanine is formed by transamination of pyruvate. Glutamate and aspartate are formed by transamination of α-ketoglutarate and oxaloacetate, respectively. Glutamate is also formed from α-ketoglutarate through the action of glutamate dehydrogenase. This important reaction converts free ammonia to an organic amino function. Glutamate then serves as an amino donor in a variety of reactions.

The biosynthesis of glutamine and asparagine requires ATP. In glutamine synthesis, ADP and P_i result. In asparagine synthesis, AMP and PP_i are formed. ***Glutamine synthetase*** catalyzes a reaction between ATP, glutamate, and ammonia to yield glutamine, ADP, and P_i (Fig. 4-46). γ-Phosphoglutamate is an activated acylphosphate intermediate that undergoes a reaction with ammonia.

In the ***asparagine synthetase*** reaction, aspartate, the amido groups of glutamine, water, and ATP reacts to form asparagine, glutamate, AMP, and PP_i. The amido group of glutamine serves the important function of nitrogen donor. The K_m of the human enzyme for ammonia is very high, and ammonia is not a physiologically important donor in this reaction.

The main pathway for serine synthesis from 3-phosphoglycerate (an intermediate in glycolysis) involves its NAD^+-dependent dehydrogenation to phosphohydroxypyruvate. Phosphohydroxypyruvate undergoes transamination reaction to form *O*-phosphoserine, which then undergoes hydrolysis to form serine and P_i Although phosphoserine is found in proteins, the amino acid is added to the nascent polypeptide chain as a seryl group. A posttranslational phosphorylation catalyzed by protein kinases mediates the phosphorylation of the protein–serine to yield the phosphoseryl residue.

Proline is derived from glutamate. Glutamate is phosphorylated by ATP, and the derivative is reduced by NADPH. A dehydration with ring formation produces Δ1-pyrroline-5-carboxylate, which is reduced by NADPH to form proline. Cysteine is derived from methionine (essential) and serine (nonessential). Methionine is converted to homocysteine, which forms an adduct with serine called cystathionine, and cystathionine is cleaved during a lyase reaction to form cysteine and homoserine. Tyrosine is formed from phenylalanine (essential) in the phenylalanine hydroxylase reaction.

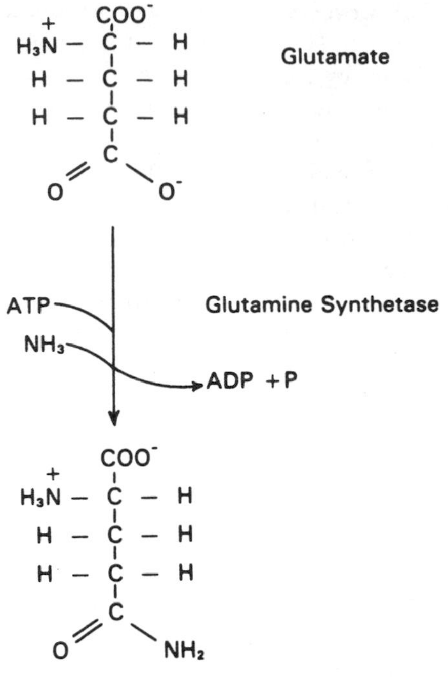

Fig. 4-46. Glutamine biosynthesis.

Porphyrins, Heme, and Bile Pigments

Porphyrins are tetrapyrroles linked by methenyl (–CH=) bridges, and ***heme*** is the iron derivative of ***protoporphyrin IX*** (Fig. 4-47). The precursors for heme in-

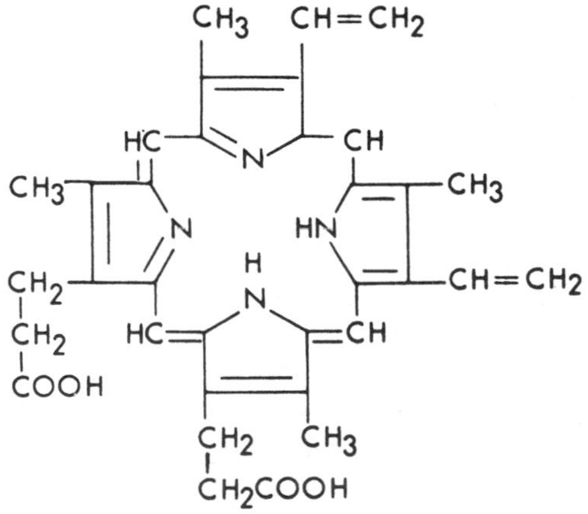

Protoporphyrin IX

Fig. 4-47. Structure of protoporphyrin IX.

clude succinyl-CoA, glycine, and iron. The rate-limiting reaction in porphyrin biosynthesis, which is catalyzed by δ-aminolevulinate synthase (ALA synthase), involves glycine and succinyl-CoA as reactants and δ-aminolevulinate, CoA, and CO_2 as products. Two molecules of δ-aminolevulinate condense to form ***porphobilinogen,*** and four of these condense to produce the tetrapyrrole. After additional decarboxylation and oxidation reactions, protoporphyrin IX is produced. The insertion of iron into protoporphyrin IX to produce heme is catalyzed by ***ferrochelatase.*** Heme combines with its apoproteins to form the heme-protein derivatives, including hemoglobin, myoglobin, cytochromes, nitric oxide synthase, and catalase. The activity of the heme biosynthetic pathway is regulated by increasing or decreasing the biosynthesis of ALA synthase by enzyme induction or repression.

After degradation of heme proteins, heme is catabolized to ***bile pigments.*** Heme oxygenase catalyzes the opening of the tetrapyrrole ring to form ***biliverdin*** (green). Carbon monoxide is a product. Moreover, there is a suggestion that carbon monoxide produced by the heme oxygenase reaction can function as a messenger molecule in signal transduction. Biliverdin is reduced to form ***bilirubin*** (red). These degradative reactions occur in the reticuloendothelial system. After transport to the liver as a complex with albumin, bilirubin reacts with two moles of UDP-glucuronate to form ***bilirubin diglucuronide*** (conjugated bilirubin). The latter is more water soluble than free bilirubin. Conjugated bilirubin is excreted in the bile. Intestinal flora catalyze the transformation of bilirubin to numerous ***bile pigments,*** most of which are excreted in the feces. The remainder are absorbed and are subsequently excreted in the urine.

One-Carbon Metabolism

The reactions of *S*-adenosylmethionine, biotin, and folate derivatives are important in the transfer of one-carbon groups in metabolism. *S*-Adenosylmethionine is important in many methyl-transfer reactions. The methyl group represents the most reduced form of carbon (Table 4-18). Biotin, covalently linked to proteins, also serves as an intermediary of one-carbon carboxyl-transfer reactions. The carboxylate represents the most oxidized form of carbon. Derivatives of tetrahydrofolate (THF) play a role in a variety of one-carbon transfers of varying oxidation states. One-carbon groups transferred by tetrahydrofolate include methyl, methylene, hydroxymethyl, methenyl, formyl, and formimino groups (Table 4-18).

Let us consider the biochemistry of *S*-adenosylmethionine (CH_3S^+[5′-adenosyl]$CH_2CH_2CH[NH_2]COOH$). It is formed in an unusual reaction between ATP, methionine, and water. In this reaction, triphosphate is displaced and is hydrolyzed to P_i and PP_i before their release from the enzyme's active site. PP_i is then hydrolyzed to two P_i molecules by a separate pyrophosphatase activity. Two high-energy bonds and a low-energy bond are consumed during the overall process.

The standard free energy of hydrolysis of the methyl group from *S*-adenosylmethionine is −30 kJ/mol, and this compound is of the high-energy variety. *S*-Adenosylmethionine represents one form of an activated methyl group. It transfers its methyl group to a variety of acceptors to yield *S*-adenosylhomocysteine and a methylated compound. Methylated products include choline, creatine, epinephrine, capped messenger RNA, and 5-methylcytosine in DNA.

Let us now consider the role of biotin in ATP-depen-

TABLE 4-18. Oxidation States of One-Carbon Groups

MOST REDUCED ⟶ MOST OXIDIZED

CH_4 Methane	CH_3^- Methyl	$^-CH_2^-$ Methylene	$^-C_4^=$ Methenyl	CO_2 Carbon dioxide
		H—C(=O)—H Formaldehyde	H—C(=O)—OH Formic acid	HO—C(=O)—OH Carbonic acid
		HO—CH₂— Hydroxymethyl	H—C(=O)— Formyl	HO—C(=O)— Carboxy
			H—C(=NH)— Formimino	
			C=O Carbon monoxide	

dent carboxylation reactions. Biotin forms a covalently linked prosthetic group in ***propionyl-CoA carboxylase, pyruvate carboxylase,*** and ***acetyl-CoA carboxylase.*** The substrate bicarbonate presumably forms an activated carbonyl phosphate (acid anhydride) intermediate and ADP in the first part of the reaction. The carbonyl phosphate reacts with the biotin prosthetic group to form an activated carbonyl-biotinyl group. The activated carboxyl group is transferred to an acceptor such as propionyl-CoA, pyruvate, or acetyl-CoA, depending on the reaction, to produce the carboxylated compound and regenerated enzyme.

Tetrahydrofolates (THF) are made up of tetrahydropterin, *p*-aminobenzoate, and glutamate. In humans the glutamyl group is covalently linked to additional glutamate residues. The one-carbon groups are linked to N^5,N^{10}, or both nitrogen atoms. Serine is the major donor of one-carbon groups in humans in a reaction catalyzed by serine hydroxylmethyltransferase. The reaction involves serine and THF and yields N^5,N^{10}-methylene-THF, glycine, and water.

Methylene-THF can be reduced by NADH to yield N^5-methyl-THF and NAD^+ in a unidirectional reaction. N^5-methyl-THF can transfer its methyl group to homocysteine in a vitamin B_{12}–dependent reaction catalyzed by methyl-THF–homocysteine methyltransferase to form methionine. With a deficiency of vitamin B_{12}, methyl-THF accumulates because it can neither be converted back to methylene-THF nor react with homocysteine. This "methyl trap" hypothesis explains some of the metabolic derangements associated with pernicious anemia and B_{12} deficiency. Methionine is the precursor of *S*-adenosylmethionine, an important methyl donor, as noted previously. Methylene-THF also serves as methyl donor and reductant for ***thymidylate*** synthesis. Thymidylate is incorporated into DNA. N^5,N^{10}-methylene-THF can be oxidized by $NADP^+$ to yield N^5,N^{10}-methenyl-THF. This serves as a one-carbon donor in purine biosynthesis. N^5,N^{10}-methenyl-THF also can be formed from formimino-THF.

Nucleotide Metabolism

PURINE AND PYRIMIDINE NUCLEOTIDE STRUCTURES

Purine and pyrimidine nucleotides are nitrogen-containing, aromatic compounds with many important biological functions. Nucleotides serve as carriers of metabolic energy (ATP) and as coenzymes in oxidation–reduction reactions (NAD^+, $NADP^+$). Nucleotides serve as metabolic second messengers (e.g., cyclic AMP) and are components of DNA and RNA.

The structures of the common purine and pyrimidine bases are shown in Figure 4-48. These compounds are called bases because they contain nitrogen, which accepts protons. Under physiological conditions, however, these nitrogen atoms rarely bear a frank positive charge as does the ammonium ion. The bases are aromatic and planar. ***Adenine*** and ***guanine*** occur in both DNA and RNA. ***Cytosine*** and ***thymine*** occur in DNA; ***cytosine*** and ***uracil*** occur in RNA. ***Nucleosides*** consist of a base and sugar. The sugar is ***ribose*** in RNA and in the common coenzymes. The sugar is ***2-deoxyribose*** in DNA. ***Nucleotides*** are ***phosphorylated nucleosides*** and consist of a base, sugar, and phosphate. AMP is a nucleoside monophosphate. This is mistakenly called "nucleotide" monophosphate; the term "nucleotide" signifies the presence of phosphate. The terminology of bases and derivatives is based on historical precedents and is an understandable source of confusion. Table 4-19 gives a list of the bases and the corresponding nucleosides and nucleotides.

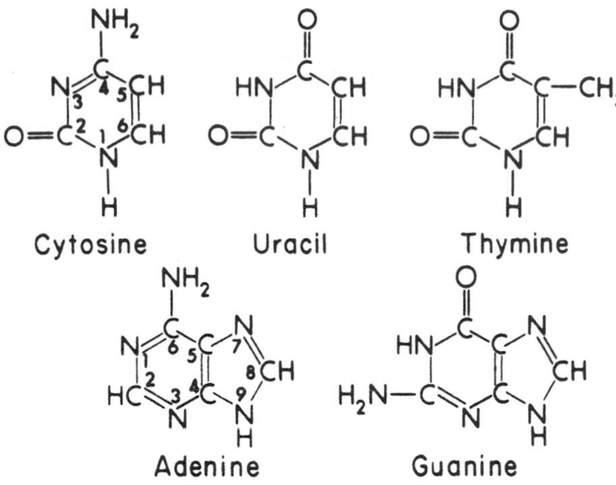

Fig. 4-48. The pyrimidine and purine bases.

PYRIMIDINE BIOSYNTHESIS

Nucleotide biosynthesis can be divided into two categories: simple and complex. Pyrimidine biosynthesis is simple when compared with purine biosynthesis. We first consider pyrimidine formation and then sketch the pathway for purine biosynthesis. The bases of the pyrimidines are derived from two precursors, namely, aspartate and carbamoyl phosphate (Fig. 4-49). We divide the pathway for pyrimidine biosynthesis into four portions: (1) formation of carbamoyl phosphate, (2) formation of the pyrimidine ring, (3) addition of pentose phosphate, and (4) formation of the various pyrimidine derivatives.

The formation of active carbamate in humans is catalyzed by ***carbamoyl-phosphate synthetase II.*** This enzyme differs in three ways from the enzyme that participates in urea biosynthesis. The pyrimidine enzyme (1) is

TABLE 4-19. Nomenclature of the Common Purines and Pyrimidines

BASE (ABBREVIATION)	NUCLEOSIDE; BASE-SUGAR	NUCLEOTIDE; NUCLEOSIDE MONOPHOSPHATE (ABBREVIATION)	NUCLEOSIDE TRIPHOSPHATE (ABBREVIATION)
Purine			
Adenine (A)	Adenosine	Adenosine monophosphate (AMP)	Adenosine triphosphate (ATP)
Guanine (G)	Guanosine	Guanosine monophosphate (GMP)	Guanosine triphosphate (GTP)
Hypoxanthine (H)	Inosine	Inosine monophosphate (IMP)	Inosine triphosphate (ITP)
Xanthine (X)	Xanthosine	Xanthosine monophosphate (XMP)	Xanthosine triphosphate (XTP)
Pyrimidine			
Cytosine (C)	Cytidine	Cytidine monophosphate (CMP)	Cytidine triphosphate (CTP)
Uracil (U)	Uridine	Uridine monophosphate (UMP)	Uridine triphosphate (UTP)
Thymine (T)	Thymidine*	Thymidine* monophosphate (TMP)	Thymidine* triphosphate (TTP)

* Refers to the deoxyribo derivative; the unusual ribose derivative is called ribothymidine; dTMP = TMP; dTTP = TTP.

found in the cytosol (Table 4-2) of all nucleated cells (and not just in liver and kidney mitochondria), (2) uses glutamine as the amido group donor, and (3) is not regulated by *N*-acetylglutamate. The reaction catalyzed by carbamoyl-phosphate synthetase II is given by the following chemical equation:

$$\begin{array}{ccc} 2\ \text{ATP} & & 2\ \text{ADP} + \text{P}_i \\ + & & + \\ \text{HCO}_3^- & \longrightarrow & \text{glutamate}^- \\ + & & + \\ \text{glutamine} & & \text{carbamoyl phosphate} \end{array}$$

Aspartate transcarbamoylase catalyzes the reaction between aspartate and carbamoyl phosphate to yield *N*-carbamoyl aspartate (Fig. 4-49). Dihydroorotase then catalyzes a condensation reaction with the concomitant removal of the elements of water to produce dihydroorotate. Dihydroorotate is oxidized by NAD^+ in a dihydroorotate dehydrogenase–catalyzed reaction to form orotate. Dihydroorotate dehydrogenase is a flavoprotein found on the outer face of the inner mitochondrial membrane.

Next, we consider the reaction responsible for adding ribose-phosphate to the pyrimidine ring. The donor is phosphoribosylpyrophosphate (PRPP), and we consider the pathway for PRPP formation. The reactants for PRPP formation include ribose 5-phosphate (from the pentose phosphate pathway) and ATP, and the enzyme is ***PRPP synthetase.*** The pyrophosphoryl group is transferred from ATP to the hemiacetal oxygen on C1; PRPP and AMP are the products.

PRPP represents active phosphoribose; the standard free energy of hydrolysis of PRPP to ribose 5-phosphate and PP_i is about -30 kJ/mol. PRPP reacts with orotate to yield orotidine monophosphate (OMP) and PP_i. The latter is hydrolyzed to two P_i molecules by a separate pyrophosphatase that helps to pull the reaction forward (Table 4-1). OMP is decarboxylated in a pyridoxal phosphate–dependent, or vitamin B_6–dependent, fashion to form uridine monophosphate (UMP) and CO_2. Uridylate kinase catalyzes an isoergonic reaction of UMP and ATP to yield UDP and ADP.

UDP is a key intermediate in pyrimidine metabolism. Nucleoside diphosphokinase catalyzes an isoergonic reaction between UDP and ATP to form UTP and ADP. UTP is a precursor for RNA biosynthesis and numerous uridine diphosphate sugar compounds used in carbohydrate metabolism. UTP is also converted to CTP. ***CTP synthetase*** catalyzes a reaction between UTP, ATP (an energy source), glutamine (an amido donor), and water to yield CTP, ADP, P_i, and glutamate. CTP is a precursor of RNA and numerous CDP derivatives important in lipid biosynthesis such as CDP-choline (Fig. 4-34).

UDP is also a precursor of thymidylate. Ribonucleotide reductase catalyzes the reduction of UDP to deoxyuridine diphosphate (dUDP). ***Ribonucleotide reductase,*** or ***ribonucleoside diphosphate reductase,*** catalyzes a reaction between nucleoside ***diphosphates*** and reduced thioredoxin to form the corresponding deoxynucleoside diphosphate and oxidized thioredoxin (Fig. 4-50). The latter is reduced by NADPH and H^+ in a reaction catalyzed by ***thioredoxin reductase.*** Ribonucleotide reductase is extremely important because of its obligatory participation in the synthesis of DNA precursors. However, uridine nucleotides are not genuine constituents of DNA. Deoxyuridine diphosphate is converted to dUTP by phosphorylation in a reaction catalyzed by nucleoside diphosphate

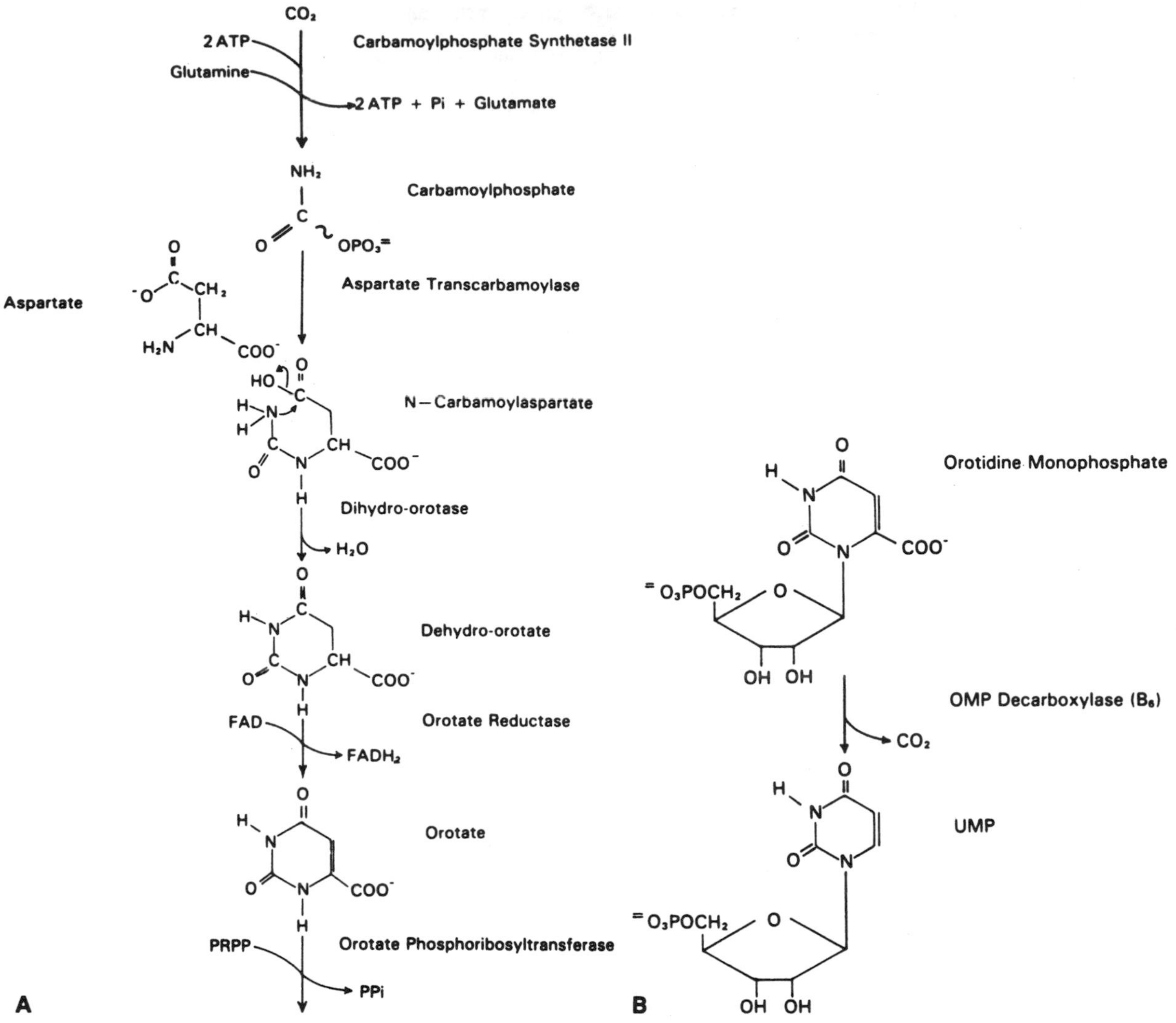

Fig. 4-49. Pyrimidine biosynthesis.

Fig. 4-50. The ribonucleotide reductase reaction.

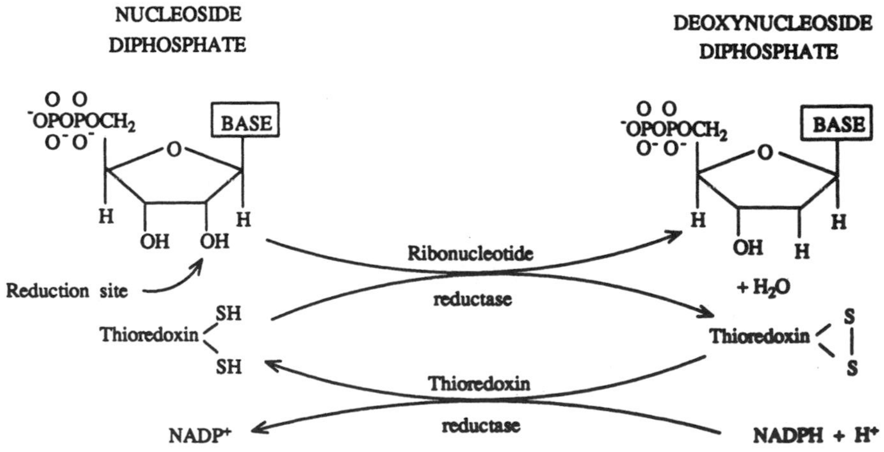

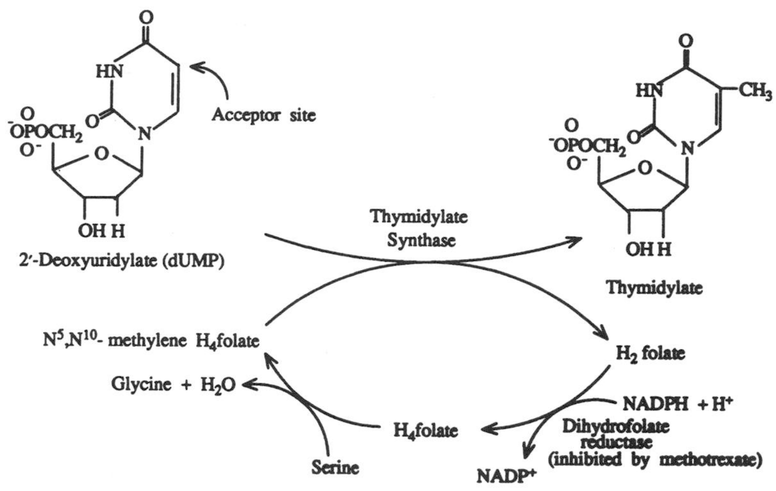

Fig. 4-51. Thymidylate biosynthesis.

kinase, and then dUTP is hydrolyzed to dUMP and PP_i in a reaction catalyzed by dUTPase.

Deoxyuridine monophosphate (dUMP) is a substrate for the important ***thymidylate synthase*** reaction (Fig. 4-51). dUMP reacts with N^5, N^{10}-methylene-THF to yield thymidylate monophosphate (dTMP) and dihydrofolate. In this reaction, N^5, N^{10}-methylene-THF serves as (1) a one-carbon donor and (2) a reductant. This sequence of reactions is important in understanding the mechanism of action of antifolates such as methotrexate. Methotrexate is a drug used in the treatment of children with acute lymphocytic leukemia and a number of other neoplastic disorders. Methotrexate is a structural analogue of dihydrofolate and binds avidly to ***dihydrofolate reductase.*** Methotrexate inhibits the conversion of dihydrofolate to THF and thereby diminishes the levels of the fully reduced and active form of folate. The therapeutic effectiveness of this and other drugs is dependent on the differential sensitivity of normal and tumorigenic cells. Although neoplastic tissues may initially be sensitive to the action of methotrexate, resistance may develop. One form of resistance is related to overproduction of the enzyme dihydrofolate reductase.

PURINE BIOSYNTHESIS

In contrast to the simple pathway for pyrimidines, that for purines is intricate. We discuss only the initial steps in detail. The purine ring is built on the ribose phosphate backbone. This contrasts with pyrimidine formation, in which the sugar phosphate is added after formation of the ring (Fig. 4-49A). The source of atoms found in the purine ring, illustrated for inosine monophosphate, is indicated in Figure 4-52.

The first and committed step in the pathway is catalyzed by ***glutamine PRPP amidotransferase.*** The reactants are PRPP, an activated form of the 5-phosphoribosyl group, glutamine, and water. The products include glutamate, PP_i, and 5-phosphoribosylamine. Note that inversion at C1 of ribose occurs (Fig. 4-52). C1 changes from the α-configuration in PRPP to the β-configuration in 5-phosphoribosylamine. Next, the carboxylate group of glycine condenses with the amino group in an ATP-dependent reaction. Glycine contributes atoms 4, 5, and 7 of the final purine structure. *N*-formyl-THF then donates C8. Glutamine contributes N3 in an ATP-dependent reaction (ATP $\rightarrow$ ADP + P_i). The five-membered ring is formed in a subsequent ATP-dependent reaction (ATP $\rightarrow$ ADP + P_i). This constitutes a mechanism for removing the elements of water from the precursor to yield the five-membered imidazole ring. C6 is next derived from CO_2 in an ***ATP-independent*** reaction. N1 is derived from aspartate in a reaction analogous to that seen in urea biosynthesis. The amino group of aspartate condenses with a carboxylate to yield an *N*-succinylamide derivative in an ATP-dependent process. Unlike the reaction in urea biosynthesis (ATP $\rightarrow$ AMP + PP_i), in purine formation ATP is converted to ADP and P_i. As in urea formation, a lyase catalyzes the elimination of fumarate. In summary, to add nitrogen, aspartate reacts with a compound in an ATP-dependent reaction and then fumarate is eliminated. Next, N^5, N^{10}-methenyl-THF donates C2. Closure of the six-membered ring occurs with the elimination of water; no ATP is required for this reaction. The product of the reaction is 5′-inosine monophosphate (IMP), as shown in Figure 4-52.

IMP is the precursor of AMP and GMP and occupies a branch point for these processes (Fig. 4-52). A two-step reaction is required to convert IMP to ***AMP.*** This conversion involves the replacement of an oxygen (or hydroxyl group of the tautomer) by an amino group. The amino donor is again aspartate using a familiar motif. IMP condenses with aspartate (as ***GTP*** is converted to GDP + P_i) to form *N*-succinyladenylate. A lyase cata-

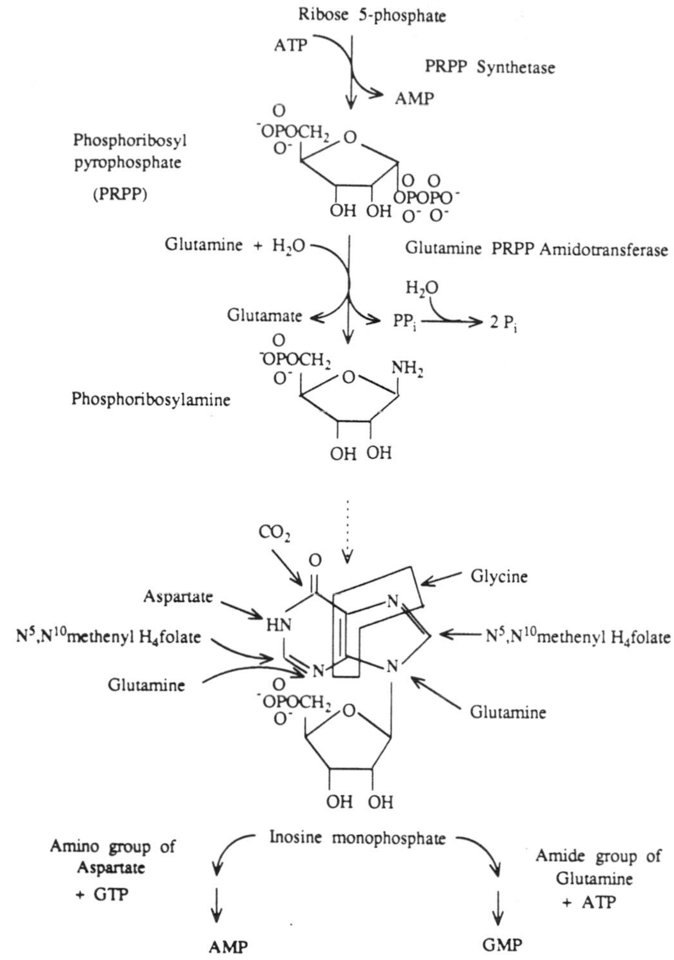

Fig. 4-52. Overview of purine biosynthesis.

lyzes the elimination of fumarate to form AMP. Two steps are also required to convert IMP to GMP. First, IMP is oxidized in a reaction involving IMP, H_2O, and NAD^+. The products are NADH + H^+ and xanthosine monophosphate (XMP). Glutamine serves as the amido donor to yield the amino group found on C2 of the purine ring. The reactants are XMP, glutamine, water, and ATP; the products are GMP, glutamate, AMP, and PP_i. Note that ATP is required for GMP formation and GTP is required for AMP formation. Kinases catalyze the phosphorylation

TABLE 4-20. Selected Enzymes of Purine Catabolism

ENZYME	REACTION	COMMENTS
5′-Nucleotidase	5′-nucleotide + H_2O → nucleoside + P_i	Will operate on all 5′-nucleotides and 5′-deoxynucleotides including IMP and XMP
AMP deaminase	AMP + H_2O → NH_3 + IMP	
Adenosine deaminase	Adenosine + H_2O → NH_3 + Inosine	Hereditary deficiency associated with fatal immunodeficiency syndrome
Purine nucleoside phosphorylase	Purine nucleoside + P_i → purine + ribose-1-phosphate or deoxyribose-1-phosphate	Generates free base
Guanine deaminase	Guanine + H_2O → xanthine + NH_3	
GMP deaminase (d)GMP + H_2O → (d) XMP + NH_3	NAD^+	
Xanthine dehydrogenase	Hypoxanthine + O_2 + H_2O → xanthine + NADH + H^+ Xanthine + NAD^+ + H_2O → urate − + NADH + $2H^+$	

of the purine nucleoside monophosphates to the corresponding diphosphates with ATP as donor. The nucleoside diphosphates are substrates for ribonucleotide reductase to yield the corresponding deoxyribonucleotides as necessary (Fig. 4-50). GTP, dGTP, and dATP are formed from the corresponding diphosphates and ATP. Several mechanisms exist for the formation of ATP from ADP by substrate-level and electron-transport phosphorylation.

In addition to the synthesis of purines from low–molecular mass precursors (*de novo* synthesis), salvage pathways exist. The preformed bases (adenine, hypoxanthine, guanine) resulting from degradative reactions are reused for anabolic pathways. Two enzymes catalyze the salvage reactions. ***Adenine phosphoribosyl transferase*** (APT) catalyzes a reaction of substrate with PRPP to form AMP and PP_i. ***Hypoxanthine-guanine phosphoribosyl transferase*** (HGPRT) catalyzes a reaction of either base with PRPP to form IMP (from hypoxanthine) or GMP. The physiological importance of salvage pathways was not fully appreciated until it was discovered that Lesch-Nyhan syndrome is due to a hereditary deficiency of HGPRT. This human genetic disorder is associated with extreme aggression and self-mutilation. It is X-linked, is recessive, occurs in males, and is (fortunately) rare.

The metabolism of PRPP is preeminent in both purine and pyrimidine metabolism and is important in metabolic regulation. The committed step in purine formation is catalyzed by ***glutamine PRPP amidotransferase.*** This amidotransferase is also allosterically inhibited by AMP and GMP. Moreover, the amidotransferase is the most important regulatory enzyme of purine biosynthesis. Pyrimidine biosynthesis in humans is regulated as ***carbamoyl-phosphate synthetase II.*** Synthetase II is inhibited by UTP and is activated by ATP and PRPP. The regulatory step of pyrimidine biosynthesis in *E. coli,* in contrast to humans, is at the level of the aspartate transcarbamoylase reaction, which is inhibited by CTP. Aspartate transcarbamoylase from *E. coli* is historically important in biochemistry because it was one of the first allosteric enzymes to be characterized. The conversion of IMP to AMP and GMP is differentially regulated. AMP inhibits its own synthesis, and GMP inhibits its own synthesis in the first step of the pathway from IMP.

PURINE AND PYRIMIDINE CATABOLISM

The end product of purine metabolism in humans is ***uric acid*** or its salt, ***urate.*** There are multiple pathways for converting AMP and GMP into xanthine and thence urate. Some of these enzyme activities are listed in Table 4-20. Through the action of various deaminases, a general 5′-nucleotidase, and purine nucleoside phosphorylase, purine bases result. These include adenine, hypoxanthine (from adenosine via inosine [a nucleoside]), and guanine. About 90% of these bases are reused by the salvage pathway in reactions with PRPP. The remaining 10% of these purines are converted to urate. Hypoxanthine is oxidized to xanthine in a reaction catalyzed by ***xanthine dehydrogenase.*** Guanosine is deaminated (by hydrolysis) to yield xanthine. Xanthine dehydrogenase also catalyzes the oxidation of xanthine to urate.

A common derangement of purine metabolism in humans is that of gout with an incidence of about three per 1,000 persons. Gout is associated with hyperuricemia. Gout tophi in joints and urate calculi in the kidney occasionally result. Individuals are frequently treated with allopurinol, which is an inhibitor of xanthine dehydrogenase. The build-up of hypoxanthine resulting from inhibition of xanthine dehydrogenase provides substrate for the salvage pathway and the formation of IMP. IMP inhibits glutamine PRPP amidotransferase (the rate-limiting step in purine biosynthesis). Inhibition of xanthine dehydrogenase and urate formation by allopurinol and secondary inhibition of glutamine PRPP amidotransferase by IMP and by allopurinol monophosphate (also formed by salvage enzymes) account for the therapeutic effects of allopurinol. However, the biochemical mechanisms responsible for the development of most cases of gout have not been identified.

Pyrimidines are converted to ***dihydrouracil*** during their catabolism. Deaminases and nucleoside phosphorylase result in the conversion of the ribo- and deoxyribopyrimidines to uracil. Uracil is converted to dihydrouracil by NADPH and H^+ in a reaction catalyzed by dihydrouracil dehydrogenase. Dihydrouracil is hydrolyzed to β-ureido propionate, which is hydrolyzed to CO_2, ammonia, and β-alanine. Thymine catabolism yields β-aminoisobutyrate instead of β-alanine. β-Alanine is catabolized to acetyl-CoA, and β-aminoisobutyrate is catabolized to propionyl-CoA.

MOLECULAR BIOLOGY

Biology is the science of life, and it focuses on the nature of living organisms and how they reproduce, develop, function, adapt, and evolve. The goal of molecular biology is to understand biological phenomena at the molecular level. It has been known for millennia that progeny resemble their parents. During the past century the science of genetics has made prodigious advances; progress continues at an accelerating pace. The science of ***molecular biology*** concerns the structure, function, and expression of the gene. The ***gene*** is the unit of inheritance. Fifty years ago, the gene was a biological concept. As progress in science has occurred, we now know that genes are made up of DNA (Table 4-1). Genes consist of specific

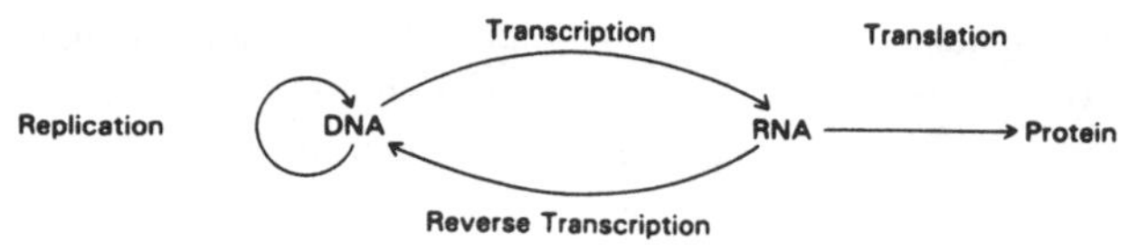

Fig. 4-53. Information transfer; the central dogma of molecular biology.

sequences of bases (A, T, G, and C), along a sugar phosphate backbone, which code for specific RNAs and proteins or which play a regulatory role in genetic expression.

In the next section we consider the structure of DNA and how it is replicated. The information present in parental DNA is used to direct the synthesis of two daughter molecules identical to the parent molecule in the process called ***replication.*** The pathway for the direction of information flow in biological systems is given in Table 4-1 and is shown in Figure 4-53. The information in the parental sequence of DNA serves as the source of information for progeny DNA in replication. It also dictates the sequence of nucleotides of RNA during gene ***transcription*** during RNA biosynthesis. RNA in turn directs the synthesis of proteins during ***translation.*** The four-letter alphabet of nucleic acids (corresponding to four bases) is translated into the 20-letter alphabet of proteins (corresponding to the 20 genetically encoded amino acids).

Messenger RNA (mRNA) dictates the sequence of amino acids found in proteins. mRNA in humans is derived from heterogeneous nuclear RNA (hnRNA) in a process involving splicing. Small nuclear RNA (snRNA) molecules play a role in the splicing process. ***Transfer RNA*** (tRNA) has two important functions. tRNA combines with its corresponding amino acid to produce a bioenergetically activated form of amino acid. Second, tRNA serves as an adapter in translating serial nucleic acid hydrogen-bonding patterns into an amino acid sequence of a protein. A third type of RNA, ***ribosomal RNA*** (rRNA), forms a scaffold for the ribosome and perhaps plays a functional role in ribosome action during protein synthesis. After ribosome-dependent protein synthesis (translation), proteins are subject to translocation to another part of the cell, exocytosis from the cell, and covalent modifications. The latter are called posttranslational, or processing, reactions and include, *inter alia,* proteolytic cleavage, glycosylation, phosphorylation, hydroxylation, methylation, carboxylation, farnesylation, and acetylation.

In addition to these physiological events, important advances in manipulating DNA and RNA in the laboratory have developed since the 1970s. It is possible to obtain considerable amounts of purified DNA for analysis and study. The techniques involve the production of ***recombinant DNA*** molecules. Recombinant DNA is often constructed from any DNA of interest ***(target DNA)*** and a ***vehicle DNA,*** which can be combined with the target DNA. The vehicle serves as a molecular handle and provides a means for amplifying DNA by cloning procedures to produce adequate amounts of DNA for study. Vehicles are often bacterial ***plasmids*** (extrachromosomal DNAs that replicate autonomously) and bacterial ***viruses.*** Sometimes animal virus sequences are added to recombinant DNA so that one can propagate the DNA in either bacterial or animal cells in culture. Recombinant DNA also can be used to produce ***chimeric genes,*** which encode products that are derived from two different organisms. The design of DNA molecules with specific properties is called ***genetic engineering.***

DNA, moreover, can be sequenced, which permits the deduction of amino acid sequences of proteins (both normal and mutant) through the use of the ***genetic code.*** The class of enzymes that revolutionized the study of DNA and permitted the production, manipulation, and analysis of recombinant DNA molecules are ***restriction endonucleases.*** These molecules cleave DNA only at specific nucleotide sequences. It is also possible to prepare radioactive or fluorescent DNA for use as probes. The probes interact with related sequences of DNA obtained from the genome by complementary base pairing or ***annealing.*** This practice has permitted the development of genetic fingerprinting techniques and is playing a role in the diagnosis of a variety of diseases through the use of ***restriction fragment length polymorphisms*** (RFLPs). The ***polymerase chain reaction*** (PCR) is a technique for amplifying target DNA molecules in an exponential fashion during 25 or more cycles of DNA synthesis *in vitro*. This procedure permits the amplification and subsequent study of minute amounts of DNA for cloning, genetic analysis, and diagnosis of infectious diseases.

It is possible to introduce human DNA into *E. coli* and other microorganisms; this process is called ***transformation.*** By appropriate genetic engineering, cells can be induced to produce large amounts of protein corresponding to the human DNA. Human insulin and human growth hormone produced by recombinant DNA technology are currently available for treatment of diabetes mellitus and dwarfism, respectively. Prokaryotic cells are unable to mediate certain posttranslational modifications such as glycosylation. When such modifications are important for stability or activity of the gene product, expression of human genes is performed in animal cells in culture. Tissue plasminogen activator, interferons, interleukins, blood-clotting factors, and erythropoietin are among the glycoprotein therapeutic agents produced by this technology. Besides having the protein with the human sequence (as opposed to that of another species), the shortcoming that only minuscule amounts can be obtained from human sources is obviated by expression systems.

DNA and RNA Structures

DNA is the molecule of heredity (Table 4-1). DNA is a long, thin macromolecule that is made up of a large number of deoxynucleotides. It can be made up of millions of deoxynucleotides depending on the species or particular chromosome of a species. The specificity and uniqueness of a DNA molecule are determined by the sequence of bases constituting each deoxynucleotide (base–sugar–phosphate) unit. The information of a DNA molecule corresponds to the sequence of bases in the same way that the information in this sentence depends on the sequence of letters of the alphabet. The structure of a tetranucleotide is shown in Figure 4-54. It illustrates the sugar–phosphate backbone with bases (A, T, G, and C) attached to the 1′-carbon of deoxyribose by a glycosidic bond. The bonds between the sugars are phosphodiesters linking a 3′ group to the 5′ group in an adjacent nucleotide unit. Linear molecules have a directionality or polarity from the 5′ end to the 3′ end. If an arrow is drawn from the 5′- to 3′-carbon of the same sugar, the direction of the arrow shows the 5′ to 3′ polarity (Fig. 4-54).

Human DNA and almost all other DNA forms a double-stranded duplex (the DNA of a few viruses exists as a single strand but forms a double strand during replication). The nature of duplex DNA was described by James Watson and Francis Crick in 1953. The double-stranded DNA forms a ***right-handed double helix;*** the strands of the helix ascend as a right hand is turned clockwise (Fig. 4-55). The two strands of the double helix are composed of ***complementary polydeoxynucleotides.*** The sugar–phosphate backbone of each strand is on the exterior and is represented by the ribbons; the bases face the interior and are represented by the horizontal lines. The hydrogen bonds between bases are represented by the vertical lines (Fig. 4-55). The crux of the Watson-Crick structure is the formation of ***complementary base pairs.*** The complementary base pairs are **A** and **T** (adenine and thymine) and **G** and **C** (guanine and cytosine) (Fig. 4-56). The complementary nature is associated with specific base pairing involving hydrogen bonds (two hydrogen bonds between A and T and three hydrogen bonds between G and C). Each complementary pair is composed of a purine and pyrimidine (and not two purines or two pyrimidines). Analysis of DNA molecules from a variety of species has shown that the mole fraction of adenine equals that of thymine; the mole fraction of guanine also equals that of cytosine. This is called ***Chargaff's rule.*** However, the G + C content varies from about 30% to 70% in all species (it is constant in a given species).

The two strands of the double helix exhibit opposite polarity. One courses in the 5′ to 3′ direction, and the complementary strand extends in the opposite direction, as indicated by the arrows in Figure 4-55. This property is called ***antiparallel.*** Besides complementary hydrogen bonding between double strands in DNA, complementary base pairing occurs between DNA and RNA (during transcription) and between RNA and RNA (intramolecularly in the tRNA cloverleaf and intermolecularly between the anticodon of tRNA and the codon of mRNA). In all

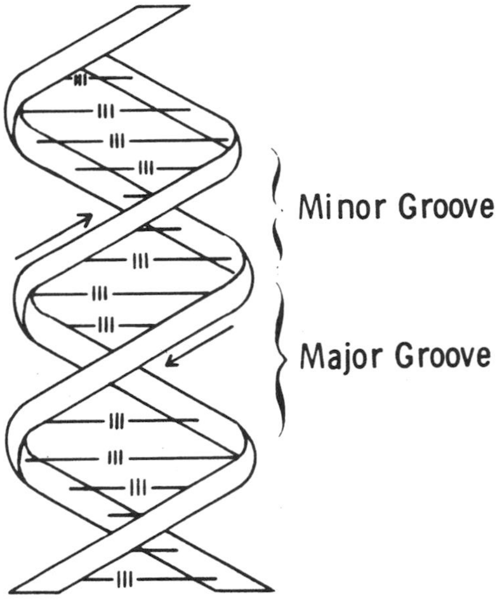

Fig. 4-55. DNA forms a double helix.

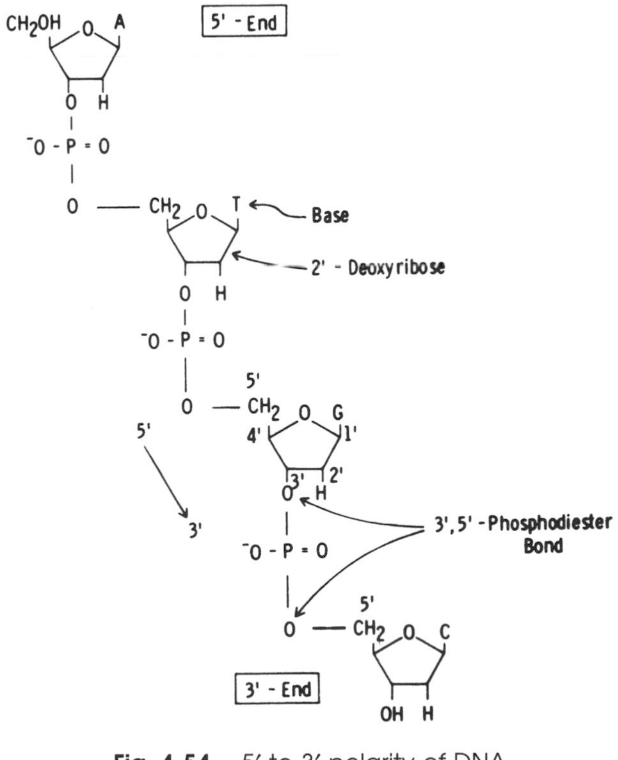

Fig. 4-54. 5′ to 3′ polarity of DNA.

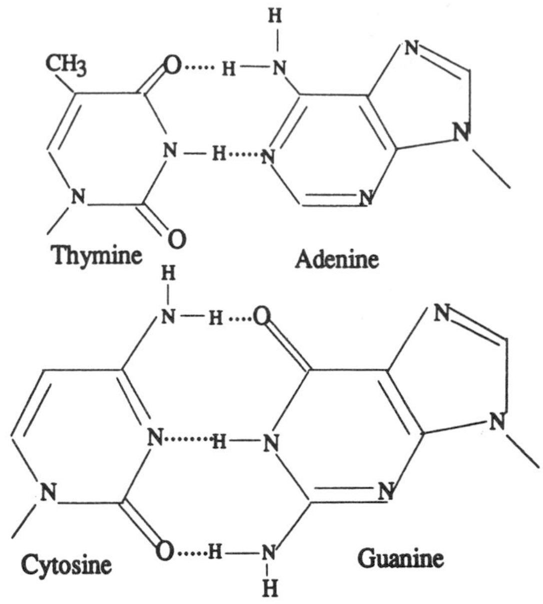

Fig. 4-56. Watson-Crick complementary base pairing.

known instances, complementary base pairing is antiparallel in nature (Table 4-1).

The existence of a double-stranded DNA structure with complementary base pairing has a number of theoretical and practical consequences. First, if we know the sequence of bases along one strand of DNA, then we can deduce the sequence of bases along the other because A base-pairs with T, and G with C. The sequence has the opposite polarity when compared with its complementary strand. Second, the duplex structure suggests a replication mechanism. If each strand serves as a template for the biosynthesis of a complementary strand, then two daughter DNA duplexes result, and each is identical with the parent duplex. Third, methods have been developed for studying the complementary interaction of natural or artificial segments of DNA or RNA with any DNA or RNA of interest. When nucleic acids form a complementary duplex, the polynucleotides are said to ***anneal*** or ***hybridize.*** The natural, functional DNA duplex exists in its native conformation. The native structure can be converted into two single-stranded polynucleotides by denaturation. The denatured form is produced by treatment with heat, alkali, or selected organic solvents such as formamide. Under appropriate conditions, the denatured DNA can reanneal to form a native duplex, and this hybridization is important in genetic diagnosis.

The familiar DNA double helix exists in the B form. The B form of DNA corresponds to a specific structure determined from its x-ray diffraction pattern. One complete turn of the double helix occurs every 3.4 nm. There are 10 base pairs for each complete turn, and each pair extends 0.34 nm. The B form of DNA also exhibits a major and minor groove when viewed from the side (Fig. 4-55). X-ray diffraction studies also have shown the existence of another form of DNA called ***Z-DNA*** (for zig zag). The major difference between the B form and Z form is that the Z form exists as a left-handed helix. The Z form still retains the Watson-Crick complementary base-pairing property. The sugar phosphates reside on the exterior, and the bases occur on the interior. The Z form is slimmer and more elongated than the B form. In Z-DNA, there are 12 base pairs per turn of the helix; one full turn is 4.6 nm in length. The physiological role of Z-DNA is unclear.

Diploid nuclear DNA of human somatic cells contains about 6×10^9 base pairs. The DNA is distributed among 23 pairs of linear chromosomes. The haploid genome consists of 3×10^9 base pairs in the 23 individual chromosomes. The DNA in each chromosome consists of a single, linear DNA duplex. Each human mitochondrion contains on the order of a hundred small, circular DNA molecules. Mitochondrial DNA codes for 13 essential genes of oxidative phosphorylation, two rRNAs, and 22 tRNAs. The ***genome*** of a cell or organism refers to its total DNA. A gene is a portion of DNA that codes for a functional unit. The gene may code for a polypeptide chain, a tRNA, or an rRNA, or the gene may play a regulatory role and not code for a macromolecule.

Let us now consider the manner in which the DNA of a cell is packaged or organized. The length of the DNA in a single human cell is about 2 m. However, the length of a typical human cell, is only 20×10^{-6} m, or 20 μm. DNA must be condensed into a compact structure. Because DNA is found in the nucleus and because the nucleus represents only a portion of the cell (Table 4-2), the condensation required is even more formidable. ***Chromatin*** is the term applied to the condensed DNA–protein complex. ***Euchromatin,*** which is transcriptionally active, is decondensed and light staining during metaphase. ***Heterochromatin*** is condensed and dark staining during metaphase. Heterochromatin, which is not transcribed, is composed of the DNA that corresponds to centromeres, telomeres, acrocentric short arms of chromosomes, and nontranscribed DNA. Chromatin in humans is about 35% DNA, 5% RNA, and 60% protein by mass. Proteins in chromatin are divided into two classes: histones and nonhistones. The mass of DNA and protein in chromatin is nearly equal. In humans, ***histones*** are the most abundant proteins associated with DNA. Histones are class of proteins that are rich in positively charged lysine and arginine residues. The positively charged residues interact with the negatively charged phosphates along the DNA backbone.

The lowest order of condensation of DNA and that which is best understood relates to the formation of nucleosomes. ***Nucleosomes,*** which resemble beads on a string when observed by electron microscopy, contain two loops of DNA containing about 150 base pairs wrapped around a protein core. The protein core consists of two molecules each of histone H2A, H2B, H3, and H4. These molecules form an octomer. Adjacent nucleosomes are connected by a 50–base pair region, associated with one molecule of histone H1, called the ***linking region.*** Higher-order fibrils and chromatin fibers have been described. These structures account for only a small proportion of packaging necessary to delimit 2 m of DNA in an 8 μm–diameter nucleus.

Nearly the entire chromosome (4×10^6 base pairs) of *E. coli* contains information corresponding to proteins or functional RNA molecules. It was a surprise to find that a significant fraction of human DNA consists of sequences that do not correspond to functional protein or RNA. The quantity of DNA in the human haploid genome is sufficient to encode for 3×10^6 proteins. However, the actual number of proteins that humans produce in their lifetime is estimated to range from 50,000 to 100,000. The function of the apparently excessive DNA, if any, is unknown.

Human DNA consists of various classes based on their copy number in a haploid genome. About 75% of human DNA is unique and occurs only once. ***Interspersed DNA*** consists of short interspersed nuclear elements (SINEs), long interspersed nuclear elements (LINEs), variable number of tandem repeats (VNTRs), and inverted repeats. Short interspersed repeats consist of a few to only several hundred base pairs. The Alu family is one example of a short interspersed repeat. (Alu is a restriction enzyme used in characterizing this family). There are 500,000 copies of the Alu family in humans, and Alu constitutes 5% of the haploid genome. Long interspersed repeats occur in unit lengths of 5,000 to 7,000 base pairs, and they also constitute about 5% of the genome. Inverted repeats are linear DNA sequences (from 100 to 1,000 bases) that can form stem loops and complementary structures with just one strand of DNA. The function of inverted repeats, if any, is an enigma.

Let us now consider the chemical structure and function of ***RNA.*** RNA is a polyribonucleotide consisting of a sugar phosphate 3′,5′-phosphodiester backbone to which either of two purine or two pyrimidine bases are attached. RNA shares many properties with DNA but also possesses some unique attributes. First, the pentose sugar in RNA is ribose. The presence of ribose confers alkaline lability to the molecule (0.1 N NaOH). This property is used to advantage experimentally. Second, although both RNA and DNA contain adenine, guanine, and cytosine, RNA contains uracil in place of thymine. Third, RNA is single stranded and does not exist as a duplex. As a corollary, the content of guanine does not necessarily equal cytosine, nor does adenine equal uracil. The ***primary structure*** of DNA and RNA refers to the sequence of bases along the molecule. By convention, sequences of each are given in the 5′ to 3′ direction from left to right unless specified otherwise. The ***secondary structure*** of RNA refers to hydrogen-bonding properties. The single-stranded RNA molecule forms intramolecular loops when segments are self-complementary. These complementary regions are prominent in tRNA.

There are three major classes of RNA in all living organisms. Humans and other eukaryotes possess two additional RNA classes. The three universal classes are tRNA, rRNA, and mRNA. Some of their properties are noted in Table 4-21. Humans also contain hnRNA. This is the precursor of mRNA. Humans, moreover, contain snRNA, some of which play a role in splicing reactions (removal of intervening sequences of RNA).

Replication

REQUIRED COMPONENTS

We first will discuss the properties of the various enzymes and proteins necessary for DNA replication and will focus on the replication process in *E. coli.* The biochemistry and genetics of this system have been extensively characterized. We also will discuss the properties of human replication enzymes. After the known components have been described, we will correlate biochemistry with cell biology and describe a working model of replication. We also will consider mechanisms for repairing DNA that has undergone an alteration resulting from the inherent instability of the bases or as a result of an environmental insult.

The classes of enzyme activity that are required for replication in *E. coli* include the DNA polymerases and DNA ligase. Another enzyme, called primase, is required for the formation of a polynucleotide primer. The 3′-exonuclease activity of *E. coli* DNA polymerases catalyzes the stepwise hydrolysis of deoxynucleotides from the 3′ end and plays a role in proofreading, or editing. Their 5′-exonuclease activity degrades DNA stepwise (or in blocks of up to 10 residues in length) and is important in excising the primer and in repairing DNA. A ***helicase*** is an ATP-dependent enzyme that separates the bases of the double strand ahead of the site of polydeoxyribonucleotide biosynthesis. A ***DNA gyrase*** is an enzyme that alters the supercoiling of DNA, which facilitates the polymerization reactions (Table 4-22). Otherwise identical molecules of DNA with different degrees of supercoiling are called ***topological isomers. Topoisomerases*** catalyze the interconversion of these various forms. DNA gyrase is one type of topoisomerase.

Let us consider the elongation reactions of DNA biosynthesis. The generic name for enzymes that catalyze

TABLE 4-21. General Classes of Eukaryotic and Prokaryotic RNA

CLASS	SIZE	COMMENTS
Eukaryotic ribosomal RNA	18S 1,900 bases	18S, 28S, and 5.8S rRNA derived from common precursor; RNA polymerase I transcript
	28S 4,700 bases	
	5.8S 160 bases	18S found in small ribosomal subunit; other three occur in large subunit
	5S 120 bases	RNA polymerase III transcript
Prokaryotic ribosomal RNA	16S 1,541 bases	Small subunit
	23S 2,904 bases	Large subunit
	5S 120 bases	Large subunit
Prokaryotic and eukaryotic transfer RNA	75–90 bases	About 40 different tRNAs in cytosol of human cells; many bases modified posttranscriptionally; products include: ribothymidine, dihydrouracil, pseudouridine, 4-thiouridine, inosine, and isopentenyladenosine among others
Prokaryotic messenger RNA	600 bases and greater	5% of total cellular RNA; short half-life (minutes); may be polycistronic (translated into more than one protein)
Eukaryotic mRNA	600 bases and greater	5% of total; half-life from minutes to days; contains 5′-7 methyl G cap and poly A 3′-tail; derived from hnRNA; monocistronic.
Eukaryotic heterogeneous nuclear RNA	May contain 100 kb of nucleotide or more	95% degraded in nucleus; precursor of mRNA; undergoes splicing reactions; RNA polymerase II transcript
Eukaryotic small nuclear RNA (snRNA)	100–300 Bases	At least 10 classes exist; each present at 10^5–10^6 copies/cell; RNA polymerase III transcript

these elongation reactions is ***DNA polymerase.*** In *E. coli*, three polymerases have been described, and they are designated I, II, and III in the order of their discovery. DNA polymerase III is responsible for the preponderance of DNA synthesis in *E. coli in vivo*. DNA polymerase I is required for replacing the primer (a mixed ribo-deoxyribonucleotide segment) and for repair synthesis. The function of DNA polymerase II is unknown. Five mammalian DNA polymerases have been described: α, β, γ, δ, and ϵ. Polymerase α mediates the synthesis of the lagging strand (see below), and polymerase δ mediates the synthesis of the leading strand. Polymerases β and ϵ function in nuclear repair synthesis (Table 4-23).

TABLE 4-22. Replication Proteins in *E. coli*

PROTEIN	ROLE
DNA polymerase III	Synthesizes DNA
DNA polymerase I	Degrades primer and fills gaps; repair synthesis
DNA ligase	Eliminates nicks in phosphodiester backbone; NAD^+ serves as a source of phosphate bond energy
Primase	Initiates polymerization with hybrid ribodeoxyribonucleotides
Helicase	ATP-dependent separation of base pairs in the replication fork
DNA gyrase	A topoisomerase that introduces superthelical twists
Single-strand binding protein (SSB)	Stabilizes single-stranded regions in replication fork

All known DNA polymerases (both eukaryotic and prokaryotic) exhibit the following properties. They catalyze the elongation of an existing polynucleotide (designated as the ***primer***) in the ***5′ to 3′ direction*** (Table 4-1). The enzyme requires all four deoxynucleoside triphosphates (as their Mg^{2+} complex) as substrates. The sequence of deoxyribonucleotides in the growing chain is determined by a ***template*** strand of DNA by the principle of Watson-Crick base pairing. If a C is present in the template strand, then G is added to the growing chain (Fig. 4-57) and vice versa. If T is present in the template strand, then A is added to the growing chain (and vice versa). The template strand is antiparallel to the growing polynucleotide chain (Fig. 4-57). The chemistry of the elongation reaction is shown in Figure 4-58. (This dia-

TABLE 4-23. Replication Proteins in Humans

PROTEIN	FUNCTION
DNA polymerase α	Synthesizes lagging strand of DNA
DNA polymerase β	Repair synthesis
DNA polymerase γ	Mitochondrial DNA synthesis
DNA polymerase δ	Synthesizes leading strand of DNA, PCNA cofactor
DNA polymerase ϵ	Repair synthesis
DNA ligase	Eliminates nicks in phosphodiester backbone; ATP serves as a source of phosphate bond energy
Topoisomerase II	ATP-dependent topoisomerase that introduces superhelical twists

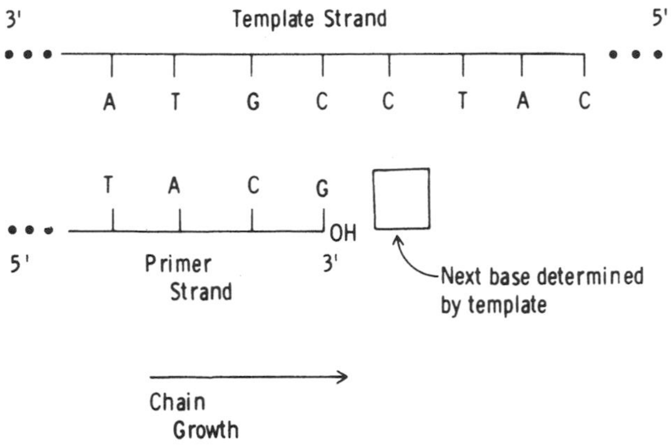

Fig. 4-57. Role of template and primer in DNA biosynthesis.

gram contains a deceptively large amount of information and should be understood by the reader). It shows that the 3′-hydroxyl group of the growing chain attacks the α-phosphorous of the incoming deoxynucleoside triphosphate. A new phosphodiester bond forms, and PP_i is displaced. From this diagram, we can readily see that chain growth is in the 5′ to 3′ direction. The polarity of the growing polynucleotide is such that the last residue added contains a free 3′-hydroxyl group.

DNA polymerases from bacteria exhibit 3′-exonuclease activity. This apparently paradoxical activity in a polymerase catalyzes the hydrolytic removal of the last nucleotide added to the growing polynucleotide chain. The product is a polynucleotide with one fewer residue and a free 3′-hydroxyl group. The best substrate for this 3′-exonuclease activity is a molecule that contains a mismatched 3′-deoxynucleotide (Fig. 4-59). For example, if

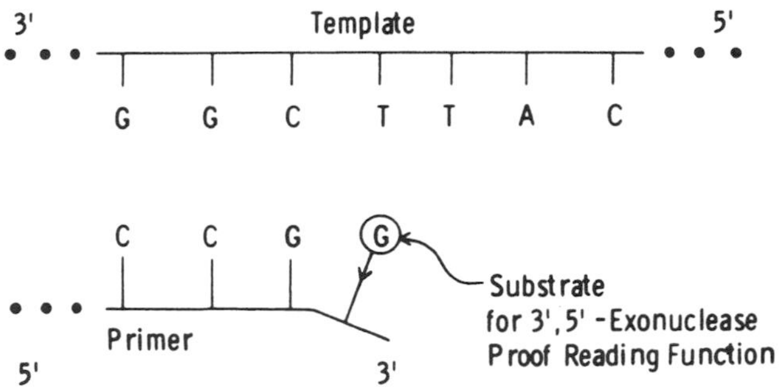

Fig. 4-59. Substrate for the 3′,5′-exonuclease proofreading activity of DNA polymerase.

G is added in a position complementary to T, then the deoxyguanosine monophosphate residue constitutes a good substrate for hydrolytic removal. The 3′-exonuclease activity is called the ***editing*** or ***proofreading*** function of DNA polymerase. After this correction, A is incorporated. Editing increases the fidelity of enzymatic DNA replication. The polymerase selects the appropriate deoxynucleoside triphosphate by the base-pairing principle. The selection is monitored a second time by the proofreading function, and the occasional mistake is eliminated. The error frequency is reduced to one in 10^8 by this mechanism.

DNA polymerases from bacteria also exhibit 5′-exonuclease activity. The enzyme can remove monomers and somewhat higher segments (perhaps up to 10) by a single hydrolytic cleavage. The enzyme can degrade polynucleotide segments by 5′-exonuclease activity and can fill in the resulting gaps by polymerase activity. These dual characteristics are postulated to be important in (1) removing the mixed ribo-deoxyribonucleotide primer

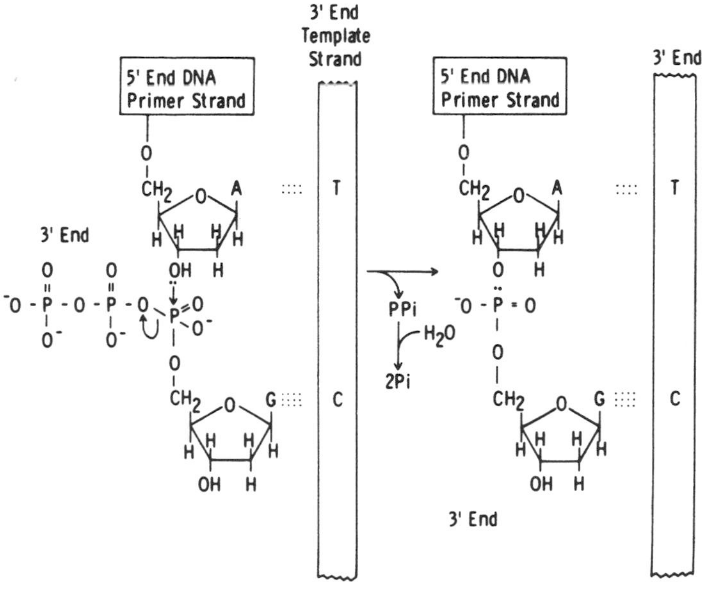

Fig. 4-58. Chemistry of the chain elongation reaction of DNA biosynthesis.

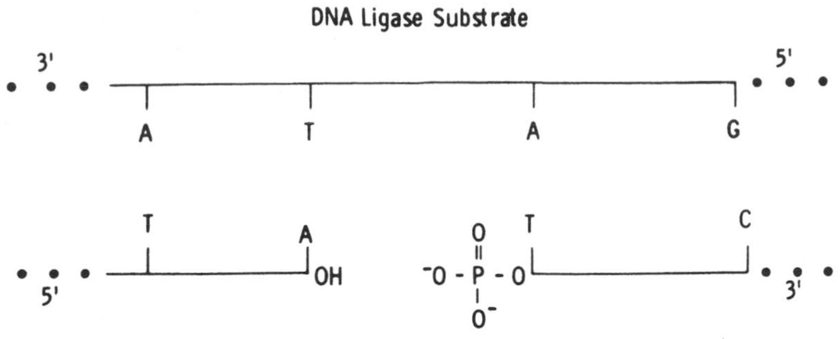

Fig. 4-60. Substrate for DNA ligase.

whose formation is mediated by primase and (2) filling the gap resulting from the excision of the primer.

Let us now consider the action of ***DNA ligase.*** DNA ligase activity is responsible for linking a free 3′-hydroxyl with an adjacent 5′-phosphate occurring in a DNA duplex (Fig. 4-60). DNA eliminates a nick from DNA. The elimination of nicks is important for both replication and DNA repair. In humans, DNA ligase catalyzes the adenylylation of the 5′-phosphate (Fig. 4-61). This results in activation of the 5′-phosphate; the molecule contains an acid anhydride, high-energy bond. The enzyme catalyzes the reaction between the nucleophilic 3′-hydroxyl with the activated phosphate to produce a phosphodiester bond (the nick is eliminated), and AMP is released. PP_1 is the other product, and PP_1 is degraded by hydrolysis by pyrophosphatase. The reaction in *E. coli* is analogous except that NAD^+ (nicotinamide-ribose-phosphate-phosphate-adenosine) is the adenylyl (phosphoryl-adenosine) donor.

We noted previously that DNA polymerase requires a prefabricated polynucleotide (primer) in order to catalyze the formation of any phosphodiester bonds. ***Primase*** initiates polynucleotide formation. Primase uses both nucleoside and deoxynucleoside triphosphates as substrates, and primase also requires a template. Chain growth is in the 5′ to 3′ direction, and the reaction catalyzed is analogous to that shown in Figure 4-58. After a primer of 10 to 50 residues is produced, polymerase III uses the resulting primer and catalyzes the template-directed synthesis of polydeoxyribonucleotide (Fig. 4-62). The primer is recognized by cellular proteins as being distinct from the product of the elongation or polymerization reaction because the primer contains ribonucleotides. The primer is removed by the 5′-exonuclease activity of DNA polymerase I; DNA polymerase I also fills the resulting gap. DNA ligase completes the process by combining a free 3′ hydroxyl with a 5′ phosphate.

DNA BIOSYNTHESIS

We consider now the process of replication from a broader perspective. Replication involves the synthesis of DNA complementary to both strands of the DNA duplex, and replication forks move in both directions from a replication origin. In *E. coli,* there is a unique sequence of DNA, named oriC, that serves as replication origin. In human cells, there are hundreds of replication origins on each chromosome occurring, on the average, about every 150 kilobases. Multiple origins of replication are illustrated in Figure 4-63.

The following components play a role in the replication process in *E. coli.* A helicase separates the strands at the cost of two ATP per base pair. DNA gyrase (a topoisomerase) introduces supercoils to relieve the torsion. Single-strand binding (SSB) proteins stabilize the single-stranded regions. Primase initiates synthesis of one strand toward the right. Polymerase III continues synthesis.

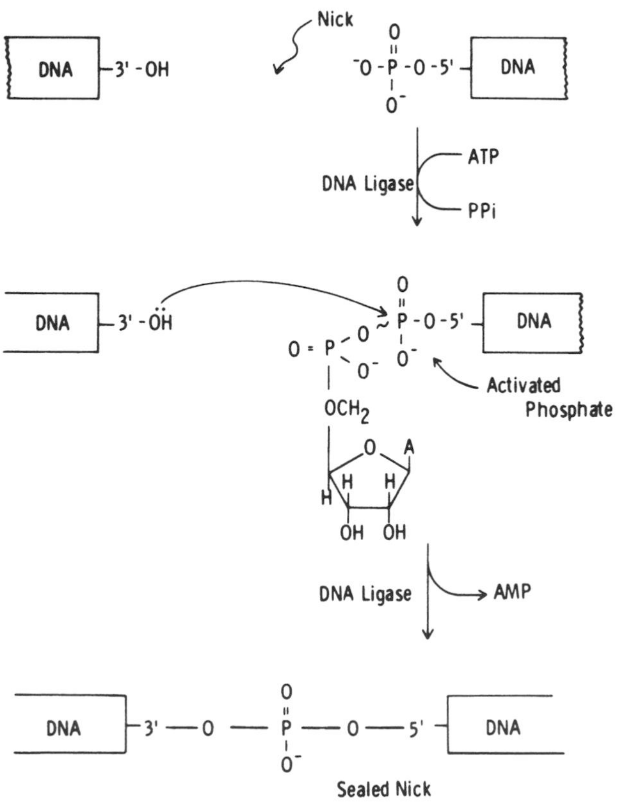

Fig. 4-61. Bioenergetics of the DNA ligase reaction.

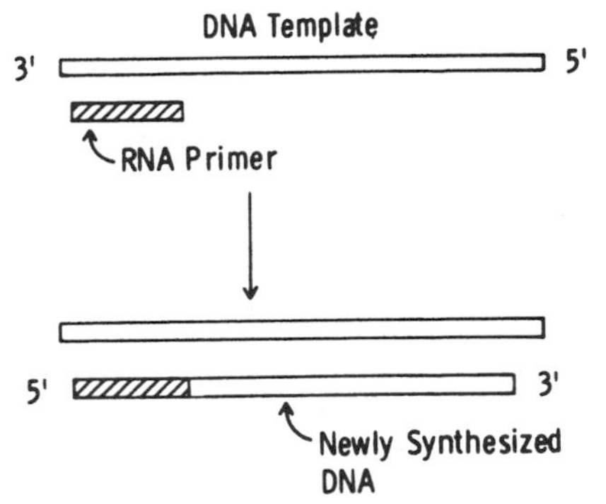

Fig. 4-62. An RNA primer is required to initiate DNA biosynthesis.

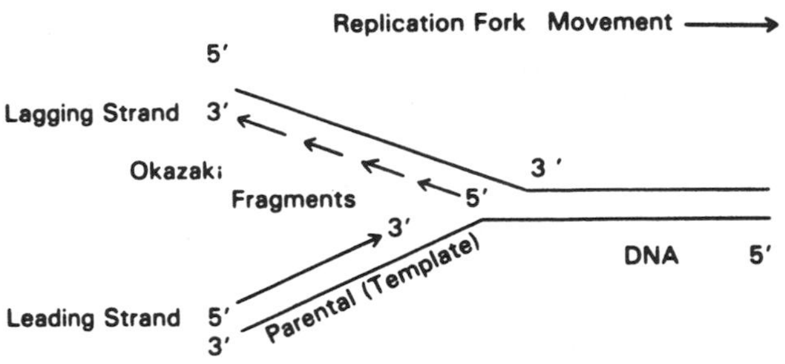

Fig. 4-64. Leading and lagging strands in DNA replication.

Elongation toward the right is in the 5′ to 3′ direction, and synthesis of the leading strand proceeds continuously (Fig. 4-64).

A major dilemma results in the synthesis of the opposite or lagging strand as the replication fork moves to the right. All DNA polymerases catalyze elongation in the 5′ to 3′ direction. The solution to this quandary emerged when it was discovered that one strand of DNA is synthesized in short segments ***(Okazaki fragments)*** in a discontinuous fashion (Figs. 4-64 and 4-65). For this to occur, primase starts on the right and polymerase III synthesizes the complementary strand toward the left. Primase then initiates synthesis of another segment farther to the right, and synthesis continues toward the left (Fig. 4-65). In this fashion both strands are elongated as the replication fork proceeds rightward. The trick used by nature is to synthesize the lagging strand in short (1,000-nucleotide) stretches to the left. This procedure emphasizes the importance of polymerase I in physiological synthesis. At the many primer sites on the lagging strand, polymerase I 5′-exonuclease activity degrades the primer portion, and the enzyme's polymerase activity fills the gap. DNA ligase then seals the nick, and a continuous strand thereby results (Fig. 4-64).

An analogous situation exists as the replication fork progresses leftward. Primase can initiate chain growth toward the left, and polymerase can keep it going in a continuous fashion on one of the two strands. Synthesis

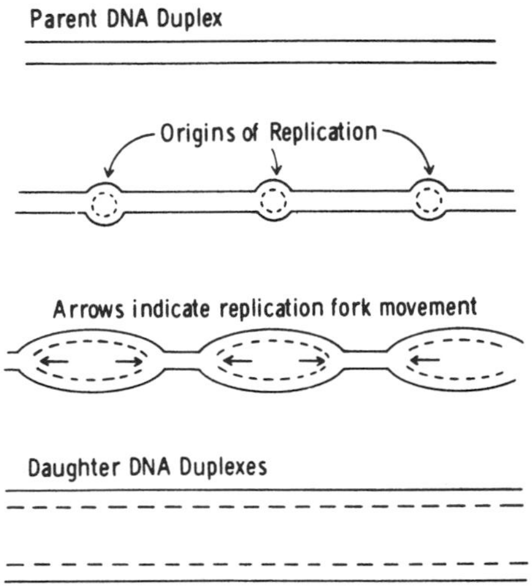

Fig. 4-63. Eukaryotic DNA exhibits multiple origins of replication.

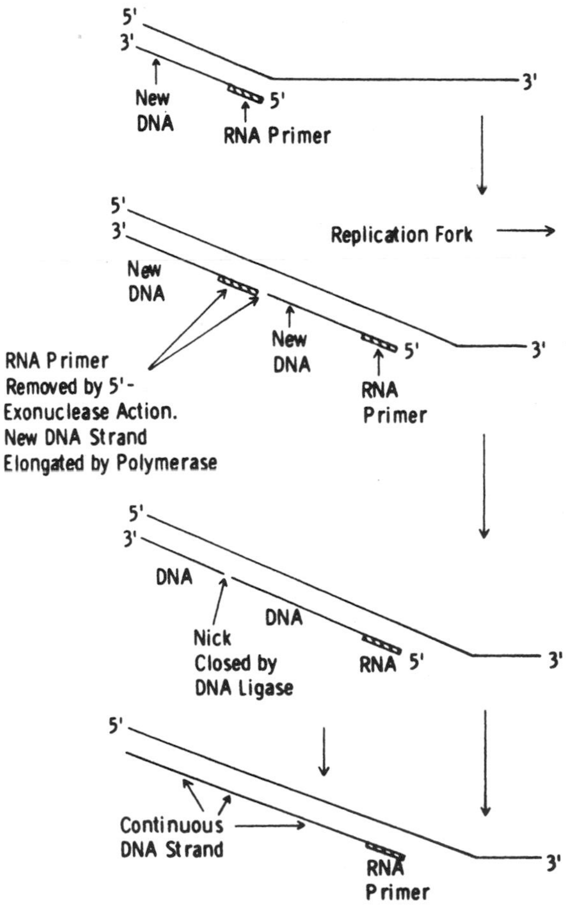

Fig. 4-65. Lagging strand biosynthesis in DNA replication.

using the opposite strand as template begins on the left and continues to the right. A second strand begins farther to the left and continues to the first strand. Then 5′-exonuclease activity of polymerase I removes the ribonucleotide-deoxyribonucleotide portion and fills the gap. DNA ligase seals the nick. As chain growth continues, the parental strands separate. The daughter DNA contains one parental strand and one newly synthesized strand. This property is referred to as ***semiconservative replication*** (conservative replication refers to the nonexistent situation where both parent strands and both daughter strands are found together). DNA gyrase aids in the process by converting the supercoiled DNA into more favorable topological isomers. It removes twists that are produced by unwinding.

The previous description reflects current knowledge of the process of replication in *E. coli* and other bacteria. Human DNA replication is similar in principle. Unlike *E. coli,* with a single origin of replication, thousands of replication origins exist. Proteins may exist that cause initiation at specific and currently uncharacterized sites. Human chromosomes also possess nucleosomes with their associated histones; bacterial chromosomes lack histones and nucleosomes. The negative charges of DNA phosphate in bacteria are neutralized by metals (Mg^{2+}, K^{+}) and organic cations such as spermine and spermidine. The histones associated with the parent human DNA duplex become associated with the leading strand and its template strand where reformation of nucleosomes occurs. Newly synthesized histones become associated with the lagging strand and its template strand. Human DNA polymerases progress along their templates with about one-tenth the velocity of that of *E. coli*. The discontinuous strands, called Okazaki fragments, in humans are 10% to 20% the length of those in *E. coli*. These differences may be related to the presence of nucleosomes and the greater degree of compactness of human DNA when compared with *E. coli* DNA.

DNA polymerase α is associated with primase activity. Primase activity is important in the initiation of DNA synthesis of the Okazaki fragments of the lagging strand. DNA polymerase α lacks 3′,5′-exonuclease activity. DNA polymerase δ contains 3′,5′-exonuclease activity but lacks primase activity. DNA polymerase δ is dependent on proliferating cell nuclear antigen (PCNA) for activity. PCNA is one type of cyclin. Cyclins are proteins necessary for replication or traversing the cell cycle, hence their name. A complex of DNA polymerase δ and PCNA mediates the synthesis of the DNA leading strand. After chain initiation, the strand is synthesized continuously and there is no need for continued primase activity. Leading strand synthesis is initiated by DNA polymerase α.

DNA Repair

DNA, which is altered by physical and chemical agents in the environment, is inherently unstable. Altered DNA is repaired by mechanisms considered in this section. These repair mechanisms rely on information originally contained in the two strands. If only one strand is modified, information residing on the other can be used to effect the repair process. If both strands of the duplex are altered, then a recombinational process involving an allele on the other chromosome of the pair may provide the information necessary for repair. If neither type of repair occurs, then the damage is retained as a mutation (an inheritable change in DNA, which is passed on to progeny cells). Such insults accumulate in humans and have been postulated to be important factors in tumorigenesis, cell death, and aging.

Let us consider the types of chemical modification that DNA undergoes and then the process of repair. The amino groups of cytosine and adenine in DNA undergo spontaneous (nonenzymatic) hydrolysis and form uracil and hypoxanthine, respectively. These structures are recognized by cellular proteins as abnormal. ***Base excision repair*** is the process used to correct such lesions. An ***AP-glycosidase*** catalyzes the hydrolytic removal of the abnormal base, leaving an intact sugar phosphate backbone. The result is an AP site, where AP is an abbreviation for apurinic (lacking A or G) or apyrimidinic (lacking C or T). Endonucleases catalyzes the hydrolysis of phosphodiester bonds on each side of the AP site removing deoxyribose. A repair polymerase, using a newly created 3′-hydroxyl group, replaces the deoxyribonucleotide. Then DNA ligase seals the nick, and the original base sequence is restored. A similar sequence of reactions results when a purine is spontaneously hydrolyzed from one of the strands.

Alterations produced by ionizing radiation, the chemical modification of bases by alkylating agents, and the formation of thymine dimers and other dimers by ultraviolet light can also be corrected by this ***nucleotide excision-repair.*** The four steps in this process include (1) hydrolysis of the affected strand on the 3′ side of the lesion by ***exinuclease,*** (2) hydrolysis on the 5′ side by exinuclease to give an oligonucleotide ($\approx$30 residues) containing the lesion, (3) DNA synthesis—using the 3′-hydroxyl group produced by exinuclease as primer—by repair polymerase, and (4) DNA ligation to seal the nick.

Transcription: RNA Biosynthesis

RNA is transcribed from DNA. The enzymes that catalyze RNA biosynthesis are ***DNA-dependent RNA polymerases.*** We discuss the reaction catalyzed by prokaryotic and eukaryotic RNA polymerases. We then consider the structural differences in enzymes isolated from *E. coli* and from humans. After biosynthesis, the primary RNA transcript may be chemically modified in processing reactions. We discuss the signals in DNA that are important in dictating the start site for transcription and the sequences that play a regulatory role in determining the frequency of initiation.

RNA polymerase, unlike DNA polymerase, can initiate polynucleotide synthesis; a primer is not required. The elongation reactions are analogous to those catalyzed by DNA polymerase. Chain growth proceeds in the 5′ to 3′ direction (Table 4-1). The sequence of nucleotides in the resulting RNA is determined by Watson-Crick base-pairing principles with the substitution of uracil (RNA) for thymine (DNA). The base-pairing rules are as follows: template A yields U, T yields A, G yields C, and C yields G. The RNA strand is antiparallel to its template. During replication, both strands of DNA serve as a template to produce two daughter duplexes. In RNA synthesis, only one of the two strands of a particular genetic DNA functions as a template. One strand of the DNA duplex serves as template in some genes, whereas the opposite strand is the template strand in other genes. However, the template strand is antiparallel to the RNA in all cases. The ***sense*** strand of DNA corresponds to the strand with the sequence that corresponds to that of the RNA (except RNA contains U in place of T). The ***antisense*** strand is complementary to the sense strand, and the antisense strand serves as a template for RNA synthesis.

Besides the DNA template, the four nucleoside triphosphates (as their Mg^{2+} complex) are required as substrates. The chemistry of the elongation reaction is illustrated in Figure 4-66. From this diagram we can see that chain growth occurs in the 5′ to 3′ direction. This scheme contains a deceptively large amount of information and should be understood by the reader. RNA polymerases lack the 3′ to 5′ proofreading exonuclease function that DNA polymerases exhibit. The physiological consequence of an error in RNA synthesis is not as great as that for DNA synthesis.

TABLE 4-24. RNA Polymerase Subunits and Transcription Factors in *E. coli*

SUBUNIT	NUMBER IN ENZYME	FUNCTION
β (Beta)	1	Catalytic site
β' (Beta prime)	1	DNA binding
α (Alpha)	2	Unknown
σ (Sigma)	1	Promotor recognition, initiation
ρ (Rho)	1	Termination

Let us consider the properties of the ***RNA polymerase*** isolated from *E. coli*. The holoenzyme consists of four different protein subunits. They exhibit the stoichiometry $\alpha_2\beta\beta'\sigma$ (Table 4-24). The $\alpha_2\beta\beta'$ component constitutes the ***core enzyme.*** The core enzyme possesses RNA polymerase activity. The ***sigma subunit*** (σ) confers the property of specific initiation to the core enzyme. After initiation at a physiological start site, the sigma subunit dissociates from the holoenzyme. The sigma subunit can combine with another core enzyme to initiate synthesis of another chain of RNA. *E. coli* contains about five different sigma subunits that recognize different promoters and are responsible for differential gene expression.

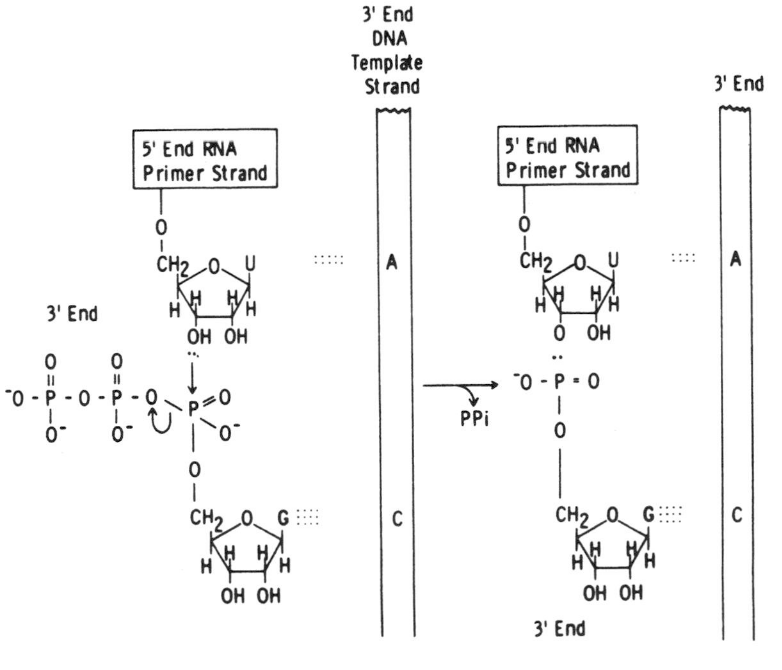

Fig. 4-66. Chemistry of the RNA polymerase reaction.

When the core enzyme approaches a transcriptional stop signal, a factor named ***rho (ρ)*** interacts with the core polymerase and results in appropriate chain termination.

In contrast to *E. coli* with its single RNA polymerase, humans have three RNA polymerases in the cell nucleus that catalyze the biosynthesis of different classes of RNA. Each of the three polymerases has more subunits (≈10) than the bacterial enzyme. However, the functions of the subunits have not yet been determined. In addition to the polymerases, several auxiliary proteins called ***transcription factors*** are required for initiation of RNA synthesis at the correct sites on DNA. The three classes of human RNA polymerase are designated by Roman numerals I, II, and III. ***RNA polymerase I*** is responsible for rRNA synthesis in the nucleolus. ***RNA polymerase II*** mediates the formation of hnRNA, the precursor of mRNA. ***RNA polymerase III*** catalyzes the formation of 5S RNA and other small RNAs (Table 4-21). RNA polymerase II has been studied extensively because it participates in the synthesis of mRNA, which codes for proteins.

The primary transcripts of all three classes of RNA in humans undergo additional modifications called processing reactions. The conversion of hnRNA to mRNA by processing is the most complex. Before completion of the primary transcript or RNA molecule, the 5′ end of the growing nascent chain reacts with GTP to form a 5′ to 5′ guanosine triphosphate terminus (Fig. 4-67A). The 5′ terminus is methylated by *S*-adenosylmethionine, and the resulting structure is called the 5′-cap. After chain termination, the 3′ end reacts with several (≈100) ATP molecules to form a polyA tail structure (a series of covalently linked adenylate residues) and PP_i. Canonical sequences in the 3′ region of hnRNA (AAUAAA) specify the site for adding the 3′ polyA tail 10 to 30 nucleotides downstream from the AAUAAA signal. The cap is probably necessary for mRNA to interact with the ribosome, and the polyA tail may stabilize the message. Occasional mRNAs, such as those encoding histones, lack the polyA tail.

Heterogeneous nuclear RNA, or hnRNA, also undergoes splicing reactions. During this process, intervening sequences are removed by excision. It is imperative that

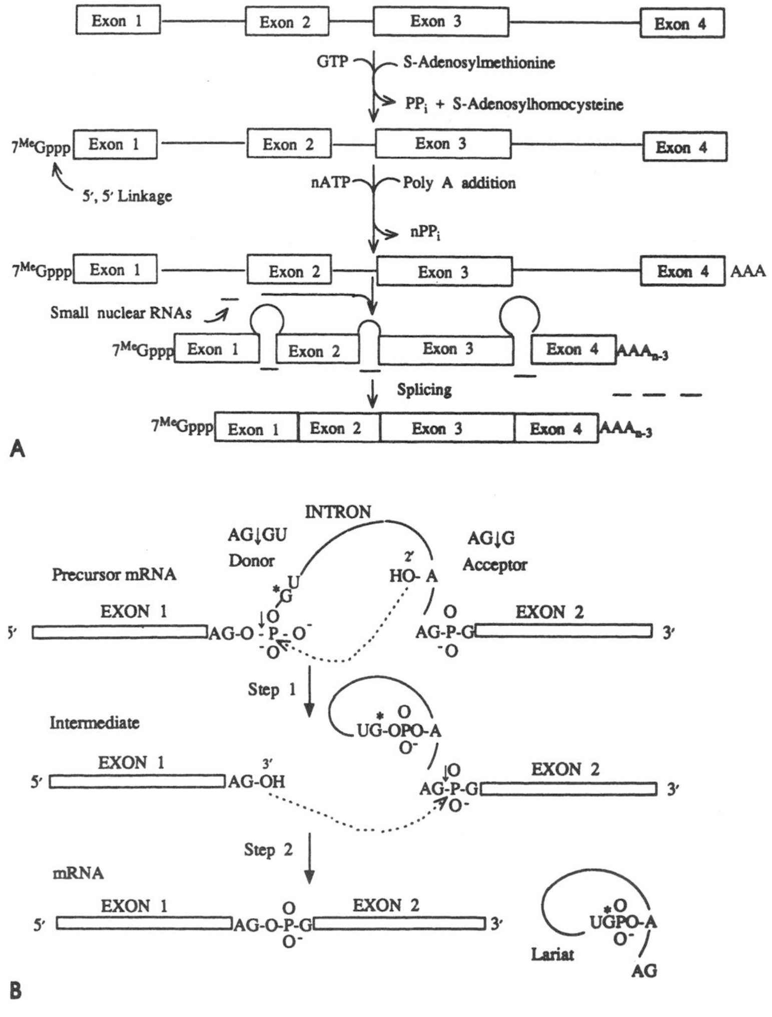

Fig. 4-67. Capping, polyadenylation, and splicing reactions are involved in mRNA formation *(A)*. Splicing involves the formation of a lariat-form of RNA *(B)*.

splicing be performed accurately; otherwise, an aberrant protein would result. (snRNAs) (or snurps) play a role in aligning hnRNA to ensure accurate splicing (Fig. 4-67A). The signals for splicing out, or excising, intervening sequences within hnRNA consist of canonical sequences of about nine bases consisting of 5′-donor and 3′-acceptor sites. The first two bases of the excised RNA are GU, and the last two are AG (Fig. 4-67B). hnRNA splicing occurs with the formation of an RNA lariat (Fig. 4-67B). A 2′-hydroxyl group contributed by an adenosine residue in the RNA segment attacks the phosphorus atom at the 5′ end of the splice junction as shown in step 1 of Figure 4-67B. A free 3′-hydroxyl group attacks the phosphorus atom at the 3′ end of the splice junction. The two exons are joined, and the lariat-shaped RNA is displaced. These processing reactions occur in the cell nucleus before transport to cytoplasmic ribosomes.

Rifamycin is a drug that inhibits the initiation, but not the elongation or completion, of RNA biosynthesis in prokaryotes. Rifamycin binds specifically to the β-subunit of RNA polymerase. This suggests that the interaction of the β- and σ-subunits is important during the initiation process. Rifamycin is currently one of the three drugs used for the treatment of persons with tuberculosis. It does not inhibit initiation of RNA synthesis in humans. ***Actinomycin D*** is a drug that binds to DNA and inhibits RNA elongation reactions in both eukaryotes and prokaryotes. This substance is used in the treatment of several types of malignant tumors. It fails to inhibit DNA elongation reactions.

Translation: Protein Biosynthesis

Crick's law of molecular biology (often called the central dogma of molecular biology) states that information flows from DNA to RNA to protein (Table 4-1). The alphabet of nucleic acids consists of four letters: A, T, G, and C in DNA and A, U, G, and C in RNA. The alphabet of proteins consists of 20 letters corresponding to the 20 amino acids that participate in ribosome-dependent protein synthesis (Table 4-5). The conversion of the four-letter nucleic acid alphabet to the 20-letter protein alphabet is called ***translation.*** Translation, or protein synthesis, requires elaborate biochemical machinery consisting of more than 150 molecular components.

Three classes of RNA are involved in translation: rRNA, tRNA, and mRNA. The rRNA constitutes about half the mass of ribosomes, and protein constitutes the remainder. Ribosomes are made up of two subunits: a small subunit and a large subunit. ***Ribosomes*** are the subcellular machines in which peptide bond formation and protein synthesis occur. ***Transfer RNA*** has two functions. tRNAs serve as adapters that recognize the nucleic acid code, and tRNAs carry activated amino acids bound through a high-energy bond. ***Messenger RNA*** carries information as a specific sequence of bases (codons), which specify the sequence of amino acids found in the corresponding protein. ***Amino acyl-tRNA synthetases*** are a family of enzymes that catalyze the attachment of the amino acids to their corresponding or cognate tRNAs (one amino acyl–tRNA synthetase per amino acid). Several nonribosomal proteins participate in protein biosynthesis. These proteins include initiation factors, elongation factors, and termination, or release, factors. Before considering the steps involved in protein synthesis, let us first consider the properties of the genetic code.

THE GENETIC CODE

A two-letter code constructed from any four letters (A, T, G, or C in DNA or A, U, G, or C in RNA) yields 4^2, or 16, different code words, or ***codons.*** This is insufficient to uniquely specify the 20 different amino acids. A three-letter, or triplet, code yields 4^3, or 64, different codons, which is more than adequate to specify the 20 different amino acids. Experiments show that the genetic code is triplet in nature; the codons and their corresponding amino acids are tabulated in Table 4-25. Based on the methodology used to decipher the code, the codons are expressed as a sequence of RNA beginning from the 5′ end of each triplet. During protein synthesis, mRNA is translated triplet by triplet in the 5′ to 3′ direction.

Of the 64 possible codons, all but three (*i.e.,* 61) correspond to an amino acid. The three exceptions (UAG, UAA, UGA) are stop codons and code for chain termination. Methionine (AUG) and tryptophan (UGG) have a single codon. ***AUG*** is the initiating codon for protein biosynthesis, and ***methionine*** is the initiating amino acid

TABLE 4-25. Genetic Code

FIRST POSITION (5′-END)	SECOND POSITION U	C	A	G	THIRD POSITION (3′-END)
U	Phe	Ser	Tyr	Cys	U
	Phe	Ser	Tyr	Cys	C
	Leu	Ser	Stop	Stop	A
	Leu	Ser	Stop	Trp	G
C	Leu	Pro	His	Arg	U
	Leu	Pro	His	Arg	C
	Leu	Pro	Gln	Arg	A
	Leu	Pro	Gln	Arg	G
A	Ile	Thr	Asn	Ser	U
	Ile	Thr	Asn	Ser	C
	Ile	Thr	Lys	Arg	A
	Met	Thr	Lys	Arg	G
G	Val	Ala	Asp	Gly	U
	Val	Ala	Asp	Gly	C
	Val	Ala	Glu	Gly	A
	Val	Ala	Glu	Gly	G

in eukaryotes and prokaryotes. AUG also codes for the methionine residues that occur in the interior of proteins. The 18 other amino acids are represented by more than one codon, and this property is called ***degeneracy.*** Nine amino acids are represented by two codons. In this group of nine, the first two bases are the same, and the third position is either a pyrimidine (Py) or a purine (Pu). The codons are XYPy or XYPu. Five amino acids are represented by four codons. In each case, the first two bases are the same, and the third can be any of the four bases (A, U, G, or C). Three amino acids are represented by six codons. These constitute a combination of (a) four codons and (b) two codons with the above-mentioned properties (Table 4-25). Isoleucine is the only amino acid represented by three codons (Table 4-5). Again, the first two bases are the same (Table 4-25).

Because of the variation in the third position of the codon and because it participates in some nonstandard Watson-Crick base pairing with the tRNA anticodon, the third codon position was designated the ***wobble*** position by Crick. As a result of this property, some tRNA molecules are able to interact with (adapt to) two or even three different codons. On the order of 40 tRNA molecules interact with the 61 codons. We do not discuss the precise nature of wobble base pairing here. The interaction of tRNA with mRNA occurs in an antiparallel orientation. The wobble position is on the 3′ end of the mRNA codon; the wobble position corresponds to the 5′ end of the anticodon triplet.

As mentioned previously, AUG codes for the first and initiating amino acid, which is methionine. The genetic code is read triplet by triplet in the 5′ to 3′ direction until a termination or stop codon is reached. No punctuation signal is required to indicate the end of one codon and the beginning of the next (the code is ***commaless***). Each base of the triplet is used only once per polypeptide synthesized (the code is ***nonoverlapping***). The genetic code is (almost) ***universal.*** The genetic code is the same in both prokaryotes (*e.g., E. coli*) and the cytosol of eukaryotes (*e.g.,* humans). This genetic code is called the standard genetic code. That for mitochondrial protein synthesis is exceptional and is somewhat different from the one shown in Table 4-25.

THE RIBOSOME

The ribosome is the biochemical machine on which protein biosynthesis occurs. The ribosome is where mRNA and aminoacyl-tRNA interact and where peptide bond formation occurs. The size of ribosomes and their subunits is expressed by their sedimentation coefficients (Svedberg, or S, values). The *E. coli* ribosome is a 70S ribosome. It is composed of a large subunit (50S) and a small subunit (30S). The composition is shown in Table 4-26. The human ribosome is 80S in nature and consists of a large (60S) and small (40S) subunit (Table 4-27). The primary structures of the rRNAs and most of the ribosomal proteins have been determined.

TABLE 4-26. Composition of the Ribosomes of *E. coli*

PROPERTY	RIBOSOME	SMALL SUBUNIT	LARGE SUBUNIT
Sedimentation coefficient	70S	30S	50S
RNA		16S	23S 5S
Protein		21 Polypeptides	35 Polypeptides

Ribosomes contain two functional sites termed the ***A site*** and the ***P site.*** Aminoacyl-tRNA binds at the A site; peptidyl-tRNA and the initiating methionine-$tRNA_I$ bind at the P site. The small and large subunits make contributions to both sites. ***Peptidyltransferase*** activity, which catalyzes peptide bond formation, resides on the large subunit and is intrinsic to the ribosome; moreover, this activity may be associated with rRNA and not protein.

AMINO ACID ACTIVATION

The enzymes that catalyze the formation of aminoacyl-tRNA are termed ***aminoacyl-tRNA synthetases*** (or ligases). There is one enzyme in *E. coli* and one cytoplasmic enzyme in humans corresponding to each of the 20 genetically encoded amino acids. These enzymes attach the specific amino acid to each of the tRNA molecules that correspond to that amino acid. The degeneracy of the genetic code necessitates the use of more than one tRNA for several amino acids. The tRNA molecules that correspond to a given amino acid are called ***isoacceptors.*** The mechanism of amino acid activation is analogous to that for fatty acid activation. It involves a pyrophosphate split from ATP to yield an aminoacyl-AMP intermediate. Aminoacyl-AMP reacts with its corresponding tRNA to

TABLE 4-27. Composition of Mammalian Ribosomes

PROPERTY	RIBOSOME	SMALL SUBUNIT	LARGE SUBUNIT
Sedimentation coefficient	80S	40S	60S
RNA		18S	28S 5.8S 5S
Protein		33 Polypeptides	49 Polypeptides

form aminoacyl-tRNA and AMP. The reaction can be outlined as follows (where aa denotes amino acid).

$$aa + ATP \rightleftharpoons aa\text{-}AMP + PP_i$$

$$aa\text{-}AMP + tRNA \rightleftharpoons aa\text{-}tRNA + AMP$$

Both steps of this reaction are catalyzed by a single enzyme. There is no loss of energy-rich bonds in this process. However, the hydrolysis of PP_i catalyzed by a separate pyrophosphatase is exergonic and serves to pull the reaction in the forward direction (Table 4-1). The 3′ sequence of eukaryotic and prokaryotic tRNA molecules ends with CCA. The amino acid is covalently linked through an energy-rich bond to the 2′- or 3′-hydroxyl of ribose on the 3′-terminal adenosine-containing nucleotide of tRNA.

PROTEIN SYNTHESIS FACTORS

Protein synthesis is divided into initiation, elongation, and termination. There are protein factors that transiently associate with the ribosome to perform specific functions. In prokaryotes, the initiation factors are designated IF, the elongation factors are designated EF, and the termination or release factors are designated RF. The factors in humans are designated similarly but with an e prefix for eukaryotic (*e.g.*, eIF for eukaryotic initiation factor). The various factors are given in Tables 4-28 and 4-29.

Three initiation factors are required in prokaryotes, and several more occur in humans. The functions of the first three initiation factors for prokaryotes and eukaryotes are similar. IF2 binds GTP and formyl-Met-$tRNA_I$ (where I refers to a special initiator molecule) in prokaryotes; eIF2 binds GTP and Met-$tRNA_I$ in humans. These factors place the initiator methionine-$tRNA_I$ into the P site of the ribosome during the initiation process. *N*-formyl-methionine-$tRNA_I$ (fMet-$tRNA_I$) is the initiating residue in prokaryotes, and Met-$tRNA_I$ (unformylated) is the initiator in humans. The formyl group in prokaryotes is added after methionine has been linked to its cognate tRNA; *N*-formyltetrahydrofolate is the formyl donor. The initiation factors do not form a complex with methionine-$tRNA^{Met}$, the latter is the source of the methionine placed into internal positions of nascent polypeptide chains. Methionine-$tRNA^{Met}$ is not formylated. EF-Tu (where T refers to transfer and u refers to unstable) in prokaryotes and eEF-1 in humans forms a complex with GTP and methionine-$tRNA^{Met}$ and all other aminoacyl-tRNAs (one at a time) required for protein biosynthesis. The complex consisting of the elongation factor, GTP, and aminoacyl-tRNA is called a ternary complex. These factors place the aminoacyl-tRNA into the A site during protein synthesis. Let us now consider the various steps of protein synthesis.

TABLE 4-28. Factors involved in Protein Synthesis in *E. coli*

FACTOR	MOLECULAR WEIGHT	FUNCTION
Initiation Factors		
IF1	9,000	Keeps ribosomes dissociated
IF2	100,000	Binds GTP and formyl-Met-$tRNA_I$
IF3	23,000	Keeps ribosomes dissociated
Elongation Factors		
EF-T is made of		Transfer
EF-Tu	43,000	unstable; binds aminoacyltRNA/GTP
EF-Ts	74,000	stable; displaces GDP
EF-G	77,000	GTPase; translocates mRNA along ribosome
Release Factors		
RF1		Recognizes UAA, UAG
RF2		Recognizes UAA, UGA

TABLE 4-29. Eukaryotic Protein Synthesis Factors

FACTOR	FUNCTION
Initiation factor	
eIF1	Assists mRNA binding
eIF2	Binds initiator Met-$tRNA^{Met}_I$ and GTP
eIF2A	Binds Met-$tRNA^{Met}_I$ to 40S ribosome via AUG in mRNA
eIF2B	Exchanges GTP/GDP
eIF2C	Stabilizes ternary complex
eIF3	Binds to 40S subunit before mRNA binding
eIF4A	Unwinds secondary structure of mRNA via ATP-dependent helicase activity
eIF4B	Assists mRNA binding
eIF4C	Assists mRNA binding
eIF4D	Plays role in formation of the first peptide bond
eIF4E	Recognizes mRNA cap
eIF4F	Is a complex made of eIF4A, eIF4E, and p220
eIF5	Promotes GTP hydrolysis and release of other initiation factors
eIF6	Dissociates subunits
Elongation factor	
eEF1	
EF1α	Binds aminoacyl tRNA and GTP
eEF1$\beta\gamma$	Assists in the exchange of GTP and GDP in EF1α
eEF2	Translocates mRNA along ribosome; hydrolyzes GTP; is inhibited by ADP-ribosylation catalyzed by diphtheria toxin
Release factor	
eRF	Promotes the hydrolysis of peptidyl-tRNA to form peptide and tRNA; the factor also binds and hydrolyzes GTP (GDP + P_i)

STEPS IN PROTEIN SYNTHESIS

To initiate biosynthesis, mRNA forms a complex with the ribosome and fMet-tRNA$_I$ (prokaryotes) or Met-tRNA$_I$ (eukaryotes). In prokaryotes, or bacteria, the small ribosomal subunit is prevented from associating with the large subunit by the action of IF1 and IF3, which are bound to the small subunit. The initiating AUG codon is not at the 5′ end of mRNA but is 50 to 100 nucleotides or more from the 5′ end. To initiate synthesis in bacteria, mRNA binds to the small ribosomal subunit at five bases (CCUCC) near the 3′ end of 16S RNA called the ***Shine-Dalgarno*** sequence in a process that is negotiated by IF3; this places the initiating AUG in the correct position relative to the ribosome. Next, IF2·GTP·fMet-tRNA$_I$ binds to the mRNA–small subunit complex, IF3 is released, and then the large subunit binds to the small subunit. After this association, GTP is hydrolyzed to GDP and P$_i$; IF2 dissociates from the complex along with IF1. At the end of this process, fMet-tRNA$_I$ is bound to the P site of the ribosome with its anticodon bound in an antiparallel fashion with the initiating AUG of mRNA.

Initiation of protein synthesis in eukaryotes, which involves an ***AUG scanning*** mechanism, is similar in outline but differs in detail. Initiation differs in that Met-tRNA$_I$ is unformylated, more initiation factors participate, and there is no comparable interaction of mRNA with a Shine-Dalgarno sequence. In contrast to bacterial protein synthesis, the ternary complex formed from eIF2·GTP·Met-tRNA$_I$ with the small subunit occurs before binding to mRNA. eIF4E recognizes the guanine cap of mRNA. The 40S subunit binds to the 5′ end of monocistronic mRNA and scans along the message until the first AUG is encountered. Several other initiation factors participate in binding the small subunit to mRNA. The anticodon of Met-tRNA$_I$ plays a role in scanning. After the first AUG is encountered, the large subunit binds to form the initiation complex. eIF5 catalyzes GTP hydrolysis and the dissociation of initiation factors from the ribosomes; ATP hydrolysis also accompanies the formation of the human initiation complex. At the end of the initiation process in both bacterial and human protein synthesis, the initiator methionine-tRNA is found in the P site. Initiator methionine tRNA is the only aminoacyl-tRNA that is delivered physiologically to the P site; the other aminoacyl-tRNAs are delivered to the A site.

After the formation of the initiation complex, a series of repetitive elongation reactions occurs. For a protein containing 300 amino acids, there is a unique initiation event, 299 elongation events, and a unique termination event. A series of ternary complexes of EF-Tu·GTP·aminoacyl-tRNAs (eEF-1α·GTP·aminoacyl-tRNAs in humans) interact, with the A (aminoacyl-tRNA) site of the ribosome. When a match between the triplet codon imme-

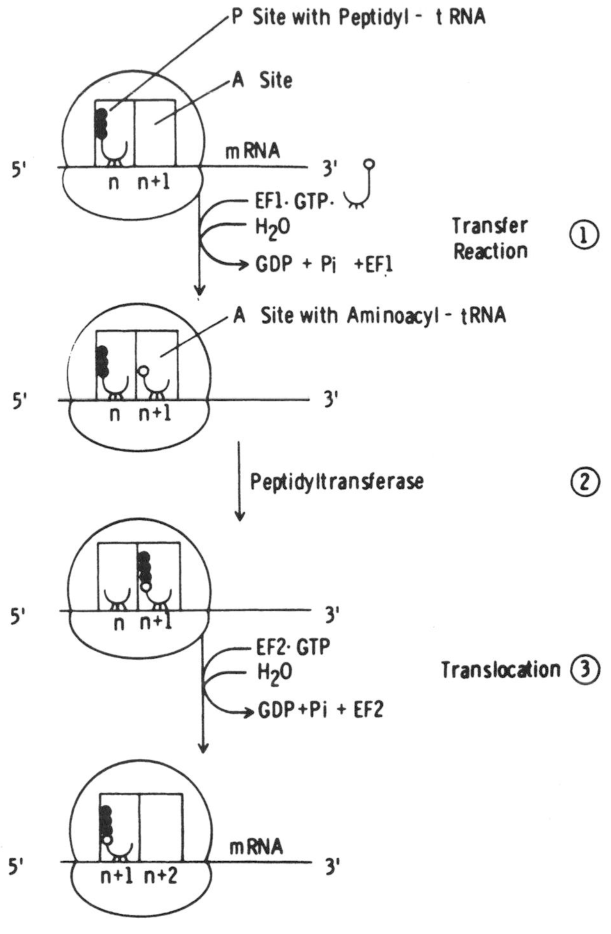

Fig. 4-68. Topography of elongation and translocation reactions in protein biosynthesis: the A and P sites.

diately after the AUG (on the 3′ side) and the corresponding aminoacyl-tRNA anticodon occurs, then GTP is hydrolyzed and EF-Tu dissociates from the ribosome. The appropriate aminoacyl-tRNA is implanted in the A site. Next, the endogenous peptidyltransferase activity of the large ribosomal subunit catalyzes a reaction between the amino group in the A site with the activated carboxyl group in the P site to form the first peptide bond. After this reaction, the dipeptidyl-tRNA is bound to the A site and free tRNA is found in the P site. Before the next elongation reaction, EFG·GTP interacts with the complex and mediates the translocation of mRNA and peptidyl-tRNA from the A site to the P site. In the process, GTP is hydrolyzed to GDP and P$_i$ and the free tRNA is ejected from the P site. This completes the first elongation cycle. The dipeptidyl-tRNA now occupies the P site. The second and subsequent cycles of elongation occur as described for the first. Aminoacyl-tRNA is brought to the A site as a ternary complex with EF-Tu and GTP. After interaction of the matching codon with anticodon, GTP hydrolysis

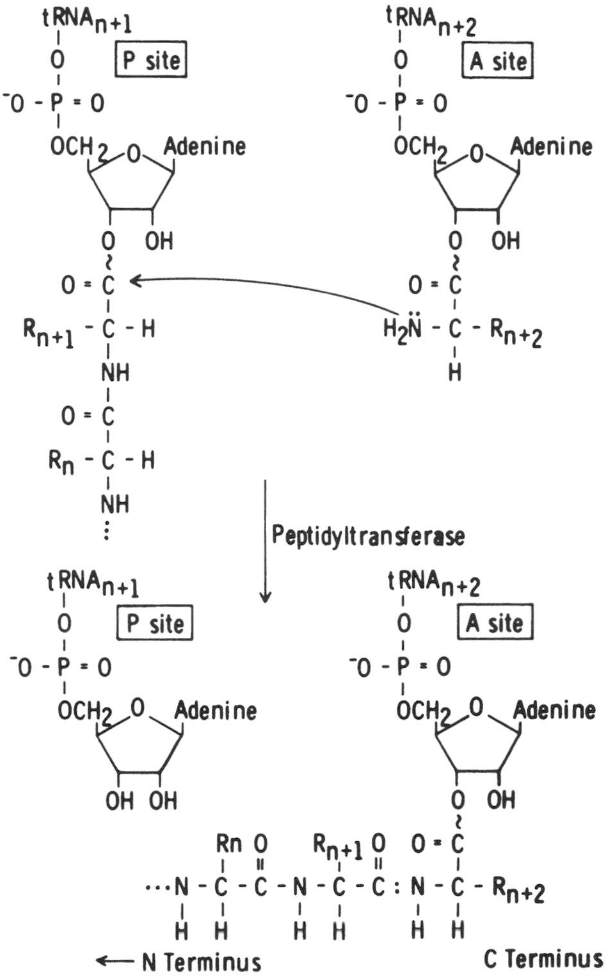

Fig. 4-69. Chemistry of the elongation reaction of protein synthesis.

occurs. Peptide bond formation and translocation follow. The process is shown in Figure 4-68.

The reaction catalyzed by peptidyltransferase is the same in prokaryotes and eukaryotes and is shown in Figure 4-69. This diagram contains a deceptively large amount of information and should be understood by the reader. From the diagram, one can determine that chain growth occurs from the amino to the carboxyl terminus. One also can see that peptidyl-tRNA occupies the A site after the peptidyltransferase reaction. This necessitates a translocation reaction as illustrated in Figure 4-68.

The elongation cycles continue until a stop codon (UAA, UAG, or UGA; Table 4-25) occupies the A site. An RF, or release factor, interacts with the complex and discharges the polypeptide from tRNA by hydrolysis. The ribosomal subunits dissociate, and the tRNA is liberated. The process in prokaryotes and eukaryotes is analogous.

Several antibiotics inhibit specific steps of translation; the actions of several of these are given in Table 4-30. Additionally, diphtheria toxin catalyzes a reaction between eEF-2 and NAD^+ to give ADP ribosyl–eEF-2 and nicotinamide. The covalently bound ADP ribosyl group inactivates the eukaryotic elongation factor. The potent toxin, made in *Corynebacterium diphtheriae,* has no effect on bacterial protein synthesis.

TABLE 4-30. Antibiotics That Inhibit Protein Synthesis

ANTIBIOTIC	SENSITIVE ORGANISMS	PROCESS INHIBITED
Streptomycin	Prokaryotes	Initiation; produces mistakes in translation
Tetracycline	Prokaryotes	Aminoacyl-tRNA attachment to the ribosome
Chloramphenicol	Prokaryotes	Ribosomal peptidyltransferase
Puromycin	Prokaryotes and eukaryotes	Causes premature chain termination
Cycloheximide	Eukaryotes	Ribosomal peptidyltransferase

Let us now consider the bioenergetic cost of peptide bond formation. Two high-energy bonds of ATP are expended to form aminoacyl-tRNA ($ATP \rightarrow AMP + 2\ P_i$), and one GTP is hydrolyzed (to GDP and P_i) in the transfer reaction, where aminoacyl-tRNA is placed in the A site. Peptide bond formation per se does not require any additional energy expenditure. The high-energy bond of aminoacyl-tRNA is converted to the low-energy peptide bond in an exergonic reaction. A fourth high-energy bond is expended as GTP is hydrolyzed (to GDP and P_i) in the translocation reaction. A total of four high-energy bonds are thus expended per peptide bond formed. The cost of peptide bond formation therefore is considerable. The chemical energy and the complex ribosomal machinery are required to convert the language of the four-letter nucleic acid alphabet to the 20-letter alphabet of proteins.

Reverse Transcription: RNA-Dependent DNA Synthesis

The direction of biological information flow was thought initially to extend from DNA to DNA (replication), DNA to RNA (transcription), and RNA to protein (translation), as noted in Table 4-1. Later work with the avian Rous sarcoma virus (one of a large number of tumor viruses) showed that the viral genetic RNA possesses a DNA intermediate during its life cycle. Furthermore, the DNA intermediate integrates into the host cell genome. The synthesis of DNA from RNA templates is termed reverse transcription, and this virus is one example of a retrovirus.

The enzyme that catalyzes RNA-dependent DNA synthesis is ***reverse transcriptase;*** it requires the four deoxynucleoside triphosphates and an RNA template. Like DNA polymerases, reverse transcriptase cannot initiate DNA synthesis *de novo*; a primer is required. Reverse transcriptase, the RNA template (the genome), and the primer (a tRNA) are carried by the infectious virus. The elongation reactions proceed in the 5′ to 3′ direction.

A large number of retroviruses produce cancer in a variety of species. However, only one human neoplasm (T-cell leukemia) is caused by a retrovirus (human T-cell lymphotropic virus, or HTLV–1). Moreover, the human disorder named acquired immunodeficiency syndrome (AIDS) is a result of infection by a retrovirus called human immunodeficiency virus (HIV). The study of retroviruses has been helpful in the study of tumorigenesis and AIDS. Moreover, reverse transcriptase is an extremely important tool in molecular biology and biotechnology.

Posttranslational Protein Modification

Two common posttranslational modifications, which occur either during or shortly after synthesis of polypeptides, include proteolytic cleavage and glycosylation. Although methionine is the universal initiating amino acid, methionine is found on the amino terminus of only a small proportion of proteins. The initiating methionine is hydrolytically removed from those proteins lacking methionine at the amino terminus by the action of an aminopeptidase. Acetylation of the resulting amino terminus by acetyl-CoA to give an *N*-acetylprotein is a common posttranslational modification in humans. Additional posttranslational modification occurs in proteins destined for secretion from the cell, insertion into the plasma membrane, or translocation into the lysosome. Proteins with these properties are synthesized on ribosomes found with the rough endoplasmic reticulum. We shall consider the properties of proteins that lead to their synthesis at this location under the rubric of the signal peptide hypothesis.

SIGNAL PEPTIDE HYPOTHESIS

Proteins destined for insertion into membranes or secretion exhibit a leader sequence of 15 to 40 amino acids at their amino terminus. The signal contains at least one positively charged residue and a hydrophobic stretch of 10 to 15 residues. Translation begins on free ribosomes and stops shortly after the leader or signal sequence has been synthesized. A ***signal recognition particle*** (SRP) is responsible for arresting biosynthesis as SRP recognizes the hydrophobic leader sequence and binds to the nascent polypeptide-ribosome complex. SRP, which is a G-protein, consists of several proteins and 7SL RNA, a 300-nucleotide RNA. The arrested complex binds to an SRP receptor and two ribosome receptors in the rough endoplasmic reticulum. This interaction allows biosynthesis to resume as the nascent polypeptide chain with its signal sequence is directed into the lumen of the endoplasmic reticulum. GTP is hydrolyzed after the formation of the SRP–SRP receptor complex, and SRP is recycled. Before translation is complete, the signal sequence is hydrolyzed from the precursor, or the preprotein, to produce the protein within the lumen of the rough endoplasmic reticulum. ***Signal peptidase*** catalyzes the hydrolytic removal of the leader sequence (Fig. 4-70).

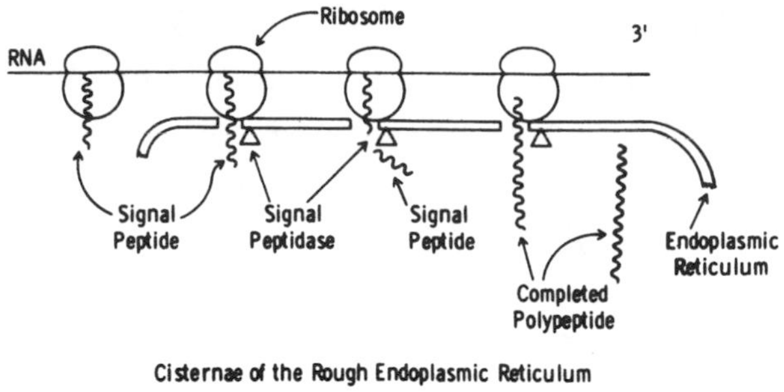

Fig. 4-70. The signal peptide directs nascent proteins to the rough endoplasmic reticulum.

Let us briefly consider the mechanism of insulin biosynthesis in the β cells of the pancreas. Insulin consists of an A chain and a B chain linked by two disulfide bonds. Insulin is synthesized from a precursor called ***preproinsulin.*** The order of synthesis of preproinsulin is leader sequence, B chain, connecting peptide, and finally A chain. All of these reside initially on a single polypeptide, preproinsulin; the discrete chains form as a result of proteolytic processing. After synthesis is initiated, preproinsulin is channeled into the lumen of the rough endoplasmic reticulum in a process involving a signal peptide sequence (the presequence of preproinsulin), the SRP, and the SRP receptor and two ribosome receptors on the rough endoplasmic reticulum membrane (as described in the previous paragraph). A signal peptidase catalyzes the hydrolytic removal of the signal sequence, and synthesis continues to yield ***proinsulin.*** The three disulfide bonds found in native insulin (two between the A and B chain, and one within the A chain) form within the single polypeptide chain constituting proinsulin as catalyzed by ***protein disulfide isomerase.*** The polypeptide is cleaved at paired basic residues at two sites by enzymes with trypsinlike specificity called prohormone convertases to yield a C, or connecting, peptide and insulin composed of its two chains (A and B). Carboxypeptidase H removes extra carboxyterminal basic residues on the B chain to yield insulin. Insulin is packaged into secretory vesicles, stored, and released upon demand. It undergoes no further posttranslational modifications. Insulin is released in response to elevated glucose within the β cell as sensed by glucokinase, the high K_m (10 mM) isoform of hexokinase that is found in liver and the β cell and is not inhibited by glucose 6-phosphate.

PROTEIN GLYCOSYLATION

Many proteins found in the plasma membrane and many circulating proteins such as antibodies and hormones (e.g., thyroid-stimulating hormone, luteinizing hormone, follicle-stimulating hormone) are glycoproteins. Glycosylation of proteins occurs within the Golgi complex and before their transport into secretory vesicles (Fig. 4-1). Albumin, the most abundant plasma protein, is synthesized in and secreted by the liver. Albumin, however, is not glycosylated. This finding indicates that glycosylation is not a requirement for secretion.

There are two major classes of glycoprotein. However, a single protein can be a member of both classes. The two classes of glycoprotein are *O*-linked (involving protein-serine or threonine) and *N*-linked (involving protein-asparagine residues). The *O*-linked class, which is the simpler of the two, is considered first. There are about 80 types of sugar linkages in glycoproteins. Each type of linkage is determined by enzyme specificity. The donor substrates are listed in Table 4-31. Formation of these oligomeric sugar derivatives is unlike that of nucleic acids because the sequence is not determined by a template mechanism.

The ABO blood group pentasaccharide is an example of a carbohydrate attached to protein by an *O*-linkage. A specific transferase catalyzes the addition of each residue to its acceptor substrate. Biosynthesis is specified and determined by enzymes acting sequentially. For the ABO oligosaccharide, *N*-acetylgalactosamine is attached to an acceptor protein-serine or threonine. Then galactose, *N*-acetylglucose, galactose, and fucose are added sequentially to yield the H antigen, which corresponds to blood type O. The addition of *N*-acetylgalactose yields A antigen, or the addition of galactose yields B antigen. There are four nucleotide differences in the genes encoding the *N*-acetylgalactosyltransferase and the galactosyltransferase that distinguish between the A and B blood types. The corresponding H antigen and the O allele result from a defect in the gene that encodes for the terminal transferase (*N*-acetylgalactosyltransferase or galactosyltransferase). There is a deletion in the gene for the O allele that produces a nonfunctional protein; as a consequence, H antigen is not further metabolized to produce the A or B antigen.

The oligosaccharides attached at *N*-linkages are larger than those attached at *O*-linkages, and the mechanism of biosynthesis is more formidable. There are three subclasses of *N*-linked oligosaccharides: ***high mannose, complex,*** and ***hybrid.*** The complex and hybrid subclasses are derived from the high mannose variety by additional reactions. The pathway for biosynthesis of high mannose chains involves the following three operations: (1) formation of a 14-member oligosaccharide linked via a high-energy bond to dolichol by a pyrophosphate group, (2) transfer of the oligosaccharide to the acceptor protein, and (3) hydrolytic removal (trimming) of specific sugars. The subsequent addition of several sugars from nucleotides to the high mannose subclass results in the formation of the hybrid and complex classes of oligosaccharide. These processes begin in the endoplasmic reticulum and are completed in the Golgi (Fig. 4-1).

Let us consider the first phase. ***Dolichol*** is a polyisoprenoid compound (17 to 20 five-carbon, or isoprenoid, units) with an alcohol at one terminus. Dolichol is found within the membranes of the endoplasmic reticulum. The alcohol group is phosphorylated by CTP to form CDP and dolichol phosphate. Dolichol phosphate reacts with UDP-*N*-acetylglucosamine to form dolichol diphospho-*N*-acetylglucosamine and UMP. Six additional sugars are transferred from nucleotide donors, and then seven sugars are transferred from dolichol phosphate derivatives. The 14-member core is transferred *en bloc* to the acceptor protein at a specific asparagine residue. Transfer occurs to sites in the acceptor protein in the sequence . . . AsnXSer (Thr) . . . , where X is nearly any amino acid. Terminal glucosyl residues (four) are removed by hydrolysis reactions catalyzed by glycosidases. A single mannose is removed. When the process stops here the product is a ***high mannose oligosaccharide.*** To form the ***complex*** and ***hybrid chain oligosaccharide,*** *N*-acetylglucosamine, fucose, galactose, and sialic acid are added from the derivatives indicated in Table 4-31. These activated monomers serve as precursors or donors for condensation or polymerization reactions (Table 4-1).

Regulation of Gene Expression

Gene regulation lies at the heart of differentiation, development, and cell maintenance. Major advances in our understanding of gene regulation have been made with the advent of gene isolation, gene sequence analysis, and recombinant DNA methodologies. Before considering gene regulation, we must introduce a few terms. As previously stated, DNA-dependent RNA synthesis is called ***transcription.*** A bacterial ***promoter*** represents the RNA polymerase binding site on genetic DNA, and the ***terminator*** is the region of genetic DNA downstream from the promoter where RNA synthesis stops. The ***transcription unit*** extends from the promoter to the terminator, and the RNA product resulting from transcription is called the ***primary transcript.***

TABLE 4-31. Carbohydrate Donors Required for *O*-Linked and *N*-Linked Glycoprotein Synthesis

DONOR	BOTH *O*- AND *N*-LINKED OR *N*-LINKED	COMMENTS
UDP-galactose	Both	
CMP-sialic acid	Both	A nine-carbon sugar acid; same as *N*-acetylneuraminic acid
GDP-fucose	Both	
UDP-*N*-acetylgalactosamine	Both	
UDP-glucose	*N*	Glucose present as an intermediate but eliminated in final product
GDP-mannose	*N*	
UDP-*N*-acetylglucosamine	*N*	

A ***cistron*** is a unit of gene expression. In prokaryotes the product of several contiguous genes may be transcribed to produce a ***polycistronic message.*** A single mRNA, for example, in *E. coli* codes for three proteins called β-galactosidase, permease, and acetylase. Initiation and termination of protein synthesis from a polycistronic message occurs independently for each of the components. In contrast to prokaryotes, messages for eukaryotes are generally ***monocistronic.***

HUMAN TRANSCRIPTION SIGNALS

Through DNA sequence analysis and functional studies, ***consensus sequences*** for functional elements of DNA have been established. These constitute the predominant base at each position of the functional unit. About 25 nucleotides upstream from the start sites of human hnRNA is an AT-rich region called the TATA box (Fig. 4-71). The TATA box corresponds to the following consensus sequence: TATAAAAG. Recall that there are two hydrogen bonds between A and T and three hydrogen bonds between G and C (Fig. 4-56). The AT-rich region is therefore thought to participate in local strand separation that allows for template-directed RNA biosynthesis. About 75 nucleotides upstream from the transcription start site is the CAAT (pronounced "cat") box with its specific consensus sequence (Fig. 4-71). Both CAAT and TATA sequences provide information on where hnRNA synthesis should originate.

Other classes of sequences called ***enhancers*** and ***silencers*** play a role in determining the ***frequency*** of transcription initiation. These sequences, which may be 50 to 100 nucleotides long, can be effective hundreds or thousands of nucleotides away from the promoter (either upstream or downstream). Moreover, they are effective in both orientations: left to right or vice versa with respect to the promoter. ***Regulatory elements*** represent DNA sequences that affect transcriptional regulation of hormones or second messengers such as cyclic AMP. Other genetic elements play a role in tissue-specific expression so that a given gene is transcribed only in the liver, pancreas, or hematopoietic system, and not in other cells. Proteins that bind to specific DNA sequences have been implicated in the overall process.

BACTERIAL TRANSCRIPTION SIGNALS AND THE LAC OPERON OF E. COLI

Bacteria such as *E. coli* have a TATA box about eight nucleotides upstream from an mRNA transcription start site. They also have a TTGACA consensus sequence 35 nucleotides upstream from start sites.

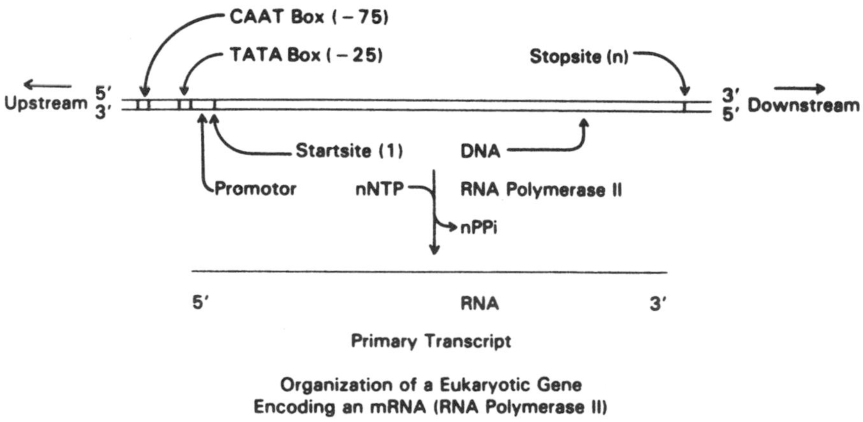

Fig. 4-71. Organization of a eukaryotic gene encoding an mRNA.

E. coli that are grown on glucose as a carbon source possess low levels of three proteins required to metabolize lactose. When the growth medium is changed to lactose as a carbon source, the levels of these three lactose-related proteins increase by several orders of magnitude. This system proved convenient for the study of the regulation of gene expression, and the concepts are briefly outlined here.

The ***lac operon*** constitutes the regulatory and structural genes that play a role in lactose metabolism. The following genes are involved. A continuous DNA segment includes an ***operator*** gene plus the ***z, y,*** and ***a*** genes, which encode for β-galactosidase, galactoside permease, and acetylase, respectively. An ***i*** gene, which is separated from these four genes, is also involved. The operator gene is a regulatory gene and does not code for a protein, but the ***z, y, a,*** and ***i*** genes are structural genes and code for proteins. A group of contiguous genes controlled by a single operator is called an ***operon.***

The *i* gene codes for a ***repressor.*** The repressor is a protein that binds to the operator (a specific 17-nucleotide DNA sequence) and inhibits transcription of the *z, y,* and *a* genes. When lactose serves as the carbon source, lactose or a metabolite (allolactose) binds to the repressor. The sugar-repressor complex is inactive and can no longer bind to the operator. Transcription and translation of the proteins of the *z, y,* and *a* genes then transpire. The corresponding proteins are synthesized, and their levels increase by several orders of magnitude. The three proteins participate in the use of lactose as a fuel to support cellular metabolism. The operator lies between the promoter and start site of the *z* gene. The binding of the repressor inhibits gene expression and is a negative regulator. Moreover, examples of positive regulators, or ***inducers,*** are known in bacterial and animal systems.

Recombinant DNA Technology and Restriction Fragment Length Polymorphisms

In the previous sections we considered the general principles of genetic chemistry. A field of recombinant DNA technology and genetic engineering was initiated in the mid-1970s. Besides advancing our understanding of physiological and pathological processes, the use of these methodologies has led to advances in the diagnosis and understanding of many genetic disorders. This section gives a general overview of progress in this rapidly developing field.

RESTRICTION ENZYMES

Scientists have isolated more than 100 enzymes, called restriction endonucleases, from several bacterial species. ***Restriction endonucleases*** catalyze the hydrolysis of a phosphodiester bond in each of the complementary strands of DNA containing a specific sequence of nucleotide bases. The great utility of these enzymes is that cleavage is sequence specific and not random. The sequence recognized by restriction endonucleases constitutes a palindrome. A ***palindrome*** is a word, sentence, or number that reads the same forward and backward. Examples include Otto, Able was I ere I saw Elba, and 2002. In the case of nucleic acids, a different definition of palindrome is used. A DNA palindrome occurs when the sequence on one strand of nucleic acid (from 5′ to 3′) is identical to its complementary strand (from 5′ to 3′). For example,

5′ GGCC 3′
3′ CCGG 5′

5′ GAATTC 3′
3′ CTTAAG 5′

In each case the sequence of the bottom strand is identical to that of the top strand. One convenient way to recognize palindromes is to identify bases where identities occur in adjacent positions on opposite strands. Then determine whether sequence identities occur when reading in opposite directions from the center of symmetry. Consider the second example. G differs from T, A differs from T, but A is identical to A. This represents a center of symmetry. To determine its extent, read in opposite directions from the point of symmetry on opposite strands. Going leftward on the top strand, we see that AAG (3′ to 5′) is the same as going rightward on the lower strand (AAG, 3′ to 5′). Similarly TTC (5′ to 3′) on the top strand is the same as TTC (5′ to 3′) on the bottom. This is easier than comparing six bases on one strand with six on the other strand one segment at a time. It is much easier to confirm the identification of these palindromes because only the relevant sequence is given; it is more difficult to identify palindromes in long sequences of DNA by inspection. Computers are used in practice to analyze sequences of many kilobases (kb) in length for palindromes and other sequence characteristics.

The sequences and positions of cleavage of a few restriction endonucleases are given in Table 4-32. Some enzymes nick or hydrolyze the DNA at staggered positions, for example, *Bam*HI; other enzymes produce blunt ends, for example, *Bal*I. The ends produced by *Bam*HI are self-complementary and are called ***cohesive*** or "sticky" ends. The product of the *Bam*HI cleavage has an extended 5′-end termed a 5′-overhang. That from the *Pst* I has a 3′ overhand. If we mixed two different DNAs (*e.g.,* human and bacterial) treated with the same restriction endonuclease that produces cohesive ends, some strands of human DNA combine at their cohesive end with the complementary ends of *E. coli* DNA. This is one of the

TABLE 4-32. Restriction Endonuclease Cleavage Sites

SOURCE	ENZYME DESIGNATION	SEQUENCE $5' \rightarrow 3'$ $3' \leftarrow 5'$
Bacillus amyloliquefaciens H	Bam HI	GGATCC CCTAGG
Brevibacterium albidum	Bal I	TGGCCA ACCGGT
Escherichia coli RY13	EcoRi	GAATTC CTTAAG
Haemophilus aegyptius	Hae III	GGCC CCGG
Providencia stuartii 164	Pst 1	CTGCAG GACGTC

important strategies used in producing ***recombinant DNA molecules.*** The restriction endonucleases yield a strand with a 5′-phosphate, and the other contains a free 3′-hydroxyl group. Annealed cohesive ends are bona fide substrates for DNA ligase, so that the recombinant strands can be covalently attached to one another.

The probability of having a tetranucleotide sequence of GGCC in a DNA molecule is $1:4 \times 4 \times 4 \times 4$, or 1:256. This sequence would occur on a random basis once every 256 nucleotides. In contrast, the probability for restriction endonuclease sites for CTGCAG is $1:4 \times 4 \times 4 \times 4 \times 4 \times 4$, or 1:4,096. The number and size of the DNA fragments produced by restriction endonucleases depend on the actual DNA sequence. SV40 DNA (from an animal virus) is 5,226 nucleotides long and contains a single *Eco*RI restriction enzyme cleavage site. Bacteriophage T7 DNA is 40,000 nucleotides long but it lacks a single *Eco*RI site.

NUCLEIC ACID RESOLUTION BY ELECTROPHORESIS

Negatively charged (anionic) DNA and RNA migrate in an electric field toward the anode. The distance of migration is inversely related to the molecular mass or number of monomeric residues in the polynucleotide; small molecules migrate more rapidly than large molecules. The matrix, or medium in which the macromolecule is electrophoresed, is synthetic polyacrylamide or a carbohydrate polymer called agarose. The concentration and composition of the matrix are varied, depending on the size of the nucleic acid of interest. In some cases, nucleic acids of 2 to 10 kilobases (kb) or larger are under study, and in others the size ranges from 30 to 300 nucleotides. Systems have been developed for resolving DNA molecules of one million nucleotides and greater. Handling large pieces of DNA is important to the proposed sequencing of the human genome.

DNA samples can be characterized by ***Southern blotting.*** A sample of DNA, (*e.g.*, human DNA), is treated with a restriction endonuclease and then subjected to agarose gel electrophoresis. The resulting fragments are resolved on the basis of size. The DNA on the gel is transferred to a thin support system such as nitrocellulose paper by capillary action. Buffer moves through the slab gel and nitrocellulose; in the process, DNA (or RNA) is transferred from the gel and is retained by nitrocellulose. The DNA (or RNA) is bonded to the nitrocellulose by treatment with heat or ultraviolet light. The mechanics are such that the relative positions of DNA (or RNA) on the gel are maintained on the nitrocellulose paper.

The resolution of DNA by electrophoresis and transfer to nitrocellulose is called a ***Southern blot*** (named after Edwin Southern, the originator). A similar analysis of RNA was dubbed a ***Northern blot.*** Electrophoresis and transfer of proteins are called a ***Western blot.*** The principles involve electrophoretic resolution of macromolecules based on size and a transfer to a bonding agent by a method that ensures maintenance of resolution. In the next section, we consider methods for identifying specific DNA or RNA segments by annealing or hybridization.

PREPARATION OF RADIOACTIVE DNA PROBES AND HYBRIDIZATION

Southern blotting of an *Eco*RI restriction endonuclease enzyme digest of a sample of human DNA might yield 850,000 different fragments. To identify the fragment of interest requires the use of a probe. This is generally accomplished by preparing a radioactive (^{32}P) DNA sample. Several strategies are used. If we can obtain the primary structure of the DNA from the literature, we can chemically synthesize a complementary DNA of 15 to 25 nucleotides in length. This oligonucleotide can be labeled at the free 5′-hydroxyl group in a reaction between radioactive ATP and the synthetic oligonucleotide catalyzed by ***polynucleotide kinase.***

$$\text{oligonucleotide} + [\gamma^{32}\text{P}]\text{ATP} \rightarrow [^{32}\text{P}]\text{oligonucleotide} + \text{ADP}$$

If we know the primary structure of a segment of protein of interest, we can synthesize corresponding oligonucleotides based on the genetic code. Because of codon degeneracy, we would have to make a family of oligomers corresponding to each possible codon.

If we possess a sample of a larger, double-stranded, or duplex DNA corresponding to a gene, we can produce labeled probes using random sequence oligonucleotides (typically six bases in length) as primers with heat-denatured genomic DNA as template. Random sequence oligonucleotides are mixtures that contain each of the four bases at each of the six positions, and the components of the mixture can base pair with complementary sequences on genomic DNA.

Next, the Southern or Northern blots are incubated with the radioactive probe under specific temperature and salt concentrations. During this procedure, the probe hybridizes or anneals to any immobilized complementary DNA (a Southern blot) or RNA (a Northern blot) present on the filter. After hybridization, the blot is washed with buffer to remove nonannealed probe. The samples are autoradiographed to locate the position of the probe and the polynucleotide(s) to which it bound. Standard nucleic acids are run in parallel so that the length or size of the DNA or RNA bands can be ascertained.

When a restriction enzyme digest of DNA from several humans is performed, the resulting Southern blots might show different patterns in response to a specific DNA probe. This might reflect ***restriction fragment length polymorphisms*** (RFLPs) or different forms of a gene ***(alleles)***. Some individuals may show a 10-kb band, and others may show a 6-kb fragment. It might be that one form is closely associated with a specific disease. For example, RFLPs associated with Huntington disease, cystic fibrosis, and Duchenne muscular dystrophy have been described. It is not necessary that the restriction enzyme cleave the defective gene; often the altered site is near the defective gene and serves as a marker. Similar tests are feasible in diagnosing hereditary diseases in cells isolated from amniotic fluid after amniocentesis. Extensive experimentation and painstaking efforts are required to establish and validate such diagnostic tests.

PLASMIDS AND DNA CLONING

Plasmids are small, autonomously replicating circular DNA molecules; we consider only bacterial plasmids. Many copies (up to 50) of small plasmids (4 kb or fewer) can be produced per bacterium. Plasmids replicate independently of the main chromosome. Many naturally occurring plasmids carry genes that confer antibiotic resistance; antibiotic resistance markers have been used in the production of genetically engineered plasmids for recombinant DNA research. Plasmids are used as vectors for cloning foreign DNA. When we allude to cloning the DNA of a gene, we are describing the process of preparing a large number of identical DNA molecules. A ***clone*** is an exact copy of an original form (DNA, cell, or organism). Plasmids can be used to clone DNA up to 4 or 5 kb in length, and other vehicles are used to produce DNAs of longer length. Bacteriophage lambda, for example, can be used to clone DNAs of 10 kb, cosmid vectors can be used to prepare DNAs up to 50 kb in length, and yeast artificial chromosomes (YACs) are used to prepare even larger DNA fragments.

Because human genes are interrupted and contain sequences that are removed by splicing from the primary transcript, the DNA corresponding to mRNA is contained in a much longer nucleotide segment. For example, the 2-kb mRNA of phenylalanine hydroxylase is derived from a DNA sequence of nearly 100 kb. The 1.8-kb mRNA of tyrosine hydroxylase is derived from a DNA sequence of 10 kb. One reason that scientists are interested in cloning large DNAs is to obtain segments that contain the entire gene, which may extend for many kilobases.

pBR322 (and many of its engineered derivatives) is perhaps the most commonly used plasmid in molecular biology. pBR322 contains 4,362 base pairs and genes that code for resistance to ampicillin and tetracycline. These genes contain unique restriction enzyme sites. If we mix a sample of target DNA previously treated with *Pst* I endonuclease with pBR322, also treated with this enzyme, a certain proportion of the pBR322 will anneal with the target DNA. After treatment with (bacteriophage) T4 DNA ligase and ATP, a covalently closed circle results. Some pBR322 reanneals (does not bind to target DNA). To minimize the yield of pBR322 without inserts, the plasmid is treated with bacterial alkaline phosphatase to remove its 5′ phosphate that was generated during *Pst* I treatment so that reannealed pBR322 lacking an insert is not a substrate for DNA ligase. Some target DNA reanneals (does not bind to pBR322 DNA); such DNA is a substrate for DNA ligase, but it is not capable of autonomous replication. Some complexes consisting of target DNA and pBR322 DNA result; these complexes are substrates for DNA ligase, and such recombinant molecules are capable of replication. Bacteria *(e.g., E. coli)* lacking antibiotic resistance genes are exposed to the recombinant plasmids (in the presence of $CaCl_2$), and some of them take up the DNA (they are transformed). The cells are grown in the presence of tetracycline. Untransformed bacteria do not grow under such conditions because they lack the antibiotic resistance gene. Individual cells with recombinant plasmids form colonies of cells containing identical copies (clones) of the original recombinant molecule.

A ***gene library*** refers to a collection of plasmids, phages, cosmids, or yeast artificial chromosomes containing the DNA corresponding to the entire genome of an organism. A bacteriophage lambda library of 250,000 different recombinant molecules is sufficient to contain the entire human genome. This library can be contained in a single drop of medium. To identify the DNA sequence or gene of interest requires ingenuity, and there are a number of successful strategies. One common procedure is to screen thousands of plasmid-containing bacterial colonies grown on several Petri dishes. The few positive colonies of the library that hybridize with the radioactive DNA probe of interest are taken for further study.

COMPLEMENTARY DNA PREPARATION

Complementary DNA (cDNA) generally denotes DNA that is complementary to RNA. It is easier to clone, sequence, and manipulate DNA in the laboratory than it is to perform these functions with RNA. A cDNA library corresponds to many clones of DNA complementary to an assortment of isolated sequences of RNA. In some instances, it is possible to enrich or purify RNA so that the cDNA produced is limited. When a cDNA corresponding to mRNA is the goal, mRNA can be resolved from rRNA and tRNA through the use of oligo-dT cellulose chromatography. Most mRNAs bind to oligo-dT by their 3′-polyA tail. However, ribosomal RNA and tRNA fail to bind. Very few mRNAs lack the 3′-polyA tail and fail to bind. However, histone mRNA is a prominent example of an mRNA lacking the 3′-polyA tail.

The first step in preparing cDNA is to incubate RNA with the four deoxynucleoside triphosphates, reverse transcriptase (RNA-dependent DNA polymerase derived from animal retroviruses), and a primer. Oligo-dT, which is complementary to the polyA tail at the 5′ end of mRNA, is often used as a primer in the preparation of an mRNA library. After synthesis of the first strand (an RNA–DNA hybrid results), the sample is treated with NaOH. RNA is hydrolyzed by alkali, but DNA is stable. After neutralization to physiological *p*H, DNA polymerase I and the deoxynucleoside triphosphates are then added to effect synthesis of the second strand of DNA. As previously noted, DNA polymerase requires a primer and will not synthesize DNA *de novo*. Apparently the first strand folds back on itself (making a hairpin loop) and serves as a primer. After synthesis of the second strand, the product is treated with S1 nuclease, which is specific for single-stranded nucleic acids. S1 catalyzes the hydrolysis of phosphodiesters constituting the non–double-stranded portions of the hairpin loop and produces linear duplex DNAs.

There are a number of procedures for combining the cDNA with plasmid or bacteriophage DNA for molecular cloning. One procedure involves the attachment of synthetic oligonucleotides to the duplex DNA in an ATP-dependent process catalyzed by bacteriophage T4 DNA ligase. The sequence of the linkers can be designed to produce cohesive ends complementary to those of a cloning vector that is treated with the appropriate restriction enzyme.

DNA SEQUENCE ANALYSIS

One of the great technical advances in biochemistry is the development of methods for rapidly determining the sequence of large molecules of DNA. It is possible to determine the sequence of thousands of residues in a day. From such sequences, one can determine the sequence of corresponding proteins by using the genetic code. What might require several years' work in protein sequencing can be accomplished in months or days by DNA sequence analysis (DNA sequence analysis may be performed in a few days, but considerable time may be required to obtain the desired DNA for analysis). Computers are essential in analyzing the sequence of DNA and the corresponding protein. Present-day cloning and DNA sequencing techniques provide vastly more protein sequence information than direct protein sequencing by chemical methods.

The ***dideoxynucleotide*** or ***chain termination*** method of DNA sequence analysis is described in abbreviated form. DNA of interest in segments of 200 to 300 bases is subcloned into a single-stranded bacteriophage (M13) adjacent to a specific sequence of nucleotides. A synthetic oligonucleotide is annealed to this specific sequence of the phage DNA, and the nucleotide serves as primer. This annealed complex is divided into four identical reaction mixtures. To each mixture is added a solution of the four deoxynucleoside triphosphates (one or more of which contains ^{32}P in the α-position or ^{35}S in place of oxygen on the α-phosphate) and DNA polymerase I. A different chain terminator is included in each of the four mixtures. These terminators include ddATP, ddTTP, ddGTP, and ddCTP, where dd indicates dideoxy. Dideoxynucleotides lack hydroxyl groups at both the 2′- and 3′-carbons of ribose. When these dideoxynucleotides are incorporated into the nascent chain at positions complementary to the cloned insert, elongation is impossible (there is no free 3′-hydroxyl group) and chain termination results. If ddATP is included, chain termination occurs randomly at every position complementary to a thymine residue, and a family of polydeoxynucleotides results. Chain extension to synthesize a family of polynucleotides ending at specific residues is possible because of the presence of dATP in the reaction mixture. The incorporation of the other dideoxynucleotides indicates the positions corresponding to their complementary base. The four mixtures are subjected to gel electrophoresis and autoradiography. The gels resolve every polydeoxynucleotide by size. For example, it is possible to resolve a polynucleotide of 197 from one of 198 bases. One can read from the shortest to longest and identify the residues terminating in A, T, G, or C by the order of their appearance on the

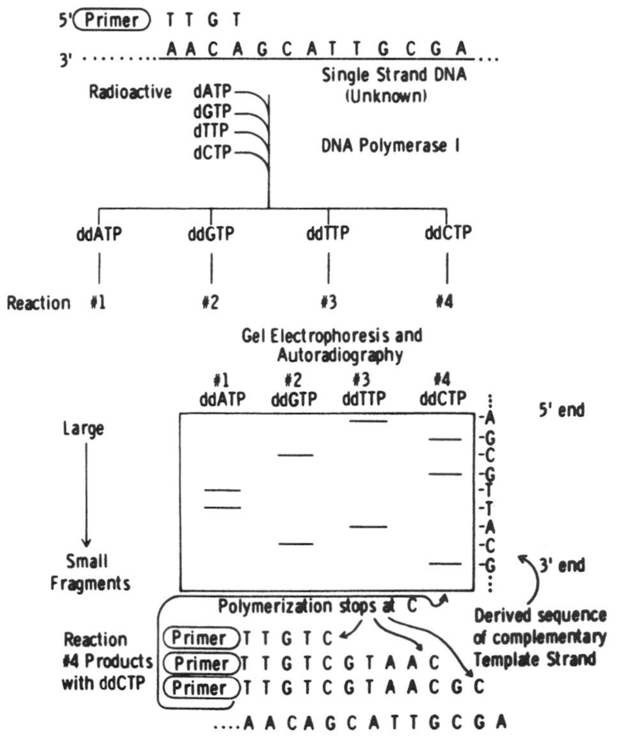

Fig. 4-72. DNA sequence analysis by the dideoxy chain termination technique.

autoradiograph. The information can be entered into a computer data bank for full analysis. The steps in preparing the four samples corresponding to a given DNA sequence are shown in Figure 4-72. The figure illustrates many fundamental aspects of DNA biosynthesis and is therefore worth all the time it takes to understand the principles outlined. These principles are more important to the reader than the DNA sequencing procedure itself.

THE POLYMERASE CHAIN REACTION

The polymerase chain reaction (PCR) represents a technique that is revolutionizing genetic biochemistry and genetic engineering. PCR is used to amplify DNA for study. For example, the minute quantities of DNA from a few hair follicle cells can be characterized. This technique finds use in forensic medicine, genetic and microbiological diagnostics, and gene manipulation and engineering. PCR technology is being used to study Duchenne muscular dystrophy, hemophilia A, the detection of human T-cell lymphoma, HIV, hepatitis B virus, and retinoblastoma. PCR technology also can be used for preparing mutant DNAs with site-specific changes.

The chain reaction refers to the use of multiple cycles (25 to 35) of primer-directed DNA elongation. The requirements include a target DNA for amplification, two DNA oligonucleotide primers complementary to the ends of each strand of the target DNA and extending toward the other primer, deoxynucleoside triphosphates, and a heat-stable DNA polymerase (Fig. 4-73). The heat-stable polymerase (called taq polymerase) is currently obtained from a bacterium, *Thermus aquaticus,* which grows in hot springs at 100° C or higher. The components of a PCR reaction are incubated in a thermal cycler. First, the temperature is elevated to about 92° C for 1 minute, which causes the two strands of a DNA duplex to dissociate. The reaction components are cooled to 50 to 65° C for 1 minute so that the oligonucleotide primers can anneal with DNA. The reaction components are heated to 72° C for 1 minute so that the primers can be elongated over the length of the target DNA. The process is repeated 25 to 35 times. Each DNA duplex present initially results in the formation of two daughter strands for a total of four strands. During the second cycle, the four strands serve as template and eight strands result. At the end of the second cycle, polynucleotides that extend from only one end to the other end of the target DNA result. Subsequent cycles result in the doubling of the amount of target DNA. This procedure can amplify the amount of DNA by several million–fold. Scientists predict that PCR technology will affect genetic biochemistry in the same fundamental way that the use of restriction enzymes has altered molecular biology.

CELL SIGNALING: NEUROCHEMISTRY

The brain and spinal cord constitute the ***central nervous system.*** The ***peripheral nervous system*** lies outside the

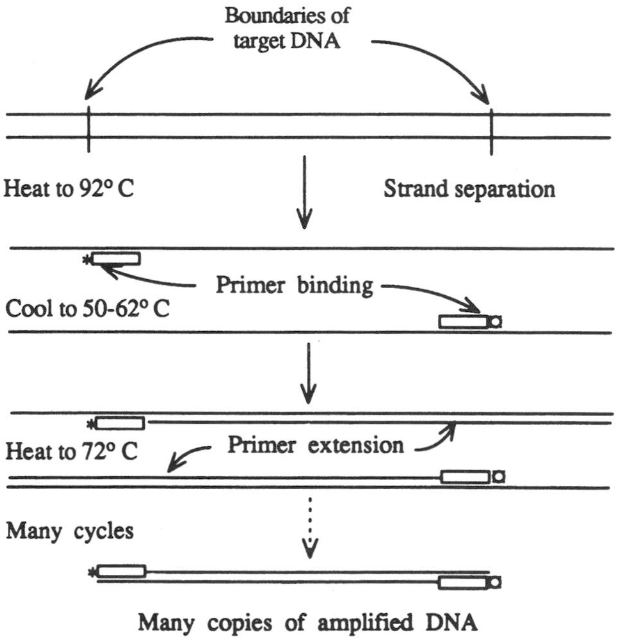

Fig. 4-73. Amplification of target DNA sequences by the polymerase chain reaction (PCR).

skull and vertebral column. The peripheral nervous system is made up of the voluntary nervous system (nerves to skeletal muscle), the autonomic nervous system (sympathetic and parasympathetic), and the sensory nervous system. The neurotransmitter of the voluntary, or motor, nervous system is acetylcholine. Acetylcholine is also the neurotransmitter of the preganglionic sympathetic and pre- and postganglionic parasympathetic nervous system. Norepinephrine is the neurotransmitter of the postganglionic sympathetic nervous system. The identity of the neurotransmitters of the sensory nervous system has not yet been definitively established.

Considerable work has been performed to ascertain the identity of the neurotransmitters of the central nervous system. These include acetylcholine, the catecholamines (dopamine, norepinephrine, and epinephrine), serotonin, glutamate, GABA (γ-aminobutyrate), and several neuropeptides. We discuss the biochemistry and metabolism of most of these agents.

ACETYLCHOLINE METABOLISM

Acetylcholine synthesis is limited, for practical purposes, to nerves that are ***cholinergic*** in nature. Mature noradrenergic nerves, for example, do not synthesize acetylcholine. The enzyme that catalyzes acetylcholine formation is ***choline acetyltransferase,*** which catalyzes the reaction between acetyl-CoA and choline as indicated:

$$\text{acetyl-CoA} + \text{choline} \rightleftharpoons \text{acetylcholine} + \text{CoA}$$

Acetyl-CoA is an energy-rich donor of the acetyl group. Acetylcholine is packaged into synaptic vesicles. When a nerve action potential invades a cholinergic nerve terminal, acetylcholine is released in discrete quanta or packets by calcium-dependent exocytosis. Acetylcholine diffuses across a synapse or a junctional region, interacts with an effector cell, and brings about the biological response.

To effect their physiological responses, acetylcholine and other neurotransmitters interact with their cognate receptor (Table 4-33). There are two major classes of ***acetylcholine receptor:*** nicotinic and muscarinic. These receptors differ in their molecular structure, anatomic location, and action. Moreover, several subclasses of nicotinic and muscarinic receptors exist. The ***nicotinic receptor*** occurs at the neuromuscular junction, on postganglionic autonomic cell bodies, and in the central nervous system. The receptor at the neuromuscular junction has been extensively studied. The form of the receptor in adults consists of four different polypeptide chains with the following composition: $\alpha_2\beta\delta\epsilon$; the embryonic form is $\alpha_2\beta\gamma\delta$. The nicotinic receptor acts as an ion channel or ion gate. After binding acetylcholine, Na^+ flows into a cell through the receptor. ***Myasthenia gravis,*** an autoimmune disease, is caused by the adventitious production of antibodies against the nicotinic receptor at the neuromuscular junction. The ***muscarinic receptor*** is responsible for the actions of acetylcholine liberated from the postganglionic parasympathetic system; acetylcholine is the postganglionic parasympathetic effector. The muscarinic receptor is specifically blocked or antagonized by atropine. Experimental evidence suggests that different subclasses of nicotinic and muscarinic receptors exist in different brain regions and in different regions innervated by the peripheral nervous system. Results from cloning the genes corresponding to various receptors indicate that the actual number of receptor subtypes is greater than the number of receptor subtypes based on pharmacological specificity.

Neurotransmitters such as acetylcholine can be ***excitatory*** or ***inhibitory;*** the physiological response depends on the receptor and its action. Activation of the nicotinic receptor at the neuromuscular junction and activation of the muscarinic receptor in the pancreas is excitatory. Activation of the muscarinic receptor in the heart, on the other hand, is inhibitory.

Inactivation of acetylcholine is mediated by metabolic degradation. ***Acetylcholinesterase,*** localized on the exterior of the cell surface of many neural and non-neuronal cells, catalyzes the hydrolysis of acetylcholine:

$$\text{acetylcholine} + H_2O \rightarrow \text{acetate} + \text{choline}$$

After its liberation in the acetylcholinesterase reaction, choline is transported into nerve cells by a sodium-dependent high-affinity transport system, and choline can be used. A circulating form of acetylcholine esterase called pseudocholinesterase also exists in humans. Its physiological function is unclear. The hereditary deficiency of pseudocholinesterase results in increased sensitivity to succinylcholine used as a muscle relaxant during surgery. Diisopropylfluorophosphate is an irreversible inhibitor of acetylcholinesterase. It forms a covalent adduct with an active site serine hydroxyl group of the esterase. Diisopropylfluorophosphate has been used in chemical warfare as a nerve gas. Related inhibitors of acetylcholinesterase are used as insecticides.

CATECHOLAMINE METABOLISM

Catecholamines are derived from tyrosine. The first, rate-limiting, and regulatory step in catecholamine biosynthesis is catalyzed by ***tyrosine hydroxylase.*** Tetrahydrobiopterin and oxygen are the other reactants. Dihydroxyphenylalanine (Dopa), water, and dihydrobiopterin are the products. Tyrosine hydroxylase is activated by through the action of protein kinase A and other protein kinases and is inhibited by the catecholamine pathway end products. ***Aromatic amino acid decarboxylase*** (a pyridoxal phosphate–dependent enzyme) catalyzes the conversion of Dopa to dopamine and CO_2 (Fig. 4-74).

TABLE 4-33. Classification of Neurotransmitter Receptors

RECEPTOR TYPE	FUNCTION
Acetylcholine	
Muscarinic	
M_1 and M_4	Inhibit adenylyl cyclase; activate potassium channels
M_2 and M_3	Activate phospholipase C
M_5	Inhibits adenylyl cyclase and may couple to phospholipase C
Nicotinic	
N_1	Forms an ion channel at the neuromuscular junction
N_2	Forms an ion channel at autonomic ganglia and in the central nervous system
Adrenoceptor	
α_1	Activates phospholipase C
α_2	Inhibits adenylyl cyclase
β_1, β_2, and β_3	Activate adenylyl cyclase
Dopamine	
D_{1A} and D_{1B}	Activate adenylyl cyclase
D_{2S} and D_{2L}	Inhibit adenylyl cyclase; open potassium channels
D_3 and D_4	Unknown
GABA	
$GABA_A$	Increases chloride conductance
$GABA_B$	Inhibits adenylyl cyclase and affects calcium and potassium channels via G-protein action
Glutamate	
Glu_1 (NMDA)	Activated by *N*-methyl-D-aspartate, a synthetic drug; functions as a cation channel and may play a role in memory
Glu_2 (AMPA)	Activated by α-amino-3-hydroxy-5-methyl-4-isoxazole propionate, a synthetic drug; functions as a cation channel and is responsible for most "fast" excitatory neurotransmission in brain and spinal cord
Glu_3 (kainate)	Activated by kainate, a synthetic drug; functions as a cation channel
Glu_4 (ACPD)	Activated by 1-amino-cyclopentane-1,3-dicarboxylate; activates phospholipase C
Glu_5 (AP4)	Activated by phosphonylglutamate; activates cyclic nucleotide phosphodiesterase in retina and hyperpolarizes cells
Histamine	
H_1	Linked to G-protein and phospholipase C activation
H_2	Linked to G-protein and adenylyl cyclase activation; blocked by cimetidine
H_3	Linked to G-protein and calcium and potassium ion fluxes
Opioid	
μ (mu)	Morphine (and β-endorphin) receptor; linked to G_i
δ (delta)	Enkephalin receptor; linked to G_i
κ (kappa)	Dynorphin receptor; linked to G_i
Serotonin	
$5\text{-}HT_{1A}$	Inhibits adenylyl cyclase and opens potassium channels; activates adenylyl cyclase in some cells
$5\text{-}HT_{1B}$	Inhibits adenylyl cyclase
$5\text{-}HT_{1C}$	Activates phospholipase C
$5\text{-}HT_{1D}$	Inhibits adenylyl cyclase
$5\text{-}HT_2$	Activates phospholipase C and closes potassium channels
$5\text{-}HT_3$	Ligand-gated cation channel depolarizes cells
$5\text{-}HT_4$	Activates adenylyl cyclase and closes potassium channels

This is the end product in dopaminergic cells of the brain including those of the nigrostriatal pathway. In other cells, dopamine reacts with oxygen and ascorbate to yield norepinephrine, water, and ascorbate radical in a reaction catalyzed by ***dopamine β-hydroxylase.*** This is the end product in noradrenergic neurons. In other brain cells and in the adrenal medulla, norepinephrine is methylated by *S*-adenosylmethionine to yield epinephrine and *S*-adenosylhomocysteine (Fig. 4-74). The corresponding enzyme is ***phenylethanolamine N-methyltransferase*** (PMNT). Epinephrine and norepinephrine are the hormones of the adrenal medulla.

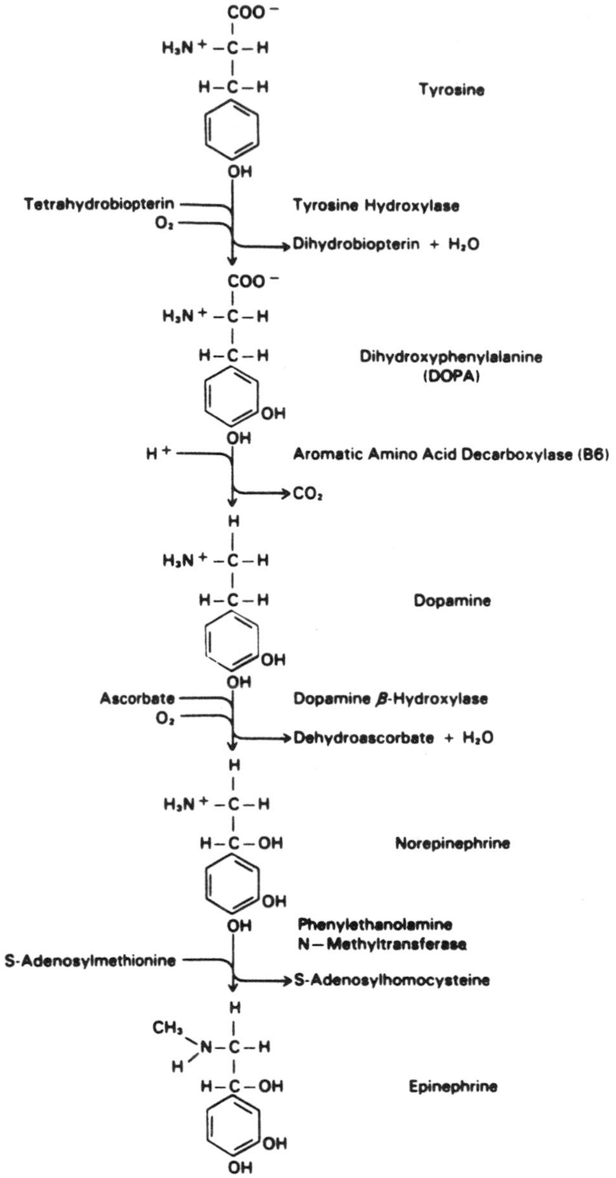

Fig. 4-74. Pathway of catecholamine biosynthesis.

Catecholamines are released from cells and interact with their specific receptor (Table 4-33) and bring about their physiological responses. The β-adrenergic receptor activates adenylyl cyclase at many locations. The action of catecholamines, in contrast to acetylcholine, is not terminated by metabolic degradation within the synaptic cleft or junctional region. Catecholamines are inactivated by sodium-dependent transport systems. The most active systems reside in the plasma membrane of the nerve cells that release the catecholamines by exocytosis.

Transport from the exterior to the interior of cells is the major mechanism for neurotransmitter inactivation. The two exceptions are acetylcholine and the neuropeptides. Inactivation of these two classes of neurotransmitter is mediated by hydrolytic cleavage catalyzed by degradative enzymes. The metabolism (not inactivation) of intracellular catecholamines is mediated by catechol-*O*-methyltransferase, monoamine oxidase, aldehyde reductase, and aldehyde dehydrogenase. The structures of the many intermediates are not considered here. The chief metabolite of norepinephrine is ***vanillylmandelate*** (VMA). VMA is often measured in the urine of patients with suspected pheochromocytoma (a tumor of the adrenal medulla or abdominal paraganglia [organs of Zuckerkandl]) to aid in diagnosis.

The nigrostriatal pathway of the brain uses dopamine as neurotransmitter. ***Parkinson disease*** is associated with a degeneration of these neurons and a decrease in dopamine content in these brain regions. The mechanism of degeneration is unknown. The oral administration of L-Dopa constitutes one treatment. L-Dopa is transported across the blood–brain barrier and is taken up by the surviving cells and converted into dopamine. Dopamine does not cross the blood–brain barrier and is ineffective in the treatment of Parkinson's disease. In addition to Dopa, an aromatic decarboxylase inhibitor that does not cross the blood–brain barrier is administered. Inhibition is based on the pyridoxal phosphate cofactor of the decarboxylase.

SEROTONIN METABOLISM

Serotonin is found in the brain and gut. In fact, many neurotransmitters and neuropeptides are found in both locations. Serotonin is derived from tryptophan in a two-step pathway. First, tryptophan hydroxylase catalyzes a reaction with substrate, oxygen, and tetrahydrobiopterin to yield 5-hydroxytryptophan, water, and dihydrobiopterin. This reaction is analogous to those catalyzed by tyrosine hydroxylase and phenylalanine hydroxylase. The three enzymes exhibit homologous primary structures and constitute a family of aromatic amino acid hydroxylases. Next, 5-hydroxytryptophan is converted to serotonin and CO_2 by aromatic amino acid decarboxylase; this is the same pyridoxal phosphate–dependent enzyme that converts Dopa to dopamine. Serotonin is packaged in synaptic vesicles and released by exocytosis; after diffusion to its receptor to bring about its effect, serotonin is inactivated by sodium-dependent uptake. Serotonin is metabolized intracellularly to 5-hydroxyindole acetate (5-HIAA) by the action of monoamine oxidase and aldehyde dehydrogenase. Quantification of 5-HIAA in urine is undertaken in patients suspected of having the carcinoid syndrome associated with the production of excessive serotonin.

EXCITATORY AMINO ACIDS

Considerable physiological and pharmacological evidence suggests that glutamate is the main excitatory neurotransmitter in the human brain. Glutamate is packaged into synaptic vesicles and released into the synaptic region to interact with its receptors to bring about its effect, and it undergoes inactivation by uptake. In contrast to the restricted cellular distribution of acetylcholine, the catecholamines, and serotonin, glutamate is present in all cells. The glutamate AMPA receptor is responsible for most ''fast'' excitatory neurotransmission in brain and spinal cord. The glutamate NMDA receptor functions as a cation channel and may play a role in memory.

γ-AMINOBUTYRATE (GABA) METABOLISM

GABA is the chief inhibitory neurotransmitter of the human brain. GABA is formed from glutamate in a one-step reaction catalyzed by glutamate decarboxylase; GABA and CO_2 are the products. As in many decarboxylase reactions, pyridoxal phosphate serves as a cofactor. In the 1950s, infants inadvertently fed formulas deficient in vitamin B_6 developed seizures. Seizures were apparently produced by a paucity of inhibitory GABA. GABA is released by exocytosis, acts on its receptor to bring about a response, and is inactivated by its specific high-affinity sodium-dependent uptake system. Its degradation is mediated by a pathway called the ***GABA shunt.*** GABA (C4) undergoes transamination with α-ketoglutarate to form succinate semialdehyde (C4) and glutamate as catalyzed by GABA transaminase. Succinate semialdehyde dehydrogenase catalyzes a reaction of substrate with NAD^+ to form succinate, NADH, and H^+. The latter donates electrons to the electron-transport chain, which results in ATP formation.

The content of the biogenic amines (acetylcholine, serotonin, and the catecholamines) in the brain is measured in micromoles/kilogram. On the other hand, the content of glutamate and GABA is measured in millimoles/kilogram.

NITRIC OXIDE METABOLISM

Nitric oxide is a gas with the formula NO. The compound was known for many years as endothelium-derived relaxation factor (EDRF). Nitric oxide is derived from a reaction of arginine, molecular oxygen, and NADPH; the products include NO, citrulline, water, and $NADP^+$. NO is an unstable free radical (it contains an unpaired electron) that self-inactivates. Nitric oxide diffuses from its site of synthesis and acts on adjacent cells; NO is not packaged in vesicles and is not released by exocytosis.

NEUROACTIVE PEPTIDES

More than 50 peptides are known to exist in the brain as demonstrated by immunochemical techniques. A selected list of neuropeptides is shown in Table 4-34. Most of these peptides are small (three to 50 amino acids). They are synthesized as polypeptide precursors in an mRNA-dependent fashion and converted to the active agent by specific proteolysis or processing. The peptides are packaged, are released by exocytosis, interact with their receptor to bring about their physiological effect, and are inactivated by proteolytic degradation. Besides their exclusive release from their own specific neurons, they may be coreleased with other low–molecular mass neurotransmitters. The list of possible coexisting neuropeptides and low–molecular mass transmitters is long. Some cortical neurons, to cite one example, contain and corelease GABA and somatostatin.

TABLE 4-34. Selected Neuroactive Peptides

Angiotensin II	Neurotensin
Cholecystokinin	Oxytocin
Dynorphin*	Secretin
Endorphin*	Somatostatin
Leucine enkephalin*	Substance P
Methionine enkephalin*	Vasoactive intestinal peptide (VIP)
Neuropeptide Y	Vasopressin

* Opoid peptide.

GENERAL ASPECTS OF NERVOUS SYSTEM METABOLISM

Under physiological conditions, the brain uses glucose as a metabolic fuel. The brain is unable to use fatty acids as a source of chemical energy. However, the brain may be able to use ketone bodies after prolonged starvation to account for nearly half of its ATP production. The brain is dependent on a continual supply of blood for both glucose and oxygen. A decrease of blood glucose to less than 40 mg/dl produces coma. Occlusion of the cerebral blood supply produces a stroke because of impaired delivery of oxygen and fuels.

The brain contains a small amount of glycogen, which may play an important function during hypoglycemia or during other forms of stress. Glycogen is clearly inadequate to sustain metabolism under conditions of severe hypoglycemia. Glycogen is stored in a hydrated state. Substantive changes of the glycogen content of the brain are prohibited because increases in volume are limited in the rigid cranium. Regardless of the underlying mechanisms, the brain is dependent on the liver to maintain adequate blood glucose levels.

Nearly all cells maintain a high intracellular potassium and a low intracellular sodium concentration. The diffusion of potassium through the plasma membrane and out of the cell accounts, in part, for the negative intracellular electrochemical potential ranging from -50 mV to -70

mV. Sodium is impermeant under resting conditions. During the propagation of a nerve action potential, sodium courses down its electrochemical gradient (from outside to inside) through sodium channels, and the polarity is briefly reversed.

The sodium/potassium ATPase is responsible for generating these ion gradients in nerve, heart, muscle, and other cells. A considerable proportion of ATP generated in nerve cells is required to maintain these ion gradients (Table 4-1). The ATPase is an integral membrane glycoprotein with a subunit composition of $\alpha_2\beta_2$. The enzyme reacts with ATP to form a phosphoenzyme intermediate and transports three sodium ions to the cell exterior. The ATPase transports two potassium ions into the cell and undergoes a hydrolytic dephosphorylation reaction. The sodium-potassium/ATPase is a receptor for cardiac glycosides such as digitalis, which interact with the α-subunit. Cardiac glycosides exert their pharmacological effects by altering sodium and secondarily calcium levels in the failing heart.

Hormones

Hormones are substances produced by ***endocrine*** cells, released into and transported by the circulatory system to their target organs where they exert their effects. ***Paracrine*** function, in contrast to endocrine action, involves the release and action of substances on neighboring cells. ***Autocrine*** function involves the release of an effector that then acts on the cell that released the substance. The latter two functions, paracrine and autocrine, do not involve transport by the circulatory system.

Hormones are conveniently classified as lipophilic (lipid soluble) or hydrophilic (water soluble). The lipid-soluble hormones listed in Table 4-35 include steroid hormones, thyroid hormones (T_3, triiodothyronine; and T_4, tetraiodothyronine), retinoic acid, and 1,25-dihydroxycholecalciferol (derived from vitamin D). Although these lipid-soluble hormones enter cells by diffusion, their sites of action are restricted to those cells that possess specific intracellular protein receptors. After interaction with the hormone, the receptor undergoes a conformational change (called transformation). The initial binding and transformation of the glucocorticoid receptor occurs in the cytosol. The hormone–receptor complex is translocated into the nucleus, interacts with the genome, and enhances or diminishes the transcription of hormone-responsive genes. Receptors for the other lipophilic hormones (Table 4-35) are located in the nucleus. Current studies suggest that the hormone–receptor complex recognizes a specific sequence of nucleotides upstream from the target genes called a ***hormone-responsive element.***

The structures of the steroid hormones are shown in Figure 4-75. Steroid hormones are synthesized from cholesterol in the appropriate endocrine cell. In contrast to the water-soluble hormones, steroid hormones are not stored to a significant extent but are synthesized and released upon demand. Steroid hormones and other hormones are effective at nanomolar (1×10^{-9} M) concentrations.

The water-soluble hormones include catecholamines, small peptides, polypeptides, proteins, and glycoproteins. The biosynthesis of norepinephrine and epinephrine (catecholamines) from tyrosine was considered in the section on neurochemistry (Fig. 4-74). The peptides and polypeptides are synthesized by ribosomes in an mRNA-dependent fashion. Removal of signal peptides and processing by prohormone convertases are required to produce the active hormone. Glycosylation may also occur. These modifications occur in the Golgi. Hydrophilic hor-

TABLE 4-35. Lipid-Soluble Hormones

HORMONE	STRUCTURAL PROPERTIES	TRANSPORT PROTEIN
STEROID HORMONES		
Pregnane Group (C21)		
Progesterone	Acetyl group attached to C17	Transcortin
Aldosterone	C18 is an aldehyde group (Ald)	None
Cortisol	II, 17-Dihydroxyl groups	Transcortin
Corticosterone	II Hydroxyl group	Transcortin
Androstane Group (C19)		
Testosterone	17-Hydroxyl group; no aromatic ring	Sex hormone–binding globulin
Estrane Group (C18)		
Estradiol	Aromatic A ring; 3,17-dihydroxyl groups	Sex hormone–binding globulin
THYROID HORMONES		
Triiodothyronine	Three iodines	Thyroxine-binding globulin
Tetraiodothyronine	Four iodines	Thyroxine-binding globulin
Cholecalciferol		
1,25-Dihydroxycholecalciferol	Vitamin D ring system	α_1-Globulin transport protein

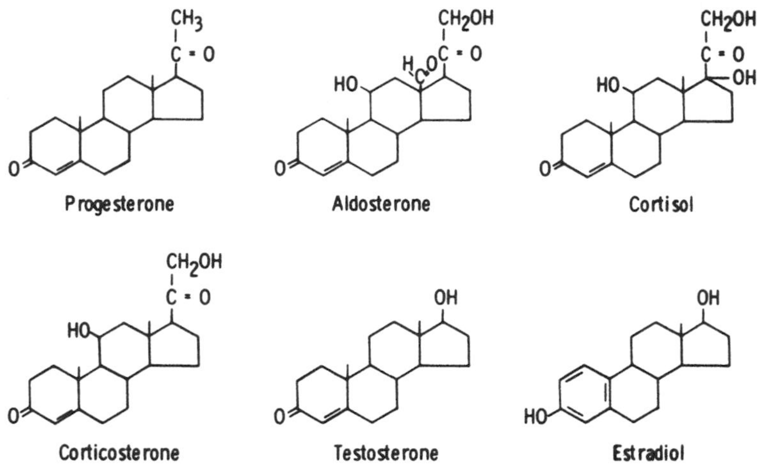

Fig. 4-75. Steroid hormone structures.

mones are stored in secretory granules and released from the endocrine cell by exocytosis.

After release into the circulation, hydrophilic hormones interact with their corresponding target cells through the action of an integral membrane protein receptor located in the plasma membrane. The receptors for lipophilic hormones, in contrast, are found intracellularly. The next step in the sequence of events that brings about the physiological response varies. In many cases the hormone, considered the ***first messenger,*** alters the levels of an intracellular ***second messenger.*** Second messengers include cyclic AMP, cyclic GMP, calcium, inositol 1,4,5-trisphosphate, and diglyceride.

THE CYCLIC AMP SECOND MESSENGER SYSTEM

After the interaction of norepinephrine and epinephrine with the β-adrenergic receptor on target cells, the intracellular concentration of cyclic AMP increases. The activated receptor does not stimulate directly the activity of adenylyl cyclase (the enzyme that catalyzes the formation of cyclic AMP from ATP). The activity of adenylyl cyclase is regulated by intermediary guanine nucleotide–binding proteins or G-proteins. The β-adrenergic receptor interacts with G_s (stimulatory guanine nucleotide–binding protein); the muscarinic acetylcholine receptor in many, but not all, instances interacts with G_i (inhibitory guanine nucleotide–binding protein).

G_s and G_i consist of three different polypeptides (heterotrimers): α, β, and γ. The α-subunits differ; the β- and γ-subunits are similar, if not identical. The epinephrine/β-receptor complex activates G_s; activation involves the exchange of GTP for GDP and the dissociation of α_s/GTP from the $\beta\gamma$-dimer. The α_s/GTP complex activates adenylyl cyclase. After hydrolysis of GTP to GDP and P_i catalyzed by intrinsic activity of the α-subunit, inorganic phosphate is released and GDP remains bound to the subunit. α_s/GDP binds to $\beta\gamma$ to form inactive α/GDP/$\beta\gamma$. The G-protein trimer can be reactivated by epinephrine/β-receptor or by other activated stimulatory receptors present in the cell's plasma membrane. The interaction of an inhibitory hormone receptor complex with G_i results in the formation of α_i/GTP and a dissociated $\beta\gamma$-dimer; α_i/GTP inhibits adenylyl cyclase activity. Hydrolysis of GTP to GDP + P_i is followed by formation of the inactive α/GDP/$\beta\gamma$ protein trimer of G_i. The hydrolysis reactions are catalyzed by intrinsic GTPase activity of α_s or α_i. Another prominent G-protein is G_p, a protein that activates phospholipase C that leads to the hydrolysis of phosphatidylinositol 4,5-bisphosphate, thus yielding diglyceride (an activator of protein kinase C) and inositol 1,4,5-trisphosphate (which leads to the release of calcium from the endoplasmic reticulum and an increase in cytosolic calcium). G_p is also a heterotrimer made of α-, β-, and γ-subunits that function in a manner analogous to that of G_s and G_i.

As noted in the discussion of glycogen metabolism, adenylyl cyclase mediates the formation of cyclic AMP, which in turn activates protein kinase A (cyclic AMP–dependent protein kinase). Activated protein kinase A catalyzes the phosphorylation of acceptor proteins, which then have altered activity (either increased or decreased, depending on the acceptor protein). To reverse the activation process, ***cyclic AMP phosphodiesterase*** catalyzes the hydrolysis of cyclic AMP to inactive 5′-AMP. Cyclic AMP dissociates from the protein kinase, and protein kinase A returns to the inactive form. ***Phosphoprotein phosphatases*** catalyze the hydrolytic dephosphorylation of the phosphorylated substrate proteins; the activity of the unphosphorylated from is again expressed.

The predominant residue phosphorylated by protein kinase A is protein-serine; in a few cases, protein-threonine is phosphorylated. A partial list of hormones that increase or decrease cyclic AMP levels in target cells is given in Table 4-36.

TABLE 4-36. Hormones That Affect Cyclic AMP Levels in Appropriate Target Cells by Altering Adenylyl Cyclase Activity

Stimulatory
Adrenocorticotrophic hormone (ACTH)
β-Adrenergic catecholamines
Follicle-stimulating hormone (FSH)
Glucagon
Luteinizing hormone (LH)
Thyroid-stimulating hormone (TSH)
Vasopressin (antidiuretic hormone or ADH)
Inhibitory
Acetylcholine (muscarinic)
α_2-Adrenergic catecholamines
Angiotensin II
Somatostatin

THE CYCLIC GMP SECOND MESSENGER SYSTEM

Most human cells contain cyclic GMP. The components of the cyclic GMP system parallel those of cyclic AMP, and these include guanylyl cyclase, phosphodiesterase, cyclic GMP–dependent protein kinase (protein kinase G), acceptor substrates, and phosphoprotein phosphatases. Adenylyl cyclase is localized exclusively in the plasma membrane. In contrast, guanylyl cyclase occurs in both a plasma membrane particulate form and a cytosolic form. The particulate guanylyl cyclase is regulated by cardionatrin I, or atrial natriuretic factor (ANF). The soluble form of guanylyl cyclase is stimulated by nitric oxide (NO). The latter functions as a messenger in the central and peripheral nervous system and other cells. NO is formed from the amino acid arginine by an oxidation process.

Cells also possess protein kinase G. It is a dimer of identical subunits. This protein kinase is activated in an allosteric manner by cyclic GMP. In contrast to protein kinase A, protein kinase G does not dissociate into separate catalytic and regulatory subunits. Activation can be expressed in the following fashion:

$$\underset{\text{(less active)}}{E_2 + 4\ \text{cGMP}} \rightleftharpoons \underset{\text{(more active)}}{E_2 - \text{cyclic GMP}_4}$$

The physiological substrates of protein kinase G are unknown. In some cases this enzyme phosphorylates the same substrates as protein kinase A. However, other protein kinase A substrates are phosphorylated poorly if at all by protein kinase G. It was hypothesized that cyclic AMP and cyclic GMP have antagonistic functions. However, this notion has fallen out of favor.

THE CALCIUM SECOND MESSENGER SYSTEM

Calcium serves as an important intracellular regulator. Calcium is required for exocytosis and muscle contraction. Calcium also plays an important role as a second messenger. A number of bioactive substances that exert their action, at least in part, by affecting intracellular calcium levels are shown in Table 4-37.

A first messenger acting through its receptor can increase intracellular calcium via at least two mechanisms. The hormone–receptor complex may enhance calcium influx through the plasma membrane in exchange for intracellular sodium. Another mechanism involves the phosphoinositide system. The initial substrate for this process is ***phosphatidylinositol 4,5-bisphosphate*** (PIP_2), and PIP_2 is present on the inner aspect of the plasma membrane. The hormone–receptor complex activates ***phospholipase C*** (Fig. 4-38), which in turn catalyzes the hydrolysis of phosphatidylinositol 4,5-bisphosphate to form 1,2-diglyceride and inositol 1,4,5-trisphosphate (IP_3). Inositol trisphosphate, liberated into the cytosol, interacts with the endoplasmic reticulum and promotes the release of stored calcium. Experiments indicate that the endoplasmic reticulum possesses a protein receptor that binds with IP_3.

To effect a response, calcium interacts in many cases with a calcium-binding protein called ***calmodulin.*** Calmodulin is a low–molecular mass protein (17,000 daltons) that binds up to four calcium ions with high affinity (binding constants are in the micromolar range). After binding with calcium, calmodulin undergoes a conformational change and alters the activity of specific effectors. Calcium/calmodulin, for example, activates one form of cyclic nucleotide phosphodiesterase. This provides reciprocal interaction of the calcium and cyclic nucleotide second-messenger systems. The activity of adenylyl cyclase is also regulated by calcium/calmodulin. The interaction of various second-messenger systems is common and is called cross talk.

The activity of several protein kinases is enhanced by calcium/calmodulin. Glycogen metabolism, for example, is but one process regulated by calcium. Phosphorylase kinase is composed of four different types of subunits: α, β, γ, and δ. The δ-subunits, tightly attached to the others, are actually calmodulin. Phosphorylase kinase is activated as calcium binds to the δ-subunit. Calcium triggers both muscle contraction and activation of phospho-

TABLE 4-37. Hormones That Affect Calcium Levels in Appropriate Target Cells

ACTH	Histamine (H1)†
Acetylcholine (muscarinic)*	Luteinizing hormone
α_1-Adrenergic catecholamines	Thyrotropin-releasing hormone
Angiotensin II	Vasopressin
Cholecytokinin	
Gastrin	

* Neurotransmitter.
† Autocrine agent.

TABLE 4-38. Some Physiological Substrates of Cyclic AMP–Dependent Protein Kinase

PROTEIN SUBSTRATE	EFFECT
Glycogen synthase	Inhibits
Hormone-sensitive lipase	Activates
Phosphatase inhibitor I	Activates
Phospholamban (muscle)	Activates
Phosphorylase kinase	Activates
Pyruvate kinase (liver)	Inhibits
Tyrosine hydroxylase (nerve)	Activates

rylase kinase in parallel. This dual regulation constitutes a part of the molecular logic of the cell (Table 4-1). Phosphorylase kinase also is activated by the phosphorylation catalyzed by protein kinase A (Table 4-38). Regulation of glycogen metabolism by calcium and cyclic AMP demonstrates the convergence of two second-messenger systems on a common function. Three enzymes have been distinguished by their substrate specificity and are called ***calcium/calmodulin-dependent protein kinases I, II,*** and ***III*** based on the historical order of their discovery. Calcium/calmodulin-dependent protein kinase II is a broad-specificity protein kinase and may play a general regulatory role in several aspects of metabolism. The other two calmodulin-regulated kinases exhibit restricted substrate specificity.

THE DIGLYCERIDE SECOND-MESSENGER SYSTEM

The hydrolysis of phosphatidylinositol 4,5-bisphosphate generates two second messengers: inositol 1,4,5-trisphosphate and diglyceride. Diglyceride, or diacylglycerol, activates its cognate protein kinase, which is called protein kinase C. Protein kinase C requires phospholipid and calcium for full expression of its activity. The C of protein kinase C refers to calcium. Diglyceride increases the affinity of protein kinase C for calcium so that the kinase can function at basal intracellular calcium concentrations (0.1 μM). One intriguing finding concerning protein kinase C is that it is specifically activated by tumor promoters including phorbol esters. Tumor promoters alone do not produce cancers. They must be added after an initiating agent such as benzo[*a*]pyrene is for tumorigenesis to occur. Protein kinase C has been implicated in the regulation of scores of processes, and its postulated actions rival those of protein kinase A.

Protein–Serine Kinases

All the protein kinases mentioned in the previous sections (protein kinases A, C, G, and calcium/calmodulin-dependent protein kinases) catalyze the phosphorylation of protein–serine residues. In many cases, the substrate proteins and even the residue(s) phosphorylated have been determined. Protein kinase A catalyzes the phosphorylation of phosphorylase kinase (and activates it) and glycogen synthase (and inactivates it). A partial list of its other protein substrates is given in Table 4-38. We know less about the identity of the physiological substrates of protein kinase G, calcium/calmodulin-dependent protein kinase (II), and protein kinase C. The vast majority of phosphate in proteins (≈99%) is attached to serine (Table 4-5). Protein–serine kinases constitute one of the most important means of enzyme and protein regulation by covalent modification in humans. A large number of protein–serine kinases are not regulated by these second messengers. One example, already considered, is pyruvate dehydrogenase kinase, which is regulated by acetyl-CoA and NADH in an allosteric fashion. After phosphorylation of pyruvate dehydrogenase, enzyme activity is decreased.

Protein–Tyrosine Kinases

Phosphorylation of protein–tyrosine residues plays an important role in the action of several hormones and growth factors and perhaps in the mechanism of tumorigenesis. The insulin, epidermal growth factor, and platelet-derived growth factor receptors, for example, possess protein–tyrosine kinase activity. These are called receptor protein–tyrosine kinases. The growth hormone receptor, not a protein–tyrosine kinase, activates a protein–tyrosine kinase. The *src* gene protein, a protein that plays a role in the pathogenesis of tumors in some animals, is also a protein–tyrosine kinase. The latter two are called nonreceptor protein–tyrosine kinases.

The insulin receptor is a tetramer of two α- and two β-chains linked by disulfide bridges as α-β-β-α. The α-chains recognize and interact with insulin on the cell exterior. The β-chains interact with the α-chains, which extend into the cell interior where protein–tyrosine kinase activity occurs. After activation of the insulin receptor, one β-chain undergoes an autophosphorylation of an intrinsic tyrosine residue catalyzed by the opposite β-chain. One mechanism of insulin action involves the binding of Grb2, an adaptor protein, to the protein–tyrosine phosphate on the insulin receptor. Grb2 contains an SH2 domain (src homology domain 2) that binds to protein–tyrosine phosphates. Guanine nucleotide exchange factor (GEF) binds to Grb2 via an SH3 domain. This domain recognizes proline-rich regions of proteins. GEF activates Ras, a G-protein. Active Ras (with bound GTP) activates Raf, a protein kinase, which catalyzes the phosphorylation of Mek. Mek is a dual-specificity protein kinase, and Mek catalyzes the phosphorylation of Erk on specific threonine and tyrosine residues. Erk, in turn, catalyzes the phosphorylation of target proteins and causes their activation. Downstream targets include Fos and Jun, transcription factors. The cascade from the insulin receptor, Ras, the Raf-Mek-Erk cascade, and transcription factor phosphorylation alter gene expression and mediate many insulin effects.

Other growth factor receptors such as that for epidermal growth factor and platelet-derived growth factor follow similar protein kinase cascade mechanisms. Growth hormone, prolactin, and several interleukins activate nonreceptor protein–tyrosine kinases. These enzymes also can activate the Raf-Mek-Erk protein kinase cascade. Other cascades exist. From this brief summary, one can see that protein kinases play a major role in metabolic and genetic regulation. Protein phosphorylation is the most common form of posttranslational modification. Moreover, life scientists estimate that the human genome encodes between 3,000 and different protein kinases.

CARCINOGENESIS

Great advances in understanding the pathogenesis of cancer have been made in recent decades, and progress continues at an accelerating rate. Epidemiologic studies have indicated that chemicals such as asbestos (lung), vinyl chloride (liver), benzo[*a*]pyrene (skin and lung), and β-naphthylamine (bladder) are carcinogenic. More recent work suggests that many agents undergo oxidation reactions catalyzed by the hepatic cytochrome P-450 system to yield the active carcinogen.

Most carcinogens are mutagens. The ***Ames*** test is one method for testing the mutagenicity and possible carcinogenicity of compounds. The test substance is first incubated with a liver extract containing the cytochrome P-450 system, followed by incubation with a histidine-requiring *Salmonella* strain. Mutagens produce revertants not requiring histidine; the mutagens can be further characterized in animal systems. The Ames test is about 90% accurate in identifying carcinogens.

Certain DNA and RNA viruses produce tumors in animals. A study of the mechanisms of tumorigenesis by viruses has been enlightening in understanding human cancer. Rous sarcoma virus, for example, contains an oncogene—a nonreceptor protein–tyrosine kinase—that is responsible for tumorigenesis. Each viral oncogene (designated v-onc) was originally derived from the host organism. The host gene is called a protooncogene. The action of ***protooncogenes*** is thought to be required for normal growth control or development.

Protooncogenes are highly conserved evolutionarily, and closely related genes occur in yeast, ***Drosophila*** (fruit flies), and humans. Oncogenes and their gene products fall into a few families. One large family, for example, possesses protein–tyrosine kinase activity (Table 4-39). This is reminiscent of plasma membrane receptors for insulin, platelet-derived growth factor, and epidermal growth factor. The *src* gene of the Rous sarcoma virus is an example of a nonreceptor protein–tyrosine kinase. Myc and Fos are nuclear proteins that function as transcription factors. The production of the neoplastic state might result from (1) abnormal expression of protooncogenes or (2) from a mutation producing an abnormal product. Evidence for both processes contributing to neoplasia is known. Mutant *ras* genes are found in about a quarter of all human cancers. Protooncogenes are dominant, and mutation of a single allele can result in tumorigenesis.

Tumor suppressor genes block abnormal growth and malignant transformation. These genes are recessive, and both copies of normal diploid suppressor genes must undergo mutation to allow for malignant transformation. One tumor suppressor gene is the retinoblastoma tumor suppressor gene called *RB1*. The gene product, RB1, appears to function at the G_1-S transition in the cell cycle.

TABLE 4-39. Oncogenes

DESIGNATION	VIRUS	GENE PRODUCT ACTIVITY OR LOCATION
abl	Abelson murine leukemia	Protein–tyrosine kinase
fes	Feline sarcoma	Protein–tyrosine kinase
fps	Fujinami sarcoma	Protein–tyrosine kinase
src*	Rous sarcoma*	Protein–tyrosine kinase*
erb B*	Avian erythroblastosis	Truncated epidermal growth factor receptor and tyrosine kinase*
sis*	Simian sarcoma	Platelet-derived growth factor B chain*
H-ras*	Harvey murine sarcoma	Binds GTP*
K-ras*	Kirstin murine sarcoma	Binds GTP*
myc*	MC29 myelocytomatosis	Nucleus*
fos	FBJ murine osteosarcoma	Nucleus
erb A	Avian erythroblastosis	Cytoplasm
ets	Avian E26 myeloblastosis	Cytoplasm

* Noteworthy.

A second tumor suppressor gene, *p53,* has a protein gene product with a molecular mass of 53 kDa. Alteration of this gene occurs in about half of all human neoplasms. p53 is usually located in the nucleus and it normally binds to DNA. p53 can put the brakes on cell growth and division, and it prevents the unruly amplification and mutation of DNA. Normal p53 can turn on the synthesis of p21, a protein that inhibits cyclin-dependent protein kinases. As a result of this inhibition, the cell is unable to pass a checkpoint in the cell division cycle.

MUSCLE AND CONNECTIVE TISSUE

Muscle Metabolism

Muscle accounts for about half the mass of humans. There are three classes of muscle: skeletal, cardiac, and smooth. The former two are striated in microscopic appearance. In this section we discuss the nature of the proteins that constitute muscle as well as the use of ATP as a source of chemical energy for muscle contraction.

MUSCLE PROTEINS

The two most abundant proteins in muscle are actin and myosin. Myosin is the chief protein of the thick filament, and actin is found in the thin filament. Some of their properties are noted in Table 4-40. Moreover, actin occurs in most nonmuscle cells, where it is a component of the thin filaments of the cytoskeleton. Myosin contains a globular head (with ATPase activity) and a rod-like tail. The two essential and two regulatory light chains of myosin interact with the two heavy chains of myosin in the globular region.

ROLE OF ATP IN MUSCLE CONTRACTION

The following is a description of the sliding filament theory of muscle contraction. ATP (with bound Mg^{2+}) interacts with an actin–myosin complex to displace actin and form a complex with myosin. ATP is hydrolyzed to yield ADP and P_i and an energized state of myosin (shown diagrammatically in Fig. 4-76). Note that ATP hydrolysis occurs before force generation. In response to a nerve impulse, calcium is released from the sarcoplasmic reticulum, and calcium triggers muscle contraction according to the following scheme. Calcium binds to troponin C, and binding produces a conformational change such that tropomyosin rotates out of the path between actin and myosin (Fig. 4-77). Actin then interacts with myosin, the energized myosin moves relative to actin by a rachet like mechanism to generate force, and myosin is converted to a deenergized state. The ATPase cycle repeats as many as eight times per second to shorten the sarcomere and generate force. After cessation of nerve impulses, calcium is sequestered into the sarcoplasmic reticulum by an ATP-dependent process. The calcium concentration decreases, and troponin reverts to its original conformation. Tropomyosin again blocks the interaction of actin and myosin.

Both skeletal and cardiac muscle, as well as brain, contain creatine phosphate. Creatine phosphate serves as a storage form of energy-rich phosphate

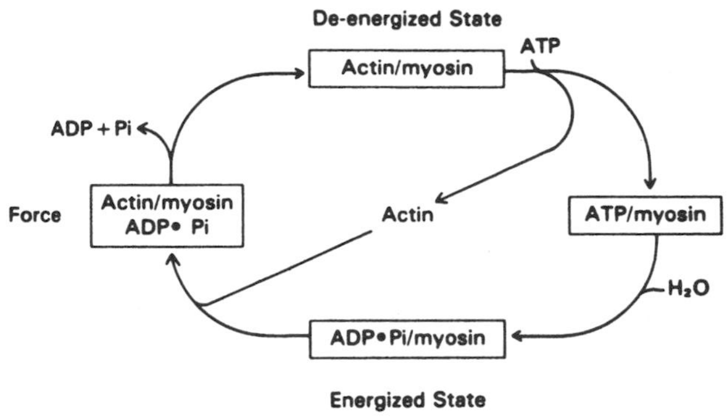

Fig. 4-76. The actin/myosin energy transduction cycle.

TABLE 4-40. Contractile Proteins

COMPONENT	MOLECULAR MASS	STRUCTURE	COMMENTS
Thick filament			
Myosin	520,000	Two heavy chains, four light chains (two essential and two regulatory)	ATPase heads
Thin filament			
Actin	42,000	Globular monomers form fibrous aggregate	Interacts with myosin to generate force
Tropomyosin	70,000	Two coiled subunits that extend the length of seven actin monomers	Blocks binding of actin to myosin
Troponin	76,000		
Troponin I	21,000		Inhibitory
Troponin T	37,000		Binds tropomyosin
Troponin C	18,000		Binds Ca^{2+}

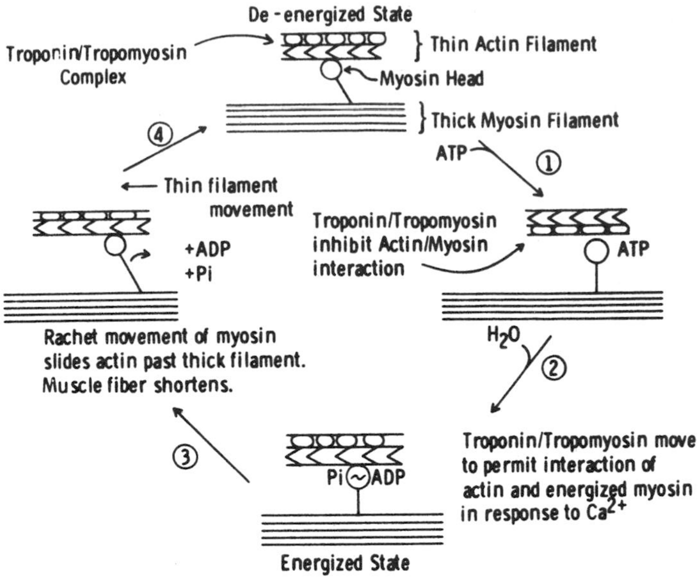

Fig. 4-77. Troponin and calcium mediate the interaction of actin and myosin during muscle contraction.

($HOOCCH_2N(CH_3)C(=NH)N(H){\sim}PO_3=$). Creatine is *N*-methylguanidinoacetate. The P~N, or phosphoramidate, bond is of the high-energy, or energy-rich variety. Creatine phosphokinase (CPK) catalyzes a reversible reaction between creatine and ATP to form creatine phosphate and ADP. After contraction and the formation of ADP, CPK catalyzes the phosphorylation of ADP to form ATP. The latter can serve as a substrate for continued muscle contraction. In exercising muscle, the level of creatine phosphate decreases before the decrease in the level of ATP. The level of creatine phosphate returns to its initial value during rest. ATP, formed from substrate level and oxidative phosphorylation, serves as the source of chemical energy for regenerating creatine phosphate. CPK is measured in serum samples in the clinical chemistry laboratory, and it is commonly elevated after a myocardial infarction as well as in people with muscular dystrophy.

Connective Tissue

The intercellular space in humans contains an organic matrix rich in proteoglycans. ***Proteoglycans*** consist of acidic polysaccharides (95% by mass) and proteins (5%). Proteoglycans form the ground substance in which collagen and cells are embedded to form tissues.

PROTEOGLYCANS

Proteoglycans are composed of a polysaccharide axis of hyaluronate. Many core proteins emanate laterally from the long, thin hyaluronate axis. A ***link protein*** stabilizes the ***hyaluronate–core protein*** complex. Many chondroitin sulfate and keratan sulfate chains are covalently attached to the core proteins and constitute the major mass of the molecule.

There are three types of bonds by which the polysaccharide is covalently linked to the core protein. These consist of (1) an *O*-glycosidic bond between xylose and serine, (2) an *O*-glycosidic bond between *N*-acetylgalactosamine and serine or threonine, and (3) an *N*-glycosidic bond between *N*-acetylglucosamine and the amide nitrogen of asparagine.

The components of the polysaccharide repeating units are listed in Table 4-41. The following generalizations can be made to simplify the subject. One component of the repeating disaccharide unit consists of either *N*-acetylglucosamine or *N*-acetylgalactosamine, or one of their sulfate derivatives. Except for keratan sulfate (with galactose), the second component consists of a uronic acid salt; it is either D-glucuronate or its 5-epimer L-iduronate. Except for hyaluronate, the polysaccharides of proteoglycans contain *O*-sulfate or *N*-sulfate esters. The donor of sulfate during biosynthesis is phosphoadenosylphosphosulfate (PAPS). The linkages connecting the disaccharides, which are not given here, are specific and determined by the biosynthetic enzyme (specific glycosyltransferases catalyze each addition from a nucleotide sugar). The sulfates and glucuronides account for the acidic nature of this group of complex carbohydrates.

Several inherited proteoglycan or mucopolysaccharide storage diseases are the result of deficient activities of lysosomal catabolic enzymes. Some of these are listed in Table 4-42.

COLLAGEN

Collagen is the major macromolecule of connective tissue and the most abundant protein in humans and the animal

TABLE 4-41. Properties of the Polysaccharide Components of Proteoglycans

CLASS	COMPOSITION OF REPEATING UNIT	COMMENTS
Hyaluronate	Glucuronic acid and *N*-acetylglucosamine	Widely distributed in animal tissues, synovial fluid, and vitreous of the eye
Chondroitin sulfate	Glucuronic acid and *N*-acetylgalactosamine as the *O*-4 or *O*-6 sulfate	Polysaccharide chains of 20,000 daltons
Keratan sulfate	Galactose and *N*-acetylglucosamine as the *O*-6 sulfate	Two forms (I and II) differ in bonding to protein
Heparan sulfate	L-Iduronate *O*-2 sulfate and glucosamine *O*-6 and *N*-2 sulfate or acetate	
Dermatan sulfate	L-Iduronate *O*-2 sulfate and *N*-acetylgalactosamine 4-sulfate; glucuronic acid and *N*-acetylgalactose	Two types of repeating subunit
Heparin	Glucosamine and L-Iduronic acid (90%) or glucuronic acid (10%)	Protein core almost all serine and glycine

kingdom. Collagen accounts for perhaps one third of human protein by mass. Collagen is secreted by fibroblasts. Collagen forms insoluble fibers of high tensile strength. The most distinguishing property of collagen is that it forms a ***triple, left-handed helix*** made up of three polypeptide chains. There are three amino acid residues per turn. Three left-handed helices combine to form a right-handed super helix, which is long (300 nm) and narrow (1.5 nm).

Another distinguishing feature of collagen is that every third residue is glycine. Glycine is the only amino acid small enough to exist at the central core of a triple helix. The sequence of the main body of collagen is thus Gly-X-Y, where X and Y are residues other than glycine. Of the 1,050 residues per chain, about 100 of the X residues are proline and 100 Y residues are 4-hydroxyproline. Collagen also contains 5-hydroxylysine residues, which serve as attachment sites for carbohydrate. The collagen helix is stabilized by multiple interchain cross links. The collagens of humans consist of more than one dozen molecules composed of more than 18 genetically distinct α-chains, some of which are given for reference purposes in Table 4-43.

The synthesis of collagen requires a number of post-translational reactions similar to those given previously. Collagen synthesis begins intracellularly, and synthesis is completed extracellularly by proteolytic processing. Collagen is synthesized as ***preprocollagen*** in the rough endoplasmic reticulum. The signal peptide is promptly cleaved, yielding ***procollagen.*** Prolyl and lysyl hydroxylation are followed by the subsequent glycosylation of several hydroxylysyl residues. The formation of the triple helical structure occurs in the Golgi. The procollagen triple helix is secreted from the fibroblast. Procollagen amino-terminal protease and procollagen carboxyterminal protease are extracellular enzymes that catalyze the hydrolytic removal of amino-terminal and carboxyterminal fragments, yielding ***tropocollagen.*** The amino-terminal and carboxyterminal fragments, the proprotein sequences, contain disulfide bonds. However, tropocollagen and collagen lack cysteine residues. The tropocollagen molecules form regular, parallel arrays and are stabilized by cross-linking reactions. Cross links occur between ϵ-aldehyde groups formed from collagen–lysine and ϵ-amino groups of other collagen–lysines.

TABLE 4-42. Proteoglycan Storage Diseases (Mucopolysaccharidoses)

NAME	ENZYME DEFECT	ALTERNATE DESIGNATION
Hurler	α-L-Iduronidase	MPS I
Hunter	Iduronate sulfatase	MPS II
Sanfilippo A	*N*-Sulfatase	MPS III A
Sanfilippo B	α-*N*-Acetylglucosamidase	MPS III B
Sanfilippo C	Acetyltransferase	MPS III C
Morquio	*N*-Acetylgalactosamine 6-sulfatase	MPS IV

BLOOD CLOTTING

Clotting Factors

There is a fine balance between initiating and retarding the formation of blood clots. The physiological purpose

TABLE 4-43. Major Types of Collagen

TYPE	MOLECULAR FORMULA	LOCATION
I	$(\alpha 1(I))_2\alpha_2$	Skin, tendon, bone
II	$(\alpha(II))_3$	Cartilage
III	$(\alpha 1(III))_3$	Skin, blood vessels, uterus
IV	$(\alpha 1(IV))_3$ and $(\alpha 2(IV))_3$	Basement membranes
V	$\alpha A(\alpha B)_2$ or $(\alpha A)_3$ and $(\alpha B)_3$	Widespread in small amounts

of blood clotting is to prevent the extravasation of blood from the circulatory system, which may result from injury or trauma. The blood-clotting scheme involves several protein components. Before considering their specific functions, we consider the general scheme of blood clotting.

Blood clotting involves a series of reactions in which the product of one process initiates a subsequent process, the product of which initiates still another. This scheme is called a ***cascade.*** Blood clotting involves at least six distinct proteases with a serine residue at the active site (factors II, VII, IX, X, XI, and XII). These serine proteases exhibit trypsinlike specificity (hydrolyzing a peptide bond on the carboxyl side of a basic amino acid residue) but of a more restricted nature. During proteolysis, an inactive proenzyme (*e.g.,* factor II) is converted to an active enzyme designated by the letter *a* after the factor number (*e.g.,* IIa). The protein substrate for clot formation is fibrinogen (factor I); fibrinogen is converted into a fibrin clot by proteolysis catalyzed by factor IIa. One of the clotting factors (XIIIa) catalyzes the cross linking of fibrin to form a more stable clot.

Four factors (III, IV, V, and VIII) function as auxiliary components in mediating specific conversions. Factor IV is calcium and factors III, V, and VIII are proteins. Ca^{2+} is necessary for at least five steps in the clotting cascade (formation of IIa, VIIa, IXa, Xa, and XIIIa). The first four of these protein factors contain γ-carboxyglutamyl residues that bind calcium. γ-Carboxyglutamate is a product of posttranslational modification and involves a vitamin K–dependent reaction. Factor VIII is the famous ***antihemophilic factor*** associated with hemophilia A. Hemophilia A is an X-linked bleeding disorder associated historically with European royalty. Factor IX is called ***Christmas factor.*** The name is based on that of a patient who had a disease resembling classical hemophilia but whose biochemical lesion was shown to be different. Christmas disease is hemophilia B. That a deficiency of either factor produces the same clinical manifestations illustrates that the two factors participate in the same step of the blood-clotting cascade. Their functions are noted later.

There are two clotting pathways: intrinsic and extrinsic. The ***intrinsic pathway,*** which may be initiated by an abnormal surface provided by endothelium *in vivo* or by glass *in vitro,* is so named because all components are present in blood; no exogenous component is required to initiate or propagate the reaction. In contrast, the ***extrinsic pathway*** requires the addition of an extravascular component (thromboplastin or factor III), which results when blood contacts any tissue as a result of injury (Fig. 4-78).

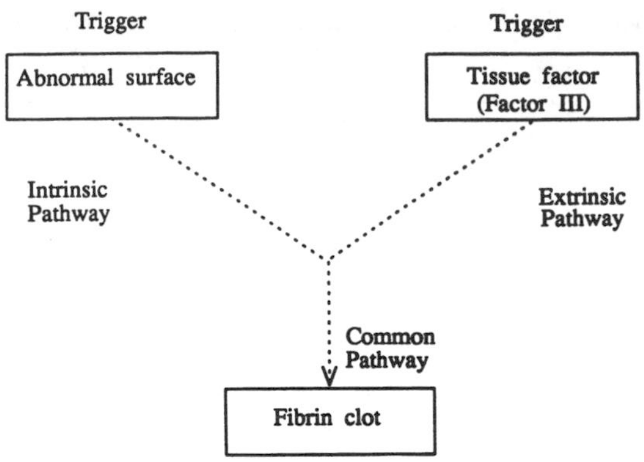

Fig. 4-78. Scheme for the intrinsic and extrinsic clotting pathways.

Blood-Clotting Cascade

The reactions involved in the intrinsic and extrinsic pathways are shown in Figure 4-79. The intrinsic pathway is the more complex. In response to a condition such as an abnormal surface, factor XII is converted to XIIa by proteolysis. Kallikrein and kininogen may participate in this reaction. Factors XI and IX become activated in succession. The coordinate action of IXa, VIII, and Ca^{2+} promote the conversion of X to Xa. Xa, V, and Ca^{2+} then lead to the conversion of prothrombin (II) to thrombin (IIa). Thrombin catalyzes the proteolytic conversion of fibrinogen to fibrin.

Fibrinogen consists of three different polypeptides found with the following stoichiometry: $\alpha_2\beta_2\gamma_2$ and molecular mass of 340,000 daltons. Thrombin catalyzes the hydrolysis of four specific Arg-Gly bonds in the α- and β-subunits to form four small fibrinopeptides (two A and two B peptides) and fibrin. Fibrin spontaneously associates to form a loose fibrin clot. Thrombin also activates factor XIII by proteolysis to yield XIIIa. XIIIa catalyzes cross-link formation between fibrin-glutamine and fibrin-lysine residues (Fig. 4-80). Although the amide bond of glutamine (Fig. 4-4) is not high energy in nature, the

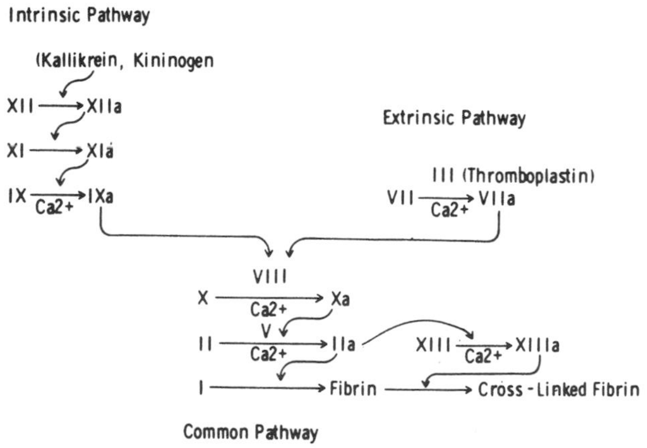

Fig. 4-79. The blood-clotting cascade of reactions.

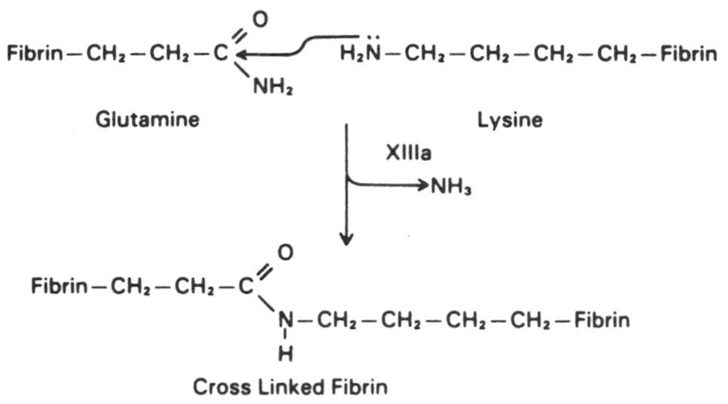

Fig. 4-80. The cross-linking reaction in blood clot formation.

amide linkage provides a modicum of activation to energize the cross-linking reaction.

The extrinsic pathway is initiated by the addition of tissue-derived ***thromboplastin*** (factor III) to blood. Although not a protease, thromboplastin participates in the proteolytic conversion of VII to VIIa in a calcium-requiring reaction; VIIa, VIII, and Ca^{2+} promote the proteolytic conversion of X to Xa. The step involving X occurs at the intersection of the intrinsic and extrinsic pathways. Properties of the blood-clotting factors are noted in Table 4-44; note that factor VI does not play a role in the current blood clotting cascade.

Fibrinolysis

After tissue repair has abrogated the need for a clot, the clot is removed by the process of fibrinolysis. ***Plasmin,*** a serine protease formed from plasminogen, is a proteolytic enzyme responsible for fibrinolysis. Plasmin catalyzes the digestion, or hydrolysis, of fibrin. Plasmin also degrades factor V and factor VIII. ***Tissue plasminogen activator*** (tPA) is a serine protease that catalyzes the conversion of plasminogen to plasmin. Tissue plasminogen activator produced by recombinant DNA methods is used for restoring coronary artery patency after coronary thrombosis. ***Streptokinase*** is a protein isolated from streptococci that initiates fibrinolysis. Streptokinase per se lacks protease activity. Streptokinase forms a complex with plasminogen and activates its proteolytic activity. Activated plasminogen catalyzes the proteolytic activation of other plasminogen molecules to form plasmin, thereby initiating fibrinolysis. Urokinase is a physiological activator of plasminogen, and studies are underway to determine its therapeutic effectiveness.

NUTRITION

The essential requirements for human growth, development, maintenance, and activity are oxygen, energy-yielding metabolic fuels (mainly carbohydrate and fat), protein, vitamins, minerals, and water.

Water

About 70% of the lean body mass is water. The distribution of water in the various compartments is given in Table 4-45. The interstitial fluid is the intercellular fluid exclusive of that in the arteries, veins, and heart (*i.e.,* it is extracardiovascular). The plasma volume, which amounts to about 5% of the lean body mass, is the extracellular fluid within the cardiovascular system. The value of 5% is important in calculating some intravenous fluid requirements.

Water balance describes the condition whereby fluid intake is equivalent to output. Representative values for water balance are given in Table 4-46. Wide variations in fluid intake in the normal range are possible. Compensating changes in the urinary output maintain balance under physiological conditions. ***Metabolic water*** is produced by oxidative phosphorylation. Protons, electrons, and oxygen react in the terminal step of respiratory chain phosphorylation in a mitochondrial reaction catalyzed by cytochrome oxidase to produce water. Humans are able to live without oxygen for only a matter of minutes. Water is the next most essential requirement for life. Death from dehydration ensues within several days in the absence of fluid intake. Massive fluid loss caused by diarrhea (*e.g.,* cholera) can lead to death within 10 hours.

Caloric and Energy Expenditure

Body weight in adults is determined by the balance between energy expended and energy consumed. If more energy is consumed than expended, then body weight (as adipose tissue) increases. Energy expenditure varies considerably among individuals. Energy expenditure is generally greater in children than in adults, in males than in females, and in young adults than in the elderly. Energy output is also increased by activity. A general formula for calculating approximate energy requirements in adults is shown in Table 4-47. The ***basal metabolic rate*** is the energy necessary for maintaining basal physiological activities (cardiac output, brain activity, renal output, body temperature, and respiratory function). The energy requirement for basal metabolism is approximately 1 kcal/kg/h or 24 kcal/kg/day. The additional energy required for activity can be much greater than indicated in Table 4-47 for athletes, lumberjacks, and those in other active occupations. The kcal of the biochemist (kilocalorie) is equivalent to the Calorie (capital C) of the nutritionist. The approximate energy requirement for a 70-kg individual with moderate activity is estimated as follows:

TABLE 4-44. Blood-Clotting Factors

NAME (DISORDER)	NUMERICAL FACTOR DESIGNATION	SITE OF SYNTHESIS	SERINE PRO-TEASE	γ-CARBOXY GLUTAMATE	Ca^{2+} REQUIRED	GENERAL PROPERTIES
Fibrinogen (afibrinogenemia)	I	Liver	–	–	–	Converted to fibrin clot by thrombin-catalyzed proteolysis; stabilized by transglutaminyl transferase (factor XIIIa)
Prothrombin (hypoprothrombinemia)	II	Liver	+	+	+	Acts on fibrinogen and factors V, VII, VIII, XIII by proteolysis
Thromboplastin	III	Most tissues	–	–	–	Auxiliary component in factor VII activation
Calcium	IV		–	–		Required for vitamin K–dependent factors (II, VII, IX, X) and activation of XIII
Proaccelerin	V	Liver	–	–	–	Auxiliary to action of Xa
Proconvertin	VII	Liver	+	+	+	Activates IX and X
Antihemophilic factor (hemophilia)	VIII	Liver	–	–	–	Auxiliary to action of IXa
Christmas factor (Christmas disease)	IX	Liver	+	+	+	Activates X
Stuart factor	X	Liver	+	+	+	Activates prothrombin
Plasma thromboplastin antecedent	XI	Liver	+	–	–	Activates IX
Hageman factor	XII	?	+	–	–	Initiates intrinsic pathway
Fibrin-stabilizing factor	XIII	?	–	–	+	Transglutaminase cross links fibrin
Protein C	XIV	Liver	+	–	–	Inactivates V and VII by proteolysis; anticoagulant
Protein S		?	–	–	–	Auxiliary to action of Protein C
Prekallikrein		Liver	+	–	–	Kallikrein activates XII by proteolysis
High molecular weight kininogen		Liver	–	–	–	Accessory to kallikrein
von Willebrand factor (von Willebrand's disease)	VIII antigen		–	–	–	Carrier of VIII

$$70 \times 24 = 1{,}680$$
$$0.4 \times 1680 = \underline{672}$$
$$\text{Total requirement} = 2{,}352 \text{ kcal or Calories}$$

Since this is an approximation, the figure can be rounded off to 2,400 kcal.

Energy Sources

The main sources of energy include carbohydrates, lipids, and proteins. The metabolic energy derived from 1 g of each is given in Table 4-48. The metabolic energy derived from carbohydrates, lipids, and alcohol is equivalent to that obtained by oxidation in a bomb calorimeter. The metabolic energy derived from proteins (4 kcal/g) is about 80% of that obtained by complete oxidation of protein in a bomb calorimeter. The explanation for this discrepancy is related to the conversion of amino nitrogen to urea *in*

TABLE 4-45. Fluid Compartments in Humans

	PERCENT OF LEAN BODY MASS	VOLUME (LITERS)/70-kg BODY MASS
Total body water	70	49.0
Intracellular compartment	50	35.0
Extracellular compartment	20	14.0
Interstitial fluid	15	10.5
Plasma	5	3.5

TABLE 4-46. Fluid Intake and Output in Humans

Output	
Expired air	800
Feces	200
Perspiration	400
Urine	1,200
	2,600 ml
Intake	
Food and beverage	2,300
Metabolic	300
	2,600 ml

TABLE 4-47. Daily Energy Requirements for Adults

Daily energy = BMR + activity Expenditure
BMR = weight (kg) × 24 kcal
Activity: Modest = 0.3 × BMR
Moderate = 0.4 × BMR
Heavy = 0.5 × BMR

1 kcal = 1 Calorie of the nutritionist.

TABLE 4-48. Metabolic Calories Derivable from Foodstuffs

CLASS	kcal/gram
Carbohydrate	4
Protein	4
Fat	9
Ethanol	7

vivo and not to nitrogen oxides as in the calorimeter. Note that the caloric value of ethanol is rather substantial. Ethanol is more reduced than carbohydrate, and this accounts for the greater energy yield of ethanol when compared with carbohydrate. Ethanol is oxidized to acetic acid in two NAD^+-dependent steps. Acetic acid is converted into acetyl-CoA and metabolized by the Krebs cycle.

When energy expenditure exceeds intake, weight loss ensues. The caloric equivalent of a pound of adipose tissue is about 3,500 kcal. This is based on a value of 85% fat, 15% water, and negligible carbohydrate and protein per pound of adipose tissue.

$$1 \text{ lb} \times 454 \text{ g lb}^{-1} \times 0.85 \times 9 \text{ Cal g}^{-1} = 3{,}500 \text{ Cal}$$

Triglyceride is the major storage form of metabolic fuel in humans.

The caloric energy derived from the average U.S. diet is as follows: carbohydrates, 40%; fats, 45%; proteins, 15%. Various health authorities suggest that decreasing fats to provide 30% of the energy requirement and increasing carbohydrates to provide 55% of the energy requirement would promote good health.

Essential Human Nutrients

Essential nutrients are those that cannot be synthesized in adequate amounts (if at all) and are required in the diet. These are listed in Table 4-49. The essential amino acids can be represented by the acronym PVT TIM *HA*LL ("private Tim Hall"). It is likely that histidine is essential in children and adults and arginine is essential in infants. Foods vary in protein quality, reflecting the proportion of essential amino acids in them, their digestibility, and their absorbability. In general, animal proteins are of higher quality than plant proteins. The recommended

(text continued on page 381)

TABLE 4-49. Essential Human Nutrients

AMINO ACIDS	FATTY ACIDS	VITAMINS	MINERALS	OTHER
		Water-soluble	***Bulk***	
Phenylalanine	Linoleic	Thiamine (B_1)	Sodium	Water
Valine	Linolenic	Riboflavin (B_2)	Potassium	Energy
Threonine		Niacin	Phosphate	
Tryptophan		Pyridoxine (B_6)	Magnesium	
Isoleucine		Pantothenate	Calcium	
Methionine		Folate	Chloride	
Histidine*		Cobalamin (B_{12})	***Trace***	
Arginine†		Ascorbate (C)	Chromium	
Leucine		Biotin†	Cobalt‡	
Lysine		Myonositol†	Copper	
			Iodine	
		Fat-soluble	Iron	
		A	Molybdenum	
		D	Selenium	
		E	Zinc	
		K	Floride§	

* Essential in infants.
† Human requirement not rigorously established.
‡ As vitamin B_{12}.
§ Promotes stronger teeth and bones; essentialness not established.

TABLE 4-50. Major Characteristics of Vitamins

VITAMIN	COFACTOR	DEFICIENCY STATE	BIOCHEMICAL FUNCTIONS	COMMENTS
Water-soluble group				
Thiamine (B_1)	Thiamine pyrophosphate	Beriberi	Oxidative decarboxylation, pyruvate dehydrogenase (pyruvate → acetyl-CoA) α-Ketoglutarate dehydrogenase (α-Ketoglutarate → succinyl-CoA) Ketoacid dehydrogenase Leucine, isoleucine, valine catabolism Transketolase	
Riboflavin (B_2)	FAD FMN		Oxidative decarboxylation reactions listed under thiamine electron transport	
Niacin Nicotinic acid Nicotinamine	NAD^+	Pellagra	Many hydrogen-transfer redox reactions	Some derived from tryptophan metabolism
Pantothenate	Coenzyme A 4′-phosphopantetheine		Acyl transfer Cofactor of acyl carrier protein in fatty acid biosynthesis	Widely distributed (pan . . .) and isolated deficiency unknown
Biotin	Biotinyllysyl		Acetyl-CoA carboxylase Propionyl-CoA carboxylase Pyruvate carboxylase	
Cobalamin (B_{12})	Methylcobalamin	Pernicious anemia	Methylmalonyl-CoA mutase 5-Methyl H_4-folate homocysteine transmethylase	B_{12} = extrinsic factor Not found in plants
Folate	Derivatives of H_4-folate		One-carbon transfer Thymidylate synthase Purine biosynthesis	
Ascorbate (C)	Ascorbate	Scurvy	Prolyl and lysyl hydroxylases (collagen) Dopamine β-hydroxylase	Effectiveness in viral disease controversial
Fat-soluble group				
A, retinol		Night blindness	Forms 11-*cis* retinal with rhodopsin	Retinal and retinoic acid may play a role in differentiation; possibly beneficial in prevention of some types of cancer
D,7-Dehydrocholesterol, (skin), ergosterol (plants, yeast)	1,25-dihydroxyvitamin D_3	Rickets in children Osteomalacia in adults	Calcium and phosphate metabolism	25 Hydroxylation in liver, 1 hydroxylation in kidney
E, tocopherol		Unknown	Unknown	
K		Bleeding diathesis	Activated blood-clotting factors II, VII, IX, and X	Mediates formation of γ-carboxyglutamyl protein residues

dietary allowance for proteins in adults is 56 g/day. The estimated average consumption of proteins in the United States is 100 g/day. The recommended daily allowance for children per kilogram is about twice that for adults.

Kwashiorkor develops in children with adequate energy but insufficient protein intake. ***Marasmus*** develops in children with both inadequate energy and protein intake; in terms of morbidity and mortality, marasmus is the most important worldwide nutritional problem in children.

Linoleate and ***linolenate*** are essential in humans. They cannot be synthesized and are therefore required in the diet. Linoleate serves as a precursor of prostaglandins, leukotrienes, thromboxanes, and prostacyclins (Fig. 4-42). The function of linolenate is a puzzle. Linoleate belongs to the ω-6 family of fatty acids. The double bond is found at carbon atom 6 when counting from the ω-, or methyl-, end of the fatty acid. Linolenate belongs to the ω-3 family of fatty acids.

Carbohydrates can be synthesized from glycogenic amino acids and from glycerol derived from triglyceride. Carbohydrates are a common and abundant source of energy. Individuals on a carbohydrate-free or -deficient diet develop ketosis associated with production of the ketone bodies by the pathway noted previously.

The general properties and functions of the vitamins are listed in Table 4-50. Vitamins are generally divided into two classes: water soluble and fat soluble. The fat-soluble vitamins are A, D, E, and K.

Pernicious anemia is associated with inadequate ***vitamin B_{12}***. Pernicious anemia is more commonly related to a failure to absorb vitamin B_{12} than due to inadequate dietary intake. Pernicious anemia develops in individuals who fail to produce a gastric glycoprotein (called intrinsic factor) required for vitamin B_{12} (extrinsic factor) absorption. The vitamin B_{12} content of plants is nil. A deficiency state may therefore occur in individuals on a strict vegetarian diet. Vegetarians and individuals with pernicious anemia often excrete methylmalonate in the urine owing to the diminished ability to convert methylmalonyl-CoA to succinyl-CoA (Fig. 4-31).

The interrelationship of B_{12} and folate metabolism is complex and incompletely understood. Individuals with pernicious anemia develop both anemia and central nervous system lesions. Folate corrects the anemia but not the neuropathology. The anemia is reversible, but the nervous pathology is not. Folate is absent from proprietary vitamins to avoid masking the symptomatology of pernicious anemia, which prompts the behavior of seeking medical attention. The advisability of limiting folate in proprietary vitamins is debatable because many people have marginally adequate folate intake. Folate deficiency during pregnancy is postulated to produce neural tube defects, and folate is often prescribed for pregnant women. In humans, vitamin B_{12} is necessary for the transfer of the methyl group from methyltetrahydrofolate to homocysteine. It is unclear whether this is the only interrelationship between folate and vitamin B_{12}.

Provitamin D (7-dehydrocholesterol and ergosterol) requires two metabolic transformations (hydroxylations) for conversion to the active form. The first step occurs in the liver and produces 25-hydroxyvitamin D_3. The second occurs in the kidney and produces 1,25-dihydroxyvitamin D_3 (1,25-dihydroxycholecalciferol). This compound is transported in the circulation to act on a variety of tissues and organs such as the kidney, bone, and intestine. Vitamin D constitutes both a vitamin and hormone.

Vitamin K is necessary for the carboxylation of protein-glutamate residues in four blood clotting factors (Table 4-44). The production of γ-carboxyglutamyl groups results in residues that bind calcium. Vitamin K antagonists such as dicumarol and warfarin are used as anticoagulants in the prevention and treatment of coronary thrombosis and pulmonary embolus. Such antagonists inhibit the formation of functional blood clotting factors.

The role of minerals in human metabolism is given in Table 4-3.

QUESTIONS IN BIOCHEMISTRY

Indicate the functions associated with each of the following: cell nucleus, mitochondrion, lysosome, Golgi, peroxisome, endoplasmic reticulum, and cytosol.

Specify the subcellular location of the following: thyroid hormone receptor, insulin receptor, β-adrenergic receptor, malate/α-ketoglutarate exchange protein, succinate dehydrogenase, pyruvate dehydrogenase, sodium/potassium ATPase, carbamoyl-phosphate synthetase II of pyrimidine biosynthesis, HMG-CoA reductase, HMG-CoA lyase, malate dehydrogenase, phosphofructokinase, phosphorylase, fatty acid synthase, RNA polymerase II, DNA polymerase α, DNA polymerase γ, catalase, adenylyl cyclase, β-ketothiolase, fatty acyl–CoA dehydrogenase.

Discuss the primary, secondary, tertiary, and quaternary hierarchical structures of proteins.

Describe the nature of the bonds important in maintaining the primary, secondary, and tertiary structures of proteins.

What is the difference between the native and denatured structures of proteins? DNA? How can the denatured forms be produced?

Name the amino acids whose side chains (R groups) are charged at physiological pH.

Name the three genetically encoded amino acids that contain a hydroxyl group.

Name the initiating amino acid of protein synthesis.

Name the aromatic amino acids.

Define (1) enzyme, (2) holoenzyme, and (3) apoenzyme.

Define (1) pH, (2) pK_a, (3) acid, (4) salt, and (5) buffer.

Calculate the ratio of $[HPO_4^{-2}]/[H_2PO_4^{-}]$ at pH 7.4 ($pK_a = 6.8$).

Calculate the ratio of $[HCO_3^{-}]/[CO_2 + H_2CO_3]$ at pH 7.4 ($pK_a = 6.1$).

Draw the double reciprocal (1/S vs. 1/v) plot associated with a (1) competitive inhibitor and (2) noncompetitive inhibitor. Which plot best describes the inhibition of succinate dehydrogenase by malonate with succinate as substrate?

An enzyme has a V_{max} of 100 μmol/min and a K_m of 1.0 mM. Calculate the velocity at the following substrate concentrations: 0.1 mM, 1 mM, 10 mM, and 100 mM.

Glucocorticoids induce the formation of hepatic tyrosine aminotransferase. Describe a plausible mechanism for this action of glucocorticoids.

Define positive cooperativity. Hemoglobin binds oxygen in a cooperative fashion. Plot the binding of oxygen to hemoglobin as a function of $[O_2]$. 2,3-Bisphosphoglycerate shifts the binding curve to the right but does not alter its shape. What type of agent is 2,3-bisphosphoglycerate?

Draw the structure of ATP. Indicate the location of its high-energy bonds.

The standard free energy of hydrolysis of ATP to ADP and P_i is -30 kJ/mol at 30° C and pH 7.0. Calculate the equilibrium constant for this reaction: $ATP + H_2O \leftrightharpoons ADP + P_i$.

Phosphoglucomutase catalyzes the following reaction: glucose 6-phosphate $\leftrightharpoons$ glucose 1-phosphate. At equilibrium at 30° C and pH 7, the concentration of glucose 6-phosphate in a sample is 19 mM and that for glucose 1-phosphate is 1 mM. Calculate the standard free energy change ($\Delta G^{\circ\prime}$). Calculate the free energy change when 1 mole of glucose 6-phosphate is converted to glucose 1-phosphate when the concentrations of each are 1 mM. When the concentration of glucose 6-phosphate is 100 mM and that of glucose 1-phosphate is 1 mM.

Which of the following contain a high-energy phosphate bond: glucose 6-phosphate, phosphoenolpyruvate, dATP, 1,3-bisphosphoglycerate, or glyceraldehyde 3-phosphate?

Draw the Haworth projection formulas for D-glucose, D-mannose, D-galactose, D-fructose, lactose (galactosyl-β1,4-glucose), and sucrose (glucosyl-α1,β2-fructose).

Name the three irreversible enzyme-catalyzed reactions in the Embden-Meyerhof glycolytic pathway. Which enzyme is the chief regulatory enzyme of the pathway? How is its activity affected by ATP, AMP, citrate, and fructose 2,6-bisphosphate? Which of the four compounds plays a predominant role in regulating enzyme activity in liver?

How is the NADH generated in the Embden-Meyerhof glycolytic pathway oxidized under (1) anaerobic and (2) aerobic conditions?

How does the conversion of glucose to lactate differ from the conversion of lactate to glucose?

How can muscle glycogen contribute to the maintenance of blood glucose? What is the Cori cycle?

Describe the pathway for converting galactose to glucose 6-phosphate. What is the enzyme deficiency in galactosemia?

Name the five cofactors required for the conversion of pyruvate to acetyl-CoA.

Name the irreversible steps in the Krebs citric acid cycle. What is the chief regulatory enzyme and its allosteric effector? Name the two enzymes of the cycle that catalyze decarboxylation reactions. Which step of the Krebs cycle is associated with substrate level phosphorylation? Which step of the Krebs cycle is inhibited by malonate?

Describe the pathway of electron transport from NADH to oxygen. Describe the effect of (1) rotenone and (2) cyanide on this process.

Describe the mechanism for ATP formation in mitochondria. What is the mechanism of action of 2,4-dinitrophenol on this process *in vivo?*

How many ATP molecules result from the oxidation of pyruvate and acetyl-CoA by the citric acid cycle and oxidative phosphorylation? Account for each molecule of ATP formed.

Name the two enzymes necessary for (1) glycogen formation and (2) glycogenolysis. Describe the action of glucagon on glycogenolysis.

Name the enzyme that catalyzes the following reaction. Identify its cofactor.

Describe the pathway for the conversion of glucose to ribose 5-phosphate.

Compare and contrast fatty acid oxidation and fatty acid biosynthesis.

Calculate the yield of ATP associated with the complete oxidation of (1) palmitate (16 carbon atoms, saturated) and (2) palmitoleate (16 carbon atoms, one double bond).

Describe the various processes by which fatty acids originating as triglyceride in adipose tissue are subsequently oxidized in the heart.

Describe the biosynthesis of (1) triglyceride, (2) phosphatidylcholine, (3) sphingosine, (4) ceramide, (5) sphingomyelin, and (6) cerebroside.

Define (1) transport, (2) symport, and (3) antiport. Give examples of each.

What is the locus of action of phospholipase A_2? Phospholipase C?

Account for the biosynthesis of ketone bodies in the liver and their use in extrahepatic tissues.

Lovastatin is a drug that inhibits the rate-limiting reaction in cholesterol biosynthesis. What is this reaction? Lovastatin is a competitive inhibitor of this enzyme. Draw a Lineweaver-Burk plot that results from this inhibition. Name the 10-, 15-, and 30-carbon intermediates in cholesterol formation.

Describe the route for (1) triglyceride and (2) cholesterol transport from liver to other tissues. Describe the function of (1) HDL and (2) LDL.

Which amino acid is entirely ketogenic? Distinguish between glycogenic and ketogenic amino acids. How do these concepts relate to the aphorism that fatty acids cannot be converted to net quantities of carbohydrate in humans?

Name the metabolic precursors of the atoms present in urea. Outline the pathway for urea biosynthesis.

Name the amino acids converted into oxaloacetate.

Name the vitamin and cofactor required for transamination reactions.

How are intermediates of the citric acid cycle maintained at adequate levels? Define (1) catabolic, (2) anabolic, and (3) amphibolic processes.

Specify the configuration of (1) amino acids that occur in proteins and (2) glucose that occurs in glycogen, relative to D- and L-glyceraldehyde.

What is the amino acid that is the chief source of one-carbon atoms used for purine biosynthesis?

Describe the two roles of vitamin B_{12} in metabolism in humans.

Describe the processes involved in the conversion of muscle alanine into hepatic glucose.

Describe the conversion of phenylalanine into tyrosine. In which organ does this conversion occur?

Name the precursors of porphyrin.

Outline the pathway for heme degradation.

Name three substances formed by transmethylation from *S*-adenosylmethionine.

Draw the common pyrimidines. Identify the precursor of each atom in the ring.

Draw the common purines. Identify the precursor of each atom in the ring system. Distinguish between nucleoside and nucleotide. Name five nucleotides. Name two polynucleotides.

Contrast the general pathways of purine and pyrimidine nucleotide formation.

What is meant by the salvage pathway for purine formation? How is it known that the salvage pathway is operational in human metabolism?

Describe the mechanism of the amination reaction during the conversion of IMP to AMP. Name two other reactions where a similar biochemical strategy is used.

Describe the biosynthesis of phosphoribosyl pyrophosphate. Describe the reaction for converting ribonucleotides to deoxyribonucleotides.

Describe thymidylate biosynthesis. What is the mechanism of action of methotrexate?

Describe two reactions catalyzed by xanthine dehydrogenase.

Describe the Watson-Crick structure of DNA. Describe or define (1) complementary base pairs, (2) antiparallel structure, (3) phosphodiester bond, (4) hydrogen bond, and (5) Chargaff's rule. If a sample of duplex DNA contains 20% A, what are the molar ratios of T, G, and C?

The diploid human genome contains 6×10^9 base pairs. Calculate the length of the corresponding DNA if it were all in the B form.

What is meant by unique DNA?

Describe the polarity of interaction of primer and template DNA and the polarity of the DNA polymerization or elongation reactions.

Describe the chemical structure of RNA. What are the main differences between the structure and function of DNA and RNA?

Define or describe (1) DNA polymerase, (2) 5′-exonuclease activity, (3) 3′-exonuclease activity, (4) DNA ligase, (5) helicase, (6) topoisomerase, (7) single-strand binding protein, (8) leading strand, (9) lagging strand, (10) template, (11) primer, (12) primase, (13) proofreading, or editing, function, (14) replication fork, and (15) semiconservative replication.

Describe base-excision repair of DNA. Describe nucleotide-excision repair of DNA.

Describe the functions of the five human DNA polymerases.

What are the chemical energy requirements for the DNA ligase reaction in humans?

Describe the reactions involved in mRNA biosynthesis in *E. coli*.

Define mRNA, rRNA, 5S RNA, tRNA, snRNA, and hnRNA. Which human RNA polymerases are involved in the biosynthesis of each?

Describe the reactions involved in mRNA biosynthesis in humans. Describe capping, polyadenylation, and the splicing reactions.

Describe the properties of the genetic code with respect to degeneracy and the wobble.

Name the initiation and termination codons.

Describe the ribosome. What are the A site and P site? Where is peptidyltransferase activity located?

Describe the mechanism of amino acid activation.

Recount the role of the soluble (nonribosomal) factors of protein synthesis. Describe how these factors exclude Met-$tRNA^{Met}$ from participation in the initiation reaction and fMet-$tRNA_I$ (in prokaryotes) or Met-$tRNA_I$ (in humans) from participation in the elongation reaction.

The mRNA for the normal α-chain of hemoglobin ends

with the following sequence: ACU UCU* AAA UAC CGU UAA GCU CGA GCC UCG GUA GCA. Specify the sequence of amino acids that corresponds to the indicated triplets. In hemoglobin Wayne, the U denoted with the asterisk is deleted. What is the consequence of this mutation? In hemoglobin Constant Spring, the underlined U is changed to a C. What is the consequence?

Describe the reactants that participate in peptide bond formation. In which direction does chain growth occur? Why is a translocation reaction required?

How many high-energy bonds are expanded in each polymerization reaction, on the average, in (1) DNA biosynthesis, (2) RNA biosynthesis, and (3) protein biosynthesis?

List several types of posttranslational modification. Describe insulin biosynthesis.

Compare and contrast the *O*-glycosylation and *N*-glycosylation reactions.

Describe the biosynthesis and secretion of a protein such as albumin.

Define (1) promoter, (2) terminator, (3) primary transcript, (4) monocistronic message, (5) polycistronic message, (6) TATA box, (7) consensus sequence, (8) enhancer, and (9) regulatory element.

How does lactose regulate the expression of the *E. coli lac* operon?

Describe the structure of a human gene and its general mode of regulation.

Define (1) restriction enzyme, (2) palindrome, (3) plasmid, (4) recombinant DNA, (5) Southern blot, (6) Northern blot, (7) hybridization, (8) gene library, (9) cDNA library, and (10) polymerase chain reaction (PCR).

Write the structures of the family of mRNA oligonucleotides corresponding to the peptide: Cys-Met-Pro. Write the structure of each DNA complementary to each of these RNA molecules. How many oligonucleotide structures correspond to the peptide Cys-Leu-Pro?

Describe the general procedure for DNA sequence analysis using the dideoxynucleotide chain termination technique. What principles in DNA synthesis are illustrated by this methodology?

What is the mechanism for terminating the action of the following neurotransmitter agents: (1) acetylcholine, (2) dopamine, (3) GABA, (4) glutamate, (5) serotonin, (6) leucine enkephalin, and (7) norepinephrine?

Describe acetylcholine biosynthesis and degradation.

Name the two major types of acetylcholine receptor.

Describe the pathway for norepinephrine biosynthesis.

What is the neurochemical basis of (1) myasthenia gravis and (2) Parkinson's disease?

Compare the ATP yield in converting α-ketoglutarate to succinate in the Krebs cycle and the conversion of glutamate to succinate by means of GABA in the GABA shunt.

What is the main metabolic fuel for brain metabolism? Which organ plays a role in maintaining adequate blood levels of this fuel? Explain.

What is meant by the Sutherland second messenger hypothesis? Name three first messengers. Name three second messengers.

Define (1) endocrine, (2) paracrine, and (3) autocrine action.

Define protein kinases. What amino acid residues accept phosphate? What is the predominant phosphorylated residue in human cells?

Describe the metabolism and action of cyclic AMP. Describe the mechanism whereby cyclic AMP regulates the activity of protein kinase A.

Name the main muscle proteins. Which has ATPase activity? How does ATP drive muscle contraction?

Describe the structure of collagen. Describe its pathway of biosynthesis.

Compare and contrast the intrinsic and extrinsic pathway of blood clotting. What is meant by cascade? Name the blood-clotting factors that are serine proteases. Which factors require Ca^{2+} for their action? Which factors contain γ-carboxyglutamate? Which factor has transglutaminase activity?

What is the function of tissue plasminogen activator (tPA)?

Give the nutritional caloric value of protein, carbohydrate, fat, and ethanol. Why does the nutritional caloric value of protein differ from that obtained by oxidation in a bomb calorimeter?

Estimate the daily caloric requirement of a 60-kg adult human with modest activity.

What is the composition of the average U.S. diet in terms of the percentage of calories contributed by carbohydrate, protein, and fat? What types of changes in dietary intake are thought by many health authorities to promote more optimal health? For an individual with a requirement of 2,000 kcal daily, calculate the number of grams of foodstuff that corresponds to 15% of total calories as protein, 55% of the total calories as carbohydrate, and 30% of the total calories as fat.

What is metabolic water? What amount is produced daily in human adults?

Name the lipids essential in humans. Define the term "essential."

What are nitrogen balance, negative nitrogen balance, and positive nitrogen balance? Describe circumstances related to each.

What is the importance of the following in humans: (1) cobalt, (2) iodide, (3) fluoride, (4) copper, and (5) iron?

What is marasmus? Kwashiorkor?

Name the vitamin deficiency associated with (1) rickets, (2) beriberi, (3) scurvy, (4) pernicious anemia, and (5) pellagra.

Name the cofactor derived from (1) thiamine, (2) riboflavin, (3) pantothenate, and (4) niacin. Identify the biochemical functions of each cofactor.

Account for the inability of extrahepatic tissues to release free glucose into the circulation.

What is the function of catalase? Where is it located within the cell?

What type of reactions are catalyzed by (1) kinases, (2) hydrolases, (3) phosphorylases, (4) mutases, (5) ligases (5) lyases, (6) synthetases, and (7) synthases?

Define (1) exergonic and (2) endergonic.

Describe the action of (1) cyanide, (2) tetracycline, (3) rotenone, (4) carbon monoxide, (5) antimycin A, (6) streptomycin, (7) actinomycin D, (8) methotrexate, (9) chloramphenicol, and (10) rifamycin.

Describe the defect associated with the following disorders: (1) von Gierke disease, (2) Christmas disease, (3) Pompe disease, (4) Tay-Sachs disease, (5) Gaucher disease, (6) familial hypercholesterolemia, (7) maple syrup urine disease, (8) phenylketonuria, (9) Hurler syndrome, (10) hemophilia, (11) Lesch-Nyhan syndrome, (12) beriberi, (13) Hunter disease, and (14) drug-induced hemolytic anemia.

Describe the role of ATP in (1) DNA synthesis, (2) RNA synthesis, (3) protein synthesis, (4) cholesterol synthesis, (5) fatty acid biosynthesis, (6) gluconeogenesis, (7) pyrimidine biosynthesis, and (8) purine biosynthesis.

Describe the role of GTP in (1) RNA synthesis, (2) protein synthesis, (3) purine biosynthesis, (4) gluconeogenesis, and (5) Krebs cycle function.

Describe the role of CTP in (1) RNA biosynthesis and (2) lipid biosynthesis.

Describe the role of UTP in (1) RNA biosynthesis and (2) carbohydrate biosynthesis.

Name a divalent cation indispensable for blood coagulation.

Name a substrate with a P/O ratio of 1.5.

What is the source of hydrogen for the reductive steps of fatty acid and cholesterol biosynthesis?

Describe Mitchell's chemiosmotic theory.

Describe Blobel's signal peptide hypothesis.

Write the structural formula for cholesterol, and indicate the numbering system for its carbon atoms.

How are nucleotides linked in (1) DNA and (2) RNA?

What vitamin is concerned with the synthesis of prothrombin in the liver?

Outline the steps in blood clotting.

Discuss the role of niacin and tryptophan in the treatment and prevention of pellagra.

Multiple-Choice Questions

Directions: *Choose the best answer.*

1. An abundant mineral that is used in the treatment of osteoporosis
   (a) calcium
   (b) sodium
   (c) potassium
   (d) cobalt
   (e) iron
2. Which of the following amino acids contains two chiral (asymmetric) carbon atoms?
   (a) tryptophan
   (b) leucine
   (c) methionine
   (d) glycine
   (e) threonine
3. The substitution of valine for glutamate in the β-chain of hemoglobin results in sickle cell hemoglobin. This mutation describes in a change in the protein's
   (a) primary structure
   (b) secondary structure
   (c) tertiary structure
   (d) quaternary structure
4. Diisopropylflurophosphate (DFP), a deadly poison, forms a covalent bond with an active site serine of acetylcholinesterase. DFP is an example of which type of inhibitor?
   (a) steady state
   (b) reversible
   (c) noncompetitive
   (d) irreversible
   (e) allosteric
5. The breakdown of complex molecules such as fatty acids to carbon dioxide and water is called
   (a) allosteric regulation
   (b) anabolism
   (c) catabolism
   (d) end-product inhibition
   (e) substrate level phosphorylation
6. Which one of the following enzymes of the Embden-Meyerhof glycolytic pathway would be expected to exhibit diminished activity in people with pellagra because of decreased substrate availability?
   (a) phosphohexose isomerase
   (b) glyceraldehyde-3-phosphate dehydrogenase
   (c) triose phosphate isomerase
   (d) enolase
   (e) pyruvate kinase
7. Which of the following is a true statement about pyruvate dehydrogenase kinase?
   (a) It is activated by coenzyme A.

(b) It is activated by NAD^+.
(c) It is activated by ADP.
(d) It inhibits pyruvate dehydrogenase by phosphorylation.
(e) It is located in the cytosol.

8. NADH is a product of which enzyme-catalyzed reaction?
(a) aconitase
(b) α-ketoglutarate dehydrogenase
(c) succinate thiokinase
(d) succinate dehydrogenase
(e) fumarase

9. Which of the following substances, which was once used for the treatment of obesity, uncouples oxidative phosphorylation?
(a) rotenone
(b) carbon monoxide
(c) antimycin A
(d) cyanide
(e) 2,4-dinitrophenol

10. 5′-AMP is an allosteric activator of which enzyme?
(a) glycogen phosphorylase
(b) UDP-glucose pyrophosphorylase
(c) glycogen synthase
(d) debranching enzyme
(e) branching enzyme

11. Thiamine pyrophosphate, whose deficiency results in beriberi, is a cofactor for which of the following enzymes?
(a) glucose-6-phosphate dehydrogenase
(b) hexokinase
(c) pyruvate kinase
(d) transaldolase
(e) pyruvate dehydrogenase

12. Vitamin B_{12}, which is not absorbed in people with pernicious anemia, is a cofactor for which enzyme?
(a) acetyl-CoA carboxylase
(b) acetoacetyl-CoA:succinyl-CoA transferase
(c) methylmalonyl-CoA epimerase
(d) methylmalonyl-CoA mutase
(e) propionyl-CoA carboxylase

13. Sphingolipids accumulate in a variety of lysosomal enzyme deficiencies. Which of the following is a true statement about sphingolipids?
(a) They contain glycerol.
(b) They contain ether linkages.
(c) They contain *N*-acyl groups.
(d) They are degraded by phospholipase A_2.
(e) They are squalene derivatives.

14. Which hormone activates hormone-sensitive lipase *in vivo* via activation of adenylyl cyclase?
(a) cortisol
(b) epinephrine
(c) heparin
(d) insulin
(e) triiodothyronine

15. Which substance serves directly as a nitrogen donor in urea biosynthesis?
(a) aspartate
(b) proline
(c) histidine
(d) alanine
(e) tyrosine

16. *N*-formimino-L-glutamate, whose formation is used as a diagnostic test for folate deficiency, is a metabolite which of the following amino acids?
(a) arginine
(b) aspartate
(c) histidine
(d) methionine
(e) tryptophan

17. A deficiency of which of the following amino acids does not result in negative nitrogen balance in adults?
(a) methionine
(b) leucine
(c) lysine
(d) proline
(e) valine

18. Which is a true statement about carbamoyl-phosphate synthetase II (which participates in pyrimidine biosynthesis)?
(a) It is located in the mitochondrion.
(b) It is the main regulatory enzyme in pyrimidine biosynthesis in humans.
(c) It requires GTP as the energy donor.
(d) It uses ammonia as the nitrogen donor.
(e) It occurs only in the liver.

19. Which enzyme is deficient in patients with the Lesch-Nyhan syndrome?
(a) AMP deaminase
(b) adenosine deaminase
(c) APT (adenine phosphoribosyl transferase)
(d) xanthine dehydrogenase
(e) HGPRT (hypoxanthine-guanine phosphoribosyl transferase)

20. Which substrate, whose synthesis is inhibited by fluorouracil, participates in the elongation reaction catalyzed by the replicative DNA polymerase of humans?
(a) TTP
(b) ATP
(c) GTP
(d) UTP
(e) CTP

21. Which of the following components is not required for the initiation of transcription by RNA polymerase?
(a) a template strand

(b) a primer strand
(c) a free 3′-hydroxyl group
(d) an incoming nucleoside triphosphate
(e) DNA

22. Inadequate absorption of which one of the following compounds, as occurs in Hartnup disease, leads to negative nitrogen balance?
(a) linolenate
(b) phenylalanine
(c) glutathione
(d) cobalamin
(e) serine

23. Which enzyme, whose activity may be decreased in people with alcoholism, contains thiamine pyrophosphate as cofactor?
(a) glucose-6-phosphate dehydrogenase
(b) lactonase
(c) 6-phosphogluconate dehydrogenase
(d) transaldolase
(e) transketolase

24. Bovine insulin, which is effective in treating humans with insulin-dependent diabetes mellitus, differs from human insulin at two of 51 amino acid residues. Which one of their structures are different?
(a) primary
(b) secondary
(c) tertiary
(d) quaternary

25. α Amylase, an enzyme whose activity in serum is elevated in pancreatitis,
(a) catalyzes the hydrolysis of α-1,6-glycosidic bonds of amylopectin
(b) catalyzes the hydrolysis of α-1,4-glycosidic bonds of amylose
(c) is most active at the *p*H of the stomach lumen (≈1)
(d) is inhibited by chloride
(e) catalyzes the hydrolysis of milk sugar (lactose) to galactose and glucose

26. The initiating amino acid in protein biosynthesis in eukaryotes and prokaryotes is
(a) valine
(b) leucine
(c) methionine
(d) serine
(e) tryptophan

27. The average number of high-energy bonds expended for the production of one peptide bond during ribosome-dependent protein synthesis is
(a) 1
(b) 2
(c) 3
(d) 4
(e) 5

28. Cyanide (CN^-), which is one of the most rapidly acting poisons in humans, blocks oxidative phosphorylation by
(a) dissipating the proton gradient between matrix and intermembrane space
(b) binding to the ferrous iron in myoglobin
(c) binding to the ferric iron of cytochrome a_3 in cytochrome oxidase
(d) lowering the oxygen-carrying capacity of the blood
(e) inhibiting ATP synthase

29. Which of the following enzymes is bypassed when people with Parkinson's disease are treated with Dopa?
(a) aromatic amino acid decarboxylase
(b) tryptophan hydroxylase
(c) tyrosine hydroxylase
(d) dopamine β-hydroxylase
(e) phenylethanolamine *N*-methyltransferase

30. The elevated blood glucose seen in diabetes mellitus is a consequence of
(a) increased activity of gluconeogenic enzymes due to enzyme induction by glucagon
(b) increased glycolytic activity in liver
(c) a failure of glucose to enter liver cells
(d) increased liver glycogenesis
(e) conversion of fatty acids to glucose

31. G-proteins that alter the activity of adenylyl cyclase are defective in Albright disease, a form of pseudohypoparathyroidism. Which of the following hormones stimulates adenylyl cyclase in target cells via interaction with a stimulatory G-protein?
(a) cortisone
(b) acetylcholine
(c) somatostatin
(d) aldosterone
(e) glucagon

32. Infants with lethargy, hypotonia, metabolic acidosis without ketosis, and very high levels of urinary β-hydroxy-β-methylglutarate in the urine suffer from
(a) HMG-CoA lyase deficiency
(b) β-ketothiolase deficiency
(c) maple syrup urine disease
(d) medium-chain acyl–CoA dehydrogenase deficiency
(e) propionyl-CoA carboxylase deficiency

33. Every third residue of mature collagen, mutations of which results in Ehlers-Danlos syndrome, is
(a) proline
(b) hydroxyproline
(c) methionine
(d) tryptophan
(e) glycine

34. The γ-carboxylglutamate found in blood-clotting factor II, whose synthesis is inhibited by warfarin and dicumarol, is derived in a oxidation process involving
    (a) ascorbate
    (b) cholecalciferol
    (c) β-carotene
    (d) vitamin K
    (e) vitamin E
35. Which of the following foods lacks cholesterol?
    (a) beef
    (b) baked potatoes
    (c) eggs
    (d) bacon
    (e) chicken
36. Which enzyme-catalyzed reaction requires biotin as a cofactor?
    (a) pyruvate dehydrogenase
    (b) glycogen phosphorylase
    (c) hexokinase
    (d) pyruvate carboxylase
    (e) succinate dehydrogenase
37. Impaired degradation of pyrimidine nucleoside monophosphates due to a deficiency of which enzyme activity can lead to orotic aciduria?
    (a) hydrolytic removal of amino groups by deaminase
    (b) hydrolytic removal of phosphate groups by nucleotidase
    (c) hydrolytic removal of sugars by nucleosidase
    (d) phosphorolytic removal of sugars by nucleoside phosphorylase
38. Which organ plays a major role in ketogenesis?
    (a) adrenal
    (b) kidney
    (c) thymus
    (d) spleen
    (e) liver
39. Hydrolysis of the amino group of 5-methylcytosine without subsequent repair leads to which type of mutation?
    (a) transition
    (b) transversion
    (c) translocation
    (d) transformation
    (e) transduction
40. A fast-food outlet cheeseburger contains 15 g protein, 15 g fat, 50 mg cholesterol, 30 g carbohydrate, 750 mg sodium, and 220 mg potassium. The percent of caloric energy that is due to fat is about
    (a) 10
    (b) 20
    (c) 30
    (d) 40
    (e) 50
41. The insulin receptor contains which one of the following enzyme activities?
    (a) protein-tyrosine phosphatase activity
    (b) protein-tyrosine kinase activity
    (c) protein-serine phosphatase activity
    (d) protein-serine kinase activity
    (e) dual-specificity protein kinase activity

Directions. *Each group of questions consists of several lettered headings followed by a list of numbered statements. For each numbered phrase, select the one lettered heading that is most closely associated with each statement.*

(a) NADH dehydrogenase
(b) coenzyme Q (ubiquinone)
(c) dolichol
(d) complex II
(e) site 1
(f) cytochrome b
(g) cytochrome c
(h) cytochrome aa_3

42. Mobile lipid-soluble electron carrier
43. Reacts with oxygen under physiological conditions to produce water
44. Peripheral membrane protein

(a) adenosine deaminase
(b) hypoxanthine guanine phosphoribosyltransferase (HGPRT)
(c) glucose 6-phosphatase
(d) hexosaminidase A
(e) phenylalanine hydroxylase
(f) argininosuccinate lyase
(g) pyruvate dehydrogenase kinase
(h) galactocerebrosidase
(i) histidine ammonia lyase
(j) phenylalanine hydroxylase
(k) sphingomyelinase
(l) uroporphyrinogen synthase
(m) homogentisate oxidase

45. Deficiency associated with Tay-Sachs disease
46. Deficiency associated with immunodeficiency
47. Deficiency associated with hyperammonemia
48. Deficiency associated with urine that darkens upon standing and with ochronosis
49. Deficiency associated with hypoglycemia, hypertriglyceridemia, and increased hepatic glycogen levels

(a) albumin
(b) chylomicrons
(c) VLDL
(d) LDL
(e) HDL

50. Transports triglyceride from the liver to extrahepatic tissues
51. Transports cholesterol from peripheral organs to the liver

(a) rotenone
(b) antimycin A
(c) carbon monoxide
(d) 2,4-dinitrophenol
(e) atractyloside

52. A site 1–specific inhibitor of mitochondrial electron transport that is used as a rat poison
53. Inhibits the transport of ATP into the mitochondrion

(a) carnitine
(b) biotin
(c) NADPH
(d) β-ketothiolase
(e) acyl carrier protein (ACP)

54. Participates in the transfer of acyl groups from outside to inside the mitochondrion
55. A secondary deficiency of this compound occurs in people with pyruvate dehydrogenase deficiency.

(a) acetoacetyl CoA
(b) oxaloacetate
(c) α-ketoglutarate
(d) succinyl-CoA
(e) pyruvate

56. Breakdown product of proline
57. Breakdown product of methionine

(a) promoter
(b) terminator
(c) transcription unit
(d) monocistronic
(e) silencer

58. RNA polymerase binding site
59. Decreases frequency of transcription

(a) kwashiorkor
(b) marasmus
(c) pernicious anemia
(d) beriberi
(e) pellagra

60. Protein-calorie malnutrition in children
61. Thiamine deficiency

(a) tryptophan
(b) serine
(c) proline
(d) cysteine
(e) glutamate

62. Deficiency leads to negative nitrogen balance in humans
63. Synthesized from α-ketoglutarate in one step

(a) asparagine	(f) leucine
(b) aspartate	(g) lysine
(c) glycine	(h) cysteine
(d) tryptophan	(i) proline
(e) isoleucine	(j) serine

For each biochemical feature, select the most appropriate amino acid.

64. Failure to hydroxylate this amino acid in collagen leads to one form of Ehlers-Danlos syndrome.
65. The R group of this amino acid is negatively charged at *p*H 7.0.
66. This amino acid is entirely ketogenic.
67. This amino acid is a precursor of serotonin and melatonin.
68. This amino acid forms disulfide bonds.

ANSWERS TO MULTIPLE-CHOICE QUESTIONS

1. a	**18.** b	**35.** b	**52.** a
2. e	**19.** e	**36.** d	**53.** e
3. a	**20.** a	**37.** c	**54.** a
4. d	**21.** b	**38.** e	**55.** a
5. c	**22.** b	**39.** a	**56.** c
6. b	**23.** e	**40.** d	**57.** d
7. d	**24.** a	**41.** b	**58.** a
8. b	**25.** b	**42.** b	**59.** e
9. e	**26.** c	**43.** h	**60.** b
10. a	**27.** d	**44.** g	**61.** d
11. e	**28.** c	**45.** d	**62.** a
12. d	**29.** c	**46.** a	**63.** e
13. c	**30.** a	**47.** f	**64.** g
14. b	**31.** e	**48.** m	**65.** b
15. a	**32.** a	**49.** c	**66.** f
16. c	**33.** e	**50.** c	**67.** d
17. d	**34.** d	**51.** e	**68.** h

Rypins' Basic Sciences Review, 17th Edition,
edited by Edward D. Frohlich. Lippincott–Raven Publishers,
Philadelphia © 1997.

5

General Microbiology and Immunology

Ronald B. Luftig, Ph.D.
Professor and Head
Department of Microbiology
Immunology, and Parasitology
Louisiana State University Medical Center
New Orleans, Louisiana

THE MICROORGANISM

Microorganisms of medical importance include various species of bacteria, protozoa, fungi, and viruses.

Bacteria are generally spoken of as ***prokaryotes.*** The cells of all other organisms, including protozoans, fungi, and higher order species, are said to be ***eukaryotic,*** that is, their nucleus is enclosed in a membrane, and the cytoplasm contains numerous organelles, including ribosomes (protein synthesis), mitochondria (energy transfer), endoplasmic reticulum (energy transfer and other enzymic functions), lysosomes, Golgi bodies, and a cytoskeleton. All bacterial and eukaryotic cells contain both DNA and RNA. In contrast, viruses may contain either, but never both.

Historical Notes

Antonj van Leeuwenhoek, in 1672, built single-lens microscopes with effective magnification of more than 100× and was the first to see bacteria and protozoa, which he called animalcules, or ''little animals.'' He is often called the ''father of bacteriology and protozoology.''

Edward Jenner, in 1796, demonstrated that inoculation with active cowpox vesical material conferred immunity to smallpox. As of 1980, smallpox was eradicated as a result of sustained worldwide immunization.

Louis Pasteur (1822–1895), a French chemist interested in the cause of spoilage (''diseases'') of beer and wines, entered the controversy concerning spontaneous generation and finally refuted the doctrine by heating infusions in flasks with long, downtwisted necks that excluded dust but were open to the air without any substance between the outer air and the infusion. Such flasks remained sterile until dust was put into them. Pasteur later became interested in the analogy between diseases of beer and wine and human disease and formulated anew the old idea that disease was caused by invasive microorganisms. He also introduced autoclaving to destroy spores and was the first to use synthetic media as well as the first to discover bacteria that can live without air ***(anaerobes).*** In 1885, Pasteur also successfully developed a vaccine against rabies.

Joseph Lister (1827–1912), an English physician and scientist, contemporary with Pasteur and well acquainted with his ideas on dust in the air as a source of contaminating organisms, conceived the idea of using phenol solutions on surgical wounds to prevent sepsis and, later, of operating in an atmosphere filled with phenol mist. This opened the door to antiseptic surgery and later to aseptic surgery. Lister is the ''father of modern aseptic surgery.''

Robert Koch (1843–1910), in 1877, provided the first demonstration that a specific bacterium could cause anthrax, an animal disease. Working with the anthrax bacillus, he developed methods for isolating pure cultures on solid media and for staining microorganisms to render them visible under the microscope. Six years later he discovered tubercle bacillus to be the cause of tuberculosis. Koch also set forth postulates that are still used today to determine whether a specific agent is the cause of a particular infectious disease.

Elie Metchnikoff, a Russian pupil of Koch, discovered phagocytosis in 1883.

H. C. J. Gram, in 1884, devised his method for differential staining of bacteria.

Emil A. Von Behring, Shibasaburo Kitasato, and **Albert Fränkel,** in 1890, discovered the phenomena of active and passive immunization against diphtheria and tetanus, which are due to the properties of serum, which we now recognize as a specific antibody.

Adolf Mayer, Dimitri Iwanowski, and **Martinus Beijernick,** in 1886–1898, played a role in developing the concept of viruses, through their studies on the first noncultivable, invisible, and filterable agent of disease—tobacco mosaic virus.

Jules Bordet, in 1895, discovered the heat-labile antibacterial properties of immune serum, which we now ascribe to complement.

F. A. J. Löffler and **Paul Frosch,** in 1898, discovered the agent of hoof-and-mouth disease, the first-described agent of a viral disease of lower animals.

Walter Reed and the U.S. Army Yellow Fever Commission at Havana, in 1899 confirmed the mosquito *(Aedes aegypti)* as vector and discovered the agent of yellow fever, the first virus to be described as the cause of human disease.

K. Landsteiner, in 1900–1901, reported the isohemagglutination reactions that formed the basis for the major (ABO) human blood groups; in 1908, he was the first to transmit poliomyelitis in monkeys by intracerebral inoculation of bacteria-free brain tissue.

Howard Taylor Ricketts, in 1909, discovered the cause of Rocky Mountain spotted fever *(Rickettsia sp.).*

Peyton Rous, in 1911, was the first to demonstrate the transmission of a malignant tumor (chicken sarcoma) by means of cell-free filtrate (Rous sarcoma virus).

Frederick W. Twort, in 1915, and **Felix H. d'Herelle,** in 1917, discovered the bacterial viruses—bacteriophages.

Alexander Fleming, the discoverer of lysozyme, in 1929 isolated *Penicillium notatum* and demonstrated antibacterial activity *in vitro* in culture filtrates. It was not until 1940, however, that **H. W. Florey, E. B. Chain,** and their collaborators at Oxford University showed experimentally that penicillin was nontoxic and highly effective systemically in treating pyogenic infection, thus inaugurating the antibiotic era.

M. Heidelberger and **F. E. Kendall,** in 1929, developed the quantitative precipitin reaction, which underlies the interpretation of most antigen-antibody reactions.

In 1931, **Max Theiler** adapted the virus of yellow fever to embryonated eggs, leading to the development of the 17D attenuated strain of yellow fever virus used in the vaccine.

A. Tiselius and **E. A. Kabat,** in 1939, demonstrated that antibodies were contained in the γ-globulin fraction of serum.

A. H. Coons and his collaborators, in 1942, developed the fluorescent antibody technique.

O. T. Avery, C. MacLeod, and **M. McCarty,** in 1944, demonstrated that the genetic information responsible for transformation of pneumococci was embodied in DNA. This discovery ushered in the era of molecular biology and molecular genetics.

In 1949, **John F. Enders, T. H. Weller,** and **F. C. Robbins** cultivated the virus of poliomyelitis in nonneural tissue explants, making possible the development of polio and other attenuated viral vaccines. The use in the early 1950s of a killed poliomyelitis vaccine developed by **Jonas Salk** and his collaborators at the University of Pittsburgh, followed by the subsequent development of an attenuated vaccine by **Albert Sabin** and colleagues, essentially eliminated paralytic poliomyelitis from the United States.

The third quarter of this century (about 1950 to 1975) saw a veritable explosion in biomedical knowledge, represented by many signal contributions. To mention only a few, **F. Lipman** and **H. Krebs** contributed fundamental knowledge in the fields of energy metabolism and synthetic pathways in living cells (pentose phosphate pathway and Krebs cycle). In immunobiology, **G. M. Edelman** and colleagues provided the first definitive indication that immunoglobulin G comprised "light" and "heavy" peptide chains; **F. M. Burnet** formulated important theories of antibody formation and the immune response (clonal selection), and **P. B. Medawar** was the first to describe induced tolerance to foreign antigens. **K. Ishizaka** and **T. Ishizaka** identified immunoglobulin E as the agent of reaginic ("immediate")-type hypersensitivity. In microbial and molecular genetics, the contributions of **J. Lederberg, G. Beadle, S. E. Luria, E. Tatum, F. Jacob, A. Lwoff, J. Monod, M. Delbruck,** and **A. D. Hershey** were seminal. **T. Akiba** and **K. Ochiai** described the phenomenon of simultaneous transfer (from *E. coli* to *Shigella dysenteriae*) of resistance to multiple antibiotics, which **T. Watanabe** subsequently showed to be due to an infectious drug resistance transfer factor (R factor), the first of many types of plasmids to be described. **F. H. C. Crick, J. D. Watson,** and **M. H. F. Wilkins** elucidated the structure of DNA, and **M. W. Nirenberg, H. G. Khorana** and **R. W. Holley** described the genetic code, setting the stage for all of the startling recent advances in "genetic engineering." **H. M. Temin** and **D. Baltimore** identified reverse transcriptase in tumor viruses. In 1975, **G. Kohler** and **C. Milstein** developed the mouse hybridoma procedure for the preparation of monoclonal antibodies, the application of which has had a profound effect in many areas of biomedical science.

Most recently, in 1983 and 1984, two groups, one at the Pasteur Institute headed by **L. Montagnier** and one at the National Institute of Health (NIH) headed by **R. Gallo,** isolated a retrovirus, now designated as human immunodeficiency virus (HIV), as the causative agent of acquired immune deficiency syndrome AIDS.

Classification of Bacteria (Prokaryotes)

Bacteria are single-celled organisms that reproduce by binary fission, have smaller ribosome(s) than eukaryotic cells, and do not contain their DNA within a nuclear membrane. They are classified primarily on the basis of morphology, and on various physiological properties such as pigment, spore formation, staining reactions, motility, enzyme content (*e.g.,* aerobic or anaerobic, proteolytic, fermentative), and DNA analysis. Immunologic properties (antigenic structure) and susceptibility to highly specific bacterial viruses (bacteriophages) are also used in their differentiation and identification.

All medically significant species of bacteria are chemosynthetic and heterotrophic (chemo-organotrophs; see section on bacterial metabolism), having diameters typically <5 μm (usually 1 to 2 μm and less in *Rickettsia* and *Chlamydia*). Unlike viruses, all except rickettsiae and chlamydiae and two or three other species of pathogenic bacteria (*e.g.,* syphilis spirochetes and leprosy bacilli) are cultivable in *inanimate* media. Viruses, rickettsiae, and chlamydiae can multiply only in living cells (cell and tissue cultures, etc.). All bacteria have cell walls of peptidoglycan or murein that contain muramic acid, a substance unique to the prokaryotes. Medically significant bacteria occur in six orders as follows:

1. *Order Pseudomonadales:* These gram-negative rods grow in simple peptone media at 10° C to 40° C; generally motile with polar flagella, strictly aerobic. Some produce blue pyocyanin, a yellow fluorescent pigment, or both. They characteristically secrete a number of exoenzymes, such as collagenase, lipase, protease, and hemolysin, which allow them to survive in unusual environments such as hot tubs, distilled water, and disinfectants. They also excrete exotoxins, which account in large part for the serious nature of their infections. Representatives: *Pseudomonas aeruginosa, P. pseudomallei.*
2. *Order Eubacteriales:* (''True Bacteria''): Gram-positive or Gram-negative rods or cocci, no helical forms; possess a rigid cell wall; motile species have peritrichous flagella; aerobic, facultative, or strict anaerobes; only two genera (*Clostridium* and *Bacillus*) product heat-resistant endospores; must grow at 37° C in peptone or meat infusion media; some also require blood, yeast extract, or serum. This order contains most of the pathogenic bacteria. Representatives: *Salmonella typhi* and related *Enterobacteriaceae, Streptococcus pyogenes, Staphylococcus aureus, Clostridium tetani, Bacillus anthracis, Neisseria gonorrhoeae.*
3. *Order Actinomycetales:* Exhibit a branching, rodlike or filamentous cell; no motile pathogens; generally Gram-positive; some species are acid-fast; others are the source of many important antibiotics. Representatives: *Mycobacterium tuberculosis, M. leprae, Actinomyces israelii, Nocardia* sp.
4. *Order Spirochaetales:* Helical; flexible; motile without flagella; generally Gram-negative, but preferentially observed with darkfield microscope; contain a central, fibrillar, elastic structure (axial filament) around which the tubular cell is wound. Representatives: *Treponema pallidum, Leptospira icterohaemorrhagiae, Borrelia recurrentis.*
5. *Order Mycoplasmatales:* No cell wall, therefore osmotically fragile and extremely pleomorphic; very small cells (0.2 μm) that pass through filters that retain bacteria; the smallest known living units capable of independent multiplication in inanimate media; nonmotile, though some have flagella; no heat-resistant endospores; colonies on special ''enriched media'' extremely minute, typically with inverted fried egg appearance (except Eaton agent); aerobic or facultative; parasitic species are rich in lipids, mostly steroids, which stabilize and strengthen the cell membrane. Representatives: *Mycoplasma pneumoniae (Eaton agent), M. hominis, Ureaplasma urealyticum.*
6. *Order Rickettsiales:* Bacteria that lack important enzyme systems characteristic of other bacteria, hence their ***obligate intracellular parasitism*** and extremely minute (0.3 μm) size; only cultivable in cell and tissue cultures, and most in viable chick embryos; prokaryotic, bacterialike cell structure.

   Family Rickettsiaceae: Lack several synthetic enzyme systems but can synthesize ATP; multiply by binary fission like other bacteria; have distinct cell walls with muramic acid; morphologically are distinct rods, cocci or filaments. Representatives: *Rickettsia prowazekii, Coxiella burnetii.*

   Family Chlamydiaceae: Lack many synthetic enzymes; unlike all other bacteria, *cannot synthesize ATP;* complex intracellular mode of multiplication; cell walls are layered and, like bacteria, contain muramic acid; spheroidal morphology. Representatives: *Chlamydia trachomatis, C. psittaci.*

Classification of Medically Important Protozoa, Fungi, Helminths (Eukaryotes), and Viruses

In addition to bacteria, other groups containing pathogenic microorganisms are listed as follows:

A. Protozoa: Unicellular animals; rarely cultivable on artificial media; five groups differentiated by type of motility:
   1. Superclass Sarcodina (move with pseudopodia): *Entamoeba histolytica;* enteric and tissue parasites
   2. Subphylum Ciliophora (move with cilia): *Balantidium coli;* enteric
   3. Superclass Mastigophora (move with flagella): Arthropod-borne: *Leishmania, Trypanosoma;* blood and tissues; *Trichomonas,* chiefly genitalia
   4. Subphylum Sporozoa (ameboid movement in some trophozoites): Alternating sexual and asexual multiplication in different hosts, *e.g.,* humans and mosquito in *Plasmodium* (malaria parasites); blood and tissues
   5. Class Toxoplasmea (gliding and flexing motility): Asexual multiplication by binary fission, endogony or sporogony, or both; trophozoites in cysts or pseudocysts. *Toxoplasma gondii, Sarcocystis lindemanni*

B. Fungi: Eukaryotic cellular structure; may grow as branching and filamentous forms (mycelia) or single cells (yeasts), or both; nonphotosynthetic (no chlorophyll); chemo-organotrophic; cultivable on inanimate media, *e.g.,* Sabouraud's agar; pathogens are mainly in the division called Fungi Imperfecti or Deuteromycetes, which are not known to reproduce sexually
   1. Superficial infections (tinea, athlete's foot, etc.) due to dermatophytes: *Trichophyton* spp; *Microsporum* spp; *Epidermophyton* spp.
   2. Deep or systemic infections (histoplasmosis, paracoccidioidomycosis, coccidioidomycosis, blastomycosis) due to yeastlike or dimorphic fungi

C. Helminths (parasitic worms): Eukaryotic cell structure; contain DNA and RNA. Adult helminths are not microscopic, but many of their developmental, infective, and diagnostically important forms are.
   1. Platyhelminthes (flatworms)
      a. Trematodes—flukes: Nonsegmented; digenetic (alternate sexual and asexual generations in different hosts); sexual stage in humans; bilaterally symmetrical; dorsoventrally compressed; hermaphroditic except dioecious (♀ and ♂) schistosomes (blood flukes); *e.g.,* liver flukes, lung flukes
      b. Cestodes—tapeworms: Hermaphroditic; consist of enlarged scolex ("head") with suckers (and hooks, depending on species) for attachment to intestinal mucosa; narrow "neck" produces, by budding, successive flat segments; these form the ribbon-like strobilia or chain of from three to several thousand hermaphroditic proglottids, *e.g.,* beef tapeworms
   2. Nematodes—roundworms: Nonsegmented; long, slender, cylindrical; dioecious
      a. Intestinal parasites: Typically no intermediate hosts; eggs, larvae, or both mature in intestine, on skin, in or on soil; *e.g.,* pinworms, hookworms, Ascaris
      b. Blood and tissue parasites (intermediate hosts necessary)
         (1) *Trichinella spiralis* (pork worm)
         (2) Filaria worms (various species and insect vectors)

D. Viruses: Visible only with the electron microscope; obligate intracellular parasites that grow in cell or organ culture, embryonated eggs, experimental animals; lack intrinsic metabolic mechanisms; contain core of genetic information as DNA or RNA, never both; nucleic acid genome associated with protein (capsid); virus structure has icosahedral, helical, or complex (bilateral) symmetry; some viruses possess an outer envelope containing lipid derived from the host-cell and virus-coded glycoproteins onto which glycosyl residues are incorporated by host-cell transferases; some virus particles contain intravirion nucleic acid transcriptases.

MICROSCOPIC METHODS

The optical microscope commonly used in medical work consists of three principal parts: condenser (with iris diaphragm), objective and ocular or eyepiece; and a source of visible light. Light enters at the lowest part of the optical system and passes upward toward the eye through the object on the stage and the magnifying lenses. Immersion oil is placed between the object and the objective lens to prevent loss of light due to refraction and reflection at the several glass surfaces. An objective lens designed to operate in oil is called an ***oil-immersion*** objective.

The objective produces a real image magnified about 90 times. The ocular or eyepiece further enlarges it about 10 times, giving a final image about 900 times the size of the object (*i.e.,* 10 × 90 or 900×).

The Electron Microscope

The ***resolving power*** of the common (optical) microscope is limited by the nature of visible light; images typically obtained in a good-quality research microscope by using a high-power oil-immersion lens are at a magnification of about 1,000×. To increase the magnification and resolution further, electrons that have a much shorter wavelength than ordinary light (about 0.5 nm or 5Å) are used. An electron microscope has a much greater resolving power and is capable of giving distinct images at magnifications of 100,000 or more.

The electron microscope uses electromagnetic "lenses" that are functionally analogous to glass lenses in the optical microscope. The electron beam is focused by varying the strength and direction of the electromagnets. Moreover, since electrons travel only in a high vacuum (the mean free path of electrons in air is about 1 cm, while under an appropriate vacuum it can be more than 10 m), the entire instrument, including the specimen chamber, is designed to be evacuated. This means that specimens, in order to retain their shape, must be chemically fixed (*e.g.*, with aldehydes and/or osmium tetroxide), stained with heavy metal salts (*e.g.*, uranyl acetate) to enhance contrast, and embedded in plastic of high density, such as epoxy resin, which can be cut into ultrathin sections, usually a fraction of a nanometer thick. Additional techniques, such as surface replication, freeze-fracturing, freeze-etching, and negative staining, are also utilized for transmission electron microscopy (TEM). Images generated by transmission of electrons are viewed on a fluorescent screen set below the specimen onto which the electron beam is focused. For micrography, the fluorescent screen is replaced by a photographic plate.

Other Optical Methods

Other optical methods are (1) ***phase microscopy,*** in which light rays passing *through* the object, and those diffracted *around* it (and therefore out of wavephase with the rays passing through the object) are integrated into a single image, (2) x-ray, and (3) fluorescence microscopy.

For ***fluorescence microscopy,*** specimens are stained with a fluorescent dye (*e.g.*, fluorescein [FITC] or rhodamine [TMR]), which, in the presence of detergent, penetrates the cell wall of microorganisms such as *Mycobacteria*. FITC preparations are viewed with an ultraviolet light source, which excites the dye to emit yellow-green light.

Darkfield Microscopy

By means of a darkfield condenser or a "stop," central rays of light (usually admitted) are prevented from passing upward through the object to the eye. Peripheral rays (usually eliminated) are refracted by the darkfield condenser to emerge so obliquely from the surface of the slide that they do not reach the eye when the field is devoid of any object. The field therefore appears dark (hence darkfield). When the oblique rays impinge on an object on the slide, *e.g.*, a spirochete or bacterium, they are reflected upward from the surface of the object of the eye through the lenses. The object is then seen brightly outlined by the rays reflected from its surface.

STAINING METHODS

In order to determine the shape of bacteria and also to provide a means of classification, several differential staining techniques have been developed to be used with the light microscope.

Gram's Stain

1. Smear the material to be stained on a slide. Allow to dry in air. Fix by gently heating, which kills the bacteria and allows it to attach to the slide.
2. Apply an appropriate solution of crystal violet. Allow to stain about 1 minute. Wash gently.
3. Apply iodine solution (a mordant, which strengthens the bond between dye and substrate) for 1 minute. Wash gently.
4. Apply 95% ethyl alcohol until all but the thickest parts of the smear are decolorized, or for not more than 10 to 15 seconds. Wash.
5. Counterstain with safranin for 1 minute. Wash. Blot dry.
6. Examine naked smear, using the oil immersion lens of the light microscope.
7. Gram-positive organisms are blue-purple and gram-negative bacteria are pink-red.

With the use of Gram's stain, bacteria are differentiated by their ability to either retain or lose the crystal violet-iodine combination in the presence of a decolorizing agent. Those that retain the violet dye are called gram-positive. Those that lose the violet dye (*i.e.*, are decolorized) will take the red safranin counterstain and are called gram-negative. The result of the Gram's stain reaction depends on the type of bacterial cell wall: gram-positive bacteria have a thicker cell wall that is highly cross-linked and can trap the crystal violet-iodine aggregate. In contrast, gram-negative cell walls are thinner and, after alcohol treatment, more easily release the initial dye complex.

Gram-Positive Bacteria

All streptococci
All staphylococci

TABLE 5-1. Antimicrobial Agents That Inhibit Cell Wall Synthesis

DRUG	CHEMICAL GROUP	PRIMARY SITE OF BINDING	ACTIVITY BLOCKED	ACTIVE ON	ADVERSE REACTIONS	SENSITIVITY TO β-LACTAMASES
Penicillin G	β-lactam ring	Periplasmic space (cross-linking enzyme)	Blocks peptidoglycan cross-linking (cidal)	Gram-positive, fastidious gram-negative	Hypersensitivity develops to all penicillins	Gram-positive and gram-negative
Penicillin V	β-lactam ring	Periplasmic space	Blocks peptidoglycan cross-linking	Gram-positive, fastidious gram-negative	Hypersensitivity develops to all penicillins	Gram-positive and gram-negative
Methicillin, Nafcillin, Oxacillin	β-lactam ring	Periplasmic space	Blocks peptidoglycan cross-linking	Staph and other gram-positive	Hypersensitivity develops to all penicillins	Resistant to penicillinase
Ampicillin	β-lactam ring	Periplasmic space	Blocks peptidoglycan cross-linking	Broad spectrum	Hypersensitivity develops to all penicillins	Sensitive to most
Carbenicillin	β-lactam ring	Periplasmic space	Blocks peptidoglycan cross-linking	Broad spectrum *(Pseudomonas)*	Hypersensitivity develops to all penicillins	Resistant to some gram-negative enzymes
Cephalothin	β-lactam ring	Periplasmic space	Blocks peptidoglycan cross-linking	Broad spectrum	Hypersensitivity to all cephalosporins	Sensitive to many gram-negative enzymes
Cefamandole, Cefoxitin	β-lactam ring	Periplasmic space	Blocks peptidoglycan cross-linking	Broad spectrum	Hypersensitivity to all cephalosporins	Resistant to most
Cycloserine	D-alanine analogue	Cytoplasmic enzyme	Inhibits conversion of D-alanine to L-alanine for subunit synthesis	Gram-positive		
Bacitracin	Polypeptide	Cytoplasmic lipid	Inhibits subunit synthesis	Gram-positive	Limited to topical use	
Vancomycin		Cell membrane	Blocks secretion of cell wall subunit	Gram-positive		

Pneumococci *(Streptococcus pneumoniae)*
Diphtheria bacillus *(Corynebacterium diphtheriae)*
All acid-fast bacilli, such as *Mycobacterium tuberculosis*
All spore-forming anaerobes (genus *Clostridium*)
Bacillus anthracis, B. cereus
Listeria, Erysipelothrix, Actinomyces, Nocardia, Streptomyces, Coxiella

Gram-Negative Bacteria

Genus Neisseria
The Enterobacteriaceae, including *Salmonella, Shigella,* the coliform group
The *Haemophilus* groups *(H. influenzae, H. ducreyi)*
Organisms of pertussis *(Bordetella pertussis),* plague *(Yersinia pestis),* cholera *(Vibrio cholerae)*
All species of *Pseudomonas, e.g., Pseudomonas aeruginosa*
Spirillum minus, Brucella spp., *Francisella tularensis, Bacteroides, Fusobacterium, Veillonella, Citrobacter, Proteus, Campylobacter, Legionella*

Differences in reaction to the Gram's stain also reflect medically important differences in properties of the organisms, chiefly susceptibility to antibiotics affecting cell wall synthesis (see Table 5-1).

Acid-Fast Stain (Ziehl-Neelsen) and Kinyoun (Cold) Methods

Organisms of tuberculosis and leprosy, and several related saprophytic species of *Mycobacterium* have the distinctive character called acid-fastness (AF), due to the presence of lipids (waxlike mycolic acid) in the cell wall. They quickly absorb red carbolfuchsin dye when in the presence of a detergent, such as Tween-80, or when warmed, and retain dye after washing with an acidified alcohol solution. All non-acid-fast bacteria, mucus, pus, cells, etc., lose the carbolfuchsin when treated with acid alcohol and take a contrasting counterstain, *e.g.*, methylene blue, yellow picric acid, or brilliant green. The acid-fast stain is performed as follows:

1. Fix the smear as for Gram's stain.
2. Flood slide with carbolfuchsin, steam gently for 5 minutes over low flame, do not allow to dry, add more stain if necessary. Cool. Alternatively, carbolfuchsin-containing phenol and alcohol (cool) may be used without heat.
3. Apply 90% alcohol containing 3 to 5% HCl until all but thickest parts of smear cease to give off color (about 1 to 3 minutes). Wash.
4. Counterstain 1 minute with methylene blue. Wash.

Tubercle bacilli are more strongly acid-fast than other members of the acid-fast group, and give a characteristic beaded appearance. Both Gram's stain and acid-fast stain depend on the integrity of the cell wall. Broken or disintegrated bacilli or their parts are neither gram-positive nor acid-fast.

Fluorescence Labelling for Detection of Antigen-Antibody Reactions *In Situ*

Antibodies, or protein antigens, can be chemically conjugated with fluorescein without significant loss of specific reactivity. For detection of surface antigens on animal cells, unfixed cells in suspension are treated with fluorescent antibody (FAb) (direct method) or with unlabelled antibody followed by fluorescent antiglobulin (indirect method) of the same species and viewed in the fresh state with ultraviolet illumination. Cells tagged in suspension with FAb can be enumerated by using a light microscope equipped with an epifluorescence accessory or by passage through a fluorescence-activated cell sorter (FACS). To detect both surface and intracellular antigen-antibody reactions, the cells (or tissues) must be fixed in a way that allows penetration of macromolecular reagents through the membrane but causes minimal disruption of ultrastructure. Frozen sections and smears (including those for bacteriological diagnosis) or cell monolayers fixed in acetone or glutaraldehyde generally meet these requirements. Appropriately fixed preparations are stained by either direct or indirect methods; the latter method has the advantage of requiring only one labeled antiglobulin, provided that all the primary antisera to be used are from the same animal species.

Labelling for Electron Microscopy

Antigen-antibody reactions can be recognized on thin-sections by transmission electron microscopy (TEM) of preparations which have previously been stained with appropriate immunological reagents. However, accurate interpretation of images requires adequate specificity controls for the putative immune reactions. Specific reactions can frequently be identified by the density and distribution of molecular aggregates, particularly on the surface of cells, or by the specific aggregation of antigen particles by antibody, as in immune electron microscopy used in virological diagnosis. Labelling antibody with ferritin greatly increases the ease with which immune reactions are detected, due to the presence of complexed electron-dense iron molecules at the reaction sites. Antibody can be labelled with an enzyme (peroxidase or phosphatase), which, at the sites of combination with antigen, yields an electron-dense chromogen by reaction with substrate. The same preparations stained with enzyme-labelled antibody and developed with chromogenic substrate can be fixed and permanently mounted for light microscopy.

THE ANATOMY AND PHYSIOLOGY OF BACTERIA

The Bacterial Genome

The genome of bacterial cells contains double-stranded deoxyribonucleic acid (DNA) predominantly in a B-type supercoiled, double helical conformation. Z-type DNA (the backbone "zigzags" down the molecule) has recently been described in certain, local regions of the DNA. A left-handed DNA helical conformation may have an important role in regulating the interaction of certain regions of genes, *i.e.*, promoters, based on their differential interaction with large proteins that bind to it and that vary in their abundance in different kinds of cells.

Upon separation, each of the two DNA strands is seen to be a long-chain polymer of deoxyribonucleotides, each nucleotide bearing either a purine base: guanine (G) or adenine (A), or a pyrimidine base: thymine (T) or cytosine (C). The nucleotides of each strand are held together lengthwise by strong, covalent, phosphodiester linkages between the sugars while the two strands themselves are held together by relatively weak hydrogen bonds between the bases:

```
      deoxyribose       deoxyribose
 ━━ phosphate ━━ phosphate ━━
         |                  |
      purine (A or G)   pyrimidine (C or T)
        ||(|)               ||(|)
      pyrimidine (C or T)   purine (A or G)
         |                  |
      deoxyribose       deoxyribose
 ━━ phosphate ━━ phosphate ━━
```

A always pairs with T; C with G. The whole structure can be seen as a helical ladder: the sides are the firm phosphosugar polymers, the rungs are the separable purine-pyrimidine base pairs. The numbers, sequence, and kinds of nucleotides and their pairing are fixed for each species and constitute its genetic code. The ends of the helix are connected, forming a twisted closed circle, an arrangement important in its replication. The twists in the circle are highly strained, as in a twisted rope. The resulting "supercoils" are released in a controlled manner, which presumably facilitates revolution of the molecule about the helical axis during replication and recombination.

The contrast between prokaryotic and eukaryotic chromosomes is not limited to physical arrangement of molecules, but extends to the organization of the genetic message. The DNA of prokaryotes has few repeated sequences, most of the DNA is transcribed, and there are no intervening sequences within structural genes. Eukaryotic DNA contains many repeated sequences; some repeat millions of times. Much of the DNA is not transcribed; portions of structural genes (exons) are separated from each other by intervening sequences (introns).

Bacterial Cytoplasm

This consists of a fluid matrix containing particulate matter, as well as various ions, enzymes, amino acids, vitamins, nucleotides, tRNA, etc., in solution. Because of the selective permeability of the cell membrane and the action of "one-way" permease enzymes in the cell envelope, many of these substances increase in concentration inside the cell so as to raise the intracellular osmotic pressure to several atmospheres. When the cell (especially a gram-positive cell) is deprived of its strong wall of peptidoglycan or murein (as by lysozyme or growth in penicillin, cephalothin, etc.), in a hypotonic solution the fragile cell membrane ruptures (see Table 5-2).

Particulate matter includes inert granules of stored food such as polymetaphosphates (volutin); lipids, principally as poly-betahydroxybutyric acid; starchlike granules, etc. The largest portion of cytoplasmic particulate matter of the bacterial cell consists of ribosomes, minute granules of rRNA with some protein. Each 70s ribosome monomer consists of two subunits, 50s and 30s. Ribosomes function in the synthesis of proteins. With the assistance of tRNA anticodons to transfer amino acids, and mRNA codons to carry the genetic code of the nuclear DNA, the se-

TABLE 5-2. Antimicrobial Agents That Affect Membrane or Nucleic Acid Synthesis

NAME	CHEMICAL FEATURE	SITE OF BINDING	ACTIVITY BLOCKED	RANGE OF ACTIVITY
Polymyxins	Polypeptide ring	Cell membrane	Osmotic properties, detergent-like action	Gram-negative
Nystatin, Amphotericin	Polyene	Cell membrane	Interact with sterols to alter permeability, detergent-like action	Fungi
Sulfanilamide	PAGA-analogue	Cytoplasmic enzyme (dihydrofolic acid synthetase)	Purine and thymidine shortages block RNA and DNA synthesis	Broad
Trimethoprim-Sulfamethoxazole (co-trimoxazole)	—	Cytoplasmic enzymes (dihydrofolic acid reductase)	Purine and thymidine shortages block RNA and DNA synthesis	Broad
Griseofulvin	Guanosine analogue	Unknown	DNA replication	Fungi
Rifampicins	Semisynthetic macrolide	Cytoplasmic enzyme (RNA polymerase)	Transcription of mRNA	Broad
Nalidixic acid, Floxacins	—	Cytoplasmic enzyme (gyrase)	Inhibits DNA unwinding needed for DNA synthesis	Gram-negative
Nitrofurantoin	—	Reduced by microorganisms and reacts with DNA	Integrity of DNA replication	Broad
Metronidazole	—	Reduced by microorganisms and reacts with DNA	Integrity of DNA replication	Anaerobes
Ketoconazole	Synthetic imidazole derivative	Cell membrane	Alters cell membrane permeability by interfering with sterol synthesis	Broad antifungal (hepatotoxic)

TABLE 5-3. Antimicrobial Agents That Block Protein Synthesis

DRUG	CHEMICAL	PRIMARY SITE OF BINDING	STEP BLOCKED	RANGE OF ACTIVITY
Streptomycin, Neomycin, Kanamycin, Gentamicin, Tobramycin, Amikacin	Aminoglycoside	30s ribosomal subunit	Binding of tRNA to ribosome	Broad spectrum
Spectinomycin	Aminocyclitol	30s ribosomal subunit	Binding of tRNA to ribosome	Broad spectrum
Tetracycline	—	30s ribosomal subunit	Binding of tRNA to ribosome	Broad spectrum
Chloramphenicol	—	50s ribosomal subunit	Formation of peptide bond	Broad spectrum
Lincomycin	Macrolide	50s ribosomal subunit	Formation of peptide bond	Gram-positive
Clindamycin	Macrolide	50s ribosomal subunit	Formation of peptide bond	Broad (anaerobes) spectrum
Erythromycin	Macrolide	50s ribosomal subunit	Translocation of ribosome on mRNA	Broad spectrum
Fusidic acid	—	Cytoplasmic soluble protein (elongation factor)	Translocation of ribosome on mRNA	Gram-positive

quence of the amino acids in the polypeptides made by the ribosomes are the points of attachment of numerous antibiotics that interfere with protein synthesis (see Table 5-3).

Mesosomes (possibly primitive endoplasmic reticulum) are saccular invaginations of the cytoplasmic membrane and, in contrast with the nuclear material, are associated with cell fission. Mesosomes are absent from mycoplasmas. Bacteria contain no mitochondria, lysosomes, Golgi bodies, or other complex organelles that characterize eukaryotic cells.

BACTERIAL SURFACE COMPONENTS

Fimbriae

Fimbriae, or common pili, are straight, rapid, hair-like microfibrillar structures extending out from the surface and visible only by electron microscopy; they are predominantly found on gram-negative bacteria, particularly those encountered in the oropharynx and the infected urinary tract. They are present in multiple copies (100 to 200) over the entire cell; they are shorter than flagella. Fimbriae allow bacteria to adhere to one another, as seen in the formation of pellicles on the surface of broth cultures. Fimbriae also by virtue of their ability to bind to sugar residues can bind to eukaryotic cell surfaces, *e.g.*, glycoproteins, and thus constitute an important pathogenic mechanism whereby microorganisms initiate infection by adhering to cell and mucosal surfaces (*e.g.*, gonococci in the genitourinary tract) through specific receptors.

F-type pili, or sex pili, are larger, longer, and less rigid than common pili and occur in gram-negative ''male'' donor, or F^+, bacteria, in which they serve as conjugation tubes during sexual reproduction (see section on conjugation). When present, F pili are randomly distributed and in fewer numbers than common pili. F pili also serve as receptors for specific bacteriophages, such as the RNA phage f1 or the DNA phage M13.

Slimes and Capsules

Some species of bacteria produce extracellular gels which adhere by noncovalent chemical interactions to the cell as ***capsules*** or as less dense macromolecular coatings, ***slimes.*** Capsules most often are polysaccharides (*e.g.*, capsules of pneumococci, meningococci), sometimes glycoprotein (*e.g.*, hyaluronic acid in *Streptococcus pyogenes* of groups A and C). Capsules protect the bacterium from dehydration and phagocytosis, thereby acting as virulence factors. Pathogenic organisms that are encapsulated when first isolated, on further cultivation lose their capsules and become avirulent (*e.g.*, ''smooth'' to ''rough'' [S-R] variation in appearance of pneumococcal colonies on agar). Vi, or virulence capsular antigens, seen in *E. coli* and *Salmonella typhi,* are similarly antiphagocytic and are readily removed by heat, or on subcultivation, which concomitantly diminishes virulence.

Bacterial Flagella

Flagella of prokaryotic cells are protein structures that extend out from the bacterial surface. They are attached to the cell membrane by a hook that in turn is bound to a basal body. The flagella impart motility by their characteristic wavelike motion that is governed by chemotactic responses to nutrients or toxic substances through chemoreceptors on the cell surface. The distribution of flagella (whether at one or both poles, over the entire surface of the cell, or in the form of axial filaments as in *Spirillum*) varies with the species of bacteria (there are no motile cocci). Among the *Enterobacteriaceae,* flagellar proteins confer species or type specificity on the cell. Flagellar antigens for these gram-negative bacteria are referred to as H antigens, in contrast to O antigens that reside in the cell wall. Specifically, O antigen specificity is conferred by the lipopolysaccharide (LPS)–protein–phosphatide complexes and this provides for the endotoxic activity characteristic of gram-negative bacteria. In practice, O and H antigens for serodiagnosis (*e.g.,* of salmonellosis) are bacterial suspensions prepared in a manner that on the one hand destroys flagella without affecting somatic (group) antigens (*e.g.,* ethanol at 37°) and on the other hand stabilizes (*e.g.,* dilute formalin) flagella to permit them to react preferentially with type-specific antibody.

Closely related species of bacteria, such as the many serotypes of *Salmonella,* may contain identical O antigens. (Not to be confused with O[H] blood-group antigens. See section on Immunohematology.) Thus, if a person is stimulated antigenically, either by injections of vaccine or by infection with any of the genus *Salmonella,* say *S. typhi,* the blood may contain O agglutinins for several other species of *Salmonella.* This is helpful in diagnosing salmonellosis retrospectively by serum agglutination titrations with any of several group-related species of *Salmonella* (Widal test). With *S. typhi,* it is customary to use both O and H (type) antigens.

Flagella of spirochetes are polar but, unlike the separate flagella of other bacteria, occur in bipolar bundles bent sharply back on the tubular cell, their ends meeting near the midlength. These bundles together form an end-to-end axial filament around which the helical cell is twined. Like other flagella they are attached in the cell wall by hooks and rings.

The Cytoplasmic Membrane

This is commonly of the three-layer, unit-membrane type: a double, inner, lipid leaflet between two outer layers of protein. It acts as a highly selective, semipermeable, osmotic barrier for the cell. In bacteria (except pathogenic mycoplasmas, which have no cell wall) sterols are not present, whereas they are present in pathogenic fungi in which they constitute points of attack by such fungicidal antibiotics as nystatin and amphotericin B (see Table 5-2).

Attached to the cell membrane are many ribosomes, and integrated with it are many enzymes of energy-mediating systems, including cytochromes and the associated oxidative phosphorylation (ATP-producing) systems.

Endospores

Some bacteria can exist either in a vegetative state or as an endospore. These are intracellular, minute, dehydrated, round or oval bodies, only one per cell, with thick, multilayered walls. They contain the essential cell contents in compact form. Endospores cannot take up any form of the Gram's stain and are highly resistant to heat, sunlight, radiation, drying, as well as chemical disinfectants. Under suitable conditions of moisture, nutrition, and warmth, they germinate, much as seeds germinate, and grow into the vulnerable, vegetative form of the organism.

The only known pathogenic organisms forming such highly heat- and disinfectant-resisting spores are species of the aerobic genus *Bacillus (B. anthracis)* and of the anaerobic genus *Clostridium,* including *C. tetani, C. perfringens, C. botulinum,* and several species associated with *C. perfringens* in gas gangrene of contaminated wounds. *Coxiella burnetii,* the causative agent of Q fever, also produces an endospore.

The Cell Wall and Periplasmic Space

Prokaryotic cell walls differ from those of eukaryotic green plants and from those of eukaryotic fungi, which contain glycans (*e.g.,* chitin, a homopolymer of *N*-acetylglucosamine). Animal cells have no true cell wall. The cell walls of gram-positive bacteria consist wholly of relatively thick layers of ***peptidoglycan*** or ***murein,*** a complex of polymers of *N*-acetylglucosamine (GlcNAc) alternating with N-acetyl muramic acid (MurNAc) and cross-linked by a tetrapeptide through the carboxyl group of MurNAc. The composition of both the glycan and the cross-linking polypeptide may vary among different bacterial species, including additional antigenic polymers (*e.g.,* teichoic acids) linked to peptidoglycan. Certain species contain proteins externally associated with the cell wall that have an important relation to pathogenetic and immune mechanisms (*e.g.,* M proteins of group A streptococci, staphylococcal protein A linked to peptidoglycan).

Gram-negative cells have a rather loosely attached outer membrane (OM) or layer with unit-membrane-type structure that contains the O (LPS, endotoxin) antigen and a relatively thin inner layer of lysozyme-sensitive peptidoglycan in contact with the plasma membrane. The OM acts as a selective permeability barrier, which excludes hydrophobic substances as well as hydrophilic substances above a critical size.

When the rigid cell wall peptidoglycan is lost (*e.g.,* by growth in hypertonic medium with penicillin, which inhibits peptidoglycan synthesis, by treatment with lysozyme, or by mutation), gram-positive bacteria become osmotically fragile ***protoplasts.*** The analogous form derived from gram-negative species are called ***spheroplasts,*** which, while retaining cell wall LPS, are less osmotically fragile than protoplasts. Formation and persistent viability of protoplasts *in vivo* (*e.g.,* in the course of penicillin therapy) are thought to have an important role in endogenous recurrence of active bacterial infection (*e.g.,* infective endocarditis, urinary tract infection).

GENETIC TRANSFER IN BACTERIA

Three mechanisms for transfer of bacterial DNA from cell to cell are known: conjugation, transformation, and transduction.

Conjugation

Conjugation, the nearest approach to true sexuality in bacteria, depends on the presence of fertility genes that are often associated with extrachromosomal elements called ***plasmids,*** some of which confer ability to produce sexual organelles. Such plasmids, through the action of transfer genes, produce sex pili and mediate the intercellular transfer of DNA by the replicative process. An autonomously replicating molecule (replicon) bearing genes for sexual organelles constitutes a self-transferable fertility factor. Furthermore, plasmids bearing transfer genes can transiently insert into other replicons, including the chromosome, and thus promote the transfer by conjugation of the entire genetic complex.

Recent rapid bacterial evolution has been mediated by plasmids and is attributable to their ability to transfer genetic information from cell to cell during conjugation. The importance of plasmids to medicine lies in the fact that they may contain genes for drug resistance and toxin production as well as the means for transferring these traits across interspecies barriers. Moreover, plasmid genes possess "*transposon*" activity, in that genetic information can be freely exchanged from plasmid to plasmid, or from plasmid to chromosome, within the same cell. This property of transposability has served as the basis for constructing new "genetically engineered" strains of bacteria.

In this regard, the emergence of plasmid-born penicillinase genes among clinical isolates of *Haemophilus* and *Neisseria* has caused much concern for the future effectiveness of antibiotic therapy. The DNA responsible has been shown to be derived from Enterobacteriaceae. Based on chronological order of acquired resistance, the information was carried by plasmids from the Enterobacteriaceae into species of *Haemophilus.*

Transformation

In bacteria, this is the transfer of DNA from one cell to another by exposing the recipient cells, *in vitro* or *in vivo,* to contact with DNA derived from a different (but related through adequate base-pair homology of their DNAs) donor cell. This is exemplified by the transformation of *Pneumococcus* serologic (capsular) types and can occur between other related species. Only fragments of DNA from the donor cell enter the recipient cell through the cell wall and membrane. The recipient cell must be in a competent state (*i.e.,* rough, R, or no interfering capsule, etc.) to receive the transforming DNA. Competence also depends on the presence of a particular surface protein.

Note: Do not confuse bacterial transformation with malignant transformation of animal cells due to the integration of oncogenic DNA from animal viruses, such as mouse polyoma viruses or monkey SV40, with the cell chromosome. Oncogenic transformation results in heritable alterations of morphology, the appearance of new tumor-specific membrane antigens, due to the release of tumor-specific growth factors, and inhibition of movement. The cells pile up, become aneuploid, and when injected into susceptible hosts, such as new-born hamsters, cause the formation of tumors.

Transduction

In early studies with the temperate or lysogenic bacteriophages, such as λ (lambda), a class of defective viruses was discovered (lambda dg) that could not replicate without helper functions supplied by normal phage. Upon subsequent study it was shown that the reason lambda dg particles were defective was because they contained host bacterial DNA in place of an essential lambda gene. Furthermore, this bacterial DNA that had been mispackaged into phage particles could be transmitted to other cells by viral infection ***(transduction).*** Since the error occurred during excision of prophage DNA from a specific bacterial location, this was known as ***specialized transduction.*** Mispackaging of bacterial DNA can also occur throughout the host genome for viruses such as P1. This is known as ***generalized transduction.***

VARIATION AND MUTATION

Phenotypic Changes

The distinguishing characteristics of any cell and its progeny are its phenotype. Because the DNA molecule is remarkably stable, phenotypic characters remain quite constant under ordinary conditions of growth. However, they may be greatly altered by environmental circumstances such as *p*H, temperature, as well as the presence or absence of certain ions or nutritional or toxic substances. Characters commonly altered by such influences are pigment, slime formation, sporulation, and filamentous growth. Changes of this nature are noninheritable; each cell reverts to its original or unaltered state immediately on removal of the altering influence; the genotype (entire sequences of nucleotides in the chromosome) has remained intact.

INDUCED ENZYMES

A particular type of phenotypic variation is seen in inducible enzyme function. The genotype may code for production of certain enzymes such as β-galactosidase, penicillinase, or certain permeases, but these are suppressed by an intracellular repressor. In the presence of the specific substrate of the enzyme, or of a chemically related substance (*e.g.*, β-galactose or lactose), the repressor is removed or inactivated, and the genetic potentiality is phenotypically expressed. Thus we see formation of lactose by β-galactosidase or destruction of penicillin by penicillinase or admission to the cell of the substrate of the particular permease involved. An important aspect of this is the development of bacteria, notably staphylococci, that, originally susceptible to penicillin, on contact with penicillin produce the enzyme penicillinase, thus becoming wholly resistant to penicillin (see section on drug resistance). The induced change appears to be permanent though it is not a genetic change. ***Inducibility*** of an enzyme represents an inherited potentiality under repression; its ***induction*** is the result of removal of the repressor by an external stimulus.

Lysogenic Conversion

This is a variation in a bacterial property that results when a temperate phage codes for a gene product that alters the host cell, *e.g.*, introduction of the property of toxigenicity into a cell of nontoxigenic *Corynebacterium diphtheriae*. The nontoxigenic cell becomes toxigenic (virulent), but only as long as the converting prophage remains in the cell genome. ''Curing'' the converted cell of its prophage DNA causes the cell to revert to nontoxigenicity (avirulence). Similar examples of phageborn toxicity are found in other bacterial species, *e.g.*, *Streptococcus pyogenes*.

Colony Variation

Bacteria of virtually any species, when grown on solid agar, may form variant colonies that have differing morphology and biological properties due to variation in their genotype, *i.e.*, alternating mutations and back-mutations.

Smooth, or S-type, colonies are of pasty or butyraceous consistency, smooth, moist-looking, glistening, domed and circular, with even, regular margins. Cells in S colonies tend to be encapsulated and may form long chains (*e.g.*, streptococci in blood broth) or even longer filaments. Growth in broth culture is said to be smooth when the growing organisms impart a more or less even turbidity to the medium.

Rough, or R-type, colonies have a dull, dry-looking granular surface, are brittle in consistency, and are rather flat, with crenated, indented, or irregular margins. Bacteria in R colonies are not encapsulated and tend not to form chains or filaments. S to R changes, which are not usually stable, often occur as a result of suboptimal conditions of cultivation. Conversely, R strains passed through an experimental animal (*e.g.*, R pneumococci inoculated into a mouse and subsequently reisolated) may regain capsules, and hence virulence. Pathogenic bacteria (*e.g.*, pneumococci, meningococci) on primary isolation from loci of disease (*e.g.*, purulent sputum, spinal fluid) are always encapsulated.

The capsular substance of S-type cells, usually but not always carbohydrate, is antigenically active and highly specific and, in species such as *Streptococcus pneumoniae, Haemophilus influenzae, and Neisseria meningitidis*, is antiphagocytic and hence associated with virulence. Accordingly, in considering strains to incorporate into a vaccine, it is advantageous to select S variants, which are most likely to produce the largest amounts of protective antigen(s), *e.g.*, capsules in the pneumococcus or meningococcus. In general, R variants, since they are deficient in capsular antigen(s), are of lower virulence than S variants of the same species and retain a broader antigenicity that is more group- than type-specific. These considerations are especially pertinent to the formulation of pertussis or pneumococcal vaccines.

Recombination

It is important to differentiate ***recombination,*** which involves formation of a new DNA molecule by breakage and joining of two DNA molecules or of two regions within a single DNA molecule and results in a rearrangement of sequences within one or more molecules of DNA, from simple ***reassortment*** of DNA molecules between cells, such as occurs with plasmid transfer.

The bacterial chromosome is not a fixed structure; all homologous sequences present within the genome will be foci of virtually constant recombinational activity. A strikingly evident example of the consequences is the phenomenon of phase variation. The antigenic specificity of the flagella of *Salmonella* alternates periodically between two states. It is now known that this antigenic alteration is due to recombination between homologous DNA sequences (insertion sequences, IS) that bracket the flagellar structural genes. With each recombinational event, the chromosomal sequence of the flagella genes is reversed: When the genes are inserted into the genome in one orientation, the H_1 antigenic phase is expressed; when they are inserted in the other orientation, the H_2 phase is expressed. Many recombinational events go undetected; it is nevertheless becoming apparent that the normal condition of the *E. coli* genome is one of dynamic flux.

Genotypic Changes

These are true genetic mutations; the actual chemical composition of the DNA molecule or genome is altered and if the change is not lethal, as often happens, the change is passed on to the progeny of the cell. Because of the stability of the DNA molecule, most types of spontaneous mutation are rare, ordinarily occurring at frequencies of about 1 in 10^6 or less, unless the frequency is increased by certain mutagenic agents.

The smallest genetic unit, the presence, absence, or alteration of which can result in a mutation, is a single nucleotide, a ***muton.*** The presence, or structure, of a single nucleotide or base pair may determine a heritable character and be a gene or recombinational unit or ***recon,*** but genes generally consist of many nucleotides. A gene is defined as any genetically functional segment of the chromosome.

Mutagenic agents may be chemical or physical. Among the most potent physical mutagens are ultraviolet and ionizing radiations. Ultraviolet irradiation, among other effects, tends especially to cause aberrant chemical linkages (dimers) to occur between pyrimidines: T to T, T to C, or C to C. Ionizing radiations can cause destructive effects due to release of free radicals, or mutations due to deletion of nucleotides.

Several chemicals are active mutagens. Alkylating agents such as N and S mustards affect guanine, causing changes that result in erroneous pairing of bases. Nitrosamines are an important possible source of some base analogues, *e.g.,* 5-bromouracil (enol form), which can cause false pairing with G instead of A; AT is thus replaced by GC. Some dyes such as acridine orange cause distortion of the secondary structure of the DNA helix, resulting in faulty replication or recombination.

Potentially lethal lesions occur repeatedly in the DNA of living organisms. Only the presence of error-free DNA repair systems prevents the loss of genetic fidelity. Bacteria continue to provide valuable insights into DNA repair mechanisms and mutagenesis. Bacteria also serve as a principal short-term screen for detection and analysis of environmental mutagens that are responsible for increasing the endogenous load of premutational lesions in mammalian DNA.

The most widely used test (Ames test) has been shown to have highly accurate predictive value for carcinogenic activity in experimental animals. Indeed, of 176 chemical carcinogens tested, 158 or 90% were mutagenic. Conversely, of 108 "noncarcinogens," only 13 were mutagenic. These 13 negatives may reflect the relative lack of sensitivity of tests in animals.

Many mutagens and carcinogens are metabolized to active forms by enzymes present in mammalian cells. Cellular extracts containing these enzymes are often included in the Ames test plates so that compounds requiring activation will not be missed.

As a point of reference, the condensate of the smoke from a single cigarette causes approximately 20,000 mutations when tested in the presence of cellular enzymes.

Auxotrophs

Auxotrophs are deficient mutants that have lost one or more synthetic properties characteristic of the original type ("wild type" or prototype) from which the mutant was derived. Mutations affect antigenic, metabolic, and morphologic properties that form the basis of many diagnostic tests and also determine virulence (*e.g.,* toxigenicity, capsule formation). Resistance to chemotherapeutic agents and, conversely, a metabolic requirement for antibiotics are particularly undesirable mutations. Some of these are transmissible by certain episomes (R or RTF) through conjugation among gram-negative bacteria (see section on antibiotics).

BACTERIAL METABOLISM; BIOENERGETICS

Metabolic Types

All living cells depend on extraneous sources of energy for growth, reproduction, and self-synthesis. Those obtaining energy from the sun, (*e.g.,* green plants, blue-green algae and a few species of nonpathogenic bacteria) are said to be ***photosynthetic.*** All microorganisms of medical significance (except viruses) obtain energy from exothermic (exergonic) chemical reactions, that is, oxidations; they are said to be ***chemosynthetic.*** Viruses obtain their energy from the cells they infect.

Some chemosynthetic bacteria of the soil, called ***chemolithotrophs,*** oxidize only inorganic substrates (*e.g.,* $2NH_3 + 4O_2 \rightarrow 2HNO_3 + H_2O$) as sources of energy. They can use CO_2 as a sole source of carbon. Organisms capable of using CO_2 as a sole source of carbon are often called ***autotrophs.*** All microorganisms of medical interest, including bacteria, protozoans, and fungi, are chemosynthetic but, unlike autotrophs or chemolithotrophs, can utilize only *organic* substrates as sources of energy *and* carbon, *i.e.,* they are ***chemo-organotrophic.*** Organisms requiring organic sources of CO_2 are often called ***heterotrophs.*** Many of these also require CO_2. The various metabolic types may be listed as follows:

Photosynthetic
- Green plants
- Blue-green algae
- Some bacteria of no medical interest

Chemosynthetic

Chemolithotrophs: oxidize inorganic substrates; use only inorganic N, S, and C (are autotrophic with respect to C source) (of no medical interest)

Chemo-organotrophs: oxidize only organic substrates; use mainly organic sources of S, N, and C (are heterotrophic with respect to C source); may also require CO_2

Although all pathogenic microorganisms are chemo-organotrophs, some, such as certain enteric species, require only a single organic compound such as glucose if furnished with a complete mineral supplement. Others, like the strict anaerobes, streptococci, and gonococci, require numerous preformed complex substances: peptones, carbohydrates, amino acids, vitamins, and others. Bacteria cannot ingest solid particles of food: their nutrition is entirely by osmosis and diffusion of nutrients in solution. They are said to be ***osmotrophic.***

Energy Metabolism of Bacteria

In all chemo-organotrophs, bacterial as well as human, the most generally used source of carbon and energy is glucose. The most common first stage in energy metabolism of glucose is glycolysis by the Embden-Meyerhof scheme. Among bacteria, other systems may also be used, depending on species: the pentose-phosphate pathway, which is thermodynamically less efficient than glycolysis, and the Entner-Doudoroff pathway, found especially in species of *Pseudomonas.* Some species of bacteria can also use numerous other sugars and organic compounds (*e.g.,* phenol and petroleum) as sources of energy and carbon, depending on the enzymic ability of the organism to convert the sugar into a form such that at some point in the metabolic process it can enter the glycolytic or other pathway. These differences are often exploited for diagnostic purposes.

Among bacteria, and depending on species, glucose may be used in one or two of three general types of exergonic reactions: (a) aerobic respiration, (b) anaerobic respiration, and (c) fermentation. In all three the prime source of energy is enzymic (dehydrogenase) removal, from a substrate, of pairs of hydrogen atoms with liberation of their electrons ($H \rightleftharpoons H^+ + e^-$). Removal of electrons is oxidation and yields energy; acceptance of electrons is reduction. In cell metabolism, when hydrogen (e^-) is removed from a substrate by a dehydrogenase, it is transferred to an agent at a higher oxidative potential, commonly nicotinamide-adenine dinucleotide (NAD), which then becomes $NADH_2$. The functioning part of the dehydrogenase is ''niacin,'' which can accept the hydrogen and yield it up. In order to continue to function, the $NADH_2$ must be reoxidized (*i.e.,* 2H removed).

In ***aerobic respiration*** the $NADH_2$ becomes reoxidized by enzymically transferring the hydrogen to a second O—R system, usually the riboflavin (or flavoprotein) system. Here the electrons are diverted and transferred to a series of four or five enzymes called ***cytochromes,*** each of greater e^--accepting (oxidizing) potency than the one before it. The co-enzymes of the cytochromes are much like heme in having an atom of iron chelated in a porphyrin ring, the iron being able to accept and transfer e^-. In aerobic respiration the final cytochrome of the series, in the presence of the enzyme oxidase and $2H^+$, transfers the $2e^-$ to $\frac{1}{2}O_2$, forming H_2O. The entire series of enzymes and reactions from flavin to, and including, oxidase is called a ***respiratory chain.*** Many bacteria are restricted to the use of O_2 as a final hydrogen (electron) acceptor; they are called strict or ***obligate aerobes.***

Many common organisms (called ***facultative***) are capable of respiration under anaerobic conditions as well as under aerobic conditions as above. In the absence of O_2 they can use, as an alternative, several readily reducible inorganic compounds like $NaNO_3$ (substances depending on species) as final hydrogen acceptor in place of O_2: $NaNO_3 + 2H \rightleftharpoons NaNO_2 + H_2O$. Nitrate reduction is a familiar ''test'' in laboratory microbiology. Nitrite (NO_2) is a toxic product. It is also mutagenic and possibly carcinogenic. Furthermore, it can react with endogenous cellular amines (particularly the ubiquitous compounds spermine and spermidine) to produce nitroso compounds of great mutagenic potency. Some species reduce the nitrite, which is toxic, to N or NH_3 in stepwise reactions.

In ***fermentation*** two (or more) parts of the same organic substrate molecule (or two similar organic molecules, *e.g.,* the Stickland reaction between two amino acids: alanine + glycine $\rightarrow$ acetic acid + NH_3 + CO_2) serve as hydrogen (electron) donor and hydrogen (electron) acceptor, respectively, a thermodynamically inefficient mechanism since much less energy is released than in either form of respiration described above.

In aerobic and anaerobic respiration the pyruvate resulting from glycolysis (or alternate pathway) is first combined with acetyl coenzyme A, with liberation of 2H, via NAD, to the respiratory chain. The pyruvate then undergoes the series of changes constituting the Krebs or citric acid or tricarboxylic acid cycle. The overall reaction in bacterial respiration (aerobic or anaerobic) is $C_6H_{12}O_6 \rightarrow 6CO_2 + 6O_2 + 6H_2O$ (plus 34 ATP) and 688 kcal not all of which is available for cell synthesis and reproduction. Some is given off as heat or otherwise lost to entropy.

In fermentation the pyruvate undergoes various alterations different from those seen in aerobic respiration depending on species. There is no respiratory chain of cytochromes; much of the energy is not used. Reoxidation of the $NADH_2$ produced by glycolysis is accomplished by the reduction of cellular metabolites (*e.g.*, pyruvate) followed by excretion of the reduced product (*e.g.*, lactate) from the cell. In this way, the $NADH_2$ is oxidized, but its reducing power is lost to that cell. Some lactic acid bacteria, for example, reduce all of the pyruvate to lactic acid; some produce mainly propionic acid; and others produce a variety of substances, some of which are distinctive: acetylmethyl carbinol (basis of the Voges-Proskauer reaction), ethyl alcohol, acetone, butyric acid, CO_2, and others. All of these products of fermentation contain much of the original energy of the glucose and can serve as energy sources for other species of bacteria and fungi.

ENERGY AND PHOSPHORYLATION

The most important result of any form of energy metabolism for the cell is the phosphorylation of certain organic compounds that, because of the strained state of the phosphate ester bond, become high-energy compounds. Among these are adenosine triphosphate (ATP), guanosine triphosphate (GTP), acetyl phosphate, 1,3-diphosphoglyceric acid, and others. The high-energy ester bond on hydrolysis yields energy to the compound temporarily associated with the high-energy compound. ATP, ADP, and AMP constitute a series of energy transfer compounds, each of the latter two absorbing energy on phosphorylation that is transferred to ATP and H_3PO_4. Together they constitute an almost universally used energy transfer system in the cell.

In the ***bacterial respiratory chain,*** energy from electrons passing along the chain of cytochromes is transferred to the cell at two or three specific points, forming, with inorganic phosphate, ATP from ADP (oxidative level phosphorylation). Two molecules of ATP are also formed (from ADP + H_3PO_4) during glycolysis, from hydrolysis of 1,3-phosphoglyceric acid (substrate level oxidative phosphorylation) and hydrolysis of phosphoenol pyruvic acid to pyruvic acid. This is almost the entire yield of energy in fermentation.

All forms of exothermic reaction in living cells are sometimes referred to collectively as ***bio-oxidations.***

Three other types of bacteria, differing in respect to oxygen requirements, deserve mention: (a) the microaerophils; (b) the indifferent organisms; and (c) the obligate aerobes.

Microaerophils require somewhat lowered oxygen pressures, neither complete anaerobiosis nor full aerobiosis. Probably certain of their enzymes are sensitive to atmospheric oxygen tension. Some pathogens are microaerophils, *(e.g., Leptospira, Campylobacter, Brucella)* when first isolated.

Indifferent species can grow in the presence of air but do not contain cytochrome or the citric acid cycle enzymes. Such species grow better in the absence of free oxygen than aerobically. They have no metabolic pathway to oxygen from glucose. They neither need nor utilize free oxygen, though they can use it for metabolizing glycerol to H_2O_2, which kills them because they do not produce catalase. Neither are they ''poisoned'' by free oxygen, as are strict anaerobes. They are indifferent to it. Examples are *Streptococcus pyogenes* and *Lactobacillus* species.

Strict or obligate anaerobes not only cannot grow but cannot survive in the presence of free oxygen. They are obliged to live in the absence of air (anaerobically). Their metabolism is entirely fermentative. Their sensitivity to free oxygen may depend on certain enzymes or coenzymes that are poisoned by oxygen or must remain in a reduced condition. Typically they do not produce catalase, which decomposes the highly toxic H_2O_2 that is produced by them in contact with O_2. Examples of strict anaerobes are *Clostridium tetani,* certain hemolytic streptococci, and *Bacteroides* species. Anaerobic enzyme systems function only at low O—R potentials (*e.g.,* -0.3 volt).

Cultivation of Anaerobes

Cultural conditions suitable for strictly anaerobic bacteria are found in the bottom of tubes filled to a depth of at least 10 cm with chopped animal tissue and covered with broth containing 1% glucose and heated to drive off air (oxygen) shortly before use, or in any organic or tissue medium from which free oxygen is excluded. A plating medium for isolating pure cultures of strict anaerobes consists of meat-infusion glucose agar containing a strong reducing substance, such as cysteine or sodium thioglycollate. In a hermetically sealed ''anerobic jar'' device, using chemicals in a plastic pack (Gaspak), a combination of oxygen with hydrogen is catalyzed at room temperature without use of electricity or exterior source of hydrogen.

Saprophytes

Not all chemo-organotrophs are pathogens. Some are of great value in the dairy and fermentation industries and in the commercial production of antibiotics. Many are effective scavengers and are called ***saprophytes*** (Gr. decay-plants). They inhabit the environment in the soil, on plants, and in the oceans and swamps, and in normal animals and humans they constitute the normal flora of the intestinal and genitourinary tracts, the oropharynx, and the external body surfaces. Saprophytes do not commonly invade living tissues or the blood stream unless introduced under circumstances favorable to their survival, such as in immunosuppression, or in contaminated wounds containing devitalized tissue (lowered redox potential) where they grow and secrete toxins (*e.g., Clostridium tetani* and tetanus toxin, or *C. perfringens,* involved in anaerobic cellulitis). Certain soil saprophytes can grow in foodstuffs in which they elaborate toxins (*e.g., C. botulinum*). Thus we may have noninvasive but highly pathogenic saprophytes.

A DESCRIPTIVE CHECKLIST OF IMPORTANT BACTERIA IN MEDICAL MICROBIOLOGY

I. Rod-shaped bacteria
A. Non-spore-forming
1. Gram-negative
a. Enteric bacteria:

The enteric bacteria include many genera, some of them normal flora and others (*Salmonella* and *Shigella*) exogenous and regularly pathogenic. Enteric organisms are aerobic, ferment a variety of carbohydrates, and possess complex antigenic structures. Because on Gram's stain they all look more or less alike, their identification rests on biochemical reactions, antigenic analysis, susceptibility to colicins (*e.g., Pseudomonas*), and DNA homology analyses. All have endotoxin (LPS); some secrete potent enterotoxins (protein exotoxins). As a group, these organisms are responsible for a large number of nosocomial infections, and many of them are resistant to multiple antibiotics because of their acquisition of drug-resistance plasmids. Most of the enteric organisms are opportunistic pathogens, particularly of the genitourinary tract and central nervous system, in burn patients, and in the compromised host. For all these reasons, careful antibiotic sensitivity testing is central to effective antibacterial chemotherapy.

The main taxonomic groups (***tribes*** and ***genera***) of enteric bacteria are:

Family: Enterobacteriaceae

Escherichieae—*Escherichia, Shigella*

Klebsielleae—*Klebsiella* (includes *K. pneumoniae* and other species; non-motile *Aerobacter aerogenes*; Friedländer's bacillus in older terminology); *Enterobacter* (includes *E. aerogenes* [older name *Aerobacter aerogenes*]); *Serratia* group

Salmonelleae—*Salmonella, Arizona, Citrobacter*

Proteae—*Proteus (P. vulgaris. P. mirabilis); Providencia (P. rettgeri, P. stuartii, P. alcalifaciens); Morganella (M. morganii)*

Family: Vibrionaceae

Vibrio (V. cholerae, V. Parahemolyticus,etc.); Aeromonas; Plesiomonas

Family: Campylo/Helicobacter spp.

Campylobacter (C. jejuni, C. fetus, etc.); Helicobacter (H. pylori, H. cinaedi,etc.)

b. Respiratory pathogens (see Table 5-4):

Haemophilus influenzae. Very small, nonmotile, pleomorphic coccobacillus; nonhemolytic; aerobic; requires hemin (X factor) and NADP (V factor) as supplied in "chocolate" agar. Infant tracheobronchitis, epiglottitis, septic meningitis, conjunctivitis (*H. aegyptius*). Virulent strains (type b most frequent) encapsulated. *H. parainfluenzae*—normal oral flora, endocarditis

Bordetella pertussis. Primary isolation on Bordet-Gengou (BG) agar containing methicillin; hemolytic, pearllike colonies; identification by immunofluorescence; contain histamine-sensitizing and lymphocytosis-promoting factors, heat-labile toxin and endotoxin (LPS); phase variation. Localized infection or pertussis syndrome; attachment to and immobilization of cilia; never invasive. Killed phase I cells in DPT. Related species *B. parapertussis*

c. Genitourinary tract pathogen (other than enterics):

Haemophilus ducreyi. Fastidious; morphologically like *H. influenzae.* Soft chancre (chancroid); in tropics, endemic and commonest cause of genital ulcerative disease

d. Blood and tissue pathogens:

Brucella suis, B. abortus, B. melitensis. Small coccobacilli or rods; nonmotile; biotyped according to metabolism, sensitivity to dyes, antigenic analysis. Primary zoonosis; erythritol (large amounts in fetal tissues of ungulates, not of humans) promotes intracellular localization, infectious abortion in animals; spectrum of acute septicemic to chronic granulomatous human multisystem dis-

TABLE 5-4. Differential Properties of *Haemophilus* and *Bordetella*

ORGANISM	COLONIES	REQUIREMENT FOR FACTORS		PRODUCTION OF			FERMENTATION OF GLUCOSE	REDUCTION OF NITRATE	MOTILITY
		X*	V†	Indole	Catalase	Porphyrins			
H. influenzae	Small, "dew drop" nonhemolytic‡	+	+	+	+	−	+	+	−
H. parainfluenzae	Small, ± hemolytic	−	+	−	+/−	+			
H. hemolyticus	Small, betahemolytic	+	+	+	+	−	+		
H. ducreyi	Small, weakly hemolytic		−	−	−	−	+/−	−	
H. aegyptius (Koch-Weeks bacillus)	Nonhemolytic	+	+	−	+ *Urease*	−			
B. pertussis	Tiny, hemolytic	niacin		−	−		−	−	−
B. parapertussis	Tiny, hemolytic	cysteine		−	+		−	−	−
B. bronchiseptica		methionine			+		−	+	+

* Hemin.

† Coenzyme 1 or nicotinamide-adenine-dinucleotide (NAD), responsible for "satellite phenomenon" when growing near colonies of *Staphylococcus aureus.*

‡ Typable distinguishable from untypable strains by opalescence (due to capsules) on Levinthal transparent agar. Primary isolation best on chocolate agar (contains free hemin and NAD).

TABLE 5-5. Properties of *Brucella*

ORGANISM	REQUIREMENT FOR CO_2 ON PRIMARY ISOLATION*	HYDROGEN SULFIDE PRODUCTION	UREASE ACTIVITY	GROWTH ON AGAR CONTAINING	
				Basic Fuchsin	Thionin
Brucella abortus	+	+	+	+	−
Brucella suis	−	++	++	−	+
Brucella melitensis	−	−	+	+	+
Brucella canis	−	+	+	−	+

* On Castañeda's double medium.

ease; serodiagnosis based on IgM/IgG agglutinins; cross-reaction with *Francisella tularensis* and *Vibrio cholerae*. Cell-mediated immunity important in recovery and resistance. Tetracycline, streptomycin, rifampin (see Table 5-5)

Francisella tularensis. Small pleomorphic bacillus; fastidious; facultative intracellular parasite. Primary zoonosis; human disease (tularemia), acquired by direct contact or via arthropod vector from diseased animals, has protean manifestations, from localized infection to septicemic pneumonia. Cell-mediated immunity primary factor in recovery and resistance; serodiagnosis by agglutination test. Streptomycin, chloramphenicol, tetracycline

Yersinia pestis (the genus *Yersinia* is in the tribe Yersinieae, included in the family Enterobacteriaceae). Short, ovoid, nonmotile bacillus with bipolar staining. Primary zoonosis in domestic and wild rodents; human disease acquired by direct contact or bites of infected arthropods; septicemic bubonic and pneumonic (100% fatal) plague. Cell-mediated immunity important in recovery and resistance. Streptomycin, tetracyclines and/or chloramphenicol

Bacteroides fragilis group, *B. melaninogenicus* group (black pigment on blood agar). Strict anaerobes; pleomorphic; gas–liquid chromatography useful in speciation. Most produce beta-lactamase. Normal intestinal and oral flora, opportunistic polymicrobic (e.g., *Fusobacterium, Propionibacterium, Peptococcus, Peptostreptococcus*) obstetric-gynecologic infections, infections of central nervous system and thoracic and abdominal cavities, necrotizing cellulitis and metastatic abscesses, septicemia. Chloramphenicol, clindamycin, cefoxitin, moxalactam, metronidazole; also newer penicillins, mezlocillin and piperacillin. Surgical drainage of primary importance (see Table 5-6)

Pseudomonas. Straight or curved rods, chemo-organotrophic; strict aerobes. Normal flora of skin and intestine, environment.

P. aeruginosa produces green pigment (pyocyanin) and is responsible for almost 20% of nosocomial infections. It can adhere to inert solid surfaces and thus causes opportunistic urinary (catheter-associated) as well as respiratory tract (respiratory-associated) infections, particularly in debilitated, immunosuppressed, or burn patients. Treatment according to antibiogram. *P. pseudomallai*—motile; characteristic nonpigmented growth; multiple antibiotic resistance. Melioidosis (acute and recrudescent). Tetracycline, chloramphenicol, trimethoprim-sulfamethoxazole

Legionella pneumophila. Major human pathogen of family Legionellaceae; faintly gram-negative; stains with silver impregnation in tissues; facultative intracellular parasite; isolation on charcoal yeast extract agar; identification with immunofluorescence. Infection acquired from environment, acute pneumonia, milder upper respiratory infection, septicemia. Erythromycin

Cat scratch disease bacillus. Found in lymph nodes of affected patients; pleomorphic, gram-negative bacillus found in almost 90% of biopsied lymph nodes examined; stainable with silver impregnation; specific reactivity with convales-

TABLE 5-6. Nonsporulating Anaerobic Bacilli*

	PREDOMINANT HABITAT(S)	MORPHOLOGY
Gram-positive		
Actinomyces (A. Israelii, A. naeslundii)	Mouth, upper respiratory tract	Long, filamentous, irregular branching
Arachnia	Mouth	Pleomorphic, pointed ends
Propionibacterium	Skin	Pleomorphic, chains
Lactobacillus	Mouth, vagina	Short, bifurcated or clubbed ends
Bifidobacterium	Colon, vagina	Pleomorphic, V-shaped arrangements
Eubacterium	Mouth, colon	
Gram-negative		
Bacteroides		
B. fragilis group	Vagina, colon (dominant species)	Long, pleomorphic, vacuoles
B. melaninogenicus group	Mouth	Short, coccobacilli; brown-black pigment formed on blood agar
Fusobacterium	Mouth	Long, tapered ends *(F. nucleatum)* Most species variable

* Account for over 90% of normal intestinal flora. Speciated by gas-liquid chromatography of metabolic products in liquid cultures (pure) and/or immunofluorescence. Direct Gram stain of exudates useful in preliminary diagnosis.

cent sera; newly classifildas Bartonella henslae; uncultivable; supportive, symptomatic treatment without use of antibiotics is recommended.

Bartonella bacilliformis. Oroya fever, verruga peruana.

2. Gram-positive
   a. Respiratory pathogens:

      Corynebacterium diphtheriae. Methylene blue stain: clublike, beaded, and barred forms; soluble exotoxin, alum-precipitated toxoid (DTP); antitoxin (despeciated horse serum) (see Table 5-24)

      Mycobacterium tuberculosis. Acid-fast, niacin +; nonmotile; obligate aerobe; slow growth on Lowenstein-Jensen egg yolk–glycerine–malachite green medium; virulent strains form ''cord factor''; usually isoniazid-sensitive, some strains resistant; distinguish from ''atypical'' or Runyon-group species; delayed (tuberculin) hypersensitivity; BCG (Table 5-7).

   b. *Mycobacterium leprae.* Obligate intracellular parasite; ''lepra'' cells; not cultivable on lifeless media. Leprosy (lepromatous, tuberculoid), erythema nodosum, deficient Tc function. Dapsone, rifampin, clofazimine

   c. Blood and tissue pathogens:

      Listeria monocytogenes. A motile ''diphtheroid,'' hemolytic on blood agar. Zoonosis; clinically protean, including amnionitis, perinatal infections, meningitis

      Actinomyces israelii. Branching, filamentous bacterium; strictly anaerobic; found only in humans (bovine species is *A. bovis*); gram-positive but not acid-fast; ''sulfur granules'' in masses of ''ray fungus'' in pus. Actinomycosis, penicillin-sensitive

      Nocardia asteroides. Branching forms that readily fragment to bacillus-like or coccoid segments; gram-positive; *N. asteroides* and some others acid-fast in exudates; strictly aerobic; some species form ''sulfur-granules'' in pus. Madura foot or systemic and pulmonary nocardiosis. Sulfadiazine

B. Spore-forming (special spore stains required; unstained areas in gram-positive bacilli)

   Endospores resist 15 minutes or longer boiling at 100° C and 1 hour or more of dry heat at 150° C.

   1. Gram-negative: none of medical importance
   2. Gram-positive:
      a. Aerobic or facultative. Sporulate only in contact with free oxygen

         *Bacillus anthracis.** Grows well on blood-free media; spores contaminate pastures, hides, wool. Pulmonary anthrax or woolsorters' disease, malignant pustule, septicemia, toxemia, toxoid

      b. Anaerobic or microaerophilic. Spores form and germinate only under anaerobic conditions (Table 5-8).

* Distinguish between the general use of the term *bacillus* in reference to any rod-shaped organism and the generic use of the term *Bacillus* in reference to the genus of aerobic spore-formers, such as *Bacillus anthracis*.

TABLE 5-7. Differential Properties of *Mycobacterium* Species of Recognized Pathogenicity for Humans

SPECIES (GROUPINGS)	GROWTH TEMPERATURE	PRODUCTION OF NIACIN	NITRATE REDUCTION	TOLERANCE TO 5% NaCl	TWEEN 80 HYDROLYSIS	CATALASE ACTIVITY	RESISTANCE TO ISONIAZID
M. tuberculosis	37	+	+	−	−	−	−
M. bovis (includes BCG strain)	37	+/−	−	−	−	−	−
M. ulcerans	30–33	−	−	−	+	+	(+)
''Atypical'' mycobacteria:							
Group I (photochromogens)*							
M. kansasii	30–37	+/−	+	−	+	+/−	+
M. marinum	30–32	−	−	−	+	+	+
Group II (scotochromogens)†							
M. scrofulaceum	30–37	−	−	−	−	+	+
Group III (nonchromogens)							
M. intracellularis (Battey)	37–44	−	−	−	−	+	+
M. avium							
Group IV (rapid growers; 3–7 days, some scotochromogens)							
M. fortuitum	25–37	−	+	+	Variable	+	+
M. chelonel							

* Produce lemon-yellow pigments on exposure to light.
† Produce yellow-orange to dark-red pigments in the dark.

Clostridium species. All inhabit soil, many occur in animal feces; cultivable in the thioglycollate media, etc.; all pathogens motile except *C. perfringens*

C. tetani fecally contaminated wounds; soluble exotoxin affects motor nerve endings; alum-precipitated toxoid prophyl vs. tetanus DTP (see Table 5-24)

C. perfringens ''gas bacillus''; associated with *C. novyi, C. histolyticum, C. septicum, and C. tetani* in fecally contaminated, deep wounds; exotoxins are various proteolytic and saccharolytic enzymes, collagenases, gas gangrene

C. botulinum. ''Snow-shoe'' sporulation; grows in soil-contaminated, improperly heat-processed canned foods, forming exotoxin that causes flaccid paralysis; toxin destroyed by 80° C in 15 minutes. Botulism (infant, endogenous)

II. Coccoid bacteria

A. Diplococci

1. Gram-negative:

Neisseria species. Diplococci; aerobic; colonies indophenol-oxidase positive

N. gonorrhoeae. Gonococcus (GC) requires chocolate agar on Thayer-Martin selective chocolate agar containing vancomycin, colistin, nystatin under CO_2; 35° C to 37° C; isolation essential for diagnosis in females and chronic cases; in smears of exudate GC typically found in polymorphonuclear neutrophils (PMN); oxidase-positive colonies do not utilize maltose. Gonorrhea and septic complications (acute endocarditis, arthritis, proctitis, pharyngitis, meningitis), ophthalmia neonatorum; penicillinase-producing strains (PPNG), chromosome-mediated resistance (CMRNG) to penicillin

N. meningitidis. Culturally and morphologically like *N. gonorrhoeae* but ferments maltose; found in leukocytes in spinal fluid; serotyping by capsular swelling, agglutination. *Epidemic* meningitis, chronic meningococcemia and septic complications. Polysaccharide vaccine for types A and C

2. Gram-positive:

Streptococcus pneumoniae. Green zone (alpha) hemolytic colonies on blood agar; lancet-shaped cocci paired in type-specific

TABLE 5-8. Differential Properties of *Clostridium* Species

ORGANISM	MORPHOLOGY (ALL GRAM-POSITIVE)	MOTILITY	METABOLIC ACTIVITY: Lecithinase Activity	Fermentation of: Glucose	Sucrose	Lactose	DISEASES
Histotoxic*							
C. perfringens	Short, thick rods; rare oval subterminal spores; double hemolysis on blood agar	−	+	+	+	+	Myonecrosis, suppuration, cellulitis, septicemia
C. septicum	Oval, subterminal spores, long thin rods	+	−	+	−	+	(*C. perfringens:* enterocolitis, food poisoning, intravascular hemolysis)
C. novyi	Oval, subterminal spores	+	+	+	−	−	
C. histolyticum	Oval, subterminal spores, pleomorphic rods	+	−	±	−	−	
Cytotoxic†							
C. botulinum	Large rods, oval subterminal spores	+	−	+	−	−	Botulism (type A, B, E, F toxins) food poisoning; wound botulism; infant botulism (honey)
C. tetani	Slender rods, terminal spores, "drumstick"	+	−	−	−	−	Tetanus (neurotoxin)
C. difficile	Oval, terminal spores. Cytotoxins A, B demonstrable in feces. Primary isolation on selective medium (egg-yolk fructose agar, with cycloserine and cefoxitin)	−	(Gas–liquid chromatography)				Antibiotic-associated pseudomembranous colitis (clindamycin, penicillin, cephalosporins) Vancomycin for treatment

* Damage to organized tissues due to local secretion of proteolytic and saccharolytic enzymes.
† Disease due to specific exotoxins disseminated via the bloodstream and reactive with target cells (e.g., tetanus toxin and synaptic junctions of anterior horn cells).

polysaccharide capsules; swelling reaction with type-specific serum; optochin-sensitive; inulin-positive. Lobar pneumonia, meningitis, otitis

S. pyogenes. β-hemolytic: clear zones in blood agar pour plates; cell wall polysaccharides determine Lancefield groups A-U; type specificity determined by M- or T-cell wall proteins. Scarlet fever (erythrogenic toxin, lysogenic streptococci), puerperal sepsis, septicemia, septic sore throat, pyoderma. Nonsuppurative sequelae to group A only: rheumatic fever, glomerulonephritis. Group B-neonatal sepsis, meningitis

Group D. Enterococci *(S. faecalis)* and nonenterococci (Table 5-9) urinary tract infections, endocarditis

Viridans group. Heterogeneous; no group-specific carbohydrate. Normal oropharyngeal flora; some secrete dextrans or levans; cause dental plaque *(S. mutans, S. salivarius);* infective endocarditis

Staphylococcus species. Irregular clusters, pairs and single cocci; facultative; catalase-positive; anaerobic use of glucose and pyruvate; grow well on blood-free media at 20° C to 40° C; bacteriophage typing

S. aureus. Golden pigment; most of the pathogenic strains produce coagulase, leukocidin, hemolysin, and other tissue-damaging factors; also ferment mannitol, produce DNase, and liquefy gelatin; penicillin resistance due to production of penicillinase. Nosocomial, pyogenic infections, endocarditis; thermostable enterotoxin causes food

TABLE 5-9. Properties of Streptococci Most Frequently Isolated from Clinical Specimens (Aerobic)

LANCEFIELD SEROGROUP (SPECIES)	GROUP-SPECIFIC CELL WALL POLY-SACCHARIDE	USUAL TYPE OF HEMOLYSIS (SHEEP BLOOD)	GROWTH AT			FERMENTATION OF			HIP-PURATE HYDROL-YSIS	SENSITIVITY TO		BE‡	TOLERANCE TO 6.5 PERCENT NaCl	DISEASES
			37°	10°	45°	Trehalose	Sorbitol	Inulin		Baci-tracin†	Opto-chin			
A (*S. pyogenes*)	Rhamnose-GNac	β	+	–	–	+	–		–	+				Pharyngitis, tonsillitis, otitis, pyoderma, systemic infections, nonsuppurative sequelae: ARF, AGN
B (*S. agalactiae*)	Rhamnose-GNH_2	β(α γ)§	+	–	–	+	–		+	–(+)		–		Ascending amnionitis, neonatal sepsis, pneumonia, meningitis, nosocomial infections
C (*S. equi, equismilis dysgaloctiae*)	Rhamnose-Gal-Nac	β	+	–	–	–	–		–	–				Mild URI, puerperal sepsis, endocarditis
D (*S. faecalis, bovis, equinus*)	Glycerolteichoic acid-D-ala-glu	Enterococcus (*S. faecalis, faecium, durans*): α β γ							v	–	–	+	+	UTI, endocarditis (Enterococci: penicillin resistant)
		Nonenterococcus (*S. bovis, equinus*): α γ							–	–	–	+	–	
F (*S. milleri, anginosus, minutus, MG*)								–		–				Respiratory infections, pneumonia
G (*S. canis*)								+		+				Puerperal, skin, wound infections
VIRIDANS		α									–	–(+)	–	Dental caries, endocarditis
S. salivarius (K)			+	–	+									
S. mitis			+	–	+									
S. mutans			+	–	+									
S. sanguis (H)		(β)	+	–	–									
S. pneumoniae (84 serotypes)	C substance (teichoic acid gal-6P-choline)	α									+	–	–	Pneumonia, septicemia, meningitis, endocarditis, otitis

* Representative species named.
† 5 to 10% of group B and C-G are bacitracin sensitive.
‡ Growth and hydrolysis of esculin on bile-esculin (BE) agar.
§ CAMP test positive.

AGN = acute glomerulonephritis.
ARF = acute rheumatic fever.
URI = upper respiratory infection.
UTI = urinary tract infection.
v = variable.

poisoning, toxic shock, and ''scalded skin'' syndromes. (Differentiate: exotoxin, endotoxin, enterotoxin)

S. epidermidis (S. albus). No pigment; coagulase not produced; culturally similar to *S. aureus.* Commensal skin organism, opportunistic endocarditis (*e.g.,* prosthetic heart valves, long-term central vascular lines)

III. Helical, flexible bacteria

Treponema species. Four to 14 close, regular spirals; tubular cell wound around an axial filament composed of bundles of modified polar flagella; best seen in darkfield; rotatory and flexing motion; pathogenic species morphologically indistinguishable; antigenically closely related; not cultivable in artificial media; the anaerobically cultivable Reiter treponeme is antigenically similar to *T. pallidum* but not virulent; *T. genitalis, T. microdentium,* and other saprophytes can be confused morphologically with *T. pallidum* in darkfield. *T. pallidum,* syphilis and bejel; *T. pertenue,* yaws; *T. carateum,* pinta. Numerous saprophytic strains are cultivable *in vitro.*

Borrelia species. Longer, coarser, more open, and irregular spirals than *Treponema;* vigorous lashing motion; stain readily; gram-negative; cultivable microaerophilically in special media. *Ixodes dammini* (nymphal stage) ticks transmit Lyme disease, caused by *B. burgdorferi.*

Leptospira species. Thinnest (<0.1 μm) and most tightly coiled (12 to 24 turns) of the spirochetes; hooked ends; unifibrillar axial filament; rapid rotatory and progressive motion; cultivable in media with serum; microaerophilic; blood and tissue parasites. Zoonoses source of human infection, ''aseptic'' meningitis

IV. Bacteria without cell walls

This group includes mycoplasma and pleuropneumonia–like organisms (PPLO). These organisms lack the enzymes that synthesize cell walls, the entire cell (except rare flagella) being enclosed within the thin, pliable, typically bacterial, cell membrane. In general, lack of the strong cell wall leaves them osmotically fragile (*i.e.,* subject to osmotic rupture) unless suspended in special PPLO medium of increased osmotic pressure (*e.g.,* 20% serum, 3% sucrose). Colonies on agar begin growth just below the surface and spread on the surface forming a foamy-looking colony with a fried-egg appearance. As a result of their pliable cell membrane, mycoplasmas are highly pleomorphic, forming cocci, branched filaments, ringforms. Some of the forms are so minute as to be filterable. Lack of cell wall makes mycoplasmas totally resistant to antibiotics that inhibit cell wall formation: penicillin, cephalosporins. They are very sensitive to surfactant substances such as soaps and bile and to tetracyclines. Except for *Mycoplasma pneumoniae,* they are nonhemolytic.

Over 30 species of genus *Mycoplasma* are recognized. These require sterols for growth. Some are associated with a variety of pathologic processes of humans and lower vertebrates: *M. hominis, M. gallisepticum, M. arthritidis, M. agalactiae, M. pneumoniae. Ureaplasma urealyticum* causes ''nongonococcal'' urethritis (NGU). Of a second genus, *Acholesplasma,* most are saprophytes or of doubtful pathogenicity. They do not require sterols for growth and are osmotically very fragile *(e.g., A. laidlawi).*

V. Minute Bacteria: Obligate intracellular parasites. All are real bacteria, nonmotile, nonsporing rods or cocci, 0.3 to 0.6 μm. by 0.8 to 2.0 μm. Two orders are now recognized: Rickettsiales and Chlamydiales.

A. Order I. ***Rickettsiales.*** Of three families containing some seventeen genera, only two (genus *Rickettsia* and genus *Coxiella*) contain human pathogens of general importance, though several are of veterinary importance.

Genus *Rickettsia.* Not filterable; normally only arthropod-borne; can synthesize their own ATP. Typhus, Rocky Mountain spotted fever (Table 5-10).

Genus *Coxiella.* Much like *Rickettsia* but filterable: raw milk, dust of barns and cattle yards, infected lochia; probably also several species of ticks. Q fever *(C. burnetii).*

B. Order II. ***Chlamydiales.*** *Chlamydia trachomatis:* trachoma, inclusion conjunctivitis, infant pneumonia (perinatal), lymphogranuloma venereum (L). Nongonococcal urethritis, salpingitis (D–K), well-defined glycogen-rich inclusions, sensitive to sulfonamide, tetracyclines.

C. psittaci. Ornithosis (many species of mammals and birds), no glycogen in inclusions, insensitive to sulfonamide, sensitive to tetracyclines.

Bartonella bacilliformis. Oroya fever, verruga peruana.

STERILIZATION AND DISINFECTION

Sterilization

In relation to microbiology, ***sterilization*** means the destruction of all life. It is often incorrectly used inter-

TABLE 5-10. Diseases Due to Rickettsiae

DISEASES	GENERA	USUAL VECTOR	WEIL-FELIX REACTION			MOLE PERCENT G + C
			OX19	OX2	OXK	
Typhus group:						
Epidemic typhus	*Rickettsia prowazekii**	Body louse *(Pediculus humanus corporis)*	+ + + +	+	–	29–30
Brill-Zinsser disease	*Rickettsia prowazekii*	Endogenous recrudescent typhus	(variable)			
Murine (endemic) typhus	*Rickettsia typhi* (mooseri)*	Rat flea *(Xenopsylla cheopis)*	+ + +	+	–	29–30
Spotted fever group:						
Rocky Mountain spotted fever. Other tickborne diseases (*e.g.*, Asian tick typhus, fievre boutonneuse)	*Rickettsia rickettsii**	Dog tick *(Dermacentor variabilis)*; rabbit tick *(D. andersoni)*	+ + + +	+	–	32–33
Rickettsialpox	*Rickettsia akari**	Mouse mite *(Allodermanyssus sanguineus)*	–	–	–	32–33
Scrub typhus group:						
Tsutsugamushi (Japanese oriental river or swamp fever; scrub typhus)	*Rickettsia tsutsugamushi**	Harvest (field) mite *(Leptotrombidium deliense, L. akamushi)*	–	–	+ + + +	
Q fever	*Coxiella burnetii†*	Aerosolized fomites; ticks	–	–	–	43
Trench fever	*Rochalimaea quintana‡*	Body louse *(P. humanus corporis)*	(Not applicable)			39

* Grows in chick embryo; cultured mammalian cells.
† Grows in chick yolk sac; eukaryotic phagolysosomes. Develops endospore.
‡ Grows in complex cell-free media and on surface of eukaryotic cells; newly classified as *Bartonella quintana*.

changeably with ***disinfection,*** which means the destruction of pathogenic organisms. Thus, milk that is pasteurized (heated at 63°C for 30 minutes and quickly cooled) is disinfected but is not sterile, since many common harmless organisms and spores resist this heating process.

Disinfection

A disinfectant is a substance that kills pathogenic microorganisms but is generally understood not to be sporicidal. A ***sporicidal*** disinfectant would also be a sterilizing agent, *e.g.*, ethylene oxide, betapropiolactone.

Chemical disinfectants are indiscriminately poisonous. They may combine in cells with a variety of chemical groups, such as carboxyl, sulfhydryl, and hydroxyl. They may act by (1) injuring cell membranes (especially lipid components), causing leakages, rupture or both (*e.g.*, lipid solvents like ethyl or propyl alcohol or emulsifying agents like cationic detergents, *e.g.*, Zephiran), and other surfactants like phenolic compounds (*e.g.*, hexachlorophene, Lysol, Creolin); (2) chemically or physically altering enzymes and other proteins and DNA by breaking hydrogen and sulfide bonds and causing denaturation, coagulation, precipitation (*e.g.*, phenolics, heavy metals like organic mercurials and $AgNO_3$); (3) oxidizing cell components, such as $KMnO_4$; chlorine free or loosely combined as chloramines ($Cl_2 + H_2O = HOCl + H^+ + Cl^-$; HOCl a potent oxidizer); (4) toxic combinations, as with I in surfactant iodophers (*e.g.*, Wescodyne) or alkylations as in the presence of ethylene oxide. In many instances the action of any agent is not clearly of one type or another but a combination of effects on different cell components. Factors that affect the action of any disinfectant are kind, numbers and age of bacterial cells present, *p*H, temperature, time of exposure, concentration. In general, within limits, increase of any of the physical factors increases disinfectant action.

Sepsis; Antiseptics

Sepsis means the presence of pathogenic organisms growing in the tissues or blood. An ***antiseptic,*** strictly speaking, is a substance that combats sepsis but is generally thought of as a microbicidal or microbistatic substance applicable to exposed living tissues without undue damage to the tissues, *e.g.*, dilute alcohol, surfactant compounds of iodine (iodophors), mild tincture of iodine, and some organic mercurials. Antiseptics are not used internally. The terms antiseptic and disinfectant are often loosely used interchangeably.

Asepsis, strictly speaking, means absence of sepsis, but generally it is used to mean the absence of any living organisms. ***Aseptic technique*** is any procedure designed to eliminate live organisms and to keep them away. Modern surgical and microbiologic procedures are based on aseptic technique.

Methods

Sterilization may be accomplished by heat, mechanical means such as filtration, and use of sporicidal chemicals, notably ethylene oxide and betapropiolactone. Less widely used are penetrating, ionizing radiations in dosages of 2.5 mrad, chiefly for sterilization of heat-labile drugs, surgical equipment. Ultraviolet (about 260 mm) light has little power of penetration and is best used to control contamination by dust in air in enclosed spaces such as laboratories.

DRY HEAT

1. *Incineration.* Useful for bandages, paper dishes, sputum cups, etc.
2. *Oven Baking.* Useful for articles not containing water or that may be injured by steam. Applied usually to laboratory glassware and to materials not readily permeable by steam, such as petrolatum, mineral oil, sand, wooden articles, and glass syringes. A temperature of 165° C for at least 2 hours is necessary to kill all spores.

MOIST HEAT

1. *Boiling* (100° C at sea level). Some bacterial spores can survive 90 minutes or more of boiling. Hepatitis viruses can survive at least 10 minutes of boiling and probably longer. Therefore, boiling is not satisfactory as a means of sterilization under ordinary circumstances. Boiling for 10 minutes is suitable for disinfection in situations from which (1) spores of pathogenic bacteria and (2) hepatitis viruses are known to be absent.
2. *Autoclaving.* Steam, when compressed, is much hotter than free steam, and at 15 pounds pressure has a temperature of 121° C. An autoclave is a vessel that may be closed hermetically so as to exclude all air but retain steam under pressure. An ordinary household pressure cooker is a miniature autoclave capable of perfect sterilization.

   In autoclaving, steam pressure of 15 to 20 pounds is usually applied from 10 to 30 minutes. All air must escape and all space be filled with steam. Air does not reach the desired temperature. Also, since steam is depended on to bring about ***hydrolysis*** of bacteria and their spores, mixture with dry air reduces the effectiveness of the process. Autoclaving is generally used for culture media, saline solutions, for surgical supplies, for solutions intended for intravenous injections, and for bandages, dressings. Glassware is often autoclaved. Autoclaving is not used for oils or petrolatum, which cannot absorb steam and therefore remain dry.

SPORICIDAL VAPORS

1. *Formaldehyde* vapor is sometimes used to disinfect (sterilize?) interiors of rooms, ships, but has the disadvantage of polymerizing (paraformaldehyde) on surfaces and being difficult to remove. In high concentration it is sporicidal. It is commonly used dissolved 37% (weight) in water as formalin or formol for tissue fixation and embalming.
2. *Ethylene oxide,* an alkylating agent, is used, diluted about 1 : 10 with CO_2 or other vapor, to reduce toxicity and inflammability, inside autoclaves under conditions of controlled concentration (around 500 mg/liter, of air), pressure (around 10 lb), temperature (around 130° F or 55° C), and relative humidity (around 40%). It is effective but expensive and is useful mainly for objects that are damaged by ordinary methods of heat sterilization.
3. *Betapropiolactone,* liquid at room temperatures, forms a sporicidal vapor in concentrations around 1.5 mg/liter of air at relative humidities around 80% and temperatures around 25° C. Potentially useful (combined with ultraviolet irradiation to remove hepatitis viruses from blood products), but a potent carcinogen.

FILTRATION

Fine-pored filters, long used for mechanical sterilization (*e.g.,* cellulose mixed with asbestos [Seitz disks]; sintered [fused] granular glass), have been supplanted by paper-thin membrane filters that depend chiefly on pore size (about 12 to 0.22 μm) for mechanical sieve action, especially if the perforations in the filters have been made by regulated nuclear bombardment. Such filters also severe to collect microorganisms from fluids for microscopic examination or cultivation directly on the filter when placed on pads saturated with culture medium, often selective media.

MICROBISTASIS (BACTERIOSTASIS)

By this term is meant nonlethal inhibition of growth of microorganisms for hours, days, or years, generally by interfering with certain enzyme functions. Microbistatic agents may be physical (*e.g.*, refrigeration, freeze-drying, pickling brines, or dehydration), or chemical (*e.g.*, various aniline dyes in media, antibodies, antibiotics, sulfonamide drugs). In selective bacteriostasis in the diagnostic laboratory, such agents are used to inhibit growth of undesired contaminants in specimens such as feces or sputum and permit the desired species to grow. Microbistasis is an inexact term, since, if microorganisms are held "static" long enough, they eventually die, though they may survive for many years under some microbistatic conditions, such as freeze-drying.

Microbistasis is characteristically reversible, for example, by chemical neutralization of the bacteriostatic agent (Hg + H_2S); mechanical removal (washing or dilution); cessation (warming of frozen cells); or rehydrating of dried cells.

Surface Disinfection

Agents that damage bacterial cell membranes may be used to disinfect inert surfaces or the skin. These include cationic (*e.g.*, Zephyran) and anionic (soaps and fatty acids) detergents; phenolic compounds (*e.g.*, tricresol) emulsified with green soap (*e.g.*, Lysol); diphenyl compounds (*e.g.*, hexachlorophene); alcohols (*e.g.*, 50% to 70% ethanol).

Protein-Denaturing Agents

Denaturing of bacterial cellular proteins, and hence germicidal action, can be achieved with acids (*e.g.*, benzoic acid as food preservative); soluble salts of heavy metals (*e.g.*, merthiolate, silver nitrate, silver sulfadiazine); oxidizing agents (*e.g.*, iodine, hydrogen peroxide); alkylating agents (*e.g.*, formaldehyde; glutaraldehyde as for cold sterilization of instruments; ethylene oxide).

ANTIBIOTICS

Antimicrobial agents used in the treatment of infectious diseases must have deleterious effects on the microorganism with little toxicity for host tissue. This difference in selective toxicity is expressed quantitatively as the therapeutic index. The concept of selective toxicity requires the binding of a drug to a microbial structure or protein that is either absent or significantly different from its counterpart in mammalian cells. The prokaryotic ribosome, which is smaller than its eukaryotic counterpart (70s versus 80s), the peptidoglycan layer of bacterial cell walls, which is unique to these microorganisms and certain special enzymatic stages in bacterial nucleic acid replication or transcription are prime targets.

Mode of Action of Cell Wall Inhibitors

The drugs that inhibit cell wall synthesis are listed in Table 5-1. The inhibition of peptidoglycan synthesis is usually a lethal event for a bacterium because the process of adding new material to the wall is coupled with autolytic digestion of the wall at the anticipated growth sites. In the absence of synthesis, the continued enzymatic digestion weakens the wall until osmotic pressure causes bursting of the cytoplasmic membrane. Cells can survive inhibition of cell wall synthesis if the autolytic enzymes are not functioning, as in nongrowing cells. They can survive also in spite of wall digestion if the osmotic pressure is not sufficient to force lysis, a condition occurring in hypertonic solutions (*e.g.*, pus). These factors support the need for wound drainage concurrent with the institution of antimicrobial therapy.

The process of cell wall synthesis must be understood to appreciate the activity of various antimicrobials. The process includes a cytoplasmic component leading to the synthesis of a peptidoglycan subunit, secretion of this subunit through the cytoplasmic membrane into the periplasmic space, and finally enzymatic addition of subunits to the growing portion of the peptidoglycan and cross-linking by pentaglycine bridges. Each of these three major sets of reactions is subject to selective interference by various antimicrobials. Synthesis of the subunit is blocked by cycloserine and bacitracin. Secretion through the membrane is blocked by vancomycin. Cross-linking of the subunit is blocked by penicillins, semisynthetic penicillins, and cephalosporins.

In Table 5-1 are listed a first-generation cephalosporin (*e.g.*, cephalothin) and two second-generation ones (*e.g.*, cefamandole and cefoxitin), all of which are parenterally administered. In addition, several other first- and second-generation oral cephalosporins are available (*e.g.*, first-generation: cephradine, cephalexin [Keflex], and cefadroxil; second-generation: cefaclor and cefuroxime axetil). Generally, the first-generation cephalosporins exhibit a broad spectrum of activity against both gram-positive and gram-negative bacterial infections (*e.g.*, *S. aureus* and non-enterococcal *S. pneumoniae,* as well as *Klebsiella* spp). The second-generation cephalosporins have been modified to exhibit an expanded activity against gram-negative bacteria *(e.g., H. influenza)* but have less activity against gram-positive bacteria. An exception is cefaclor, which works well against both. Also, cefoxitin is used for *B. fragilis* anaerobe infections. In the past 5 to 10 years there has been further expansion to a third generation of cephalosporins, including oral ones (*e.g.*, cefixime [Suprax], cefpodoxime proxetil, and loracarbef), as well as parenteral ones (*e.g.*, cefotaxamine, ceftriaxone, and ceftazidime). These now have an even broader spectrum of activity, extended to the Enterobacteriaceae, as well as in some cases (ceftazidime) *Pseudomonas aeruginosa* infections. Also with this third group of cephalosporins, there is an even greater enhanced resistance against bacterial β-lactamases. Typical uses are: loracarbef, for otitis media, lower respiratory infections, and sinusitis; cefpodoxime proxetil, for uncomplicated gonorrhea, urinary tract infection; and ceftriaxone, for *H. influenzae* meningitis.

In addition to the third-generation cephalosporins, a number of other new antibiotics have been developed in the past 5 or so years. For example, as a potential substitute for erythromycin, a macrolide antibiotic that has been available for almost 50 years to treat community-acquired respiratory tract, as well as skin and soft-tissue infections (see Table 5-3), one now has available clarithromycin and azithromycin. These two have fewer side effects (*e.g.*, less diarrhea) and a longer tissue half-life than erythromycin. Clarithromycin is useful in treating *Legionella pneumophila* and MAC (*M*ycobacterium *a*vian-intracellulare *c*omplex) opportunistic infections in AIDS patients. Azithromycin is recommended for treatment of gonorrhea.

Other new antibiotics are improved quinolones in the floxacin family (see Table 5-2), such as lomafloxacin (to treat chronic bronchitis) and enoxacin (single-dose therapy for gonorrhea). The latter is less expensive than the currently used ciprofloxacin, and as managed care becomes a bigger issue in this country, decisions regarding cost-effectiveness, as well as toxicity, effectiveness, and pharmacokinectic considerations need to be made in prescribing newer versus older antibiotics.

Finally, it should be noted that attempts at combination antibiotic therapy are being made to improve effectiveness. Two examples of this are (a) amoxicillin/clavulanic acid or augmentin and (b) piperacillin/tazobactam. In each case β-lactamase inhibitors are combined with a penicillin.

PROBLEMS OF INSENSITIVITY AND RESISTANCE RELATED TO ANTIMICROBIALS THAT AFFECT CELL WALL SYNTHESIS

No single antimicrobial agent has effects on all types of microorganisms. There are entire genera in which no species of organism is ever found to be inhibited by a particular drug, that is, these organisms are considered to be inherently *in*sensitive to that drug because of physiological or structural traits common to all members of the group. Accordingly, the degree to which an antibiotic might inhibit such microbes is entirely predictable. On the other hand, most isolates of a given genus or species may be susceptible to a drug, only occasional strains being found to be less sensitive than the majority. These exceptions are generally designated as being ***resistant,*** that is, insusceptible to concentrations of drug that inhibit other strains of the same organism. Such resistant strains occur at rates that cannot always be predicted, and in such cases, careful *in vitro* susceptibility testing of each isolate is required as a guide to choice of chemotherapeutic agents.

Most gram-negative organisms are insensitive to clinically attainable levels of penicillin G and V. This insensitivity is determined by the impermeability of the lipopolysaccharide layer of the cell wall. Most gram-positive organisms and some of the fastidious gram-negative bacteria allow the penicillins to reach the periplasmic space and exert their lethal action. Some strains of these normally sensitive species resist penicillin because they lack certain proteins in the periplasmic space or because they produce penicillinase. Penicillinase cleaves the β-lactam ring of the penicillin molecule to form penicilloic acid, thereby completely eliminating the activity of the drug. The penicillinases of gram-positive organisms tend to be inducible exoenzymes, whereas the penicillinases of gram-negative organisms remain in the periplasmic space and can be constitutive. Each penicillinase has a range of substrates, most semisynthetic penicillins and cephalosporins being subject to digestion by penicillinases. Chemical substitutions that lead to the protection of the β-lactam ring are partial solutions to the chemotherapeutic problems posed by penicillinase. Nafcillin, methicillin, and oxacillin are resistant to penicillinases common in *Staphylococcus aureus*. Carbenicillin resists some penicillinases of gram-negative rods. Some of the new cephalosporins, for example, cefoxitin and cefamandole, resist a wide variety of penicillinases.

The similarity between penicillins and cephalosporins includes their mechanisms of action but fortunately excludes to a large degree their haptenic properties. Penicillin, like almost all antimicrobial agents, following combination with host proteins, can induce hypersensitivity to the penicillin molecule. A person allergic to penicillin G produces an allergic reaction when exposed to semisynthetic penicillins (*i.e.*, nafcillin, oxacillin, ampicillin). Fortunately, such hypersensitive individuals fail in most cases to react with cephalosporins. Atopic individuals, however, can become hypersensitive to cephalosporins as well as to any of the other drugs.

Vancomycin inhibits cell wall synthesis by blocking the secretion of peptidoglycan subunits into the periplasmic space. Vancomycin should be held in reserve as a valuable drug for use against gram-positive organisms resistant to penicillins and other antimicrobial agents.

Bacitracin and cycloserine, in the bacterial cytoplasm, inhibit cell wall synthesis by different mechanisms. Bacitracin limits the availability of a lipid carrier, the functions of which include binding of newly formed subunits to the internal surface of the cytoplasmic membrane. Cycloserine inhibits synthesis of subunits by blocking the enzymatic conversion of L-alanine to D-alanine.

Mode of Action of Drugs Affecting Nucleic Acid Synthesis

During synthesis, DNA may be cleaved at specific points by endonucleases, which thus allow modifications to be introduced, provided that normal repair mechanisms can act to reconstitute the integrity of the molecule. If normal DNA repair mechanisms are blocked, the nicks caused by endonucleases are lethal to the microorganism.

The inhibitors of nucleic acids act either at the macromolecular level or on the synthesis of nucleic acid bases (Table 5-2).

Several drugs that function at the macromolecular level are ***nalidixic acid,*** the new quinolones ***(floxacins),*** and ***rifampicin.*** Nalidixic acid exerts a bactericidal effect on gram-negative organisms by blocking one enzyme required for normal DNA synthesis. Nalidixic acid binds to the enzyme gyrase, the functions of which include the unwinding of tightly coiled regions of DNA during DNA synthesis. Gyrase-mediated unwinding of DNA is induced by cutting the DNA and allowing relaxation of supercoils and then repair of the nicks. Nalidixic acid binding to this bifunctional enzyme allows the DNA nicking to continue but inhibits repair of the nicks. It is used for gram-negative, non-*Pseudomonas* urinary tract infections. Quinolones, such as norfloxacin and ciprofloxacin, also block gyrase action. They are effective on gram-negative organisms, including *Pseudomonas* and gram-positive organisms, except streptococci. The frequency of mutation is very low ($\leq 10^{11}$).

The action of rifampicin requires its binding to DNA-dependent RNA polymerase of bacteria. This enzyme is composed of a core of four protein subunits plus a separate soluble regulatory protein, sigma *(σ)*. Synthesis of messenger RNA (mRNA) by this enzyme begins when the core binds to the promoter region of a bacterial operon. However, construction of the mRNA requires the binding of protein to the core portion of the enzyme. Rifampicin binds to the core portion of the enzyme, inhibiting the core-sigma interaction required for initiation of mRNA synthesis.

Ansamycin is a new derivative of rifampicin with improved properties for clinical use.

The synthesis of nucleic acid bases in bacteria requires the addition of single carbon units, a reaction mediated by folic acid. Folic acid is synthesized *de novo* in bacterial cells but not in eukaryotic cells, in which it is only consumed or enzymatically modified. Two important enzymatic reactions involved in the synthesis of bacterial folic acid are sensitive to chemotherapeutic agents. The conversion of para-aminobenzoic acid to dihydrofolic acid, a reaction mediated by dihydrofolic acid synthetase, is sensitive to competitive inhibition by "sulfa" drugs, such as sulfanilamide. These drugs do not affect the mammalian cell, which, because it lacks mechanisms for primary synthesis, has a nutritional requirement for dihydrofolic acid.

The second enzymatic reaction in folic acid synthesis that is sensitive to antimicrobial agents is the conversion of dihydrofolic acid to tetrahydrofolic acid. Dihydrofolic acid reductase mediates this reaction in both eucaryotic and bacterial cells. The drug trimethoprim binds about 50,000 times more avidly to the bacterial than to the mammalian enzyme because of differences in structure between the two species of protein. Bacteriostatic concentrations of the drug are therefore well tolerated by the eukaryotic cell. Both sulfonamides and trimethoprim effect a folic acid deficiency, but because they act at different stages in the pathway, a mixture of the two drugs generates a synergistic antibacterial effect and is used for treatment of urinary tract infections, acute otitis media, as well as acute inflammatory diarrhea.

Griseofulvin is an analogue of the purine base guanosine and inhibits DNA synthesis by a mechanism that is not clear. It is an antifungal, used for chitin-containing fungi, especially those in nail infections.

Mode of Action of Drugs Directly Affecting Cell Membranes

Microbial cell membranes resemble those of eukaryotic cells in general organization and chemistry. This fact makes it likely that drugs designed to act directly on cell membrane structure would be unacceptably toxic. However, there are subtle differences that permit selective binding of certain antimicrobial agents (*e.g.,* lack of sterols in bacterial membranes) (see Table 5-2). Polymyxins and gramicidin bind to bacterial membranes and cause reorganization of phospholipids around the drug, thereby introducing sites of ionic leakage. Unlike many other bactericidal agents, the polymyxins exert an almost immediately lethal effect, in this respect resembling the action of detergents.

Nystatin (Mycostatin) and amphotericin interact in a detergentlike manner with the membrane of susceptible fungi. The toxicity of nystatin for host tissue and its relative insolubility limit its application to treatment of surface infections.

Mode of Action of Drugs Affecting Protein Synthesis

Protein synthesis in bacteria begins when the 30s portion of ribosomes, through the action of soluble initiation proteins, binds to mRNA (Table 5-3). The amino acids to be linked into a protein are each bound to species of transfer RNA (tRNA) that in turn recognize specific sequences in mRNA. The binding of tRNA, charged with amino acids, to the 30s portion of the ribosome-mRNA complex is the first stage of protein synthesis susceptible to antibiotic action. Drugs that bind to the 30s subunit and block tRNA recognition include aminoglycosides, spectinomycin, and tetracycline (see Table 5-3).

The formation of peptide bonds requires both 30s and 50s portions of the ribosome. The actual formation of peptide bonds may be blocked by certain drugs, such as chloramphenicol, lincomycin, and clindamycin, which bind to the 50s subunit.

In the normal process of protein synthesis, the ribosome moves relative to the mRNA (*i.e.*, translocates), a reaction that requires soluble proteins and GTP for energy. Erythromycin blocks translocation by binding to proteins that form the 50s subunit. Fusidic acid blocks translocation by binding to one of the soluble proteins (elongation factor G) involved in energizing the movement.

The consequences, to the bacterium, of inhibition of protein synthesis, vary depending on the manner in which the process is inhibited. Inhibition by chloramphenicol is completely reversible and is therefore only bacteriostatic. This implies that continuous protein synthesis per se is not absolutely required for bacterial survival. An antibiotic such as streptomycin binds irreversibly to the ribosome, thereby causing nearly complete inhibition of protein synthesis, and hence causing death of the bacterium. The killing effect is related to the production of ''mis-sense'' proteins, which are synthesized in the presence of the drug and that misfunction because of incorrect amino acid sequences caused by drug-induced alterations of the ribosome. Mis-sense proteins in the cell lead to changes in internal structures or enzymes, thus accounting for the death of the cell.

Major Mechanisms of Antibiotic Resistance

Changes in the structural or physiologic components of an organism that occur by mutation can result in resistance to antibiotics. Significant levels of resistance may occur after a single mutation or after a series of mutations. Antimicrobial drugs do not themselves induce mutation(s), but select out those organisms that have undergone mutation. This sequence is the most common mechanism of resistance to vancomycin, rifampicin, nalidixic acid, and polymyxins. Although resistance to other drugs can emerge as a result of bacterial mutation, acquisition of specific plasmids more often accounts for observed changes in sensitivity to drugs (Table 5-11).

Resistance plasmids (R) govern their own replication and confer resistance on the bacterial host cell. Plasmids that in addition contain a set of transfer genes are called resistance transfer factors (RTF) because they mediate conjugation. The R and RTF plasmids thus differ in size

TABLE 5-11. Major Mechanisms of Specific Antibiotic Resistance

DRUG	MECHANISM OF RESISTANCE	GENETIC BASIS OF RESISTANCE
Penicillin	β-lactamase	Plasmid*
Ampicillin	β-lactamase	Plasmid*
Cephalothin	β-lactamase	Plasmid*
Methicillin	Impermeability	Plasmid
Vancomycin	Membrane alteration	Chromosome (mutation)
Sulfanilamide	Novel dihydrofolic acid synthetase	Plasmid*
Trimethoprim	Novel dihydrofolic acid synthetase	Plasmid
Rifampicin	Altered RNA polymerase	Chromosome (mutation)
Nalidixic acid	Altered gyrase enzyme	Chromosome (mutation)
Polymyxins	Altered membrane components	Chromosome (mutation)
Aminoglycosides	Antibiotic-modifying enzyme	Plasmid*
Spectinomycin	Antibiotic-modifying enzyme	Plasmid
Tetracycline	Permeability barrier	Plasmid*
Chloramphenicol	Antibiotic-modifying enzyme	Plasmid*
Lincomycin	Ribosome-modifying enzyme	Plasmid
Clindamycin	Ribosome-modifying enzyme	Plasmid
Erythromycin	Ribosome-modifying enzyme	Plasmid

* Resistance may be part of a transposon.

and in ability to initiate conjugation. One bacterium can accommodate a variety of plasmids, and it is not uncommon to encounter mixtures of R and RTF plasmids in a single organism. The R plasmids, although unable to initiate conjugation, can be transferred by conjugation mediated by an RTF in the same organism. In the absence of an RTF, the R plasmid can be transferred only when the organism is infected with a bacteriophage capable of generalized transduction. Because RTF plasmids are not encountered in *Staphylococcus,* the transfer of R plasmids in this organism is dependent on phage. In enteric bacteria, *Haemophilus,* and a variety of other organisms, transfer of R plasmids occurs by either RTF-mediated conjugation or by transduction.

The resistance to antibiotics that is mediated by R and RTF plasmids is determined by a protein product of the plasmid. In the case of penicillins and cephalosporins, this protein has β-lactamase activity and destroys the antibiotic in the periplasmic space or outside of the cell wall. Chloramphenicol, aminoglycosides, and spectinomycin are inactivated because the plasmid protein in the periplasmic space mediates the enzymatic attachment of acetyl, phosphate or adenyl groups. Lincomycin, clindamycin, and erythromycin are inactivated because the plasmid protein mediates the enzymatic methylation of an RNA molecule in the ribosome, methylation inhibiting the binding of drug to the ribosome. The plasmid product in some way reduces the uptake of tetracycline drug into the bacterium. In the case of folic acid inhibitors, the plasmid product is a pathway enzyme that is not competitively inhibited by the drug as is the chromosomally produced enzyme.

The single product of a plasmid in some cases reacts with a variety of compounds, that is, a given β-lactamase may destroy ampicillin, penicillin G, and cephalothin, or a given aminoglycoside-modifying enzyme may react with kanamycin, gentamicin, and tobramycin. Thus the expression of resistance to several related drugs is often mediated by one gene product of the plasmid. A single plasmid may contain multiple genes each mediating resistance(s). Because a bacterium can harbor numerous plasmids, the emergence of genetically complex and highly resistant strains is encountered in environments subject to the powerful selective pressure of multiple antibiotics (*e.g.,* a hospital).

One further complication introduced by R and RTF plasmids is that the plasmid gene responsible for resistance may form a transposon. A transposon is capable of ''hopping'' from the plasmid on which it entered a bacterium to another plasmid, to the chromosome, or even to the DNA of a phage that infects the same cell. Hopping of transposons accounts for the spread of resistance to organisms that are otherwise unable to support the replication of the plasmid originally harboring the resistance gene. This process accounts for the spread of β-lactamase genes from plasmids of enteric bacteria to species of *Haemophilus* and *Neisseria.*

Methods for Testing Bacterial Sensitivity to Antibiotics

Because of occasional adverse side effects and increasing emergence of antibiotic-resistant organisms, chemotherapeutic agents must be used in critical fashion to safeguard their clinical efficacy. The purpose of testing an organism for sensitivity to several antibiotics is to allow the physician some latitude in the ultimate choice of therapy. This consideration may be important in avoiding undesirable complications attending the use of a particular drug in a given patient (*e.g.,* allergy) and to offer a choice of potentially effective substitutes. The selection of drugs to be tested is based primarily on knowledge of the infection, that is, whether it is in the urinary tract, blood, localized pus, or spinal fluid. In this connection, a carefully done Gram's stain, particularly of pus, spinal fluid, and unspun urine correctly collected, yields vital information about the initial choice of antibiotics that will then be confirmed or modified on the basis of results of sensitivity testing of the organism(s) in question.

The widely used Kirby-Bauer method is based on the inhibition of surface bacterial growth under standard conditions. Several colonies of the organism to be tested are inoculated into Todd-Hewitt broth and grown to a standard optical density. Inoculum from this culture is then spread across the surface of a nutrient agar plate in a manner that gives heavy confluent growth. Disks containing antibiotics are then placed on the agar. After incubation, the diameter of the zone of growth inhibition around each antibiotic disk is measured. Each organism is then scored as sensitive, intermediate or resistant, according to the size of the zone of inhibition, which is a direct function of the sensitivity of the organism to the antibiotic. However, other factors also affect the zone size (*e.g.,* diffusion, stability and concentration of the drug, characteristically of the particular organism, size of inoculum) that collectively impose upper and lower limits within which variations in sensitivity among individual strains of a bacterial species can be judged. Infections due to organisms designated as sensitive to a given antibiotic are more likely to yield clinically to that antibiotic than are infections with strains designated as intermediate or resistant.

It is sometimes important to determine accurately the concentration of an antibiotic that must be achieved to inhibit a particular microorganism. For such determinations, the tube dilution method is used in addition to the Kirby-Bauer method. In this procedure, an antibiotic is serially diluted in growth medium and inoculated with relatively small numbers (10^5/ml) of a particular organism. The lowest concentration of antibiotic that prevents bacterial growth (turbidity) is the minimal inhibitory concentration (MIC).

For antibiotics that are bactericidal, the bactericidal endpoint can be determined by subculturing the tubes in which there is no turbidity and in which viable organisms from the inoculum may have survived. The bactericidal concentration is higher than the bacteriostatic. The MIC refers to the bacteriostatic endpoint. The minimal lethal concentration (MLC) refers to the bactericidal endpoint.

BACTERIAL INFECTIONS

Gram-Negative Enteric Bacteria

For classification, refer to A Descriptive Checklist of Important Bacteria in Medical Microbiology, earlier in this chapter. All but the exogenous pathogens, *Salmonella, Shigella, Yersinia,* and *Vibrio,* are usual members of the normal intestinal flora. Along with *Pseudomonas,* anaerobes, etc., they are important causes of opportunistic infections.

SALMONELLOSIS

This term covers infection by any of the several hundred serotypes or bioserotypes of *Salmonella* and covers a wide range of clinical manifestations, including acute gastroenterocolitis (inaccurately referred to as food poisoning), various localized infections (arthritis, myocarditis, abscesses), and typhoid (enteric) fever. The latter is usually regarded as a distinct entity because, unlike common enterocolitis, *S. typhi* is first isolated from the blood and only later from the lower intestinal tract; the disease carries a relatively high morbidity, and despite chemotherapy occasional fatalities occur.

Salmonellae are classified according to their H and O antigens by agglutination reactions with appropriately specific antisera. On this basis (Kauffman-White schema) the genus is divisible into three major species: *S. choleraesuis,* the prototype, *S. typhi* and *S. enteritidis;* the latter makes up the largest number of subspecies. In usual hospital laboratory practice, clinical isolates of *Salmonella* are reported as belonging to groups A, B, C, or D (*S. typhi* only); for final species identification isolates are sent to a central laboratory (*e.g.,* state health department or Centers for Disease Control).

While *Salmonella* grows readily on the usual bacteriologic media, procedures for primary isolation differ according to whether the specimen is a sample of feces, pus, or urine, in which relatively few *Salmonella* might be mixed in with predominant normal flora (cultured on enrichment and selective media), or whether it is from a normally sterile body fluid, such as blood or spinal fluid (cultured directly on blood agar and differential media). Once isolated in pure culture, preliminary identification is achieved on the basis of biochemical reactions (*e.g.,* nonutilization of lactose, selective fermentation of other sugars, motility, hydrogen sulfide formation, lack of urease activity, etc.) and serogrouping with polyvalent antisera (to O antigens).

Excepting typhoid fever, salmonellosis is commonly (but not invariably) localized in the intestinal tract, is mild or acute and self-limited. Occasional cases resemble typhoid fever, dysentery, or even cholera, especially in debilitated patients. Neither species nor clinical picture is constant. *S. typhi, S. paratyphi A, S. paratyphi B* (now *S. schottmueller*), and *S. paratyphi C* are especially invasive.

Meningitis, pneumonia, osteomyelitis, septicemia (especially *S. choleraesuis*) may occur. *Salmonella* infection not infrequently is found in association with debilitating conditions, such as sickle cell anemia, bartonellosis (verruga peruana), or immunosuppression and/or malnutrition.

In typhoid fever, intestinal perforation may occur at necrotic lymphatic areas (Peyer's patches) that are the site of initial localization of *S. typhi.* In typhoid fever, stubborn residual infection of the gallbladder sometimes develops, resulting in cholelithiasis and its complications, one of which is a persistent carrier state, usually curable by cholecystectomy, and especially dangerous in public food handlers (''typhoid Mary'').

S. typhimurium, S. choleraesuis, S. oranienburg, and *S. enteritidis* are among species commonly involved in *Salmonella* infection through ingestion of contaminated food. They and others (not *S. typhi,* which is restricted to humans) commonly infect a wide range of wild and domestic animals and poultry, which thus become reservoirs of infection of man via foods: raw meats of infected birds and animals, raw dairy products, raw eggs. All *Salmonella* species are transmitted in human feces (*S. typhi* sometimes also in urine following pyelonephritis and cystitis), hence in sewage and in sewage- or feces-polluted water, food and dairy products; by coprophagic arthropods (flies, ants, roaches, etc.); and by fomites.

In typical *Salmonella* food infection, symptoms commonly begin more than 10 hours following ingestion, that is, long enough for bacterial multiplication to occur, in contrast with food poisoning, especially the common staphylococcal food poisoning, in which symptoms of intense gastroenteritis commonly begin within about 10 hours following ingestion, since the toxin is preformed and growth of staphylococci in the alimentary tract does not ordinarily occur.

Diagnosis. In food infection by *Salmonella* (except *S. typhi*) the organisms occur in the stool early during the enteritis and may be isolated and identified on appropriate media. They usually do not invade the bloodstream.

In typhoid fever, on the contrary, the incubation period may be 2 to 3 weeks, symptoms delayed, and the bacilli appear in the blood (2% bile infusion broth and plain infusion broth) during the first 10 days and in the stool or the urine only after the first week. They often persist in the stools up to 12 weeks, and in about 3% of cases they persist more or less intermittently for years. In overt typhoid fever, splenomegaly and rose spots on the trunk are distinctive. Lifelong immunity to *S. typhi* follows documented typhoid fever.

In ***serologic diagnosis*** of salmonellosis, patients' sera are examined for antibodies against *Salmonella* using standard strains of *S. typhi* as antigen in titered agglutination tests. A significant (greater than 1:160) level or a rise (fourfold or greater) in titer with O antigen (*S. typhi* treated so that primarily the somatic antigens are exposed) denotes active infection. A significant rise in antibody to H antigen (*S. typhi* treated to preserve the flagellar antigens that will then be the primary reactants with antibody) was usually found to follow immunization with typhoid vaccine, which is little used nowadays. Antibodies to a surface (capsular) antigen (Vi) characteristic of some strains of *S. typhi* are thought to be associated with the presence of *S. typhi* in asymptomatic carriers.

Phage Types. Strains of *S. typhi* possessing Vi antigen and antigenically indistinguishable from one another can be further subdivided on the basis of differential sensitivity to bacteriophages. At least 50 phage types are known. This differentiation by phage typing is useful in epidemiologic studies; for example, in tracing possible different sources of infection during a supposedly single-source epidemic. Similar systems of phage typing have been developed for several other groups of bacteria: *Salmonella paratyphi A* and *S. paratyphi B; Shigella; Escherichia coli; Vibrio cholerae; Staphylococcus aureus.*

Treatment. Ampicillin and chloramphenicol are the drugs of choice in the treatment of typhoid fever and systemic infection with other strains of *Salmonella.* Strains resistant to either or both of these antibiotics occur. An alternative choice is trimethoprim-sulfamethoxazole. Uncomplicated *Salmonella* gastroenteritis is usually self-limited; antibiotics are therefore unnecessary and only promote the emergence of drug-resistant strains. Resistance plasmids are extensively shared between human and animal strains of bacteria. Close to half the antibiotics sold in the United States are fed to domestic herd animals and are therefore unwittingly ingested by humans. It is not surprising, therefore, that strains of *Salmonella* isolated from these two sources should show similar antibiograms. Antibiotics fed to livestock thus have a direct role in the rising incidence of multiple drug resistance among members of the Enterobacteriaceae. These multiple resistant strains now represent 20% to 25% of identified cases, in which the fatality rate is much higher than in cases due to sensitive strains.

Prevention of salmonellosis as well as of other communicable diseases of the intestinal tract centers primarily on adequate sanitation and thorough cooking of foods containing animal products or eggs and foods susceptible to contamination by sewage or excreta by avian or mammalian carriers, including humans. Human carriers should not serve as food handlers or nurses. Typhoid carriers are generally registered with, and supervised by, health departments.

Active immunization against typhoid is justified for persons in intimate continued household exposure to a documented typhoid carrier or for travelers to areas in which there is a recognized risk of exposure to typhoid because of poor sanitation practices. The appropriate dosage for adults and children over 10 years of age is 0.5 ml subcutaneously on two occasions 4 weeks apart, and for children younger than 10 years of age, 0.25 ml subcutaneously on two occasions 4 weeks apart. Under conditions of continued or repeated exposure or for indications if more than 3 years after primary immunization, booster (single doses administered subcutaneously as recommended above for each age group) should be given. Only monovalent *Salmonella typhi* vaccine should be used; previous formulations of "TAB" vaccines (combining typhoid and "paratyphoid A and B" antigens) should not be used.

SHIGELLOSIS (BACILLARY DYSENTERY)

Clinical dysentery may be caused by a variety of agents: certain protozoa, viruses, unripe apples, *Salmonella.* Shiga, a Japanese scientist, in 1896 first isolated the bacterium now called *Shigella dysenteriae* during outbreaks of severe dysentery in Japan. Flexner later (ca. 1900) isolated a different species from cases of dysentery in the Philippines. Many varieties were afterward described elsewhere. The various strains were named according to names of discoverers of places where found.

The genus *Shigella* is now classified into four major groups, each with several numbered serotypes based on O antigens:

Group A. *S. dysenteriae*
Group B. *S. flexneri*
Group C. *S. boydii*
Group D. *S. sonnei*

Biochemical reactions serve to differentiate *Shigella* from *Salmonella.* Shigellae do not ferment lactose (except *S. sonnei,* a slow lactose fermenter); are nonmotile; and do not produce H_2S, or gas (except *S. flexneri*) during carbohydrate fermentation. Further species identification depends on numerous additional biochemical reactions and on reactions with group-specific antisera.

Multiplication of dysentery bacilli occurs in the mucosa and the lymph nodes of the lower ileum and colon, with ulceration and sometimes pseudomembrane formation. Acute gastroenteritis is common. Bacteremia is rare. Stools typically contain mucus, pus, and blood. All of the gram-negative enteric bacilli possess lipopolysaccharide (endotoxin) in their cell walls. *Shigella dysenteriae* and *S. flexneri* produce antigenically similar toxins, the former in larger amounts than the latter. The enterotoxin is probably responsible for the watery, small-bowel diarrhea, often severe, that is characteristic of the first few days of shigellosis. *S. dysenteriae* infections cause higher fatality rates (20%) than infections by other *Shigella* species and occur chiefly in epidemic form. They are rare in the United States. In this country *S. flexneri* and *S. sonnei* are the most commonly encountered as the cause of both sporadic and epidemic disease. The fatality rate for shigellosis is relatively low in adults; it is higher in infants, particularly in developing countries, in which it is a leading cause of acute diarrhea in young children. Endemic shigellosis is associated with malnutrition and other concomitants of poor economic and sanitary conditions. Malnutrition-associated complications include hemolytic-uremic syndrome and Reiter's syndrome; in poorly nourished children the organisms may persist for long periods, with clinical relapses. Under ordinary circumstances, the infection is self-limited, and chronic carriers are rare. Control of shigellosis depends primarily on improving sanitary conditions to minimize fecal contamination of food and water sources. A safe or effective vaccine is not yet available.

In laboratory diagnosis, fecal samples and tissue swabs of the rectal mucosa should be cultured and examined microscopically for erythrocytes and leukocytes. Serum agglutinins for *Shigella* when present are of no diagnostic value. Chemotherapy is unnecessary in the usual self-limited form of shigellosis. In severe enteric disease in the presence of malnutrition and dehydration, ampicillin is the drug of choice; when ampicillin-resistant strains are involved, trimethoprim-sulfamethoxazole is used; tetracycline should be reserved for severe disease due to strains resistant to the other two drugs. Transferable multiple drug resistance in *Shigella,* mediated by plasmids, is widespread; complete antibiograms should therefore be done to guide the choice of antibiotic.

INFECTIONS DUE TO ENTEROBACTERIA (*E. COLI* AND OTHER INTESTINAL GRAM-NEGATIVE BACTERIA)

The enteric bacteria are readily cultivable on ordinary media (blood agar; eosin methylene blue agar, which inhibits gram-positive bacteria; and selective media such as McConkey's agar) and are differentiated on the basis of their biochemical reactions in pure culture; all (except for *Proteus* species and *Pseudomonas aeruginosa*) ferment lactose. All may cause opportunistic infection. *E. coli* is responsible for about 85% of cases of cystitis and is the commonest cause of pyelonephritis. The remaining 10% to 15% are accounted for by other *Enterobacteriaceae* (*e.g., Proteus* species, *Klebsiella* species, and *Enterobacter* species) and *Pseudomonas aeruginosa.* Colonization of the urinary tract by certain (pyelonephritogenic) strains of *E. coli* is mediated by attachment of bacterial fimbriae to specific tissue cell receptors. Bacteria defective in cell wall material (so-called L-forms) appear to be important in chronic relapsing pyelonephritis; L-forms do not grow on ordinary culture media and so may escape detection unless specifically searched for. Most of the strains of *E. coli* causing neonatal meningitis carry the K_1 capsular antigen, which is related to the polysaccharide antigen of Group B *Neisseria meningitidis* and is similarly antiphagocytic (*i.e.,* a virulence factor). Infections due to strains resistant to multiple antibiotics carry a relatively high mortality rate. Any of the Enterobacteriaceae (as well as *Neisseria meningitidis, Haemophilus influenzae*) may cause life-threatening septicemia (gram-negative sepsis) in which endotoxic shock is ascribed to lipid A (attached to LPS core polysaccharide common to most gram-negative bacteria). Successful treatment of potentially fatal endotoxic shock with human antiserum to LPS core antigen has been reported. Besides being a frequent cause of nosocomial infection, *Klebsiella pneumoniae* is one of the few gram-negative bacilli that can cause primary lobar pneumonia, particularly in compromised patients in whom the upper lobes are usually involved and undergo cavitation due to the necrotizing infection. Therapy is sometimes successful with a combination of an aminoglycoside and a cephalosporin. Prevalence of multiply resistant strains in a hospital environment is directly related to unregulated and injudicious use of antibiotics.

Certain (enteropathogenic) strains of *E. coli* cause acute diarrheal disease (particularly severe in infants) because of the elaboration of either a heat-labile toxin (LT) or a heat-stable (ST) toxin, both of which are coded for by plasmids. The mechanism of action of LT resembles that of choleratoxin in stimulating the production of adenosine 3′,5′-cyclic monophosphate (cAMP) in small bowel epithelial cells. Certain enteroinvasive strains have been recognized that cause true dysentery (diarrhea with blood and pus) with invasion of the mucosa, in contrast to the choleralike clinical picture caused by enterotoxin. The invasive character of these strains is probably also plasmid coded. Serogrouping of *E. coli* outbreaks is of value only as an epidemiologic tool and not in the routine analysis of nonepidemic isolates. Travelers' diarrhea, frequently due to toxigenic *E. coli,* may be prevented (but not treated) by administration of doxycycline (100 mg/day), a long-acting tetracycline analogue.

INFECTIONS DUE TO VIBRIONACEAE

The family Vibrionaceae comprises three genera: *Vibrio, Aeromonas,* and *Plesiomonas.*

The principal agents of cholera are *V. cholerae* and *V. eltor. V. cholerae* resembles *Salmonella typhi* in many respects but is comma-shaped (*V. comma* in older literature). Whereas all motile Enterobacteriaceae have peritrichous flagella, those of *V. cholerae* are polar. In contrast to *S. typhi, V. cholerae* is proteolytic and grows well in alkaline (*p*H 9) medium (*e.g.,* TCBS agar).

V. cholerae resembles *S. typhi* in being an intestinal pathogen restricted to humans, and in modes of transmission, surviving for long periods in polluted water. Also like *S. typhi,* it contains heat-stable O antigens, lipopolysaccharide endotoxin and a heat-labile flagellar antigen.

Antigenic groupings (I to VI) are based on at least three type-specific O antigens: A, B, and C. The Inaba group is designated AC; Ogawa group, AB; Hikojima group, ABC. The Inaba and Ogawa antigenic types are included in vaccines. For diagnosis, an O-group serum with Inaba and Ogawa immunoglobulins is sufficient since all *V. cholerae* and El Tor vibrios are agglutinated by these.

V. eltor causes endemic and epidemic choleralike disease (El Tor cholera), generally with lower death rates than in *V. cholerae* outbreaks. It is of importance in Malaysia and adjacent areas. Both *V. cholerae* and *V. eltor* agglutinate with cholera serum of O group I (A). All may be variants of a common stock. Cholera vibrios also share O antigens with *Brucella,* so that persons who have received cholera vaccine may show significant levels of serum agglutinins for *Br. abortus,* the standard test antigen (see below). The El Tor vibrio produces hemolysin (Greig positive) and its cultures agglutinate chick erythrocytes. Unlike *V. cholerae,* it kills chick embryos, resists polymyxin and group IV choleraphage.

There are saprophytic species of vibrios and some that are pathogenic for lower animals: *V. metschnikovi* (pigeons); *V. proteus; V. fetus* (sheep, cattle, goats, sometimes humans).

In *V. cholerae,* multiplication of the vibrios is entirely in the gut, with the endotoxin producing intense gastritis and nausea and irritation of the bowel, chiefly the ileum. The exotoxin produced by *Vibrio* is the prototypic enterotoxin, which causes fluid secretion through the activation of tissue adenylcyclase to increase intestinal cAMP concentration. Similar LTs are produced by *E. coli* and all are coded for by transmissible plasmids. Ingestion of contaminated water leads to the penetration of the mucous layer and colonization of the lining epithelium of the small intestine by the vibrios. The epithelium remains intact, but it passes immense quantities of water fluid, turbid with mucus (''rice water'' stools), with resulting dehydration, hemoconcentration, electrolyte imbalance, toxemia, and shock. Administration of fluids and electrolytes is of critical importance and is dramatically effective in therapy. Without treatment, mortality in *V. cholerae* outbreaks may range from 5% to 75%.

Epidemic cholera is largely water borne, but sporadic cases may be transmitted by any raw foods contaminated with feces or vomitus of patients or of temporary carriers. Chronic carriers of *V. cholerae* seem to be rare, but convalescent carriers and mild, ambulatory cases seem to be common. The disease has recently reached epidemic proportions in Peru. It is endemic and epidemic in India and mainland Southeast Asia. Isolated outbreaks in Louisiana have been associated with ingestion of raw oysters taken from contaminated coastal waters.

Control measures are basically as in other enteric bacterial disease. Rigid inspection and control of travelers from endemic and epidemic areas are important in preventing the international spread of cholera.

Vaccines are required for United States travelers to the epidemic or endemic areas. Modern cholera vaccine consists of killed *V. cholerae* suspensions, 10^8 cells per ml, half Inaba, half Ogawa. Studies and experience in the Orient indicate the desirability of including El Tor vibrios. Protection begins about 10 days after vaccination and lasts only about 6 months. It is not very solid and should be reinforced by booster doses each 6 months. The vaccine also evokes antibodies that agglutinate *Brucella* organisms. Toxoid derived from the ''permeability factor'' or exotoxin is currently under field trial.

Laboratory Diagnosis. Liquid (rice water) stools of patients may be examined microscopically for typical vibrios, blood, mucus, and pus. Cultivation of stools or suspect water in selective (*p*H 9.0) alkaline peptone water often yields prolific growth of the vibrios in a surface pellicle after 6 to 8 hours at 37° C. This pellicle may be examined microscopically and used to inoculate plates of a special thiosulfate-citrate-bile-salts (T-C-B-S) medium containing 1:200,000 KTe for selectivity, for isolation of colonies, also for a rapid, preliminary, slide agglutination test. Colonies resemble those of *Shigella.* Final identification depends on morphology, cultural properties, and serologic tests.

Neither serum nor chemotherapy is of recognized value in cholera.

Vibrio parahemolyticus is an inhabitant of saline, estuarine, coastal waters and is very similar to *V. cholerae.* It causes a severe form of gastroenteritis associated especially with consumption of insufficiently cooked or raw shellfish. In the summer months, it causes about 50% of all bacterial food poisoning in Japan. It differs from *V. cholerae* in requiring 3% to 7% NaCl in the culture medium, growth at 43° C, ability to metabolize chitin, and positive Greig reaction. Infectious strains are associated with production of a heat-stable hemolysin (Kanagawa). It is transmitted by the fecal-oral route and by sewage-contaminated foods and water.

Vibrio vulnificus can produce a primary septicemia after ingestion of raw oysters by individuals with elevated serum iron levels, such as in chronic liver or renal disease, thalassemia, as well as in an immunocompromised state. Fatality of greater than 50% can occur despite use of tetracycline therapy.

Infections Due to Campylobacter/Helicobacter

Based on 16s rRNA sequencing, the Campylobacter spp. were reclassified from the Vibrios into a loosely defined new group of microaerophilic, motile, helical/vibroid, gram-negative bacteria. They had originally been classified in the Vibrionaceae, due to their curved (Gr. Campylo, curved) shape.

Campylobacter infections are important in veterinary medicine; and animal disease (cattle, dogs, fowl) may be an important source of human infection, which may also spread from person to person (*e.g.,* small children with diarrhea in day-care centers). *Campylobacter jejuni* causes enteric disease in any age group. *C. fetus* is a cause of opportunistic infection in debilitated patients and pregnant women; fatal septicemic infections of newborns may be endogenous from the mother.

Also, *C. pylori* (now reclassified as the leading example of a new genera and called *Helicobacter pylori*), originally isolated in 1982, is currently being touted as a cause of 77% of duodenal and gastric ulcers. Thus, antimicrobial treatment together with acid antagonist therapy may prove to be the treatment of choice in the future for these ailments.

Pathogenic, Gram-Positive, Pyogenic Cocci

STREPTOCOCCI

For convenience, three subdivisions of streptococci may be made on the basis of types of hemolytic zones produced around colonies on sheep or rabbit blood agar plates incubated aerobically at 37° C, as follows:

Hemolytic

1. Beta type (''Strep hemolyticus,'' ''beta hemolytic strep,'' etc.). With one or two exceptions, these comprise the pyogenic group of streptococci. They form a clear, colorless zone of hemolysis, devoid of intact erythrocytes around small colonies.
2. Alpha type (''Strep viridans,'' ''green strep''). These form a greenish zone of intact erythrocytes around small colonies, with varying degrees of hemolysis at the periphery. The group includes *S. mitis, S. mutans, S. salivarius, S. bovis, S. thermophilus, S. faecium, S. pneumoniae,* and others.

Nonhemolytic

3. Gamma type (''indifferent strep,'' ''nonhemolytic strep''). These produce no visible change in the blood around their colonies. The group includes *S. lactis,* some of the Enterococcus group: *S. faecalis, S. liquefaciens,* etc. (Table 5-9).

Serologic Subdivisions of Streptococci. Lancefield subdivided the ***beta-type*** hemolytic streptococci into immunologic groups on the basis of cell wall polysaccharide antigens. Grouping is done with highly specific antisera as a precipitin reaction or with counterimmunoelectrophoresis (CIE), using streptococcal extracts, as a coagglutination reaction with antibody-coated staphylococcal cells (protein A) or latex particles, or by ultraviolet light microscopy of bacterial cells stained with fluorescein-labelled antibody (see Table 5-5). The Lancefield groups are lettered A to U and, with a few exceptions, are beta hemolytic.

Over 90% of strains isolated from human disease are members of group A, including the classic *Streptococcus pyogenes* from human sources. *S. pyogenes* is the principal human pathogen, causing scarlet fever, septic sore throat, erysipelas, puerperal sepsis, empyema, meningitis. Group A strains are sensitive to bacitracin; most other beta-hemolytic streptococci are resistant. All group A strains are sensitive to penicillin, the drug of choice for therapy and/or prophylaxis of acute rheumatic fever.

Group B strains are a frequent cause of neonatal infections (especially type 3) and are distinguished from all others in producing double-zone (''hot-cold'') beta hemolysis, hydrolyzing sodium hippurate, and positive CAMP test. These are mainly *S. agalactiae* strains.

Group D streptococci include enterococci *(S. faecalis)* and are found in miscellaneous human infections such as arthritis, sinusitis, endocarditis, and cystitis, probably as opportunistic invaders. Group D streptococci, although usually indifferently hemolytic (γ), may be viridans or, less frequently, beta-hemolytic. All group D streptococci grow on bile-esculin (B-E) agar with a positive reaction; only enterococci grow in broth containing 6.5% NaCl, which allows one to distinguish them from nonenterococci.

Other groups, through K, Q, and T, occur in lower animals or in dairy products. A few alpha-type and gamma-type *(e.g., S. lactis)* streptococci contain Lancefield group N antigens.

The determination of the Lancefield group of a beta-hemolytic streptococcus is of diagnostic and prognostic value as well as an index to epidemiology and therapy.

A further subdivision of group A streptococci is made into more than 60 numbered serologic types on the basis of precipitin tests with type-specific soluble protein antigens (M proteins) in these streptococci. M proteins are antiphagocytic and therefore are essential to virulence. M protein is the only streptococcal antigen that is protective to the host, in that it protects against reinfection with the same serological type. The M types of group A streptococci are related to certain clinical conditions; for example, types 1, 3, 4, 6, 12 and 25 have been found to predominate in certain epidemics in which acute hemorrhagic nephritis was a prominent complication of acute pharyngitis. Type 2 and a few higher serotypes (49, 55, 57, 59, 60, 61) have been reported as the cause of pyoderma-associated acute glomerulonephritis (AGN). This fact accounts for the sporadic occurrence and geographic localization of AGN in contrast to the relatively constant seasonal incidence of ARF without evident geographic localization in temperate climates. There is little or no cross-immunity between M types. Therefore, repeated group A streptococcal infections may occur in the same individual, each caused by a different M type of streptococcus.

Other cell wall fractions of group A streptococci include acid- and heat-labile but trypsin-resistant T proteins. These can be used as antigens to prepare specific antisera that differentiate some 45 T-agglutinin types. T-agglutination typing is useful in epidemiologic studies on group-A *Streptococcus* infection, especially when M antigens are ill-defined.

Fibrinolysin or ***streptokinase*** is a protein elaborated by streptococci of groups A, C, and G that activates a serum enzyme, plasmin, able to digest supposedly protective, retaining, fibrin clots that may be formed around infected lesions. ***Antifibrinolysin*** or ***antistreptokinase*** appears in the blood of patients recovering from infections with streptococci of these groups and, if increasing in titer, is of diagnostic value.

Beta-type streptococci of group A also produce at least two kinds of soluble hemolysin: S and O. *Streptolysin O* is readily oxidized and appears, in blood agar plates, only around subsurface colonies unless anaerobically incubated. *Streptolysin S* is sensitive to heat, acid, or both, but *not* to oxygen. A significant increase in titer of antistreptolysin O (ASO) or of other antienzymes (streptozyme test) during beta-hemolytic streptococcal infection, especially respiratory infections, is of diagnostic significance in relation to the subsequent emergence of acute rheumatic fever (ARF). *Streptolysin S* is not antigenic.

Capsules and Hyaluronidase. Group A streptococci, especially M types 4 and 22, form protective capsules of hyaluronic acid, a slimy polysaccharide. These capsules may be hydrolyzed by ***hyaluronidase,*** produced in varying amounts by the streptococci themselves. Although this may offset the antiphagocytic effect of the capsules, it can also digest the ground substance of the connective tissues and has therefore been regarded by some as a spreading factor, permitting invasion of the tissues by the streptococci.

Streptodornase is an enzyme found in cultures of beta-type streptococci that digests deoxyribonucleic acid (hence strepto-*dorn*ase). Much of the slimy, fibrinous exudate in empyema and other conditions consists of fibrin and DNA from lysed leukocytes. Streptokinase and streptodornase have clinical use in chemical debridement of such highly viscous exudates. Antibodies to hyaluronidase and/or to deoxyribonuclease B have the same significance as ASO. In the absence of a significant elevation in one or more of these antienzymes (titer greater than 1/100), a diagnosis of ARF is most unlikely. In streptococcal pyoderma, little or no ASO response may occur, but anti-DNase titers rise.

Infections by Streptococci

Scarlet Fever and Septic Sore Throat. The surface of group A beta-hemolytic streptococci contains lipoteichoic acid residues by which the bacterial cells adhere to specific receptors on mucosal cells in the oropharynx; additional virulence factors (*e.g.,* M protein, numerous extracellular enzymes) interfere with phagocytosis and activation of the alternate complement (C) pathway and allow the bacteria to invade the host more deeply. Many strains of *S. pyogenes* (group A) produce an exotoxin (erythrogenic or scarlet-fever toxin) that, when absorbed by the susceptible host, produces the nausea, chills, fever and rash of scarlet fever.

Like the toxin of *Corynebacterium diphtheriae,* erythrogenic toxin is produced only by lysogenic streptococci ***(lysogenic conversion).***

Scarlet fever and septic sore throat are two manifestations of the same infection. In both, a septic sore throat is present. Persons susceptible to the erythrogenic toxin also develop a rash and are said to have scarlet fever. Persons insusceptible to the toxin, that is, with antitoxic immunity, have no rash, and such cases are diagnosed as septic sore throat. Reinfections and septic sore throat without rash, due to different M types of toxigenic streptococci, are possible.

Transmission of streptococcal infections is as for respiratory infections in general: oronasopharyngeal secretions and contact.

For diagnostic cultures, swabbings from nose or throat

are streaked on blood agar, and undercut or, better, emulsified in broth that is then used to inoculate blood agar pour plates to obtain subsurface colonies. Beta-type hemolytic colonies found after 24 hours at 35° C are fished to blood broth and incubated. Pure cultures may be subjected to appropriate differential tests shown in Table 5-5.

In severe cases septicemia may develop, and blood cultures (10 ml of blood in 150 ml of tryptose broth) are of utmost importance as a guide to treatment.

Acute rheumatic fever is a nonsuppurative sequel to group A streptococcal infection only (acute pharyngitis and tonsillitis and inapparent infection). There is a relatively constant level of incidence up to 3% following all untreated cases regardless of the serotype. Clear delineation of the pathogenesis of ARF has thus far eluded investigators and is made even more difficult by the lack of a suitable experimental animal model. Several factors are thought to have a role in producing tissue damage (*e.g.*, Aschoff bodies characteristically seen in the myocardium, preceded by ''rheumatic inflammation'' of connective tissue). The most important factors are immunological, primarily the incontrovertible role of antecedent upper respiratory tract infection with group A streptococci and the production of antibodies and cell-mediated immune responses to streptococcal antigen(s) (*e.g.*, M protein, protoplast membrane?) cross-reactive with host tissue; some form of autoimmunity has been proposed but remains unproven. Patients with a history of ARF are about 10 times more at risk of recurrence of ARF with each successive acute group A streptococcal infection than are persons without known previous history of streptococcal infection. ARF can be effectively prevented by prompt and adequate penicillin treatment of acute streptococcal pharyngitis.

The pathogenesis of AGN revolves primarily around the subepithelial deposition of immune complexes, containing immunoglobulin and streptococcal antigens, in the glomerular basement membrane, where the C cascade is triggered locally to cause an acute inflammatory reaction and transient impairment of renal function. AGN is usually completely reversible; chronic nephritis rarely if ever results. Circulating immune complexes are also encountered in patients with poststreptococcal AGN. Prompt penicillin treatment of acute pharyngitis caused by nephritogenic strains reduces the incidence of AGN.

Other Streptococcal Infections. Beta hemolytic streptococci of any Lancefield group, but especially groups A, C, and G, may cause various nonepidemic infections, such as otitis media, empyema, sore throat, erysipelas, and meningitis. Puerperal sepsis may be transmitted to parturient women by carriers of beta hemolytic streptococci, which are common, and by unsterile hands, instruments, gloves, dressings, dust.

Group B streptococci (*S. agalactiae,* four serotypes) are found in 25% of normal vaginas and from this source may cause severe and often fatal neonatal infection. ''Early onset'' disease, due to any of the four serotypes and fatal in up to 60% of cases, occurs during the first postnatal week in association with prematurity and/or obstetric complications; it is characterized chiefly by ''respiratory distress syndrome'' (pneumonia) and septicemia. ''Delayed onset'' disease, with lower mortality, is caused usually by type III (either maternally acquired or nosocomial) and is characterized by meningitis, septicemia, and/or more localized infections.

Maternal antibody to group B streptococci protects infants at risk from ascending infection by B streptococci. About 5% of the group B strains are nonhemolytic and may therefore be missed. Up to 30% of the strains may be bacitracin sensitive and thus may be mistaken for group A streptococci. Definitive identification is made by fluorescent antibody techniques and by the CAMP test. Penicillin and related antibiotics are effective in the treatment of these infections in which early diagnosis is lifesaving.

Group G beta-hemolytic streptococci may normally inhabit the vagina, oropharynx, gastrointestinal tract, or skin, and from any of these sites (most often the skin) can be introduced into the bloodstream and cause serious infection, particularly in patients with neoplastic disease. Maternally derived group G streptococci also may cause neonatal sepsis and respiratory distress syndrome. All strains of group G streptococci are sensitive to penicillin.

Alpha-hemolytic (viridans) streptococci fall into several serogroups and some are untypable. *S. mutans,* by virtue of its capacity to produce high-molecular-weight dextran, is a prime cause of dental plaque formation that, if unchecked, leads directly to dental caries. *S. mitis* and *S. sanguis* are the viridans streptococci most commonly causing endocarditis. All viridans streptococci are universally found in the normal oropharynx and from this site may gain transient entrance into the blood following minor trauma to the supporting periodontal tissues. In patients with damaged endocardial surfaces (healed rheumatic fever, congenital deformities, prostheses), these otherwise noninvasive bacteria of low intrinsic virulence are the primary cause of endocarditis initiated at the site of endocardial discontinuity or denudation. In the same way, group D streptococci account for up to 10% of endocardial infections. If endocarditis is suspected, a persistent effort should be made prior to therapy to recover organisms from the blood. To this end, bidaily cultures should be made until at least three separate blood samples yield the same organisms, for which the minimal inhibitory concentrations of penicillin and streptomycin should be determined. Upon primary isolation, most group D and many viridans streptococci are relatively resistant to penicillin *in vitro* but still yield clinically to adequate dosage of combined antibiotics, usually penicillin and streptomycin with the adjunctive administration of probenecid.

Streptococcus pneumoniae, distinguished from viridans streptococci by sensitivity to optochin, is the most common cause of lobar pneumonia and a frequent cause of meningitis. There are 84 serotypes determined by the capsular swelling reaction with type-specific rabbit antisera. Types 1, 2, 3, 4, 7, 8, 12, and 14 are most virulent. The capsular polysaccharide is antiphagocytic (*i.e.,* the chief virulence factor) and is also the protective antigen.

C polysaccharide is a cell wall group-specific antigen (as opposed to type-specific capsular polysaccharides) which has the unique property of reacting, in the presence of calcium, with a beta-globulin (C-reactive protein, CRP) present in small amounts in normal serum. Serum CRP levels increase in response to any kind of tissue inflammatory reaction (*e.g.,* ARF). CRP in serum is detected and measured by reactivity (precipitin tests, CIE, ELISA) with specially prepared rabbit antisera to CRP (which is readily isolated and purified from human serum). CRP levels are accorded the same significance as other nonspecific ''acute phase reactants'' (*e.g.,* erythrocyte sedimentation rate). The binding of CRP to C substance in the bacterial cell wall activates complement and promotes phagocytosis; CRP can thus be considered a nonspecific host-protective factor. Certain extracellular pneumococcal enzymes (*e.g.,* neuraminidase) may contribute to virulence.

A vaccine is now available composed of purified capsular polysaccharides of 23 pneumococcal types that account for over 90% of infections. The vaccine is effective in preventing pneumococcal pneumonia in selected high-risk populations in which the case fatality rate of treated bacteremia exceeds 25% (*e.g.,* patients compromised by kyphoscoliosis, diabetes, cellular immune deficiencies, sickle cell disease, splenectomy). Vaccine should not be given to children under 2 years of age or to pregnant women. Most strains of *S. pneumoniae* are sensitive to penicillin at levels easily achieved in the bloodstream. Since 1967, however, strains resistant to penicillin have been encountered with increasing frequency. Resistance to multiple antibiotics has been reported (strain 19A), suggesting that antibiograms should be done on significant clinical isolates.

Respiratory infection with *S. pneumoniae* is not highly contagious. In contrast to lobar pneumonia, which almost always yields to appropriate antibiotic treatment, pneumococcal meningitis carries a high mortality despite what appears to be adequate treatment. Counterimmunoelectrophoresis is an important aid in diagnosis of meningeal infection when viable organisms cannot be recovered in cultures of the spinal fluid.

PEPTOSTREPTOCOCCI

Strictly anaerobic streptococci are grouped together in the genus *Peptostreptococcus,* in which there are at least six species, identifiable by gas-liquid chromatography of metabolic products. Peptostreptococci are commensal inhabitants of the oral cavity, the lower intestinal tract, and the female genitourinary tract, from any of which sites they can be hematogenously disseminated (by trauma, surgery, etc.) to cause foul-smelling purulent infection in various organs (*e.g.,* lung, paranasal sinuses, brain, liver, pelvic organs) and septicemia. Localized infections are usually polymicrobial, including, besides anaerobic streptococci, other commensal anaerobes such as *Bacteroides, Propionibacterium, Fusobacterium,* and *Peptococcus. Peptococcus* species are similar to peptostreptococci in that both are anaerobic, gram-positive cocci. They differ in that peptococci tend to grow in clumps, while peptostreptococci grow in chains of cocci. Both are uniformly sensitive to penicillin.

STAPHYLOCOCCI

Staphylococcal Infections. Staphylococci cause numerous types of suppurative inflammatory conditions in any part of the body. They commonly form abscesses and furuncles of the skin and produce a number of metabolites of varying degrees of toxicity. *Staphylococcus aureus* is now a leading cause of frequently fatal endocarditis, particularly in intravenous drug users. In the course of staphylococcal endocarditis, cryoglobulins and circulating immune complexes (CIC) are found, the latter being the triggering mechanism for glomerulonephritis. CIC levels decline when the infection is arrested by chemotherapy. Most pathogenic strains produce β-type hemolysis (but not α type) on blood-agar plates. Staphylococci are much hardier than streptococci (resist drying, can survive a wide temperature range of 4° C to 60° C), grow vigorously on media like those used for streptococci, but are somewhat less fastidious as to temperature (15° C to 40° C) and requirements for blood or serum, though they also require organic N and glucose. Like streptococci, they are facultative anaerobes. Blood agar with mannitol, 7% NaCl, and tellurite is a useful selective medium.

Staphylococci differ from streptococci in producing catalase, having cytochrome systems, and in producing, at 25° C, large opaque, white, cream-colored, or butter-yellow colonies. *S. aureus* tends to produce more yellow pigment than *S. epidermidis,* especially in pus. Resistance of staphylococci to penicillin is transmissible by plasmids that code for penicillinase. Most strains of *S. aureus* pathogenic for humans are characterized by the production of the enzyme coagulase (*bound* or *free*), which induces clotting of citrated or oxalated human or rabbit plasma. Other characteristics often associated with (but not necessarily the cause of) pathogenicity of *S. aureus* are: fermentation of mannitol; elaboration of acid phosphatase, β-lactamase (penicillinase), protease, hyaluronidase, lysozyme, catalase, deoxyribonuclease; protein A (in cell wall), which binds to Fc portion of immunoglobulins, is antiphagocytic and anticomplementary; several hemolysins or toxins, including exfoliatin (which causes the "scalded skin syndrome") and enterotoxins (causing acute gastroenteritis). In *Staphylococcus aureus,* species-specific polysaccharide A is composed of *N*-acetylglucosamine residues attached alpha or beta to a polyribitol phosphate backbone and is associated with cell-wall peptidoglycan. Antibodies to teichoic acids become markedly elevated in staphylococcal septicemia and endocarditis. Measurement of antiteichoic acid antibody (by CIE) is valuable in gauging antibiotic therapy. Exaggerated hypersensitivity to staphylococcal components develops in certain individuals with persistent staphylococcal infections, particularly chronic furunculosis; in these cases cell-mediated immune responses may contribute to the accentuated inflammatory reactions usually observed. *Staphylococcus epidermidis* species-specific polysaccharide B is composed of polyglycerol P-teichoic acid with beta-linked glycosyl residues.

S. epidermidis and nonpathogenic micrococci are ubiquitous on the human skin. Infections by *S. epidermidis* are typically superficial and rarely severe, except for occasional opportunistic infections (*e.g.,* urinary tract infections resulting from catheterization) and postoperative endocarditis associated with cardiac valve prostheses.

Phage Types and Antibiotic Resistance. Differential sensitivity to 20 or more staphylococcal bacteriophages (divided for convenience into lytic groups I to IV) provides a means of identifying the source and distribution of pathogenic strains, for example, nosocomial infections. Most strains of *S. aureus* in the community, and all hospital strains (*i.e.,* carried asymptomatically by personnel), are resistant to penicillin. Beta-lactamase-resistant drugs (*e.g.,* methicillin, oxacillin, nafcillin, cephalosporins) are used in therapy. Some staphylococcal strains exhibit a type of genome-encoded resistance unrelated to penicillinase, that is, intrinsic resistance (*e.g.,* to methicillin). These MRSA strains, if at high prevalence in the hospital, dictate initial treatment with vancomycin. Also, patients allergic to penicillin can be treated with vancomycin or trimethoprim-sulfamethoxazole. Recent reports that *S. epidermidis* can transfer vancomycin-resistant genes *in vitro* to *S. aureus* have raised concerns.

Food Poisoning. Some strains of coagulase-positive staphylococci produce a thermostable exotoxin (enterotoxin) that, when ingested, causes acute staphylococcal food poisoning or gastroenteritis. There are at least five antigenic types of staphylococcal enterotoxin (SEA to SEE).

Heat-stable enterotoxin is preformed in contaminated food that has been allowed to stand at 20° C to 38° C (room or incubating temperature) for some hours. A wide variety of foods is suitable for growth of staphylococci.

Contamination of foods, resulting in staphylococcal food poisoning, often is traced to food handlers who have abscesses or boils on hands or arms or in the nose. Foods exposed openly in shops and cafeterias may be infected by coughing and sneezing workers or customers.

Intoxication is characterized primarily by the sudden onset of nausea and vomiting after a short incubation period (2 to 6 hours) and is unaccompanied by fever. Dehydration may be severe and even life-threatening, particularly in infants and elderly or debilitated patients. True enterocolitis (bloody diarrhea, necrotizing lesions of small and/or large bowel) as contrasted with acute upper gastroenterointoxication may be caused by antibiotic-resistant strains that colonize the colon, overgrowing the normal flora and producing enterotoxin in situ. Another soluble exotoxin (exofoliatin or exfoliative dermatitis toxin [ExFT]) produced particularly by strains of phage group II causes the scalded skin syndrome, bullous impetigo, and scarlatiniform rash.

ExFT as well as the serologically distinct staphylococcal enterotoxins SEA to SEE also belong to a class of molecules called ***superantigens*** (SAgs). These are bivalent, highly potent mitogens that stimulate certain subsets of T cells by directly binding to the outer surface of both a class II MHC molecule on an antigen-presenting cell (APC) and to the V_β-CDR_4 region on the T-cell receptor (TCR) (see Fig. 5-11, in the immunology section). SAgs are not proteolytically processed, so that the binding to class II molecules is not through the peptide-groove structure. Superantigens provide for enhanced proliferation of specific subsets of V_β-expressing T cells; that is, SED stimulates human T cells with $V_\beta5$ and 12 specificity, while SEE stimulates T cells with $V_\beta6$, 8, and 18 specificity.

Toxic Shock Syndrome. Toxic shock syndrome (TSS) is an acute and occasionally fatal illness resulting from infection with *Staphylococcus aureus* (usually of phage group I); it is characterized by signs of acute intoxication (fever, hypotension, scarlatiniform rash) and is usually, but not invariably, associated with the use of specific types of vaginal tampons. The product most regularly elaborated by TSS-associated strains of *Staphylococcus* is also an exotoxin, referred to as toxic shock syndrome toxin-1 (TSST-1), which was renamed from SEF. As with the other SEs, TSST-1 is a superantigen, and it is this ability to overstimulate T_H cells, accompanied by overproduction of several cytokines (IL-2, IL-4, IL-6, TNF α, INF γ), that leads to acute systemic illness, clinical shock, and potentially, even death. It is ironic that among survivors, the acute phase of T-cell activation seen in TSS is followed by a period of immunosuppression, where the SAg reactive T cells become anergic. This is evidenced by depressed reticuloendothelial system (RES) clearance and IgM synthesis, increased sensitivity to endotoxin (from indigenous gram-negative flora), and enhanced delayed type acquired hypersensitivity possibly accounting for the exfoliation seen in TSS.

Gram-Negative Cocci

INFECTIONS DUE TO NEISSERIA

This genus, found only in humans, is named for Neisser, first to recognize (in 1879) the causative agent of gonorrhea.

Gonorrhea. Although no demonstrable *exo*toxins are produced, the organisms contain endotoxin (LPS) and are highly pyogenic. Gaining entrance to suitable tissues such as glandular or mucosal surfaces of the genitalia, especially those covered by columnar epithelium, they produce an intense inflammatory exudate. Usually within less than 10 (1 to 31) days of infection there is a rapid formation of thick, mucopurulent exudate from the posterior urethra of males or from the cervix. Invasion of neighboring tissues (*e.g.*, prostate and fallopian tubes) often occurs and uncommonly there is bacteremia with arthritis and endocarditis. The gonococci in an infected mother may gain entrance to the conjunctival sac of the infant during birth, causing severe ophthalmia ***(ophthalmia neonatorum).*** Thus, in males urethritis is most common with a heavy urethral discharge and dysuria, while in females cervicitis with a light to heavy discharge and abdominal pain is commonly seen.

Gonococcal ophthalmia of adults may occur as a result of autoinfection. Gonococci may be found in the urethra, prostate, Bartholin's glands, cervix, vagina, rectum.

N. gonorrhoeae can cause meningitis with septicemia. Disseminated gonococcemia may result in arthritis and/or acute endocarditis. The organism may also be found in the posterior nasopharynx and can cause tracheitis and pneumonitis. *N. meningitidis* can likewise be found in the genital tract and cause essentially all of the same syndromes as *N. gonorrhoeae*. Gonorrhea continues to increase in prevalence, especially among teenagers, in company with syphilis and chlamydial infection. The latter currently exceeds gonorrhea in epidemiological importance.

In the diagnosis of gonorrheal urethritis, gram-stained smears are made of fresh exudate; detection of "gram-negative intracellular diplococci" resembling *N. gonorrhoeae* is good presumptive evidence, which should be confirmed by culture on Thayer-Martin agar (containing vancomycin, colistin, nystatin) incubated in a candle jar or CO_2 incubator. In females, smears are not reliable (many vaginal commensal organisms resemble *N. gonorrhoeae* morphologically); endocervical culture is mandatory. Oxidase-positive colonies detected on primary culture are inoculated into semisolid agar with differential sugars (glucose, maltose, sucrose). *N. gonorrhoeae* ferments only dextrose, *N. meningitidis,* dextrose and maltose; commensal organisms, all three. Definitive identification can be made with fluorescent antibody on appropriately fixed smears of exudate or of cultures. *N. gonorrhoeae* of the small colony types (T1, T2) usually isolated from fresh gonorrheal exudates possess pili that mediate initial attachment to cells and have inherent antiphagocytic (virulence) properties. Pili are the protective antigen of gonococci: antibodies to pili have been shown to protect against experimental infection in primates.

Penicillin is the drug of choice in treatment of gonorrhea; blood levels achieved with high dose (4.8 million units of procaine penicillin G) regimens may be enhanced by the administration of benemid. However, because of the high incidence of concurrent chlamydial infection (in heterosexual as well as homosexual patients), trimethoprim plus sulfamethoxazole and tetracycline are currently recommended to reduce the risk of persistent postgonococcal chlamydial disease (nongonococcal urethritis, NGU, pelvic inflammatory disease, PID). Penicillin-producing *N. gonorrhoeae* (PPNG) (these are mostly strains imported from the Far East, and not indigenous strains that have acquired penicillinase plasmids) as well as indigenous strains showing chromosomally mediated resistance (CMRNG) to penicillin are being encountered with increasing frequency. Infection due to PPNG or CMRNG is best treated with spectinomycin, resistance to which, although reported, is still infrequent; tetracycline may be added to treat coexistent chlamydial infection. Spectinomycin-resistant gonorrhea should be treated with cefoxitin plus probenecid; for pharyngitis due to PPNG, trimethoprim plus sulfamethoxazole should be used. Norfloxacin (a relative of nalidixic acid) has been used successfully in uncomplicated urethritis due to these resistant strains. Causes of NGU include *Chlamydia trachomatis* and *Ureaplasma urealyticum.* Rapid diagnosis of chlamydial infection is achieved on freshly smeared exudate by staining with specific anti-chlamydial fluorescent antibody (or indirectly with specific monoclonal antibody and fluorescent antiglobulin) and detecting the presence of specifically stained elementary bodies of *C. trachomatis.* Neisserial ophthalmia neonatorum may be prevented by the instillation (mandatory in most states) of 1% silver nitrate solution; neonates born to mothers with known gonococcal infection should receive systemic penicillin therapy. Neonatal infection due to PPNG should be treated with cefotaxime or gentamicin.

Meningococcal Disease. *Neisseria meningitidis* colonizes the posterior nasopharynx in about 5% to 30% of normal individuals; in epidemics carrier rates can approach 95%. From this site; meningococci may spread to cause pneumonia or may invade the bloodstream to cause meningitis, purpura, and endotoxic shock. Chronic meningococcemia should suggest itself as a possible cause of unexplained recurrent generalized petechial hemorrhages. Overwhelming meningococcemia with widespread intravascular coagulation and adrenal cortical hemorrhage (Waterhouse-Friderichsen syndrome) may result. Serum antibody to the meningococcus tends to increase with age beyond 6 months to 1 year, as a result of colonization with different species of cross-reactive nonpathogenic *Neisseria*. Maximum incidence of meningitis is from 6 months (no maternal antibody) to about 2 years. (The same general incidence pattern obtains with *Haemophilus influenzae* type b and *Streptococcus pneumoniae*.) Asymptomatic carriers of *N. meningitidis* are the source of infection of contacts via droplets of respiratory secretion. As the carrier rate in a given population increases, the potential for epidemic meningitis intensifies proportionally. The carrier state itself is an immunizing process; carriers rarely if ever contract overt disease. The risk of secondary cases among household contacts of a case of meningitis (meningococcal or *Haemophilus*) is more than 600 times greater than in the general population.

N. meningitidis is divisible into nine serogroups (A, B, C, D, X, Y, Z, W135, 29E) on the basis of capsular polysaccharides. Group B polysaccharide is identical to the K_1 antigen of *E. coli*. Organisms of groups A, B, and C account for most meningococcal disease. Group B meningococci, currently the prevalent type in the United States, are sensitive to sulfadiazine; groups A and C are resistant. Primary isolation is made on chocolate agar; oxidase-positive colonies are transferred to semisolid differential sugar media (*N. meningitidis* ferments glucose and maltose, but not sucrose or lactose). Serotyping is done by agglutination or immunofluorescence. Examination of the cerebrospinal fluid reveals depressed sugar levels (compared with simultaneously drawn and measured blood sugar), and a polymorphonuclear leukocyte count that may be very high. In the absence of cultivable bacteria, spinal fluid should be examined by counterimmunoelectrophoresis (CIE) for polysaccharides of *Meningococcus, H. influenzae* type b, *Pneumococcus,* and *Cryptococcus*.

Treatment and Control. Penicillin G is still the drug of choice; chloramphenicol is an effective alternative in penicillin-sensitive patients. Currently an increasing number of sulfadiazine-sensitive strains are being encountered; sulfadiazine may therefore again become useful in treating meningococcal infection. Intimate household (or other) contacts of proven cases of meningococcal meningitis should be carefully watched for early signs; chemoprophylaxis may be undertaken with rifampicin or sulfadiazine (especially group B). Polysaccharide vaccines against groups A, C, Y, and W-135 are available, and their use should be considered in community outbreaks according to individually assessed risk. Vaccines, however, are not effective in infants under 18 months of age.

INFECTIONS DUE TO BRUCELLA

Brucellosis (Undulant Fever). Undulant fever (Malta fever, Mediterranean fever, Bang's disease in cattle) may be caused by any of three species of the genus *Brucella: B. abortus, B. melitensis* (Melita, Malta), and *B. suis* (Table 5-5). The species names refer to geographic origin or affinities for respective animal hosts in which infectious abortion is prominent (*B. abortus,* cattle; *B. suis,* swine; *B. melitensis,* goats) and which are the sources of human infection. Brucellosis is contracted by ingestion of raw milk from infected cattle or goats, or by direct contact with effluvia or decidua of infected animals. Brucellosis is therefore an occupational hazard for farm, dairy, and abattoir workers; person-to-person transmission does not occur. Fetal tissues from infected animals contain high concentrations of erythritol (not present in significant amounts in human decidua), which serves as a growth factor for *Brucella,* thus accounting for the predilection of the organisms for animal fetal tissues. *Brucella* have potent endotoxic activity but do not form any exotoxin. These organisms invade the bloodstream and localize in lymph nodes, liver, spleen, and glandular tissues; all are facultative intracellular parasites. *B. abortus* tends to form poorly organized granulomata; infections with *B. melitensis* or *B. suis* tend to cause the severest and most protracted clinical illness, which is protean in its manifestations and may include suppurative granulomata with central caseation. Relapses are not uncommon; and serious neurological sequelae have been reported.

A prolonged and variable antibody response characterizes most of these infections and is readily detectable as serum agglutinins for *B. abortus* (broadly cross-reactive with *B. melitensis* and *B. suis*). Agglutinins may be present in the absence of positive blood cultures and, above a certain level (usually about 1:160), are diagnostic. *Brucella* organisms cross-react with *Francisella tularensis* and *Vibrio cholerae,* a fact that must be born in mind in the interpretation of agglutination tests for brucellosis. Primary diagnosis is best made by repeated attempts at recovery of *Brucella* from the blood, from exudates, or from liver biopsy tissue. Blood cultures are taken under CO_2 (required for primary isolation of *B. abortus*) and incubated and periodically subcultured for up to a month. Isolates are speciated by biochemical reactions (Table 5-6) and immunofluorescence. Delayed hypersensitivity is a prominent feature of brucellosis and is concordant with the prolonged intracellular survival of the organisms and with the cell-mediated immune mechanisms involved in pathogenesis and containment of the infection. Diagnostic skin tests with brucellergen, a crude extract of the organism, are no longer recommended because of the risk of severe local and constitutional reactions.

Treatment and Control. Antibiotics of choice in treating proven brucellosis are tetracyclines, with streptomycin. For patients intolerant of tetracyclines, trimethoprim-sulfamethoxazole is used. Therapy should be prolonged well beyond recovery from acute clinical illness. In control of brucellosis, products and tissues of infected animals should be avoided; only pasteurized dairy products should be consumed. Farm animals, particularly cattle, should be tested for brucellosis (Bang's disease) periodically. In the face of threatened infection of a herd, immunization should be undertaken with live attenuated vaccine (attenuated *B. abortus,* strain 19), which itself, however, is the occasional cause of accidental infection in veterinarians and farm personnel. No vaccine is available for human use.

INFECTIONS DUE TO BORDETELLA

Pertussis and Related Diseases. *Bordetella pertussis* is the etiologic agent of pertussis (whooping cough). Syndromes much like classic pertussis, but milder, may be produced by *B. parapertussis* and, rarely, *B. bronchiseptica* (see Table 5-4). All these organisms are related antigenically, and all are easily killed by heat, standard disinfectants, and sunlight.

In the initiation of infection in a susceptible individual, organisms enter the upper respiratory tract in droplets of saliva and mucus from patients with active pertussis. The organisms attach by fimbriae to epithelium, immobilizing the cilia. (The bacterial fimbriae also embody the hemagglutinin characteristic of organisms in young cultures and are part of the protective antigen of *B. pertussis.*) Once the respiratory tract has been colonized, there is damage to superficial epithelial layers by both endotoxin (pyrogenic LPS) and a heat-labile exotoxin, as well as by other biologically active substances elaborated by the organism (lymphocytosis-stimulating and histamine-sensitizing factors). As a result of these changes, the mucous membrane of the respiratory tract becomes hyperesthetic, thereby accounting for the persistent and often strangling cough and stridor characteristic of full-blown pertussis. Obstructive edema and some degree of anoxia occur. With intractable coughing, anoxia may become severe and in infants and young children may trigger convulsions. Large numbers of organisms are found in the viscid, mucoid material coughed up during the first 2 to 3 weeks of the disease, but disappear after the fourth week. Carriers are unknown or very rare; bacteremia does not occur. Infection confers lasting immunity, in which both antibody and cellular factors are important.

Control. Infected children should be isolated from susceptibles for 5 weeks after onset. Susceptible children should be isolated for 3 weeks after last exposure unless examined daily by a physician or school nurse. Young children should never come in contact with infectious cases, since postpertussis pneumonia is a frequent cause of mortality in children under 5.

Three rough variants or phases 2, 3, 4 of low virulence and antigenicity occur in cultures undergoing S to R variation and are not associated with human disease. The vaccine in current use is made of phenol-killed encapsulated smooth (S) phase 1 *B. pertussis,* alum precipitated, and usually combined with alum-precipitated diphtheria and tetanus toxoids (DTP). Presently recommended schedules (CDC Advisory Committee on Immunization Practices) call for routine immunization of infants and children by subcutaneous inoculation with DTP at 2, 4, 6, and 18 months of age, with boosters at 4 to 6 years. Adult type D and P toxoids (Td) should be used after the seventh year. Infants and young children who have previously had convulsions (febrile or nonfebrile) are more likely to have seizures following initial pertussis immunization than those without this history. There is no evidence to suggest that seizures temporally associated with vaccine administration predispose to central nervous system damage. However, deferral of pertussis immunization in patients with any seizure history is recommended; severe reactions (*e.g.,* collapse, shock, persistent screaming episode, fever, or any neurological sign) are strong contraindications to the further administration of pertussis vaccine; this does not apply to diphtheria and tetanus toxoids, which can be independently administered.

Laboratory Diagnosis and Treatment. Plates of Bordet-Gengou blood agar, which may be made more selective by inclusion of methicillin and cycloheximide (to inhibit gram-positive organisms and fungi), are inoculated with fresh respiratory secretions obtained by pernasal swab. Plates are incubated at 35° C for at least 6 days and examined frequently for minute, pearly, hemolytic colonies. Colonies are fished to B-G and blood agar, gram-stained, and identified with immunofluorescence. The same material from the swab, smeared and examined directly by immunofluorescence, may yield an early presumptive diagnosis. Lymphocytosis is a frequent and diagnostic sign in the acute ''whooping'' stage. Antimicrobials have no effect on the clinical course once it has entered the paroxysmal stage. Erythromycin significantly reduces the number of *B. pertussis* in the respiratory tract; corticosteroids may favorably influence severe pertussis.

INFECTIONS DUE TO HAEMOPHILUS

The haemophilic group includes *H. influenzae* (meningitis), *H. parainfluenzae* (endocarditis), *H. aegyptius* (conjunctivitis), and *H. ducreyi* (chancroid) (Table 5-4).

Haemophilus influenzae is a common resident of the normal upper respiratory tract; it does *not* cause the disease influenza, although formerly thought to do so; hence, the species misnomer. *H. influenzae* causes several diseases, including ''pink-eye'' conjunctivitis *(H. aegyptius),* purulent pansinusitis, and severe obstructive epiglottitis and tracheolaryngitis with septicemia. *H. influenzae* type b is the most frequent cause of bacterial meningitis in children 2 months to 5 years of age. This form of meningitis still carries an appreciable mortality, about 35%, and recovery is associated with a substantial incidence of neurological sequelae with 3% to 50% of survivors demonstrating some form of learning disability.

The several serotypes of *H. influenzae* (a to f) are recognized on the basis of capsular polysaccharides (polyribitol phosphate in type b) demonstrable by swelling reactions with type-specific antisera, as with pneumococci; the capsular polysaccharides have antiphagocytic properties and hence are a prime virulence factor. *H. influenzae* produces IgA protease, also possibly an additional factor in virulence. Blood cultures and sputum cultures on chocolate agar are usually positive in acute epiglottitis and laryngotracheobronchitis; blood and spinal fluid cultures are positive in meningitis. On Levinthal transparent agar, typable colonies of *H. influenzae* are immediately recognizable by their characteristic opalescence caused by the massed capsular material. Free capsular polysaccharide can also be detected in cerebrospinal fluid and urine by CIF, an important diagnostic adjunct in the absence of cultivable bacteria. Untypable *H. influenzae* is associated with otitis media in children and with bronchitis and bronchopneumonia in adults suffering from chronic pulmonary disease.

Up to 10% of strains of *H. influenzae* isolated from patients with severe disease are resistant to ampicillin; this resistance is coded for by a plasmid originally derived from *E. coli*. Treatment of meningitis, always life-threatening, should be promptly instituted with chloramphenicol alone or along with ampicillin pending results of the antibiogram. Immunization (after the age of 18 months) with purified capsular polysaccharide of *Hemophilus influenzae* type b has been found to reduce the incidence of meningitis in children between the age of 18 months and 10 years.

Chancroid. Chancroid (soft chancre) is an acute, inflammatory, localized and self-limited necrotizing disease, due to *Haemophilus ducreyi,* occurring on or near the genitalia. It begins as a small pustule, which soon ruptures, leaving an irregular, painful ulcer with undermined edges and a necrotic, erosive, soft base (soft chancre) that spreads rapidly. Like syphilis it usually produces buboes, but, unlike syphilis, these buboes are soft, painful, and often suppurate. Chancroid also differs from syphilitic chancre in the absence of induration and in its violent inflammatory nature. Chancroidlike lesions are sometimes due to (or involve) Herpes simplex virus type 2 and must be differentiated from syphilitic lesions.

Haemophilus ducreyi is typically seen with leukocytes, sometimes in small clusters (''school of fish'' pattern) in direct smears, and morphologically resembles *H. influenzae*. *H. ducreyi* resembles *H. influenzae* also in being very fragile and susceptible to environmental conditions (see Table 5-7).

Diagnosis is based largely on clinical findings and history of exposure. Smears of exudate in chancroid, or of pus aspirated from closed buboes, may reveal the organisms. Rabbit blood (25%) infusion agar (3%) under 10% CO_2 is essential for initial isolation of *H. ducreyi.*

Transmission is typically by sexual intercourse, rarely by fomites. The infection is autoinoculable; pus and exudates are infectious. Although broadspectrum antibiotics (erythromycin) are effective in treatment, the use of antibiotics in any venereal disease entails the danger of masking syphilis, the diagnosis of which should always be excluded by darkfield examination of lesion scrapings and by serology. For this reason, trimethoprim-sulfamethoxazole is considered the treatment of choice.

INFECTIONS DUE TO YERSINIA AND FRANCISELLA

Plaguelike Diseases. This term includes plague, due to *Yersinia pestis;* tularemia, due to *Francisella tularensis*; and hemorrhagic septicemia, due to *Pasteurella multocida.*

All of the above are primarily ***zoonoses*** (animal diseases transmissible to humans) and are fundamentally alike in pathogenesis. All are, in varying degrees, generalized, hemorrhagic, and septicemic, with localization in various organs and tissues and in lymph nodes that become suppurative, painful buboes. In each disease the organisms occur in pathologic exudates (respiratory, ulcers, draining buboes, etc.).

P. multocida infection is neither common nor serious in man but is highly fatal in animals.

Bubonic Plague and Tularemia. In the advanced, septicemic stage in animals these diseases are transmissible to humans by the bites of arthropods: *Yersinia pestis* by rat fleas (*Xenopsylla cheopis* and others) and by arthropod parasites of ground squirrels and other rodents of forest and prairie (***sylvatic*** and ***campestral*** plague, respectively). Plague-infected household pets, particularly cats, can be the source of infection via cat fleas. *Francisella tularensis* is transmitted by deer flies *(Chrysops discalis)* and various ticks (*Dermacentor variabilis, D. andersoni,* etc.). Human-to-human transmission may also occur via fleas, *Pulex irritans.* In either disease an infectious pustule develops at the site of the bite. Local buboes develop (hence, ''bubonic'' plague); in many cases septicemia follows. Tularemia is also transmitted to humans by handling of carcasses of infected animals, notably wild rabbits, resulting in rabbit fever in hunters, market workers, cooks, and others. Lakes and streams contaminated from decaying infected animal carcasses may also be a source of infection by ingestion or inhalation.

The fatality rate in bubonic plague may range from 50% to 80% in untreated cases, but it is much less with early treatment. The less common septicemic plague, which if untreated may go on to pneumonia, is almost invariably fatal. Pneumonic plague may also be contracted by inhalation of respiratory droplets laden with *Y. pestis* from infected patients and is marked by deep cyanosis (the Black Death); when unrecognized and untreated the mortality is 100%.

Tularemia is often very severe, prolonged, and debilitating though rarely fatal if treated early with streptomycin and other broad-spectrum antibiotics. Fatality may range to 5% if untreated. Pulmonary tularemia is especially serious.

Rat flea-borne bubonic plague is prevented by measures that diminish contact between humans and rats (live or dead) and rat fleas. Elimination of open garbage dumps and rat-proofing of buildings are important measures. Dusting rat runways with insecticides to control the fleas, and antirat-poisoning campaigns are often effective. Pneumonic plague is controlled only by prompt diagnosis, immediate and rigid segregation of patients, and expert communicable-disease nursing. Streptomycin, chloramphenicol, and tetracycline are the drugs of choice for the tularemia. Uncomplicated bubonic plague responds to streptomycin, tetracycline, chloramphenicol, or sulfadiazine if treatment is begun early. Streptomycin or tetracyclines are preferred for septicemic plague. A living attenuated vaccine is recommended under special circumstances involving high risk of exposure (*e.g.,* laboratory workers). Chemopropylaxis of plague contacts (*i.e.,* close household contacts) with either tetracycline or sulfadiazine is recommended.

Recovery from both tularemia and bubonic plague confers high-grade, durable immunity, evidenced by sustained levels of agglutinins, which are cross-reactive with *Fr. tularensis* and *V. cholerae.* Cell-mediated immune responses are important in containment of these infections.

In diagnosis, pathologic material stained with Wayson's stain (methylene blue and carbon fuchsin) reveals the organisms as ovoid rods. *Yersinia pestis* is distinguished by having well-marked bipolar staining, most of the cells resembling a closed safety pin. The other species show this character to a lesser degree. The polar granules tend to disappear in cultures.

Yersinia pestis grows well on any media, is motile, and produces an exotoxin and soluble protein antigen (fraction 1) that is antiphagocytic. The lipopolysaccharides of both *Francisella* and *Yersinia* contribute to clinical manifestations of disease. *Yersinia* exhibit capsules and bipolar staining and can be readily identified with fluorescent antibody. *Francisella tularensis* is difficult to recover on primary isolation, for which blood glucose cysteine agar or other media containing sufficient SH compounds are required; the organism is identified by specific agglutination or by fluorescent antibody. Phagocytized by polymorphonuclear leukocytes, *Y. pestis* is killed; in monocytes it survives, multiplies, forms capsules, and gains virulence. *Y. enterocolytica* is an increasingly recognized cause of diarrheal disease, mesenteric adenitis, and self-limited reactive arthritis (associated with HLA-B27).

Legionellaceae. A group of related bacterial pathogens are now subsumed in a newly established family, *Legionellaceae,* the most important member of which is *Legionella pneumophila,* the cause of legionnaires' disease. This was originally described as a fulminant pneumonia with high morbidity and mortality. It has generally been seen in either apparently healthy older patients (mean age of 55 years) or in high-risk renal dialysis and transplant patients as a nosocomial infection.

''Pontiac fever,'' a milder form of the disease, is characterized by pleuritis without pneumonia. The etiologic agent of both these entities was identified as a fastidious unencapsulated, aerobic, pleomorphic, motile, nonsporulating rod, capable of surviving intracellularly as well as in the environment, such as aquatic ecosystems. It is the source of human infection by inhalation of infectious droplets or dust. The organism has a worldwide distribution. Person-to-person transmission has not been documented. The organism *(Legionella pneumophila)* is cultivable on buffered charcoal yeast extract (BCYE) agar and identified by direct immunofluorescence. *Legionella* organisms, albeit gram-negative, stain weakly with Gram's stain; the bacterial cells can be demonstrated in tissues and smears of body fluids with silver impregnation stains and by direct immunofluorescence. By the latter technique, six serogroups of *L. pneumophila* are currently recognized. There are at least 23 other species within the genus, some of which cause milder forms of disease.

"Pittsburgh fever," caused by *L. micdadei* is a pneumonic form that to date has been described only in immunosuppressed patients. Specific antibody response can be demonstrated by indirect immunofluorescence with paired sera; the duration of immunity to reinfection is unknown. *L. pneumophila* multiplies in human blood monocytes. Cell-mediated immunity is of prime importance and humoral immunity of relatively little importance in the containment of this infection. Antibiotics (erythromycin, rifampicin) that penetrate macrophages inhibit but do not kill *L. pneumophila,* a fact that probably helps explain the relapses that may follow antibiotic therapy. Erythromycin is the drug of choice in the treatment of any form of legionellosis, combined with rifampicin in the severest cases.

Actinomycetes and Related Organisms

INFECTIONS DUE TO CORYNEBACTERIUM

Diphtheria. *Corynebacterium* shares cell wall and other characteristics (cord factor, glycolipid, enzymes) with *Nocardia* and *Mycobacteria*. *C. diphtheriae,* the cause of diphtheria, occurs on the oropharyngeal mucosa and in active diseases may spread to larynx, trachea, bronchi, nares, and lips. Strictly aerobic, it is not invasive. However, at the sites of primary infection in the mucosa of the respiratory tract, or on the skin, pathogenic strains produce toxin that has both local and systemic effects on the host. In the respiratory tract, the toxin causes local irritation, an acute inflammatory reaction, and necrosis contributing to pseudomembrane formation. Acute airway obstruction may have to be relieved by intubation or tracheotomy. Toxin absorbed from the local lesion into the lymphatics and bloodstream causes myocardial degeneration and peripheral neuritis.

Transmission from person to person occurs via infected respiratory secretions. Patients with active diphtheria should be isolated until two or three successive daily negative posterior nasal cultures have been obtained. If antibacterial chemotherapy has been employed, negative cultures are of no significance until 1 week after the last dose of drug. The age of incidence of diphtheria has shifted in recent years to involve those 30 to 50 years of age. Skin diphtheria is seen not infrequently, especially in the tropics where fungal infections of the skin may become secondarily infected with toxigenic *C. diphtheriae*.

The ***Schick test*** (undertaken to determine immunity or susceptibility to diphtherial toxin) consists of an intracutaneous injection of active toxin (0.02 guinea pig MLD). A positive reaction, appearing in 24 to 36 hours, consists of slight infiltration surrounded by a red areola 1 to 5 cm in diameter and is caused by the direct dermonecrotic action of the toxin; it is *not* in itself a hypersensitivity reaction. A typical positive reaction does not reach maximal intensity for at least 5 days and may be accompanied by necrosis and sloughing; it indicates that there is less than about 0.01 unit of circulating antitoxin per milliliter, that is, not enough to neutralize either the test toxin or any toxin that might emanate from naturally acquired diphtherial infection. A negative reaction (no erythema) indicates antitoxic immunity. A pseudoreaction, denoting delayed type hypersensitivity to diphtherial protein (engendered by colonization with commensal *Corynebacteria*), recedes after 36 to 48 hours, well before a positive reaction peaks. Persons giving pseudoreactions are immune to the toxin, but allergic to diphtherial protein. Such persons are at risk of having severe adverse reactions to the administration of toxoid. Adults who have a negative Schick test and who are therefore candidates for immunization should be tested first for type IV allergy to diphtherial protein (Moloney test: 0.1 ml. of 1 : 100 fluid toxoid intracutaneously). Positive Moloney reactors may already have antitoxic immunity or will develop it in response to the Moloney test itself. Only those with negative reactions to the Moloney test should be given adult (Td) toxoid.

Laboratory Diagnosis. On slants of Löffler's coagulated-serum medium or Pai's coagulated-egg medium the organisms grow readily at 35° C when inoculated with swabbings from local lesions. Stained with alkaline methylene blue, *C. diphtheriae* has a very distinctive beaded, barred, club-, spindle-, and dumbbell-shaped morphology readily recognized by the experienced bacteriologist. *C. diphtheriae* is readily isolated by streaking throat swabs on blood agar containing about 0.04% of potassium tellurite as a selective agent. Suspicious block colonies are fished to slants for pure culture study, including determinations of type and toxigenicity on freshly prepared Tinsdale (tellurite) agar. *C. diphtheriae* grows in black colonies surrounded by a brown "halo." Staphylococci and commensal *Corynebacteria* (diphtheroids) produce similar black colonies, but without halos. *Listeria monocytogenes* may be misdiagnosed as a "hemolytic diphtheroid."

Suspected diphtheriaelike organisms should be tested for toxigenicity by immunodiffusion (*in vitro* toxigenicity test). A simple form of the latter consists of embedding, in special serum-agar medium in a Petri dish, a strip of filter paper saturated with diphtheria antitoxin. After the agar hardens, the suspected culture is heavily streaked linearly across the agar surface at right angles to the paper. A precipitin reaction, visible as a white line in the agar, develops where toxin diffusing from virulent cultures meets antitoxin diffusing from the paper strip.

All pathogenic (toxigenic) strains of *C. diphtheriae* elaborate antigenically identical toxin. All toxigenic strains of *C. diphtheriae* carry a specific bacteriophage (corynephage beta) that codes for the toxin; strains that are not lysogenic are not toxigenic. The toxin is synthesized as a single polypeptide chain, which can be cleaved by trypsin (and probably tissue enzymes) to yield two portions: fragment A (which, once it is internalized, exerts toxic activity by blocking elongation factors in protein synthesis) and fragment B (which, about twice the size of fragment A, binds whole toxin to cell surfaces and facilitates internalization of toxin molecules). There is striking similarity between diphtherial toxin and other bacterial toxins (*e.g., Shigella* and cholera toxins, *E. coli* enterotoxin, pseudomonas exotoxin A, pertussis, anthrax, tetanus, botulinus toxins) in three general respects: An A-B enzyme-binding structure, receptor-mediated endocytotic penetration into target cells, and ADP-ribosylating activity.

Diphtheria antitoxin is produced commercially by immunization of horses with toxin or toxoid. The globulin fraction is concentrated by standard methods of serum fractionation and is "despeciated" by digestion with pepsin, which reduces its antigenicity by removing most of the Fc portion of the immunoglobulins. The final antitoxin product contains 20,000 units per milliliter and is still allergenic. To be effective (*i.e.,* prevent the effects of toxin on myocardial and neural tissues), antitoxin must be given by intramuscular injection as soon as the diagnosis is established, in order to neutralize free toxin in the circulation; toxin already fixed to tissues can no longer be neutralized. Administration of antitoxin should be preceded by a skin test for hypersensitivity to horse serum (0.1 ml of a 1:1,000 dilution of antitoxin), and epinephrine should be at hand. Whenever antitoxin is administered, in the absence of demonstrable horse serum sensitivity, the development of serum sickness within a week or 10 days should be anticipated. Antibiotics (erythromycin and/or penicillin) are given to treat the upper respiratory tract infection and eliminate the organism, and hence prevent the carrier state. Tonsillectomy and adenoidectomy may be necessary to eliminate the carrier state which persists despite adequate antibiotic therapy.

Recommended immunization schedules (CDC Advisory Committee on Immunization Practices) for normal infants and children call for DTP at 2 to 3 months of age, followed by two boosters, respectively, at 2-month intervals, and a third at 18 months. DTP may be used through the seventh year, after which only adult toxoids (Td) should be administered in order to avoid severe reactions (see Table 5-24).

INFECTIONS DUE TO ACTINOMYCETALES

Tuberculosis. *Mycobacterium tuberculosis,* var. *hominis,* is the principal pathogen of the genus and the etiologic agent of human tuberculosis (TB), which as recently as 1980 was the leading cause of death among 38 notifiable diseases. More than 10 million persons in the United States are infected, with about 30,000 active cases reported yearly. This number is bound to increase with the arrival of immigrants from other areas of the world in which the infection rate is high and because of the recent appearance of drug-resistant strains. These new *M. tuberculosis* strains are increasingly seen in prisons and hospitals. This may be a reflection of higher numbers of immune-suppressed HIV-1-infected, homeless people living under unsanitary conditions. In particular, AIDS patients can get fulminant tuberculosis, which spreads rapidly and is almost uniformly fatal, within several weeks after exposure. Overall, 15 million active cases exist worldwide and 3 million people die annually of TB. Many of the unusual characteristics of the organism are attributable to the extraordinarily high (40%) lipid content of the cell and cell wall, for example, resistance to staining, acid-fastness, slow growth rate, resistance to the action of antibodies plus complement, virulence, and resistance to the action of drying, as well as physical and chemical agents.

A primary infection that follows the inhalation of airborne tubercle bacilli induces in the patients a cell-mediated immune response, detectable by the tuberculin skin test. Delayed or tuberculin-type allergy is directly referable to intracellular persistence of tubercle bacilli and greatly affects the course of the disease in either reinfection or reactivation type seen in adults. Resistance to reinfection, which is usually endogenous, depends on the capacity of the host to contain the organism by the same cell-mediated mechanisms that produce the inflammatory response in delayed dermal hypersensitivity, that is, T lymphocytes and lymphokines such as MIF and MAF.

Consequences of infection depend upon the immune status of the host, size of the inoculating dose, and virulence of the bacilli. Progressive tuberculosis is a chronic granulomatous process that may eventually involve multiple organ systems. The concept of tuberculous infection is to be distinguished from that of tuberculous disease. Both generate cell-mediated immune responses.

Specimens collected for smear and culture include 24-hour sputa, gastric washings (especially desirable for infants, for some adults who swallow their sputum, and for sputum-negative individuals with minimal activity), 24-hour urines, cerebrospinal fluid, and other appropriate materials. Microscopic examination of direct smears stained with either the Kinyoun acid-fast or the fluorescent dye techniques may not reveal any acid-fast bacilli. Sediments of specimens concentrated by centrifugation following digestion using one of several standard techniques provide better material from which to isolate tubercle bacilli. Cultures are an absolute necessity for speciation of mycobacteria because identification cannot be accomplished using only microscopic morphology.

Growth on solid media such as coagulated egg proteins (*e.g.*, Lowenstein-Jensen medium) or oleic acid-albumin (*e.g.*, Dubos-Middlebrook medium) permits observations regarding colonial morphology, thermal tolerance, and growth rate and also provides organisms for various biochemical tests, for example, niacin production, nitrate reduction, Tween-80 hydrolysis, catalase activity; for virulence tests, for example, serpentine cord formation or presence of cord factor, neutral red binding, guinea pig inoculation; and drug-susceptibility assays (see Table 5-7).

M. tuberculosis grows best at 37° C and requires 2 to 4 weeks to produce typical, dry, crumbly, cornmeal-like colonies. The organism is niacin positive, reduces nitrate to nitrite, does not hydrolyse Tween-80, is negative for catalase activity after heating at 68° C for 20 minutes, produces cord factor (serpentine cords), binds neutral red dye, and is virulent for guinea pigs.

Antigens used in the tuberculin skin test are standardized based on milligrams of tuberculoprotein and expressed as tuberculin units (TU), old tuberculin (OT), or purified protein derivative (PPD). One milligram standard PPD contains 50,000 TU. Intermediate strength PPD equals 5 TU (OT $\frac{1}{2000}$). The greatest value of the tuberculin skin test is in the detection of those individuals whose reactions have converted from negative to positive. Equivocal reactions may be seen in patients infected with a mycobacterial species other than *M. tuberculosis,* in which instances, species-specific antigens may be used to aid in the differentiation process. Antituberculous drugs are prescribed for converters with clinical symptoms and may be prescribed for prophylaxis for asymptomatic converters. The latter should be distinguished by their age and the chronology of their responses to PPD-testing from persons who show a "booster" response and who may therefore be presumed to have long-standing infection and should not be treated.

A vaccine (BCG, bacille Calmette-Guérin), prepared from an attenuated strain of *M. bovis,* is available for prophylactic immunization. The vaccine should be administered only to those who are nonreactive to tuberculin. Although the vaccine is widely used in Europe and other countries, its use in the United States is highly restricted to certain high-risk groups, such as young children in a household in which there is an open case of tuberculosis. Immunization vitiates the usefulness of the tuberculin test. BCG should not be given to anyone with a positive tuberculin (PPD) skin test.

Many BCG vaccines are available, all derived from the original strain, but varying widely in immunogenicity, efficacy, and reactogenicity. Lasting protection cannot be assured by vaccination. Therefore tuberculosis must be included in the differential diagnosis even in vaccinees.

Treatment usually consists of a combination of drugs (at least two) to increase therapeutic effectiveness and to minimize the emergence of drug-resistant mutants. When the patient's bacterial population is thought to be particularly large, three drugs are frequently used during the early phase of therapy, for instance when there are extensive infiltrates or cavitary lesions and thus bacilli can be found on direct smears of unconcentrated sputum.

Isoniazid (INH), rifampicin, ethambutol, and streptomycin are generally considered first-line drugs. The most frequently used regimen in the United States is a combination of the first two. Prevention of infection secondary to open cases is effectively achieved by isoniazid, especially if the tuberculin test is negative, indicating maximal susceptibility, or in cases in which tuberculin tests have converted recently from negative to positive. In the latter instance, whether or not roentgenographic evidence of tuberculosis is present, INH is indicated to prevent progression of active disease. With short-course chemotherapy (twice weekly isoniazid and rifampin for 9 months), a 95% success rate has been reported. When drug-resistance is identified, streptomycin and pyrazinamide are added. When there is reason to suspect isoniazid resistance, residence in a developing country or past exposure to antituberculous drugs, therapy should be started with four drugs initially (streptomycin, INH, rifampin, pyrazinamide). However, as noted above there is an increasing appearance of multiresistant strains, some of which are resistant to more than 50% of the most frequently used drugs. In part, this reflects the fact that patients do not always take the full course of drugs (up to 18 months) they have been prescribed, so that all bacteria are not killed.

Other mycobacterial species, although less pathogenic for man than *M. tuberculosis,* are capable of causing human tuberculous disease and therefore present diagnostic and therapeutic problems. *M. bovis* causes bovine tuberculosis and at one time was a leading cause of human tuberculosis. *M. avium,* the cause of avian tuberculosis, has been isolated from human pulmonary lesions. In particular, *M. avian-intracellulare,* which is normally found in soil and water, has become a significant opportunistic pathogen among AIDS patients. *M. ulcerans* is the etiologic agent of chronic cutaneous tuberculosis. Species classified in the Runyon groups I–IV, sometimes called the "atypical mycobacteria," cause both pulmonary disease and chronic cutaneous lesions. Identification of these less virulent mycobacterial species is necessary because many of them exhibit responses to chemotherapeutic drugs, which are different from those of *M. tuberculosis.* The close antigenic relationships that exist among the mycobacteria make immunologic differentiation difficult or impossible. Identification therefore depends upon accurate observations regarding colonial morphology, nutritional and environmental influences on growth and growth rate, and precise performance of the variety of biochemical tests described in other literature (Table 5-8).

Leprosy. *Mycobacterium leprae,* the etiologic agent of human leprosy, has never been cultured either on lifeless media or in tissue explants. A generation time of 20 to 30 days has been obtained from serial passages in mouse foot pads. Lesion distribution suggests a diminished ability to multiply in body areas where temperatures exceed 30° C. In tissues, the acid-fast organism closely resembles *M. tuberculosis*. Athymic (''nude'') mice offer a good host cell medium for propagation of *Mycobacterium leprae*. The nine-banded armadillo has been shown to develop a chronic infection in which *M. leprae* multiplies to high numbers and with little harm to the animal.

M. leprae is probably as communicable as *M. tuberculosis*. However, the portal of entry, method of spread, genesis of lesions, and manner of dissemination are still unclear. Children are infected more readily than adults. Disease usually occurs in individuals who live in endemic areas, such as Africa, Asia, Pacific islands (in a recent survey, more than 1,100 cases in Micronesia, twice the 1977 total), and certain areas of the United States and who have a history of long and close contacts with leprosy patients. An increasing number of new cases are reported annually in the United States, all thought to have been imported from Southeast Asia and Latin America. The usually prolonged incubation period varies from several months to 30 years. Regardless of the portal of entry and incubation period, the bacilli eventually find their way to the mucous membranes, skin, and peripheral nerves, giving rise to cutaneous lesions and peripheral anesthesias.

The tuberculoid or mild form and the lepromatous or progressive form are the two recognized types of leprosy. Tuberculoid leprosy lesions are usually localized and confined to the skin, mucous membranes, and area nerves. Histologically, they resemble tubercles and are comprised of epithelioid cells, lymphocytes, and plasma cells; there is usually no caseation, and organisms are rare. In contrast, lepromatous leprosy lesions appear as cutaneous nodules called lepromas that occur principally on the face and extremities, but may involve the liver, spleen, bone marrow, viscera, and other areas. Histologically, the lepromas are composed of lymphocytes, plasma cells, and lipid-laden macrophages and giant cells (called lepra cells) containing numerous bacilli arranged in bundles or globular masses (globi).

The status of the patient's cellular immune system and the ability to mount a competent cell-mediated immune response determines to a large degree the type of leprosy that will develop. Tuberculoid leprosy is seen in the more resistant patients whereas lepromatous leprosy is seen in patients with T-lymphocyte defects.

Patients with tuberculoid leprosy react positively to intradermal injections of lepromin, an antigen derived from homogenized leprous tissue, and to tuberculin. Lepromatous leprosy patients give a negative response to lepromin, indicating a defect in the cell-mediated immune responses. This absence of a cutaneous delayed type hypersensitivity reaction reflects a lack of $CD4^+$ T-cell infiltration into the lesion. Normal individuals, persons immunized with BCG, and tuberculosis patients also give a positive reaction to lepromin, indicating cross-reactivity with tuberculoproteins and tissue antigens. The only real value of the lepromin test rests in its ability to identify anergic leprosy patients.

Excepting injuries stemming from peripheral anesthesias, complications of leprosy appear to have an immunologic origin, such as erythema nodosum, erythema necroticans, and others.

Sulfone drugs are most effective in treatment, especially dapsone (DDS, 4′-4′-diamino-diphenyl-sulfone). Rifampin kills *M. leprae* and shows promise as a useful drug. Clofazimine has been shown to suppress the erythema nodosum reaction in the lepromatous form.

INFECTIONS DUE TO ACTINOMYCES AND NOCARDIA

Actinomyces and *Nocardia* species are gram-positive bacilli that grow slowly, producing delicate, branching filaments that tend to fragment into bacillary elements. These organisms and the infections they cause are usually grouped and studied with the fungi for the reasons stated previously and because they cause chronic infections characterized by suppuration and abscess and granuloma formation. The two genera are classified into separate families, Actinomycetaceae and Nocardiaceae, respectively, based on oxygen requirements, catabolic activities, and cell wall composition. *Actinomyces* species, part of the normal oral flora, are anaerobic, ferment carbohydrates, are non-acid-fast, and their cell walls do not contain diaminopimelic acid (DAP). *Nocardia* species are soil inhabitants, are aerobic, produce acid from carbohydrates oxidatively, are partially acid-fast, and contain meso-DAP and nocardiomycolic acid in their cell walls.

Among the *Actinomyces* species, *Actinomyces israelii,* and *Actinomyces bovis* are the principal etiologic agents of actinomycosis, the former in humans, the latter in cattle. Differentiation of the two species is dependent upon biochemical tests such as nitrate reduction, starch hydrolysis, carbohydrate fermentations; upon serologic tests such as immunofluorescent tests (FA) and immunodiffusion tests (IG); upon the appearance of micro- and macrocolonies; and upon microscopic morphology.

The disease is seen more frequently in cattle than in humans. The organisms are indigenous in humans and probably in cattle, initiating infection following oral tissue trauma. Bovine infections, called "lumpy jaw," usually involve the mandible with the formation of tumefactions, abscesses, fistulas and sinus tracts, producing soft-tissue and bone destruction and marked cicatrization. The disease is chronic, spreading to contiguous tissues rather than involving blood and lymph vessels. The animal's general health is not affected unless mastication or breathing is impaired.

Human actinomycosis occurs as cervicofacial, abdominal, and thoracic infections. Similar to the bovine counterpart in its initiation and clinical picture, the cervicofacial type is the most common and has the best prognosis. Abdominal actinomycosis is thought to arise from swallowing *A. israelii* bacilli or from abdominal trauma and may occur concurrently with or in the absence of a preexisting cervicofacial infection. Abdominal disease often involves the appendix with spread to nearby tissues. Symptoms are referable to the organ systems involved. Thoracic actinomycosis is thought to arise as an extension through the neck from a cervicofacial infection or as an extension through the diaphragm from hepatic infection or as a primary infection initiated by aspirating organisms present in the mouth. Symptoms are those of a subacute pulmonary infection, often resembling tuberculosis. Disseminated infections may occur, and death may supervene as a result of secondary bacterial infections. Rarely are pure cultures of *Actinomyces israelii* (or *Actinomyces bovis*) obtained from lesions or exudates.

In purulent discharges from the sinus tracts, minute yellow-white granules are found ("sulfur granules"). The granules, crushed under a coverslip and examined microscopically, are composed of tangled, branching filaments with peripheral ends radially arranged and clubbed. After being washed to remove contaminants, the granules should be cultured in a broth medium containing a reducing agent or on blood agar and incubated anaerobically at 37° C. Examination of cultures for microcolonies at 48 hours and macrocolonies at 14 days facilitates identification.

Penicillin, the drug of choice, is administered intravenously in doses that vary from 3 to 20 million units per day, depending on the severity of the disease. Energetic surgical intervention to incise and drain lesions and to excise lesions and devitalized tissues is highly recommended. Other drugs used for therapy are tetracycline, chloramphenicol, streptomycin, and sulfadiazine. Antibiotic therapy should be continued for 12 to 18 months following surgical procedures.

Nocardiosis is an acute or chronic disease usually caused by *Nocardia asteroides*. It most often begins as a primary pulmonary infection characterized by suppuration, less frequently by granuloma formation. Bacilli are hematogenously disseminated to subcutaneous tissues and other organs, particularly the central nervous system where they produce multiple abscesses in the brain and meninges. Delicate, branching filaments that are gram-positive and acid-fast are seen in sputum, infected tissues, and exudates from abscesses. Granules are not produced.

Nocardiosis is a term usually reserved for primary pulmonary infections or systemic infections resulting from dissemination from a pulmonary locus. Other infections caused by the *Nocardia* are mycetoma, a localized, chronic process characterized by the development of tumefactions, abscesses, fistulas, and sinus tracts, and the lymphocutaneous syndrome characterized by the progression of abscesses along a lymphatic channel, producing a clinical picture similar to that seen in lymphocutaneous sporotrichosis. Granules, composed of fine, radially arranged, branching, acid-fast filaments with or without terminal clubbing, are produced and found in exudates from mycetoma lesions. Granule morphology facilitates a presumptive diagnosis by permitting differentiation between bacterial and fungal etiology. Mycetoma is usually caused by *Nocardia brasiliensis* or *Nocardia caviae*. *N. brasiliensis* is the usual etiologic agent of the lymphocutaneous syndrome. All are soil microbes, initiating infections following inhalation or traumatic cutaneous implantation of the bacilli.

Sputum from nocardiosis patients and deep-tissue biopsies (preferred because fewer contaminants are present) or granules (processed as are actinomycosis granules) from mycetoma patients are cultured on Sabouraud's dextrose or blood agar without added antibiotics and incubated aerobically and anaerobically at 22° C and 37° C. All three species produce similar colonies that appear as dry, brittle, orange or yellow, cauliflowerlike, or cerebriform growths that are often covered with a short-napped mycelium. Speciation of nocardia is based on biochemical reactions, principally casein, tyrosine, and xanthine hydrolysis and oxidative acid production from carbohydrates.

Sulfadiazine, the drug of choice for nocardiosis, is administered in doses of 3 to 10 g/day to achieve a blood level of 9 to 20 mg/100 ml (depending upon the severity of the infection) for 3 to 6 months. Sulfamethoxazole is also effective. Therapy for mycetoma depends upon the etiologic agent; bacterial or actinomycotic mycetoma responds to antibiotic or antibacterial drugs, whereas eumycotic mycetoma is extremely refractory to antibiotics or antimycotic drugs. Early actinomycotic mycetoma lesions (before bone involvement) respond to sulfadiazine. More advanced cases respond to high doses of penicillin. Surgical intervention to drain abscesses and remove devitalized tissues augments healing.

Pathogenic Anaerobic Bacilli

Improved techniques with prereduced media and specialized apparatus have greatly enhanced our capability to isolate strictly anaerobic bacteria from blood, exudates, and affected tissues; the application of gas-liquid chromatography (GLC) has been central to elucidating the distinctive biochemical patterns of these organisms. Their often rigid requirements for anaerobiosis depend on lack of cytochrome respiratory chains, despite the presence of flavoprotein enzymes that transfer hydrogen to free oxygen to form H_2O_2, a very toxic product; and failure of strict anaerobes to form peroxidase or catalase to destroy H_2O_2, or of superoxide dismutase to destroy superoxide radicals. Prominent among the anaerobes are endospore-forming rods, *Clostridium* species (see Table 5-8), various species of gram-negative, nonsporulating pleomorphic rods (see Table 5-6), and *Peptostreptococcus* and *Peptococcus* (see earlier sections). On initial isolation, these organisms (especially the gram-negative rods) require strictly anaerobic conditions and rich organic media, such as cooked chopped meat, or special anaerobic media. Diseases caused by clostridia are primarily intoxications; those caused by anaerobic gram-negative organisms are always endogenous metastatic pyogenic infections.

DISEASES CAUSED BY CLOSTRIDIA

Tetanus. *Clostridium tetani,* the cause of tetanus or lockjaw, has the general properties of the genus (see Table 5-9). It is not invasive but grows well in dead tissue; there it can produce its soluble exotoxin. It normally inhabits superficial layers of the soil, especially of cultivated and manured fields, because of its regular presence in the feces of domestic and wild animals and sometimes of man. The spores of *C. tetani* resist dry heat at 150° C for 1 hour, autoclaving at 121° C for 5 to 10 minutes and 5% phenol for 12 to 15 hours. Protected from sunlight (ultraviolet light), the dried spores remain viable for many years. Toxin interferes with neuromuscular transmission by inhibiting release of acetylcholine from nerve terminals in muscle. Muscle spasms are due to interference, by the toxin, with spinal cord synaptic reflexes, leading to inhibition of antagonists (strychninelike action). Secondary disturbances of autonomic functions occur.

Tetanus Toxin. Tetanus neurotoxin, the structural gene which is on a plasmid, has marked affinity for nervous tissue and reaches the central nervous system (spinal cord) via the blood and lymphatics, especially those associated with nerve trunks.

Tetanus bacilli or spores are doubtless frequently introduced into wounds. The nature of the wound determines whether the bacilli can proliferate. Deep (anaerobic), soil-contaminated wounds in which there has been considerable tissue destruction are especially likely to supply these conditions.

Tetanus neonatorum occurs especially when filthy conditions surround parturition with infection of the umbilical stump by feces and soil containing *C. tetani* spores.

In the acute form of tetanus the incubation time ranges from 3 to 14 days; in the chronic form the incubation period may exceed a month.

Recognition of conditions favoring development of tetanus should prompt measures to prevent it, that is, adequate surgical debridement of contaminated wounds supplemented by administration of systemic antibiotics (penicillin or alternative). In individuals without known prior immunization, tetanus immune globulin (TIg, human) should be infiltrated around the wound and given systemically, up to a total of 10,000 units; one dose is usually sufficient. In individuals with known prior immunization, 0.5 ml of tetanus toxoid should be given if the time of injury is more than 3 to 5 years after the last booster. Previously immunized individuals begin to produce adequate levels of antitoxin within 2 to 4 hours after a booster dose of toxoid. Basic primary immunity is achieved by routine immunization of infants with DPT at 2, 4, and 6 months of age (see Table 5-23). Boosters are given at 18 months and at 4 to 6 years of age. After the 6th year, 0.5 ml alum-precipitated toxoid boosters need be given only at 10-year intervals or whenever tetanus-prone injury is sustained more than 3 to 5 years after a booster.

The diagnosis of tetanus is made entirely on clinical grounds and once established (mortality up to 40%) requires intensive supportive care: muscle relaxants, neuromuscular blocking agents (in collaboration with the anesthesiologist), respiratory assistance, attention to fluid balance.

Gas Gangrene (Clostridial Myositis). Gas gangrene may occur when deep (anaerobic), contused wounds are contaminated with soil that contains spores of one or more of several species of clostridia. Devitalized tissue provides an environment with lowered redox potential that favors the germination and multiplication of anaerobic bacteria. *Clostridium perfringens,* the principal agent in gas gangrene, inhabits the mammalian intestine and female genital tract and soil and is nearly always accompanied in infected wounds by one or more other soil clostridia that act synergistically with *C. perfringens: C. putrificum, C. histolyticum, C. novyi, C. fallax, C. septicum,* and others; the bacteriology is rather variable and heterogeneous. *C. tetani* is also commonly present. As in tetanus, whether or not gas gangrene develops depends on the nature of the wound and the virulence of the bacteria present. Approximately 30 species of *Clostridium* have been isolated from human infections. Taxonomic differentiation, usually impractical for the routine diagnostic laboratory, is based on morphologic and cultural characteristics and on gas-liquid chromatography to identify fermentation products.

Clinical manifestations of clostridial infections are highly varied. Clostridial food poisoning ranks second or third on the list of common forms, usually involves ingestion of meat contaminated with *C. perfringens*; and has an attack rate of 50% to 70%. Diarrheal disease is caused by heat-labile protein enterotoxin associated with the spore coat that is released as the ingested vegetative cells are lysed in the intestine. Maximum activity occurs in the ileum. The toxin inhibits glucose transport and causes protein loss into the intestinal lumen. Diagnosis is made by isolation of toxigenic *Clostridium perfringens* from food and/or feces of afflicted patients. Enteritis necrotans is caused by ingestion of meat contaminated with *Clostridium perfringens* type C, the β-toxin of which is the cause of an acute ulcerative process, restricted to the small intestine in which the mucosa is denuded and sloughed. It is accompanied by acute abdominal pain, bloody diarrhea, vomiting, shock, and a high incidence of peritonitis by direct extension; it is frequently fatal. A somewhat similar process has been recognized as occurring in association with prolonged broad-spectrum antibiotic therapy, most often clindamycin, in the presence of which *Clostridium difficile,* a member of the normal flora, overgrows to produce a potent necrotizing toxin, which is heat labile and acid sensitive. Vancomycin is effective in suppressing *C. difficile. Clostridium perfringens* and *Clostridium ramosum* together represent almost half of the total isolates from clostridial infections of soft tissue, which can occur in almost any region of the body and in which devitalization of tissue and polymicrobial contamination promote anaerobic conditions. These include intra-abdominal and abdominal sepsis, carcinoma, empyema and pelvic, brain, pulmonary, prostatic, and perianal abscesses. Localized infection of the skin and subcutaneous tissue occurs, particularly in compromised patients such as diabetics and heroin addicts (suppurative myositis), and may develop into diffuse spreading cellulitis and fasciitis, with widespread gas formation, toxemia, shock, renal failure, and intravascular hemolysis, ending in death. *C. perfringens, ramosum,* and *septicum* may be recovered in blood cultures. In contrast to the foregoing, clostridial myonecrosis (gas gangrene) is a process in which muscle destruction is prominent, in association with crepitance and systemic toxemia, and usually follows trauma or a surgical procedure (*e.g.,* elective colon resection, biliary tract surgery). Gram-stained water discharges show myriad gram-positive rods and relatively few inflammatory cells. Blood cultures frequently yield *Clostridia. C. perfringens* accounts for 80% of cases, the remaining being attributable to *C. novyi, septicum,* and *bifermentans.*

Diagnosis rests on the characteristic appearance of affected muscle, which initially is pale, edematous, and devitalized, progressing inward to frank gangrene. The same condition may occur in the absence of evident trauma (nontraumatic myonecrosis) and is occasionally associated with silent colonic carcinoma. Septic abortion and, less frequently, normal delivery may be complicated by uterine myonecrosis, usually signaled by jaundice, massive intravenous hemolysis (due to the α-toxin lecithinase) and renal failure with hemoglobinuria, and hypotension. Uncomplicated clostridial bacteremia may occur in the absence of clear-cut localizing signs of infection.

Central to treatment is adequate debridement, along with judiciously selected antimicrobial therapy, particularly of suppurative infections in which broad-spectrum antibiotics can serve to suppress aerobic as well as anaerobic bacteria in this invariably polymicrobial infection (aerobes: aminoglycosides such as gentamicin, tobramycin, amikacin; anaerobes: clindamycin, chloramphenicol, metronidazole, cefoxitin). Penicillin G is maximally effective against *C. perfringens.* The use of pentavalent clostridial antitoxin is controversial and should be limited to those patients clearly exhibiting toxemia (hemoglobinemia, disseminated intravascular coagulation, shock, renal failure). The decision to use it must be weighed against the hazards of serum sickness or anaphylactic shock. Skin tests should precede the administration of antitoxin (horse serum). Exchange erythrocyte transfusion to remove damaged erythrocytes has adjunctive therapeutic value. Hyperbaric oxygen, also a controversial topic, has its proponents. Substantial risks are involved and the number of centers with hyperbaric chambers is limited. It cannot replace other modalities of therapy focused on containing and obliterating the source of infection according to good surgical principles.

Botulism (Food Poisoning). Botulism was first described in cases of poisoning by meat sausage (botulus is Latin for sausage). *C. botulinum* may grow in sausages, hams, and canned foods of any sort not too dry and not too acid (limiting *p*H 4.5) for growth, that are contaminated with soil or marine sediment (E spores); anaerobically packed; and heat processed at a temperature inadequate to kill spores of *C. botulinum,* which are highly resistant to heat and drying. In storage at room temperatures the spores germinate and the growing bacilli form the potent exotoxin. Under commercial canning conditions in the United States, botulism is uncommon.

The ability of organisms to produce botulinus toxin (the most neurotoxic substance known) is mediated by specific bacteriophage. In contrast to most exotoxins, botulinus toxin is not actively secreted into the tissues or growth medium; rather it is produced inside the bacterial cell and released only on the death and lysis of vegetative *C. botulinum.* Types A, B, and, less commonly, E and F affect humans; types C and D affect ungulates, and type E affects avian species. The toxins are antigenically distinct polypeptides with a molecular weight of about 140,000 daltons. The toxins spread hematogenously to the motor nerves, where the large subunit of the toxin molecule binds to specific acceptors on nerve terminal membranes. Toxin is then internalized by the acceptors in an energy-dependent step and, by antagonizing the effects of Ca^{2+}, irreversibly inhibits release of acetylcholine from peripheral nerves. Botulinus toxin is inactivated by boiling for 10 minutes or by heating to 80° C for 30 minutes and by ultraviolet light.

Botulism presents as an afebrile neurological disorder, characterized by symmetrical descending weakness or paralysis (diplopia, photophobia, fixed pupils, dysphonia, dysarthria, dysphagia, respiratory muscle weakness), diminished salivation, oropharyngeal desiccation, ileus, and urinary retention. Any or all of these signs and symptoms may occur beginning 6 hours to 8 days after ingestion of toxin-containing food. Specific diagnosis rests on a demonstration of toxin in the blood or in the stool and/or food, in which *Clostridium botulinum* may also be found (mouse bioassay for toxin). Death is from respiratory failure. Polyvalent antitoxin (horse serum) preceded by a skin test is recommended, 1 vial intravenously, 1 intramuscularly. Expectant supportive care is essential, particularly respiratory care, and may be lifesaving, because intoxication is self-limited. Contamination wounds have been reported as a primary source of botulin. Infantile botulism (the hypotonic or ''floppy'' infant) and sudden infant death syndrome (SIDS) can both be caused by botulin (types A and B) emanating from organisms that colonize the gastrointestinal tract from some unknown source, *e.g.*, bee honey.

INFECTIONS DUE TO NONSPORULATING ANAEROBIC BACILLI

The indigenous microbiota of humans is heavily weighted in favor of the anaerobes: by factors of 10:1 on the skin and in the vagina, 100:1 in the oral cavity, and as much as 1,000:1 in the large intestine (see Table 5-6). Life-threatening infections (*e.g.,* lung or brain abscess, peritonitis, septicemia, septic abortion, etc.) caused by endogenous pyogenic anaerobes are now more frequently recognized than disease due to the clostridia. ***Kawasaki disease*** (mucocutaneous lymph node syndrome), a multisystem disease of young children, may be caused by an unknown human retrovirus or by *Propionibacterium acnes,* a common intestinal and skin inhabitant in older age groups. The disease is not favorably influenced by antibiotics. Recovery of fastidious pyogenic anaerobes from clinical specimens requires correct use of prereduced transport medium for sample collection and, in the laboratory, appropriate anaerobic environmental systems and special media for primary isolation. Speciation of isolates is accomplished by GLC of metabolic products, which gives elution patterns characteristic of each strain of bacteria. The most accessible natural source of these organisms is the oral cavity, where they constitute a major portion of the normal flora, but where they may also be directly related to pathology of periodontal disease, root canal infections, and other localized lesions destructive of teeth and supporting tissues. Each of these pathologic conditions, while of immediate concern for the dental surgeon, may be the source of metastatic systemic infection at distant sites. It may seem paradoxical that strict anaerobes, highly sensitive to oxygen, should normally inhabit the oral cavity, which is constantly exposed to hot air. However, anaerobic conditions (anaerobiosis, lowered redox potential) are maintained by the presence of necrotic tissue in periodontal and crevicular spaces as well as through the utilization of oxygen by commensal aerobic bacteria inhabiting the same microenvironment.

A presumptive diagnosis of anaerobic infection is suggested by foul-smelling putrid exudate or discharge from sites in which anaerobes normally occur, by evident tissue necrosis and gas formation (crepitus), by failure to recover potential pathogens on routine aerobic culture (culture under CO_2 is *not* anaerobic), and, most importantly, by Gram's stain of exudate or pus from the lesion. The latter may be the only clue on which to base therapy pending results of anaerobic culture and GLC analysis.

Pathogenic Aerobic Bacilli

DISEASES DUE TO AEROBIC BACILLI

Anthrax. Anthrax, due to *Bacillus anthracis,* a strict aerobe, is primarily a disease of domestic herbivora grazing on spore-infested pastures. It is contracted by humans usually via skin abrasions, mainly from tissues or body fluids of infected animals and handling spore-contaminated hides or wool from infected animals or fertilizer made from infected bone meal. Spores sometimes occur in dust on sheep's wool or other animal hair, and inhalation of the infectious dust produces a dangerous pneumonic form of anthrax (called wool-sorters' disease). Gastrointestinal anthrax, highly fatal, may also occur. Infection of the face through improperly sterilized shaving brushes and analogous accidents have occurred. A skin lesion (malignant pustule) is most typical.

Most species of *Bacillus* are harmless, motile, ubiquitous saprophytes of the soil and environment. *B. anthracis* is distinctive, being highly pathogenic, nonmotile, and nonhemolytic. *B. cereus* is a hemolytic, harmless species closely similar to *B. anthracis*. Most species of *Bacillus* are more or less strict aerobes or facultative and readily cultivable on simple peptone media or blood agar at 25° C to 40° C. Oval spores occur near the middle of anthrax bacilli without swelling the rod. Anthrax spores are long lived and unusually resistant to heat and chemicals. In infected tissues *B. anthracis* forms a large polypeptide capsule that is antiphagocytic and therefore associated with virulence.

In ***cutaneous anthrax,*** the most common form, the characteristic ulcer appears within about 24 hours after infection, teeming with bacilli. Its center soon changes into a black, central necrotic area with markedly edematous areola, spreading eschar (''malignant pustule'') and painful local lymphadenopathy. With severe local reactions, especially around the head and neck, toxemia may occur (''malignant edema''). Anthrax in any form, but especially pulmonary and gastrointestinal forms with toxemia, is accompanied by bacteremia and may be the source of hematogenous meningitis. Penicillin is the drug of choice in therapy. Cortisone is indicated in cases of malignant edema. Penicillin-allergic patients can be successfully treated with erythromycin, tetracycline, or chloramphenicol.

A potent and complex protein exotoxin consisting of three distinct factors was first discovered in tissues and exudates of infected animals and was later demonstrated in cultures rich in serum and bicarbonate ions, which also increase capsule production. Virulence of *B. anthracis* depends on production of both capsules and toxin. Infection evokes antibodies against both. Nontoxigenic, encapsulated variants occur.

Control. Careful incineration or deep burial of dead animals, their exudates, and contaminated straw is necessary. Animal autopsies should not be performed on farms, as all body fluids and tissues are highly infectious, and exposure to air induces anthrax organisms to sporulate. Legislation requires disinfection of hides, wool, bone meal fertilizer, and brush bristles in commercial use.

During an outbreak, unaffected animals should be immunized with a spore vaccine available for veterinary use and/or a ''protective antigen'' (PA) vaccine (alum-precipitated toxoid). The latter can be used to immunize persons who may be at particular risk.

Diagnosis. Gram-stained smears of pus or exudate, body fluids, tissues, or blood (from animals moribund or dead of anthrax) show characteristic encapsulated rods. Cultures on ordinary blood agar of these materials readily yield large nonhemolytic colonies, and the diagnosis can be confirmed by immunofluorescence or mouse inoculation.

Pathogenic Spirochetes

The order Spirochaetales (spirochetes) includes spiral, flexible bacteria (contrast with rigid *Spirillum*). Although procaryons, the spirochetes are structurally the most complex of bacteria, consisting of three principal parts: an outer envelope or periplast probably containing murein, on which marked susceptibility of some species to penicillin presumably depends; the cell proper, an elongated cylindrical tube with cytoplasmic membrane; a fibrillar, axial filament arising, like flagella (and, seemingly like them, contractile), from basal granules at one end of the tubular cell and gathered into a bundle constituting an axial filament around which the cell is wound helically. In general, spirochetes are not readily stained and are commonly examined in the living state in moist material by means of the darkfield microscope. (See also Fluorescent Antibody-Staining Technique.)

The order contains numerous saprophytes, and only a few genera are of medical importance.

All pathogenic spirochetes are quite fragile and readily killed by drying, heat, and disinfectants. However, they can survive for years at $-76°$ C.

TREPONEMAL DISEASES

Syphilis. *Treponema pallidum,* the cause of syphilis, is from 4 μm to 20 μm in length and 0.2 μm in diameter. The cytoplasm is surrounded by a trilaminar cytoplasmic membrane, a delicate inner mucopeptide layer (periplast), and an outer lipoprotein membrane containing lipopolysaccharides. Three fibrils are inserted into the tapered ends of the cell. The organism has 4 to 14 coils and differs from *Borrelia* (see below) in the tightness and regularity of its coils. Its distinctive movements consist of occasional rotation about the long axis, slow to-and-fro gliding and occasional sedate bending.

For diagnostic darkfield examination fluid should be taken from a cleanly scraped chancre or, better, punctured bubo and should contain as little blood and solid material as possible. Dried smears, negatively stained with India ink, nigrosin, or other stains in lieu of darkfield for diagnosis can lead to error because distinctive motility permits some degree of differentiation from saprophytic treponemes of the genitalia.

Spirochetes are demonstrated in tissues by the silver impregnation method of Levaditi or Fontana. *Treponema pallidum* has never been cultivated in a virulent state on artificial media, though several readily cultured nonpathogenic strains (notably the Reiter strain) morphologically identical with, and antigenically very closely similar to, *T. pallidum* are well known.

Demonstrable immunity appears in 2 to 4 weeks after appearance of the primary lesion (chancre) when standard serologic tests (SST or STS) become positive. Specific antitreponemal tests also become positive.

Primary (2 to 6 weeks) and secondary stages (4 weeks to 4 months) subside with developing specific resistance. Years later, tertiary gummatous lesions of arteries, central nervous system, bones, viscera, and other organs, with intense cytologic response and necrosis, probably related to allergy, develop. Transplacental transmission leads to congenital syphilis, which continues at a constant level as a cause of neonatal morbidity. A healthy neonate of a syphilitic mother may have syphilitic IgG globulins in its blood since IgG molecules pass the placenta. Syphilitic IgM cannot pass the placenta and appears in the neonate only as a result of active fetal syphilitic infection.

If effective antispirochetal therapy (*e.g.*, penicillin) is instituted early in the disease (before immunity has developed) reinfection can occur. High-grade immunity develops in 2 to 6 weeks. Relapse may occur if the early therapy is not totally effective.

Transmission is by sexual contact (vaginal or oral) or, rarely (0.01%), by contact with *fresh* exudates from any open lesions at any stage; direct blood transfusion or insufficiently aged (less than 4 days) blood-bank blood can transmit during any septicemic stage. Freshly infected needles, syringes, etc., can also transmit the disease to nonimmune persons.

Diagnosis

1. *Darkfield examination* of material from open lesions at any stage, including secondary lesions on mucosal surfaces of oropharynx and vagina.
2. *Nontreponemal standard serologic tests (SSTs)* or serologic tests for syphilis (STS) depend on the presence in the serum of immunoglobulins (IgM or IgG) reactive with a lipoidal antigen prepared from bovine heart muscle (cardiolipin). This antibody (referred to as ***reagin*** or ***reaginic*** or ***Wassermann*** antibody) results from the interaction of the host with *Treponema pallidum* and has nothing to do with IgE, which is also referred to as reagin or reaginic antibody, but is associated with atopic allergy. Wassermann antibody, although also mainly IgG in syphilitic infection, is distinct from antibody to *T. pallidum* and is measured by flocculation with cardiolipin-cholesterol-lecithin antigen in the venereal disease research laboratory (VDRL) test, the rapid plasma reagin (RPR), or the automated reagin test (ART). A positive nontreponemal serologic test may occur in many conditions other than syphilis, from which they must be distinguished by a negative specific test for treponemal antibody (FTA-ABS). "Biological false-positive" STSs occur frequently in infectious mononucleosis, malaria, granulomatous disease of many etiologies, some viral and chlamydial infections, dysgammaglobulinemias, autoimmune diseases such as rheumatoid arthritis and systemic lupus erythematosus, and malignancies.
3. *Tests for specific antitreponemal antibody.* These antibodies are evoked by and are *specific* for *T. pallidum* and persist throughout the duration of syphilitic infection, including latent syphilis, even when SSTs are negative. Treponemal antibody is detected with the fluorescent treponemal antibody absorption (FTA-ABS) test, in which the indirect or "sandwich" FAb staining procedure is used. Patients' sera and known positive and negative control sera are inactivated at 56° C for 30 minutes and absorbed with material (sorbent) from Reiter spirochetes to remove antibody to commensal spirochetes that cross-react with *T. pallidum. T. pallidum* (Nichols strain) grown in rabbit testis, lyophilized and fixed to slides are used as antigen substrate. The microhemagglutination-*Treponema pallidum* (MHA–TP) test, more recently developed, is just as specific and sensitive as the FTA–ABS and is cheaper and simpler to perform. In the MHA–TP test, tanned erythrocytes coated with treponemal antigens are agglutinated in microtiter plates by specific antibody in the test sera. False-positive treponemal antibody tests (FTA–ABS, MHA–TP), due mainly to IgM, are unusual, but may occur in connective tissue disorders (systemic lupus erythematosus, rheumatoid arthritis), leprosy, and infectious mononucleosis; these discrepancies may be resolved by application of the *Treponema pallidum* immobilization (TPI) test, the first specific treponemal test introduced, but also the most difficult because it requires the use of living treponemes. The TPI test now serves chiefly as a standard of reference available at the Centers for Disease Control. It should be remembered that nonsyphilitic treponemal diseases (yaws, bejel, pinta) give *bona fide* positive treponemal antibody tests and must therefore be distinguished from syphilis on clinical and epidemiological grounds.

   In the diagnosis of neurosyphilis, the treponemal tests are unreliable, and serodiagnosis is made on the basis of the VDRL test carried out on spinal fluid. VDRL-CSF, however, may be negative in late neurosyphilis. False-positive VDRL reactions on spinal fluid are rare.

Yaws, Pinta, Bejel. These nonvenereal, tropical treponematoses are caused by *Treponema pertenue, T. carateum,* and *T. pallidum,* respectively. Bejel is endemic (nonvenereal) syphilis. The infections are usually acquired in childhood by direct body contact. As with venereal syphilis, all of these diseases are characterized by self-limited primary and secondary lesions, a latent period apparently disease-free and late lesions that frequently are destructive, particularly of bone and skin. In all three diseases, there are at some stage positive VDRL or RPR and/or treponemal antibody (FTA–ABS) tests indistinguishable from those accompanying sexually transmitted syphilis. In yaws, the distinctive "framboise" (French

TABLE 5-12. Zoonoses As Sources of Human Infection

PROTOZOA	BACTERIA	RICKETTSIAE/CHLAMYDIAE	VIRUSES
Babesiosis (2)	Anthrax (2,P)		
Cryptosporidiosis (2,4)	Brucellosis (2m,3,Te + Sm)	Rocky Mountain spotted fever (1,Ch,Te)	Contagious ecthyma (Orf) (2,4)
Echinococcosis	Erysipeloid (2,P)	Q fever (5,Te)	Dengue fever (1)
Larva migrans (2) (cutaneous; visceral (Th))	Listeriosis (?2,P,Am,Er)	Typhus (1,Te,Ch)	Encephalitides (1) (Western esquire, St. Louis, Venezuelan, California, Powassan)
Schistosomiasis (2)	Leptospirosis (3,Te)		
Taeniasis (3)	Plaque (2,4,Sm,Te,Ch,Tr/S)		Hemorrhagic fevers (2)
Taenia solium (Pr) (cysticercosis)	Salmonellosis (2,3,Am,Ch)	Psittacosis (5,Te) (ornithosis)	Rabies (2) (5,Te)
Taenia saginata (Ni,Pr)			
Toxoplasmosis (2,3,Py,Tr/S)	Tularemia (1,2,3,5,Sm,(Te,Ch))		Yellow fever (1)
Trichinosis (3,Th)	Relapsing fever *(Borrelia duttoni)* (1,Te)		

Mode of transmission:
1 = Arthropod vector.
2 = Direct contact with infected animal, tissue, discharges.
3 = Ingestion of, or contact with, contaminated material.
4 = Human-to-human transmission possible.
5 = Inhalation.

Chemotherapeutic agent(s) used:
Am = ampicillin.
Ch = chloramphenicol.
Cl = clindamycin.
Er = erythromycin.
Ni = niclosamide.
P = penicillin.
Pr = praziquantel.
Py = pyrimethamine.
Sm = Streptomycin
Te = tetracycline.
Th = thiabendazole.
Tr/s = trimethoprimsulfamethoxazole.

for *raspberry*) lesion is diagnostic. Yaws confers solid immunity to syphilis. All three of the nonvenereal treponematoses can be diagnosed by darkfield examination, the organisms being morphologically indistinguishable from one another. Unlike syphilis, the diseases are commonly transmitted by fomites and nonvenereal contact, as between mother and child; in addition, yaws is transmitted (probably mechanically) by small flies.

A single injection of long-acting penicillin G (benzathine penicillin G) is effective in the treatment of each of these treponematoses.

ZOONOSES

Zoonoses are diseases that are communicable from animals to humans and may be caused by any of a variety of protozoa, bacteria, intermediate forms and viruses (Table 5-12). In general, the risk to humans is directly proportional to the degree of contact, direct or through vectors, with diseased animals or their discharges (*e.g.*, veterinarians, hunters, farmers). In this section we will confine ourselves to those zoonoses caused by spirochetes of the *Lepstospira* or *Borrelia* genera.

Leptospirosis. Leptospirosis is a zoonotic infection caused by any of approximately 150 serotypes of a single species *(Leptospira interrogans)*. About 40 cases were reported in the United States in 1986. Morphologically and culturally, the pathogenic types are distinguishable from one another. The general properties of leptospires are listed elsewhere. There are numerous free-living saprophytic species, often collectively referred to as the *L. biflexa* group. These are commonly found in wet, decomposing materials or domestic drain pipes. They differ markedly from pathogenic species in their resistance to azaguanine, their survival in contaminated cultures and sewage, and their capacity to grow at temperatures from 5° to 15° C.

Pathogens (generally referred to as the *L. interrogans* complex) grow well only between 30° and 37° C and are readily overgrown by contaminants in culture. Like *Treponema pallidum,* these organisms are extremely sensitive to detergents and acid conditions, although they will survive in urine-contaminated water if not too acid. They will traverse ordinary bacteriostatic filters. The various pathogenic types can be differentiated from each other antigenically.

Leptospirosis is primarily a disease of wild and domestic animals and is readily transmissible to humans (Weil's disease, Fort Bragg fever, rice field fever) by water contaminated with urine from infected rats, dogs, cats, cattle, and humans or through direct contact with infected animal carcasses in abattoirs or infected fowl in poultry-dressing plants. Person-to-person transmission occurs rarely. Leptospires enter the blood mainly via abrasions in the skin or via the oral mucosa during ingestion of contaminated foods or water. Neither endotoxins nor exotoxins have been demonstrated. Following an incubation period of 1 to 2 weeks, a spectrum of systemic symptoms (high fever, chills, headache, generalized myalgias) may supervene, during which the organisms are found in the blood, spinal fluid, and most organs, particularly kidneys and liver. With the development of antibodies, the organisms are cleared and symptoms subside. Subsequently, the organisms may appear in the urine, and meningitis or hepatitis (with or without icterus) may develop. In most cases, the disease is entirely self-limited; immunity is type specific.

Diagnosis can be made presumptively early in the disease by darkfield examination of urine and blood and confirmed by culture of blood in special semisolid media and by darkfield microscopic agglutination tests for antibody in acute and convalescent sera. Because of the presence of lymphocytes in the spinal fluid, this disease may be mistaken for aseptic (viral) meningitis, making darkfield microscopy essential. Penicillin and/or tetracycline is recommended for clinically severe leptospirosis.

Relapsing Fever (Borreliosis). There are up to 19 recognized species within the genus *Borrelia,* all of which are arthropod-borne, and 10 of which cause relapsing fevers (do not confuse with undulant fever, brucellosis) and one that causes Lyme disease (see below). *Borrelia* are distinguished morphologically from treponemes by their course irregular coils and are cultivable, though with difficulty, on Kelly's semisolid medium. *Borrelia* are best observed with darkfield microscopy in blood of febrile patients, or in blood of rats that have been injected for diagnostic purposes and in which infection may develop rapidly with marked borrelemia. Blood films stained with Giemsa also reveal the organisms.

Transmission is by body lice *(Pediculus humanus)* in south central Europe, India, Asia, and North Africa, and other areas where pediculosis occurs. In these geographical areas, epidemic relapsing fever is due principally to *B. recurrentis,* for which humans are the only hosts. In South Africa, the Balkans, eastern Mediterranean regions, South and Central America, and the western United States, other species, notably *B. duttoni,* are transmitted in the bites, joint (coxal) fluids and feces (depending on the species) of various *Ornithodoros* soft ticks. The tick-borne disease is a true zoonosis (endemic relapsing fever), the animal reservoirs being principally wild rodents, monkeys, armadillos, and opossums, the sources of tangential human infection. If contracted during pregnancy, *Borrelia* may cause intrauterine infection that is fatal to the fetus.

After inoculation into the human host, the organisms multiply in the bloodstream, as well as in the tissues. After an initial acute, febrile episode with headache, chills, hepatosplenomegaly, and macular rash, the fever ends by crisis in 1 to 2 weeks, due to the appearance of serum antibody. Examination of blood at this point may reveal agglutinated *Borrelia* in "rosette" formation. The organisms persist in lymphoid tissues, become resistant to antibody, presumably due to the appearance of antigenic mutants, and again invade the bloodstream for 1 to 3 weeks, repeating the clinical cycle, though usually with diminished severity. Relapses may occur from 2 to 10 times (depending on the type of *Borrelia*).

Prevention depends on active louse control in areas of epidemic disease prevalence and avoidance of tick-infected rodents and other carriers of endemic borreliosis. Antibiotic treatment (tetracycline and/or chloramphenicol) is effective; if it is given during a febrile attack, Jarisch-Herxheimer-like reactions may occur.

Lyme Disease. Lyme disease is a syndrome that was first recognized in 1975 through a clustering of affected children in Lyme, Connecticut; it is now known to occur in at least 14 states, in Europe, and in Australia. The disease is characterized by a unique red skin lesion (erythema chronicum migrans, ECM) and by arthritis, which appears about a month after onset of acute symptoms, affects one or more joints, and may be recurrent. Erosive and proliferative synovitis may develop that resembles rheumatoid arthritis. Persons with HLA-DR2 histocompatibility antigens are also prone to develop meningoencephalitis and peripheral neuropathies in association with other manifestations of Lyme disease. Disease activity is correlated with serum IgM levels; there is also lymphopenia and lowered response of mononuclear cells to mitogens (*e.g.,* phytohemagglutinin). Immune complexes are found in the blood simultaneously with the skin lesions. The infectious origin of ECM was deduced by the transmission of ECM between human volunteers by injection of tissue of active lesions. Lyme disease, or Lyme borreliosis, is caused by the spirochete *Borrelia burgdorferi,* which is carried by several species of hard ticks from the *Ixodes ricinus* complex, including *I. dammini* and *I. pacificus.* In 1986 there were 1,500 cases, predominantly seen in the Northeast. Currently, several thousand new cases are reported each year from Europe and the United States. The organism is cultivable in special medium, in which it grows slowly; it is highly sensitive to high-dose penicillin, which is essentially curative of the infection. However, in some patients the spirochete can persist despite antibiotic therapy. Because of increased T-suppressor-cell activity, late manifestations of the disease may mimic any of a number of disorders of immune origin (*e.g.,* rheumatoid arthritis, Reiter's syndrome, multiple sclerosis) either because of autoimmune phenomena or exaggerated immune responses to the spirochete. Arthritis appears more commonly in U.S. patients.

MYCOPLASMAS AND L FORMS

Infections Due to Mycoplasmas. *Mycoplasma mycoides,* the first of this group to be discovered (1898), was found to be the cause of contagious bovine pleuropneumonia. Subsequently, similar forms, called pleuropneumonialike organisms (PPLO), were found in cases of mastitis in sheep and goats and in rodents, often associated with arthritis and lesions of eyes and ears. Mycoplasmas are the smallest known free-living forms of life, with no cell wall and a variable morphology; most inhabit the normal upper respiratory and genitourinary tracts. Only three are of clinical importance: *M. pneumoniae, M. hominis,* and *Ureaplasma urealyticum.*

Mycoplasma pneumoniae. *M. pneumoniae* (Eaton agent), the first of the mycoplasmas proven to be a cause of human disease, is the etiologic agent of ''primary atypical pneumonia'' (PAP), so called because of its clinical dissimilarity to lobar (typically pneumococcal) pneumonia and its failure to respond to sulfonamides and penicillin. Because of this, PAP was at first thought to have a viral etiology, in accord with the ability of the infectious principal to pass through bacteriostatic filters. However, unequivocal clinical response to broad-spectrum antibiotics in the earliest cases reported, and ultimately the cultivation of the causative organism on lifeless media, clearly substantiated the bacterial nature of the Eaton agent.

M. pneumoniae is a significant cause of lower respiratory tract infection (tracheobronchitis to interstitial pneumonia) characterized by nonproductive cough, persistent fever, absence of leukocytosis, and ''walking pneumonia.'' The infection occurs primarily in temperate climates and may become epidemic, most frequently affecting school-age children and young adults; it is spread by respiratory droplet and close contact. The clinical disease must be distinguished from Q fever, legionnaires' disease, ornithosis (chlamydial), and interstitial pneumonia of viral etiology. Being a surface infection, *M. pneumoniae* colonizes the respiratory epithelium, interrupting normal ciliary motion; the organism is not invasive and is never recovered from the blood. Recovery and immunity to reinfection are due to local accumulation of secretory IgA and serum IgG antibody. Treatment with tetracyclines or erythromycin is effective; penicillin is ineffective because *M. pneumoniae* lacks a cell wall. Rarely, central nervous system and other systemic complications may follow proven *M. pneumoniae* infection.

To establish the diagnosis, *M. pneumoniae* can be recovered from sputum on special selective agar enriched with animal serum and yeast extract, on which colonies of *M. pneumoniae* are recognized by their ability to adsorb erythrocytes (hemadsorption) and by direct immunofluorescence. The organisms are too small and fragile to stain with Gram's or Giemsa stain. The clinical diagnosis is confirmed retrospectively by a rise in serum antibody demonstrated by complement fixation or tetrazolium-reduction-inhibition (TRI, metabolic inhibition) tests. In addition to specific antibody, up to 40% of patients with mycoplasmal pneumonia develop serum ''cold'' agglutinins, that is, their serum agglutinates human O erythrocytes at 4° C, frequently to very high titer, but not at 37° C. This transient cold agglutinin is an IgM antibody with cross-reactive specificity for the I antigen in erythrocyte glycophorin and membrane antigen(s) of *M. pneumoniae.*

Mycoplasma hominis. *M. hominis* in adults is a cause of prostatitis, pelvic inflammatory disease, as well as postpartum or postabortal sepsis. In newborns it is a cause of sepsis, lymphadenitis, meningitis, pericarditis, and conjunctivitis. Diagnosis is difficult and mainly by exclusion of other sexually transmitted or neonatal diseases. There is a typical purulent infection with polymorphonuclear leukocytes in the cerebrospinal fluid and joint fluid. Treatment is with lincomycin or clindamycin.

Ureaplasma urealyticum. *U. urealyticum* normally inhabits the oral and/or genitourinary tract and comprises eight serotypes (formerly referred to as T or ''tiny'' mycoplasma because of their small colony size). *U. urealyticum* infection is sexually transmitted and is an important cause of nonchlamydial, nongonococcal urethritis (NGU) in both sexes and of pelvic inflammatory disease. Antibodies to *U. urealyticum* rise during many pregnancies, suggesting that maternal infection with mycoplasma may contribute to perinatal morbidity. Under such circumstances, treatment with erythromycin during the third trimester has been reported to reduce the incidence of low-birthweight infants born to women colonized with genital mycoplasmas. Diagnosis is based on recovery and identification of urease-producing mycoplasma *(U. urealyticum)* on special media and metabolic inhibition with specific antibody. Tetracycline is the drug of choice in treatment.

L Forms of Bacteria. Many common gram-positive bacteria, cultivated in the presence of penicillin in media with increased osmotic pressure (*e.g.,* 3% sucrose), grow without their cell wall and are therefore called ***protoplasts;*** in many respects they are much like PPLO. Gram-negative bacteria retain the lipoprotein portions of their cell wall in the presence of penicillin and are therefore not wholly naked and are called ***spheroplasts.*** These cell-wall-less or cell-wall-defective forms are called L forms (from the Lister Institute, where they were first described) of the particular bacterium involved. Removed from the osmotically protective medium they undergo plasmolysis, that is, they are ''osmotically fragile.'' With the removal of penicillin they revert to true bacteria. PPLO also not uncommonly revert to well-known species of bacteria, and vice versa. It is suggested that nonreverting PPLO are genetically stabilized bacterial L form mutants with decreased osmotic fragility. The possible development of L forms of pathogens *in vivo,* especially during penicillin therapy, with establishment of latent and antibiotic-resistant infections, is of obvious clinical importance.

A number of other species of PPLO, also bacterial L forms, are of importance in diagnostic work with viruses, since they can contaminate tissues used as sources of cell cultures for diagnostic virology as well as animal products used for cell culture.

Streptobacillus moniliformis is a bacterial species, bacillary and streptobacilly in form, that produces minute PPLO called L_1 bodies, that revert in turn to *S. moniliformis*. Both forms may occur in the same culture. *Streptobacillus moniliformis* is related to one form of rat-bite fever and to Haverhill fever.

Minute Bacteria

FAMILY RICKETTSIACEAE

Rickettsia. Rickettsiae are pleomorphic cocci and rods, the latter often containing bipolar granules of unknown significance. The organisms can grow in cell cultures but are commonly propagated in cells of the yolk sac of embryonated hens' eggs. Machiavello's stain is commonly used. In spite of their minute size, rickettsiae do not pass through bacterial-retaining filters (but see *Coxiella* of Q fever, the exception). Their cell structure is prokaryotic, and their cell walls contain muramic acid, a substance found only in bacteria. They are obligate intracellular parasites and contain both DNA and RNA. Rickettsiae contain a potent endotoxin but produce no exotoxin. Cellular substances are antigenic and species specific, except the antigen that is shared with *Proteus* (see Weil-Felix reaction).

Habitat. Most rickettsiae are primarily parasites of insects and only secondarily of animals. They are transmitted from insects to humans and from person to person by the bites of insects or by being rubbed into scratches and cuts when infected insects are crushed on the skin.

Antibiotic Susceptibility. Rickettsiae possess bacterium-like, though limited, enzyme systems, including those of the Krebs cycle and those necessary to the synthesis of ATP, cell wall, and some proteins. Hence rickettsiae are susceptible to enzyme-inhibiting chemotherapeutic drugs, especially the tetracyclines and chloramphenicol, which are effective therapeutically. Relapses occur during therapy because the organisms survive intracellularly.

Diagnosis. Laboratory diagnosis of rickettsial disease is made by agglutination tests using purified yolk sac antigens to reveal group-specific antibodies in patient sera. Adult guinea pigs or white mice are inoculated with appropriate specimens (most often blood) and evaluated for febrile reactions; tissues from inoculated animals are examined at autopsy and put into cell culture for recovery of rickettsiae. Cell culture, however, is not appropriate for direct diagnostic inoculation of clinical specimens.

The ***Weil-Felix test*** depends on the differential agglutination of strains of *Proteus vulgaris* by the serum of patients with suspected rickettsiosis (see Table 5-10). *Proteus* has no etiologic relationship to rickettsial diseases, but the O antigen in *Proteus* cross-reacts with a minor rickettsial antigen. Misleading positive reactions may occur in patients who are free of rickettsiae but who have urinary tract infections due to *Proteus* and a significant homologous antibody response.

Diseases Due to Rickettsiae. Three main groups of diseases are recognized as due to rickettsiae: (1) the ***typhus*** group, (2) the ***spotted fever*** group, and (3) the ***scrub typhus*** group. The first group includes European or "classic" epidemic typhus and Brill's disease (recrudescent typhus), in which the transmission is human–louse–human, the lice being killed by the infection, and murine or endemic typhus, in which transmission to humans is by the rat flea. Diseases of the second group are mainly tick-borne within animal reservoirs, the ticks maintaining infection transovarially and by sexual transmission and incidentally infecting humans. The one exception is rickettsialpox, transmitted by a mite from domestic murine reservoirs. Diseases of the third group are larval-mite borne. Q fever differs from all of the foregoing with respect to both etiology and clinical aspects.

Clinically, all rickettsial diseases (except Q fever, which resembles influenza, and rickettsialpox, which resembles chickenpox) have certain cardinal features in common: stupor and other neurological signs, rash, and invasion of reticuloendothelial cells by the rickettsiae. Usually there are both clinical and pathologic diagnostic differences between these rickettsioses, such as chronology, intensity, and distribution of the rash, development of eschar at site of arthropod bite, and so on.

In nature, epidemic typhus occurs only in humans, the other rickettsioses being primarily zoonoses (*i.e.,* enzootic in lower animals, occurring only secondarily in humans). The rickettsiae of typhus and tsutsugamushi fevers remain in the cytoplasm of infected cells, while those of Rocky Mountain spotted fever and of rickettsialpox also invade the nucleus. In severe Rocky Mountain spotted fever the smooth muscles of peripheral vascular walls are destroyed. In rickettsialpox and tsutsugamushi there is a definite ulcer or eschar at the site of the infecting bite. Rickettsialpox is distinguished by its poxlike vesicles. Tsutsugamushi, Rocky Mountain spotted fever and epidemic typhus are generally more severe than murine typhus or rickettsialpox.

Brill-Zinsser disease is epidemic or classic typhus occurring sporadically in the total absence of body lice, as a relatively mild recrudescence of latent infection years after the initial attack. In the febrile stage the disease is transmissible by body lice. Apparently the rickettsiae can remain viable but quiescent in the tissues for many years after initial infection. Occasionally, this disease appears in the United States, especially in immigrants from central Europe, Asia Minor, and eastern Mediterranean areas.

Coxiella. This genus contains only one species, *Coxiella burnetii,* named for H. L. Cox and F. M. Burnet, simultaneous discoverers. It is immunologically distinct from other rickettsiae. *C. Burnetii* causes Q fever (Q for "query") first observed and named by Derrick in Australia. *C. burnetii* has most of the properties of *Rickettsia* but differs in being (1) filterable; (2) quite resistant to environmental conditions (probably due to endosporelike forms) such as drying, diffuse sunlight, disinfectants, heating at 62° C for 30 minutes; (3) mode of transmission: improperly pasteurized contaminated milk; dust, from barns housing infected sheep, cattle, goats, rodents; tissues and parturition fluids from infectious animals; several species of ticks.

In ***Q fever*** the respiratory tract is most commonly affected. There is no rash. The disease clinically resembles influenza, often with interstitial pneumonitis. Mortality is low or nil. Q fever appears to be disseminated widely, especially among persons in the animal industries, having been reported from more than 31 states and 50 countries on 5 continents. The organisms may be isolated from the blood by animal inoculation. Diagnosis also may be made by serologic methods but *not* by the Weil-Felix test. Milk can be made safe only by pasteurization for 30 minutes at a temperature of 63° C (145° F). Tetracycline and chloramphenicol are the drugs of choice in treatment. An experimental Q fever vaccine for human and veterinary use has shown promise.

FAMILY CHLAMYDIACEAE

Chlamydia. Formerly classified with "filtrable viruses," *Chlamydia,* like *Rickettsia* and *Coxiella,* are bacteria modified to obligate intracellular parasitism because of their lack of certain protein-synthetic and oxidative enzyme systems. Chlamydiae are distinctive in lacking enzymes that synthesize ATP; they must use host-derived energy. These organisms exhibit a complex intracellular developmental cycle. Elementary bodies, the infectious units, attach to susceptible cells, penetrate by phagocytosis, and develop into reticulate bodies. The latter increase in number, some developing into intermediate forms, which end up as new infectious elementary bodies released by disruption of the cell.

The genus is divided into two main groups, *C. trachomatis* and *C. psittaci*. The first group (previously referred to as TRIC agents) is the most important because it includes classic ocular trachoma (serogroups A, B, and C), genital infections (particularly nongonococcal urethritis; NGU), inclusion conjunctivitis and pneumonitis of infants (serotypes D to M), and lymphogranuloma venereum (LGV serotypes I, II, and III). The second major group *(C. psittaci)* comprises the agents of psittacosis and ornithosis. *Chlamydia* possess a common group-specific antigen; individual serotypes can be distinguished by immunofluorescence using type-specific antisera. Members of both groups are readily isolated and propagated either in the yolk sac of chicken eggs or in cell culture systems (*e.g.,* McCoy cells treated with IUDR and cycloheximide to prevent cellular mitosis). The cytopathology induced by *C. trachomatis* is readily identified because of large intracytoplasmic inclusions. These are composed of glycogen and therefore stain readily with iodine (Lugol's solution) and autofluoresce in ultraviolet light without the addition of labelled antisera. Similar inclusions are diagnostic when discovered in tarsal scrapings from clinically suspected neonatal inclusion conjunctivitis. In adults, *C. trachomatis* is an important and frequent cause of sexually transmitted disease, manifest as NGU, proctitis and attendant complications in the male, and cervicitis and pelvic inflammatory disease in the female. In both sexes, it also occurs asymptomatically, but is still infectious. Chlamydial infection ranks with gonorrhea as a major cause of sexually transmitted disease and accordingly also accounts for a substantial number of cases of acute pharyngitis. The likelihood of coexistent chlamydial infection (estimated to occur in up to 20%) should therefore be kept in mind in the management of primary gonococcal infection. Rapid diagnosis of chlamydial infection is readily accomplished by direct immunofluorescence with monoclonal antibodies applied to smears of urethral or cervical secretions. In view of the possibility of dual infection, some form of combined therapy (*e.g.,* sulfamethoxazole-trimethoprim or penicillin, plus tetracycline, rather than penicillin alone with probenecid) should be considered in treating men with these infections. For women with probable combined infection, the current recommendation is to treat the gonococcal infection first (single dose of ampicillin, amoxicillin, or penicillin) and then give tetracycline for chlamydial infection, which may not be demonstrable but is probably present.

Lymphogranuloma venereum (LGV) (not to be confused with granuloma inguinale due to *Calymmatobacterium granulomatis*) is a sporadically occurring sexually transmitted disease, worldwide in distribution, commoner in blacks and males than in whites and females. Three serotypes of *C. trachomatis* (LCV, I, II, and III, cross-reactive with serotypes D and E) are distinguished by microimmunofluorescence. Clinically, an initial painless superficial genital ulcer progresses to lymphadenopathy, draining bubo formation, and finally scarring of rectal mucosa and stricture. The diagnosis is made more often serologically (complement fixation tests on paired sera) than by isolation of the agent, which may be difficult. The Frei test, once the mainstay of diagnosis, is no longer much used. Treatment with tetracycline or sulfonamides is usually effective.

Chlamydia psittaci is the cause of psittacosis, or parrot fever, named for psittacine birds that are the natural reservoirs of the organism. Domestic fowl and park pigeons may harbor the infection, and person-to-person transmission occurs. Human ornithosis, more frequent in occurrence than previously thought, is contracted by inhalation of dust harboring dried feces and respiratory secretions of infected birds. The disease occurs as a primary interstitial pneumonia with a patchy lobular distribution and is accompanied by variable constitutional signs and symptoms and normal leukocyte count. It must be distinguished from influenza, mycoplasmal pneumonia, legionellosis, and Q fever. *C. psittaci* can be isolated from the sputum in modified cell culture, as with *C. trachomatis;* however, no iodine-staining glycogen inclusions are formed. Diagnosis is made or confirmed retrospectively by complement fixation tests on paired sera. Tetracycline is considered to be effective in therapy.

VIRUSES

Viruses must be distinguished on the one hand from the smaller macromolecules of which they are constituted (DNA or RNA, proteins) and on the other hand from the larger bacteria or other parasitic microorganisms. Viruses are much smaller than bacteria or animal cells that they infect and can pass through filters that trap such cells.

General Concept of Viruses

A virus may be defined as a strictly particulate intracellular entity with an infectious phase, possessing only one type of nucleic acid (called the genome) and replicating or multiplying in the form of their genetic material, although in some virus families there may be an intermediate stage in nucleic acid replication involving another nucleic acid type. For example, retroviruses such as human immunodeficiency virus (HIV), the causative agent of acquired immune deficiency syndrome (AIDS), are RNA viruses that replicate through a DNA intermediate, and hepatitis B virus (HBV), a DNA virus, utilizes an RNA intermediate. Viruses are unable to grow by themselves or undergo binary fission, and finally, they are devoid of an energy-producing enzyme system.

Nomenclature and Structure

Animal viruses can be classified as either naked or enveloped: ***Naked viruses*** contain *only* RNA or DNA and a protein coat, while ***enveloped viruses*** contain *only* RNA or DNA + protein coat + lipid-containing membrane (also called an envelope).

The nucleic acid or ***genome*** as the hereditary material serves an absolutely necessary function; for some viruses, like poliovirus, the RNA after modification serves as mRNA on entry into the cell.

The ***protein coat*** protects the nucleic acid from nucleases. For naked viruses it also serves as an attachment vehicle to cells—the major determinant of host range. For enveloped viruses, glycoprotein spikes embedded in the envelope serve as the attachment site to specific host cell receptors. Thus, in AIDS, the HIV virus attaches by the gp120 spikes to cells with the CD4 receptors, such as T_h (helper) cells or certain monocytes.

In recent years, there have been breakthroughs made in the discovery of a smaller class of infectious agents than even viruses. These agents are called ***viroids.*** They are not viruses but appear to be covalently closed single-stranded RNA circles about 300 to 400 nucleotides in length, which are resistant to ultraviolet (UV) radiation, as well as to denaturing chemical agents. Viroids do not encode proteins. They replicate *in vitro* via the rolling circle model of replication. *In vivo* the pathogenesis caused by viroids may be a result of their interference with normal transcription inside host cells. Recently, the delta agent that causes a virulent form of hepatitis B disease (''fulminant hepatitis'') has been isolated and characterized. It is a viroidlike RNA packaged into the hepatitis B virus capsid shell.

Terminology

Before undertaking a detailed discussion of viruses, it is important to define certain basic terms.

1. ***Virion:*** The complete virus particle
2. ***Capsid:*** The protein coat surrounding the nucleic acid or genome
3. ***Capsomers:*** The repeating protein subunits that make up the capsid
4. ***Protomers:*** The polypeptide chains that make up the capsomers. Note: Noncovalent bonds between protomers are usually stronger than those between capsomers.
5. ***Symmetry*** of the virus, which can be:
    a. ***Icosahedral:*** A virus particle with 20 triangular faces, exhibiting 5 : 3 : 2 rotational symmetry, for example, adenovirus
    b. ***Helical:*** Exemplified by the measles virus, which contains a helical nucleocapsid inside the envelope
    c. ***Bilateral:*** A vaccinia virus is morphologically symmetrical when viewed by thin section electron microscopy.

The first known virus (tobacco mosaic) was discovered in 1892 by Iwanowski, regarded as a living contagious fluid *(contagium vivum fluidum)* by Beijerinck in 1898, and purified as protein in crystalline form by Stanley in

1935. The first known virus of vertebrates (foot-and-mouth disease) was discovered by Löffler and Frosch in 1898; the first known virus of humans (yellow fever), by Walter Reed and his associates in 1899. Studies of animal viruses were laborious, cumbersome, and expensive and progressed slowly until the discovery of bacteriophage (phage) by Twort in 1915 and d'Herelle in 1917. Because phage could be cultivated easily, quickly, safely, and inexpensively in test-tube cultures by allowing them to infect cells of a harmless bacterium (generally *Escherichia coli*), they became a principal experimental subject of virologists. Although bacteria are prokaryotes, studies of phage have yielded much information directly applicable to virology of animal cells. The development of practical means of cultivating animal tissue eliminated the drudgery and expense of using live animals and provided a relatively simple means, now widely used, of studying animal viruses.

Bacteriophage

Studies of phages have provided the foundation for studying mammalian viruses and are therefore discussed in some detail here.

Although phage have been found for many species of bacteria, blue-green algae, and some yeasts, the most studied phages are certain types that infect *Escherichia coli*, or *Bacillus subtilis*. They are identified by number(s) and letter(s), such as the "T-even" phages: T2, T4, T6; the "T-odd" phages: T3, T7, etc., λ, ϕX174, each with distinctive form, antigenic proteins, capsomers, and dimensions. Some have genomes of DNA, some of RNA, some single-stranded, some double. Some have 5-hydroxy-methylcytosine in place of cytosine; some have uracil or 5-hydroxymethyluracil in place of thymine; some have tails, others do not. Small, tailless phages (24 to 60 nm, *e.g.*, ϕX174, M12) are icosahedral in form; some (*e.g.*, fl, M13) are filamentous (800 nm long) with helical symmetry; larger phages (50 to 90 nm) have tails up to 210 nm long attached to the "head" or nucleocapsid. The tails of T-even phages are of very complex structure with terminal spikes and long thin fibers for attachment of the phage to its host cell. Other phage tails are relatively simple. Unlike animal viruses, few phages are enveloped. Small, RNA-containing phages are much like picornaviruses (animal) (see Table 5-13), though they contain RNA only equivalent to about five genes. The RNA of such viruses acts in the host cell as its own mRNA.

PHAGE ACTIVITY

Phages attach to specific receptors on susceptible cells, using structures such as tail fibers. By means of enzymic mechanisms located at the tip of the tail, an opening is made through the bacterial cell wall and cell membrane. Through this, the nucleic acid (NA) core from the head of the phage enters the cell. The capsid is now an empty shell that may remain attached to the exterior of the cell.

Some phages attach only to bacterial F pili and are therefore said to be male specific. Filamentous phages attach at the tip of the F pili, while male specific icosahedral phages adsorb at various specific sites along the F-pilus. Once inside the bacterium, all phages, whether male specific or not, can no longer be demonstrable as phage ***(eclipse phase).*** In some instances the phage NA becomes integrated with the genetic mechanism of the cell as though a part of the bacterial genome ***(prophage),*** replicating with the bacterial chromosome. There it may remain in a latent stage for many generations, doing no evident harm. Phage in this form is said to be ***temperate.*** The cell containing it is said to be ***lysogenic.*** The lysogenic cell is sometimes called a ***lysogen.*** The term *lysogeny* applies only to phage-infected bacteria. However, analogous relationships are found between some transforming or oncogenic viruses and their animal host cells.

As a result of various chemical or physical stimuli (*e.g.*, ultraviolet or x irradiation) to the lysogenic bacterium, the prophage can be ***induced*** or ***activated.*** The temperate phage then multiplies vegetatively, injuring the host bacterium and takes control of the synthetic mechanisms of the cell to replicate itself.

In the active state (lytic or vegetative) the phage genome codes for enzymes that cause prompt disintegration of the host DNA to nucleotides, with resulting immediate cessation of cell synthesis, the synthesis of new DNA precursors and "early" replication of phage NA, as well as transcription of the phage genome. Functioning of host-specific mRNA stops, and "late" phage mRNA forms phage materials (NA, enzymes, capsids, etc.) using cell ribosomes. Similar events occur in animal cells infected by animal viruses, with modifications depending on the characteristics of each specific cell-virus system.

Once replicated, the new phage NA is ***encapsidated;*** nucleocapsids and the tails, if present, then combine and the intracellular virions are assembled as ***mature*** virions (end of the eclipse period). The bacterial cell wall is soon disintegrated by a phagecoded lysozyme ***(lysis from within),*** liberating new virions. The various periods usually take about 30 minutes for phage and about 1 to 2 hours for analogous naked viruses.

A lysogenic cell containing prophage has ***prophage immunity,*** that is, it cannot be superinfected by another virion of that phage type, although NA of other lysogenic phage types may infect the cell.

When bacterial cells undergo phage lysis, they suddenly liberate many intact virions, producing a "one-step" increase in the number of virions or ***plaque-form-***

(Text continues on page 454)

TABLE 5-13. Classification of Viruses

FAMILY	VIRUSES	DISEASES
DNA Viruses:		
Naked (Unenveloped)		
Parvoviruses	Parvoviruses (Kilham rat virus, minute virus of mice, H viruses)	(Animals only)
ss positive strand; complementary (+ or −) in separate virions, icosahedral symmetry	Adenosatellite viruses (4 serotypes)	Indigenous, no recognized disease
	Densoviruses (insects)	
	B19 virus	Bone marrow failure; ''fifth disease'' in young children
Papovaviruses ds, circular DNA naked, icosahedral symmetry	Papillomavirus	Verruca vulgaris, condyloma acuminatum (?HPV16 precancerous)
	Simian virus 40 (SV 40)	
	JC virus	Progressive multifocal leukoencephalopathy (PML)
	BK virus	
	Polyomavirus	(Multiple tumors in hamsters)
Adenoviruses ds, icosahedral	Adenoviruses (49 serotypes)	URTI
	Common CF antigen (hexon), type-specific antigens (penton), H (Animal adenoviruses)	Gastroenteritis, conjunctivitis, lymphadenitis (certain types oncogenic in hamsters)
Hepatitis virus ds	Hepatitis B (HB) virus (Surface (s), core (c) and e antigens; Dane particle = virion)	Acute, chronic and inapparent infection (''long incubation,'' ''serum''), hepatocellular carcinoma
Enveloped		
Herpesviruses		Herpes labialis, herpes genitalis, encephalitis, keratoconjunctivitis
ds, icosahedral capsid	Herpes simplex, types 1, 2	Latent, recurrent infection (oncogenic transformation in animals)
	Simian herpesvirus (herpes B)	Type 2: sexually transmitted Encephalitis
	Epstein-Barr (EB) virus	Infectious mononucleosis, (non-Forssman heterophile antibody) Burkitt lymphoma (lymphoma, malignant neurolymphomatosis), (?nasopharyngeal carcinoma), hepatitis
	Varicella-zoster (VZ) virus	Chickenpox-shingles; VZ pneumonia, postinfectious encephalitis (?Reye's syndrome)
	Cytomegalovirus (CMV)	Congenital, neonatal systemic infections; compromised host, hepatitis, mononucleosis (no heterophile antibody)
	Pseudorabies	(Equines)
Poxviruses ds, complex, lateral bodies, separate HA	Variola virus	Smallpox (variola major, minor; alastrim)
	Vaccinia virus	Eczema vaccinatum, generalized vaccinia, postvaccinal encephalitis (rare complications of vaccination) Cowpox
	Parapoxviruses	Milkers'nodes, Orf (sheep)
	Molluscum contaglosum	Multiple skin lesions
	Yaba virus	Localized skin lesions (monkeys)

TABLE 5-13. *(continued)*

FAMILY	VIRUSES	DISEASES
RNA Viruses:		
Naked (Unenveloped) Picornaviruses ss, positive, icosahedral symmetry	Enteroviruses (poliovirus (3 serotypes), echovirus and coxsackievirus (70 + serotypes), hepatitis A virus)	Meningitis, meningoencephalitis, poliomyelitis, inapparent infection (lower GI tract), herpangina, URTI, pleurodynia, myocarditis, exanthemata
	Cardioviruses (encephalomyocarditis (EMC) virus)	
	Rhinoviruses (100 + serotypes)	URTI, CCS
Caliciviruses	Norwalk agent	Gastroenteritis in infants and children
Reoviruses ds, segmented, linear icosahedral symmetry, double shell capsid inner icosahedron	Reoviruses (3 serotypes), H	Lower gastrointestinal trace, ?disease
	Orbiviruses (all are arboviruses)	Colorado tick fever, (various ungulates)
	Rotavirus (2 serotypes)	Infantile diarrhea (winter)
Enveloped Togaviruses ss, positive, icosahedral symmetry	Alphaviruses (formerly group A arboviruses), H	Encephalitis
	Flaviviruses (formerly group B arboviruses), H	Hemorrhagic fever, yellow fever, dengue fever, encephalitis
	Rubivirus (rubella), H	Rubella, with arthritis in adults, congenital rubella syndrome
Bunyaviruses helical symmetry, genome ss, 3 circular segments	Bunyamwera virus, H	Mild encephalitis, Crimean-Congo hemorrhagic fever, sandfly fever, Rift Valley fever
	California encephalitis viruses	Sin Nombre Virus among Navajo Indians
	Hantaviruses	
	Formerly group C arboviruses	
Orthomyxoviruses ss, segmented; negative, helical symmetry	Influenza viruses	Epidemic (group A) and sporadic influenza, CCS, (Reye's syndrome, group B)
	Serologic groups A, B (H-N types), C (H only)	
Paramyxoviruses ss, unsegmented, negative, helical symmetry	Parainfluenza viruses (4 serotypes), HN	URTI, croup, bronchiolitis, pneumonia
	Mumps virus, HN	Parotitis, orchitis, meningitis
	Respiratory syncytial virus (no H or N)	URTI, bronchiolitis, pneumonitis
	Measles (rubeola) virus, H (no N)	Measles, subacute sclerosing panencephalitis
Rhabdoviruses ss, helical symmetry, bullet shaped	(Vesicular stomatitis virus) (Kern Canyon (bat) virus)	
	Rabies	Rabies
	?Marburg virus (simian) ?Ebola virus	Hemorrhagic fever (?nosocomial spread) Newly classified as Filoviruses

(continued)

TABLE 5-13. (*continued*)

FAMILY	VIRUSES	DISEASES
Retroviruses ss, RNA-dependent DNA polymerase (reverse transcriptase) in virion, inner icosahedral shell, helical core	Oncoviruses, leukoviruses (Foamy virus) (Maedi-visna group of viruses)	Host-specific leukemias, sarcomas, mammary tumors (Persistent infection in different mammalian species) (''Slow'' viral diseases in sheep: panleukoencephalitis, multiorgan involvement, nononcogenic)
	Human T-cell leukemia viruses (HTLV)	Human T-cell leukemia (HTLV I)
	HIV (human immunodeficiency virus)	AIDS
Arenaviruses Spherical virion, genome ss, 2 negative segments, host ribosomal particles	Lymphocytic choriomeningitis virus Lassa virus (?rats)	Choriomeningitis Lassa fever (nosocomial spread)
	Tacaribe complex (?rodents)	Hemorrhagic fevers
Coronaviruses ss, enveloped, positive, helical symmetry	Coronavirus (3 serotypes) different animal species	Respiratory infections, CCS

Abbreviations

ss = single stranded; ds = double stranded; DNA = deoxyribonucleic acid; RNA = ribonucleic acid; URTI = upper respiratory tract infection; LRTI = lower respiratory tract infection; CCS = common cold syndrome; H = hemagglutinin; N = neuraminidase.

Definitions

Virion: The intact (infectious) viral particle.

Genome: Nucleic acid core, embodying genetic information required for viral replication.

Capsid: Protein associated with the genome in cubic or helical symmetry or in complex configuration. Capsids of unenveloped viruses contain protective antigens.

Capsomers: Structural subunits of the capsid.

Nucleocapsid: Viral nucleic acid combined with capsid protein. Intact nucleocapsid of unenveloped viruses is the infectious unit.

Envelope: Lipoprotein coat that surrounds noninfectious nucleocapsid, contains virus-coded protective antigens, and is essential for infectivity.

ing units. (Distinguish this type of growth curve from that of bacteria.)

Most nonlysogenic phages, on entering their susceptible bacterial host, proceed immediately to multiplication (vegetative activity) and destruction of the cell as described above. Such phages are said to be ***lytic*** or ***virulent.***

PLAQUE FORMATION BY BACTERIOPHAGE

To demonstrate plaque formation with bacteriophage, a broth culture of bacteria is mixed with an appropriate number (50 to 500) of bacteriophage virions in semisolid agar. The mixture is spread over the surface of nutrient agar in a Petri dish, which is then incubated. Small clear areas of lysis are seen that are called plaques. Each plaque is initiated by a single, infected bacterial cell in which phage has multiplied and from which progeny virions have been released to infect adjacent cells in the bacterial ''lawn.'' Thus the infection spreads by diffusion from a single bacterium to involve many other adjacent cells. Several cycles of infection are required before a plaque becomes visible. A count of the plaques then gives an idea of the number of particles in the original phage suspension. The term plaque-forming unit (PFU) is used to describe the number of infective phage particles in the suspension.

Replication of Animal Viruses

In a manner similar to bacteriophage, animal viruses replicate in appropriately sensitive eukaryotic cells by a process in which separate components are synthesized in the infected cell and then are assembled into virions before release. To initiate the process, virions attach to susceptible cells by interaction of discrete components on the viral surface (*e.g.,* H protein in orthomyxoviruses, fiber antigen on adenoviruses) with specific receptors on the cell. Several of these have been isolated in recent years. They are normal cellular surface components the virus has adapted for its use. Examples of human viruses and receptors are: HIV-CD4 molecule on T cells; rhinovirus-ICAM (intercellular adhesion molecule) -1; EBV-C3d receptor on B-lymphocytes. There is also a species specificity of cell receptors for certain viruses; polio binds only to primate (human, monkey) cells. This means other cells, such as chick cells, are not "susceptible" to poliovirus. However, if intact polio RNA is introduced into the chick cells, polio virus *is* produced. Thus, the chick cells are still permissive for polio virus production, although not "susceptible." In general, once the animal virus has attached to its receptor, the virus penetrates (either by viropexis or, in the case of enveloped viruses, by fusion of viral envelope with cell membrane) into the cytoplasm where the genome is uncoated and interacts with the synthetic apparatus of the cell. In most DNA viruses, the nucleic acid is double-stranded and, through mRNA, codes for synthesis of early proteins (enzymes required for synthesis of new viral DNA) and for late proteins (viral structural proteins). Naked DNA viruses (*e.g.*, adenoviruses) accumulate in the nucleus and are released by ultimate disintegration of the cell. Herpesviruses are enveloped, DNA viruses. They are also assembled in the nucleus; however, as they emerge the nucleocapsid acquires from the nuclear membrane a lipid-containing envelope into which virus-coded glycoproteins have been inserted. Poxviruses are synthesized and assembled in the cytoplasm. Parvoviruses contain only single-stranded DNA; some are defective such as adenoassociated virus (AAV) and require helper virus for replication. Certain DNA viruses (*e.g.,* adenoviruses, herpesviruses) can transform nonpermissive cells (*i.e.,* cells unable to support the complete viral replicative cycle), and viral DNA integrates into the host cell genome in a manner analogous to lysogeny by bacteriophage.

In RNA viruses with a single-stranded genome, the RNA may be "positive" (*i.e.,* have the same sequence of nucleotide bases as viral mRNA as in poliovirus) or "negative" (*i.e.,* require an intravirion transcriptase-RNA polymerase to synthesize mRNA, utilizing virion RNA as a template, as in influenza or parainfluenza virions). It is particularly of interest to note that with influenza virus, there is a cannibalization of 5′ caps (7-methyl inverted dGTP) from newly synthesized host mRNAs to serve as a primer for synthesis of the mRNA by the intravirion transcriptase. This is accomplished by a virus-encoded endonuclease. Also, note that the single-stranded RNA genome in orthomyxoviruses such as influenza is segmented, which accounts for the genetic reassortment of these viruses and hence the unique epidemiology of the disease influenza. In most other single-stranded RNA viruses (*e.g.,* paramyxoviruses), the genome is unsegmented and therefore cannot undergo intratypic reassortment; such viruses are antigenically stable. Enveloped RNA viruses (including RNA tumor viruses) are released by budding through the cell membrane, which, at the sites of viral morphogenesis, acquires the proteins (*e.g.,* H and N of influenza virus) subsequently found in the viral envelope. Newly synthesized surface components (*e.g.,* H protein of orthomyxoviruses, capsid proteins of naked viruses) evoke antibodies that block attachment and penetration by subsequently introduced virus of the same type. Viral surface components therefore include the "protective" antigens that account for the efficacy of viral vaccines in stimulating specific antiviral immunity in susceptible individuals, and for the sustained immunity to reinfection following the primary disease (*e.g.,* H antigen of measles virus, HN antigen of mumps virus). Antibody to internal antigens (*e.g.,* nucleocapsid) does not neutralize infectivity but is useful for classifying viruses such as influenza A or B. Some viruses have a double-stranded RNA genome (*e.g.,* reoviruses, rotaviruses); their replication is even more complex.

Laboratory Cultivation and Analysis of Animal Viruses

A number of animal viruses, notably orthomyxoviruses, can be propagated in embryonated chicken eggs. For primary isolation, amniotic inoculation is best. Serial passage is done by chorioallantoic inoculation, virus being shed into the chorioallantoic fluid, from which it can be concentrated and purified (as for influenza vaccines). Cell and tissue culture is the mainstay of laboratory virology. Cells for culture are dissociated initially from tissue by digestion with trypsin and EDTA ***(versene),*** washed in balanced salt solution, and suspended in growth medium containing serum and necessary minerals, amino acids, vitamins, glucose, and a bicarbonate-CO_2 buffer system to equilibrate with ambient gases. Phenol red (phenolsulfonphthalein, PSP) is the usual indicator because its color change (alkaline to acid, red to yellow) is in the physiological range (around *p*H 6.8). Dissociated cells attach readily to the surface of glass or plastic and grow out in a spreading sheet one cell thick (monolayer). Cells derived from neoplastic tissue (aneuploid) can usually be serially passaged (*i.e.,* trypsinized off the glass, divided and dispensed to new vessels) an indefinite number of times and are called cell lines. Cells derived from normal tissue (*e.g.,* human foreskin, embryonic lung, kidney) are diploid and have a finite life *in vitro,* that is, they will survive only a few serial passages. However, certain diploid cell "strains" (*e.g.,* WI 38 human embryonic lung cells) can be passaged many times before dying out and are therefore valuable for production of viruses in bulk for vaccine preparation.

The presence of virus in inoculated monolayers is signaled by the appearance of cytopathic effects (CPE) manifested as rounding, separation and necrosis of cells (*e.g.,* enteroviruses), nuclear enlargement and clumping (*e.g.,* adenoviruses), or cell-to-cell fusion with formation of syncytia or polykaryons (*e.g.,* respiratory syncytial virus). These changes are usually visible in fresh unstained cultures when examined under low power with reduced light, or by phase-contrast microscopy. Monolayers prepared and infected on coverslips can be fixed and stained (Giemsa, H&E) to reveal so-called inclusion bodies, which are frequently pathognomonic of certain viruses. The site of these changes, whether cytoplasmic (*e.g.,* respiratory syncytial virus, which, besides being syncytiogenic, produces large eosinophilic cytoplasmic inclusions) or nuclear (*e.g.,* herpesviruses produce eosinophilic nuclear inclusions; adenoviruses produce Feulgen-positive nuclear inclusions, often in crystalline array), gives an indication of the class of infecting agent involved. DNA viruses, with the exception of poxviruses, mature in the nucleus; RNA viruses mature primarily in the cytoplasm. The composition of inclusions can be determined by cytochemical (*e.g.,* Feulgen, acridine orange for NA, lipid stains) and immunochemical techniques (FAb, enzyme-labelled antibody) and by electron microscopy of ultrathin sections of infected cells. Inclusions are found to be aggregates of virions (mature and incomplete particles, as with herpesviruses) or of viral subunits (*e.g.,* paramyxoviral nucleocapsid).

Viral Hemagglutination (HA)

Many animal viruses, such as myxoviruses, paramyxoviruses, adenoviruses, some of the enteroviruses, agglutinate erythrocytes of different species *in vitro,* thereby providing a useful and relatively uncomplicated method for quantitating (titering) these viruses and for measuring antibody to them (hemagglutination inhibition, HI). In enveloped viruses, HA is mediated by an envelope glycoprotein (H in orthomyxoviruses, HN in paramyxoviruses). In orthomyxoviruses, a second glycoprotein (neuraminidase, N) is responsible for elution of the virus from the erythrocyte surface in vitro, as well as for the liberation of virions from the surface of infected cells. During elution from the erythrocyte, receptors for myxoviruses are destroyed with accompanying release of free *N*-acetylneuraminic acid (NANA). Cells in monolayer cultures infected with myxoviruses or paramyxoviruses adsorb erythrocytes (hemadsorption) owing to the presence of hemagglutinin glycoprotein in the cell membrane. This is a useful procedure to detect the presence of these viruses in diagnostic cell cultures. HA by poxviruses is mediated by a lipoprotein that is separate from the virion and is liberated into the medium during viral replication. Adenoviral HA is mediated by a capsid protein complex (penton fibers). Enteroviral HA is mediated by a specific capsid protein.

Viruses can be quantitated by plaque counts (in a manner analogous to bacteriophage). After inoculation of replicate monolayers with dilutions (usually decimal) of virus preparation, the cells are overlaid with semisolid agar containing nutrients and neutral red (a vital dye). The gel formed by the agar immobilizes any free virus remaining from the inoculum or progeny virus, thereby limiting subsequent cycles of infection to centrifugal spread from initially infected cells directly to others in immediate contact. After appropriate incubation, plaques are revealed as clear unstained areas of viral cytolysis. Intervening areas of remaining normal cells are stained. In plates inoculated with sufficiently dilute virus, each plaque represents the progeny of a single infectious unit. From the plaque count, the number of infectious viral particles (or more accurately, PFU) contained in the original preparation of virus can be estimated. With viruses that are not rapidly cytocidal, foci of infection can be revealed with special stains, immunofluorescence, or hemadsorption.

THE LABORATORY IN THE DIAGNOSIS OF VIRAL INFECTION

For the laboratory to be of maximal utility to the clinician, specimens submitted for diagnostic analysis must be accompanied by relevant clinical information regarding the patient's illness and what type of viral infection is suspected on the basis of signs, symptoms, and epidemiological data (*e.g.,* the type of infection "going around," age groups involved). The manner in which a specimen for primary isolation is handled will often depend on such data; specimens submitted with a request simply for "virus studies" are useless. For primary viral isolation, antibiotics are added (to suppress bacterial and/or fungal contaminants) and cell cultures are directly inoculated (primary human embryonic kidney and lung, WI 38 cells, HeLa, or other cell lines are those most frequently used) and subsequently observed periodically for CPE and/or hemadsorption. Detection of virus may be hastened by direct electron microscopic examination of culture fluid or of vesicular fluid (*e.g.*, herpes, vaccinia, varicella), of cells in urinary tract sediment or sputum (cytomegalovirus, measles virus) or of fecal samples (*e.g.*, rotaviruses). For direct electron microscopy, samples are stained with phosphotungstic acid (''negative'' stain), which reveals the configuration and hence the identity of intact virions of each of the major groups. Specific agglutination with sera of known specificity or with patient sera is often demonstrable (immune-electron microscopy). Serologic diagnosis, even though of necessity retrospective, should always be undertaken whenever possible by submitting to the laboratory acute and convalescent serum samples to be tested concurrently (most frequently by complement fixation) with viral antigens of known specificity. The final identification of viruses isolated in cell culture or in embryonated eggs rests on neutralization tests (HI; neutralization of CPE) with antisera of known specificity. Recently developed monoclonal antibodies with greatly sharpened specificity will have increasing utility in serodiagnosis and identification of viral isolates.

Classification of Animal Viruses

The classification of animal viruses is based on (1) the morphology of the virion as revealed by negative staining and morphogenesis in infected cells; (2) the type and size of nucleic acid (NA), DNA or RNA, constituting the viral genome, whether single-stranded or double-stranded, and genetic relatedness (homology) among individual members of a group; (3) the presence or absence of a lipid envelope as reflected in morphology and by stability of viral infectivity to lipid solvents (ether, chloroform) or detergents; (4) configuration of nucleocapsid (cubic, helical, or complex); (5) the number and immunochemical identity of viral proteins (see Table 5-13).

DNA VIRUSES

Parvoviruses. These are the smallest DNA-containing viruses known to infect vertebrate cells, with a diameter of 18 to 26 nm. Virions are highly stable and resistant to inactivation at pH 3 or at 56° C for 60 minutes. The viral genome is a single strand of DNA, either + or −. Parvoviruses are pathogenic to many animals; in rodents they are oncogenic and immunosuppressive (*e.g.*, minute virus of mice). One genus of parvovirus requires a helper virus in order to undergo a complete replicative cycle (hence named ***dependovirus***), and includes human adeno associated virus (**AAV**). AAV is not associated with any known human disease, although 40% to 80% of humans have antibody to it. The ability of AAV to establish a stable latent state in cells has kindled interest in it as a vector for human gene therapy.

The human parvovirus, B19, has been recently described as the probable cause of bone marrow failure due to a specific cytotoxic relationship with erythroid precursor cells resulting in a transient aplastic crisis for children with homozygous sickle-cell anemia. The cytopathic effect of B19 on these cells is seen as giant pronormoblasts in bone marrow aspirates. It is also the agent that causes ''fifth disease'' (erythema infectiosum) in young children, which is characterized by a ''slapped cheek'' rash. This is very common; 65% of adults have antibody to B19. In naive adults B19 can cause a rheumatoid arthritis condition, be asymptomatic, or lead to a flu-like illness. Further, individuals who are co-infected with HIV-1 and B19 have a greater risk of aplastic anemia due to the immunosuppressive nature of HIV-1. Finally, B19 infection of the fetus is associated with non-immune hydrops fetalis, where infant death is attributable to severe anemia.

Papovaviruses. The group name is derived from *pa*pilloma, *po*lyoma, and *va*cuolating viruses. Recently, the latter family has been condensed into the polyoma viruses. This group now includes rabbit or human papillomaviruses (HPV), mouse polyoma, and simian vacuolating virus 40 (SV40). The viruses can be lytic, where they undergo complete replication and kill their host (permissive) cell, in such cases as mouse polyoma (mouse fibroblast) and SV40 (African green monkey kidney cells), as well as exist in a transforming mode where they can cause tumor formation in their nonpermissive hosts (*e.g.*, newborn hamsters).

The molecular weight of the double-stranded, superhelical twisted DNA genomes of polyoma viruses is 3–5 $\times$ 10^6 daltons, and normally would be expected to have the coding potential for four polypeptides. However, it is known that the ''transforming'' gene of this virus (*e.g.*, T-antigen gene) alone codes for at least three different proteins. This is because of three potential reading frames and differential mRNA splicing. Polyoma viruses have been intensively studied as models for understanding the mechanisms of viral carcinogenesis and cellular transformation in tissue culture. Recently, the observed association of polyoma middle T antigen with normal gene products such as p53 and Rb (retinoblastoma gene product) has opened our awareness to the fact that ''tumor suppressor'' gene products such as these can be inactivated during transformation of cells and enhance progression to cancer (see below). The name polyoma refers to the fact that when large amounts of such virus are injected into newborn mice or hamsters, a wide variety of histologically different tumors is produced. However, in nature the virus is apparently not tumorigenic. Thus wild mice trapped in some (but not all) apartment buildings in New York City as well as on farms in Georgia were both found to be infected with mouse polyomaviruses; however the mice had no pathologic symptoms. SV40, a simian polyomavirus, can also be isolated from apparently normal cultures of rhesus monkey kidney cells, but only cause tumors (*e.g.*, usually sarcomas) in baby hamsters. Also, several human polyomaviruses related to SV40 have been isolated from patients with progressive multifocal leukoencephalopathy (SV40 PML and JC viruses) or from the urine of immunosuppressed patients (BK virus) and have been shown to induce brain tumors in newborn hamsters, although there is no evidence to indicate that they have a causative role in human tumor formation. PML caused by JC occurs mainly in immune-deficient hosts, as a complication of CLL (chronic lymphocytic leukemia), Hodgkins, or AIDS. As a sidelight it is of interest to note that millions of U.S. residents were exposed to SV40 between 1955 and 1961 when they were immunized with contaminated polio vaccines, yet no SV40-related tumor has appeared. Thus, at this time the oncogenic potential of polyomaviruses appears of interest more in a laboratory than a clinical setting.

In contrast to polyoma, the family of papilloma viruses has become increasingly important in recent years because of their association with a number of human cancers. In general, though most of the 65 HPVs infect surface epithelia and cause benign rather than malignant epithelial tumors or warts at the site of entry (*e.g.*, on the skin or mucous membranes: genital and laryngeal papillomas). The virus is localized to the lesion and no viremia is observed.

Although virus particles can be seen in the electron microscopy of biopsy material, they have not yet been propagated in the lab. However, since papilloma viral DNA can be isolated, it has served as a useful diagnostic marker. The virus persists in the proliferating basal cell layer of the skin in the form of free DNA and matures into virions as tissue moves upwards and outward to form the keratinized layer at the surface. Degenerating cells and cell debris shed from the surface contain large amounts of virus particles. Virus can be transmitted from human to human by inoculation of a cell-free extract of wart tissue. Of the 65 different human papilloma viruses (HPV), most have been classified based on comparison of restriction DNA patterns or by the use of DNA hybridization techniques.

1. ***Verruca vulgaris:*** This most common family of warts has three known types (HPV-1, -2, -3) and may occur anywhere on the body but usually on fingers and hands. The warts are small (1 to 2 mm) epidermal tumors that are rough, elevated, firm to palpation, and occur in groups. They are stable for years of disappear spontaneously. Plantar warts ***(Verruca plantaris)*** are a clinical subvariety that occur in weight-bearing points of the body (usually beneath a callous), grow in depth, and cause acute pain (HPV-1) and (HPV-4).
2. ***Condyloma acuminatum*** or urogenital warts: Consists of two different papilloma viruses (HPV-6 and -11). These warts occur in warm, moist areas of the external genitalia. The lesions appear as large, soft, red masses that may coalesce and are transmitted as a venereal disease. In women, HPV-6 and -11 are commonly present in cervical condylomas and early-grade CIN-1 (CIN = cervical intraepithelial neoplasia) but rarely progress to CIN-3 or invasive cancer.
3. ***Verruca plana*** (juvenile warts): The flat, smooth lesions are always multiple, and occur on face, neck, dorsal surfaces of hands or arms. Lesions may remain unchanged for months or years, or disappear spontaneously.
4. ***Juvenile laryngeal papillomas*** (HPV-11): These occur predominantly in the 2- to 5-year age group, and mothers of these children frequently have a history of genital virus warts. By molecular cloning of HPV-11 DNA from laryngeal papilloma, partial (25%) identity was shown of HPV-11 with HPV-6.
5. ***Epidermodysplasia verruciformis*** (EV): HPV-5, HPV-8, and now HPV-38b lesions are seen in patients with the disease epidermodysplasia verruciformis (EV) and can become malignant (about 60% of the time). Malignant tumors of the skin develop at an early age in EV patients, predominantly in exposed areas of the skin. The time from onset of skin lesions to the onset of cancer suggests that interaction of HPV-38b with UV light and host factors are associated with development of the skin carcinoma.
6. ***Cervical cancer:*** HPV-16, -18, as well as HPV-31, -33, -35, have recently been associated in up to 85% of CIN-3 cases, as well as two-thirds of invasive squamous cell carcinomas of the uterine cervix. A probe utilizing fragments of these DNAs is being developed as a supplementary test to do with the Pap (Papanicolaou) smear. Pap test screening has greatly (70%) reduced mortality from cervical cancer; however, improvements, such as including a mixed HPV probe, will enhance this percentage. As a caveat, it should be noted that although infection by viruses such as HPV-16 and -18 can contribute to the development of cervical carcinoma, other risk factors (smoking, hormonal imbalance, integration state, and site of viral DNA) appear needed for progression to invasive cancer. Epidemiological studies suggest a latent period of as long as 20 to 25 years.

As noted earlier, it is difficult to study viral growth and replication for papillomaviruses because there is no readily available tissue culture system (other than differentiating epithelial cells) for propagation of the viruses.

Adenoviruses. Their morphology is unique in that the icosahedral capsid comprises 240 ***hexons*** (one capsomer has six neighbors) and 12 ***pentons*** composed of one apical capsomer (with five neighbors) bearing a knobbed ***fiber.*** The penton fiber mediates attachment to cells and hemagglutination.

Adenoviruses have enabled researchers to recognize biological concepts of great significance, including splicing, viral hybridization, associated helper viruses, cell transformation, and viral oncogenesis. In terms of disease, those types most commonly associated with respiratory infections, such as types 1, 2, and 5, are nearly ubiquitous, infect most children very early in life (0 to 6 years), and their DNA may persist indefinitely in tonsillar tissues. Types 3, 4, 7, 14, and 21 are more likely to cause acute respiratory disease (ARD) in adults. Also, pharyngoconjunctival fever can be a major expression of infection with any of several types of adenovirus. However, in general, adenoviruses do not cause more than 5 to 8% of ARD in civilian populations. The highest attack rates (50% to 80%) are among military recruits.

More than 40 human adenovirus serotypes have been identified and classified into 4 different groups based on their oncogenic potential for newborn hamsters. In general, the virus reaches susceptible tissue, mostly by aerosol or direct skin contact, and multiplies there. Although there is no viremia, the virus multiplies in the GI tract and can be recovered from stool up to 18 months after infection. For most of the serotypes, adenoids may be latently infected for life after primary infection. In any case, a type-specific immunity remains for life, with no recurrent infection by the same serotype.

Most adenovirus infections are inapparent and result in a self-limited illness, followed by recovery and development of type-specific immunity. However, as indicated above certain types give a more serious illness.

1. ARD: types 3, 4, 7, 14, and sometimes 21; occurs in adults. Influenzalike fever, headache, chills, malaise, which last 2 to 4 days. Usually no complications. In young children, these viruses have been implicated in occasional cases of fatal nonbacterial pneumonia.
2. Pharyngoconjunctival fever: symptoms like ARD, with inflammation of throat and tonsils, and conjunctivitis. It is mostly associated with type 3, and sometimes with types 7, 14, and 21. The pharyngitis lasts 4 to 5 days; conjunctivitis can last as long as 3 weeks. No complications ensue.
3. Acute follicular conjunctivitis: caused mainly by type 3 or 7; can involve one or both eyes, with lacrimation and a serous exudate that lasts several weeks.
4. Epidemic keratoconjunctivitis: this is highly infectious; caused primarily by types 8 and 19. There is a sudden onset with edema of the conjunctiva accompanied by a mononuclear cell exudate, a low-grade fever, and periauricular lymphadenopathy. The keratitis consists of small opacities (0.01 to 0.3 mm) that may ulcerate. It may last weeks or months with no permanent damage.
5. Hemorrhagic cystitis and gastroenteritis without respiratory disease have also been seen in young children. Adenovirus types 40 and 41 have been isolated as the causative agents.

Herpesviruses. The human herpesviruses include herpes simplex virus (HSV) (types 1 and 2), varicella-zoster virus (VZV), cytomegalovirus (CMV) and Epstein-Barr virus (EBV). Over the past ten years, two new viruses were discovered, human herpesviruses 6 and 7 (HHV 6, 7). Most recently, sequences of a new virus (HHV 8) have been found, associated with both endemic and AIDS-associated forms of Kaposi's Sarcoma (KS). HHV 8 itself has recently been isolated.

While the clinical manifestations of infection vary, all herpesviruses have the capacity to establish latent infection after primary replication in tissues at the site of entry (*e.g.*, HSV in trigeminal or presacral ganglia, VZV in dorsal root ganglia) from which endogenous recurrences emanate (*e.g.*, shingles is recrudescent varicella). The exact molecular mechanism of latency is not known, but there appears to be a correlation for HSV latently infected neuronal cells with RNA species generated from the ***LAT*** (latency) gene. Genital herpes (usually due to HSV-2) is sexually transmitted. Herpetiform genital lesions can also be caused by EBV or CMV. These two viruses, which can be found in semen and cervical secretions, must now be added to the list of sexually transmitted disease (Table 5-14). Several of the herpesviruses have oncogenic properties. EBV, which is the etiological agent for infectious mononucleosis (''kissing disease'') in young adults (15–25 yrs) in the U.S., apparently acting with other cofactors also causes African Burkitt's lymphoma (immortalization of B cells), nasopharyngeal carcinoma (epithelial cells affected in Southeast Asia elderly men), and lymphoproliferative disorders in immunodeficient hosts. HSV, CMV, and EBV can also transform certain cells *in vitro*. A live attenuated varicella viral vaccine, first developed in Japan (Oka strain grown in human diploid fibroblasts), has been shown to be 70% to 90% effective in preventing childhood varicella, even in leukemic children who are in remission and stopped chemotherapy. In 1995, the U.S. FDA licensed and the American Academy of Pediatrics endorsed this vaccine to be given to children between 12 and 18 months of age, as well as to older children who have not had chicken pox. The potential for acquiring zoster (shin-

TABLE 5-14. Sexually Transmitted Diseases*

DISEASE	CAUSATIVE AGENTS	DIAGNOSIS	IMMUNE RESPONSE	TREATMENT
Gonorrhea	*Neisseria gonorrheae* (colony types 1,2)	Gram stain, culture, Fab	Antibody to pili	Penicillin (PPNG, CMRNG, spectinomycin)
	(*N. meningitidis*)			
Syphilis	*Treponema pallidum*	Darkfield (1°, 2°)	RPR, FTA-ABS	Penicillin
Vaginitis (nontrichomonal)	*Gardnerella vaginalis*	Gram stain, "clue cells"		Tetracycline (sulfonamide)
Chancroid (soft chancre)	*Hemophilus ducreyi*	Gram stain		Sulfonamide
Lymphogranuloma venereum (LGV)	*Chlamydia trachomatis* Immunotypes $L_{1,2,3}$	Smear and Giemsa stain, inclusions, Fab	CF antibody	Tetracycline (sulfonamide)
Cervicitis	Immunotypes D, E		Mycoplasmacidal test (metabolic inhibition)	
Nongonococcal urethritis (NGU)	D,E *Ureaplasma urealyticum* ("T" mycoplasma)	Culture		
Granuloma inguinale (donovanosis)	*Calymmatobacterium granulomatis*	CF antibody		
Pelvic inflammatory disease (PID)	Polymicrobial: *Bacteroides* and other anaerobes, Chlamydiae	Culture (endocerv.) & culdocentesis		Depends on cultures; penicillin
Herpes genitalis	Herpes simplex, type 2 (CMV, EBV)	Primary isolation	Neutralizing antibody	
Anogenital warts (condyloma acuminatum)	Papovavirus (HPV6, 11)	EM of tissue cells		Podophyllin (fetal toxicity)
Genital molluscum contagiosum	Poxvirus (Molluscum contagiosum virus)	Giemsa stain, eosinophilic inclusions		
Hepatitis	Type A (B)	B: Immunodiffusion RIA HBs ag, ab		
Intrauterine and Perinatal Infections	**T**oxoplasma			
	(**O**ther—*e.g.*, group B step. GC lues)	Fab, CF test		
	Rubella	HI (IgM)		
	Cytomegalovirus	Inclusion bodies		
	H*erpes genitalis*		Primary vs. secondary	

* Also shigellosis, amebiasis, giardiasis in homosexual men; ectoparasites (lice, scabies); trichomoniasis (vaginitis, urethritis, balanitis).

gles) from virus harbored in nerve cells and reactivated later in life is unlikely, according to the FDA.

About ten years ago, a new human herpes virus, HHV-6, was isolated from patients with immune or lymphoproliferative disorders. Although there is no *in vivo* evidence for HHV-6 enhancing progression to AIDS, *in vitro* it and HIV-1 can co-infect $CD4^+$ cells. Serological studies show that HHV-6 infection begins early (<2 yrs) in life, with up to 90% of individuals being infected by age 40. Recently, it has been associated with "roseola" or exanthem subitum, a benign febrile illness of infants.

Poxviruses. These are the largest of the animal viruses (200 to 350 nm), the tightly structured lipoprotein enveloped virion having complex bilateral symmetry. The virus develops in the cytoplasm, where it produces characteristic eosinophilic inclusions (Guarnieri bodies). This family of DNA viruses is unique in that it replicates in the cytoplasm and carries its own transcriptase to make early mRNA. There is a two-stage uncoating process; after complete uncoating, viral DNA is replicated in excess (20,000 DNA/cell) with only 25% of the DNA used for progeny. Then late mRNA begins, with a switchoff of early mRNA, synthesis of capsid proteins, and of the transcriptase. Assembly then occurs in the cytoplasmic factories, which appear as inclusion bodies.

It has recently been shown that during infection of the host, large DNA viruses, such as poxviruses, also encode proteins that specifically interfere early with components of the immune system. Among these poxvirus immune defense molecules is a secreted protein that, by binding

C4B and C3B complement components, inhibits both classical and alternative pathways of complement activation. Other poxvirus inhibitors block interferon transduction as well as IL-1 and TNF activity (see Immunology section).

The following poxviruses affect humans.

1. ***Variola (smallpox):*** Humans are the only natural hosts; the last case as determined by the WHO was diagnosed about 20 years ago. Because of the tightly structured envelope, the virus is resistant to drying. It can persist in bedclothes and is airborne from skin lesions.
2. ***Cowpox*** (cattle, humans): Vaccination was discovered by Jenner in the 1790s, using serum from a cowpox lesion on a milkmaid. He inoculated an 8-year-old boy, who became resistant. Vaccinia virus, which is the current vaccine strain being used for recombinant DNA technology, is a variant of cowpox adapted to infect humans efficiently with a low-grade infection. Until 1971, all infants received vaccina virus vaccine to provide variola immunity. This was discontinued because of the absence of endemic and imported disease, as well as concern about complications, for example, immunosuppressed patients or those with anti-IgG antibodies develop a progressive fatal vaccinia disease; infants scratching could get the virus in the eyes leading to keratitis; and patients with eczema were likely to develop diffuse vaccinial lesions over the skin.
3. ***Paravaccinia*** and ***orf virus:*** The cause of nodules on the hands of animal handlers.
4. ***Molluscum contagiosum:*** Causes the formation of benign epidermal tumors in children and young adults that ordinarily disappear within a few months. They may be removed to prevent autologous spread.

RNA VIRUSES

Picornaviridae (*L. pico* + RNA). This group includes viruses of three genera pathogenic for humans: *Enterovirus, Rhinovirus,* and *Cardiovirus.*

Enterovirus. There are four categories of enteroviruses:

1. *Polioviruses* (three serotypes): These cause enteric infection, from which the viruses spread hematogenously to the central nervous system to cause poliomyelitis (infection of anterior horn cells, motor paralysis) or "non-paralytic poliomyelitis" (so-called aseptic meningitis); both syndromes are also occasionally due to other enteroviruses. True paralytic poliomyelitis is now a rarity thanks to effective vaccines.
2. *Coxsackievirus:* Group A viruses (23 serotypes) are distinguished from those of group B (six serotypes) on the basis of type-specific neutralization tests and selective tissue damage in suckling mice. These viruses cause a wide spectrum of disease: aseptic meningitis, encephalitis, pleurodynia (mostly group A), myocarditis (mostly group B).
3. *Echo viruses:* Originally called *e*nteric *c*ytopathic *h*uman *o*rphan viruses. They are no longer "orphan" viruses; many agents of this group produce a wide spectrum of disease, including aseptic meningitis with neuronal injury and paralysis, acute respiratory disease, infantile diarrhea, summer febrile illness with rubeoliform exanthem.
4. *Hepatitis A:* This virus is type 72 enterovirus.

Rhinovirus. More than 100 serotypes of rhinovirus are known. Most are cultivable in human embryonic kidney cells, human diploid lung cells, or tracheal organ culture at 33° C. They are rarely found in the lower intestinal tract. Rhinoviruses are the most frequent causes of the afebrile common cold syndrome in adults; immunity to reinfection is type-specific.

Cardiovirus. This group includes pathogens for various animal species. ***Encephalomyocarditis*** (EMC) virus, the only human pathogen in the group, causes relatively undifferentiated mild febrile illness.

Caliciviridae. Members of this group differ from the picornaviruses because of their larger size and the fact that they possess but a single structural protein. The only human pathogen in the group (***Norwalk agent,*** of which there may be at least four serogroups as determined by immune electron microscopy) has not yet been propagated in cell culture, but is readily seen by direct electron microscopy of negatively stained fecal extracts. The Norwalk agent is an important cause of acute epidemic gastroenteritis in all age groups. Recently, a specific NA probe has been developed for it that should aid both in diagnosis and detection of the virus in polluted estuarine or shellfish-growing waters.

Reoviridae. ***Orthoreoviruses*** (three serotypes) are widely distributed in humans and in lower animals, their role in human disease still not being clearly defined (*re*spiratory *e*nteric *o*rphan viruses). Originally grouped with the echoviruses, they subsequently were found to differ significantly in being larger than picornaviruses and in having a double-stranded segmented RNA genome. Structurally similar but antigenically distinct viruses are ***orbivirus,*** the cause of Colorado tick fever (encephalitis) and therefore operationally an arbovirus, and ***rotavirus,*** the cause of acute infectious gastroenteritis in infants and young children. Two serotypes of rotavirus are distinguishable by immune electron microscopy of virions that appear in large quantity during active diarrheal disease. Efforts are under way to develop a vaccine against this important cause of enteric disease.

Togaviridae and Flaviviridae. These include viruses previously designated as *arboviruses* (*ar*thropod *bo*rne), four genera being distinguished primarily on the basis of antigenic analysis (CF, HI, N). Arboviruses typically infect mammals and avian species and are maintained in animal reservoirs by hematophagous arthropods. To become infectious, the arthropod vector must bite the animal during the viremic stage of infection. True arboviruses actually multiply in, or migrate from the stomach to the mouth parts of, the insect vector. The geographic distribution of arthropod-borne diseases depends on climate, which, in turn, determines the distribution of animal reservoirs and vectors. Human disease due to arboviruses takes many forms, including encephalitis as well as subclinical infection. ***Alphaviruses*** (formerly group A arboviruses) cause eastern, western, and Venezuelan equine encephalitides. ***Flaviviruses*** (formerly group B arboviruses) include viruses causing yellow fever, dengue (four serotypes), encephalitis, both mosquito-borne (Japanese B, St. Louis, Murray Valley, West Nile encephalitides) and tick-borne (Russian spring-summer and other animal encephalitides). ***Rubella*** virus, the cause of German measles, is now classified in the Togaviridae as ***rubivirus.*** Rubella contracted during the first trimester of pregnancy causes severe fetal damage and results in the congenital rubella syndrome in surviving infants. Maternal HI antibody (resulting from prior infection or immunization with vaccine) connotes solid immunity to reinfection and hence fetal protection if exposure occurs during pregnancy. Although there is no evidence that the RA 27/3 vaccine can cause congenital rubella syndrome, the virus nevertheless can cross the placenta and infect the fetus. Pregnancy, therefore, remains a contraindication to vaccination. Inadvertent administration of rubella vaccine during pregnancy, however, should not be construed as a reason for artificial termination.

Bunyaviridae. This group (formerly group C arboviruses) includes the California encephalitis virus group, Rift valley and sandfly fevers, and Congo-Crimean hemorrhagic fever viruses as well as the Atlanta viruses.

Myxoviruses. The term is derived from the affinity of these agents for glycoproteins that are found in secretions and that are similar to if not identical with cell ''receptors'' for viral hemagglutinin and infection. Characteristically these viruses mature by budding at the cell surface where they are enclosed by a lipid-containing membrane (envelope) into which structural subunits (hemagglutinin, H, neuraminidase, N), are inserted. Viral glycoprotein and lipids are host-specific; the polypeptide portions and the enzymes required for glycosylation are virus-coded.

Orthomyxoviruses (Influenza Virus). These are smaller (80 to 100 nm) than the paramyxoviruses (100 to 150 nm) and are divisible into three major serogroups based on the specificity of the ribonucleoprotein (NP) antigens with complement-fixing antibody that is not protective (the ribonucleoprotein is internal). Each group, particularly group A, is subdivisible into many serotypes based on the separate antigenic identities of H and N glycoproteins. The latter are subject to antigenic drift and shift resulting from complex genetic reassortments (the viral genome comprises eight segments) in response to immunologic pressures in the individual and herd environments. Group A viruses include swine, equine, and avian viruses; the human strains have hitherto been the cause of all epidemic influenza. Group B strains cause continuing sporadic incidence of influenza and are peculiarly related to the serious and often fatal complication of Reye's syndrome, although recently some cases have been linked to type A flu. Because of the role of salicylates in exacerbating this syndrome, the use of aspirin has been contraindicated in treatment of influenza. Group C viruses are of apparently low intrinsic virulence and account for an unknown, but probably appreciable, proportion of minor respiratory illness, particularly in young children and the elderly. Antibodies to all the major groups are widespread in the adult population.

For diagnosis, orthomyxoviruses are readily recovered by the inoculation of throat washings into primary monkey kidney or human embryonic kidney cells. Hemadsorption indicates the presence of virus, which is then typed by hemagglutination inhibition with sera of known specificity.

Retrospective serodiagnosis is achieved by complement fixation with group-specific ribonucleoprotein antigens or with hemagglutination inhibition with standard viruses. Nonspecific inhibitors (non-immunoglobulin sialoprotein receptor analogues) universally present in normal sera must be inactivated with receptor-destroying enzyme (RDE), which leaves specific antibody present to account for any HI activity in the serum.

Active immunization with killed virus vaccine is the single most important measure to prevent and/or attenuate the disease influenza. Vaccine currently in use is grown in chicken eggs (chorioallantoic fluid), inactivated with formalin, and partially purified to reduce the content of egg protein. When the virus in the vaccine has been disrupted by detergent (subunit, subvirion, or ''split'' vaccine), the content of H and N (protective antigens) is relatively enhanced, with correspondingly less total protein per dose. Split virus vaccine, reactions to which are less than to whole virus, should be used to immunize infants and children up to 12 years of age. H and N antigens of virus in the vaccine should match the antigens of strains prevalent in the community as closely as possible. The current variable influenza type A antigens are H1N1 and H3N2. No one with known allergy to egg protein should be immunized. Although pregnancy per se is *not* a contraindication to administration of influenza virus vaccine, immunization should be deferred until the second or third trimesters. The target groups with highest priority are (1) adults and children with chronic cardiopulmonary disorders, chronic metabolic diseases, renal dysfunction, anemia, immunosuppression, or asthma; (2) residents of chronic care facilities; (3) individuals over 65 years of age; (3) health care personnel who have extensive contact with high-risk patients. Amantadine hydrochloride (Symmetrel) is an alternative to active immunization. It is effective (by interfering with uncoating of virus during replication) in mollifying disease due to group A strains, but is *not* effective against group B strains. Amantadine is also effective prophylactically when influenza A outbreaks are anticipated.

Paramyxoviruses. These are large enveloped viruses in which the genome is a single strand of unsegmented RNA. This accounts for their antigenic stability. In parainfluenza, mumps, and Newcastle disease (of fowls) viruses, one glycoprotein in the envelope contains both H and N activities. Measles (also called rubeola, or ''red measles''), canine distemper, and rinderpest (a disease of cattle) viruses, which are antigenically related to one another, lack N activity; respiratory syncytial virus has neither H nor N. A second separate glycoprotein (F) in the viral envelope accounts for the cell-fusing activity which characterizes the cytopathology of these viruses, particularly measles and respiratory syncytial viruses. Measles vaccine is an attenuated strain (Edmonston) of the virus grown in chicken embryo fibroblast culture.

Current efforts are being directed at developing a recombinant vaccinia virus vector to ***human respiratory syncytial virus*** (RSV), a major cause of viral lower respiratory tract illness in infants and young children worldwide. Previous attempts to develop a safe and effective RSV vaccine have met with failure. A formalin-inactivated vaccine tested 20 years ago not only failed to protect but also led to an enhancement of disease during infection by RSV. The live recombinant vaccinia virus vector currently being developed expresses the glycoprotein fusion protein F, which mediates viral penetration and cell-cell spread by membrane fusion.

Rhabdoviridae. Viruses of this group are elongated, bullet-shaped particles (Gr. rhabdos, rod). The chief pathogen is rabies virus *(Lyssavirus)* and antigenically related viruses in various parts of the world. The virus has a lipoprotein-glycoprotein envelope containing a single (protective) antigen, and the helical nucleocapsid contains the genome as a single strand of negative (nonmessenger) RNA. The virion carries an RNA transcriptase and is cultivable in a variety of cells *in vitro.* The virus replicates in the cytoplasm, forming inclusions (Negri bodies), and matures by budding at the cell membrane. Virus grown in human diploid cells and inactivated constitutes the vaccine used for prophylaxis, in conjunction with human immune globulin from hyperimmunized individuals. Marburg and Ebola agents (hemorrhagic fevers transmissible from person to person without an intermediate vector) are probably in this biologic group; classification of these agents in the family *Filoviridae* has been approved. Rabies is enzootic in rodents (bats, skunks, foxes, raccoons), which are the major sources of human infection. Infection of domestic animals is derived from infected endemic foci. Virus travels along nerve trunks from the sites of entry (usually an animal bite) and localizes in the central nervous system, salivary glands and, occasionally, viscera. Diagnosis is based on clinical and epidemiologic data and on demonstration of Negri bodies by immunofluorescence in smears of hippocampal tissue of the rabid animal.

Retroviruses. Retroviruses are enveloped icosahedral viruses with glycoprotein peplomers on their surface that contain two identical strands of RNA (~8,500 nucleotides) and the unique enzyme reverse transcriptase inside an icosahedral shell. Retrovirus replication, in brief, begins with adsorption of the virus by the spikes or peplomers to specific receptors on host cells, followed by uncoating of the icosahedral core in the cytoplasm, synthesis of a DNA intermediate by the reverse transcriptase, and subsequent integration of this double-stranded proviral DNA into cellular DNA. Transcription of this proviral DNA then provides both viral RNA (vRNA) and mRNA for the following three groups of viral proteins:

1. Group-specific antigens (***gag*** proteins), which make up the icosahedral viral core and enclose the vRNA.
2. ***pol*** polyprotein includes the reverse transcriptase, a viral specific protease, needed for cleavage of the *gag* polyprotein, and an integrase needed for integration of the viral DNA into cellular DNA.
3. ***env*** proteins are inserted at the membrane surface into the budding virus particle.

The ***viral reverse transcriptase*** (RT) is a unique enzyme in that vRNA is converted first to single-stranded DNA (minus strand) and then to double-stranded DNA (minus and plus strand). In the initial replication step, RT binds to a site at the 5′ end of the genomic RNA where a specific cellular tRNA has also bound. Synthesis of the minus strand continues back through the tRNA binding site and, as this process occurs, RNase H activity of the RT degrades the vRNA. In the final stage, both a long terminal repeat (LTR) and double-stranded DNA are formed.

The retroviruses fall into two large families of viruses that cause serious disease in man and other vertebrates. One, the ***oncogenic RNA viruses*** or ***RNA tumor viruses,*** are the major cause of leukemias, lymphomas, and sometimes sarcomas in many species of animals, including chickens, mice, cats, cattle, and gibbon apes.

The principal morphology of the RNA tumor viruses is type C, in which an immature (uncleaved) particle is initially formed and then after cleavage of the *gag* and *pol* polyproteins, a mature (central dense nucleoid) infectious particle results. Among avian type C viruses are both nondefective leukosis viruses (low oncogenic potential), which cause lymphomas or leukemias in chickens, after 4 to 8 months, and the ***Rous sarcoma virus*** (RSV) family (high oncogenic activity because they contain the viral *src* gene).

The other family of retroviruses, the ***lentiviruses,*** which includes HIV, the causative agent of AIDS, has a different morphology. These viruses, such as visna (virus of sheep), are cytopathic rather than oncogenic. In lentiviruses, the particles have a ''C'' type budding or ''immature'' form of the particle, but once matured the particle develops a cylindrical or prolate nucleoid core.

For many years no retrovirus had been linked to a human disease; however, about 15 years ago, a human adult T-cell leukemia virus (HTLV-I) was isolated both in the U.S. and Japan from about 200 patients who had a rare type of T-cell lymphocytic leukemia called adult T-cell leukemia/lymphoma (ATL). Recently, HTLV-I has also been isolated from patients with tropical spastic paraperesis (TSP) and a rare form of myelopathy (HAM). Another human T-cell retrovirus was isolated from several patients with ''hairy'' cell leukemia and named HTLV-II. Antibodies to HTLV-I are found early in life in 10% to 12% of the population in villages of Southwest Japan. HTLV-I lymphocytes have been found as well in the milk of antibody-positive mothers. An increased positivity with age is consistent with sexual and/or blood transmission of the virus. By age 60, 20% of individuals are positive in endemic areas. Incidence of the disease ATL among HTLV-I seropositive individuals is relatively low (<0.1%) at this time, with an incubation period of more than 30 years. Recently, seropositive HTLV-I individuals are being detected among intravenous drug abusers in inner-city areas of New York. The link is thought to be through Caribbean area carriers. The U.S. FDA has approved a test kit for HTLV-I antibody detection to be used by blood banks. The rate of infection among U.S. blood donors is 0.015%. Thus far, only 42 cases of ATL have occurred in the U.S. These patients have all been socioeconomically deprived minority individuals. Since there is no specific antiviral treatment for ATL, a combination of cytotoxic chemotherapeutic regimens are used with moderate, if any, success. The mean survival for ATL patients is 11 months.

The other human T-cell retrovirus, isolated from several patients with ''hairy'' cell leukemia, is named HTLV-II. It may be implicated in the etiology of some human lymphomas; however, at this time no disease has been specifically associated with HTLV-II. Cell lines established from infected patients produce giant cells when co-cultivated with BJAB, an EBV-infected virus negative producing B cell line. In HIV-1 (see below) co-infected individuals there is a 6 times higher risk of Kaposi's sarcoma (KS). In co-infected patients, HTLV-II selects $CD8^+$ cells for infection, leading to an unusual lymphadenopathy. HTLV-II is bloodborne and sexually transmitted. Both HTLV-I and HTLV-II were able to be isolated only because of the development of T-cell growth factors (interleukin-2) to keep T-cells from HTLV-infected patients growing in tissue culture for multiple generations.

In 1983 to 1984, the retrovirus HIV was isolated in France (LAV), as well as the U.S. (HTLV-III) and was shown to be the causative agent of AIDS. In contrast to HTLV-I and II, HIV is cytopathic. This is of interest, since early attempts to isolate the AIDS virus involved long-term culture of cells, anticipating that they were like other oncogenic retroviruses. Instead, it appears that HIV is cytotoxic for lymphocytes with CD4 on their surface ($CD4^+$) and this specificity apparently explains the widespread damage to cell-mediated immunity in AIDS patients. The virus is transmitted through blood or other body fluids, such as semen. Direct physical contact appears to be required. Serologic tests have been developed to screen hospital blood supplies for the AIDS virus and vaccine developments using inactivated whole virus particles, as well as viral glycoprotein subunits are currently under development. At present there is no known cure for AIDS. As discussed above, HIV, although a retrovirus, does not belong to the same viral subfamily as the oncogenic retroviruses such as Rous sarcoma virus, or HTLV-I. Instead it shares homology with the *Lentivirus* subfamily, which are nononcogenic, but cytocidal for lymphocytes, such as Visna virus.

In particular, HIV encodes several regulatory proteins in addition to those coded by *gag, pol,* and *env*. Among these are the *tat, rev, vif,* and *nef* gene products. Specifically, *tat* is a transactivator; *rev* controls regulation of expression of virion proteins and allows transport of single spliced mRNA for *gag* and other proteins from nucleus to cytoplasm, whereby they are translated; *vif* is a virion factor for enhanced infectivity and *nef* is a negative factor postulated to reduce virus expression *in vitro;* however its role *in vivo* is still not defined.

Although HIV itself is not oncogenic, one in five homosexuals who contract AIDS also have an unusual form of Kaposi's sarcoma (purple skin lesions). Overall, one in six people with AIDS has cancer, Kaposi's sarcoma, or non-Hodgkin lymphoma. AIDS is discussed in greater detail in the section Immunodeficiencies and Gammopathies later in this chapter.

Arenaviruses. In this group of viruses, the virion contains characteristic electron-dense granules (*L. arena,* sand), which are now known to be host cell ribosomes. One of the group is the cause of lymphocytic choriomeningitis characterized by infiltration of meninges and choroid plexus, the first-recognized viral, aseptic meningitis. The symptoms are varied, and the disease is usually mild, rarely involving the central nervous system, being mainly referable to the respiratory and enteric tracts. The virus is enzoötic in domestic mice, the source of tangential human infection.

More serious diseases of the hemorrhagic fever type, with neurotropic involvement and hemorrhagic necrosis, and frequently fatal, involve the worldwide Tacaribe group of arenaviruses. Many are arthropod borne. Lassa fever virus is an arenavirus.

Coronaviruses. These agents are named for the "crown" of large, club-shaped projections from the envelope, which encloses a helical nucleocapsid. They are the cause of upper respiratory tract disease and common cold syndrome in adults. Coronaviruses grow poorly in anything but ciliated epithelial organ culture or in particularly sensitive human diploid cells. Twenty strains of coronavirus have been isolated, which by N and CF tests can be classified into three broad serogroups.

Hepatitis Viruses. Hepatitis A (HA) virus purified from human feces is a 27-nm particle that contains RNA and is now classified as a picornavirus (enterovirus 72). It is propagable in a variety of cells in culture, the way thus being opened toward development of an attenuated live viral vaccine. However, the FDA has just recently licensed a safe, effective inactivated HAV vaccine (HAVRIX), which is recommended for individuals at high risk—travelers to endemic areas, IV drug users, individuals in resident institutions, attendants at day care centers, and certain food handlers. HA viruses are worldwide in distribution, with four demonstrated genotypes, which are identical at the serotype level. Introduction of the virus is usually followed rapidly (15 to 45 days) by liver disease of varying severity, which is indistinguishable clinically from infection with hepatitis B virus or with so-called non-A, non-B viruses. Spread of HA is by the fecal-oral route and is related to socioeconomic status and crowded living conditions with poor sanitation. The most common age of incidence is childhood/young adulthood. Antibody is prevalent in a high percentage of most population groups. Percutaneous transmission of HA virus is infrequent. Diagnosis rests on the identification of A particles in feces and/or serodiagnosis with RIA. Specifically, IgM HAV appears after the onset of disease and can be detected by a modified competitive binding RIA. This is important since IgG anti-HAV has limited diagnostic value because it persists for life and it is difficult to see a fourfold rise over such a background. In patients diagnosed with HAV, a dose of 0.02 ml/kg pooled immune serum globulins (IgG) administered intramuscularly within two weeks after exposure can be 80% to 90% effective.

Hepatitis B (HB) virus, contains DNA. The complete virion or Dane particle is surrounded by the surface (S) antigen (originally identified as Australia antigen) containing at least five antigenic specificities (a group antigen, two pairs of subtypic determinants, d/y, w/r, which are mutually exclusive). A variety of subtypes have been recognized. HBs antigen may appear free in the blood early after infection. The Dane particle contains a core that is circular and partially (60 to 85%) double-stranded DNA, as well as two additional antigens (c and e). HBV infection is acquired percutaneously (transfusions, blood-contaminated injection apparatus), or by contact with body effluvia (*e.g.,* semen, saliva). The disease has a relatively long incubation period (40 to 180 days) and insidious onset showing a prolonged elevation of liver enzymes, such as serum glutamic oxaloacetic transaminase (SGOT). Although the disease is most frequently self-limited (virus and HBs antigen disappear, antibody appears) in 5% to 10% of cases, it may evolve into persistent hepatitis (HBs antigen and/or Dane particles and/or HBc antigen persist, little or no antibody appears). Hepatic injury in persistent HB infection may be immunogenic, including both cell-mediated responses and antigen-antibody complex disease. Chronic HBV infection is implicated in the causation of hepatocellular carcinoma (HCC). Diagnosis of HB is by detection of HBs antigen and/or antibody and HBc antigen in the serum by radioimmunoassay. The Delta agent is a viroid (see earlier section) contained in an HBs coat. It was first described in Italy in 1977 and has since then been encountered worldwide. Superinfection with Delta or coprimary infection (HB + Delta) causes particularly fulminant disease. Since Delta never occurs in the absence of HB infection, immunization against the latter will protect against both agents. Pooled normal immunoglobulin affords effective postexposure or preexposure prophylaxis against both A and B viruses. Active immunization with HBs (hepatitis B surface antigen) purified from the plasma of persistently infected patients is noninfectious and is an effective prophylactic agent.

This vaccine was approved in 1981 by the FDA and is recommended for high-risk populations such as dialysis patients and health care professionals. Since there are about 100,000 new cases of HB disease each year in the U.S. with a 1% to 2% fatality rate, this vaccine or one made by recombinant DNA technology (using yeast cells to produce HBs antigen) is extremely important.

No active immunization against other forms of hepatitis is available. Control measures are obvious from the known modes of transmission of both A and B viruses.

Most (estimated at up to 80%) posttransfusion hepatitis is caused by so-called non-A, non-B virus(es) (NANB). Diagnosis in the past was made by exclusion; that is, no IgM anti-HAV, no HBs, and no IgM anti-HBc (in the absence of anti-HBs). Recently, a newly identified virus, Hepatitis C virus (HCV), a positive-strand RNA virus belonging to the Flavivirus (pestivirus) family has been shown to account for more than 60% of NANB in the U.S. and Europe, as well as Japan. Some patients with chronic HCV also develop HCC. In Japan, this has doubled in the past 25 years, while HBV-associated HCC has remained the same. This may be related to a Japanese-specific strain of HCV, as well as a high percentage (>50%) of patients infected (chronic) with HCV who go on to have cirrhosis of the liver. Currently, several second-generation EIA serological tests are available to test blood supplies for HCV, so that a major cause of NANB can be eliminated. Almost 100% of individuals show antibody detection within 20 weeks of exposure. However, there may yet be other agents involved in the cause of this disease.

Chronic Infectious Neuropathic Agents (CHINA Group). This group includes the unconventional agents causing ***kuru*** and ***Creutzfeldt-Jakob*** disease (presenile dementia with myoclonus), both degenerative diseases of the central system (spongiform encephalopathies) with exceptionally long (months to years) incubation periods and usually a fatal outcome. Neither agent has been seen, let alone isolated, although both have been transmitted experimentally to primates. The agent of ***scrapie,*** a similar neuropathy of sheep, has similar properties. Recent evidence, based on resistance of infectivity to ionizing radiation, suggests that the scrapie agent (for which the term *prion* has been introduced), as well as the two human slow encephalopathy agents, may not contain nucleic acid and be classified as agents "subviral" in size. No immune response develops to either human agent. These "slow agent diseases" are to be distinguished from those caused by conventional viruses, that is, subacute sclerosing panencephalitis (SSPE), associated with antecedent rubeola infection or congenital rubella syndrome, and progressive multifocal leukoencephalopathy (PML), caused by a papovavirus (JC virus).

Chemotherapy of Viral Infection

Each of the relatively few agents presently available for antiviral chemoprophylaxis and chemotherapy has restricted application. The amantanes, amantadine (Symmetrel) and rimantadine, by inhibiting uncoating and thereby primary transcription of virus, prevent infection with group A influenza viruses and mollify the disease once it has become clinically evident; these drugs are ineffective against infection with group B or C viruses. DNA analogues are effective in certain infections due to herpesviruses. Topical IUdR (5′-iododeoxyuridine), by blocking viral replication, inhibits the progression of early prestromal stages of keratitis caused by HSV, but cannot be used systemically. Trifluoridine (trifluorothymidine, TFT) is similarly active by topical administration. Adenosine arabinoside (ara-A, vidarabine) and 9-(2-hydroxyethoxymethyl)guanine (acycloguanosine, ACV, acyclovir) are useful in topical treatment of genital herpes simplex. ACV given by mouth markedly reduces, but does not prevent, recurrences of genital lesions; it is effective in systemic (intravenous) therapy of HSV encephalitis proven by brain biopsy as well as of severe herpetic disease in the immunocompromised host. Both these nucleoside analogues are effective in limiting the spread of VZV in the immunocompromised host. Ribavirin (Virazole), an analogue of the purine precursor 5′-aminoimidazole-4-carboxamide, has a wider antiviral spectrum and is active against RNA- and DNA-containing viruses; it is currently undergoing clinical trials in herpesvirus 1 and 2 and VZV infections. Inosine pranobex (Immunovir), a new drug that acts by stimulating the immune system rather than by acting directly against the virus, significantly reduces genital shedding of HSV. Human interferons are receiving increasing attention as potential chemotherapeutic agents. Human leukocyte interferon (HUIFN α 1) has been found to limit systemic varicella infection in immunocompromised (lymphoma) patients. With recent advances in genetic engineering, large-scale production of interferon in cloned bacterial culture is now possible because interferon has been rigorously purified and the human genes coding for its synthesis have been isolated. Isatin-beta-thiosemicarbazone, one of the first antiviral drugs described, was found useful in prophylaxis of variola, which has now been eliminated globally.

Oncogenes and Proto-oncogenes

These RNA tumor virus-associated genes have previously been introduced in the subsection on carcinogenesis (see Table 4-39) and retroviruses (above). ***Oncogenes*** are viral genes responsible for tumorigenesis (v-*onc*). In tissue culture they cause transformation of cells, since they alter cellular growth control. This is because the homologous cellular oncogenes (c-***onc***) or ***proto-oncogenes*** from which they are derived by one or more mutations, recombination or deletion events normally encode factors, such as growth hormone receptors, protein kinases, GTP binding proteins or nuclear DNA binding proteins that regulate transcription. A detailed description is given for about 15 of more than 60 oncogenes in Table 5-15. Some specific examples also discussed below are the ***sis, ras,*** and ***neu*** oncogenes.

TABLE 5-15. Oncogenes

ONCOGENE ACRONYM	ANIMAL RETROVIRUS	SUBCELLULAR LOCATION OF PROTEIN	NATURE OF ENCODED PROTEIN
Class I: Protein Kinases			
src	Rous avian sarcoma (RSV)	Plasma membrane	Tyrosine-specific protein kinases (phosphorylate tyrosine residues)
abl	Abelson murine leukemia	Plasma membrane	
erbA *erbB*	Avian erythroblastosis (AEV)	Plasma membrane	Thyroid hormone (TH) receptor (erbA) can block TH induced regulation; Tyrosine-specific protein kinase derived from EGF receptor (erbB)
mos	Moloney murine sarcoma	Cytoplasm	Protein kinases specific for serine or threonine; regulation of cell cycle progression through G_2/M; homology to cytostatic factor (CSF) that can arrest oocytes at metaphase II of meiosis
Class II: p21 Proteins			
Ha-*ras*	Harvey murine sarcoma	Plasma membrane	Guanine nucleotide-binding proteins with GTPase activity
Class III: Nuclear Proteins			
myc	Avian MC29 (myelocytomatosis)	Nucleus	Proteins involved in regulating transcription
myb	Avian myeloblastosis (AMV)	Nucleus	Proteins involved in regulating transcription
ski	Avian Sloan Kettering virus (SKV)	Nucleus	Stimulates rapid proliferation of myogenic cells (muscle differentiation) by activation of myoD expression
fos	Murine osteosarcoma virus (FBJ)	Nucleus	c-fos and c-jun form a heterodimeric complex that interacts with the DNA regulatory element AP-1 binding site. Dimerization occurs via interaction between leucine zipper domains.
jun	Avian sarcoma virus	Nucleus	
rel	Avian reticuloendotheliosis	Nucleus/cytoplasm	Homology with NFκB—encodes a κB enhancer-binding protein; inhibits NFκB function
Class IV: Growth Factors			
sis	Simian sarcoma (SSV)	Secreted	Derived in part from PDGF gene B chain
HER2, *neu* erbB2	AEV or chemical carcinogen derived	Plasma membrane; transmembrane glycoprotein (185 kD); homology to EGF receptor	Growth factor receptor—extra copies show high predictability for relapse in human breast/ovarian cancer patients

v-*sis*, Ha-*ras* and Breast Cancer-associated Oncogenes *(neu)*. The gene product coding for v-*sis*, the transforming gene of simian sarcoma virus (SSV), an acute transforming primate retrovirus has an extensive homology with PDGF (human platelet-derived growth factor B chain). Thus, transformation of cells by SSV can be explained by overstimulation of infected cells with a biologically active mitogen or growth factor.

The *ras* gene family was originally identified as v-*ras* genes from several acute transforming mouse viruses, such as Harvey sarcoma virus. By using DNA from v-*ras* as a hybridization probe, c-*ras* genes were then found in many eukaryotic organisms, including yeast. Further, it has been shown that such wildtype, normal c-*ras* genes are not able to transform mouse fibroblasts (NIH 3T3 assay) *in vitro*. However, they can acquire transforming potential by a single point mutation within their coding sequences. Such mutated c-*ras* genes have been found in a variety of human cancers. Further, when a recombinant DNA was constructed between mutant c-*ras* + elastase promoter sequences, pancreatic tumors developed in adult mice from embryos microinjected with the recombinant DNA. Little is known about how the *ras* gene products cause malignant transformation. All *ras* genes code for a family of proteins called p21 that exhibit the capacity to bind guanosine nucleotides covalently, have GTPase activity and are located on the inner surface of the plasma membrane. They differ from $pp60^{src}$ since they do not induce tyrosine kinase activity; however, they may like other GTP-binding proteins act as coupling factors and thereby modulate hormone-mediated signaling within cells. This function may explain how v-*ras* genes, such as Ha-*ras,* causes transformation and act as one of the stages in carcinogenesis.

One in 9 women will develop breast cancer in her lifetime. The American Cancer Society estimates 175,000 new cases in 1991, and 45,000 women will die from this disease. Aside from risk factors such as family history, alcohol consumption, fat in the diet, and cigarette smoking, several changes in genetic alterations are observed in breast malignancies. These are amplification of the proto-oncogenes, c-myc, HER2/neu and INT 2, as well as loss of heteroyzygosity (LOH) in 6 chromosomal arms that reflect recessive mutations in tumor suppressor genes, such as 17p for p53 (70% of breast tumors have deletions here) and BRCA-1.

Tumor Suppressor Genes

In contrast to the above positive-acting oncogenes, which lead to transformation as a result of overexpression of growth control elements such as growth factor receptors, there is a newly found family of negative-acting proto-oncogenes, such as wildtype p53 and the retinoblastoma (Rb) gene. Both encode tumor suppressor factors. The two copies of RB gene located on chromosome 13, when dually inactivated by mutation (germline or somatic), lead to the eye tumor retinoblastoma. This dual loss in many cases is evidenced by the existence of two identically mutated alleles. As a means of detecting potential homozygosity of mutant alleles, one examines whether or not flanking DNA sequences exhibit loss of heterozygosity (LOH). The repeated observation of LOH of a specific chromosomal marker suggests that there is a closely mapping tumor suppressor gene, whose loss of function is involved in tumor pathogenesis, *i.e.,* a chromosome 18q DNA highly heterogeneous in most genomes had a 70% homozygous state in 70% of advanced colon carcinoma. We are at the threshold of identifying large numbers of tumor suppressor genes, many of whose gene products act in tumor surveillance.

The wildtype p53 product has been best studied. As noted above it was found initially in association with polyoma middle T, as well as SV-40T-antigen. It is expressed in the nucleus of most cells and has a rapid turnover time (20 minutes). Normally, it is believed to serve a role in oncogene surveillance. For example, the E7 gene product of HPV-16 associates with both p53 and Rb, removing these products from their protective role. If there is also an activated H-*ras* (mutant form of c-*ras*) oncogene present in these cells, it will become transformed.

PROTOZOA

These are eukaryotic unicellular microorganisms, a number of which are human pathogens, and some of which require insect vectors for transmission.

Blood and Tissue Protozoa

Development stages of these parasites occur in vertebrate hosts and in sanguivorous arthropod vectors; some are true zoonoses and cause tangential human infection.

TRYPANOSOMES (GENUS *TRYPANOSOMA*)

Protozoa of this genus may occur in one or more of four forms: ***trypomastigote, epimastigote, promastigote,*** and ***amastigote,*** depending on the species and whether in the arthropod vector or mammalian host. Mature trypanosomes are spindle-shaped, with an undulating, keel-like membrane, edged with an anteriorly projecting flagellum. They are from 15 to 30 nm in length and exhibit active lashing motility. The trypaniform stages occur in the blood, tissues, and spinal fluid of febrile victims of infection, thus furnishing a means of microscopic diagnosis. The epimastigote form occurs in the arthropod vectors.

Trypanosoma brucei gambiense is endemic in west and central Africa; *T.b.rhodesiense* is enzootic in a number of wild and domestic animals. Both cause ***African sleeping sickness*** and are transmitted by infected tsetse flies of the genus *Glossina.* Although thcsc infcctions occur primarily in Africa, the increasing intensity of world travel brings the heightened possibility of importation of these afflictions to other geographic areas. Infection with *T.b.gambiense* is a more protracted and chronic disease than infection with *T.b.rhodesiense,* which may be rapidly fatal without central nervous system involvement. Both go through three successive stages: parasitemia; lymphadenitis and invasion of the central nervous system, accompanied by increasing degrees of toxemia, wasting, and torpor; and ending in death. Trypomastigote forms are found in blood, lymph nodes, and, in protracted cases of encephalitis, spinal fluid. Trypanosomes evade the host's immune response by undergoing antigenic variation. FAb and ELISA provide useful diagnostic information, in conjunction with measurement of IgM levels. Intravenous suramin is the chemotherapeutic agent of choice, but its administration must be carefully monitored because of its major renal toxicity; in central nervous system involvement, melarsoprol (a toxic arsenical) is added to therapy.

American trypanosomiasis (Chagas' disease) is caused by *T. cruzi,* which differs from African trypanosomes in having an amastigotic intracellular (cells of the reticuloendothelial system [RES], myocardium and endocrine glands, and glial cells) phase. Trypomastigotes of *T. cruzi* bind specifically to surface "receptors" (identified as fibronectin) on the surface of cells which they subsequently penetrate. The predominant symptoms stem from myocardial failure, also the principal cause of death. Many species of triatomid (cone-nosed) bugs serve as vectors. Diagnosis is made in acute stages by blood smear, culture (both lifeless media and cell cultures), animal inoculation, and xenodiagnostic blood tests (using parasite-free triatomids). Limited therapeutic success is achieved with nifurtimox, which eliminates the trypomastigotes from the blood, but not tissue amastigotes; relapses therefore occur.

GENUS *LEISHMANIA*

These protozoa cause various forms of ***leishmaniasis.*** They are ovoid, about 3 by 1 nm in size, and occur circumterrestrially in warm, moist areas. The amastigote form (no free flagellum) occurs in macrophages of the mammalian host; the promastigote form, in the arthropod vector. Canines are the major animal reservoir, and bites of infected sand flies (50+ species of *Phlebotomus*) are the principal vectors. Laboratory diagnosis is by microscopic examination of ulcer scrapings, bone marrow, or blood smears, depending on the species. Striking polyclonal hypergammaglobulinemia (chiefly IgG) is frequent. Skin tests with leishmanin (killed promastigotes) reveal varying degrees of delayed-type hypersensitivity. Parasites may also be isolated in the promastigote stage in pure culture on special media at 20° C to 25° C. Serologic tests (*e.g.,* complement fixation, indirect fluorescent antibodies [IFA]) are of limited value in diagnosis because of cross-reactions with other parasites, notably trypanosomes. Although morphologically identical, species may be differentiated antigenically. Pentavalent antimony compounds (sodium stibogluconate [Pentostam] and *N*-methylglucamine antimonate [Glucantime]) have replaced trivalent antimonials in therapy. Amphotericin B is effective in dermal leishmaniasis refractory to antimonials. Secondary bacterial infections of leishmanial ulcers are frequent and call for appropriate antibacterial treatment. Variations within the following imprecise nosological classification of leishmaniasis depend on the species of infecting parasite, immunological reactions of the host, geographic location and animal reservoirs. Human-to-human transmission occurs (*e.g.,* kala-azar), especially in crowded urban settings.

Cutaneous leishmaniasis is caused by *Leishmania tropica, L. major* (oriental sore), *L. mexicana,* and *L. peruviana* (American leishmaniasis, uta, seen in Central and South America). The lesions are limited to the skin, where they evolve from initial maculopapular lesions to painless nodules which ulcerate. Macrophages laden with parasites are found at margins of ulcers. The ulceroglandular form of the disease mimics sporotrichosis.

Mucocutaneous leishmaniasis (espundia) is mostly associated with *L. brasiliensis.* Infections initiated in the skin metastasize to involve mucous membranes and ultimately cartilagenous nasal and tracheal structures in a destructive granulomatous process.

Visceral leishmaniasis (kala-azar) is caused mainly by *L. donovani* and results from hematogenous dissemination of parasites to cells of the RES in liver, spleen, lymph nodes, and bone marrow. Untreated kala-azar carries a high mortality rate.

GENUS *PLASMODIUM*

Each year, about 500 million people develop malaria and over 1 million (mostly children in Africa) die. In the United States, there are about 1,000 cases annually.

In nature the malarial parasites of humans are transmitted only by infected females of certain species of *Anopheles* mosquitoes. They can also be transmitted by blood transfusion or by the use of common injection apparatus, as occurs among drug addicts, who serve as a reservoir for mosquito-borne infections. The life cycle of *Plasmodium* sp. is complex and involves asexual phases in humans (***schizogony*** and early ***gametogony***) and sexual stages in the mosquito.

Asexual development in humans begins with the entrance of ***sporozoites*** from saliva in the proboscis of a mosquitoe. These first invade liver cells, undergoing replicative schizogony, the ***exoerythrocytic stage.*** In infections by *P. vivax* and *P. malariae* these may become latent and account for long delayed relapses. Recrudescences may occur in inadequately treated *P. falciparum* infections. Many ***merozoites*** are liberated from the liver cells. The merozoites enter erythrocytes and become ***trophozoites,*** which undergo further schizogony. The erythrocytes rupture, liberating many new merozoites that either enter new erythrocytes to undergo further schizogony or develop into young ***gametocytes*** awaiting necessary maturation in an *Anopheles* mosquito. Massive destruction of erythrocytes produces anemia, pigmentation of phagocytic cells by ***hemozoin*** (iron-bearing malarial pigment), anoxia of tissues, and consequent difficulties. The cyclical destruction of erythrocytes during schizogony periodically releases pyrogens causing quartan, tertian (see below) chills, and fever. The cycles are often quite irregular. The time from the mosquito bite to the first febrile attack is called the ***intrinsic incubation period.*** Hepatomegaly and splenomegaly are typical of malaria.

The sexual cycle occurs only in the mosquito, and the period from infection of the mosquito to infectivity comprises the period of ***extrinsic incubation*** (10 to 14 days). As soon as blood enters the mosquito, male gametes exflagellate and fertilize female gametes, each pair producing a ***zygote*** that develops into a motile ***ookinete.*** This invades a cell of the stomach wall and forms an ***oocyst*** containing many sporozoites. These are liberated on rupture of the oocyst and migrate to the proboscis, ready to infect humans.

Laboratory diagnosis of malaria is most often based on Giemsa-stained blood smears (thick or thin or both) and recognition of the parasites.

***Plasmodium falciparum* (Malignant Tertian or Estivoautumnal Malaria).** Mainly tropical in distribution, and accounts for up to 85% of infections, as well as practically all malaria-associated deaths. The cycle of schizogony in humans varies in duration from 36 to 48 hours. Falciform gametocytes are diagnostic; schizonts are rarely seen. Clinically, this is the severest and most dangerous form of malaria, largely because the parasites invade erythrocytes of all ages, often in multiples, resulting in very extensive parasitemia. Marked capillary obstruction occurs, probably because of adherence of parasites to capillary endothelium. The resulting tissue edema when it involves the brain (cerebral malaria) is life-threatening.

***Plasmodium malariae* (Quartan Malaria).** This is mainly subtropical. The usual cycle of schizogony is 72 hours but is subject to variations in clinical effect. Morphologically, *P. malariae* resembles *P. vivax* and *P. ovale* (see below), except that no Schüffner's stippling is present, the erythrocyte is not enlarged, and the parasite is more compact. Pigment is darker and more conspicuous than that of *P. vivax*. There is very little ameboid activity. *P. malariae* attacks only mature erythrocytes, with consequent relatively mild parasitemias. Chronicity is frequent, and glomerulonephritis may occur.

***Plasmodium vivax* (Tertian Malaria).** This is found in temperate zones as well as in the tropics. The cycle of schizogony is 48 hours, but the clinical periodicity of chills and fever is quite variable. Active ameboid motion of the trophozoites and enlargement of the erythrocytes are diagnostic. Schüffner's stippling is conspicuous and may represent pits in the membrane. Gametocytes are large and appear early. *P. vivax* attacks only reticulocytes, with consequently limited parasitemias.

Plasmodium ovale. Similar in most respects to *P. vivax,* but there is more Schüffner's stippling; erythrocytes are much enlarged and distorted; *P. ovale* infection is clinically milder than tertian malaria.

Treatment of malaria has been complicated by the emergence of drug-resistant strains of plasmodia in widely scattered geographic areas of the world. Choice of drugs will therefore be influenced by knowledge as to the source of infecting strains. Chloroquine is the drug of choice for infections by sensitive strains. In treating malaria originating in areas where chloroquine resistance is prevalent, quinine, pyrimethamine, and sulfisoxazole or sulfadiazine should be given. Mefloquine is a new antimalarial effective against chloroquine-resistant *P. falciparum.* Development of antimalarial vaccines is under active investigation. The most promising experimental approach is the elucidation of the structural gene encoding the immunodominant surface antigen (circumsporozoite protein) of *P. falciparum,* thereby paving the way toward development of a recombinant vaccine.

Intestinal Parasites

THE AMEBAE

The intestinal amebae multiply only by binary fission. The life cycles of many species alternate between very fragile, vegetative ***trophozoites,*** intermediate precysts and dormant cysts. Some do not form cysts. Many species are minor pathogens or commensals: *Entamoeba coli, Endolimax nana, Iodamoeba bütschlii, Dientamoeba fragilis.* These are of importance mainly because of possible confusion with *Entamoeba histolytica,* the only important pathogenic ameba of humans, during microscopic examination of stools.

Entamoeba histolytica causes amebiasis, including amebic dysentery. The fragile, pleomorphic, motile trophozoites, around 8 to 60 nm in size, are seen *only* (except when cultivated in special media) in acute diarrheic (or purged) stools and in invaded tissues. They sometimes contain ingested erythrocytes. The more resistant, diagnostically distinctive cysts (5 to 20 nm) are the forms most commonly seen in normal feces: round, quadrinucleate (when mature), with chromatoids (not always seen) and thick cyst membrane. Stained with iodine the nuclei are diagnostically distinctive in appearance.

The trophozoites secrete histolytic enzymes and penetrate the mucosa of cecum and colon, producing undermining ulcers and sometimes intestinal perforation. The amebae sometimes enter the portal venules or lymphatics, invading other tissues, notably liver and brain, with expanding abscess formation. There is rapid necrosis of liver parenchymal cells and lymphocytic infiltration of the abscesses. Symptoms then depend on the location of the lesion. Clinically, intestinal amebiasis ranges from subclinical (carriers) to severe dysentery characterized by bloody, mucoid stools, anemia, and dehydration. The so-called small-race of *E. histolytica* may or may not be pathogenic.

Transmission of amebiasis is only by cysts: fecal–sewage–food–oral; ''hand-to-mouth.''

Diagnosis is commonly by microscopic examination of stools for cysts. The ***cysts*** of the harmless *Entamoeba coli* are recognizable by their larger size and five or more distinctive nuclei (when mature). *Entamoeba coli* ingests few if any erythrocytes. Although it is a harmless commensal in the lower levels of the large intestine, its presence indicates that fecal material has been ingested.

GENERA TRICHOMONAS AND GIARDIA

Trichomonas hominis. The trophozoites of these pear-shaped flagellates are 7 to 15 nm by 5 to 15 nm with three to five anterior flagella and a keellike, laterally attached, undulating membrane with marginal flagellum. A prominent axostyle extends from the anterior (large) end through the center and projects posteriorly as a spike. *T. hominis* occurs in the lumen of the cecum. Transmission is fecal-oral. Pathogenicity is debatable. Diagnosis is by microscopic examination of the stool for the trophozoites. No cysts are formed.

Giardia lamblia. This flagellate is endemic in most parts of the world, and infection occurs frequently as a water-borne common source epidemic. In children, it may cause illness resembling the celiac syndrome, with steatorrhea, anemia, marked weight loss, and retardation of growth. Giardiasis in individuals with immune deficiency (*e.g.,* AIDS) may be severely debilitating. The diagnosis rests on finding *G. lamblia* trophozoites and cysts in diarrheic stools. The trophozoites, which survive mainly in duodenal mucosal crypts, are flattened dorsoventrally and have two large, eyelike nuclei, eight active flagella, and a ventral sucking depression for attachment to intestinal epithelial cells. A number of drugs are effective in therapy: metronidazole (Flagyl), tinidazole, furazolidone, and quinacrine (mepacrine).

GENUS BALANTIDIUM

Balantidium coli is the largest of the protozoan parasites of humans. It is a pear-shaped ciliate about 75 to 55 nm, with a ciliated mouth ***(cytostome),*** anal opening, prominent pulsating vacuole and macronuclei and micronuclei. Multiplication is usually by transverse binary fission. There are many saprozoic and commensal ciliates that may be morphologically confused with *B. coli,* the only ciliate of importance as a human pathogen.

B. coli occurs in the large intestine, where it feeds on host cells, bacteria, and other nutrients. It produces dysentery, which can vary from a fatal one with profuse diarrhea to one that is very mild. *B. coli* also produces openings in the mucosa and can penetrate into the submucosa, causing the formation of ulcers that resemble, but are less penetrating than, those due to *Entamoeba histolytica.* Transmission is fecal-oral, chiefly among hogs, occasionally to humans. In humans, clinically, balantidiasis ranges from (usually) asymptomatic to (rarely) fulminating and fatal.

Genitourinary Parasites

Trichomonas vaginalis, a cause of vulvovaginitis, is slightly larger than *T. hominis,* but otherwise closely resembles it. No cysts are known. *T. vaginalis* occurs in the human vagina and prostate, occasionally in urine. Transmitted usually by coitus, trichomoniasis may also be transmitted by moist, freshly contaminated clothing, washcloths, and other agents.

Genitourinary trichomoniasis is usually asymptomatic in males and sometimes in females, but in the latter often causes mild to severe vulvovaginitis. Diagnosis is by microscopic examination of exudates for the trophozoites. Cysts have not been seen.

Toxoplasmosis

The worldwide protozoan that causes this disease was observed originally in North African rodents called gondi, hence its name, *Toxoplasma gondii.*

Toxoplasma gondii has a multiphasic life cycle, somewhat like that of the malaria parasites, to which it is distantly related. The sexual stage develops in the intestine of cats; the asexual stage, in the muscles and other tissues of numerous feline and nonfeline mammals, including humans. The crescentic, pear-shaped asexual trophozoite is motile by bending and gliding movements.

In the cat, the sexual stage of the parasites results in production of drought- and starvation-resistant infective oocysts that are passed in the cat's feces. The oocysts may be ingested by many different warm-blooded vertebrates. If ingested by a cat, new trophozoites develop, the sexual process is repeated, and more oocysts are produced. If ingested by humans or any animal other than cats, the oocysts develop into trophozoites. These multiply asexually by fission and invade the tissues, where they may produce an inflammatory reaction of greater or lesser severity, commonly subclinical. They may eventually form cysts (not sexually produced oocysts as in the cat) and remain encysted in the tissues, causing chronic toxoplasmosis, also usually subclinical, which remains chronic, probably for life. Animals eating them in any forms, cyst, oocyst, or trophozoite, may become infected. Humans become infected most often by ingestion of undercooked meat containing cysts.

A large proportion of persons (50% of adults in the United States) when tested show serologic evidence of having (had) subclinical toxoplasmosis. Any mammal or bird eating raw or "rare" flesh containing the asexual cysts will contract the infection. Birds and mammals (except cats) do not pass infective oocysts so far as is known. Their flesh is infective but not their feces. Infected pregnant women can infect the fetus, sometimes with serious results: hydrocephalus, eye and brain damage. The disease appears to be worldwide in distribution and generally unnoticed.

Diagnosis of chronic toxoplasmosis is based on serology as well as on finding the pear-shaped parasites in tissues. Definitive identification of parasites can be made by indirect fluorescent antibody tests on biopsy material. Rising antibody titers, measured by ELISA or FAb, are suggestive. IgM antibody to *T. gondii* in cord blood establishes the presence of fetal (congenital) infection.

Cryptosporidiosis

Cryptosporidium (a coccidian parasite cultivable *in vitro* and related to *Toxoplasma*) was once thought to be a parasite primarily of bovine species. It has since been encountered in humans as the cause of explosive diarrhea, which in healthy individuals is self-limited; in immunologically compromised individuals, cryptosporidiosis may become chronic and debilitating and contribute to the lethal effects of other parasites, such as *Toxoplasma*. Cryptosporidiosis (for which there is no chemotherapy) and toxoplasmosis, along with infection with *Pneumocystis carinii*, have recently come into prominence as severe and often overwhelming opportunistic infections in persons with AIDS.

HELMINTHS

The term ***helminth*** is commonly used to mean parasitic worms. There are two principal groups: phylum Platyhelminthes, or ***flatworms,*** which include class Cestodea (tapeworms) and Trematoda (flukes); and phylum Nemathelminthes, class Nematoda or ***roundworms,*** which includes hookworms, pinworms, etc.

Flukes (Class Trematoda)

The life cycles of all flukes parasitic in humans are complex, details varying with species. In general, fertilized eggs are produced by sexually mature adults in the definitive host, that is, the host that harbors the sexually mature stage of any parasite. All flukes are hermaphroditic except schistosomes, which are diecious.

Eggs are discharged in feces (in *Schistosoma haematobium,* mainly in urine). Eggs hatch in polluted fresh water, each liberating a free-swimming ciliated larva ***(miracidium)*** that penetrates an intermediate host, usually a species of snail, in which it becomes a sporocyst and (except in schistosomes) produces numerous ***rediae*** and daughter rediae or sporocysts. These finally become minute, tadpole-like ***cercariae*** (with forked tails in schistosomes) that penetrate the definitive host (see below), losing their tails and becoming ***metacercariae*** (incomplete in schistosomes). They enter the definitive host by (1) direct penetration of the skin of swimmers, waders, rice planters, and others (schistosomes); (2) encysting on aquatic plants such as, water cress, water chestnuts, and lotus, which are eaten raw (liver flukes: *Fasciolopsis buski; Fasciola hepatica*); (3) penetration of, and encystment in, tissues of aquatic animals (fish, crustacea) that are eaten raw (liver fluke *Clonorchis sinensis* and lung fluke *Paragonimus westermani*).

After ingestion by the definitive host and excystation (except schistosomes, which penetrate skin and do not form cysts), migration to specific organs occurs via blood and lymph channels and penetration through intestinal walls and other tissues. Diagnostically distinctive eggs of all species occur in stools, but those of *Schistosoma haematobium* appear mainly in urine and those of *Paragonimus westermani* also in sputum.

Pathogenesis by all flukes is due principally to obstruction of various vessels and ducts, to trauma due to tissue penetration and burrowing, to abscess formation around dead worms, to intense inflammatory reaction with fibrosis and stricture, and to more or less toxic action depending on species. Symptoms depend largely on tissue of localization.

BLOOD FLUKES (GENUS *SCHISTOSOMA*)

These are distinguished from other human flukes by their slender, cylindrical form, separate sexes, and the prominent, longitudinal, copulatory canal of males, which enfolds the female during copulation. Males range in length from 10 to 20 mm. Adults most commonly live in the mesenteric, the portal, or the vesical venules, whence eggs enter the intestine or the urinary bladder and appear in feces or urine, depending on species. Intradermal tests for specific allergy with schistosomal antigens are useful in diagnosis. Eggs are not operculate. Biopsy of intestinal mucosa may be necessary for definitive diagnosis if eggs are not found in fecal samples.

***Schistosoma japonicum* (Oriental Blood Fluke).** This causes intestinal and hepatic schistosomiasis, chiefly in Japan, North China, and adjacent lands and islands. Eosinophilia is marked. This is the most dangerous form of schistosomiasis, as the worms are widely disseminated in the body. Distinctive eggs, with rudimentary lateral spikes covered with adherent fecal material, appear in the stools.

Schistosoma mansoni. This causes schistosomiasis mansoni or Manson's schistosomiasis in Africa and adjacent lands, the Caribbean islands, and Brazil. The diagnostically distinctive eggs are laterally spiked and appear mainly in stools. Recently, it was discovered that one of the surface antigens of *S. mansoni* contains an epitope identical to one on vif, a regulatory protein of HIV-1. This suggests a possible relationship between the function of these two proteins.

***Schistosoma haematobium* (Vesical Blood Fluke).** This causes vesicle bilharziasis or urinary schistosomiasis in Africa and adjacent lands. Eggs with one polar spike appear mainly in urine.

Schistosomal Dermatitis, or Swimmers' Itch. This is due to preliminary penetration, into the skin only, by cercariae of various species of avian and mammalian flukes other than human. These do not develop further in humans. Swimmer's itch is annoying but self-limited.

Control of schistosomes involves elimination of vector snails: *Bulinus* and *Physopsis* for *S. haematobium; Biomphalaria glabrata* for *S. mansoni; Oncomelania* for *S. japonicum.* Praziquantel is the newest drug found to be effective in therapy.

Tapeworms (Class Cestodea)

Adult tapeworms are typically intestinal parasites of vertebrates. They are attached to the lining of the small intestine of the host by the worm's head or scolex, which is equipped with suckers, and by multiple hooklets in some species. The scolex narrows posteriorly to form a neck from which are produced, by budding, a series of new "segments" or flattened, roughly rectangular proglottids that remain attached to the neck and to each other to form a ribbonlike strobila, which may be millimeters to meters in length, depending on species.

Each proglottid later becomes a sexually mature, hermaphroditic, egg-producing parasite. The older (most distal, and gravid with eggs) proglottids break off and are carried out in feces along with ova (except *Taenia* sp. and *Dipylidium canium*). Most ova and proglottids have diagnostically distinctive morphology. The scolex remains attached to produce more proglottids. Neither flukes nor tapeworms have alimentary systems. Nutrition is osmotropic, that is, occurring by absorption through the surface structures. The life cycles and the intermediate hosts vary with species.

Taenia saginata. The beef tapeworm, 4 to 9 m in length, is found in peoples that eat raw beef, almost never in the United States. Herbivores acquire the embryonated eggs, each containing a six-hooked ***onchosphere,*** in sewage-polluted pasturage. The freed embryos invade the muscles and remain as encysted larvae *(Cysticercus bovis)* until eaten uncooked by humans. The scolex is about 3 mm in diameter and has four sucking disks but no hooklets (although hooklets are present in the egg). The eggs (*not* species-distinctive) are found free by microscopic examination of human feces and in the proglottids that appear in the stools. Neurocysticercosis is a life-threatening complication of this infestation, for which praziquantel is effective when combined with steroids to reduce the inflammatory response.

Taenia solium. The pork tapeworm occurs in the encysted larval (cysticercus) stage in pork. Infection is rare in the United States. The distinctive scolex has four sucking disks and a ***rostellum*** with a double row of 26 to 28 hooklets. The species is recognized by counting the number of uterine branches, which in *T. saginata* range from 15 to 20 (average 18) on each side; *T. solium* has 7 to 13 (average 9) on each side. The ova are not distinguishable from those of *T. saginata.* The life history and human-pork relationship are analogous to the human-beef relationship of *T. saginata.* In addition, humans may ingest eggs via fecally polluted foods and develop cystercerci in the muscles. Hogs acquire eggs from foods polluted by human feces.

Hymenolepsis nana. The dwarf tapeworm (about 2 to 4 cm long and 1 mm wide) is the smallest and most common tapeworm affecting humans in the United States, occurring most frequently in children. The head has a rostellum with 24 to 30 hooklets and four suckers. There are from 150 to 200 segments.

No intermediate host is necessary. The diagnostically distinctive eggs are passed in feces and are transmitted to the mouth of the same host ***(autoinfection)*** by soiled hands, underclothing and unclean habits in regard to feces. The ***cysticercoid*** larvae develop in the intestinal villi and the adults and then fasten to the duodenal or the jejunal mucosa and repeat the cycle. Personal cleanliness and sanitary disposal of feces are the best prevention.

Diagnosis depends on the discovery of ova in the feces.

Diphylibothrium latum. The fish tapeworm may reach 12 m in length, with thousands of proglottids. The head, about 1 mm by 2 to 3 mm, has no hooklets but has two longitudinal sucking grooves. Each diagnostically distinctive egg has a small hinged lid or operculum at one end, suitable for hatching in water, and demonstrable by pressure on the coverglass on a slide.

Eggs from human feces in cool fresh water produce

free-swimming embryos. These are swallowed by copepods ("water fleas" [*Cyclops* or *Diaptomus*]), where a larva forms. The copepod is eaten by a plankton-eating fish and forms a ***sparganum*** in the muscles. When the fish is eaten undercooked by a human host, the larval tapeworm matures and attaches in the proximal jejunum. Competition with the host for vitamin B_{12} may cause profound anemia. Eosinophilia is frequent.

Control involves avoidance of sewage pollution of waters in which the intermediate hosts breed and the cooking of all fish to be eaten.

Echinococcus granulosus* and *E. multilocularis*.** These cause unilocular and multilocular or alveolar echinococcosis respectively; hydatid disease. The definitive hosts of these tapeworms are not humans but other carnivorous mammals, especially canines. Dogs are infected when fed discarded organs of slaughtered sheep or cattle. Cattle, sheep, swine, and people are intermediate hosts; these species harbor the larval cyst stage ***(hydatid cyst) that is analogous to the cysticerci of *Taenia* sp.

Adult *Echinococcus* tapeworms are 2 to 6 mm long. In dogs, they produce *Taenia*-like eggs that appear in the animal's feces and are swallowed with polluted fodder by a wide variety of intermediate hosts. In the case of humans, they are acquired from accidentally soiled hands, food, or both, especially among persons closely associated with dogs: Eskimos, sheep herders, and others.

The eggs produce larvae that penetrate through venules to liver, brain, lung, and other organs, where they usually slowly form either unilocular hydatid cysts *(E. granulosus),* often amenable to surgery, or alveolar or multilocular cysts *(E. multilocularis),* rarely amenable to surgery. The cysts may become very large and destructive and usually contain many infective daughter scolices that become adults when the cyst is ingested by a carnivore. In humans, a large proportion of the cysts of *E. multilocularis* are sterile: they do not have daughter cysts or scolices.

Diagnosis of echinococcosis or hydatid disease in humans may be made with hydatid-cyst-fluid antigen by complement-fixation or precipitin tests; cutaneous allergic reaction; or the finding of hooklets or scolices in the cyst fluid if surgical procedures are feasible. Praziquantel is recognized as an excellent drug for removal of tapeworms in all hosts. Medicated bait tablets are used to treat dogs in endemic areas.

Phylum Nematoda

Adult roundworms parasitic in humans generally attach to the intestinal mucosa except *Ascaris,* which remains free in the intestinal lumen, and filarial worms, which inhabit blood, tissues (especially skin), and lymph spaces. Female nematodes usually are larger than males.

Hookworms *(Necator americanus* and *Ancylostoma duodenale).* Male hookworms average around 8 by 0.4 mm in size. Hookworm infection is widely endemic in the tropics and subtropics, especially in extraurban populations. Adults, attached to duodenal and jejunal mucosa by suckers and cutting plates, digest the mucosa and blood and produce diagnostically distinctive eggs that appear in feces. On warm, moist soil the eggs hatch and undergo 10 to 15 days of development through four larval stages. The last larvae are filariform and penetrate exposed skin of bare feet, causing ground itch.

The larvae migrate through blood vessels and lymphatics to the lungs with relatively little pneumonitis; thence, after further development, by the trachea, esophagus, and stomach to the intestine where, as adults, they attach and renew the cycle.

Pathogenesis involves continuous intestinal irritation and hemorrhage, with resultant anemia, and debilitation, both physical and mental.

Control is based mainly on sanitary disposal of feces and avoidance of direct contact with feces-polluted soil. As in any control program, elimination of sources of infection by treatment of infected persons is essential.

Giant Roundworms *(Ascaris lumbricoides).* These are worldwide in distribution and among the most prevalent nematodes of humans, except in cold, dry climates.

Male *A. lumbricoides* may attain lengths of over 30 cm and diameters of 8 mm. Adults live mostly in the small intestine and may migrate *post mortem* into various parts of the gastrointestinal tract (bile and pancreatic ducts, stomach, etc.). They do not attach to the intestinal mucosa. They may perforate the intestinal wall or migrate out of anus, mouth, or nares. They die out after about a year but, in endemic areas, are replaced constantly.

Diagnostically distinctive eggs, passed in stools, mature in warm, moist soil in 2 to 3 weeks. Ingested, the mature eggs hatch in the small intestine. (Compare with hookworms, the eggs of which hatch on the soil, not in the intestine.) The larvae migrate actively to the lungs by way of blood, lymphatics, or both, with accompanying pneumonitis, possibly allergic, get into the alveoli and thence to pharynx and esophagus, where they are swallowed. In the small intestine they mature, produce eggs, and recommence the cycle. Large numbers can cause serious difficulties due to mechanical obstructions. General symptoms of gastrointestinal irritation and malnutrition are common. Severe infestations may require surgical intervention and are sometimes fatal.

Whipworms *(Trichuris trichiura).* Males are about 40 by 5 mm. Infection is circumterrestial, mainly tropical. Adults attach to the cecal mucosa and produce diagnostically distinctive eggs in the feces. The eggs do not hatch, but on warm, moist soil the intraoval embryos become larvae. Under unsanitary conditions they are ingested by humans. The eggs hatch in the intestine, and the freed larvae migrate to the cecum, mature, and repeat the cycle. A heavy burden of worms causes mucosal inflammation and erosion, diarrhea, and hemorrhage, mostly in children. A light worm burden may not cause symptoms.

Diagnosis depends on recognizing the species-distinctive eggs in the stool.

Control is dependent on sanitary disposal of feces and avoidance of feces-polluted soil, food, or objects contaminated with such soil or feces and is potentiated by adequate treatment of infested patients.

Pinworms or Seatworms *(Enterobius vermicularis).* Males are about 3 by 0.2 mm. The worms are circumterrestrial in temperate areas. Adults are attached in cecum and colon. Gravid females migrate to the anal and perianal area and deposit diagnostically distinctive eggs that are highly infectious and may be picked up for microscopic examination on clear adhesive tape. Sometimes the adult worms may be seen on the skin. Eggs are carried to the mouth on hands or on contaminated dust from clothing to the same *(autoinfection)* or another host. The eggs hatch in the intestine, and the freed worms attach and repeat the cycle.

Occurring mainly in children under unsanitary conditions, *E. vermicularis* causes perianal pruritus, local irritation, and scratching that invites transmission via hands and secondary bacterial infection. Eosinophilia is marked.

Control involves personal cleanliness and eradication of the worms by chemotherapy.

Trichina Worm or Pork Worm *(Trichinella spiralis).* These worms cause trichinosis. Most carnivorous animals are susceptible, and the disease is enzootic in rats, swine, and wild animals (bear, wild boar, walrus, and cougar). Both rats and swine eat infected pork as municipal garbage or slaughterhouse offal. Trichinosis occurs in humans as a result of eating undercooked pork or wild game containing live, encysted larvae.

Once ingested, the larvae excyst and mature in the crypts of duodenum and jejunum as small, slender worms about 1.5 mm long (males). After copulation the males die, and the females penetrate deeply into the mucous membranes where they produce large numbers of larvae (larviparous) that migrate through veins and lymphatics to the striated muscles. There the larvae grow and, about 3 weeks after ingestion of the infected meat, become encapsulated, coiled in the distinctive arrangement from which the species name is derived. In this condition they can remain viable for 12 years or more, although usually the cysts become entirely calcified in 10 to 12 months.

The early period of invasion by the newly ingested larvae is accompanied by local inflammation and gastroenteritis for several days and sometimes also by hemorrhage. The period (1 to 3 months) during which the newly produced (''second generation'') larvae are migrating through the tissues and muscles is marked by fever, edema (especially of the face; periorbital), myositis or ''muscular rheumatism,'' and general symptoms, including pain, as well as fatigue. Eosinophilia of up to 50% total white blood count is marked. Severity depends on the numbers of larvae. Many mild, unrecognized cases occur; others may be fatal.

Diagnosis depends on finding the encapsulated larvae in bits of teased-out muscle after sectioning or digestion with trypsin. Immunologic tests are useful and include precipitin and complement-fixation tests using trichina extracts as antigen and the agglutination of antigen-coated latex particles. Intradermal tests for allergy with similar antigens are also valuable.

Control depends on cooking all garbage fed to swine, eliminating rats from garbage dumps and piggeries; adequate veterinary condemnation of infected swine (difficult); freezing of pork for at least 36 hours at $-27°$ C and thorough cooking to a temperature of 170° F (77° C); addition of thiabendazole to swine fodder.

Filarial Worms. Various species of these worms and their microscopic larvae (*microfilariae,* c. 275 by 7 μm) cause various forms of filariasis in tropical and some subtropical areas. Geographic distribution of the various species depends on distribution of the arthropod vectors (various mosquitoes, gnats, and biting flies) specific for each.

Although distinctive clinical features and epidemiology depend on the species of filarial worm involved, all forms of filariae and of filariasis have some basic similarities. In general, adult filariae inhabit fibrous subcutaneous or deep lymph nodules or other tissues of humans where they produce long, thin microfilariae. In some species these migrate into peripheral capillaries at hours (diurnal or nocturnal periodicity) when the arthropod vector specific for that species of worm bites.

After a series of maturation changes in the arthropod, the microfilariae migrate to the proboscis of the arthropod, ready to infect the next person bitten.

Active and extensive migrations of the microfilariae in the human host, their gathering together in large masses, and the allergic reactions consequent to chronic infection, result in pain, blindness *(Onchocerca volvulus),* and various distinctive types and locations of swellings.

Diagnosis before microfilariae appear in the peripheral blood is based on history of exposure, clinical picture, and intradermal sensitivity tests with filarial antigens. Later, microfilariae of some species are demonstrable microscopically in the peripheral blood during hours of periodicity or in ''skin snips'' macerated in saline solution *(O. volvulus) O. volvulus* does not circulate in the blood stream.

Chemotherapy against *O. volvulus* is not universally employed because of intense reactions that occur in the skin to the sudden release of large quantities of antigen. In Central America, nodules containing the adults are periodically removed as a means of control. Elimination of arthropod vectors is not always practicable, because the larvae grow in fast streams in which pesticides wash away quickly. Diversion of streams is often impossible, because coffee-growing areas are dependent on them.

Opportunistic Zoonotic Helminthic Infections

Toxocara canis, the canine ascarid, is the cause of a zoonotic disease in humans, ***visceral larva migrans*** (VLM), contracted by ingestion of developed eggs of the nematode, usually in soil contaminated by dog feces. The larvae are disseminated from the intestine to various tissues and organs, the number and distribution of larvae and the immune response to them determining to large extent the symptoms and severity of disease. Marked eosinophilia (over 50%) and hypergammaglobulinemia (IgM) are the rule, and eosinophilic granulomata around larvae are found in liver biopsies. Larvae do not return to the intestine through a pulmonary cycle and eggs are therefore not found in the stool. ELISA is useful in serodiagnosis; attempts at chemotherapy (with thiabendazole) have not been successful.

Ancylostoma braziliense and *A. caninum,* both hookworms of dogs, cause ***cutaneous larva migrans*** (CLM) or creeping eruption, another zoonotic opportunistic infection contracted by penetration of the skin (most often on the feet) by filariform larvae in soil contaminated with dog and cat feces. Intense pruritus, edema, and inflammation are seen at the sites of penetration, from which the larvae burrow through the layers of the skin, causing linear raised inflammatory tracts and marked eosinophilic infiltration. Larvae do not mature in the human host, but survive for long periods in subcutaneous tissues. There are no serodiagnostic tests for CLM; skin lesions may heal with oral and/or topical thiabendazole.

FUNGI (EUMYCETES)

Fungi pathogenic for humans may cause one of three general types of fungal disease (mycosis):

1. Cutaneous mycoses ***(dermatophytoses).*** These are superficial and generally not dangerous per se. They involve only the skin, hair, and nails, alone or in combination. These mycoses are due to keratin-metabolizing, filamentous ***dermatophytes*** and sometimes to yeastlike *Candida albicans.*
2. Deep or ***systemic mycoses.*** These are usually serious, sometimes fatal.
3. ***Subcutaneous mycoses.*** These are usually chronic, localized infections of the skin, underlying dermis and occasionally the deep tissues, such as bones and muscles, principally of the extremities but also occasionally involving any exposed body surface. A variety of fungi, both dimorphic and monomorphic, are responsible.

Pathogenic fungi were previously grouped together under the term *Fungi Imperfecti* because a sexual or perfect mode of reproduction was not known. The discovery of a sexual reproductive cycle for many of these fungi prompted the adoption of Deuteromycetes (Gr. *deutero,* second) as their class name. Although identification of the sexual cycle resulted in a reclassification of the fungus according to the type of sexual spores produced, the name of the asexual form was retained and the organism in this form remained in the class Deuteromycetes. A sexual stage has been identified for several *Microsporum* species, assigned to the genus *Nannizzia,* several *Trichophyton* species, assigned to the genus *Arthroderma, Histoplasma capsulatum,* assigned the name *Emmonsiella capsulata, Blastomyces dermatitidis,* assigned the name *Ajellomyces dermatitidis,* and *Cryptococcus neoformans,* assigned the name *Filobasidiella neoformans.* Excepting *Filobasidiella neoformans,* which is placed in the class Basidiomycetes, all are grouped in the class Ascomycetes. Recently, *Pneumocystis carinii,* which had previously been classified as a protozoan, has been reclassified as a fungus, similar to other yeast. A detailed characterization of it is provided at the end of this section on fungi.

In general, diagnostic mycology is largely an exercise in morphology, supported secondarily by metabolic and immunochemical analysis (including the search for fungal polysaccharide antigens by CIE or ELISA). Infective agents are recovered in cultures of clinical material (scrapings, sputum, pus, tissue samples). The medium most widely used for general purposes of primary isolation and passage is Sabouraud's glucose (or maltose agar, *p*H 5.6), with added antibacterial drugs (usually chloramphenicol); in certain cases cycloheximide is also added to inhibit nonpathogenic fungi. Cultures are incubated for 1 to 4 weeks at 22° C and in special circumstances at 37° C. Pathogenic fungi are identified microscopically by characteristic mycelial formations (*e.g.,* spirals, favic chandeliers, racquet hyphae), distinctive asexual spores (*e.g.,* conidiospores, aleuriospores, chlamydospores), and color, texture and topography of colonies. For direct examination, scrapings, nail pairings, pus, and biopsy material can be macerated in 10% potassium hydroxide (KOH), or stained with lactophenol-cotton blue. Yeast cells are gram-positive; other structures do not stain well with Gram's stain. Periodic acid-Schiff stain is used to demonstrate fungal cell wall material in tissues (*e.g.*, hyphae, yeast cells). Although the primary immunologic defense against mycotic infection rests on cell-mediated mechanisms (indicated by delayed-type skin sensitivity), antibodies to fungal antigens are evoked, particularly in the deep-seated mycoses, and are useful diagnostically in certain instances. The serologic techniques used most widely are immunodiffusion and complement fixation. Skin tests with certain fungal antigens (notably histoplasmin) evoke specific antibody in persons already sensitive; anergy to fungal antigens suggests the presence of immunosuppression.

Cutaneous Mycoses

Dermatophytoses are caused principally by species of three closely related genera of keratin-metabolizing filamentous fungi called dermatophytes. Dermatomycoses are caused by a variety of yeasts and filamentous fungi, such as *Candida albicans* and *Pityrosporon furfur*.

Typically the dermatophytes grow in cutaneous tissues or in cultures in moldlike, branching, mycelial form. Asexual spores of dermatophytes, though little more thermostable than vegetative cells, survive for long periods in soil, shower-bath mats, floors, and hair brushes. Some dermatophytes *(Microsporum canis, Microsporum gypseum, Trichophyton mentagrophytes, Trichophyton verrucosum)* infect domestic animals and are directly transmissible to people. Some species can at times cause any of the conditions listed below subject only to restrictions as to skin, hair, or nails as noted. Person-to-person or animal-to-person transmission is common.

COMMON DERMATOPHYTES

1. Involve skin and hair; nails rarely.
   Microsporum audouini, M. canis, M. gypseum cause various forms of tinea (ringworm), especially in preadolescents; *M. canis* causes it in domestic animals also. The first two fluoresce yellow-green in ultraviolet light (Wood's light); *M. gypseum* fluoresces poorly or not at all. These species produce spores and hyphal elements outside the hair shaft, and hence are called ***ectothrix infections.***
2. Involve skin and nails; not hair.
   Epidermophyton floccosum causes tinea pedis (athlete's foot), tinea cruris (jock itch), and tinea unguium.
3. Involve hair, skin, and nails.
   Trichophyton mentagrophytes, T. rubrum, T. tonsurans, T. schoenleini cause tinea pedis, favus sycosis, tinea unguium. The last two produce ***endothrix infections*** and the first two ectothrix infections of hair.

COMMON DERMATOMYCOSES

1. ***Candidiasis***
   Candida albicans and other *Candida* species can cause otomycosis, onychomycosis, thrush, perlèche, vulvovaginitis, and skin lesions; *Candida* infections are among the most frequently encountered mycoses.
2. ***Tinea versicolor***
   Pityrosporon furfur causes common superficial skin infection characterized by the formation of white-, brown-, or fawn-colored lesions.

Orally administered griseofulvin is effective against dermatophytoses. Topical agents such as miconazole nitrate, clotrimazole, and the nonprescription tolnaftate are effective against skin lesions, but less effective against nail infections. Nystatin (Mycostatin) is the drug of choice for dermatomycoses caused by *Candida* species. Keratinolytic ointments and scrupulous personal hygiene are recommended for tinea versicolor.

Deep or Systemic Mycoses

These diseases are caused chiefly by soil-inhabiting, dimorphic or ***diphasic fungi,*** that is, fungi capable of existing in two phenotypically distinct forms. In general, the free-living or ***saprobic form*** is a filamentous mold whereas the pathogenic, tissue-invading form is unicellular and yeastlike. Exceptions are *Candida albicans,* which is indigenous in humans and forms mycelia and pseudomycelia when it becomes invasive, *Coccidioides immitis,* which produces sporangiospores in mammalian tissues, and *Cryptococcus neoformans,* which is a monomorphic yeast. The two forms of each of these fungi may be reproduced on artificial media in the laboratory by manipulating environmental conditions such as pH, temperature, CO_2/O_2 ratios, humidity, and nutrients-amino acids, carbohydrates, and vitamins.

As would be expected in the case of soil-inhabiting organisms, infections are acquired by inhaling spores, resulting in primary pulmonary lesions, or by traumatically implanting spores into the skin, resulting in relatively localized infections involving the cutaneous and deeper tissues and occasionally the lymphatics of the affected areas. Systemic mycoses are slowly evolving, chronic diseases characterized by granulomatous reactions, abscess formation, necrosis, and the development of a cell-mediated immune response. Agglutinins, precipitins, and complement-fixing antibodies are formed and are useful in diagnostic and prognostic procedures, including latex agglutination, immunodiffusion, complement fixation and immunofluorescent staining techniques.

In contrast to dermatophytoses, person-to-person transmission of systemic mycoses is rare.

Systemic mycotic infections may also be caused by diverse, saprobic, monomorphic, filamentous fungi, such as *Aspergillus* species, aspergillosis; *Mucor* and *Rhizopus* species, phycomycoses; and others less frequently encountered. Modern medical practice sometimes requires the use of immunosuppressants, antibiotics, hormones, and other drugs in conjunction with certain types of surgical and therapeutic procedures, thus compromising the patient and providing a target for these opportunistic fungal pathogens. In systemic pulmonary aspergillosis, early antigenemia is detectable by RIA.

CANDIDIASIS

Candida albicans, more frequently the etiologic agent of this mycosis than any other *Candida* species, is a common commensal of the human alimentary tract and vagina. Although *Candida* infections may involve any area of the body, those that involve the deep tissues and organs may be life-threatening and are therefore the most serious. Candidiasis is always endogenous.

Candida albicans is a nutritionally dependent dimorphic fungus growing as a yeast in its natural habitat or *in vitro* in the presence of glucose and as pseudomycelia and mycelia when it invades tissues and organs or in vitro in the presence of dextran, glycogen, or starch. Pathologically it is usually a secondary invader of injured, moist, superficial tissues, causing thrush (oral or vaginal), intertriginous dermatomycoses, perlèche, and paronychia. Rarely, deep invasions may occur producing pneumonias and meningitides. *C. albicans* may produce a serious enteritis as a result of suppression of the normally competitive intestinal bacterial flora by antibiotics following surgery. *C. albicans* is also a significant cause of endocarditis in surgical patients following cardiac valve replacement and in mainline drug addicts. Oral ketoconazole is effective in treating superficial candidiasis and other surface fungal infections.

COCCIDIOIDOMYCOSIS

Coccidioides immitis, the etiologic agent of this mycosis, reproduces in tissues as a sporangium, exhibiting endogenous sporulation, that is, a nucleus undergoes many divisions inside a thick-walled diagnostically distinct sporangium or spherule that ruptures in the tissues at maturity, liberating the spores to repeat the process. The soil-inhabiting, saprobic phase is truly mycelial, producing many highly infectious arthrospores on special hyphal branches from the vegetative mycelia. When disturbed, these arthrospores become airborne and, commingled with dust, are inhaled by animal and human hosts. *C. immitis* is common in hot arid areas of the United States and northern Mexico.

As in tuberculosis, most primary infections are short, asymptomatic, and pass unnoticed; however, they are both immunizing and sensitizing. Symptomatic pulmonary coccidioidomycosis with allergic hypersensitivity has been called ***San Joaquin Valley fever*** and ***desert rheumatism.*** Arrested pulmonary lesions seen in roentgenograms may be confused with those of tuberculosis. A generalized, chronic, progressive, and often fatal form of coccidioidomycosis called ***coccidioidal granuloma*** occurs, especially in dark-skinned peoples.

Coccidioidin, an antigen prepared from culture filtrates of *C. immitis,* is used in the coccidioidin skin test, which is analogous in all respects to the tuberculin test. A positive coccidioidin test in patients with significant shadows on chest roentgenograms is extremely suggestive, especially if they have been in the southwest United States or other endemic areas, if there is no clinical evidence of tuberculosis, and if the tuberculin test is negative. The presence of active disseminated disease is suggested by a rising complement fixation titer accompanied by a reversion of the skin test from positive to negative.

Primary pulmonary coccidioidomycosis, whether asymptomatic or symptomatic, has a high recovery rate, and therapy usually consists of bed rest or activity restriction and judiciously administered steroids to control the allergic manifestations of erythema multiforme and erythema nodosum. Amphotericin B is the drug of choice when antifungal therapy is indicated. There is no effective method of artificial immunization.

HISTOPLASMOSIS

The etiologic agent of this mycosis, *Histoplasma capsulatum,* is commonly found in the Ohio and Mississippi River valleys in soil of damp, fertile areas polluted by birds (especially chickens), bats, dogs, and skunks. This disease is unique among the systemic mycoses in that it primarily involves the reticuloendothelial system in which the yeastlike, oval parasite is found almost exclusively within macrophages and histiocytes. Parasitic phase cells may be grown *in vitro* under CO_2 at 36° C on artificial media enriched with blood, glucose, and cysteine. Diagnostically distinctive infective tuberculate macroconidiospores are produced in soil and *in vitro* on artificial media at 22° C. Inhaled spores give rise to primary pulmonary infections that, like coccidioidomycosis, are often silent, immunizing, and sensitizing. In overt or progressive disease, pneumonitis occurs, and lymphadenopathy may be generalized, with splenomegaly and skin lesions. Roentgenograms of arrested pulmonary lesions may be confused with those of tuberculosis and coccidioidomycosis. Progressive disease is severe and often fatal.

Dermal reactivity to histoplasmin is in all respects analogous to that seen with tuberculin and coccidiodin, indicating cell-mediated immunity to the respective agents. Diagnostically, the histoplasmin skin test is of relatively little value, because of the prevalence of inapparent infection. However, a negative reaction is consistent with deficiency in cell-mediated immunity and hence may indicate development of disseminated disease, especially in previously positive reactors.

Serologic tests with diagnostic and/or prognostic value are latex agglutination, immunodiffusion and complement-fixation, and counterimmunoelectrophoresis. The immunodiffusion test is particularly useful because the development and presence of certain precipitin bands, H and M, are indicative of active and chronic or healed histoplasmosis.

Most cases of primary pulmonary histoplasmosis heal uneventfully, with bed rest and supportive therapy prescribed for the moderately severe cases. Chronic, cavitary, or progressive systemic disease is treated with amphotericin B.

A clinically distinct form of histoplasmosis, ***African histoplasmosis,*** is caused by a large species of the genus *H. duboisii*. This mycosis is characterized by the development of granulomatous and suppurative lesions in the cutaneous, subcutaneous and osseous tissues. The lungs are rarely involved. Untreated cases can progress to cause death. Amphotericin B is the drug of choice.

There is a close antigenic relationship between the two *Histoplasma* species.

BLASTOMYCOSIS

Blastomyces dermatitidis, the etiologic agent of this mycosis, appears in lesions as large, ovoid to spherical, thick-walled, single budding, multinucleated (8 to 12 nuclei), yeastlike cells. This organism is thermally dimorphic; therefore, the tissue phase may be obtained *in vitro* by inoculation onto most laboratory media and by incubation of the culture at 36° C. At 22° C in soil or on artificial media, thc organism is filamentous. Infections are probably acquired by inhaling dust-borne spores. The endemic area, as with *Histoplasma,* includes southeastern, south central, and midwestern states, exemplified by Mississippi, Arkansas, and Wisconsin. Exposure to soil is common in many reported outbreaks.

Blastomycosis most often begins as a primary pulmonary infection when conidia are inhaled, and in most cases is eliminated by natural cellular immune processes involving polymorphonuclear leukocytes and/or macrophages. However, if conidia are converted to yeast, then the pulmonary infection has a greater chance to ensue and, unlike histoplasmosis and coccidioidomycosis, if untreated, progresses to a severe, disseminated, often fatal disease. Cutaneous lesions are common and probably result from the hematogenous metastasis of organisms from a pulmonary or abdominal site. These skin lesions begin as small papules and progress to confluent, granulomatous, verrucous ulcerations and swellings to abscesses. Rare primary cutaneous infections develop from indurated ulcers that necrotize into chancriform lesions accompanied by lymphangitis, lymphadenitis, and regional lymphadenopathy. In contrast to paracoccidioidomycosis, the mucocutaneous tissues and viscera are usually spared.

Dermal reactivity to blastomycin is not specific, and serologic tests are generally unsatisfactory for the same reason. Diagnosis is dependent upon finding the organism in a pathologic specimen and on clinical and roentgenographic evidence.

Blastomycosis responds quickly to therapy with amphotericin B at a total dose of 1.5 to 2.5 g, which is recommended for all forms of the disease. Recently ketoconazole or traconozole, taken with meals, has been recommended for nonimmunocompromised patients with mild disease and no CNS involvement.

CRYPTOCOCCOSIS

Cryptococcus neoformans, the etiologic agent of this mycosis, is a monomorphic, spherical, thin-walled, encapsulated yeast found in debris and accumulated guano in pigeon roosts. The yeasts, which are virtually unencapsulated in their saprobic existence, quickly acquire a demonstrable capsule following entry into a mammalian host; therefore, it appears that virulence is more closely associated with the potential for encapsulation than with the degree of encapsulation. Infections that progress to symptomatic diseases are most often seen in compromised patients.

It is well accepted that the primary lesions are probably pulmonary; however, these are usually silent and asymptomatic. Central nervous system cryptococcosis, particularly cryptococcal meningitis, is by far the most frequently diagnosed form of the disease, and *C. neoformans* exhibit a distinct predilection for this area. The yeasts elicit a feeble immune response in infected patients producing a histologic reaction consisting of numerous histiocytes, in which the organisms multiply profusely, and occasional giant cells, lymphocytes, and fibrosing stroma. Encapsulated organisms may be demonstrated by staining tissue preparations with mucicarmine or alcian blue stains.

C. neoformans may be detected in direct slide preparations of clinical specimens, especially spinal fluid, by mixing a drop of specimen with a drop of nigrosin, placing a cover glass over the preparation, and observing microscopically for encapsulated yeasts. When yeast cells are too few in number to be found readily, the spinal fluid is examined by CIE, ELISA, or latex agglutination (latex particles coated with antibody to cryptococcal polysaccharide) to detect the presence of free capsular polysaccharide. The organisms may be readily isolated from clinical specimens by inoculating Sabouraud's glucose agar or any good bacteriologic media incubated at 37° C. Because of the prevalence of nonpathogenic *Cryptococcus* species, isolates should be subjected to further identification procedures: mouse pathogenicity and urease production, and carbohydrate fermentation and utilization tests. Serologic tests are virtually valueless; immunofluorescent staining using rabbit antiserum to *C. neoformans* has a specificity paralleling that of the mucicarmine stains.

Amphotericin B, given parenterally, is the drug of choice for central nervous system cryptococcosis. Dermal or pulmonary disease may respond to the less toxic 5-fluorocytosine (flucytosine, 5 FC), administered by the oral route. Clinical studies indicate that optimal therapy may be a combination of these two antimycotics. Untreated cryptococcosis is often fatal.

PARACOCCIDIOIDOMYCOSIS

Paracoccidioides brasiliensis, the etiologic agent of this mycosis, is a thermally dimorphic fungus, appearing in tissues and *in vitro* at 37° C as a spherical, multiple-budding, yeastlike cell and in nature and on agar as a filamentous mold. The organism is endemic in Central and South America. Inhalation of dust-borne spores produces a mild, often asymptomatic pulmonary infection. Dissemination produces secondary lesions of the oronasal mucosa and skin, with lymphangitis of the involved area, and viscera, including liver, spleen, intestines, and lymphatics.

Untreated cases are often fatal. Amphotericin B and miconazole are recommended for all forms of the disease.

Subcutaneous Mycoses

SPOROTRICHOSIS

Lymphocutaneous sporotrichosis is the most common form of this disease, and the cutaneous form without lymphatic involvement is second in frequency for this reason. Sporotrichosis is sometimes grouped with chromomycosis, maduromycosis, and rhinosporidiosis as localized infections of the skin and subcutaneous tissues that rarely metastasize to distant sites. Primary pulmonary sporotrichosis, once extremely rare, is being reported with increasing frequency especially from large urban hospitals, probably because of increased awareness and improved diagnostic procedures. The rare disseminated form, which has a grave prognosis, involves multiorgan systems and is usually seen in compromised patients.

Typically, infection is initiated following the traumatic implantation into the skin of spores found on the bark and thorns of trees and shrubs and in garden mulches. An ulcerated, chancriform lesion develops at the inoculation site followed by the development along the lymphatic chain of multiple subcutaneous nodules that in turn become necrotic and ulcerate. The infection usually does not extend beyond the regional lymph nodes.

The etiologic agent, *Sporothrix schenckii,* is dimorphic, reproducing in tissues and *in vitro* at 36° C on blood agar enriched with glucose and cystine as oval, round, or elongated yeastlike cells and in nature and on agar at 22° C as a mold composed of septate mycelia bearing typical rosettes of small pyriform microconidiospores. There is usually a paucity of demonstrable organisms in biopsy material, even when special histologic stains are used; however, positive cultures of the same material are readily obtainable. Organisms have been demonstrated in tissues by immunofluorescent staining when none were seen using conventional techniques.

Infections are immunizing and sensitizing and elicit a cell-mediated immune response detectable by the intradermal sporotrichin test. Serologic tests using the yeast-cell antigen were found to be more specific than those in which sporotrichin was used; titers greater than 1:40 are considered significant.

Orally administered potassium iodide is used to treat lymphocutaneous and cutaneous forms of the disease. Local heat applications have been shown to promote healing. Amphotericin B is recommended for relapsed lymphocutaneous disease and disseminated sporotrichosis. 5-Fluorocytosine at a dosage of 100 mg/kg/day has been used with some success.

CHROMOMYCOSIS (CHROMOBLASTOMYCOSIS)

This mycosis, caused by a variety of dematiaceous, soil-inhabiting fungi belonging to the genera *Phialophora, Fonsecaea,* and *Cladosporium,* is usually seen as an infection of the subcutaneous tissues, that is, verrucous dermatitis, but cases of cerebral chromomycosis (*i.e.,* cladosporiosis) have been reported.

Verrucous dermatitis is a chronic, painless disease characterized by marked pseudoepitheliomatous hyperplasia. Granulomas with neutrophils, lymphocytes, plasma cells, and giant cells containing the sclerotic brown bodies of the tissue form of the fungus or strands of pigmented hyphae constitute the histologic picture. Secondary bacterial infection with resulting lymphostatis and elephantiasis is a complication.

Cerebral chromomycosis is characterized by single or multiple brain lesions, usually encapsulated abscesses formed around masses of brown pigmented hyphae.

Symptoms are diverse, depending on the location of the lesions.

Surgical excision of lesions in the early stages of verrucous dermatitis is the most reliable treatment. However, most cases are not seen until the disease is well advanced and more refractory to antimycotics. Amphotericin B, used topically or by intralesion injection, thiabenzadole, used orally and topically, and 5-fluorocytosine have been used with varying degrees of success.

MADUROMYCOSIS

This disease, clinically identical to mycetoma caused by actinomycetes, is characterized by the development, usually on the extremities, of tumefactions, abscesses, fistulas, and sinuses that involve the deep tissues and bones. The lesions contain granules or grains composed of spores and hyphal strands of the offending fungus. A variety of fungi have been isolated as etiologic agents, among them *Madurella* species and *Allescheria boydii.* The disease is extremely refractory to antimycotic therapy; amphotericin B, griseofulvin, and nystatin have had limited success even in early cases (mycetoma, on the other hand, responds to sulfa drugs, penicillins, and tetracyclines). Excision of early localized lesions is recommended for those cases that do not respond to antimycotics. Amputation of the affected extremity may be necessary.

RHINOSPORIDIOSIS

Rhinosporidium seeberii, the etiologic agent of this infection, appears in tissues as large, thick-walled sporangia, producing, by successive nuclear divisions, endogenous sporangiospores that, at maturity, exit the sporangia through a ''pore'' (actually a thinned area of the sporangium wall). The organism has not been cultured *in vitro.* Rhinosporidiosis is a chronic granulomatous disease principally of the mucocutaneous tissues characterized by the formation of friable, sessile, and pedunculated polyps. As the name implies, the disease most often involves the nose. Obstruction of passages by large, unsightly polyps may be relieved by careful surgical excision. Superficial lesions may be removed completely; recurrence of surgically removed deep lesions is not uncommon. Local injection of amphotericin B is used as an adjunct to surgery to prevent spread. Other antimycotics are generally ineffective.

Newly Classified Fungi

Pneumocystis carinii, while previously regarded as a protozoan, is now classified (based on 16s ribosomal RNA sequence) as a fungus similar to yeast. The organism is widespread in the animal kingdom; antibody is found in the majority of healthy adults, indicating that subclinical infection is almost universal. In immunocompromised individuals, particularly those with AIDS, it produces a massive generalized pulmonary infection in which large numbers of the organisms are found in bronchoalveolar lavages, needle aspirates, or transbronchoscopic biopsies of the lung; when sufficiently numerous, they may be present in sputum. As of yet, these organisms have not been cultured. Pentamidine and trimethoprim–sulfamethoxazole are currently used as chemotherapeutic agents; however, new antifungal drugs are being developed. Recently, extrapulmonary infections have been found in treated patients with very low (<100) CD_4^+ counts. Mortality may approach 50% and higher in AIDS patients. This is increased by the presence of other concurrent opportunistic infections.

MECHANISMS OF RESISTANCE TO AND RECOVERY FROM INFECTION

Nonspecific factors that aid the human host in resisting invasion by pathogenic microorganisms include mechanical barriers (intact integument; hairs in anterior nares and auditory canal; secretions such as saliva, tears, respiratory, and vaginal mucus; ciliated epithelium in the lower respiratory tract); nonspecific chemical factors (gastric and vaginal acidity, lysozyme in tears; fatty acids in sweat, bile salts in the intestinal tract; alternate pathway of complement activation and secretory IgA) (see below).

Induction and Regulation of the Immune Response

The induction of both specific humoral and cell-mediated immune responses protects the human host from invasion by disease-causing bacteria, viruses, parasites, and fungi. Generally, it requires macrophages for ''antigen processing'' for optimal results. When small amounts of an antigen on the surface of macrophages are presented to T-helper cells that have receptors for that antigen, blastogenesis and clonal expansion occur. The release of soluble factors from these cells that are specific for this antigen induces a specific B-cell response to the same antigen (*i.e.,* clonal expansion). Both cells may or may not respond to the same antigenic determinant on the antigen molecule; however, if different antigenic determinants are involved, they must be located on the same molecule. In the case of a ''hapten'' conjugated to ''carrier'' protein, B cells may recognize the hapten, whereas T-helper cells may recognize an antigenic determinant on the carrier protein. Antigens that require this process are called T-dependent (Fig. 5-1 [1]). Most complex antigens fall into this category. Antigens that bear identical repeating

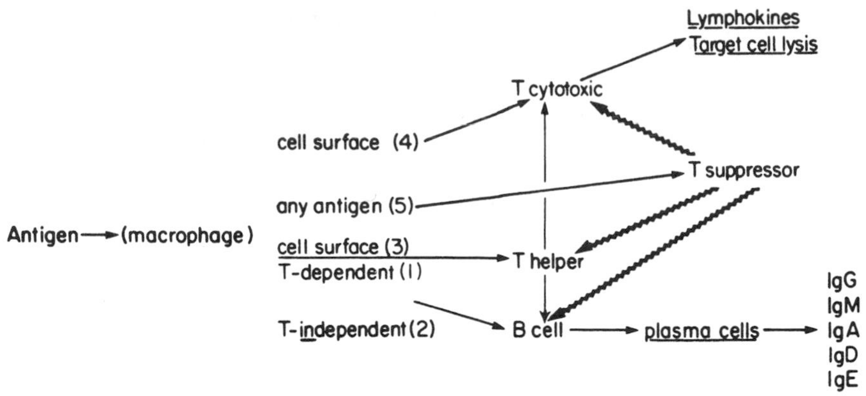

Fig. 5-1. Induction and regulation of the immune response.

antigenic determinants may stimulate B cells without T-helper cells (Fig. 5-1 [2]). Examples of these T-*in*dependent antigens include gram-negative bacterial lipopolysaccharide, pneumococcal polysaccharide, and viral capsids (protein coats). Unlike the T-dependent process, only IgM immunoglobulins are formed without T-cell help. Cell surface antigens (*e.g.*, viral antigens, tumor-specific antigens, HLA-D alloantigens (Fig. 5-1 [3]) can induce T-helper cells to provide amplification of the T cytotoxic cell response (Fig. 5-1 [4]) to the same (viral, tumor) or other antigens on the cell surface (HLA-A,B,C alloantigens). T-cell helper factors may be both specific and nonspecific in this instance.

The character of the immune response to infection in the normal host is dictated in large measure by the nature of the parasite (used in the broadest sense) (Table 5-16). Microorganisms that are obligate extracellular parasites, that is, do not penetrate into normal cells and do not survive phagocytosis, evoke specific antibodies that are protective chiefly through neutralization of the pathogen (*e.g.*, enhancement of phagocytosis and intracellular killing, as in pneumococcal, meningococcal meningitis). In acute and chronic infections with facultative intracellular parasites (*e.g.*, brucella, mycobacteria) cell-mediated immune (CMI) responses (evidenced in delayed-type hypersensitivity) come to the fore as important resistance and recovery mechanisms, although the humoral response plays a secondary role and is useful in serodiagnosis, particularly when the offending microorganism cannot be readily isolated. With obligate intracellular parasites (*e.g.*, all viruses, *Chlamydia*), CMI responses are the primary basis for containment of infection, the parasites being inaccessible to antibody except when transiently present in the bloodstream (*e.g.*, spread of poliovirus from primary sites of infection in the gut to the central nervous system). The effectiveness of vaccines is consistent with the foregoing concepts. Accordingly, killed antibacterial vaccines (*e.g.*, pneumococcal, pertussis) evoke protective antibody but no CMI against obligate extracellular parasites, and, by analogy, toxoids (*e.g.*, diphtheria, tetanus) evoke antitoxin that can neutralize toxin only when it is free in the bloodstream. In contrast, living attenuated agents (*e.g.*, measles vaccine, BCG) must multiply in cells of the host in order to evoke both antibody and CMI, the latter being the chief mechanism of resistance and recovery. In certain infections, "abnormal" antibodies are elicited that have antigenic specificities distinct from those of the microbial agents involved (*e.g.*, Wassermann, heterophile antibodies) or that may relate to host autoimmune reactions (*e.g.*, rheumatic fever, mycoplasmal pneumonia).

The chief categories of ***phagocytic cells,*** which represent the first line of defense, particularly in acute bacterial infection, are:

1. ***Polymorphonuclear leukocytes.*** Neutrophils are a major component in acute inflammatory reactions, being actively phagocytic. They also have Fc and C3 receptors through which they mediate antibody-dependent cellular cytolysis (ADCC) (see below). Eosinophils are mobilized by eosinophil-chemotactic factor (ECF-A) from IgE-activated basophils and mast cells and are particularly associated with type I hypersensitivity and with helminthic infection (*e.g.*, direct antiparasitic effect of eosinophilic degranulation). Basophils and tissue mast cells, on binding IgE through specific surface receptors, are degranulated with concomitant release of vasoactive substances (histamine, slow-reacting substance A).
2. ***Macrophages*** (blood monocytes and fixed histiocytes) are central to the initiation of primary immune responses by B and T lymphocytes (see below) and also have Fc and C3 receptors important in ADCC. Macrophages are activated by lymphokines (*e.g.*, macrophage-arming factor) elaborated by the T lymphocytes mediating delayed-type hypersensitivity (T_{dth}). Macrophages are capable of supporting replication of some viruses and certain species of bacteria

TABLE 5-16. The Immune Response in Relation to Infection and Immunoprophylaxis

			IMMUNE RESPONSE:	
IMMUNOGEN	**EXTRACELLULAR**	**INTRACELLULAR**	**Humoral**	**Cell-mediated**
Parasites (active infection)	*Obligate*—acute Pyogens* Mycoplasma Facultative acute-chronic *Brucella* *Francisella* *Mycobacteria* *Listeria* Fungi		Protective antibody, opsonins Type III HS Agglutinins CF antibody, not (?) protective	Cellular immune mechanisms, T_C, NK, K (ADCC) Type IV HS
		Obligate acute-persistent *Chlamydia* *Rickettsia** Viruses*	Neutralizing and CF antibody TYPE III HS	
Nonreplicating antigens	*Toxins* (toxoids)* Tetanus Diphtheria Botulinum Enterotoxins Anthrax		Antitoxin	
	Killed vaccines* Pertussis Influenza Rabies		Protective antibody	
Abnormal responses associated with infection	*Enzymes* Clostridial Streptococcal		Antienzymes	
	Autoimmune-crossreactive (?)			
	Mycoplasma pneumoniae		Cold agglutinins	
	SSPE, ?PRP		Antiviral	Cellular immune mechanisms
	Infectious mononucleosis		Heterophilic antibody	
	Rheumatic fever			
	Lues and other (*e.g.*, IM, malaria, SLE)		Wassermann, antibody, (BFP)	

* See Table 5-24 for immunoprophylactic reagents.

Abbreviations

ADCC = antibody-dependent cellular cytotoxicity.
BFP = biologic false-positive.
CF = complement-fixing.
HS = hypersensitivity.
IM = infectious mononucleosis.
K = killer cells.
NK = natural killer cells.
PRP = progressive rubella panencephalitis.
SSPE = subacute sclerosing panencephalitis.
T_C = cytotoxic T lymphocytes.

that are facultative (*e.g.*, mycobacteria) or obligate (viruses) intracellular parasites.

INTERFERON

Interferons (IFNs) are host-coded proteins synthesized by normal cells in response to various stimuli. Alpha and beta IFNs are produced in leukocytes or fibroblasts, respectively, in response to viral infection or inactivated virus, isolated double-stranded RNA (not dsDNA), synthetic polyribonucleotides, or endotoxin. Gamma IFN is synthesized in unsensitized T lymphocytes in response to mitogens, and in sensitized T lymphocytes in response to specific antigen(s). Beta and gamma IFNs are glycoproteins; alpha IFN is not. The antiviral protective effect of IFNs is due to the induction, in normal cells, of new protein(s) with activity that inhibits replication (probably translation) of virus, thus aborting infection. IFNs are broadly species-specific, that is, mouse IFN is inactive in humans, but IFNs are nonspecific with respect to inducing viruses; human interferon may protect against several different viruses. For example, IFN limits the spread of VZV in immunocompromised hosts, and it has had extensive clinical trial (particularly gamma IFN) in treating certain neoplasms. The mechanism of observed antitumor effects is still wholly obscure. It is clear that IFNs are to be considered not only as antiviral agents but also to have profound cytoregulatory effects (*e.g.*, on cell growth and differentiation, on the immune system in modulating T-cell cytotoxicity and macrophage activity, on expression of histocompatibility antigens on cell surfaces). The antiviral activity of all three IFNs is comparable, but the anticellular activity of gamma IFN, in fact a lymphokine, is the most potent. Interleukin 2 (T-cell growth factor, IL 2) regulates the expression of its own receptors on T lymphocytes as well as the synthesis of gamma IFN by the same cells. The quantity of human interferons available for clinical trial has been limited by availability of human leukocytes and fibroblasts in which to produce it. With the advent of cloning techniques, production of IFNs in quantities large enough for adequate clinical trials can be realistically anticipated.

Specific Immunity

Specific immunity is the result of effector mechanisms directly involving antibodies and specific cellular elements of the lymphoid system. The immunologically specific host responses to infections as well as to stimulation by other chemical or biologic molecules involves two basic effector mechanisms: ***humoral*** (antibody) and ***cell-mediated*** (lymphocytes and macrophages). Both specific immune responses originate in the lymphoid system, each effector mechanism being primarily associated with a distinct subset of lymphocytes. For example, the production of antibody involves lymphocytes called B cells, whereas the cell-mediated response involves lymphocytes designated T cells.

ANTIGEN

Antigen may be any chemical or biologic molecule that under the proper circumstances is capable of inducing a humoral or cell-mediated response. The product of that response (antibody or T lymphocytes) will react specifically with the original antigen. Antigens may vary in their capacity to induce an immune response. This degree of effectiveness is called immunogenicity. The most immunogenic antigens are usually molecules that are completely "foreign" to the host such as microbial products or components. Tissue components from animals or another species ***(xenoantigens)*** are in turn much more immunogenic than equivalent components derived from members of the same species ***(alloantigen).*** An exception to the latter statement is the extremely strong cell-mediated allograft rejection observed in immunologically unrelated members of the same species. Under certain conditions, even one's own tissue components can be immunogenic ***(autoantigens).*** For example, individuals with collagen diseases may make a variety of antibodies to their own DNA (*s*ystemic *l*upus *e*rythematosus, SLE), immunoglobulins (rheumatoid factor), and various other components (smooth muscle).

Very low molecular weight substances (including chemicals) that are not immunogenic by themselves can induce an immune response if combined with immunogenic complex molecules (protein) of higher molecular weight. The low-molecular-weight substance or chemical compound is called a ***hapten,*** whereas the immunogenic complex molecule to which it is bound is called ***carrier.*** Antibody made in response to a hapten-carrier complex binds specifically to the free hapten in the absence of the carrier. In a similar manner, certain small sequences of amino acids (proteins) or saccharides (carbohydrates) that are an innate part of complex immunogenic molecules can elicit an immune response to those specific areas of the molecule except that the remainder of the complex molecule acts as its own carrier. These integral small groupings of amino acids or saccharides are called ***antigenic determinants*** and, like haptens, determine the specificity of antibodies reacting with that particular antigen.

Some drugs, cosmetics, antibiotics, and industrial chemicals appear to act as haptens and utilize the host's own plasma or tissue proteins as carriers. These combinations can give rise to specific allergic reactions involving IgE antibody in immediate-type hypersensitivity. These must be distinguished from drug idiosyncrasies that have no immunologic basis, but in which signs suggestive of hypersensitivity may appear (rash, arthralgias). In addition to the formation of antibody, other haptens (such as heavy metals and certain chemicals) when bound to host tissue elicit cell-mediated responses to the combined antigenic determinant of hapten and adjacent host amino acids. In this case, free haptens are *not* able to react specifically with T lymphocytes in the absence of host carrier proteins. Examples that can give rise to cell-mediated, delayed-type hypersensitivity reactions include contact dermatitis and poison ivy.

Heterophile antigens contain cross-reactivity or similar antigenic determinants occurring in certain tissues, organs, or erythrocytes, and shared by a wide variety of phylogenetically unrelated species of plants and animals: dogs, sheep, turtles, spinach, cell walls of gram-negative bacteria *(e.g., Salmonella),* guinea pigs, and hamsters.

These Forssman heterophile antigens do not normally occur in pigs, frogs, or humans; antibodies to them are found in most human sera as agglutinins for sheep erythrocytes. Forssman heterophile antibodies can be absorbed out with guinea pig kidney tissue (rich in Forssman antigen). The heterophile antibody (sheep cell agglutinin) found in infectious mononucleosis (EBV) reacts with equine erythrocytes (Monospot test) and cannot be absorbed with guinea pig kidney tissue. The mononucleosis observed in CMV infection is not associated with a heterophile antibody response.

Soluble Factors in the Immune Response

ANTIBODY

In the electrophoretic analysis of serum, the major proteins are segregated into four principal portions: the alpha, beta, and gamma globulins, and albumin. Antibodies appear almost exclusively in the gamma portion and are commonly spoken of as gamma globulins or, more exactly, since they are not absolutely restricted to the gamma portion, as ***immunoglobulins*** (Ig). The immunoglobulins occur in five major molecular forms, designated as IgG, IgA, IgM, IgD, and IgE. There are several subclasses: $IgG_{1,2,3,4}$, $IgA_{1,2}$, $IgM_{1,2}$. The basic structure of IgG exemplifies the unit structure of all immunoglobulins (Fig. 5-2).

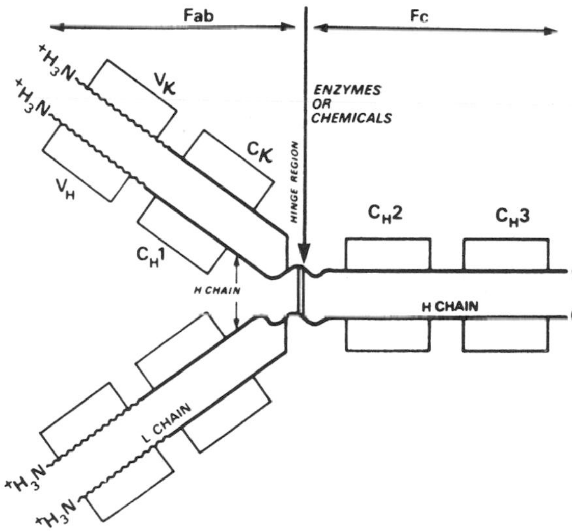

Fig. 5-2. A simplified model for an IgG1 (*κ*) human antibody molecule showing the 4-chain basic structure and domains. V indicates variable region; C, the constant region; and the vertical arrow, the hinge region. Thick line represents H and L chains; thin lines represent disulfide bonds. (Goodman JW, Wang A: Immunoglobulins: Structure and diversity. In Fudenberg HH, Stites DP, Caldwell JL, Wells JV (eds): Basic and Clinical Immunology, 2nd ed. Los Altos, CA, Lange Medical Publications, 1978)

Each molecule of IgG is Y-shaped, consisting of part of a pair of identical polypeptide chains intertwined and held together by covalent disulfide bonds. Near the midlength, each chain bends away from the other to make the arms of the Y (hinge region). Each of these chains consists of about 440 amino-acid residues, whose sequence (primary structure) is determined genetically. The total molecular weight of each chain is from 53,000 to 75,000, depending on the class. These chains are called the ***heavy*** (H) ***chains.*** Attached to each of the divergent arms of the Y-shaped molecule is a shorter polypeptide chain of about 220 amino-acid residues, with a molecular weight of about 22,000 per chain. These are called the ***light*** (L) ***chains*** and are identical in any given molecule and may be of a κ or λ type. The entire structure (including tertiary) of each immunoglobulin molecule or unit is maintained by disulfide bonds.

On both L and H chains, the distal portion (N-terminal ends) is variable in amino acid sequence from one immunoglobulin to another, which enables it to conform to the antigenic determinant for which it is specific. Within the variable regions are primary sequences of amino acids that show even greater variability in sequence composition and that are called hypervariable regions. The primary structure of the rest of the L and H chains (COO^- terminal end) is constant except for differences between IgG, A, M, D, and E heavy chains or κ and λ light chains as well as some alloantigenic differences (Inv on light chains and Gm on IgG heavy chains). The "arms" of the molecule are flexible through a "hinge" region at the point of divergence of the arms to allow better binding for each antigen binding site. The hinge region is also vulnerable to enzymatic digestion with papain, which yields two Fab (ab for antigen binding) fragments and one Fc (c for crystalizable) portion. The Fc fragment binds to certain cells that have ***receptors*** for this portion of the immunoglobulin molecule such as mast cells (IgE), K cells (IgG), macrophages (IgG and IgM), and others. Components of serum ***complement*** are "fixed" or activated by regions in the Fc fragment. (Complement is discussed in more detail later.)

IgG as described previously is representative of the various classes of antibody molecules. It is a relatively small, bivalent monomer and is late in appearing in response to initial infection. It is the most plentiful immunoglobulin and is active in agglutination, precipitation, and complement activation. It is the only form of antibody that can pass the placenta. IgA occurs as a monomer or dimer of the IgG form, the units being held together at the C ends by covalent bonds of an extra component called J chain (Fig. 5-3). Secretory IgA is the primary defense against surface infections (*e.g.*, cholera, influenza, mycoplasmal disease). The molecule is equipped with a supple-

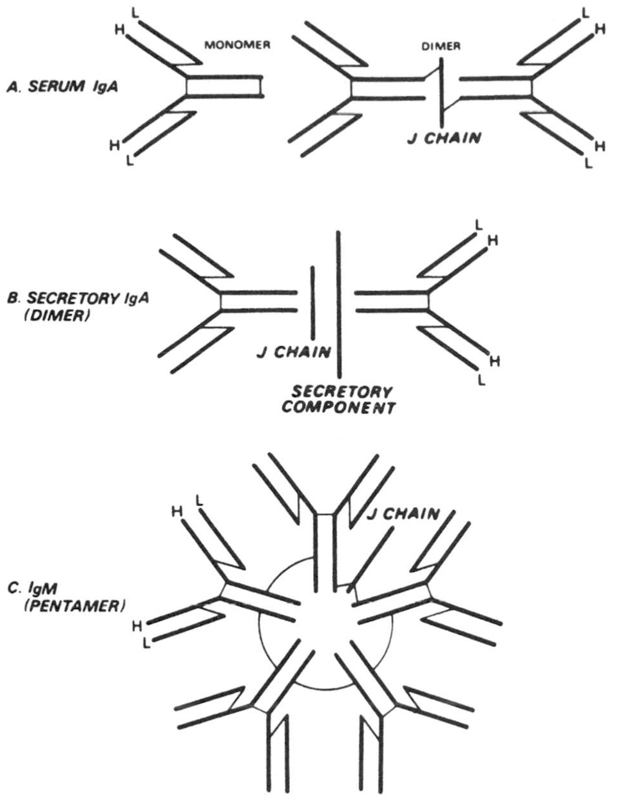

Fig. 5-3. Highly schematic illustration of polymeric human immunoglobulins. Polypeptide chains are represented by thick lines; disulfide bonds linking different polypeptide chains are represented by thin lines. (Goodman JW, Wang A: Immunoglobulins: Structure and diversity. In Fudenberg HH, Stites DP, Caldwell JL, Wells JV (eds): Basic and Clinical Immunology, 2nd ed. Los Altos, CA, Lange Medical Publications, 1978)

mentary secretory piece that facilitates its transportation across membranes.

IgM is a pentamer of subunits linked together by covalent bonds initiated by interaction with J chain. Because of its polyvalency, IgM is especially effective in forming lattices with antigens. It is also active in complement activation and is the first to appear in response to infections. IgE is functional in antibody-mediated (anaphylactic type) of hypersensitivity reactions.

IgD on the surface of B cells is co-expressed with IgM, but appears later during ontogeny and is thought to be an indicator of the mature (*i.e.*, competent) but still uncommitted resting B cell. On pre-B lymphocytes, membrane IgD is required for antigen binding and has the same specificity toward antigen as IgM, but on antigenic stimulation, IgD is shut off and only IgM continues to be synthesized. IgD may be involved in interactions between T and B cells and in regulation of resting B-cell populations.

The reciprocal structural relationship between molecules of antigen and antibody is the basis of immunologic specificity. The antigenic determinant of a molecule and its corresponding specific antibody must "fit" accurately together in order for a specific and effective antigen–antibody reaction to occur. In effect, the better the "fit" is, the stronger are the bonds between antigen and antibody molecules. Antigen–antibody interactions do not involve covalent bonds but depend upon hydrogen bonds, ionic bonds, and Van der Waals forces, all influenced by ionic concentrations, *p*H, and temperature.

Since an antigen molecule may contain more than one type of antigenic determinant, an immune response directed against the antigen consists of a group of heterogeneous antibodies, each reacting with its own antigenic determinant on the antigen molecule. As previously discussed, antibody is at least bivalent, and now antigens (especially complex molecules) may also be polyvalent with multiples of the same antigenic determinant or an assortment of different antigenic determinants.

The recent introduction of ***hybridoma techniques*** has permitted the immunochemical dissection of polyvalent antigens (*e.g.*, cell membranes, viral proteins, etc.) at the molecular level. The basic technique calls for the fusion (originally with inactive Sendai virus, currently with polyethylene glycol) of dissociated splenocytes (from immunized animals) with mutant myeloma (plasmacytoma) cells deficient in hypoxanthine-guanine-phosphoribosyltransferase (HGPRT). After cell-cell fusion, remaining single plasmacytes die out in medium containing hypoxanthine, aminopterin, and thymidine (HAT medium); hybrid cells continue to multiply, using the HGPRT gene from the splenocyte moiety, which continues to synthesize its own brand of antibody (single isotype and idiotype) against a single antigenic determinant in the antigen used in the original immunization. The hybrid cells are ***cloned*** (*i.e.*, isolated as single cells and grown up in culture) and used to produce malignant ascites tumors (hybridomas) in mice, the resulting ascitic fluid providing a rich source of ***monoclonal antibody.*** "Monoclonal" in this context refers to the original single B lymphocyte represented in the hybridoma. Monoclonal antibody (mAb) is much more restricted in specificity (*i.e.*, single antigenic determinant) than the usual polyclonal antibody, even when the latter is directed against rigorously "purified" antigen. Hybridomas made with alloactivated normal T cells have been found to secrete functional lymphokines (*e.g.*, T-cell growth factor, allogeneic effect factor, macrophage arming factor).

Precipitation. This involves molecules of soluble antigen in optimal concentration in relation to concentration of antibody molecules (*i.e.*, neither in great excess of the other). A "lattice" is formed consisting of several molecules of polyvalent antibody, such as IgM or IgG, joined to several molecules of polyvalent antigen. Such complexes may form large, visible precipitates whose size and form depend in part on the relative concentrations of antigen and antibody, the ionic content, temperature, and other properties of the fluid in which the reaction occurs.

When antibody and antigen are present in ratios of 1 : 1 or slightly higher, for example, 3 : 1 or 3 : 2 ("optimal proportions"), aggregation of antigen and antibody is maximal and lattice formation is most rapid and copious.

Agglutination. This involves intact cells or antigen-coated particles (latex agglutination) and optimal electrolyte concentration. Agglutination is best achieved with IgM through multipoint binding of the pentameric antibody, but IgG and IgA can also agglutinate particles. Because of the large size of certain cellular antigens (*e.g.*, erythrocytes), IgM antibodies, being large and pentavalent, are most effective in their agglutination. IgG molecules, being small and only divalent, often fail to "bridge the gap" between large cells, and lattice formation therefore fails. However, they (IgG) may combine with receptors on the cells, preventing the combination of IgG antibodies, thus acting as "blocking" antibodies (see Coombs test).

Neutralization. Neutralization of soluble toxins (and viruses) basically involves the blocking of reactive sites on the toxin (or virus) by antibody, thereby preventing expression of its toxic quality (or virus binding to host cells).

Opsonization. Microorganisms or foreign cells that have reacted with and retain specific antibody at their surfaces are said to have been ***opsonized,*** that is, rendered susceptible to phagocytosis by macrophages and polymorphonuclear leukocytes. The latter two cell types possess specific receptors for the Fc portion of immunoglobulins, particularly IgG, as well as for complement components (particularly C3) which, after binding to antigen-antibody complexes, contribute to opsonic activity by immune adherence (IA). Erythrocytes, neutrophils, lymphocytes, and monocytes possess receptors for IA, which is therefore important in clearing immune complexes from the circulation. This is also the basis for ADCC.

COMPLEMENT

Complement (C) is a system of 20 proteins and glycoproteins in the serum. When activated by Ag-Ab reactions, it mediates such diverse biologic functions as cytolysis of mammalian cells and gram-negative bacteria, increased vascular permeability, release of chemotactic factors, and increased opsonization for phagocytosis. Binding of antibody to an antigenic determinant, whether on a cell surface or soluble molecule, causes distortion and unveiling of a site on the Fc portion of immunoglobulins (IgG, IgM); this event in turn starts the "classic" cascade effect with the binding of the first component (C1) (Fig. 5-4). The C cascade is in its simplest terms a series of enzyme precursors that are acted on in succession and converted to active enzymes. In addition to classic activation, C may be activated by aggregated IgA, lipopolysaccharides, and yeast cell walls (zymosan). This process is called "alternate" activation and includes the components properdin (P), B factor and D factor (Fig. 5-5). Both types

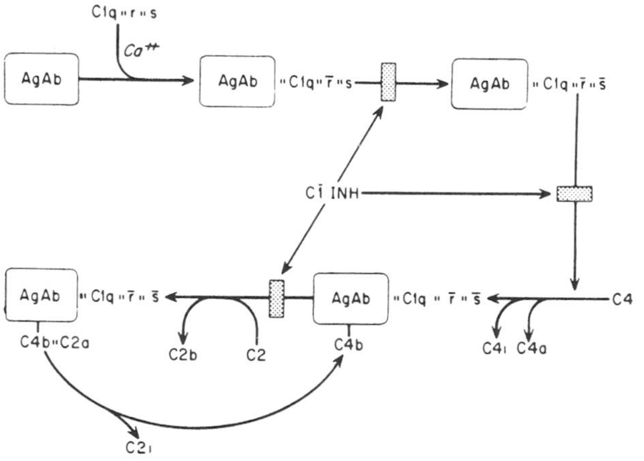

Fig. 5-4. Classic pathway of complement activation. This pathway is initiated by antigen-antibody (Ag-Ab) complexes and is controlled by the C1INH. (Austen KF: The classical and alternative complement sequence. In Benacerraf B, Unanue ER (eds): Textbook of Immunology, 2nd ed. Baltimore, Williams & Wilkins, 1984)

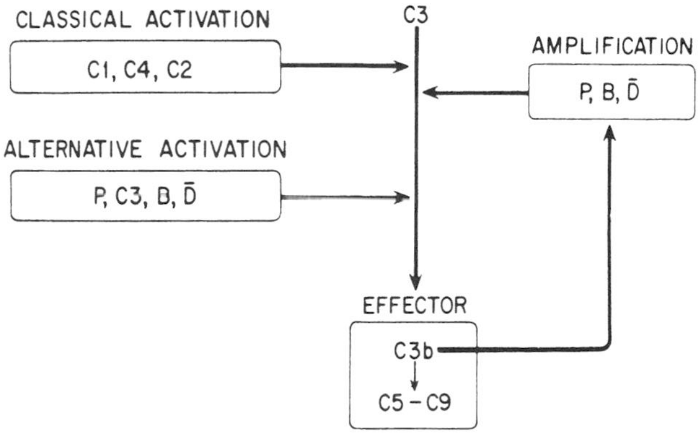

Fig. 5-5. Segregation of the complement proteins into four functional units: two pathways for initial cleavage of C3, the classic and alternative, the C3b-dependent amplification pathway for augmentation of C3 cleavage, and the effector sequence, from which are derived most of the biologic activities of the complement system. (Austen KF: The classical and alternative complement sequence. In Benacerraf B, Unanue ER (eds): Textbook of Immunology, 2nd ed. Baltimore, Williams & Wilkins, 1984)

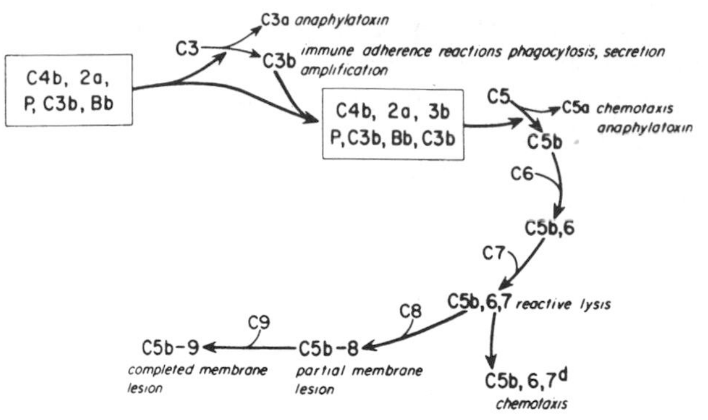

Fig. 5-6. The effector sequence of the complement system. The biologically active fragments and complexes are generated as a result of cleavage of C3 and C5 by the classic pathway and amplification of C3 and C5 convertases, respectively. (Austen KF: The classical and alternative complement sequence. In Benacerraf B, Unanue ER (eds): Textbook of Immunology, 2nd ed. Baltimore, Williams & Wilkins, 1984)

of activation lead to the "effector" series of components C3 to C9. The split products of C3 to C7 with biologic activity are shown in Figure 5-6.

Cytolysis requires the interaction of C8 and C9, which cause lesions in the membranes. Complement is regulated by extrinsic inhibitors (C1 inhibitors) and by the intrinsic short half-life of the activated components. The absence of C1 esterase inhibitor is the cause of the disease, angioedema.

Deficiency of one or more components of complement (in the classic pathway all except C1a, C15 and C9) occurs in association with a number of disease processes (*e.g.*, systemic lupus erythematosus). Lack of C3b inactivator is found in patients with recurrent pyogenic bacterial infections. Deficiency of C1 inhibitor is associated with hereditary angioneurotic edema. Some of these deficiencies are heritable.

C-REACTIVE PROTEIN (CRP)

Found in small quantities in normal serum, this beta globulin, which is not an antibody, is evoked in response to almost any acute inflammatory reaction (viral or bacterial infection, rheumatic fever). In these cases, increased serum levels of CRP have the same significance as other "acute phase reactants," for example, ESR. CRP in human serum is measured by immunoprecipitation with rabbit antibody to CRP, and the strength of the reaction is graded from 1+ to 4+; CIE and ELISA can also be used. CRP binds to phosphocholine determinants in C polysaccharide (group-specific pneumococcal antigen) thereby activating complement and enhancing phagocytosis. (See discussion of *Streptococcus pneumoniae*, previously.)

Cells of the Immune Response

It is apparent that an individual has a diverse number of both T and B lymphocytes that are capable of recognizing a large number of antigenic determinants. In a modification of Burnet's original theory, Jerne has proposed that each cell has a limited number of genes that code for appropriate allotransplantation antigens including (one's own) antigens (germ line theory). Because we cannot tolerate cells that would recognize our own antigens, these cells are suppressed as they appear by the overwhelming amount of our own antigens (immunologic tolerance). Diversification for recognition of all foreign antigens may come from somatic mutation of these cells so that mutant genes code for a variety of new antigenic determinants (somatic mutation theory). The combination of the two theories seems best to fit the evidence of immunologic tolerance, strong graft rejection, and that fact that cells are available that recognize synthetic antigens not involved in evolution. (This is considered to be an extreme oversimplification.) The interaction of a cell with its specific antigen leads to blastogenesis and replication (clonal expansion).

As indicated earlier, the specific immune response is mediated by lymphoid cells of two basic types, B and T lymphocytes. The cell surfaces of B lymphocytes contain about 10^6 antibody receptor molecules per cell, with a variable number (10 to 10^7) of different specificities built into each type of receptor molecule. The generation of antibody diversity comes from recombination between multiple germline genes for (a) light chains encoded by variable (V_L) and joining (J) gene segments, and (b) heavy chains encoded by V_H, J, as well as diversity (D) gene segments from separate locations on chromosome 14. Pre-B cells contain recombination activating genes (RAG-1 and RAG-2) that encode gene products, which control this recombination process. Binding of an antigen molecule to antibody combining site then initiates the humoral response pathway.

Similarly, T lymphocytes have about a million receptors per cell that are heterodimeric surface glycoprotein composed in about 90% to 95% of T cells of α, β chains (TCR2) and in 5% to 10% of T cells (mucosal immunity) of γ-δ chains (TCR1). Normally, TCR2 cells recognize peptide antigens presented in the context of MHC class I (predominantly CD_8^+) or class II (predominantly CD_4^+) (see Fig. 5-11) molecules. These peptide antigens are fixed on the surface and occur on a variety of cells, such as APC (antigen presenting cells), virus-infected cells, and tumor cells. TCR2 is associated with a CD_3 complex on the cell surface (see Table 5-17), and it assists in signal transduction of the message initiated when the TCR binds to the peptide antigen. T cells then proliferate and differentiate after this stimulation. Diversity, (as with immuno-

TABLE 5-17. Description of Selected Cluster of Differentiation (CD) Surface Markers on Leukocytes

T-Cell Markers (see Figs. 5-7 and 5-8)

CD_1: Three isoforms (CD_1a, CD_1b, CD_1c); found on thymocytes or dendritic cells. CD_1a, the major marker in the thymus cortex, is diminished in the medulla during T-cell maturation.

CD_3: A marker for all T cells, is comprised of five polypeptide chains δ (delta), ϵ (epsilon), γ (gamma), ζ (zeta), and η (eta). Usually, there are equal amounts of γ-ϵ and δ-ϵ heterodimers. Also, ζ-ζ (zeta-zeta) homodimer is the major (90%) species, relative to the ζ-η (zeta-eta) heterodimer (10%). Most CD_3 antibodies recognize the ϵ chain. CD_3 is closely associated with the TCR (T-cell receptor) and assists in signal transduction.

CD_4: This glycoprotein with four extracellular domains is the major marker on the surface of all T_H (helper T cells), but is also found to a lesser degree on macrophage/monocyte lineage cells. CD_4 is the major receptor for HIV-gp 120 binding. It binds to MHC class II (β chain) molecules on antigen-presenting cells (APC) and helps in the initiation of immune responses.

CD_8: This glycoprotein binds to MHC class I (α chain) molecules on APC. It is the major marker for $T_{c/s}$ (cytotoxic/suppressor T cells).

CD_{11}: This glycoprotein can be found in three isoforms; $CD_{11}a$, $CD_{11}b$, $CD_{11}c$. All are involved in mediating cell-cell adhesion. $CD_{11}a$ is found on resting or activated T cells, as well as CD_4^+ and CD_8^+ subsets of T cells. It is also found on peripheral blood NK cells. This adhesion molecule binds to ICAM-1, 2, and 3 (ICAM is intercellular adhesion molecule, which is found on vascular endothelial cells). $CD_{11}a$ is also called LFA-1. $CD_{11}b$ and $CD_{11}c$ are found primarily on neutrophils/monocytes and mediate their adhesion to endothelial cells during extravasation.

CD_{18}: This molecule forms heterodimers with $CD_{11}a$, $CD_{11}b$, or $CD_{11}c$ and mediates adhesion of T cells, as well as neutrophils/monocytes, to the endothelium. Lack of expression results in LAD (leukocyte adhesion deficiency, an autosomal-recessive genetic disease associated with frequent bacterial infections).

CD_{28}: Found in highest amounts in activated T cells. It is a T-cell costimulatory molecule that binds to a corresponding B7 (CD_{80}) ligand on APC. It enhances lymphokine secretion and plays a major role in T-cell activation. If CD_{28} and B7 do not ligate, this could lead to T-cell anergy.

$CD_{45}RA$: This is an isoform of CD_{45}, associated with naive T cells, that responds poorly to recall antigen and can induce CD_8^+ cells to suppress IgG synthesis.

$CD_{45}RO$: This isoform is associated with memory T cells, responds well to recall antigen, and stimulates B-cell IgG synthesis.

CD_{95}: This glycoprotein, also known as Fas, will bind Fas ligand and mediate apoptosis of activated T cells.

B-Cell Markers

CD_{19}: Glycoprotein found on peripheral, as well as activated splenic B cells, that is involved in B-cell activation and proliferation.

CD_{21}: B-cell glycoprotein that can bind complement (called CR_2, complement receptor 2) and Epstein-Barr virus. It is also involved in B-cell activation.

CD_{35}: Receptor for complement components C3b and C4b. Also found on activated granulocytes, where it mediates phagocytosis.

$CD_{45}RB$: Isoform of CD_{45} found on B cells; has a role in signal transduction.

CD_{54}: This Interferon γ–induced molecule is also found on endothelial, follicular dendritic, T, and NK cells. It is known as ICAM-1 and mediates adhesion by binding to the complex of $CD_{11}a/CD_{18}$. ICAM-1 is also a receptor for rhinoviruses, and on endothelial cells in the cerebrum, is a receptor of the malarial parasite *P. falciparum.*

Other Markers

CD_{30}: This is a marker found on Reed-Sternberg cells, which are bi-nucleated, large cells associated with Hodgkin's lymphoma. They are TNFR (tumor necrosis factor receptor)-like surface glycoproteins, normally associated with T-cell activation.

CD_{56}: Adhesion molecule seen on NK, but not B or T cells.

globulins) for α, β chain T-cell receptors (TCR2) is generated by recombinational V and J segment gene rearrangements (α chain), as well as V, D, J gene segment rearrangements (β chain).

Precursor, immunologically uncommitted lymphocytes of both types originate from bone marrow stem cells (precursor stem cells, PSC) and migrate to either of two primary lymphoid organs (Fig. 5-7). For B cells, the primary organ in mammalian species is the bone marrow and diffuse lymphoid structures of the gut (*i.e.*, Peyer's patches, appendix), which are functionally analogous to the bursa of Fabricius in avian species. In this microenvironment, lymphocytes are influenced to differentiate into immunologically competent B cells. In the earliest stage at which B cells can be recognized as such (pre-B cells), Ig is found in the cytoplasm. IgM then appears in the membrane and is soon joined by IgD. B lymphocytes migrate to populate the secondary lymphoid tissue: germinal centers in lymph nodes and spleen, and more mature B cells then appear with surface Ig markers of single or multiple isotypes. IgG-producing cells may be derived from IgM-producing cells by a switch in genetic control of heavy-chain synthesis. Immature B cells without cytoplasmic IgM bear surface IgM and IgD markers. On stimulation by antigen recognized by the IgM, IgD is turned off, and these cells differentiate further into plasma cells, which synthesize any of the four classes of immunoglobulin, each cell producing a single class of antibody.

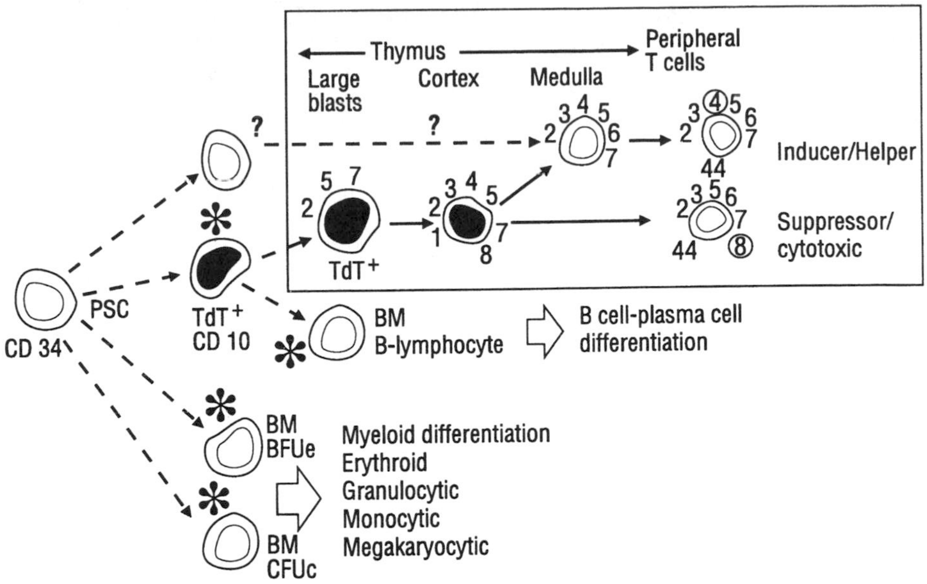

Fig. 5-7. The reactivity of cell surface cluster of differentiation (CD) reagents and other corresponding monoclonal antibodies in relation to differentiation of blood cells. CD 3, 4, 6, 7, and 8 are restricted to T lineage cells. Another marker for T cells (not shown above) is the T-cell antigen receptor (TCR), which is of 2 types. TCR-2, the major one (95% of T cells), as noted in Fig. 5-8, is an α, β heterodimer, while TCR-1 is similar but has γ, δ chains. Both receptors are complexed with CD_3, which is made up of 5 more polypeptide chains. CD_{44} is found on T-cells, as well as other leukocytes (monocytes, neutrophils), and functions as a homing receptor, mediating adhesion to endothelial cells. One other marker shared by naive (nonprimed) T_H and $T_{C/S}$ not shown above is CD 45RA. This is to be contrasted with the isoform CD45RO which is found on the surface of memory (primed) T cells. All identifiable bone marrow precursor cells tested (indicated by asterisks), and presumably also the human pluripotential stem cell (PSC), which cannot be tested *in vitro*, are unreactive with these reagents. The differentiation pathways are still hypothetical. (BM, bone marrow; BFUe, erythroid burst forming unit *in vitro;* CFUc, granulocytic-monocytic colony-forming unit *in vitro;* TdT, terminal deoxynucleotidyl transferase present in the nucleus of putative lymphoid precursors of BM and immature thymocytes (shown) by black nucleus)). (Janossy G, Goldstein G, Cosimi AB: Monoclonal anti-human lymphocyte antibodies: Their potential value in immunosuppression and bone marrow transplantation, Chap 4. In McMichael AJ, Fabre JW (eds): Monoclonal Antibodies in Clinical Medicine. New York, Academic Press Inc (London) Ltd, 1983). Updated to reflect changes in notation from OKT (monoclonal antibody) series to CD terminology.

''Memory'' B cells bear surface Ig of the same class and differentiate to plasma cells on encountering homologous antigen. The class of immunoglobulin synthesized depends on the state of ontogeny, and the specificity of immunoglobulin (variable region) is determined during exposure of the stem cell to the conditioning microenvironment (bursal equivalent).

The thymus gland is the other primary lymphoid organ serving as the microenvironment in which precursor stem cells differentiate into thymus-dependent lymphocytes, or T cells. The several subpopulations of T lymphocytes are identified by reactivity of surface markers with highly specific monoclonal antibodies to cluster determinants (CD) and terminal deoxynucleotidyl transferase (TdT) (Fig. 5-8). The term CD also refers to cluster designation and replaces terms such as OKT or Tn ($n = 1$ to 35), which were the previous T-cell surface markers determined by monoclonal antibodies raised in different laboratories. During recent international workshops, patterns of staining and molecular weights of leukocyte surface

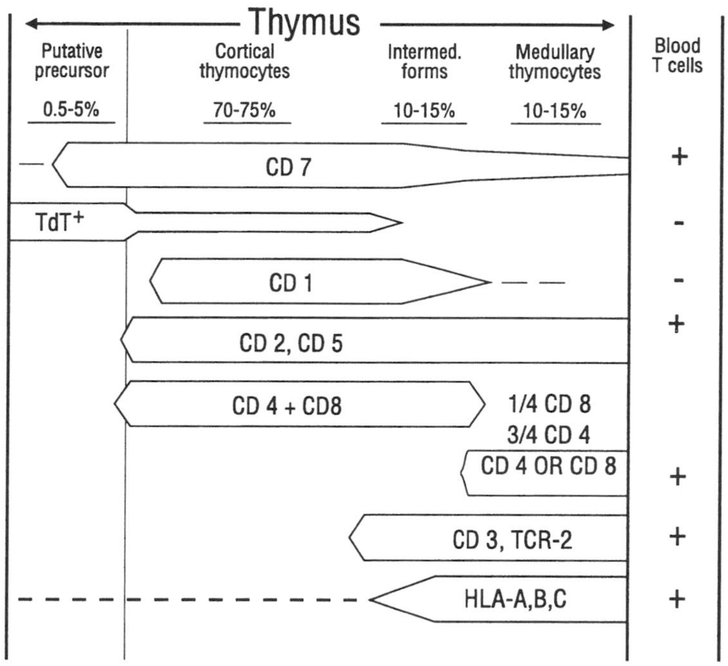

Fig. 5-8. Scheme of human lymphocyte differentiation based on reactions of monoclonal antibodies with membrane antigens and terminal deoxynucleotidyl transferase activity. Positivity of reactions among the cell populations is shown by horizontal bars; dotted lines indicate barely detectable or very weak positivity of a few cells. Putative precursors refers to large TdT^+ blasts that possess CD38. CD1, the first human leukocyte differentiation marker, appears to play a role in presentation of self antigens to T cells in the cortex. CD1a, a glycoprotein of MW about 50kD, is the predominant isoform. It is found associated with β2-microglobulin, similarly to the MHC class I surface antigen. Cortical CD2, CD5 cells simultaneously express both CD4 and CD8 resembling bone marrow TdT+ cells; medullary thymocytes are segregated into inducer/helper (CD4 majority) and suppressor/cytotoxic (CD8 minority) cell types. A number of forms are identifiable, which are intermediate between cortical and medullary thymocytes. (Data from Tidman N, Janossy G, Bodger M, et al: Clin Exp Immunol 45:437–467, 1981.) (Goldstein G, Lifter J, Mittler R: Immunoregulatory changes in human disease detected by monoclonal antibodies to T lymphocytes, Chap 3. In McMichael AJ, Fabre JW (eds): Monoclonal Antibodies in Clinical Medicine. New York, Academic Press Inc (London) Ltd, 1983). Data have been updated and altered to reflect changes in notation from OKT series to CD series of monoclonal antibodies.

molecules precipitated by the antibodies were grouped together and provided over 130 specific CD designations. Among these are several that have been well characterized as to specific cellular expression and function (see Table 5-17). They are grouped into T-cell, B-cell, and other cell markers.

Thymocytes differentiate into mature lymphocytes that have various biologic functions (T inducer/helper, T_i or T_h; T cytotoxic/suppressor, T_c; T delayed-type hypersensitivity, T_{dth}) and that populate the deep cortex of lymph nodes, and the periarterial sheaths of the spleen. T cells make up the major cellular component of the lymph and are the most numerous lymphocyte normally found in the blood. T lymphocytes also have class I HLA antigens, an important fact in recognition of antigen by T_c cells. The normal ratio of T_h ($CD4^+$) to $T_{c/s}$ ($CD8^+$) is about 2. The receptor on $T_{c/s}$ cells for antigen and MHC is a heterodimeric structure (m.w. 90,000) deduced from cDNA sequences, comprising two glycosylated chains, alpha and beta, each with two extracellular Ig-like domains, an amino-terminal variable domain and a carboxy-terminal constant domain. Each of these domains is stabilized by

TABLE 5-18. Properties of Selected Cytokines

IL-1	IL-1 refers to both IL-1α and IL-1β, which are structurally related. They are secreted proteins, cleaved from a larger precursor. After an inflammatory response, IL-1 greatly increases production of IL-1 by macrophages. IL-1 has multiple cellular as well as system responses. In particular, it induces prostaglandin synthesis, which induces fever. IL-1 also initiates the acute-phase response in the liver and plays an important role in immune functions.
IL-2	IL-2 is primarily synthesized and secreted by CD_4^+-T_H lymphocytes that have been stimulated by mitogens or a peptide antigen/MHC class II complex on APC. It was previously called T-cell growth factor. IL-2 can act as an autocrine or paracrine factor on B as well as NK cells. IL-2, along with Interferon-γ and TNF-β, push T_H cells along the TH1 pathway; involved in delayed-type hypersensitivity/cellular cytotoxicity.
IL-3	Synthesized by activated CD_4^+-T_H cells, IL-3 facilitates proliferation/differentiation/maturation of other T lymphocytes, as well as pluripotent stem cells (PSC, see Fig. 5-7).
IL-4	Formerly called B-cell stimulatory and differentiation factor. IL-4 binding to the IL-4 receptor has been useful in studying signal transduction involving the Janus family kinases (JAK) and STAT proteins. It also exhibits an antiinflammatory effect on macrophages and suppresses cytokine production by TH1-like cells. Thus, it pushes T_H cells toward the TH_2 pathway for B-cell proliferation and humoral immunity. Produced by CD_4^+-T_H lymphocytes and activated mast cells.
IL-6	IL-6 has multiple functions dependent on cell type. It leads to B-lymphocyte differentiation into plasma cells and induces hepatocytes to secrete acute phase proteins. IL-6 has additional growth factor stimulatory effects on T lymphocytes, plasmacytoma cells, and thymocytes.
IL-10	IL-10 is a cytokine synthesis inhibitor of TH1 cells and is expressed by macrophages, as well as CD_4^+ and CD_8^+ T lymphocytes. Among many pleiotropic effects, it suppresses cell-mediated immunity and stimulates B-lymphocyte responsiveness, pushing cells toward the TH_2 pathway.
IL-12	IL-12 was originally known as NK cell stimulatory factor and is produced by monocytes/macrophage cells. It promotes growth of activated NK and CD_8^+ T cells. In particular, it is being researched as a cancer immunotherapy reagent because of its ability to enhance LAK cell generation.

an S—S bound between cysteine residues, and the two chains are held together by a single interchain S—S bond located close to the outer cellular membrane, in which the protein is anchored by one hydrophobic transmembranal peptide in each chain. The alpha chain may recognize primarily HLA molecules; the beta chain may react primarily with foreign antigens. Stimulation of T lymphocytes by specifically recognized antigen (or other mitogen) results in blastogenesis and elaboration of soluble factors (lymphokines), which modulate various aspects of the immune response, particularly interaction with B lymphocytes.

For many years it was thought that these factors were only specific to T lymphocytes; but now it appears that these "B-cell factors" influence a wide variety of cells. The original division was into two functional groups of B-cell growth factors (BCGF), involved in B-cell proliferation from early precursor B cells and B-cell differentiation factors (BCDF), needed for maturation of activated B cells into Ig-secreting cells. These factors are now renamed interleukins-4 through 6, and in some cases (IL-4) can have both BCGF and BCDF activities. These, as well as other lymphokines (IL-1 through -3 and γ-IFN), which were originally thought to work on target cells other than B cells, are all known to modulate B-cell functions at different developmental stages. Currently, as many as 17 interleukins have been identified. A brief description of some selected lymphokines is presented in Table 5-18.

As noted above, the initial step in B-cell proliferation involves primary interaction of antigen with specific receptors on T lymphocytes; the lymphokines are wholly nonspecific with respect to antigen. These important lymphokines include gamma IFN, chemotactic factor, T-cell growth factor (interleukin 2), and macrophage inhibitory/activating factor (MIF/MAF). Interleukin 1 (IL-1) (previously known as lymphocyte-activating factor) is a protein (monokine) released by monocyte-macrophages undergoing an immune response, usually as a result of inflammation. As indicated, IL-1 has a wide range of biological activities, all previously recognized on a functional basis, but now known to be due to this one macromolecule. IL-1 stimulates T cells, regulates B-lymphocyte differentiation (see below), controls growth of bone marrow cells and effects generation of cytotoxic T lymphocytes. Some of these properties are doubtless interconnected with release of IL-2 from T_h cells. IL-1 may be identical to macrophage endogenous pyrogen because *in vivo* it causes fever and an increase in circulating neutrophils and stimulates release of acute-phase reactants by liver cells, and *in vivo* IL-1 stimulates release of prostaglandin and collagenase from synovial cells as well as the growth of fibroblasts. There is evidence that symptoms of TSS appearing in connection with staphylococcal infection may be due to release of IL-1 in large quantities from cells of the immune system stimulated by staphylococcal "toxic shock protein" (see TSSE in section on TSS).

IL-1 is reactive to B-cell lymphocytes at two stages; the pre-B cell and activated mature B cell. IL-2, enhanced by IFN-γ in addition to its role in stimulating Th cells, also now appears to influence activated B cells. Considering the currently discovered pleiotropic nature of these as well as the other lymphokines, homeostasis likely will involve the multiple effects of these factors on other than hemopoietic cells. To date, 17 interleukins have been identified.

The Major Histocompatibility Complex

The genetic control of graft rejection resides on the sixth chromosome in a complex of closely linked genes that is now called the major histocompatibility complex (MHC) (Fig. 5-9) coding for human leukocyte antigens (HLA). The known allelic forms for each locus in this extremely polymorphic system number at least 20 each for HLA-A, B and D, and 8 for HLA-C. These genes are autosomal as well as codominant and segregate in progeny with one set of linked (on the same chromosome) alleles (haplotype) from each parent. HLA antigens resulting from class I genes (A, B, and C loci) are found on cells in every body tissue except brain. Products of class II genes (D and D-related, DR) are restricted to B lymphocytes, macrophages, sperm, epithelial, and myeloid precursor cells, and are collectively known as ''Ia-like'' antigens (*i.e.*, like murine B-cell antigens, referred to as Ia). HLA-A, B, and C locus antigens are detected by reacting alloantiserum (usually from multiparous women) with peripheral blood lymphocytes in the presence of complement. HLA-D and DR antigens are detected by mixing peripheral blood lymphocytes of one individual (containing some B lymphocytes) with those of another (mixed lymphocyte reaction). Differences at the HLA-D locus on stimulator B lymphocytes cause blastogenesis of responder T-''helper'' lymphocytes. If the HLA-A, B, and C locus antigens are also different, responder T ''cytotoxic'' lymphocytes are induced that will lyse target cells bearing the same HLA-A, B, or C antigens as the stimulator cells. The induction of cytotoxic T lymphocytes is greater if HLA-D locus disparity occurs and T-''helper'' lymphocytes are produced. These *in vitro* processes are the basis of primary graft rejection. The MHC also contains genes controlling B factor, the fourth component of complement (Bf,C4), certain ''private'' blood-group factors (*e.g.*, Chido, Roger) related to C4, immune response (Ir) genes (*e.g.*, ragweed atopic IgE antibody), and others.

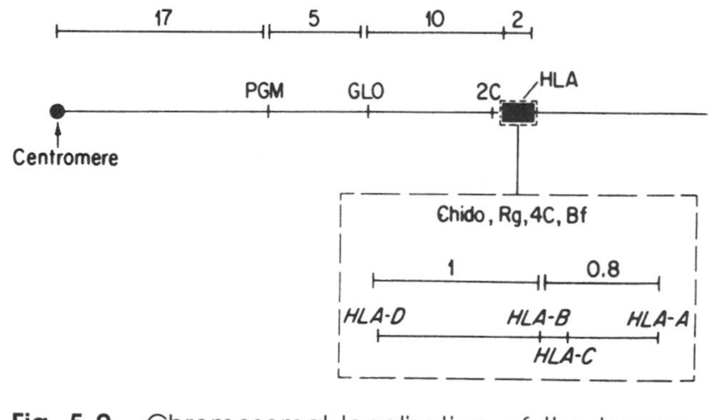

Fig. 5-9. Chromosomal localization of the human major histocompatibility complex (MHC). (Benacerraf B, Unanue ER: Transplantation Immunology. In Benacerraf B, Unanue ER (eds): Textbook of Immunology, 2nd ed. Baltimore, Williams & Wilkins, 1984)

The products of HLA-A,B and C genes consist of a transmembranal 44,000-dalton glycoprotein that binds noncovalently to beta-2-microglobulin. Products of the DR gene consist of a 34,000-dalton alpha-chain and 29,000-dalton beta-chain noncovalently bound to each other and inserted into the membrane with cytoplasmic carboxyl terminal ends. In both classes of antigen, alloantigenic specificity is contained in noncarbohydrate areas of the molecule, and not in the beta-2-microglobulin, which is the same in all members of a species.

Important linkage exists between disease states and specific HLA-B and HLA-D phenotypes. Some of the strongest linkage occurs between the allele HLA-B27 and ankylosing spondylitis, Reiter's syndrome and acute anterior uveitis. *Salmonella* and *Yersinia* enterocolitis, arthritis, and *Shigella* arthropathy have strong associations with HLA-B27. Several diseases have significant association with HLA Dw3 including juvenile onset diabetes, dermatitis herpetiformis, and idiophathic Addison's disease. These strong associations are mostly limited to HLA-B and D loci (see Fig. 5-9), which may indicate the existence, in this area of the MHC, of numerous Ir genes controlling immune regulatory mechanisms.

Immunologic Tolerance

The acquired inability of an individual to express an immune response to a molecule that would normally evoke active cell-mediated or humoral responses is called ''tolerance'' or ''immunologic unresponsiveness.''

1. Antigens that stimulate an immune response in adults can induce a state of tolerance in newborns with undeveloped immunologic competence. In 1945, Owen observed that during fetal life of dizygotic (heterozygous) twin calves, blood and erythrocytes of each fetus circulated freely in both and, though nonself (foreign), were tolerated throughout adult life as if they were ''self'' (native); each twin was an erythrocyte chimera. This exemplifies permanent, antigen-specific immunologic tolerance under natural conditions. The studies of Burnet and Medawar extended Owen's work. They injected

viable spleen cells of one strain of mice (A) into neonates of another strain of mice (B), thus artificially inducing in adult (B) mice complete, permanent and strain-specific immunologic tolerance to skin grafts from adult (A) mice.

2. T-*in*dependent antigens in extremely large doses can induce a state of "paralysis" or tolerance in an individual. Pneumococcal polysaccharide at 10 to 100 times the immunizing dose induces tolerance in animals. Challenge with immunizing doses does not induce an immunologic response. Because pneumococcal polysaccharide is a T-independent antigen, the tolerance is probably due to B-cell unresponsiveness.
3. T-dependent foreign protein antigens can be tolerogenic under the following circumstances: if the host is newborn or an immunosuppressed adult; if very low or very high doses of a lowmolecular-weight molecule in soluble, monomeric physical form are used; if introduction is by the intravenous route; and if antigen is inherently a weak immunogen in its native form. High doses of antigen probably involve tolerance by both B and T cells. Low-dose tolerance apparently involves T-suppressor-cell induction in the absence of a response by T-helper or B cells, which effectively prevents the induction of an immune response by excessive negative regulation.
4. Tolerance can be induced to new antigens if they are bound to the surface of the host's own cells. It has been demonstrated that haptens or glycoproteins covalently bound to the surface of autologous cells, when reintroduced into the host, can induce a state of functional tolerance with respect to the induction of the humoral response. T-suppressor-cell induction evidently is the main reason for unresponsiveness in this case, although T-helper tolerance may be involved under certain conditions.

Immunosuppression

This may be produced by various immunosuppressive measures, several of which are used in connection with organ "transplants" because there is as yet no generally acceptable and feasible means of inducing antigen-specific immunologic unresponsiveness to allografts. In general, they suppress proliferation and remove or destroy all clones of T and B lymphocytes nonspecifically and indiscriminately. Most of these measures have undesirable, often dangerous, side effects and also greatly enhance vulnerability to infection:

1. Whole body x-irradiation may be made specific under certain conditions and depends on injury to macrophages rather than to small lymphocytes.
2. Cannulization of the thoracic duct for mechanical removal of lymphocytes.
3. Beta-irradiation of blood; destruction of lymphocytes only.
4. Potent, equine, cytolytic, antihuman-lymphocyte globulins (ALG), especially in conjunction with thymectomy to delay regeneration of all antibody-producing lymphoid cells.
5. Drugs such as azathioprine, prednisone (and other corticosteroids), and cyclophosphamide.

Immunodeficiencies and Gammopathies

HUMAN IMMUNODEFICIENCY DISEASES

These are rare diseases, occurring at frequencies of 0.05% to 0.2%. The primary specific immunodeficiency diseases result from an absence or lack of maturation of T and/or B cells. A known familial predisposition or history of recurrent infections is a first sign that there may be an immunodeficiency. Upon further examination one finds for ***B-cell defects*** that there is low serum immunoglobulin present and no seroconversion to vaccines. For ***T-cell defects*** there is a reduced response to skin antigens and reduced response to viral or fungal infections as well as certain bacterial pathogens, such as *Mycobacteria tuberculosis.* A complete list of lymphocytic defects is shown in Table 5-19.

B-Cell Deficiencies. An example is ***X-linked agammaglobulinemia*** (congenital agammaglobulinemia, Bruton's disease). There is a family history of brothers or maternal male relatives with recurring infections. Infants generally present with infections caused by encapsulated, pyogenic bacteria at 5 to 6 months of age: often pneumonia, otitis media, dermatitis, or meningitis-type diseases. Affected males have no B lymphocytes, no detectable IgM, IgA, IgD, IgE, and only 10% of normal IgG, as well as no response to immunization. There is little development of lymph-node germinal centers, and tonsils are abnormally small. These individuals do have a normal cell-mediated response with respect to delayed-type hypersensitivity and allograft rejection. Patients can be treated with gamma globulin. With increased age, patients are at increased risk of developing neoplasias and chronic sinopulmonary disease (due to lack of secretory IgA). The cause of the defect is not certain. Pre-B cells are present with cytoplasmic μ chains, but there is a severe decrease in the number of mature B cells possessing surface immunoglobulin. This suggests that there is a block in differentiation after B cells have undergone Ig heavy chain rearrangement, but before light chain expression.

Two other examples of B-cell deficiencies showing reduced Ig levels are ***transient hypogammaglobulinemia*** and ***selective IgA deficiency.*** The former is similar to Bruton's disease in onset and features. However, in this disease patients who survive gradually develop significant antibody responses. In selective IgA deficiency, patients have reduced serum and secretory IgA levels but

TABLE 5-19. Lymphocyte Defects and Genetic Aspects of Selected Primary Immunodeficiency Syndromes

DISORDER	AFFECTED LYMPHOCYTE POPULATIONS				MODE OF INHERITANCE
	T Cells		B Cells		
	STAGE 1*	STAGE 2*	STAGE 1	STAGE 2	
B-Cell Deficiencies					
Congenital hypogammaglobulinemia (Bruton type)	No	No	Yes	Yes§	X-linked
Congenital hypogammaglobulinemia	No	No	Yes	Yes	Autosomal recessive
Common variable immunodeficiency	No	(No)	No	Yes§	? Autosomal recessive
IgA deficiency	No	(No)	No	No§	Variable
IgM deficiency	No	No	No	?	Unknown
IgG subclass deficiency	No	No	No	?	X-linked
Immunodeficiency with elevated IgM	No	No	No	(Yes)	X-linked
X-linked immunodeficiency with normal globulin count or hyperglobulinemia	No	No	(No)	(Yes)	X-linked
Hypogammaglobulinemia with thymoma	No	No	No	Yes§	Unknown
T-Cell Deficiencies					
Thymus hypoplasia Nezelof's syndrome	Yes	Yes	(No)	(No)	Variable
DiGeorge syndrome	Yes	Yes	No	No	Variable
Purine nucleoside phosphorylase deficiency	Yes	Yes	No	No	? Autosomal recessive
Chronic mucocutaneous candidiasis (CMC) with endocrinopathy	No	Yes	No	No	? Autosomal recessive
Combined B and T Cell Deficiencies					
Reticular dysgenesis	Yes	Yes	Yes	Yes	Unknown
SCID† (thymic alymphoplasia)	Yes	Yes	(Yes)‡	(Yes)	X-linked
SCID (Swiss type)	Yes	Yes	(Yes)	(Yes)	Autosomal recessive
SCID with ADA deficiency	Yes	Yes	(Yes)	(Yes)	Autosomal recessive
SCID with ectodermal dysplasia and dwarfism	Yes	Yes	Yes	Yes	? Autosomal recessive
SCID (sporadic)	Yes	Yes	Yes	Yes	Unknown
Wiskott-Aldrich syndrome	Yes	Yes	No	(Yes)	X-linked
Ataxia telangiectasia	(Yes)	Yes	No	(No)	Autosomal recessive

* Indicates first or second stages of lymphoid cell differentiation.
† SCID = severe combined immunodeficiency.
‡ Statements enclosed in parentheses indicate defects that are variable in severity or expression.
§ Recent evidence indicates the presence of excessive suppressor cell activity.

normal IgG, IgM, and cell-mediated immunity. This is the most common (1:500) immunodeficiency disorder known. Many individuals do not have overt disease and are healthy; others experience frequent respiratory infections or recurrent bronchitis and enteropathy. No IgA-producing plasma cells are found in the lamina propria, yet about 40% of patients have circulating anti-IgA Ab.

T-Cell Deficiencies. An example is ***congenital thymic aplasia*** (DiGeorge syndrome). Thymic aplasia results from a congenital defect and is not hereditary. Most patients present with intractable hypocalcemia or severe cardiac disease in the first few weeks of life. A classic facial appearance of notched or folded ears, and a small fishlike mouth is present at birth or will develop later. These individuals have no T cells and hence no delayed-type hypersensitivity or allograft rejection capability. Germinal centers are normal with normal numbers of plasma cells in lymphoid tissue. Serum immunoglobulins are normal, the result most likely of T-independent antigen stimulation from infectious agents. The lack of a cell-mediated response makes these individuals susceptible to fatal infections with viruses (measles and chickenpox), fungi, and acid-fast bacilli.

Two other T-cell deficiencies are ***Nezelof's syndrome*** and ***purine nucleoside phosphorylase deficiency.*** In the former a patient will have both a hypoplastic thymus and impaired cell-mediated immunity. Serum levels of antibody may be near normal, but the requirement for B-T cooperation means that some humoral immune responses will also be depressed. A number of bacterial, as well as viral infections occur in these individuals. In purine nucleoside phosphorylase deficiency, there is a defect in conversion of inosine and guanosine to hypoxanthine and guanine. The accumulation of deoxyguanosine and dGTP is selectively toxic for T cells. Thus, although serum immunoglobulin levels may be near normal, the decreased cell-mediated responses lead to viral and fungal infections, as well as increased tumor incidence. ***Chronic mucocutaneous candidiasis*** (CMC) is yet another cellular immunodeficiency characterized by chronic *Candida* infections of the skin, nails, and mucous membrane. It represents a highly specific disorder of T-cell function, since T-cell numbers are normal. Since these patients have antibodies that react with various endocrine tissues, this suggests that there is an autoimmune nature to the disease. Treatment involves use of ketoconazole as the drug of choice.

Combined B- and T-Cell Deficiencies. An example is ***severe combined immunodeficiency*** (SCID) (Swiss-type agammaglobulinemia). This disease is characterized by a lack of both T and B lymphocytes. It is hereditary, being transmitted by X-linked or autosomal recessive genes. Individuals with SCID are agammaglobulinemic and are incapable of rejecting allografts or of developing delayed-type hypersensitivity. An absence of stem cells in the bone marrow is thought to be the cause of this disease. Without a bone marrow transplant, the disease is usually fatal. Thymopentin, a synthetic pentapeptide that corresponds to the active moiety of thymopoietin, has, in conjunction with bone marrow transplants, had limited success in treatment.

Adenosine Deaminase (ADA) Deficiency. About 50% of all individuals with this disease have acquired it as a sex-linked disorder. In the absence of the enzyme (which catalyzes conversion of adenosine to inosine) deoxyadenosine and dATP accumulate and are lethal to B and T cells, leading to a SCIDS-like condition. It is characterized by recurrent serious infections in infancy and bone abnormalities. If untreated, affected children die in early childhood. Transfusions with irradiated normal erythrocytes provide a source of enzyme and temporary improvement. Bone marrow transplants, if marrow from siblings or half-matched donors is used, is the preferred treatment. Most recently an experimental enzyme replacement therapy using the bovine ADA enzyme linked to polyethylene glycol (PEG) shows promise for patients who do not have bone marrow donors.

Other examples of combined immunodeficiencies are ***ataxia-telangiectasia (AT)*** and ***Wiskott-Aldrich syndrome.*** Both of these diseases are very rare, with AT having an incidence of 1 : 100,000. It is characterized by progressive cerebellar ataxia and oculocutaneous telangiectasia. The primary defect is one of DNA repair. At about 5 years of age, patients present with recurrent upper respiratory tract infections due to a depression in both humoral (IgA) and cell-mediated responses.

Wiskott-Aldrich Syndrome. This is an X-linked disorder characterized by thrombocytopenia with bleeding, eczema (in the first year), and immunodeficiency. Recurrent bacterial infection occurs leading to pneumonia and chronic otitis media, as well as viral (herpes family) and parasitic *(Pneumocystis carinii)* infections. Malignancy develops in more than 10% of patients. The mechanism of this disorder involves a defect in cell-mediated immunity and low IgM production. Poor response to polysaccharide (thymus-independent) antigens of pneumococci and cell membrane glycoprotein abnormalities suggest that the defect might involve the absence of specific glycoproteins on T-cell surfaces.

In addition to the primary immunodeficiencies described above, several secondary immunodeficiencies can result in severe recurrent infections. Among these are ***chronic granulomatous disease*** (CGD) and ***Chediak-Higashi syndrome.*** CGD is an X-linked recessive disease, characterized by a susceptibility in childhood to pyogenic infections by catalase-positive bacteria (*Staphylococcus aureus, Aerobacter aerogenes,* and enterobacteria) but not other bacteria, such as streptococci and pneumococci. This is because the latter provide the neutrophil with H_2O_2 (they are catalase-negative), which is then used to kill the microorganism, since myeloperoxidase can function normally in the neutrophil if it is provided with H_2O_2. The defect in this disease is both in neutrophil and macrophage phagocyte oxidative killing, apparently due to a deficiency of a superoxide-forming enzyme (NADPH oxidase) and/or a subunit of cytochrome-b needed for NADP recycling. In CGD bacterial infection leads to severe lesions that are slow to heal, followed by granuloma formation. The disease is often fatal by seven years of age, despite the use of antibiotics.

Chediak-Higashi syndrome is an autosomal recessive condition characterized by neutrophils and platelets with abnormally large lysosomes. There is an inability of neutrophils to kill both catalase-positive and negative bacteria (in contrast to CGD); chemotaxis in these lymphocytes is defective due to an inability to rearrange microfilaments. Bacterial infection and development of lymphoid neoplasms lead to an early death. Also, there are recurrent infections due to lowered phagocytic activity caused by a lack of opsonins (antibody or complement).

Acquired Immunodeficiency Syndrome (AIDS). Since 1981, this newly recognized syndrome has been encountered worldwide with increasing frequency, until at the present writing more than 300,000 cases with about 220,000 deaths have been reported in the United States, with the greatest concentrations in New York City, Los Angeles, San Francisco, Miami, and other major urban centers. What is even more frightening is that worldwide there are over 20 million cases of AIDS, with 550,000 annual deaths. The syndrome is characterized by lymphopenia and marked impairment of T-lymphocyte function due to profound depression in numbers of helper/inducer (Th, Ti, $CD4^+$) cells and consequent inversion of the ratio (normally about 1.7–2.0) of Th to cytotoxic/suppressor (Tc, Ts, $CD8^+$) cells. Clinically, there is generalized lymphadenopathy. A prodromal complex referred to as AIDS-related complex (ARC) may last many months and is characterized by fever, weight loss, leukopenia, and severe infection with opportunistic pathogens (bacterial, viral, fungal, parasitic). The most frequently fatal are *Pneumocystis carinii,* herpesviruses, cryptosporidium, *Cryptococcus, Toxoplasma gondii, Candida* (oral candidiasis may be a signal of impending AIDS), and various pyogenic bacteria. An unusual form of Kaposi's sarcoma (KS) with facial as well as lower trunk lesions is seen in AIDS patients. KS had only rarely been seen in North America or Europe but was known to occur endemically in equatorial Africa and among older Jewish men in some Mediterranean locales. Recently, a new herpes virus (HHV 8) has been associated with all forms of KS. Major groups at risk continue to be homosexual and bisexual men and intravenous drug users. However, there has been a sharp increase in heterosexual transmission among teenagers and young adults. Previously, patients with hemophilia who relied on human blood products (Factor VIII) for survival were at high risk. Although a number of cases were caused by transfusions of whole blood prior to testing, the risk of contracting AIDS by this route is currently negligible. AIDS has also been documented in female sexual partners of AIDS patients, and in neonates born to IV drug users who were seropositive.

Asymptomatic virus-positive carriers continue to constitute a significant proportion of high-risk groups and are doubtless important in the dissemination of HIV through sexual contact. The mean interval between infection with HIV and the onset of AIDS is about 7 years for such high-risk groups: homosexual and bisexual men, intravenous drug abusers, and hemophiliacs infected before the advent of serologic testing.

It appears that the overall prevalence of HIV antibody among Red Cross blood donors who have not previously been tested is about 0.04%. It is estimated that between 1 and 1.5 million Americans are infected with HIV. There is no evidence that the virus can be transmitted through casual contact; intimate sexual contact, sharing of contaminated needles, and transfusion of contaminated blood or blood products are the real hazards. Antibody to core protein (p24) declines late in infection. As noted earlier, AIDS-related complex (ARC) (lymphadenopathy, fever, weight loss) in which circulating immune complexes are prominent along with the aforementioned T-cell abnormalities, polyclonal hypergammaglobulinemia and autoantibodies, is a prodrome to the full-blown disease, capped by overwhelming opportunistic infections. A "wasting syndrome," characterized by weight loss and fatigue, but without recognized opportunistic infection or lymphadenopathy, is also seen. Non-Hodgkins' lymphoma, like KS, is a serious manifestation of AIDS and ARC in high-risk groups. As to the origin of HIV, current theory suggests that it may have appeared first in Africa (several thousand AIDS cases occur annually in Zaire alone) and thence have spread through migrant populations to Europe and the Caribbean area, and from the latter to the east and west coasts of the United States. Azidothymidine (AZT) had been the primary drug used to prolong life, albeit for only a relatively short period, of those AIDS patients with *P. carinii* pneumonia. The drug appears specifically to block the HIV reverse transcriptase (RT), but it also has side effects in damaging bone marrow cells. Recently, a similar RT inhibitor, ddI (2′, 3′-dideoxyinosine) has been approved for use. Other traditional drugs such as pentamidine were also used to treat *P. carinii,* until the occurrence of resistant organisms precluded its effectiveness.

In 1993, it became clear from the Concorde Patient Trial that AZT, despite its initial promise, did not enhance survival of patients who received it before developing symptoms of AIDS. Additional nucleoside inhibitors, such as ddI, fared no better. However, in 1996, the recent development of several new inhibitors that block a different enzymatic step—the protease inhibitors—looks very promising. Among them are drugs with names such as saquinavir, ritonavir, and crixivan (indinavir). All have been FDA approved and in particular, the latter two greatly decrease the level of viremia in peripheral blood mononuclear cells, as measured by HIV-1 RNA, using quantitative RT-PCR. These compounds are all aspartyl protease inhibitors and prevent cleavage of the large HIV-1 Gag as well as Gag-pol precursor proteins, leading to the production of defective, immature particles that cannot replicate. Combinations of protease and reverse transcriptase inhibitors look very impressive in clearing HIV-1 viremia for at least six months. It is hoped that these combinations will provide longer lives for HIV-1–infected patients.

Precautions to be taken by clinical and laboratory staffs should be as rigorous as those for hepatitis B. Any discussion of a vaccine for prevention of AIDS is premature, not only for ethical reasons but also because of already evident variations among strains of HIV, which would pose significant problems. However, there may be some hope with several novel approaches. The most promising appears to be immunization with a form of the outer viral envelope glycoprotein gp 120 obtained using recombinant DNA technology in one of several expression vector systems: *E. coli,* yeast, mammalian cells, or vaccinia virus. This is a reasonable approach, since AIDS patients uniformly possess antibodies against the *env* proteins at all stages of infection, whereas antibodies against other HIV proteins, such as *gag* diminish during the course of the disease. As noted, difficulties may arise with this vaccine, due to antigenic variation; however, there do appear to be a few regions on gp120, which are relatively constant. Also, vaccinia/AIDS recombinant viruses are currently being constructed to use as vaccines, since these viruses show evidence for shedding of gp120 from infected cells; if a variant gp120 arises, it can also be easily incorporated into the recombinant virus. Finally, another approach being tried is to synthesize peptides to constant regions of both gp120, as well as gp41 and utilize them in combination to elicit neutralizing antibodies. Studies are under way with all of these approaches in chimpanzees as well as, in some cases, human volunteers to test their efficacy.

GAMMOPATHIES

Gammopathies are the opposite of deficiencies, being characterized by the abnormal proliferation of cells involved in the humoral response. The result is that excessive amounts of immunoglobulin are produced. Table 5-20 shows the more important monoclonal gammopathies with their associated immunoglobulin classes.

Multiple Myeloma. This is a malignant proliferation of plasma cells with the following characteristics: cell-mass expansion; immunoglobulin protein elaboration; and the concomitant suppression of normal antibody synthesis. The whole immunoglobulin (M component) may be found in the serum with or without "free" light chains in the urine (Bence Jones proteins). The disease involves osteolytic lesions and pathologic fractures, anemia due to displacement of myeloid elements in the bone marrow by plasma cells, renal failure and nervous system involvement.

Macroglobulinemia (or Waldenström's Macroglobulinemia). This is characterized by the production of a homogeneous single immunoglobulin (IgM). Clinically, increased viscosity of the blood caused by large amounts of IgM results in thrombosis and bleeding (petechiae) in the skin, nasal mucosa, and gastrointestinal tract. Retinal hemorrhages may eventually cause blindness.

TABLE 5-20. Monoclonal Gammopathies

DISORDER	CLASS OF PROTEIN	LIGHT CHAIN
Multiple myeloma	IgG, IgA, IgD or IgE	κ or λ
Macroglobulinemia	IgM	κ or λ
Heavy-chain disease	IgG, IgA or IgM	None

* Found in secretions and plasma of "secretors"; adsorbed to erythrocytes from plasma.

† Based on reactivity with 5 commonly available antisera: anti-D (anti-Rh 1), anti-C (anti-Rh 2), anti-E (anti-Rh 3), anti-c (anti-Rh 4), anti-e (anti-Rh 5)

‡ Se gene function required.

§ SXIV = type XIV peneumococcai polysaccharide cross-reactive with blood group substances because of the core common to both classes of antigen.

"Heavy Chain Disease." This was first described as being caused by the elaboration of a protein (55,000 daltons) apparently consisting of an incomplete IgG heavy chain and having the antigenic determinants of IgG, but no detectable light chains. Subsequently, IgA and IgM heavy chain diseases have been described. The syndrome is characterized clinically by frequent infections due to impairment of antibody production.

LYMPHOPROLIFERATIVE SYNDROMES

The X-linked lymphoproliferative syndrome (Duncan's syndrome) is characterized by an abnormal increase of lymphoid cells involved in the cellular immune response to EBV infection. Affected males (½–22 years) fail to limit the infection by not developing an increase in the appropriate class of $T_{c/s}$ cells that normally would kill target EBV infected B cells. Patients with this symptom die of lymphoma (non-Hodgkins) or aplastic anemia.

Allergy and Hypersensitivity

Allergy (Gr. *allos,* changed; *ergon,* action) or hypersensitivity is an altered state of reactivity of cells and tissues manifest through specific pathogenic immune reactions occurring *in vivo* (Table 5-21). Most of the manifestations of hypersensitivity are now explicable in terms of molecular and cellular interactions. The principal mechanisms underlying the clinical manifestations of allergy can be grouped conveniently under four principal headings.

- Type I: anaphylactic atopic allergy, entirely mediated by IgE
- Type II: cytotoxic type, dependent on antibody and complement
- Type III: immune complex disease (serum sickness)
- Type IV: cell-mediated immune reactions

Types I, II, and III are all referred to as "immediate hypersensitivity," being mediated by specific antibody. Type IV hypersensitivity is essentially independent of antibody, all reactions being mediated by specifically sensitized T lymphocytes. Types I and IV are independent of complement. It will be evident that more than one of the four types may be operating in a given clinical situation. Moreover, implicit in each type of hypersensitive manifestation is a first experience with a given set of antigens constituting the primary immunization or sensitization. Subsequent exposure to the same or related sets of antigens evokes tissue reaction(s) in the previously "sensitized" host. The manner and route of primary sensitization are not always evident and may be respiratory (*e.g.,* hay fever), contact (poison ivy), or oral (food allergies). Atopic persons are those who inherit (MHC) a tendency to become allergic very easily to many different antigens by synthesizing abnormally high levels of IgE.

TABLE 5-21. Hypersensitivity: Pathogenic Immune Reactions *in vivo*

DESIGNATION, TYPE*	ROUTE OF PRIMARY ANTIGENIC STIMULATION	SPECIFICITY	SKIN TEST	CLINICAL EXAMPLES	MECHANISM	PREVENTION
I. Anaphylactic, "immediate"	Respiratory GI tract Subcutaneous	IgE (reaginic antibody; distinguish from Wassermann ab)	(Intradermal) "immediate" wheal/flare sec.-min. Transferable with serum	Allergic rhinitis (hay fever); insect venom sensitivity (phospholipase A) DRUGS (e.g., penicillin). Hives (urticaria), asthma	Histamine SRS-A, ECF-A from sensitized mast cells, basophils, ?platelets. No tissue damage	"Blocking" IgG
II. Cytotoxic, ADCC	Parenteral, Infection, Drugs as haptens, Altered "self"	IgM, IgG (systemic)	(Systemic reaction, transferable with serum)	Transfusion reactions Hemolytic disease of the newborn (HDN) Hemolytic anemia (DRUGS) Viral infection (ADCC) Autoimmune diseases Thrombocytopenic purpura	C ("immune") lysis of sensitized cells (rbc, platelets) (tissue damage) Destruction of sensitized virus-infected cells by T_c lymphocytes (MHC restriction)	HDN: Rhogam prophylaxis against primary sensitization (not desensitization)
III. Antigen–Antibody complex disease, "Serum sickness"	Foreign protein, parenteral, infection	IgG, IgM ("Gatekeeper" IgE)	Arthus type (experimental passive)	Poststreptococcal AGN Rheumatoid arthritis SLE, hepatitis B Drugs, infections	Deposition of Ag/Ab/C in tissues evokes acute inflammatory reaction (pmn, platelets) Tissue damage	None specific
IV. "Delayed," tuberculin type, CMI	Persistent chronic intracellular infection (bacterial, fungal, viral, protozoal) Tumors Tissue grafts	T lymphocytes	(Intradermal) "Delayed" tuberculin type (PPD) 24–48 hours	Tuberculosis, other bacterial infections All mycoses, some viruses Contact dermatitis (e.g., drugs, poison ivy) Tumor and graft rejection	T lymphocytes specifically stimulated to release lymphokines (nonspecific) Transfer factor (specific) Tissue damage	None

* Types I, II, and III are all referred to as *Immediate-type hypersensitivity*, and all are mediated by specific antibody. Type IV is essentially independent of antibody, and all reactions are mediated by specifically sensitized T lymphocytes.

TYPE I HYPERSENSITIVITY

"Immediate"-type hypersensitivity refers to atopic allergy, manifested by a rapidly developing (minutes) wheal and flare (hives, urticaria) reaction in the skin in response to the intradermal injection of specific antigen(s), exemplified by hay fever (*e.g.*, ragweed allergy). There is no perceptible local cytotoxicity or leukocytic response. The same antigen given systemically (usually inadvertently) causes anaphylactic shock. IgE formed in response to primary (sensitizing) immune responses attaches, by the Fc portion, to specific Fc receptors on mast cells, basophils, and platelets, that is, become tissue-fixed and remain *in situ* for months or years. Reactions of homologous antigens with this fixed antibody trigger transmembranally the release of the vasoactive amines responsible for all of the manifestations of "immediate" hypersensitivity, namely, histamine, bradykinin, slow-reacting-substance of allergy (SRS-A), all of which cause smooth-muscle contraction, vasodilatation, and increased capillary permeability. Increased coagulation time is due to heparin released from mast cells. Liver damage occurs, and cartilage and collagen tissues are affected. Edema and smooth-muscle contractions in large blood vessels, air passages, and elsewhere are frequently the immediate cause of death. Commonly, the active substances are quickly decomposed in the body and the manifestations of immediate allergy are therefore short-lived (2 to 48 hours). Fatal anaphylaxis, which is not unusual, can result from bee stings or from injection of avianized vaccines and antibiotics (especially penicillin), particularly in an atopic individual. Histamine release is under the control of AMP. Falling levels (blockade of adenylcyclase) promote histamine release; promotion of cAMP synthesis by increased adenylcyclase activity (stimulated by epinephrine) reduces histamine release. Xanthines (used in therapy of type I hypersensitivity) block phosphodiesterase, which is responsible for the destruction of cAMP. Eosinophil-chemotactic factor A (ECF-A) is among the products released by basophil-mas cell activation. Eosinophils secrete their granular enzyme (arylsulfatase), which splits SRS-A, providing a feedback control mechanism. These reactions are summarized in Figure 5-10.

TYPE II HYPERSENSITIVITY

This type usually results from the cytotoxic or cytolytic action of complement on cells (tissue cells, erythrocytes) to which specific antibodies to cellular components (*e.g.*, blood group antigens) have attached. These cells are said to be "sensitized" to immune lysis, which is the mechanism underlying hemolytic disease of the newborn (HDN) (q.v.) and incompatible transfusion reactions. Some drugs (*e.g.*, Sedormid, penicillin) bind to tissue proteins and thereby become antigenic, the resulting antibody being specific for the drug (hapten). The same or related drugs adsorbed nonspecifically to cells make them the target for cytotoxic antibody (hemolytic anemia, thrombocytopenic purpura) (Figure 5-11).

TYPE III HYPERSENSITIVITY

The term ***"serum sickness"*** refers to the older observation of anaphylactic and immediate allergic manifestations in persons receiving foreign serum therapeutically (*e.g.*, diphtheria antitoxin as horse serum). The term as now used connotes type I or III allergy caused by any foreign antigenic substances, which may include low-molecular-weight compounds (haptens) bound in the circulation to serum or to tissue proteins to become complete antigens. Classically, "serum sickness"-type hypersensitivity (type III) in a previously unsensitized individual follows 7 to 10 days after systemic injection of foreign antigen, that is, the period necessary to mount a primary antibody response. At a critical level of antigen, enough excess antigen–antibody complexes (IgM, IgG) are found deposited in the tissues, especially in the renal glomerular basement membrane, to cause accretion of complement and initiation of the complement cascade and inflammatory response, accompanied by release of anaphylatoxins (C3b, C5b), which activate directly (degranulate) basophils and mast cells to release vasoactive amines. Some IgE is inevitably formed in this primary immune response. This IgE sensitizes mast cells and basophils to react with circulating antigen with the same result. At its peak, serum sickness is a constellation of reactions resulting from the relatively protracted systemic release of vasoactive amines. Symptoms and signs subside as antibody appears in excess. Anaphylactic shock occurs in a person already sensitized (*e.g.*, to penicillin) who may or may not have had clinically evident serum sickness but in whom all basophils and mast cells have previously been sensitized (*i.e.*, IgE antibody may remain attached to basophils and mast cells for years following primary sensitization with the offending antigen). The sudden union of massive amounts of antigen with widely scattered sensitized mast cells effectively provides a sudden large systemic charge of histamine, with all of its consequences.

DESENSITIZATION

A severe immediate-type allergic reaction may be avoided in foreign serum injections (e.g., equine diphtherial antitoxin) if desensitization is carried out. This consists of a series of minute (0.001 to 0.01 ml) subcutaneous doses of the serum given at intervals of half an hour for several hours before the main dose. This, in effect, gradu-

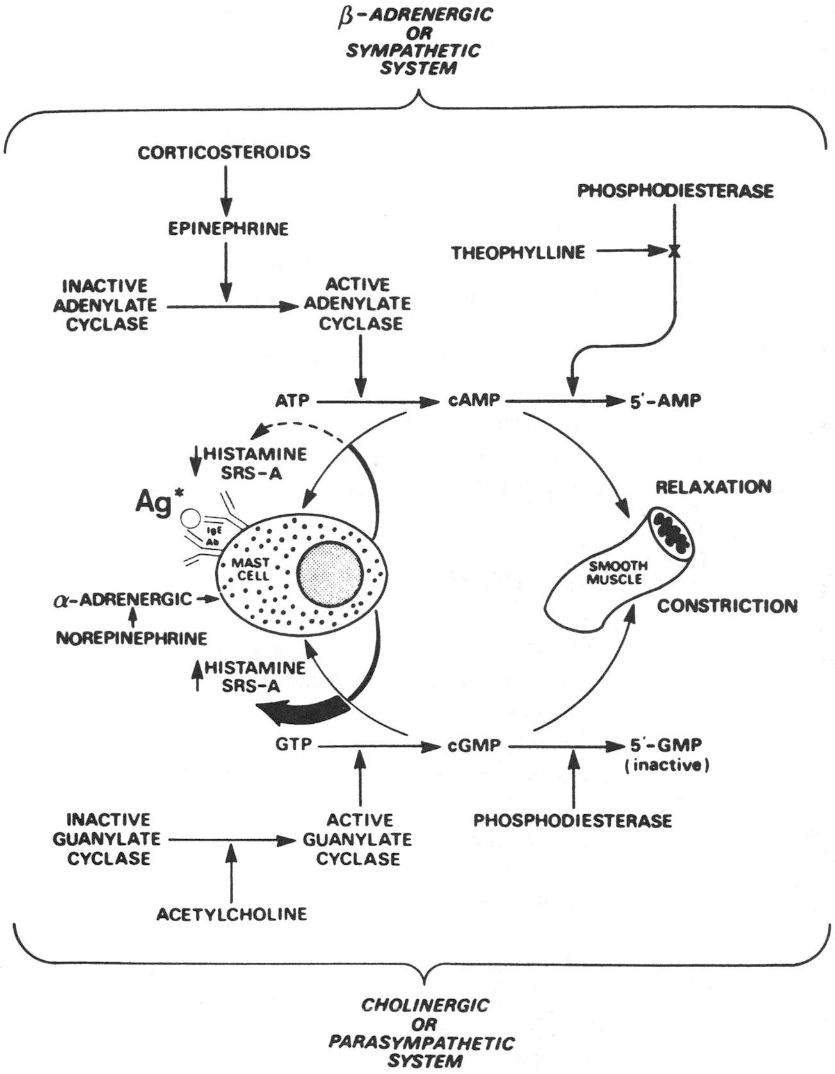

Fig. 5-10. The balance theory of sympathetic and parasympathetic regulation, indicating points of pharmacotherapeutic attack. (*Union of antigen with cell-fixed IgE antibody can be blocked by reaction with homologous IgG (blocking) antibody produced in response to "desensitization.") (Modified from Frick OL: Immediate hypersensitivity. In Fudenberg HH, Stites DP, Caldwell JL, Wells JV (eds): Basic and Clinical Immunology, 2nd ed. Los Altos, CA, Lange Medical Publications, 1978)

ally saturates all IgE antibody already attached to mast cells, thus blocking access by antigen subsequently administered in therapeutic amounts. However, new IgE antibody eventually is formed and perpetuates the state of hypersensitivity so that there can be no permanent amelioration of the atopic state. By the subcutaneous administration of carefully graded doses of antigen (active desensitization), sufficient IgG and IgA antibody can be produced to compete with antigen for fixed IgE antibody and thereby prevent or reduce the triggering of histamine release (e.g., prophylactic treatment of hay fever allergy during the "off" season) (see Fig. 5-10).

Cell-Mediated Immune Response (CMIR) and Delayed Hypersensitivity

In the CMIR, "afferent" and "efferent" limbs serve, respectively, to bring the antigen(s) into the immunologic mechanism and to mediate the responses. When exposed to antigen processed by macrophages, a proportion of T lymphocytes in the afferent limb becomes sensitized, that is, has the potential to activate the efferent limb of the CMIR when reexposed to the same antigen. Antigens involved in the CMIR include certain microorganisms (*Mycobacteria, Listeria, Brucella, Chlamydia,* fungi, viruses) and tumor and transplantation cell surface antigens; and simple chemicals (contact hypersensitivity). In the efferent limb of the CMIR, sensitized T lymphocytes reexposed to the sensitizing antigen may undergo blast transformation and then proliferate. The subsequent progeny of sensitized lymphocytes produce a variety of lymphokines that mediate the associated inflammatory response. The lymphokines themselves are nonspecific with respect to antigen, in contrast to antibody, which is antigen specific. These lymphokines include chemotactic factor, which attracts monocytes and macrophages to the scene

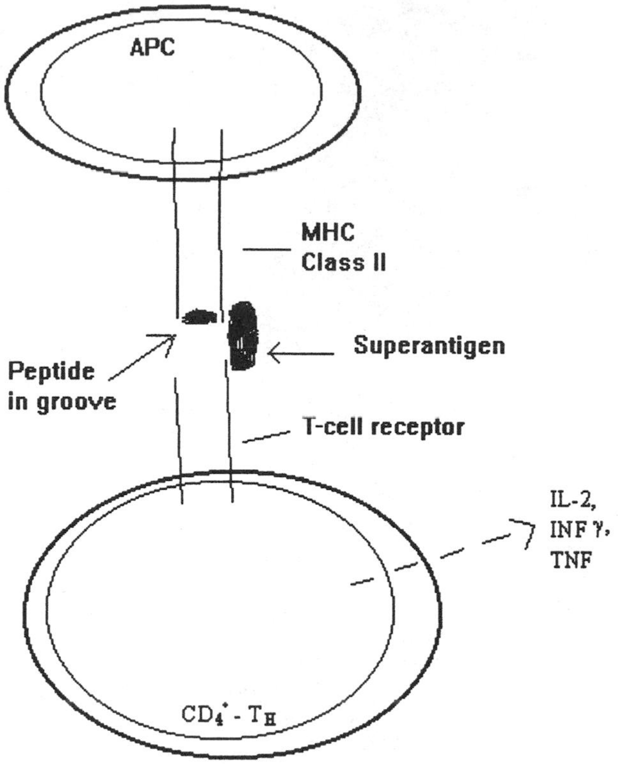

Fig. 5-11. Mode of action for superantigens by binding to the outer surface of both a Class II MHC molecule and the V_B region on the TCR, causing enhanced production of cytokines. Normally, a 13–18 amino acid peptide antigen is presented to the TCR in a groove of the Class II MHC, which in turn initiates proliferation of T_H cells. As an aside, we note these peptides are slightly larger than those of 8–9 amino acids seen in the groove of MHC Class I molecules.

of action, migration inhibition factor (MIF) and macrophage-activating factor (MAF), which hold and "activate" macrophages in the area, and lymphablastogenic factor, which stimulates nonspecifically other lymphocytes in the area to undergo blast transformation. The release of lymphokines from stimulated T lymphocytes is extremely important in "activating" macrophages toward enhanced microbicidal activity with those organisms resistant to intracellular killing *(e.g., M. tuberculosis).* Some of these specifically sensitized lymphocytes become long-term "memory" cells that circulate in blood and lymph, retaining reactivity for years. Sensitized T lymphocytes (T cytotoxic) exposed to the appropriate antigen may also produce certain lymphokines (*e.g.*, MIF or interferon) without undergoing transformation or proliferation. These nontransforming cells may lyse target cells that have an appropriate antigen on their surface (*e.g.*, viral, transplantation).

The prototypic "delayed" type CMIR is the positive reaction to the injection of tuberculin in patients or animals affected with *M. tuberculosis*. In response to the injection of antigen, there is an accumulation of T cells at the site of injection during the ensuing 24 to 48 hours, resulting in the formation of a palpable area of induration. This is in contrast to the "immediate" wheal and flare reaction caused by histamine release (type I) from IgE-sensitized tissue mast cells or basophils that follows within seconds or minutes the exposure to antigen. The tuberculin (type IV) CMIR accounts for the predominantly round-cell histologic appearance of tuberculous and other chronic infectious lesions (*e.g.*, mycoses). Contact hypersensitivity results from constant exposure of the skin to simple chemicals or heavy metals. These materials form antigenic complexes with host proteins that evoke a delayed hypersensitivity reaction whenever the host is exposed to the chemical or metal.

IMMUNOHEMATOLOGY

Human erythrocytes (rbc) have at their surfaces a variety of genetically determined and usually dominant antigens (alloantigens, isoantigens, Table 5-21). Among the many clinically important rbc antigens are those discovered by Landsteiner in 1902 and called A and B. Numerous others (*e.g.*, A_1) have been discovered since. The A and B antigens are enzymically formed from a precursor antigenic substance that is cross-reactive with type XIV pneumococcal polysaccharide (SXIV). The basic antigenic structure is contained in a branched oligosaccharide. Addition of fucose to both branches confers H (heterogenetic) specificity. Addition of *N*-acetylgalactosamine (Gal-Nac) to the terminal galactose (Gal) of both branches confers A_1 specificity. Addition of Gal only to the terminal Gal of branch II confers A_2 specificity. Alternatively, an additional Gal at the end of both branches confers B specificity (see diagram in Table 5-22). Inheritance of glycosyl transferases provides the basis for phenotypic expression of blood-group antigens. In the absence of A or B genes, H remains an unaltered antigen. Persons having both A and A_1 antigens are assigned to blood group A; those with A antigen only, to group A_2; those with B antigen, to group B; those with A, A_1 and B, to group AB; those with A and B antigens but not A_1, to group A_2B; those without A, A_1, or B but with H antigen, to group O (*i.e.*, cells are inagglutinable by anti-A or anti-B).

Rarely, persons originally found in Bombay, India, have none of the above antigens; they are assigned to the Bombay or Oh group. For preliminary and routine clinical purposes only the major groups of the ABO systems are determined, commonly by direct slide agglutination tests.

A or B antibodies (generally IgG) are continuously evoked by contact with specific A- or B-specific oligosaccharides from foods, and microorganisms and may be

TABLE 5-22. Immunohematology

Blood Group System (Genes)	Genotype	MAJOR BLOOD GROUPS Phenotype		Frequency (%)	Antibody In Serum
			Ags on RBC membrane & secretions		
ABO	O(H) O(H)	O(H)		44	Anti-A, anti-B
	A_1A_1	A		42	Anti-B
	A_1A_2				
	A_10				
	A_20				
	BB	B		10	Anti-A
	BO				
	A_1B	AB		4	None
	A_2B				
Lewis		Le^a		22	
		Le^{b*}		78	
Se	SeSe	secretors		80	
	SeSe				
	sese	nonsecretors		20	
		Ags in RBC only			
MH	MM	M		27	
	NN	N		24	
	MN	MN		50	
S	SS	S		55	
	Ss				
	ss	s		45	
Rh†		DCe,DCE,DcE,Dce		85 ("Rh+")	
		dce,dCe,dcE,dCE		15 ("Rh−")	

Minor Blood Groups
Lutheran (Lu^a, Lu^b), Kell (K^+, K^-), Duffy (Fy^a, Fy^b)
Kidd (JK^a, Jk^b)
P (P_1,P_2,p) Paroxysmal cold hemoglobinuria (Donath-Landsteiner antibody, "cold" IgG)

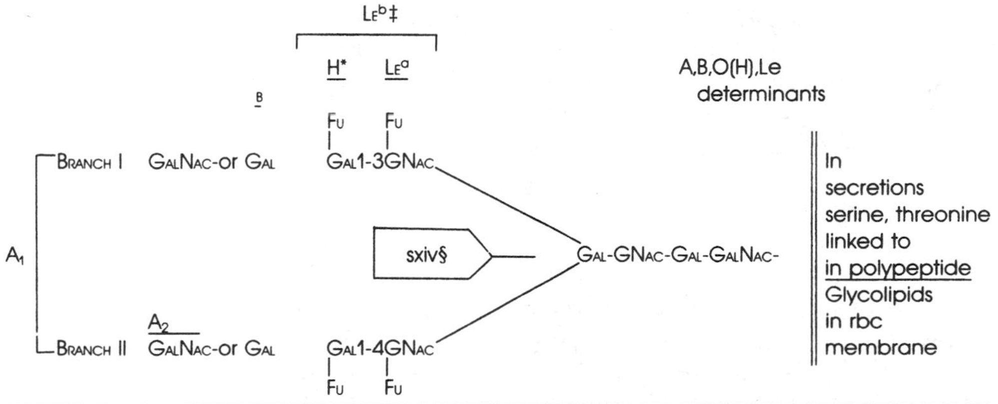

* Found in secretions and plasma of "secretors"; adsorbed to erythrocytes from plasma.
† Based on reactivity with 5 commonly available antisera: anti-D (anti-Rh 1), anti-C (anti-Rh 2), anti-E (anti-Rh 3), anti-c (anti-Rh 4), anti-e (anti-Rh 5)
‡ Se gene function required.
§ SXIV = type XIV pneumococcal polysaccharide cross-reactive with blood group substances because of the core common to both classes of antigen.

actively induced by transfusion with blood of the opposite group (A versus B; B versus A) or, in some cases, by pregnancy with a fetus of the opposite (incompatible) group.

Subdivisions (A_1, A_2, A_1B, A_2B and others) within each group account for unexpected occurrence of transfusion reactions. With specially prepared, adsorbed, monovalent sera containing ***agglutinins*** against group A or against group B erythrocytes, all four major groups may be identified.

In addition to A, B, and H antigens there are a score or more of other blood-group antigenic systems, some common, some very rare, all genetically and independently determined: Duffy, Kell, P, Kidd, Luthcran MNSs. Though occasionally involved in transfusion reactions and certain other conditions, most are of more importance in resolving problems of paternity and in genetic studies. The Lewis (a and b) antigens, when present, are found in plasma and in the saliva of secretors (SeSe, Sese) and are adsorbed to erythrocytes without contributing to the structure of the cell membrane.

Antigens of the ABO(H) system occur in soluble form in sputum, colostrum, secretions of the gastrointestinal tract, semen, tears, and sweat. They appear there in response to a secretor gene (Se) that is present in about 80% of persons and that is required for expression of the Le^b gene.

Rh Antigens: Erythroblastosis Fetalis

In 1940 Landsteiner and Wiener found agglutinogens on *Rhesus*-monkey red blood cells (RBC) that evoked agglutinins against RBC of about 87% of whites and about 95% of blacks, Native Americans, and Chinese. The same antigen was found in many human RBC and is known as Rh agglutinogen. Persons with such RBC antigens are said to be Rh positive (Rh+); those lacking it, Rh negative (Rh−). Unlike the ''natural,'' exogenously stimulated agglutinins of the ABO system, agglutinins against Rh antigen occur only if an Rh- person is actively sensitized by transfusion with Rh+ blood or by pregnancy with an Rh+ fetus.

Fetal erythrocytes from the placental circulation may gain access to the maternal blood during the late stages of pregnancy and parturition and in a first heterospecific pregnancy thus sensitize the mother. On subsequent pregnancies, the mother produces IgG antibody that crosses the placenta to react with the homologous antigen in fetal erythrocytes. Maternal Rh antibodies cause extensive agglutination and hemolysis in the fetus or neonate, resulting in death due to erythroblastosis fetalis or hemolytic disease of the newborn (HDN).

Erythroblastosis fetalis occurs in an estimated 1% of all pregnancies. Of these about 66% are said to be due to ABO incompatibilities and are usually mild. About 30%, due to Rh incompatibility, are usually severe and are often fatal unless promptly treated by exchange transfusion. A small percentage is due to other incompatibilities. Rh erythroblastosis fetalis is entirely preventable by the administration of ''Rhogam,'' which is obtained from Rh- males immunized with Rh+ erythrocytes. The globulins are given to Rh- mothers within 3 days after the birth of an Rh+ infant or fetus. The antibodies combine with and eliminate Rh+ erythrocytes of fetal origin that have passed into the maternal circulation, thus preventing the primary maternal immune response (sensitization). This must be done after each subsequent Rh+ pregnancy to avoid risk of maternal sensitization.

Two systems of nomenclature, each based on a different genetic interpretation, are used for the Rh antigens. One, the Wiener system, is based on the view that some 10 or more genes or gene complexes (multiple allelic genes) occupy a single locus (Rh locus), coding for some 28 or more antigen mosaics or complexes on RBC. Another system (Fisher and Race) assumes the existence of three linked loci with two alleles each, coding for six antigens (C, D, E, c, d, e). Numerous variants and ''compound'' antigens, e.g., C^wdE, C^wDE, ry^w, R^{zw}, also are found (Table 5-23). Rh_o and D are identical.

From a clinical standpoint the RH_o antigen and a variant of D, D^u (''weak D'') are most important because, being both the most common and the most potent antigenically, they are most often involved in HDN. Administration of D^u cells should be restricted to D+ (RH+) recipients because D^u cells can evoke anti-D (Rh_o) antibodies. Conversely, D^u persons should receive only D− (Rh−) cells.

Because the complex Rh antigenic pattern is genetically controlled its determination has great significance in resolving questions concerning parentage and other relationships. For example, two Rh+ persons, one or both heterozygous, may have an Rh− child but two Rh− persons (always homozygous) cannot have an Rh+ child. Transfusions into Rh− females should always be with Rh− blood.

The Direct Coombs Test

Immunoglobulin molecules evoked by RBC antigens are commonly IgG (relatively small, monomeric, bivalent); less commonly they are IgM (relatively large, pentameric, usually pentavalent). Both, especially IgM, can cause agglutination. However, the IgM molecules are often present in low concentration. They are found in the fetal circulation only in response to fetal infection, and they do not pass the placental barrier in either direction. The relative ineffectiveness of IgG molecules in hemagglutination is due, in great part, to their small size; they have difficulty

TABLE 5-23. Relations of Wiener and Fisher Nomenclatures

ANTIGENS		GENES		
Wiener Blood Factors	Fisher Agglutinogens	Wiener Genes		Fisher Gene Linkages
rh′	C	Rz	CDE	D present = RH+
Rh_o	D	R^1	CDe	
trh′′	E	R^2	cDE	
hr′	c	R^o	cDe	
hr′′	e	r^y	Cde	D absent = Rh−
		r′	Cde	
		r	cde	
		r′′	cdE	

in attaching simultaneously in two RBC that are (as is commonly the case) widely separated by negatively charged ions (zeta potential) when suspended in saline. Direct agglutination by IgG antibody can sometimes be made to occur if the effect of the zeta potential is reduced by mechanical force (centrifugation) or by suspending the cells in high concentrations of salt or protein. These measures often bring the RBC sufficiently close together to permit lattice formation by the IgG molecules.

When IgG antibodies attach to erythrocytes without causing lattice formation, they occupy cell receptors (antigens) and block the action of agglutinating IgM or IgG. The attached, nonagglutinating antibodies are called ''blocking'' antibodies, because they interfere with agglutination and can be detected only with the Coombs test.

Immunoglobulins are antigenic in heterologous species, in which antibody to human immunoglobulin can be easily produced. Antiglobulin (Coombs serum, named for R. R. A. Coombs, who first described the principle) agglutinates erythrocytes coated with blocking antibody that does not by itself agglutinate the cells. This is the direct Coombs test used to detect sensitization of fetal (cord) erythrocytes by maternal antibody.

The Indirect Coombs Test

Antibody to Rh and other minor blood group antigens can be detected by the indirect Coombs test, in which the serum is mixed with erythrocytes of known antigenic specificity and then with antiglobulin. Agglutination indicates the presence, in the first serum, of antibody to the suspected blood group antigen. The test may be reversed by using ''known'' serum with ''unknown'' red blood cells.

It should be noted that in the foregoing discussion the term ''sensitization'' has been used in two distinct contexts. Erythrocytes to which antibodies are specifically adsorbed (*e.g.,* Rh+ cells coated with anti-Rh) are said to be sensitized to the lytic action of complement, that is, immune cytolysis, the basis for HDN, or to agglutination by antiglobulin (Coombs serum). Sensitization is also used as the functional equivalent of the primary IR, as in a first untreated heterospecific pregnancy. In the latter instance, subsequent exposure of the maternal immune system to the same fetal (*i.e.,* paternal) antigens evokes antibody in an anamnestic response, mostly IgG (type II hypersensitivity).

IMMUNOPROPHYLAXIS

I. Active immunization (Table 5-24)
   A. *Natural:* due to infection (clinically apparent as well as subclinical or inapparent) or exposure and sensitization to noninfectious ''foreign'' antigens (*e.g.,* as in atopic allergy).
   B. *Artificial:* due to antigenic stimulation by vaccines
      1. Live attenuated microorganisms (*e.g.,* oral poliomyelitis [Sabin] vaccine, measles, mumps, rubella vaccines, BCG) BCG is the only living bacterial vaccine used in the United States. The live vaccine used in veterinary medicine against Bang's disease (*i.e., Brucella abortus* strain 19) is a source of occasional accidental human infection. Vaccination (*i.e.,* immunization against smallpox with vaccina virus) is no longer required in the United States, because smallpox has been eliminated globally. However, thanks to advances in recombinant techniques, vaccinia virus is being actively investigated as a potential ''vector'' vaccine, in which discretely selected coding sequences for protective antigens (*e.g.,* influenza viral

TABLE 5-24. Immunoprophylaxis of Infectious Diseases

Disease	Vaccine	INDICATIONS & AGE GROUP
	ROUTINE UNIVERSAL IMMUNIZATION	
Active		
Diphtheria, tetanus, pertussis	DTP (APtoxoids, killed *B. pertussis* phase I)	Normal infants & children:
Poliomyelitis (paralytic)	Trivalent oral (Sabin) live attenuated viruses (human diploid cell culture) (oral polio vaccine, OPV)	DTP, OPV at 2, 4, 6, 18 months 4–6 years
German measles (rubella)	Live attenuated virus (RA 27/3, human diploid cell culture)	Over 1 year. Contraindicated in pregnancy even though risk to fetus minimal
Measles (rubeola)	Live attenuated virus (chicken embryo fibroblast culture)	Over 1 year
Mumps	Live attenuated virus (chicken embryo fibroblast culture)	Over 1 year
Active	RESTRICTED IMMUNIZATION	
Tuberculosis	BCG, attenuated *M. tuberculosis (bovis)*	Susceptible (tuberculin-negative) individuals at particular risk (*e.g.*, medical personnel). Converts tuberculin reaction.
Poliomyelitis	Killed trivalent (Salk)	Adults at risk and without history of childhood immunization
Pneumonia	Multivalent pneumococcal polysaccharide	Individually assessed risk, compromised patients
Meningitis	Meningococcal A,C polysaccharides	Not effective under 2 years
Typhoid fever	Acetone-killed *S. typhi*	Special circumstances
Influenza	Influenza virus (groups A,B) of current H-N formulation grown in chicken embryos and formalin-inactivated	Infants (split virus) and 65 years and over; also compromised (*e.g.*, immunosuppressed, metabolic-renal disease, asthma) patients and special-risk groups (whole or split virus, annually) (*e.g.*, physicians, hospital personnel, chronic care facility residents)
Rabies	Rabies virus grown in human diploid cells, inactivated with tri-n-butyl phosphate, subunit	Individually assessed risk; combine with human hyperimmune globulin
Yellow fever	Attenuated 17D strain, grown in chicken embryos	Individually assessed risk of exposure
Smallpox (variola)	Live vaccinia virus (lyophilized)	Not required in United States (except armed forces, laboratory personnel at risk). Individually assessed risk of exposure
Hepatitis B	HB antigen from pooled carrier plasma, cloned HB,Ag	Individually assessed risk of exposure
Anthrax	AP toxoid	Individually assessed risk of exposure
Passive	*Preparation*	
Hepatitis A,B	Pooled normal human immunuglobulin	Individually assessed risk of exposure
Tetanus	Tetanus Ig (human)	Tetanus-prone injury in non-immunes
Diphtheria	Diphtheria AT (''despeciated'' horse serum)	Early proven diphtheria
Varicella-zoster pneumonia	Zoster immune globulin (ZIG)	In severe proven infection in high-risk patients
Rabies	Human rabies hyperimmune globulin (RIG)	In conjunction with vaccine

AP = alum-precipitated.
DTP = *D*iphtheria, *T*etanus (toxoids), *P*ertussis bacterial (killed) vaccine.
OPV = *O*ral *P*oliomyelitis *V*accine.
H = hemagglutinin.
N = neuraminidase.
BCG = *B*acille *C*aimette-*G*uérin

hemagglutinin) are inserted into the vaccinia viral genome.

2. Killed or inactivated microorganisms (*e.g.*, pertussis and influenza vaccines, Salk poliomyelitis vaccine) or microbial fractions (*e.g.*, pneumococcal, meningococcal polysaccharide vaccines).
3. Toxoids (*e.g.*, diphtheria and tetanus toxoids) or nonmicrobial antigens (as in "desensitization" to ragweed or other atopic allergens by injection of the offending antigen to produce IgG-blocking antibody). Toxoids are bacterial exotoxins that have been concentrated from culture fluids, treated with formalin under alkaline conditions to abolish toxicity but retain antigenicity, and precipitated on (*i.e.*, adsorbed to) $Al(OH)_3$. When injected subcutaneously, the insoluble alum retains toxoid at the site, retarding its release and enhancing immunization (*i.e.*, adjuvant effect). Killed *Bordetella pertussis* in DTP has an additional adjuvant effect on production of tetanus and diphtheria antitoxins. Natural sensitization to products of commensal corynebacteria increases with age, with concomitant risk of severe hypersensitivity reactions (both immediate and delayed) to injection of DTP. This risk is lessened by use of adult-type diphtheria toxoid (Td contains less diphtherial protein than DTP) in susceptible (Shick-positive) individuals over 12 years of age, who should be skin tested with dilute Td (Moloney test) before being immunized.

II. Passive immunization: by acquisition of preformed antibodies contained in serum "gamma globulin" or immunoglobulin fraction(s).

A. *Natural:* transplacental passage of maternal IgG antibodies (*e.g.*, protection of fetus against neonatal group B streptococcal infection; pathogenesis of HDN)

B. *Artificial:* administration of antibodies produced in another host (*e.g.*, diphtheria antitoxin is hyperimmune horse serum and its use incurs the risk of anaphylaxis and/or serum sickness; tetanus immune globulin is Ig fraction of human subjects hyperimmunized with tetanus toxoid; zoster immune globulin, [ZIG] is Ig from pooled sera of patients convalescing from varicella-zoster infection; anti-Rh, anti-D, Rhogam, is Ig from sera of men hyperimmunized with Rh+ erythrocytes). So-called normal human globulin (gamma globulin) is immunoglobulin from pooled sera containing high titers of naturally acquired antibodies against common infectious agents (*e.g.*, hepatitis viruses, poliovirus, measles virus). All human Ig fractions are free of hepatitis and other known viruses; use of human Ig avoids risk of heterospecific sensitization and reactions to animal sera.

QUESTIONS IN MICROBIOLOGY AND IMMUNOLOGY

The following questions are designed as a guide to reviewing microbiology and immunology. The student will have to consult additional sources in order to respond adequately to some of the items, which are for the most part designed to stimulate correlative thought rather than regurgitation of facts. As an additional aid, a list of suggested readings is appended to the end of this chapter.

Define and explain the mechanism of "serum sickness" as it relates to treatment of diphtheria, prophylaxis of tetanus, treatment with penicillin. How can potential serum sickness be avoided? Once manifest, how is it treated? What is its relation to atopic allergy? To acute poststreptococcal glomerulonephritis?

Define hemolytic disease of the newborn (HDN) and erythroblastosis fetalis in terms of (1) genetic predisposition; (2) risk to the fetus; (3) risk to the mother. How can HDN be prevented? What is the source of the prophylactic agent? When HDN is manifest at birth, how can the infant with HDN be treated? What, if any, may be the permanent residua in infants surviving HDN?

Explain immunological tolerance and the roles of T and B lymphocytes in induction and maintenance of tolerance.

Describe the cellular mechanisms, including biochemical sequences, involved in phagocytosis and intracellular killing of encapsulated bacteria; nonencapsulated bacteria; rickettsiae; viruses. By what immunological mechanisms is phatocytosis of pathogenic bacteria promoted? Inhibited?

Outline the mechanism of complement fixation (CF) as used, for example, in virologic serodiagnosis. How can CF be used to *identify* a viral agent isolated from a sample of sputum from a patient with bronchopneumonia? What is meant by "group-specific CF antigen" in adenoviruses? What is meant by the term "anticomplementary (AC) serum"?

Define *immune adherence,* and describe the mechanism involved and its relation to resistance to infection.

What is *anaphylaxis?* What is the immunological basis for anaphylactic reactions? Describe in detail how an anaphylactic reaction is brought about, using a specific antigen as an example (*e.g.*, bee venom).

What is the Coombs test and under what circumstances

is it used? What reagents are required? Explain the difference between the ''direct'' and ''indirect'' Coombs test as the terms are used in blood-bank jargon.

Define the following terms: cestode, AP toxoid, endotoxin, exotoxin, virus, bacterium, *Rickettsia, Chlamydia,* zoonosis, enzootic, procaryotic cell, microaerophilic bacterium, virion, capsomer, nucleocapsid.

Discuss the role of plasmids in antibiotic resistance. What are resistance transfer factors (RTF) and how do they relate to the bacterial genome?

What is *lysogenic conversion* and how does it relate to the *virulence* of certain bacteria? Give specific examples.

List the principal structural features of bacteria *(e.g., Bacillus subtilis)* and indicate the function of each.

Define in molecular terms *lipopolysaccharide* (LPS) as found in gram-negative bacteria *(e.g., E. coli, N. meningitidis).* What is the relation of LPS to pathogenicity? What *in vitro* tests are commonly used to detect LPS (*e.g.*, in solutions used for intravenous administration)?

Why are gram-positive bacteria commonly susceptible to penicillin and why are most gram-negative bacteria much less so? Explain the occurrence of resistance to penicillin in strains of gram-positive bacterial *pathogens,* citing specific examples. What measures have been successful in circumventing acquired bacterial resistance to therapeutic levels of penicillin G?

Why are viruses insusceptible to antibiotics commonly used to treat bacterial infections?

Compare and contrast SST (*e.g.*, VDRL) and FTA-ABS tests with respect to reagents, technique and specificity in the diagnosis of infection by *Treponema pallidum* (including, besides syphilis, yaws, bejel). What is the significance of the commonly used term ''biological false-positive (BFP) test''? In what conditions may a BFP test occur?

Describe BCG vaccine, how it is administered, the reactions it evokes, and the principal indications or contraindications for its use in the United States.

List four diseases in which serum therapy or prophylaxis is of proven value. Name the species of animal in which each of the sera you mention is produced.

Discuss the initiation of an immune response in a normal individual to a protein antigen, a polysaccharide antigen. What is meant by an *anamnestic* response? What is the cellular basis for a ''booster'' response to tetanus toxoid?

Discuss present-day methods for isolation of anaerobic bacteria from clinical specimens, including the procedures used for identification of individual species. Indicate the molecular basis underlying the requirement of some species of bacteria for strict anaerobiosis.

List pathways involved in, and products of, glucose energy metabolism by strictly aerobic bacteria; by facultative bacteria; by strictly anaerobic bacteria. Draw comparison with analogous aspects of human muscle metabolism.

Describe the physical concepts underlying transmission (TEM) and scanning (SEM) microscopy, drawing comparisons with light microscopy. Include a consideration of resolving power and the limitations of the respective techniques. How does the preparation of specimens differ for each? How are antigen-antibody reactions recognized by TEM? How is TEM used in *rapid* diagnosis of viral infection?

Describe the principles underlying fluorescence microscopy and the use of antibody labelled with fluorescein. What other fluorescent labels can be used? How is fluorescence microscopy used in virological diagnosis? In bacteriological diagnosis? Cite specific examples. How does the use of antibody labelled with peroxidase or phosphatase differ from the use of fluorescent antibody? What are the advantages and disadvantages of each type of label?

Define the term *antibiotic*. What is the most common source of antibiotics? Outline the principal modes of action of several widely used antibiotics (*e.g.*, tetracycline, chloramphenicol, penicillin, streptomycin, polymyxin), as well as the mechanism(s) whereby certain species of bacteria *acquire* and *express* resistance to them. Indicate which antibiotics are mainly bactericidal and which are mainly bacteriostatic.

How does penicillin G differ from the semisynthetic penicillins? From cloxacilin? From oxacillin? From cephalosporins?

Discuss the indications for and limitations of sensitivity testing (antibiograms) of bacteria isolated from clinical specimens.

Outline the principal features of the major histocompatibility complex (MHC) and its role in allograft rejection, delayed hypersensitivity, and the activity of cytotoxic T lymphocytes. What is the relation of MHC to human disease(s)?

List three vaccines involving living attenuated microorganisms. How have recent discoveries in molecular biology greatly advanced the design of viral vaccines? Of bacterial vaccines? On what objective criteria are attenuated living viral and bacterial vaccines judged to be attenuated in virulence? What, if any, adverse reactions follow the use of any of the vaccines you have listed?

What are some of the factors that determine (1) whether or not infection occurs following exposure to a given agent; (2) the virulence of infectious agents. What is meant by the ''carrier state''?

What is the role of histamine in allergic reactions? In which types of allergy are antihistamines likely to be of value? Why? What is SR-A? Where do histamine and SR-A originate? What is the role of eosinophils in allergy?

Outline the development of prophage, lysogeny, and

bacterial lysis by phage. In the bacteriophage replicative cycle, what is the latent period? The eclipse period? The "burst size"?

What are viral plaques *(in vitro)?* What is the utility of plaque formation in animal virology?

Explain the mechanism(s) of viral hemagglutination and how it is used in diagnostic virology. Cite a specific example. What does the term "nonspecific serum inhibitor" mean when used in connection with viral serodiagnosis? Define and cite specific examples of the use of complement fixation and neutralization tests in diagnostic virology. What is ELISA? RIA? For what purposes are they used, and what are the mechanisms of each?

Explain the etymology of *picornavirus; myxovirus; arbovirus; echovirus; papovavirus; reovirus; rhabdovirus; coronavirus; arenavirus; parvovirus; calicivirus; togavirus; retrovirus.*

Name four species of pathogenic spore-forming bacteria. Explain how bacterial spores (not necessarily pathogenic) can be used to monitor the preparation of operating room sterile supplies and equipment.

What are bacterial capsules? What relation do they have to virulence? To immunologic specificity of the organism?

Define pathogenicity; virulence. Indicate the factors on which each depends. What is the role of the host in determining virulence? Give specific examples of microorganisms and the "virulence factors" of each.

Describe three pathogenic, strictly (obligate) anaerobic, nonsporulating bacteria; indicate how they cause disease, including sources of infection, prevention, and treatment. Under what circumstances do commensal organisms become pathogenic? Cite specific examples.

Give the minimal time and temperature for sterilization by compressed steam (autoclave); hot air oven. Explain the mechanisms of microbicidal or microbistatic action of cresols; $HgCl_2$; penicillin; trimethoprim-sulfamethoxazole.

Discuss viral cytopathology in relation to propagation of viruses *in vitro.* Give specific examples of viral cytopathology indicating the molecular basis of each.

List five diseases of viral etiology for which effective immunoprophylaxis is available. In each case, indicate the source of the immunizing agent, how and when it is administered, how susceptibility to the corresponding disease may be determined, and what if any adverse reactions to immunization should be expected.

List the immunizing agents presently available against diseases of bacterial etiology, indicating which of the vaccines are composed of bacterial component(s) rather than whole bacteria. What is the rationale for their use?

Discuss the biological, medicoepidemiological, and ethical problems attending the development and ultimate application of immunizing agent(s) against infection with herpesviruses; HIV.

Define interferons; indicate the principal categories of interferon, their induction and purification, and problems attending their use in clinical medicine.

Discuss hepatitis viruses and indicate the preventive measures, if any, which are available against each category of virus. Which is the most frequent cause of post-transfusion hepatitis? What diagnostic procedures are available for screening blood donors for hepatitis viruses? What prophylactic (active or passive) agents against hepatitis are available?

Discuss the molecular epidemiology of the disease influenza, with particular reference to current immunization practice and chemoprophylaxis.

Discuss immunoprophylaxis against rubella, including indications and contraindications for administration of vaccine.

List six sexually transmitted diseases in the order of current epidemiologic importance. Indicate what therapeutic agents, if any, are available for each. What diagnostic procedures are used for each disease you have mentioned?

Describe three mechanisms for the transfer of genetic information in bacteria, in each instance indicating the actual or potential clinical significance.

Name three diseases transmitted by the fecal–oral route, and for each name the etiologic agent and indicate the pathogenetic mechanism. How can each of the diseases you mention be prevented? Give two examples of bacterial food poisoning–infection, and outline the diagnostic procedures you would undertake to identify the causative agent.

Discuss the viridans (alpha-hemolytic) streptococci and the diseases they cause. Under what circumstances would you undertake antibacterial chemotherapy or chemoprophylaxis against organisms in this category?

What is "gram-negative sepsis"? What microorganisms are the most frequent cause, and how are they recognized? Explain the clinical manifestations of this condition. What therapeutic agents are used in proven cases? How would you monitor the course of therapy?

Discuss the spectrum of diseases caused by group A streptococci, and the measures you would take toward therapy and/or prevention of infection. Discuss infections caused by group B beta-hemolytic streptococci. On what bacterial component(s) is this group classification based? On what antigen(s) is the *type* specificity of group A streptococci based?

Define dimorphism as it applies to fungi. Give at least three examples of dimorphic fungi that are pathogenic in one form or the other. Define asexual reproduction in fungi and discuss its significance with respect to the mycoses. What chemotherapeutic agents are presently available for treatment of fungal infection? With each drug named, indicate its mode of action and the infections against which it is most effective.

List two pathogenic protozoa (one intestinal and one that invades the bloodstream); pathogenic and opportunistic helminths; cestodes. For each outline the life cycle, vector (if any), pathogenesis, immune response, diagnostic methods, and epidemiology.

Describe the etiologic agents of filariasis and outline the usual clinical manifestations of the disease, including diagnostic methods and immune response. How do the clinical manifestations relate to the life cycle of the parasite?

Discuss toxoplasmosis with respect to pathogenesis, diagnosis, and treatment. What is the prevalence of toxoplasmosis?

Discuss infection caused by *Neisseria gonorrhoeae:* diagnosis in males and females, virulence factors, clinical picture including complications and sequelae, immune response, chemotherapy, and chemoprophylaxis. Discuss problems of drug-resistant *N. gonorrhoeae*. What is currently the leading sexually transmitted disease in the United States and how is it diagnosed? Treated?

Discuss infection caused by *Neisseria meningitidis,* including age incidence, epidemiology, clinical and laboratory diagnosis, treatment, immunoprophylaxis, and chemoprophylaxis. Include a consideration of resistance/sensitivity to available chemotherapeutic agents.

What is ''undulant fever''? Name the specific cause(s) and outline the pathogenesis of the disease, and procedures for making the specific diagnosis. What chemotherapeutic agents are most effective?

Name the most frequent cause(s) of neonatal meningitis, and outline the diagnostic and therapeutic procedures most appropriate to each. What, if any, immunoprophylactic reagents are available?

On what basis would you suspect a diagnosis of botulism, and how would you arrive at the *specific* diagnosis? With respect to tetanus (''lockjaw''), is recovery of the organism in culture from any body source diagnostic? If so, why? If not, why not? Discuss both active and passive immunoprophylaxis against tetanus. For each, describe briefly the reagents used and what reactions (in the patient), if any, should be anticipated. Does one attack of tetanus in a previously unimmunized individual confer subsequent immunity?

Describe the ''pertussis syndrome'' and discuss the etiologic agent(s) and the epidemiology relative to each. What, if any, immunoprophylactic agents are available, how and when are they used, and what are the consequences of their use? What are some of the virulence factors in the organism(s) you mention?

Discuss the pathogenesis of diphtheria, including a description of the causative organism, possible factors related to a fatal outcome, immunoprophylactic (active as well as passive) measures to take against diphtheria, the role of antibiotics in treatment of the disease. Discuss problems attending immunization of adults.

Review the major sexually transmitted diseases against the panorama of current epidemiology, including socioeconomic factors that tend to perpetuate/increase the incidence of the diseases you mention.

Discuss the disease tuberculosis as opposed to infection with *Mycobacterium tuberculosis*. What are the species of microorganism that must be taken into consideration in the differential clinical diagnosis of pulmonary disease? What are the most important sites of extrapulmonary tuberculosis? Discuss chemotherapy of infection proven to be due to *M. tuberculosis*. Discuss the immunologic basis of diagnosis, and mechanisms of immune resistance to tuberculous infection. Outline the principles underlying immunoprophylaxis and chemoprophylaxis against infection with *M. tuberculosis*. Indicate the current problems of drug-resistant strains.

Discuss plaque and plaquelike illness with respect to etiology, epidemiology, diagnosis, and chemotherapy. What is the nature of the immune response to tularemia? To brucellosis?

Discuss the rickettsioses that may be encountered in the United States. For each one you name, indicate the vector (if any), the main clinical features and appropriate chemotherapy.

Discuss infection with nonsporulating anaerobic bacteria. Name principal species involved in the disease process, where they originate and how they are identified. What is ''anaerobic cellulitis''?

Discuss anthrax with particular reference to sources of infection and microbial virulence factors and how the latter relate to pathogenesis and immunoprophylaxis. What antibiotics are effective in treatment?

Describe the rubella syndrome: causative agent, diagnosis, epidemiology, and prevention.

Outline the principal spirochetal diseases. For each, name the causative organism, indicate how the diagnosis is established, and what if any therapeutic agents are available. Discuss in detail the bacteriological and serological diagnosis of syphilis.

What are ''L'' forms of bacteria? How do they relate to pathogenesis of disease? Compare and contrast them to Mycoplasmatales. Name the known human pathogens in the latter group, and for each indicate the disease(s) caused, including epidemiology, specific diagnostic procedures, and appropriate therapy. What are ''cold agglutinins''? Are they always due to infection? For what antigen(s) are they specific? Of what kinds of pathological processes are they a sign?

Discuss the immune response to the deep-seated mycoses (*e.g.*, histoplasmosis). Include a consideration of diagnostic problems, cross-reactions, resistance, and recovery. In what general type of immune deficiency do opportunistic mycotic infections occur? Give specific examples of immune deficiencies and opportunistic infections (of any type) to which they predispose. What antifungal antibiotics are currently available? List several mycoses which can be successfully treated with antibiotics.

What is *transfer factor?* Define its function in terms of the pathobiology of infection. Give specific examples. Is transfer factor of any use therapeutically? How is it prepared?

How is *Entamoeba histolytica* identified in diarrheal stools? In formed stools? How is amebic dysentery differentiated from bacillary dysentery both on clinical grounds and by laboratory methods?

Define the life cycle of a tapeworm commonly found in humans. Why is it necessary to recover the head of the worm in order to ensure a cure? What chemotherapy is available for this infestation?

Compare *Taenia saginata, Taenia solum, Echinococcus granulosus,* and *Diphyllobothrium latum* with respect to morphology, life cycle, diagnosis, and therapy.

What laboratory procedures are useful in the diagnosis of hydatid disease?

Describe the life cycle of *Necator americanus,* including the route taken by the parasite from the site of infection to its final location in the body. Briefly describe two laboratory procedures for diagnosis of this infection.

What is ancylostomiasis and how is it prevented?

What is the cause of trichinosis in humans? How may it be diagnosed? Prevented? Describe the life cycle of the parasite and the lesions it causes.

Describe the pathogenesis of filariasis, including epidemiology. What are the sequelae of chronic filariasis? How is it treated?

Outline the life cycle of the parasites that cause human malaria, distinguishing (if possible) their various developmental stages. Outline briefly what you know about cell receptors for malaria and how the parasite gains entrance into the erythrocyte. What factors predispose to resistance to malaria? Include a discussion of the vectors of malaria and current therapeutic practice. What approach would you consider potentially fruitful in developing a vaccine against malaria? Are there any good animal models? What is the global prevalence of malaria today?

Discuss the general principles underlying rapid diagnosis of viral infection, giving the most frequently used laboratory procedures and the interpretation of results.

Discuss the significance of bacterial pili with respect to morphology and function.

What is "smooth" to "rough" variation in bacteria and how is it recognized? Relate this phenomenon to problems of virulence and immunization against specific bacterial diseases.

What is bacterial recombination? Viral recombination? Viral genetic reassortment? Give specific examples. What are restriction enzymes and how are they used in classification of viruses? What are some of the practical applications of genetic mapping and restriction analysis?

Discuss the disease(s) caused by members of the family Legionellaceae, including the names of the species involved, laboratory diagnosis, and treatment of infection. What is the usual source of infection? Can legionellosis ever arise as a nosocomial infection? Is it directly transmissible from person to person?

Discuss the clinical manifestations, specific etiology, epidemiology, and treatment of Lyme disease.

Describe the molecular basis for the clinical manifestations of cholera. How is epidemic cholera treated? Prevented? What is the character of the immune response to cholera vaccine? How is cholera vaccine prepared?

Discuss the pathogenesis of rheumatic fever, including bacteriological and immunological aspects. Compare with the pathogenesis of acute glomerulonephritis, including epidemiology, treatment, and prevention.

What is "C-reactive protein"? What is its significance with respect to mechanisms of *resistance* to bacterial infection? What is the significance of CRP in the serum? How is it measured?

Discuss several clinical syndromes caused by exotoxins of coagulase-positive *Staphylococcus aureus.*

Describe the spectrum of disease caused by *Mycobacterium leprae,* including details of the immune response, both humoral and cellular, and any deficiencies that contribute to pathogenesis. What therapeutic agents are currently available and effective in combating leprosy? What is the current incidence of leprosy in the United States and what epidemiologic factors underlie the continuing importance of the disease?

Using specific examples, outline the main molecular events in the replication of RNA and DNA viruses. Indicate the points at which the clinically useful antiviral agents act, that is, inhibit viral replication. What are the currently available antiviral agents (besides interferon) and for which diseases are they used?

Discuss the rationale for the use of living, attenuated viral vaccines. Give several examples of diseases that are preventable with vaccines, how the vaccines are produced, and what the basis and criteria for attenuation are. What, if any, adverse reactions to immunization may be expected? What are the contraindications to using any of the presently available live attenuated viral vaccines?

Discuss the general properties of retroviruses, and indicate their significance to human disease.

Discuss the structure and function of each of the five classes of immunoglobulin.

What are the principal *sub*populations of T lymphocytes and how are they recognized *in vitro?* What is the function of each?

Outline the principles underlying the production of *monoclonal antibodies.* To what, specifically, does the "-clonal" refer? On what basis do monoclonal antibodies sharpen (*i.e.,* narrow) the specificity of immunological reactions? What are the advantages or disadvantages of such "sharpening" of specificity? Compare monoclonal antibodies to polyclonal antibodies in this respect, using a highly purified protein antigen (*e.g.,* crystalline serum albumin) as an example. How have monoclonal antibodies enhanced the precision of serodiagnosis? Give specific examples.

What is meant by "acute phase reactant"? Give several examples and indicate the clinical significance of each.

Define *antibody-dependent cellular cytotoxicity* and give several examples, citing the components of the reaction.

What does the term *heterophil antibody* signify? In what clinical conditions do heterophil antibodies appear and how are they measured? What is their clinical significance?

Discuss "slow viral disease" with respect to known agents, clinical course, analogous animal diseases, and diagnosis.

Make a list of agents known to be responsible for nosocomial infection; include viruses. Indicate how you would diagnose and treat each infection you have named.

What is the significance of circulating immune complexes (CIC)? Describe their molecular composition and how they are detected, citing specific laboratory tests. How are they removed from the circulation in the normal individual? In what diseases are CIC particularly indicative of active infection? In what tissues are they most often deposited and what reaction(s) do they evoke there?

Compare and contrast the human retroviruses, HTLV-I, HTLV-II, and HIV. What can be said about their morphology, replication, epidemiology, and pathogenesis?

Multiple Choice Questions

Many of the following multiple-choice questions, all cast in formats used by the National Board of Medical Examiners, have been drawn from the computerized national *Microbiology and Immunology Test Item Bank,* through special arrangement with the Association of Medical School Microbiology Chairmen. The AMSMC, which owns and operates the MITIBANK, represents over 80 departments of microbiology and immunology throughout the United States and Canada. Questions submitted by participating departments for inclusion in the bank are accompanied by item analysis statistics and are subjected to rigorous initial review as well as periodic updating by the Editorial Committee of the AMSMC.

Section A

For each of the following (1 to 57), select the *single best answer* to the question or the *single item* that best *completes* the statement.

1. Cells specifically involved in cutaneous delayed hypersensitivity reactions:
   (a) Are B lymphocytes from germinal centers of the spleen white pulp
   (b) Probably recirculate from lymph nodes through the thoracic duct to the blood and back to the lymph nodes by the postcapillary venules
   (c) Migrate from germinal centers to the medullary cords of lymph nodes and red pulp cords of the spleen
   (d) Originate in the bone marrow and differentiate in the "bursa equivalent" microenvironment
   (e) Are derived from bone marrow precursors and reside in the germinal center caps
2. The immunologic mediator of type I (atopic hypersensitivity) is:
   (a) Cytotropic IgG (IgG2) fixed to mast cells by the Fc portion
   (b) Cytotropic antibody of the autoimmune type (as in SLE) fixed to "self" antigens on leukocytes
   (c) IgE attached to mast cells and basophils, which fixes complement and triggers the complement cascade
   (d) IgE (reaginic) antibody fixed to tissue mast cells
3. Type I (atopic) allergy to ragweed antigens is passively transferable from a sensitive to a nonsensitive subject:
   (a) By either serum heated to 56° C for 30 minutes in order to destroy complement or peripheral lymphocytes
   (b) By serum and peripheral lymphocytes combined, but by neither alone
   (c) By serum alone
   (d) By washed peripheral blood lymphocytes in the absence of serum
4. In the pathogenesis of type III disease, the complexes that are most likely to be trapped in the renal glomerular basement membrane are:
   (a) Those formed in moderate antigen excess
   (b) Those formed in large antibody excess
   (c) Complexes of antibody (particularly IgM) with complement and no antigen
   (d) Those composed of antigen with IgE

5. In attempting to ''desensitize'' a person suffering from hay fever due to ragweed, graded injections of antigen are given subcutaneously over a period of weeks during the time of year in which the air is free of pollen. The mechanism underlying the amelioration of symptoms during the subsequent ragweed season is thought to be:
   (a) Elaboration of broadly specific IgE that ''saturates'' all potential binding sites, leaving none free to bind inhaled pollen
   (b) Stimulation of IgG antibody of the same specificity
   (c) Competitive suppression of the IgE locus of the Ir gene
   (d) Stimulation of IgM (primary immunization) that would bind to mucosal cells and act as blocking antibody
6. Mother is group O, Rh-negative; father is group B, Rh-positive; and the infant is group B, Rh-positive. In this situation, the ABO incompatibility between the parents:
   (a) Enhances the chances of maternal elaboration of anti-D antibody
   (b) Lessens the chances of maternal iso(allo) immunization with Rh antigen(s)
   (c) Increases the changes of isoimmunization with minor blood-group antigens (*e.g.*, Kell, Duffy)
   (d) Increases the risk of hemolytic disease of the newborn, particularly because there is also maternal-fetal Rh incompatibility
7. The ''convertase'' most closely resembling $\overline{\text{C3bBb}}$ of the alternate pathway is:
   (a) $\overline{\text{C1}}$
   (b) $\overline{\text{C42}}$
   (c) $\overline{\text{C567}}$
   (d) $\overline{\text{C89}}$
   (e) $\overline{\text{C56789}}$
8. Enhanced intracellular levels of cAMP, induced by agents such as prostaglandins, will:
   (a) Have no effect on phagocytic processes
   (b) Retard phagocytosis
   (c) Enhance phagocytosis
9. The antigenic determinants that define antibody class (isotype) would be best described as occurring:
   (a) In constant regions
   (b) In the variable region
   (c) In the hinge region
   (d) In Fab
   (e) In the carbohydrate moiety
10. Histamine, which is a vasoactive amine initially involved in immune complex disease tissue destruction, is released from:
   (a) Polymorphonuclear neutrophils
   (b) RBCs
   (c) Platelets
   (d) Lymphocytes
   (e) Macrophages
11. The presence of cryoglobulins in a patient's serum may indicate that the patient has:
   (a) Anemia
   (b) Circulating immune complexes
   (c) Hashimoto's thyroiditis
   (d) Pernicious anemia
12. A Coombs test is the most important laboratory aid for the diagnosis of:
   (a) Myasthenia gravis
   (b) Autoimmune hemolytic anemias
   (c) Waldenström's macroglobulinemia
   (d) Rheumatoid arthritis
   (e) Systemic lupus erythematosus
13. The most important antibody playing a role in the pathogenesis of systemic lupus erythematosus is:
   (a) Antibody to thyroglobulin
   (b) Antibody to DNA
   (c) Antibody to mitochondria
   (d) Rheumatoid factor
   (e) Antibody to smooth muscle
14. The currently available vaccine pneumococcal infection contains:
   (a) Heat-killed pneumococci of the 14 serotypes most frequently encountered
   (b) Cell wall antigen(s), chiefly C substance
   (c) Type-specific polysaccharide of 14 serotypes
   (d) Attenuated pneumococci of the 14 serotypes most frequently encountered
15. In the syndrome of poststreptococcal glomerulonephritis:
   (a) Streptococcal nucleases and streptolysin accumulate in the glomerular basement membrane.
   (b) Streptococcal capsular antigen (hyaluronic acid) and glucuronic acid subunits precipitate with antibody and are deposited in the glomeruli in ''lumpy'' patterns.
   (c) Immunoglobulin and complement localize in the glomerular basement membrane.
   (d) Hematuria is due to the action of streptolysin O.
16. In group A beta-hemolytic streptococci, types are determined by the antigenic specificity of:
   (a) The capsule
   (b) The mucopeptide layer
   (c) The M and/or T proteins
   (d) The extracellular products, such as streptolysin O, which is produced only by group A streptococci
17. Prompt and adequate treatment of acute streptococcal pharyngitis constitutes prophylaxis of acute rheumatic fever because:

(a) The immune response is enhanced.
(b) The immune response to streptococcal antigens is aborted.
(c) Viable streptococci do not persist in the early rheumatic lesions.
(d) There is an antibody response to streptolysin and other streptococcal exoenzymes.

18. In the test for C-reactive protein (CRP) in patients' sera, the reagent used to precipitate the protein is:
(a) Group-specific cell wall antigen in *Streptococcus pneumoniae*
(b) Group-specific C antigen of beta-hemolytic streptococcus
(c) Factor C3 in the alternate complement pathway
(d) Rabbit antiserum

19. Recurrent staphylococcal infection in children with "chronic granulomatous disease" occurs because:
(a) The responsible organism almost always is found to produce penicillinase.
(b) No antibodies to staphylococcal teichoic acids are formed.
(c) There is a heritable defect in intraleukocytic killing of bacteria.
(d) These patients are prone to diabetes mellitus, which predisposes to bacterial infection.

20. The triple vaccine (DTP) routinely used in childhood immunization contains:
(a) Killed *Corynebacterium, diphtheriae, Bordetella pertussis* "toxoid," tetanus toxoid
(b) Diphtherial toxin exactly neutralized with antitoxin, *Bordetella pertussis,* tetanus toxoid
(c) Diphtherial toxoid, killed phase 1 *Bordetella pertussis,* tetanus toxoid
(d) Diphtherial toxoid, avirulent *Bordetella pertussis,* tetanus toxoid

21. Congenital rubella can be diagnosed in a week-old infant by:
(a) Demonstration of maternal IgM antibodies to rubella virus
(b) Testing for HI antibodies specific for the virus in the infant's serum
(c) Demonstration in the infant of circulating IgG antibodies to rubella virus
(d) Demonstration of rubella IgM antibodies in the infant
(e) The presence of infant IgA antibodies to rubella virus

22. Caesarian-section has been found to eliminate neonatal complications due to which of the following viruses?
(a) Varicella-zoster
(b) Cytomegalovirus
(c) Poliovirus
(d) Echovirus
(e) Herpes simplex virus

23. To prevent hemolytic disease in a newborn with an A-positive mother and an O-negative father, one would:
(a) Administer Rhogam to the mother after the birth of her first child
(b) Administer Rhogam to each of her subsequent children
(c) Administer Rhogam to the mother after her first A-positive daughter
(d) Administer Rhogam to her first O-negative child
(e) Do nothing—there is no danger to any of her children

24. Dermatophytes that infect special keratinized areas of the body, skin and nails only, are likely to belong to which genus?
(a) *Epidermophyton*
(b) *Trichophyton*
(c) *Microsporum*
(d) *Trichosporum*
(e) *Pitysporum*

25. In the currently accepted immunization schedule for children over the age of 6 years, one is advised to give "adult strength toxoid" instead of DTP. This is done:
(a) To prevent severe reactions to tetanus and/or pertussis antigens, to which children of that age already have developed antibody
(b) Only as a booster in children who have already had primary immunization with DTP at an earlier age
(c) To avoid hypersensitivity reactions to corynebacterial protein(s)
(d) Because susceptibility to diphtheria increases with age

26. In 1977, a U.S. Navy ship experienced a sudden outbreak of acute respiratory disease three days out of Manila, with 67% of the crew and 100% of those age 18 to 25 showing signs of respiratory disease in a 24-hour period. Armed forces epidemiologists flown to the scene isolated virus from transtracheal aspirates but not from the feces of those severely ill. The most likely agent of this outbreak was:
(a) Adenovirus, type 7
(b) Measles virus
(c) Respiratory syncytial virus
(d) Influenza of group A
(e) Influenza of group C

27. Most respiratory and intestinal infections by picornaviruses result in:
(a) Localized acute disease
(b) Latent infections
(c) Inapparent infections

(d) Recurrent infections
(e) Disseminated disease

28. Which one of the following is a binding site for amphotericin B?
(a) Cell wall mucopeptide
(b) 50s ribosomal subunit
(c) 30s ribosomal subunit
(d) Sterol-containing site in the membrane
(e) DNA

29. Rickettsiae differ from free-living bacteria in that the former:
(a) Contain DNA but no RNA
(b) Contain RNA but no DNA
(c) Are too small to be seen with the light microscope
(d) Customarily have arthropod vectors
(e) Cannot generate their metabolic energy requirements

30. The lipid envelop characteristic of some animal viruses:
(a) Contains proteins specified by the host-cell genome
(b) Contains lipids specified by the viral genome
(c) Is resistant to extractions by ether or detergents
(d) Contains lipids and carbohydrates determined by the host cell

31. Which of the following immunoglobulin classes are capable of complement fixation by the classical pathway?
(a) IgM and IgE
(b) IgM and IgA
(c) IgM and IgG
(d) IgM and IgD
(e) All of the above

32. The idiotype of an immunoglobulin molecule is determined by the amino acid sequence of the:
(a) Constant region of the H chain
(b) Constant region of the L chain
(c) Variable region of the H chain
(d) Variable region of the L chain
(e) Variable region of the H and L chain

33. A hapten is a substance that:
(a) Induces cellular immune responses but not antibody production
(b) Does not induce any immune response when given alone but does elicit an immune response when coupled to a larger molecule
(c) Induces tolerance when given alone
(d) When coupled to a larger molecule can be recognized by B lymphocytes but not by T lymphocytes
(e) Does none of the above

34. The antifungal activity of the polyene antibiotic amphotericin B is related to its:
(a) Accumulation in keratinized tissue
(b) Intercalation in mitochondrial DNA
(c) Interaction with membrane sterols
(d) Inhibiting cross-linking in fungal cell walls
(e) Inhibition of DNA-dependent RNA polymerase

35. Which of the following are detected by mixed lymphocyte culture (MLC) reactivity?
(a) HLA—A, B, C determinants
(b) HLA—D determinants
(c) HLA—Dr determinants
(d) Immune response genes
(e) All of the above

36. Abnormal neutrophil function is most often associated with recurrent infections caused by:
(a) *Mycobacterium tuberculosis*
(b) *Staphylococcus aureus*
(c) *Legionella pneumophila*
(d) *Streptococcus pneumoniae*
(e) *Streptococcus pyogenes*

37. Rh-incompatible matings are not of concern where an ABO-incompatible situation also exists. This is based upon:
(a) The fact that Rh antibodies are IgM
(b) The fact that Rh antibodies cannot cross the placenta
(c) The ability of the blood agglutinins to clear fetal RBCs rapidly before sensitization can occur
(d) The fact that maternal antibodies, although in the fetus, will only cause minor agglutination but not lysis since complement levels are low in fetal circulation
(e) The fact that fetal agglutinins will suppress maternal response to fetal RBC antigens

38. T (H) cells
(a) Proliferate in response to free antigens
(b) Bear CD4 and CD8 cell-surface markers
(c) Help convert CTL precursors into active killer cells
(d) Are restricted in their response to exogenous antigen by the requirement that they coordinately recognize HLA-A, B or C molecules
(e) Are easily differentiated from T (DTH) cells

39. The MLR test can measure:
(a) A proliferative response to $CD8^+$ cells
(b) DNA synthesis in a population of cells which influence CTL precursors
(c) Disparity of HLA-A, B, C antigens
(d) The activity of CTLs
(e) Capacity of the potential recipient of a marrow graft to mount a graft-versus-host response

40. In a sensitized subject, what cell specifically triggers delayed-type hypersensitivity?
(a) Monocyte
(b) NK cell

(c) $CD4^+$ T cell
(d) Macrophage
(e) Basophil

41. In a recombinant generated by generalized transduction, which of the following would be present?
(a) DNA sequences of the virus
(b) Proteins coded for by the virus
(c) DNA sequences from the donor
(d) Proteins coded for by the host cell

42. Actinomycin D inhibits DNA-dependent RNA synthesis. Which of the following viruses can replicate in the presence of actinomycin D?
(a) Parainfluenzae (single-stranded RNA, antimessenger)
(b) Poxvirus (double-stranded DNA)
(c) Adeno-associated virus (single-stranded DNA)
(d) Retrovirus (single-stranded RNA, messenger)

43. Which of the following is characteristic of ''positive strand'' RNA viruses?
(a) A polymerase contained in the virion is necessary for replication.
(b) The virion RNA can act as its own messenger RNA.
(c) The virion RNA cannot be extracted in an infectious form.
(d) Viral messenger RNAs are complementary to the virion RNA.
(e) All of them are nonenveloped.

44. The end of the eclipse period is marked by:
(a) The appearance of extracellular virions
(b) Viral protein synthesis
(c) Viral nucleic acid synthesis
(d) Lysis of the cell
(e) The appearance of complete virions

45. Reverse transcriptase:
(a) Makes double-stranded RNA from single-stranded DNA template
(b) Is not required for cell transformation by RNA
(c) Is activated by sigma factor from host cell
(d) Is found in RNA oncogenic viruses
(e) Is found in DNA oncogenic virions

46. Respiratory–syncytial virus differs from other paramyxoviruses in that it:
(a) Has a segmented genome
(b) Lacks envelope fusion protein
(c) Lacks envelope glycoprotein(s) with hemagglutinin and/or neuraminidase activity
(d) Has icosahedral nucleocapsid symmetry
(e) Replicates its genome in the cell nucleus

47. Which of the following components (viral antigens or specific antibodies) in the serum is most diagnostic of a past hepatitis B virus infection from which an individual has acquired immunity to subsequent hepatitis B virus infections?
(a) HBsAg
(b) HBcAg
(c) HBeAg
(d) Anti-HBsAg
(e) Anti-HBcAg

48. In malaria, the infective stage is injected into human subjects by the mosquito is:
(a) Sporozoite
(b) Gametocyte
(c) Cryptozoite
(d) Merozoite
(e) Oocyst

49. Antigenic shift within the influenza virus population:
(a) Is associated with major changes in the amino acid sequence of the nucleocapsid (NP) antigen
(b) Is the result of a mutation in the viral tRNA
(c) Involves antigenic changes in the hemagglutinin or the neuraminidase
(d) Results in a change in the amino acid sequence of the M protein of the virus
(e) Does all of the above

50. Which ONE of the following statements concerning dental plaque and caries is true?
(a) Bacteria form less than 10% of the total mass of dental plaque.
(b) Mutants of *Streptococcus mutans* lacking the enzyme invertase are noncariogenic.
(c) Gnotobiotic or germ-free rats fail to develop caries even when fed a cariogenic diet.
(d) *Streptococcus sanguis* is a major component of subgingival plaque.
(e) *Streptococcus mutans* synthesizes a water-insoluble polypeptide that enables it to adhere to the enamel pellicle found on the surface of teeth.

51. Which one of the following antimicrobial agents inhibits bacterial cell wall synthesis at a step prior to the synthesis of UDP-MurNAc-pentapeptide?
(a) Vancomycin
(b) Bacitracin
(c) Cycloserine
(d) Penicillin G
(e) Streptomycin

52. Antibiotic-associated colitis has been linked to a toxin produced by which one of the following organisms?
(a) *Clostridium perfringens*
(b) *Bacteroides fragilis*
(c) *Bacteroides corrodens*
(d) *Clostridium difficile*
(e) *Campylobacter fetus*

53. One prokaryotic organism that is always resistant to penicillin is:

(a) *Mycoplasma pneumoniae*
(b) Group A streptococcus
(c) *Treponema pallidum*
(d) *Neisseria meningitidis*
(e) *Histoplasma capsulatum*

54. Which of the following types of cells are *not* infected by HIV-1?
(a) $CD4^+$ T cells
(b) $CD8^+$ T cells
(c) Peripheral blood monocytes
(d) Lung macrophages

55. Which of the following pertains to HPV (human papilloma virus)?
(a) Plantar warts can become malignant if exposed to too much sunlight.
(b) *Epidermodysplasia verruciformis* (EV) lesions can become malignant.
(c) Cervical cancer is associated to a high degree with anogenital warts present in patients with condylomas (HPV types 6, 11).
(d) Keratinocytes that are terminally differentiated serve as a culture system for growing HPV.

56. The hepatitis agent with similarities to plant viroids is:
(a) Hepatitis A
(b) Hepatitis B
(c) Hepatitis C
(d) Hepatitis E
(e) Delta agent

57. The following best describes the antiviral action of AZT or ddI:
(a) Induces an oligonucleotide polymerase and protein kinase that interferes with the translation of viral mRNA
(b) Specific inhibitor of HIV-1 reverse transcriptase
(c) Prevents the uncoating of influenza A viruses
(d) An unusual base is responsible for its activity

Section B

Using the key shown below, answer questions 1 to 35 by selecting the best choice in each case according to the letters.

A: a, b, and c are correct.
B: a and c are correct.
C: b and d are correct.
D: d only is correct.
E: all are correct.

1. Virulence is attributable to the antiphagocytic properties of the capsules of:
(a) *Neisseria meningitidis,* groups A and C
(b) *Yersinia pestis* with V/W and F1 antigens
(c) *Hemophilus influenzae,* type b
(d) *Neisseria gonorrhoeae,* Arg^-

2. Which of the following is/are true regarding the mode of action of diphtheria toxin?
(a) The combined fragments of the toxin molecule act as an enzyme and bind to translocation factor EF-2.
(b) NAD is required to split the toxin molecule into two fragments.
(c) Fragment A attaches to receptors on the cell membrane.
(d) Antibodies to fragment B block the action of the toxin.

3. Which of the following are characteristic(s) of *Nocardia asteroides?*
(a) The organism is normally found among the oral flora of humans.
(b) Benign pulmonary lesions often precede the development of metastatic brain abscess.
(c) Nocardiosis often manifests as a necrotizing infection of the extremities.
(d) Nocardiosis response best to treatment with sulfadiazine or sulfamerazine.

4. Characteristics of actinomycosis include which of the following?
(a) Infection may follow a tooth extraction.
(b) Abdominal infection may simulate appendicitis.
(c) Sulfur granules with peripheral clubbing may be present in exudates.
(d) Penicillin is the drug of choice.

5. The following are characteristics of the genus *Clostridium:*
(a) Ability to grow in the presence of oxygen ranges from aerotolerant to obligate anaerobes
(b) Ability to utilize a wide variety of carbohydrates for energy
(c) Production of large amounts of carbon dioxide (CO_2) by most species
(d) Production of some species of exotoxins that aid in the spread of organisms in tissue

6. Optimal recovery of anaerobic bacteria from clinical specimens may be promoted by:
(a) Addition of reducing agents and growth factors to media
(b) Addition of aminoglycosides to the media
(c) Prompt transport of specimens to the laboratory
(d) Use of candle jar to increase the level of CO_2 required for growth of obligate anaerobes

7. Anaerobic bacteria would *not* be expected to play a major role in which of the following?
(a) Nongonococcal pelvic infections
(b) Septic arthritis and osteomyelitis
(c) Lung abscess and empyema
(d) Urinary tract infections

8. Anaerobic bacteria should be considered in which of the following conditions?
   (a) Myonecrosis
   (b) Septic thrombophlebitis
   (c) "Sterile pus" (no growth on blood agar in a candle jar)
   (d) Debrided decubitus ulcer
9. Specimens that would be acceptable for culture of anaerobic organisms from infection of the female genital area are:
   (a) Vaginal
   (b) Cervical
   (c) Urethral
   (d) Culdocentesis aspirate
10. Which of the following apply to *Staphylococcus aureus?*
    (a) Normal flora of nasal passages of most humans
    (b) A frequent cause of nosocomial infections
    (c) Usually susceptible to specific phage
    (d) Of strains seen in family practice and outpatient populations 20% or less are sensitive to penicillin G
11. Cytomegaloviruses are:
    (a) Usually acquired before age 15
    (b) Usually acquired as an inapparent infection
    (c) Capable of causing fatal generalized infections in neonates
    (d) Oncogenic in several animal hosts
12. "Nonspecific" effector mechanisms against infections (in contrast to the specific immune response) include:
    (a) Interferon
    (b) Lymphokines
    (c) Lysozyme of tears and saliva
    (d) Alternate complement pathway
13. Which of the following are associated with the immune response to a primary infection by *Mycobacterium tuberculosis?*
    (a) Forty-eight to 72 hours after an intradermal injection of purified tuberculoproteins, an induration of 5 mm or more will appear at the inoculation site.
    (b) A tubercle or granuloma will eventually form at the sites of bacillary proliferation.
    (c) Tubercle bacilli survive and multiply within host macrophages.
    (d) The host develops a relatively high antibody titer to tuberculoproteins.
14. The mode of action of diphtherial toxin on mammalian cells is analogous to the action of fusidic acid on bacterial cells at which of the following stages of macromolecular synthesis?
    (a) Reversible inhibition of DNA synthesis
    (b) Binding to the ribosome resulting in inhibition of mRNA synthesis
    (c) Inhibition of membrane integrity
    (d) Inhibition of mRNA translation mediated by inactivation of an elongation factor
15. A patient is diagnosed by the physician as having a deep abdominal abscess. The laboratory report identifies the causative agent as *Bacteroides fragilis.* Which of the following antibiotics could be used for therapy?
    (a) Chloramphenicol
    (b) Penicillin G
    (c) Clindamycin
    (d) Erythromycin
16. Chemotherapeutic agent(s) that is (are) safe and effective for systemic treatment of herpetic meningoencephalitis is (are):
    (a) Adenine arabinoside
    (b) Iododeoxyuridine
    (c) Acyclovir
    (d) Isatin-β-thiosemicarbazone
17. Cell-mediated immunity is most important in recovery from primary infections with:
    (a) Herpes simplex virus
    (b) *Streptococcus pyogenes*
    (c) *Mycobacterium tuberculosis*
    (d) *Corynebacterium diphtheriae*
18. Which of the following organisms exhibit a yeastlike form in infected tissues and in culture at 35° C and a mycelial form in the environment and in culture at 22° C?
    (a) *Blastomyces dermatitidis*
    (b) *Coccidioides immitis*
    (c) *Sporothrix schenckii*
    (d) *Cryptococcus neoformans*
19. The source of infection leading to a case of chickenpox may be:
    (a) Vesicular fluid from another child with chickenpox
    (b) Respiratory secretions from another child with chickenpox
    (c) Vesicular fluid from an elderly patient with herpes zoster
    (d) Respiratory secretions from an elderly patient with herpes zoster
20. Regarding hemolytic disease of the newborn:
    (a) It is a cytotoxic type II allergic reaction.
    (b) The mother forms Ab against fetal erythrocyte antigens which she lacks.
    (c) Anti-Rh globulin can suppress sensitization of Rh mothers soon after Rh-positive cell introduction into the mother.
    (d) The fetus forms Ab against maternal erythrocytes and destroys its own red blood cells.
21. Neutrophil membrane constituents that aid in phagocytosis include receptors for:
    (a) Endotoxin

(b) C3b
(c) Phytohemagglutinin
(d) Fc

22. The assembly of human secretory IgA and its transport to secretions is thought to depend on:
(a) Presence of J-chain in the IgA molecule
(b) Existence of a disulfide-interchanging enzyme in the mucosal cells
(c) Presence of secretory component on the surface of epithelial cells
(d) Presence of secretory component in secretions

23. The major histocompatibility complex (MHC) has genes that code for:
(a) Serologically detectable cell surface antigens
(b) Antigens that cause rapid rejection of tissue grafts
(c) Immune responsiveness
(d) Blood-group antigens

24. Enzymes involved in the assimilation of ammonia (in the form of ammonia) include:
(a) Transaminases
(b) Glutamine synthetase
(c) Glutamate synthetase
(d) Glutamate dehydrogenase

25. Vaccines containing only capsular polysaccharide(s) are effective in inducing type- or group-specific immunity in humans against:
(a) Acute rheumatic fever
(b) Meningitis due to group C *Neisseria meningitidis*
(c) Staphylococcal food poisoning
(d) Pneumonia due to *Streptococcus pneumoniae*

26. Antibiotics that inhibit bacterial growth by interfering with protein synthesis include:
(a) Streptomycin
(b) Chloramphenicol
(c) Erythromycin
(d) Tetracycline

27. Which of the following mechanisms are known to account for the inactivation of aminoglycoside antibiotics?
(a) Phosphorylation
(b) Adenylation
(c) Acetylation
(d) Glycosylation

28. Ketoconazole is:
(a) Antiprotozoal
(b) Useful in treatment of some *Bacteroides* infections
(c) Useful in treatment of trichomoniasis
(d) Antifungal

29. Segmented RNA genomes are characteristic of members of which of the following virus group?
(a) Arenaviruses
(b) Reoviruses
(c) Bunyaviruses
(d) Orthomyxoviruses

30. Interferon:
(a) Is species specific
(b) Reacts directly with virus particles to inactivate them
(c) Reacts with cells, and the affected cells then become resistant to a number of different viruses
(d) Is constitutively produced at high levels in cells but requires an inducer for activity

31. Which of the following viruses induce nuclear inclusions in infected cells?
(a) Cytomegalovirus
(b) Adenovirus
(c) Papovaviruses
(d) Smallpox virus

32. The life cycles of the following parasites include stages that normally pass through lung tissue:
(a) *Ancylostoma duodenale*
(b) *Giardia lamblia*
(c) *Strongyloides stercoralis*
(d) *Diphyllobothrium latum*

33. Which of the following statements is (are) true about the protozoan parasite *Pneumocystis carinii?*
(a) It causes widespread disease of many organs in infants.
(b) As many as two thirds of children have antibody evidence of infection by school age.
(c) It has a narrow species host range.
(d) It is pathogenic almost exclusively for immunosuppressed individuals or severely debilitated infants.

34. What immunologic mechanisms may be involved in killing virus-infected cells that display viral antigens on the cell surface?
(a) Antibody-dependent cell-mediated cytotoxicity
(b) Complement-dependent immune cytolysis
(c) Specifically immune T cells
(d) Secretory IgA

35. Activation of lymphocytes in type IV hypersensitivity (DTH) may result in the release of
(a) Opsonins
(b) Interleukins
(c) Anaphylatoxins
(d) Mitogenic factor

Section C

Select one (1) of the lettered items that best relates to each of the subsequent words or statements (1–83).
(a) Mycoplasma
(b) L forms
(c) Spheroplast
(d) Protoplast
(e) All of the above

1. Can be described as insensitive to antibiotics affecting cell wall synthesis
2. Can be produced from gram-positive or gram-negative bacteria by β-lactam antibiotics
3. Cannot revert to a bacterium with a cell wall

(a) *Klebsiella pneumoniae*
(b) *Proteus mirabilis*
(c) *Escherichia coli*
(d) *Pseudomonas aeruginosa*

4. The leading cause of urinary tract infections among hospitalized patients
5. Kidney stones possibly induced by alkaline *p*H of urine associated with urinary tract infections
6. Responsible for respiratory infections in cystic fibrosis patients

---

(a) *Shigella dysenteriae*
(b) Enterotoxigenic *E. coli*
(c) *Salmonella typhi*
(d) *Salmonella enteritidis*
(e) *Vibrio cholerae*

7. Infectious dose may be less than 500 bacteria
8. Often produces (ST) heat stable type of enterotoxin
9. Variations in O antigen produced by lysogenic conversion

(a) Temperate phage
(b) Virulent phage
(c) Neither
(d) Both

10. Produces enzymes mediating phage DNA insertion into the bacterial chromosome
11. Useful in phage typing of *Salmonella typhi* Vi antigen
12. Employable for gene isolation techniques

(a) Mumps virus
(b) Rabies virus
(c) Measles virus
(d) Rubella virus
(e) Hepatitis B virus

13. Australia antigen
14. Koplik spots
15. Orchitis
16. Congenital cardiopathies

(a) Inhibition of viral DNA synthesis
(b) Inhibition of viral attachment
(c) Inhibition of viral RNA and/or protein synthesis
(d) None of the above

17. Iododeoxyuridine
18. Interferon
19. Acyclovir

(a) Penicillin V
(b) Cephalothin
(c) Oxacillin
(d) Carbenicillin
(e) Any of the above

20. Allergic reactions occur in less than 10% of individuals who are allergic to ampicillin.
21. Drug most likely to cure the ''scalded-skin syndrome''
22. Drug most likely to cure conjunctivitis involving *Pseudomonas* or *Enterobacter*

(a) Spectinomycin
(b) Gentamicin
(c) Tetracycline
(d) All of the above

23. Binds to the 30S portion of the ribosome inhibiting the binding of tRNA to the ribosome-mRNA complex
24. Effect is more bacteriostatic than bactericidal
25. Employed for control of penicillinase-producing strains of *N. gonorrhoeae*
26. Capable of inducing an allergic state

(a) Sulfone
(b) Amphotericin
(c) Rifampicin
(d) Polymyxin
(e) Lincomycin

27. Drug that has a detergentlike action on bacterial membrane
28. Drug that has a detergentlike action on fungal membrane
29. Drug used for *M. leprae*
30. Drug that is used for treatment of *M. tuberculosis*
31. Inhibitor of protein synthesis used for gram-positive infections

---

(a) Penicillin V
(b) Ampicillin
(c) Carbenicillin
(d) Oxacillin
(e) Cephalosporin

32. Designed for use against penicillinase-producing staphylococci
33. Designed for use against gram-negative bacteria but sensitive to many β-lactamases
34. Designed for use against gram-negative bacteria that produce β-lactamase, such as *Pseudomonas*
35. Individuals allergic to penicillin G are not necessarily allergic to this drug

---

(a) *Chlamydia trachomatis*
(b) *Rickettsia rickettsii*
(c) *Coxiella burnettii*

(d) *Chlamydia psittaci*
(e) None of the above

36. Associated with eye infections
37. Associated with urethritis, thin discharge, and genital elephantiasis
38. Can cause high fever and rash with 90% mortality rate in untreated cases
39. Etiologic agent of ornithosis

(a) Reagin of syphilis
(b) Anti-*Treponema pallidum* antibodies
(c) Both
(d) Neither

40. Are present in the serum of patients with secondary syphylitic lesions
41. Decline in titer as the patient responds to treatment
42. Are identified in sera of patients with biologic false-positive reactions in screening tests for syphilis
43. Are measured by the VDRL and RPR screening tests
44. Are measured by the FTA-ABS test

(a) F(+) cell
(b) Hfr cell
(c) F′ cell
(d) F(−) cell
(e) None of the above

45. Transfers all bacterial genes more efficiently than plasmid genes
46. Efficiently transfers only plasmid genes
47. CanNOT transfer bacterial genes
48. Contains an integrated plasmid

(a) IgE antibody
(b) IgA antibody
(c) IgM antibody
(d) IgG antibody
(e) IgD antibody

49. Associated with the release of histamine and slow-reacting substance of anaphylaxis (SRS-A)
50. Functions primarily as an opsonin
51. Most effective in the lysis of certain gram-negative bacteria when complement is present

---

(a) Cell-mediated immunity
(b) Humoral immunity
(c) Both cell-mediated and humoral immunity
(d) Neither cell-mediated nor humoral immunity

52. Demonstrates immunological memory
53. Memory cells may express surface IgD molecules
54. May be passively transferred from an immune to a native recipient
55. Responses may involve lysis of target cells
56. Most of the inflammatory cells at the site of this reaction exhibit specificity for the inducing antigen.

(a) Permissive cells
(b) Nonpermissive cells
(c) Semipermissive cells
(d) Resistant cells
(e) Transformed cells

57. Transformed without virus production
58. Some cells transformed and some yield virus
59. Do not permit expression of any viral genes
60. Lose contact inhibition

(a) *Bacteroides fragilis*
(b) *Peptostreptococcus* species
(c) *Clostridium tetani*
(d) *Propionibacterium acnes*
(e) *Clostridium perfringens*

61. A common anaerobic species usually resistant to penicillin G
62. Produces an enterotoxin as well as numerous toxic enzymes that contribute to its pathogenic potential as an exogenous causative agent of disease
63. A normal skin flora organism found as an invader in the production of endocarditis in patients following open heart surgery
64. A gram-negative rod that is the most common causative agent of anaerobic disease
65. Aerotolerant and/or microaerophilic gram-positive organism that is a common cause of disease frequently in association with other organisms in mixed infections

---

(a) HIV-1
(b) HTLV-1
(c) Both
(d) Neither

66. Belong to the retrovirus family
67. Virus replicates in T cells and requires IL-2
68. Causative agent of adult T-cell leukemia
69. Virus isolated from patient with hairy cell leukemia

(a) Vaccinia
(b) B-19
(c) Rubella
(d) HTLV-1
(e) Rotavirus

70. Idiopathic red cell aplasia
71. Tropical spastic paraparesis
72. Member of the poxvirus family
73. Virus that causes intestinal diarrhea in young children
74. Virus that causes German measles

(a) Extra copies seen in relapsed breast/ovarian cancer patients
(b) Homology with NF$\kappa\beta$
(c) Allows transport of singly spliced mRNA from the nucleus
(d) Tyrosine specific kinase; viral form causes mesenchymal neoplasias in chickens
(e) Tumor suppressor

75. Wildtype p53
76. *rev*
77. *neu*
78. *src*
79. *rel*

(a) Reoviruses
(b) Retroviruses
(c) Both
(d) Neither

80. mRNA has a 5′ cap and 3′ poly A
81. Contains intravirion transcriptaselike enzymes
82. RNA genome is in 2 or more pieces or segments
83. Maturation involves extensive proteolytic cleavages

ANSWERS TO MULTIPLE-CHOICE QUESTIONS

Section A

1. b	**16.** c	**30.** d	**44.** e
2. d	**17.** b	**31.** c	**45.** d
3. c	**18.** d	**32.** e	**46.** c
4. a	**19.** c	**33.** b	**47.** d
5. b	**20.** c	**34.** c	**48.** a
6. b	**21.** d	**35.** b	**49.** c
7. b	**22.** e	**36.** b	**50.** c
8. b	**23.** e	**37.** c	**51.** c
9. a	**24.** a	**38.** c	**52.** d
10. c	**25.** c	**39.** b	**53.** a
11. b	**26.** d	**40.** c	**54.** b
12. b	**27.** c	**41.** c	**55.** b
13. b	**28.** d	**42.** a	**56.** e
14. c	**29.** d	**43.** b	**57.** b
15. c			

Section B

1. A	**6.** B	**11.** A	**16.** B
2. D	**7.** C	**12.** E	**17.** B
3. C	**8.** B	**13.** E	**18.** B
4. E	**9.** C	**14.** D	**19.** A
5. E	**10.** E	**15.** B	**20.** A

21. C	**25.** C	**29.** E	**33.** C
22. A	**26.** E	**30.** B	**34.** A
23. A	**27.** A	**31.** A	**35.** C
24. E	**28.** D	**32.** B	

Section C

1. e	**22.** c	**43.** a	**64.** a
2. b	**23.** d	**44.** b	**65.** b
3. a	**24.** c	**45.** b	**66.** c
4. c	**25.** a	**46.** d	**67.** c
5. b	**26.** d	**47.** d	**68.** b
6. d	**27.** d	**48.** b	**69.** d
7. a	**28.** b	**49.** a	**70.** b
8. b	**29.** a	**50.** d	**71.** d
9. d	**30.** c	**51.** c	**72.** a
10. a	**31.** c	**52.** c	**73.** e
11. b	**32.** d	**53.** b	**74.** c
12. a	**33.** b	**54.** c	**75.** e
13. e	**34.** c	**55.** c	**76.** c
14. c	**35.** e	**56.** d	**77.** a
15. a	**36.** a	**57.** b	**78.** d
16. d	**37.** a	**58.** c	**79.** b
17. a	**38.** b	**59.** c	**80.** b
18. c	**39.** d	**60.** e	**81.** c
19. a	**40.** c	**61.** a	**82.** c
20. b	**41.** a	**62.** e	**83.** b
21. b	**42.** a	**63.** d	

SUGGESTED READINGS

Barrett JT: Medical Immunology: Text and Review. FA Davis, 1991

Hoeprich PD (ed): Infectious Diseases 4th ed. Philadelphia: JB Lippincott, 1989

Joklik WK, Willett HP, Amos DB, Wilfert CM (eds): Zinsser Microbiology, 20th ed. Appleton & Lange, 1992

McLean DM, Smith JA (eds): Medical Microbiology Synopsis. Philadelphia: Lea & Febiger, 1991

Murray PR, Kobayashi GS, Pfaller MA, and Rosenthal KS (eds): Medical Microbiology, 2nd ed. St. Louis: Mosby, 1994

Peter JB: Use and Interpretation of Tests in Medical Microbiology, 2nd ed. Specialty Laboratories, 1990

Roitt I, Brostoff J, Male D (eds): Immunology, 4th ed. St. Louis: Mosby, 1996

Schaechter M, Medoff G, Schlessinger D (eds): Mechanism of Microbial Disease. Baltimore: Williams & Wilkins, 1989

Rypins' Basic Sciences Review, 17th Edition,
edited by Edward D. Frohlich. Lippincott–Raven Publishers,
Philadelphia © 1997.

6

Pathology

Ivan Damjanov, M.D.
Professor and Chair
Department of Pathology
University of Kansas
Kansas City, Kansas

Peter J. Goldblatt, M.D.
Professor and Chair
Department of Pathology
Medical College of Ohio
Toledo, Ohio

Philip B. Conran, D.V.M., Ph.D.
Professor
Department of Pathology
Medical College of Ohio
Toledo, Ohio

The goal of this chapter is to help candidates prepare for the pathology sections of the medical licensing examination. It is meant to build on and review the knowledge gained from a good course in pathology and from a comprehensive textbook in pathology, and not to replace either one. Pathology is the study of disease (Gr. *pathos,* disease). If *disease* is taken to mean a perturbation of the normal state in any plant or animal, then the breadth of the discipline can be appreciated. It is both a science basic to the study of medicine, and a clinical discipline. It derives its investigative methods from all of the other biological sciences and applies them to the study of tissues and fluids obtained postmortem, at surgical operations, and from experimental animals. Increasingly, it will depend on molecular techniques, as will other biological sciences. Clinically, pathology is divided into anatomic pathology (autopsy, surgical pathology, clinical cytology, and electron microscopy) and clinical pathology (hematology, clinical chemistry, immunology, microbiology, and the blood bank). Each of the latter now represents a subspecialty within the broad field of laboratory medicine.

THE CONCEPT OF DISEASE AS A REACTION TO INJURY

The student of pathology should consider illness as the reaction between disease and the patient. It thus becomes obvious that one must know about disease to study and treat illness.

Disease, at least in its initial stages, is only a slight departure from the normal. Although students usually learn by studying advanced disease, they should always keep in mind that the disease process is a condition that arose from normal or healthy tissue and cells, and that even in a severe disease many of the cells or portions of an affected organ system are still within ''normal'' limits.

Forbus' concept of ''reaction to injury,'' which suggests that diseased states are nothing more than reactions of the body, tissues, or cells to alterations in their natural environment, is as important as the classic proposal of Virchow, which states that all diseases could be understood ultimately in terms of cellular changes (''Cellular Pathologie''). If one recognizes that cells are able to shift from their normal level of activity within a narrow range to either hypometabolic (down-regulation) or hypermetabolic (up-regulation) states, and that these altered levels of function may be reflected in structural alterations that are visible grossly or with the aid of the light or electron microscope, then disease can be defined in terms of the functional and structural alterations that occur immediately (acute) or sequentially over time (subacute, chronic). As stated, illness is a clinical concept that relates an individual to a disease. It is the accumulated effects that determine whether a disease will be transient, long lasting, or ultimately fatal.

THE CONCEPT OF ETIOLOGY AND PATHOGENESIS OF A LESION

The meaning of *etiology* is *cause*. An etiologic agent may be physical, chemical, biological, or even chronological. There is usually a dose relationship and a time factor. A brief exposure to sunlight may produce a beneficial effect, whereas a prolonged exposure to even a low level, or a brief exposure to an intense level, can be injurious. We usually conceive of biological agents as microbial; however, one could describe an attacking tiger as a biological agent—it produces *physical* injury! The point is, some injuries are multifactorial.

The ***pathogenesis*** of a disease refers to the sequence of events that leads from the initial contact with an injurious agent to the final outcome of the illness.

A ***lesion*** is the morphologic change in a tissue or organ by which we can identify a specific disease process. It is often possible to induce from the morphologic changes the specific etiologic agent and to obtain some indication of the duration, or stage, of the disease. Thus, mycobacteria cause granulomatous lesions that start as small collections of epithelial macrophages, develop central necroses, and give rise to daughter tubercles. Over time, macrophages fuse to form giant cells, particularly of the Langerhans type. Fibrosis and hyalinization occur as the lesion heals, and there is usually deposition of calcium. The evolution of the lesion can be correlated with the elimination of the offending organism.

GENERAL PATHOLOGY

A course in pathology is usually divided into two sections, general and systemic. The general portion of the course is concerned with processes that affect various organs in a similar way. These include cell death and degeneration, adaptive responses such as hypertrophy, inflammatory processes, and neoplastic transformation. Specific diseases of a given organ are considered in the systemic pathology portion of the course. We will follow this general organizational approach in the discussion that follows. Because general pathologic processes are best understood at the cellular level, we will begin with a brief review of the normal cell and proceed to a description of some of its adaptive responses.

Cell Injury and Response

All diseases can be considered responses to injury. The elements that determine the intensity and the nature of this adaptive response include (a) the cell type, (b) the nature of the injurious agent, (c) the level of exposure (dose), and (d) the duration of exposure (time). Time itself can produce injury (*e.g.*, aging), but the mechanism is not completely understood.

The adaptive response can be immediate or gradual. Deprivation of oxygen and nutrients in ischemia demands an immediate response if it is complete, or it may be accommodated over time if it is partial. Thus, complete occlusion of a vessel exposes the cells distal to the blockage to a potentially lethal situation. The adaptation is therefore to ***acute, lethal*** cell injury. Stenosis, on the other hand, may permit a slow reduction in cellular activity, which allows some or most of the cells to survive and is therefore a ***sublethal*** adaptive response that can be maintained for a short period (subacute) or a long period (chronic). During the initial phases after a potentially lethal injury, the cell goes through a phase that is reversible. However, at some point it reaches the limit of its adaptive capabilities and then the injury becomes ***irreversible***. The ***reversible phase*** has been termed *the process of cell death*. This proceeds to *the point of no return* (cell death), beyond which lies the irreversible phase, which is the *process of necrosis*. This will be described more fully below.

CELL TYPE

There are several different populations of cells in the human body. They include (a) continuously dividing cells, such as those of the bone marrow and those that line the intestinal tract; (b) stable cells that divide only slowly under normal conditions, but which can be stimulated to divide, such as parenchymal cells of the kidney and liver, which can undergo ***tissue regeneration*** after nephrectomy or partial hepatectomy; and (c) cells such as skeletal muscle, cardiac muscle, and neurons, which are more or less permanent and which cannot divide at all or do so only to a limited degree. Mesenchymal cells can proliferate and lay down excessive extracellular matrix. Lymphocytes appear to have some unique susceptibilities to specific injurious agents, such as corticosteroids, which are relatively innocuous to other cell types. This cellular specialization conveys different susceptibilities; for example, neurons can survive complete ischemia for only 5 minutes or so, and cardiac muscle for only 10 ± 5 minutes, whereas liver cells can recover after 30 minutes or more of complete deprivation of oxygen and substrate. Continuously dividing cells are clearly more susceptible than stable cells to x-irradiation and cytotoxic drugs that are radiomimetic or become incorporated into DNA.

NATURE OF THE INJURIOUS AGENT

As stated, many cells show selectivity in their response to a given noxious agent. Dividing cells are killed by radiation, whereas fibroblasts and parenchymal liver cells are relatively resistant. This susceptibility may result from the presence of metabolic pathways that ***increase*** or ***decrease*** (detoxify) a given agent. Other factors include specific cell surface receptors for a particular virus, and other trophic factors. The different classes of injurious stimuli have been mentioned previously; they include:

1. ***Physical agents*** such as heat, cold, physical trauma, x-irradiation, and electrical and radiant energy.
2. ***Chemical agents*** such as acid, alkali, and cytotoxic agents, which can interfere directly with specific metabolic pathways or which can be metabolized to toxic intermediates.
3. ***Biological agents*** such as bacteria, viruses, and parasites.
4. ***Deprivations***, such as insufficient caloric intake, or lack of specific nutrients, such as essential vitamins or amino acids. Nutritional excesses can also be injurious.
5. ***Immune*** responses, which are in general protective, can sometimes be excessive or inappropriate (as in autoimmunity) and result in serious injury.
6. ***Genetic*** or inherited diseases can result from inappropriate genetic expression or the lack of an essential genetic trait, which makes the individual vulnerable.
7. ***Ischemia***, which is a specific example of a deprivation (blood supply—oxygen and substrate—plus accumulation of waste products).
8. ***Aging*** is incompletely understood and could be the result of a genetic program or simply the accumulation of more or less random injuries that occur inevitably over a lifetime. Both probably play a role.

LEVEL OF EXPOSURE

Many, but not all injurious agents show a dose dependency. Some cells show particular sensitivity, and at times this is unpredictable (idiosyncratic). Some agents, such as radiation, illustrate a "memory" phenomenon, meaning that the result of several small sublethal doses may be accumulated. There are also agents that show a "threshold" response; in these cases, there is relatively little toxicity up to a certain level of exposure, and then suddenly a small increment in dose produces a dramatic effect.

DURATION OF EXPOSURE

Clearly, length of exposure is a complex variable that depends on the nature and the intensity (dose) of the agent in question. Short exposure to even a high dose may be well tolerated under some circumstances and lethal under others.

Acute, Lethal Cell Injury

Two models of acute, lethal cell injury have been particularly well studied: ischemia and exposure to carbon tetrachloride. In both, there is a progression from a ***reversible*** to an irreversible stage. Each involves changes in membrane constituents and cell swelling, and in both, calcium ion (Ca^{2+}) appears to play an important role. ***Lipid peroxidation*** is also an important common thread.

In ischemic cell injury, the deprivation of oxygen and substrate leads to a shift from aerobic to anaerobic metabolism, and thus to a less efficient production of ATP, which rapidly becomes depleted. Lactic acid, ADP, and phosphate accumulate. There is a drop in intracellular pH, nuclear chromatin clumps, and production of RNA and protein slows and ultimately stops. More important, the active extrusion of sodium (with retention of potassium) slows, and with the influx of sodium, water is drawn into the cell. Initially, there is blebbing of the cell membrane and submembranous cytoplasm, and later other compartments, including the endoplasmic reticulum and mitochondria, swell. Early swelling of the mitochondria is *low amplitude swelling,* with contraction of the matrix compartment, loss of matrix granules, and swelling of the envelope space. This appears to be reversible. When the whole mitochondrion swells *(high amplitude swelling)*, and the outer membrane breaks and flocculent densities appear in the matrix, the changes are thought to be irreversible (past the ***point of no return***). The cell swelling is manifested at the light microscopic level as *hydropic degeneration* (hydropic change) and is even visible grossly as what was called *cloudy swelling*. Loss of cytoplasmic basophilia results from the disaggregation of polysomes and the degranulation of rough-surfaced endoplasmic reticulum. At about this time, lysosomes swell and their membranes break down, releasing hydrolytic enzymes. This probably initiates the cellular degradation of the process of necrosis in the final, irreversible phase. Phospholipid breakdown by phospholipases is an important process that probably begins in the reversible phase and may be triggered by calcium ion. Calcium moves out of mitochondria and into the cytoplasm from the extracellular fluid. Membrane changes, particularly in the plasma membrane, play a central role in determining irreversibility.

The injury that results from carbon tetrachloride exposure is similar to ischemic injury, but it probably stems from a direct attack on the membranes as a consequence of ***lipid peroxidation***. This may play a role in many other types of acute, lethal cell injury, including irradiation. The peroxidative reactions result from the generation of free radicals, in particular oxygen species, which have an unpaired electron in the outer shell. The most important of these are superoxide (O_2^-), hydrogen peroxide (H_2O_2), and hydroxyl radical (OH). These can be produced intracellularly at various sites such as mitochondria, lysosomes, and cytosol, and they are normally inactivated by the enzymes superoxide dismutase (SOD), catalase, and glutathione reductase. Iron is an important factor in free radical cell injury. Unmodified oxygen free radicals are extremely reactive species that produce, among other things, lipid peroxides which are also reactive species and can propagate the reaction. Proteins are modified, and neutral protease action is enhanced. Cell swelling, inhibition of protein synthesis, and many of the other reactions common to lethal cell injury ensue. Calcium is also thought to play an important role. The cells swell as a result of loss of fluid and volume control, and also fat appears in the cytoplasm. The injury becomes irreversible and is followed by the changes of ***necrosis***.

A third type of lethal cell injury that is receiving increasing attention is termed *apoptosis*, often referred to as ***programmed cell death.*** Histologically, the apoptotic cell is characterized by intense eosinophilia, accompanied by condensation of chromatin. Ultimately, there is loss of nuclear material (acidophilic body, Councilman-like body). This type of cell death is seen normally during embryonic development and is also associated with viral infections such as viral hepatitis. There is increasing evidence that it is under genetic control, and therefore there is interest in this process as an important component of such things as embryonic differentiation, neoplasia, and regulation of T and B lymphocytes.

NECROSIS

The ***process of necrosis*** is the irreversible phase that occurs after the point of no return, by which the cell is converted to a lump of debris. Usually, it is difficult to identify lethally injured cells with the light microscope before they become necrotic. However, cells can die without becoming necrotic (*e.g.*, fixed tissue). Recognition of necrotic cells depends mostly on certain characteristic nuclear changes including ***pyknosis*** (densification), which involves condensation of the chromatin which is intensely basophilic; ***karyolysis***, which involves loss of nuclear basophilia with the appearance of a hollow nuclear structure within an intact nuclear membrane; and ***karyorrhexis***, which is fragmentation of the nucleus into small pieces of chromatin. These patterns may be characteristic of the cell type. Thus, necrotic lymphocytes show pyknosis, necrotic polymorphonuclear leukocytes show karyorrhexis, and necrotic liver cells show karyolysis. Cytoplasmic changes in necrosis are more subtle and include loss of basophilia (ribonucleic acid) and increased acidophilia. Finally, the cell disintegrates.

In addition to the nuclear characteristics, there are typical gross patterns of necrosis that often correlate with the cause of the necrotizing event. Thus, ***ischemic necrosis*** is referred to as ***coagulation necrosis*** because of its resemblance to a clot or to boiled egg albumin. ***Liquefactive necrosis*** is characteristic of ischemic change in the brain and the necrotic center of an abscess with its high hydrolytic enzyme content. ***Caseation necrosis*** is seen in association with tuberculosis and may reflect high lipid content of the necrotic material. ***Gummatous necrosis*** is associated with the tertiary stage of syphilis. ***Fat necrosis***, seen most often in pancreatitis, reflects enzymatic digestion of fat; it has a chalky gross appearance and microscopically it often shows a blue tinge from calcium that combines with the fat to produce soap-like deposits.

Another term often associated with necrosis is *gangrene*, which can be *dry* when it results from ischemia and appear like mummified flesh, or *wet* when it is associated with clostridial infection. Necrosis may be classified as ***generalized***, ***zonal***, or ***focal*** depending on the extent of injury.

SUBLETHAL CELL INJURY

Not all cells die when exposed to an injurious stimulus. Some are able to adapt and to assume a new functional state, usually at a lower level than previously. Following a toxic injury that produces significant amounts of cell death within an organ, surviving cells may also become more active or enlarge to take over the function of lost cells. Sometimes the surviving cells are able to proliferate and restore the lost functional units. At other times, scarring replaces the necrotic cells and may further compromise the ability of the surviving cells to function. Thus, the continuing function of the individual, the organ, or the cell is the result of these multiple factors after an acute, lethal injury. There are a number of characteristic adaptive responses that can be recognized grossly and microscopically in the sublethally injured organs and cells.

Adaptive Responses. When a number of cells are lost, the organ shrinks (atrophy). Individual cells can lose protein and undergo autophagic (self-eating) processes and become ***atrophic***. Such cells often show accumulation of ***residual bodies***, which are lysosomes containing undigested lipid materials, usually colored various shades of brown. These ***lipochrome*** pigments, including ***lipofuscin***, may impart a brown color to the organ, especially the heart, which is said to show ***brown atrophy***. Atrophy may also be a physiological process, part of the aging or involutional phases of life (*e.g.*, the uterus after menopause).

When a number of cells die, the remaining cells, if they are uninjured, attempt to take over the function of the lost cells. If they simply enlarge as an adaptive response, they are said to ***hypertrophy***. If they proliferate, the process includes ***hyperplasia*** (increase in cell number). Hypertrophy usually precedes hyperplasia. An enlarged organ, such as the heart of a hypertensive person, is said to be hypertrophic, and its individual cells also are enlarged (hypertrophic). Cellular ***organelles*** can enlarge (*e.g.*, ***megamitochondria*** in certain liver diseases), and proliferation of the endoplasmic reticulum can occur in response to enzyme induction. This is usually referred to as hypertrophy of the endoplasmic reticulum.

Hyperplasia, an increase in cell number, can be a physiological process, for instance in response to hormonal stimulation, or a pathological process, when it is not the direct result of an identifiable appropriate stimulus. Hyperplasia is a reversible phenomenon, and the cell number returns toward normal when the stimulus is removed.

Some other responses that are not entirely adaptive deserve mention. The failure of an organ or tissue to form can result in ***hypoplasia***; in this case, the organ is present but smaller than expected. If it is entirely absent, the term *aplasia* or *agenesis* is more appropriate. If an organ achieved its expected size and then became smaller, the hypoplasia is acquired ***(acquired hypoplasia)*** rather than congenital. Atrophy is also an appropriate designation of this phenomenon.

Metaplasia is a cellular adaptive response in which one *adult* cell type becomes replaced by *another* adult cell type. This can occur both in epithelial tissues (*e.g.*, the replacement of columnar cells of the endocervix by squamous cells) and in mesenchymal cells (as in the formation of bone in fibrous connective tissue or muscle).

Fatty change (fatty degeneration, fat phanerosis) is a common adaptive response to sublethal cell injury. Many organs (*e.g.*, the heart) use fat preferentially as a source of calories, or they are involved in fat metabolism (*e.g.*, the liver). These are prone to accumulate fat under conditions that are relatively mild forms of injury. Fat can appear in the supporting framework of an organ such as the heart, in which case it is designated ***fatty stromal infiltration***. Fat droplets can accumulate in the cytoplasm of parenchymal cells of the liver as ***microvesicular*** or macrovesicular granules under a variety of circumstances. Increased ***uptake*** or ***intake*** of fat, ***mobilization*** from stores, ***decreased*** intracellular ***breakdown*** (oxidation), and increased ***synthesis*** or ***decreased transport*** out of cells can result in accumulation ***(steatosis)***. Fat must be coupled to protein before it can be secreted into the aqueous medium of the blood for transport to the organs that use it or store it. Thus, interference with transport protein synthesis is a common mechanism of fatty change.

Hyaline change or hyaline degeneration is the time-honored designation for a cellular and intercellular response to sublethal injuries of various kinds. *Hyaline* is simply a descriptive term that denotes deposition of homogeneous, "glass-like," or amorphous deposits of acidophilic material that can be seen microscopically in cells, or, more often, between them. There are specific types of hyaline substance such as ***fibrin*** or ***amyloid***, and the appearance of hyaline can result from such things as overproduction of type IV collagen or increased cross-linkage of mature fibrous collagen as part of the aging process. Hyaline change is particularly frequent in the walls of arteriosclerotic blood vessels in association with hypertension and diabetes. An example of intracellular hyaline is so-called alcoholic hyaline, in which fibrils the size of ***intermediate filaments*** accumulate in liver parenchymal cells in response to alcohol abuse. These filaments represent cytokeratin accumulation, a metaplastic response.

A specific type of hyaline, designated ***amyloid***, consists of extracellular deposits of fibrils; this can represent a primary disease or be secondary to chronic infectious disease. The peptides are variable, often related to immunoglobulin, but share the physicochemical property that a sequence within the chain can assume the beta-pleated conformation that conveys an ability of the deposits to bind dyes such as Congo red. Most types of hyaline are fibrillar. ***Zenker's hyaline*** is seen in the skeletal muscle of individuals who have had typhoid fever. Although the fibrillar nature of hyaline is not always obvious on light microscopic examination, it can usually be demonstrated by electron microscopy.

Mucinous degeneration, ***mucoid*** degeneration, and ***myxomatous*** degeneration all refer to microscopic changes in cells and tissue that convey a more edematous, amorphous, and slightly slippery look. The actual accumulation of mucopolysaccharides has not been demonstrated in all of these conditions.

Calcification is another adaptive response. Calcific deposits may be seen frequently in sites of previous cellular injury, inflammation, or necrosis *(dystrophic calcification)*, or in widespread foci in relationship to hyperparathyroidism and hypercalcemia *(metastatic calcification)*. As noted previously, calcium probably plays a central role in several of the processes related to cell death, so it is not surprising that it accumulates in sites of necrosis as a sort of gravestone.

CONSEQUENCES OF NECROSIS

Depending on the extent, necrotic foci may be completely reabsorbed or they may result in extensive tissue changes. The necrotic debris may evoke an inflammatory response and become organized as scar tissue. Usually, pulmonary infarcts are virtually completely obliterated by the surrounding alveoli, which expand into the space. Foci of necrosis in the kidney and liver can evoke proliferation of adjacent parenchyma, which completely replaces the lost cells. Calcium deposits and scarring are frequent consequences of necrosis, particularly those involving connective tissue.

SOMATIC DEATH

Although this is somewhat peripheral to our present discussion, it is worth noting that somatic death is the ultimate result of cell, tissue, and organ injury. Death is literally the absence of life, and as life defies a simple definition, death may at times be difficult to establish with certainty. However, there are characteristic changes that take place in a reasonably orderly fashion following the death of the individual that help to establish the circumstance and timing of the somatic death. Pooling of blood produces ***livor mortis,*** which occurs in dependent portions of the body and establishes how it was lying. ***Rigor mortis***, the stiffening of the muscles, proceeds from the jaw to the extremities in an orderly fashion and recedes in the opposite direction. This can help to establish how long the person has been dead if the ambient temperature is known. The cooling of the body post mortem is called ***algor mortis***.

Inflammation

Inflammation is a process typical of vascularized living tissues whereby fluid and white blood cells accumulate at a site of injury. It is caused by physical, chemical, and/or microbial agents. The cardinal signs of inflammation include redness, swelling, heat, pain, and loss of function. It is a double-edged sword that on the one hand is a defense mechanism that helps to restore damaged tissue to a normal or near-normal state, but on the other can cause additional or new tissue destruction through the release of leukocyte enzymes or oxygen radicals. Inflamed tissues are described by using the suffix *-itis* (*e.g.*, carditis and cholecystitis). Some exceptions to this terminology include *pleurisy*, used interchangeably with *pleuritis*, and *pneumonia*, used interchangeably with *pneumonitis*.

Inflammation is classified as acute or chronic. ***Acute inflammation*** is characterized as the initial event in most inflammatory processes. It is of short duration, its exudates are rich in protein, and neutrophils are the cell type present in greatest number. ***Chronic inflammation*** is of longer duration and is characterized by mononuclear inflammatory cells.

The acute inflammatory process is characterized by the exudation of fluids, proteins, and cells from intravascular locations to extravascular locations. ***Exudation*** is the escape of fluids, proteins, and cells from the vascular system, implying increased vascular permeability. An ***exudate*** is an extravascular inflammatory fluid with high protein concentrations, much cellular debris, and a specific gravity above 1.020. Exudates are classified as serous, purulent, suppurative, fibrinous, and hemorrhagic.

ACUTE INFLAMMATION

Acute inflammation is characterized by changes in vascular flow and caliber. An initial, inconsistent, transient vasoconstriction is followed by arteriolar vasodilatation that opens new capillary beds and increases blood flow. This is followed by slowing of the circulation, concomitant with increased vascular permeability and fluid and protein leakage into extravascular tissues. Stasis of flow with concentration of red blood cells and increased viscosity ensues. Increased vascular permeability can be caused by endothelial cell contraction mediated by histamine, bradykinin, or leukotrienes; junctional retraction mediated by interleukin-1 (IL-1), tumor necrosis factor (TNF), and/or interferon gamma (INF-γ); direct injury to endothelial cells; leukocyte-dependent leakage resulting from the release of oxygen radicals or enzymes; or leakage from regenerating capillaries in angiogenesis (*e.g.*, granulation tissue).

As the circulation slows and fluid and proteins leak into adjacent tissues, neutrophils migrate toward the periphery of the vessels, they roll along the endothelial surface, and eventually they adhere to the endothelial surface (a process called *margination*), and they transmigrate between endothelial cells, through the basement membrane, and into interstitial tissues. Once they arrive in the tissues, the neutrophils phagocytize organisms and/or necrotic debris by a three-step process: (a) recognition and attachment via opsonins or IgG, (b) engulfment via extending pseudopodia, and forming a phagosome, and (c) intracellular killing and/or degrading through a variety of oxygen-dependent enzyme systems (*e.g.,* peroxide-myeloperoxidase, OH^-, O_2^-) and oxygen-independent enzyme systems (*e.g.,* acid hydrolases, lysozyme, and arginine-rich cationic proteins).

Because leukocytes play a significant role in the inflammatory process, defects in leukocyte function can alter the outcome. There are both genetic and acquired leukocyte defects. Some of the more significant genetic disorders include defects in adhesion molecule receptors, defective chemotaxis, and defective killing capabilities (*e.g.,* chronic granulomatous disease, myeloperoxidase deficiency). Some acquired defects in chemotaxis are noted in thermal injury, diabetes, and sepsis. In addition, defects in adhesion and phagocytosis are observed in diabetes.

Inflammation is a chemically mediated process. The most important mediators of vascular permeability include the vasoactive amines (histamine and serotonin), the anaphylatoxins (C3a and C5a), bradykinin (which also produces pain), leukotrienes C_4, D_4, and E_4, and platelet activation factor (PAF). Leukocyte adhesion is mediated by C5a, leukotriene B_4, IL-1, and TNF, all of which activate adhesion molecules (integrins, selectins, and/or super-immunoglobulin class molecules). Leukocyte chemotaxis is most likely mediated by C5a, leukotriene B_4, bacterial products, and cytokines (*e.g.,* IL-8). Prostaglandins play a significant role in producing vasodilatation, fever, and pain, and IL-1, TNF, and IL-6 also promote fever. Nitric oxide is a potent vasodilator and, when released from macrophages, produces tissue damage. Finally, the acute-phase reaction is promoted by IL-1 and TNF.

CHRONIC INFLAMMATION

The acute inflammatory response usually terminates by (a) complete resolution, (b) healing by connective tissue replacement, or (c) abscess formation, or it proceeds to chronic inflammation. Chronic inflammation is characterized by a predominance of mononuclear inflammatory cells (*e.g.,* macrophages, lymphocytes, plasma cells, fibroblasts, and, on occasion, eosinophils). It persists for long periods of time, and, finally, there is little remaining fluid (transudate or exudate). It is a result of (a) a continuum of acute inflammation, (b) repeated bouts of acute inflammation, or (c) low-grade inflammatory processes without an acute phase (*e.g.,* persistent intracellular organisms or prolonged exposure to nondegradable substances). ***Granulomatous inflammation*** is a modified form of chronic inflammation characterized by the presence of collections of modified macrophages called epithelioid cells, giant cells, and admixtures of lymphocytes, plasma cells, and fibroblasts. It is generally a result of persistent stimuli, such as intracellular organisms *(Mycobacterium tuberculosis)* or products that are not easily digestible (foreign bodies). Granulomas may or may not have caseous centers.

MORPHOLOGIC PATTERNS IN ACUTE AND CHRONIC INFLAMMATION

The cause, severity, tissue, and site of the inflammatory response determine basic patterns of acute and chronic inflammation. ***Serous inflammation*** is characterized by thin watery fluid exudation exemplified by thermal injury (blisters), certain viral infection (herpes), or effusions. ***Fibrinous inflammation*** results from greater vascular injury that allows fibrin to escape, or from a procoagulant state. It is exemplified by pneumococcal pneumonia, uremia, and some cancers. ***Suppurative or purulent inflammation*** is characterized by the production of large amounts of pus. Pyogenic organisms are responsible for much of this, and abscesses (localized collections of pus) are representative of this type of inflammation. Finally, ***ulcers*** are local defects, or excavations of a surface of an organ that are produced by sloughing of necrotic debris.

SYSTEMIC EFFECTS OF INFLAMMATION

Acute inflammation gives rise to a series of systemic events collectively called the ***acute phase response***, which is mediated by the cytokines IL-1 and TNF. This response is characterized by fever, increase in slow-wave sleep, decreased appetite, increased degradation of proteins, hypotension, and other hemodynamic changes; synthesis of acute phase proteins (C-reactive protein, ***serum protein***, complement, coagulation proteins); and leukocytosis.

WOUND HEALING

The healing of an uncomplicated wound (*e.g.,* a surgical incision) is referred to as ***healing by first intention (primary union)***. Briefly, relatively few epithelial and connective tissue cells are damaged and the defect is quickly filled with clotted blood, the surface of which forms a scab. Within the first day, neutrophils emigrate into the wound, and the epidermis begins to regenerate within 24 to 48 hours. By 72 hours, macrophages replace neutrophils, and granulation tissue, fibroblasts, and angioblasts invade the defect. By the end of the first week, the epidermis covers the defect and granulation tissue fills the defect, with collagen fibers becoming more abundant. The process continues, with collagen becoming more abundant and inflammatory cells and vascularity diminishing until scarring is complete. ***Healing by second intention***

(secondary union) occurs when a large defect is involved and regeneration of parenchymal cells cannot completely reconstitute the region. In these instances, the inflammatory reaction is more intense, there are larger amounts of granulation tissue, and wound contraction plays a major role in reducing the size of the wound. The latter is accomplished, in large part, by myofibroblasts in the granulation tissue.

Wound healing is a carefully orchestrated process that combines the following: (a) acute inflammation, (b) regeneration of parenchymal cells, (c) migration and proliferation of both parenchymal and connective tissue cells, (d) synthesis of extracellular matrix proteins, (e) remodeling of parenchymal and connective tissue components, and (f) collagenization for wound strength. There are many intrinsic and extrinsic factors that can interfere with and delay wound healing. These include infections (the most important), nutritional deficiencies (e.g., of vitamin C, zinc, and copper), glucocorticoids, impaired vascularity, foreign bodies, and lack of stability of wound margins. Aberrant growth of connective tissue can give rise to ***hyperplastic scars*** or ***keloids***. In addition, there may be exuberant growth of granulation tissue (proud flesh). Finally, additional aberrations of fibroblast growth may yield connective tissue elements that have aggressive growth patterns and may recur after surgical excision (desmoids or fibromatosis).

CIRCULATORY DISORDERS, INCLUDING THROMBOSIS AND SHOCK

An intact circulatory system assures an orderly flow of blood and a consistent supply of nutrients and oxygen to the organs. The essential elements are a system of connected ***conduits*** through which fluid can ***flow*** without major loss, and a sufficient ***pressure*** to propel the fluid. It is not a requirement that the conduits (vascular system) be impermeable; quite the opposite, it is desirable that the fluid, at least, be able to leave, but it must also be able to return. There must be a mechanism to plug large holes in the vascular system, or the system will collapse. The force involved in the circulation, the repair of leaks, and what happens when there is collapse are considered here; the vascular system is discussed in another section.

The circulating blood represents only a small part of the total fluid volume. A 70-kg person is about 60% water (roughly 40 liters), of which about 60% is intracellular (about 25 liters), and the remainder is distributed as roughly two thirds ***extravascular*** extracellular fluid (about 10 liters) and one third ***intravascular*** fluid (about 5 liters). The principal determinates of the compartmentalization of the fluid are fixed and exchangeable ions, the extracellular one being mainly sodium (Na^+), and serum protein, largely albumin, which for the most part remains within the vascular compartment and provides the osmotic force that draws water back into the vessels.

EDEMA

The term *edema* applies to the accumulation of excessive fluid in extracellular tissue compartments or body cavities. The latter is exemplified by serous cavities lined by mesothelium, such as the pleura *(hydrothorax, pleural effusion)*, pericardium *(hydropericardium, pericardial effusion)*, and peritoneal cavity *(hydroperitoneum, ascites)*. Fluid accumulates in these cavities or in the tissue under a variety of circumstances, but principally when there is increased hydrostatic pressure, decreased osmotic (oncotic) pressure of the plasma, sodium retention, and lymphatic obstruction. Under normal circumstances, there is a drop of some 20 mmHg, or more, in the pressure between the arterial end of the capillary and the venous end. Fluid leaks out at the arterial end of the capillary bed and is drawn back largely by the oncotic pressure generated by albumin; this pressure is similar at about 20 to 25 mmHg (Starling's principle). Increased hydrostatic pressure results from congestive heart failure, constrictive pericarditis, cirrhosis of the liver, and multiple causes of venous obstruction such as thrombosis, compression, or even gravitational effects such as dependent posture, particularly in the lower extremities. Increased arteriolar dilation, such as occurs with thermal injury, may cause increased fluid leakage. Reduced oncotic pressure results from decreased production (or increased loss) of serum proteins. Protein loss through the kidneys results in generalized massive edema *(anasarca)*, or it may cause ascites and localized edema. Cirrhosis can also result in ascites because the liver makes albumin and other serum proteins. Ascites in this case is multifactorial, with venous obstruction, decrease in intravascular oncotic pressure, and weeping of protein-rich lymph into the peritoneal cavity each playing a role. Sodium concentration of the ascitic fluid is low, but total body sodium is increased, reflecting altered responsiveness to the renin–angiotensin–aldosterone system as another contributing factor. Sodium retention also plays a role in the edema of heart failure, with low renal perfusion and increased renal tubular reabsorption. Increased intake of salt may also be a factor. Lymphatic obstruction can be the result of scarring as a consequence of surgery, inflammation, or irradiation. Profound lymph edema is seen in some cases of breast cancer after surgical removal of the lymph nodes or irradiation of the axillary area.

HYPEREMIA AND CONGESTION

Hyperemia and congestion simply mean an increase in the volume of blood in a given tissue or organ. This accumulation can occur and resolve rapidly or persist for weeks or months *(acute or chronic congestion)*. Hyperemia can result from an ***active*** pumping in of blood, as in an acute inflammatory process, or it may be ***passive***, as when the failing heart is unable to clear the venous return and blood accumulates in the liver. Acute congestion, for instance in the liver or spleen, is manifested clinically by enlargement of the organ, which is often tender to palpation. Grossly, there is rounding of the edges and the parenchyma bulges when the organ is cross sectioned. There is a purple or bluish-red color, and blood oozes from the cut surface. Active hyperemia is sometimes redder than passive hyperemia, which has a bluer tinge because it contains more undersaturated hemoglobin. Microscopically, the blood is usually contained within capillaries or sinusoids. In marked acute passive congestion in the liver, there is central venous congestion with distended sinusoids radiating around the vein. As the severity and duration increase, there is atrophy of the adjacent parenchymal cells and some extravasation of the blood cells (hemorrhage) occurs. In long-standing hyperemia *(chronic congestion)*, there may be actual necrosis of the cells surrounding the central veins with fibrous replacement *(central sclerosis)*. This leads to the gross appearance termed nutmeg liver or cardiac sclerosis. It is not a true cirrhosis, because regenerative nodules are generally lacking.

HEMORRHAGE

The presence of blood, principally red blood cells, outside blood vessels in the extracellular spaces is hemorrhaging. Accumulation of blood in a body cavity such as the chest or abdomen is referred to as hemothorax or hemoperitoneum, and when a mass of clotted blood accumulates in a tissue or organ it is termed a hematoma. Bleeding into the skin, visible as a bluish-red discoloration, is variously referred to as *petechial* hemorrhage (small), *purpura* (larger) or *bruising* or *ecchymosis* (still larger). The evolution of bruises from blue-black to brown discoloration and their ultimate disappearance is well known to all of us. Hemorrhagic areas can be more or less permanently marked when, as the red blood cells break down and release their hemoglobin, tissue macrophages ingest the iron and retain intralysosomal deposits of ***hemosiderin***.

COAGULATION CASCADE, THROMBOSIS, AND THROMBOEMBOLISM

An intact endothelium prevents intravascular clotting, and therefore there are anticoagulants on the cell surface such as a heparin-like glycoprotein. When the endothelium is damaged, and particularly when the collagen beneath is exposed, the coagulation cascade may be set in motion with potentially disastrous consequences. Briefly, the altered surface sets in motion the ***intrinsic*** coagulation system, whereas tissue damage releases tissue factors that trigger the ***extrinsic*** pathway. The important elements in initiating a clot by the intrinsic pathway are (a) injury to endothelium; (b) adherence of platelets with release of ADP, generation of thromboxane A_2, participation of other factors such as nitric oxide (NO) and 5-hydroxytryptamine (5-HT), and further recruitment of platelets; and (c) the initiation of the conversion of proenzymes to active enzymes, with the generation of thrombin, which converts fibrinogen (soluble) to fibrin (an insoluble fibrous protein). The initial steps involve conversion of factor XII (Hageman factor) to XIIa, which triggers the conversion of factor XI to XIa, which, in turn, converts the inactive substrate factor IX to the active enzyme factor IXa. The extrinsic pathway can enter at this point through the generation of factor VIIa from factor VII by the cellular protein called ***tissue factor***. Subsequent steps involve the action of VIIa or VIIIa with calcium ions as a cofactor to convert factor X to Xa, the generation of thrombin (IIa), and finally the conversion of fibrinogen to fibrin. There are also anticoagulants that help to prevent propagation of the clot, and the fibrinolytic system, principally the plasminogen–plasmin system. Without these, the entire circulatory system might clot every time there was local tissue injury or endothelial damage.

Once a clot forms on a vessel wall, it can grow by entrapment of red and white blood cells and additional platelets and become an occlusive ***thrombus***. Unless circulation is promptly restored or the occluded vessel is bypassed by the collateral circulation, there will be ischemic damage, sooner or later, to the organ or tissue distal to the clot. Ultimately, this leads to coagulative necrosis, or so-called infarction, which is usually *pale* or *white*, as it is in myocardial or renal tissue, but which may be hemorrhagic or *red* in organs that have a rich collateral blood supply like the intestine or lung. The thrombus itself may undergo one of several fates: it may be dissolved by the fibrinolytic system; it may undergo ***organization*** by the ingrowth of endothelial cells and fibroblasts from the vessel wall; it may ultimately be ***recanalized*** by the formation of endothelium-lined vascular channels, although this is rarely effective in establishing blood flow; and finally, pieces of the clot may break off or the entire clot may be dislodged and carried to another site by the process of ***embolization***. Once it lodges in the new site, it may perpetuate the process by initiating a new clot, and thus it becomes a ***thrombo-embolus***. Blood clots are not the only things that can embolize. *Fat* embolism can occur subsequent to such injuries as fractured bones with dislodgement of marrow fat; *air* embolism can occur after puncture of vessels, including after administration of intravenous solutions; *bone marrow* can embolize under circumstances similar to fat embolization; and *amniotic fluid* can enter the maternal circulation especially at the time of delivery.

Factors that favor thrombus formation include alterations in blood flow, such as stasis, turbulence, and eddying at vascular branch points; atheromatous plaques; external compression of vessels; and more subtle changes, such as hypercoagulable states, which can be inherited (***primary***) or acquired (***secondary***). The best defined of these is lack of anticoagulants such as antithrombin III, protein C, or protein S.

SHOCK

The circulatory collapse that may accompany massive hemorrhage, loss of fluid volume from extensive burns, elaboration of endotoxin in sepsis with consequent vasodilatation and pooling of blood, or parasympathic discharge as a result of multiple trauma is referred to as ***shock***. Clinically, the patient is pale, the skin is cold and clammy, there is perspiration, and mental confusion may progress to coma. The pulse is rapid, weak, and thready. The blood pressure is low, and sometimes this hypotension is so severe that the diastolic pressure may be virtually undetectable. The maximal sympathetic response that supervenes in an attempt to counteract the loss of effective circulating volume also produces local vasoconstriction, which can produce localized hypoperfusion in many organs in the body. If prolonged, this results in lack of function, followed by ischemic damage. The kidneys, for instance, which normally receive as much as 25% of the cardiac output, shut down. The lack of urine production is understandable when one considers that the kidney is meant to regulate volume and composition of the extracellular fluid, but the shunting of blood to other organs such as the brain may ultimately prove disastrous: the proximal tubules of the kidney, and other constituents that are particularly sensitive to oxygen and substrate deprivation, may be irreversibly damaged.

Shock can be classified as *cardiogenic*, *hypovolemic*, *septic*, or *neurogenic*. The complex interaction of various mediators in the pathogenesis of shock is increasingly being delineated. For example, in septic shock, the infection, particularly with gram-negative organisms, leads to the release of endotoxin (lipopolysaccharide) or exotoxins, which stimulate plasma cells, macrophages, and neutrophils as well as endothelial cells to release various mediators, including cytokines such as TNF and various interleukins (including IL-1, IL-2, IL-6, and IL-8), NO, prostaglandins, kinin, leukotrienes, and coagulation factors, as well as a myocardial depressant substance. This, in turn, affects the myocardium, the coagulation system [disseminated intravascular coagulation (DIC)], and the vasculature, effecting multiorgan failure.

Shock proceeds through three phases: a ***nonprogressive phase***, during which organ perfusion is maintained by compensatory mechanisms; a ***progressive phase***, during which tissue and organ hypoperfusion creates a progressively increasing series of circulatory and metabolic problems; and last, an ***irreversible stage***, leading to severe organ failure and ultimately death of the individual.

GENETIC AND DEVELOPMENTAL DISORDERS

Many human diseases have a genetic basis, and even those that have exogenous causes are critically influenced by the genetic constitution of the affected person. Here we shall limit our discussion to diseases that are inherited or can be traced to genetic or developmental disturbances operating during the prenatal life *in utero*.

The cause of most ***developmental disorders***, over 75% of those recognized at birth or in later life, remains unknown. The remaining malformations can be traced to hereditary traits, genetic mutations, and various exogenous factors.

The best known ***teratogens*** are drugs, such as antiepileptic drugs, thalidomide (a sleeping pill removed from the market because it caused numerous abnormalities of fetal arms and legs in the 1960s); alcohol, which causes an identifiable set of lesions known as *fetal alcohol syndrome*; viruses, such as rubella, which causes a typical triad including microcephaly, microphthalmia, and cardiac defects; and x-rays and gamma rays, which have been blamed for an increased incidence of defective births after the atomic bomb explosion in Japan in 1945 and the meltdown of the Chernobyl atomic power station in the Ukraine in the 1980s. Severe developmental malformations are incompatible with normal life and most affected fetuses are aborted during early stages of pregnancy. Those that are born represent just a small fraction of all those that were conceived.

Genetic disorders can be classified for practical clinical purposes into two groups: those linked to demonstrable *chromosomal abnormalities* (known also as karyotypic or cytogenetic abnormalities), and those for which the genetic defect cannot be demonstrated on chromosomal analysis but can be documented by analyzing the genealogy of the family, or by biochemical and molecular biological testing. These abnormalities are known as *single gene defects*, and they are classified as new mutations or hereditary disorders that are inherited as autosomal dominant, autosomal recessive, X-linked dominant, or X-linked recessive traits.

Chromosomal Abnormalities

Chromosomal abnormalities are divided into two groups: those affecting one of the 22 autosomes (numbered 1 to 22) and those affecting the sex chromosomes (X and Y). The chromosomal abnormalities can be further classified as *numerical* or *structural*. ***Numerical abnormalities*** are deviations from the normal diploid number of chromosomes (46,XX, or 46,XY). These include *aneuploidy* (any number of chromosomes above or below the normal number of 46) and *triploidy* [three sets of normal haploid complements (*e.g.*, $3 \times 23 = 69$)]. Each human chromosome occurs in duplicate, except for the X and Y chromosomes, which are paired to each other, and if one of these chromosomes is lost, a monosomy develops. Additional chromosomes in excess of the normal two in the pair are called trisomy if there are three chromosomes, tetrasomy if there are four chromosomes, and so on. ***Structural chromosomal abnormalities*** include deletions or translocations of parts of the chromatids, and formation of abnormal chromosomes known as ring chromosomes or isochromosomes. All autosomal monosomies are lethal. Monosomy of sex chromosomes resulting in the retention of an X chromosome (45,X) (Turner's syndrome) occurs at a rate of 1:3000, whereas 45,Y is lethal early in pregnancy. Trisomy of sex chromosomes [47,XXY (Klinefelter syndrome)] occurs at a rate of 1:850 newborn males. Trisomy X, which occurs at a rate of 1:1200, results in normal 47,XXX females. Trisomy of several autosomes results in severe malformations, the most important of which is Down syndrome (trisomy 21), which occurs at a rate of 1:800. Trisomy 13, or Patau's syndrome, occurs in 1 of 6000 births, and the trisomy 18, or Edwards's syndrome, occurs in 1 of 8000 births. Structural chromosomal anomalies are of less clinical significance. Most often they are found in Turner's syndrome. Deletion of the short arm of chromosome 5 (46,XX-5p) results in cri-du-chat syndrome, a rare condition that has a high mortality in infancy.

Turner's syndrome, complete or partial monosomy of chromosome X, is characterized by hypogonadism and a variety of other somatic abnormalities that occur at a variable rate. Chromosomal analysis shows that approximately 50% of patients have a 45,X karyotype, whereas the remaining 50% have one normal and one abnormal X chromosome, such as an isochromosome X or a ring chromosome X. As a result of this chromosomal defect, the ovaries do not develop normally but transform into a connective-tissue band ("streak gonads") that does not respond to gonadotrophic stimulation and is incapable of producing estrogens. These patients never develop secondary sex characteristics, do not enter puberty, never menstruate, and are infertile. Other somatic features of Turner's syndrome include short stature, web neck (pterygium coli), coarctation of the aorta, and broad chest with widely spaced nipples. Hormonal substitution therapy may be used to stimulate the development of secondary sex characteristics, but it cannot restore fertility.

Klinefelter syndrome is in most cases related to a 47,XXY karyotype, although some patients may have more than two X chromosomes. Phenotypically males, these patients are tall, have small testes and penis, and never achieve sexual maturity. Testes show no spermatogenesis and accordingly these patients are infertile.

Down syndrome is characterized by a typical constellation of signs and symptoms, including mental deficiency; characteristic facial features such as low bridge of nose with everted nares and effaced philtrum, close-set eyes that are slanted and show palpebral epicanthus, and macroglossia; and abnormal extremities with clinodactyly and a simian crease on the palms. Approximately 40% of patients have congenital heart disease and most of them are at risk of developing acute leukemia. Immunologic deficiencies predispose these children to infections and autoimmune disorders. With good care, Down syndrome patients may live an almost normal life span. Almost all of those who die after puberty show pathologic signs of Alzheimer's disease, which apparently develops at an accelerated rate in these individuals. Most Down syndrome patients have 47 chromosomes (47,XX plus 21, or 47, XY plus 21). The third chromosome 21 can be in most instances traced to abnormal meiotic division during the maturation of the maternal germ cells in the ovary. These meiotic abnormalities occur more often in older women, and the incidence of Down syndrome increases among women who become pregnant after the age of 35 years. Therefore, prenatal diagnosis is offered routinely to all pregnant women older than 35 years. In a small number of cases (5%), Down syndrome is related to a translocation of the long arm of chromosome 21 to another chromosome. Such translocation may already present in otherwise normal mothers of these Down syndrome patients. Accordingly, the translocation form of Down syndrome could be hereditary.

Single Gene Defects

All human genes located on autosomes occur in duplicates known as alleles, which are classified as either dominant or recessive. A person with two dominant or two recessive genes is called a homozygote, whereas those who have one dominant and one recessive allele are called heterozygotes. Thus, some X-linked recessive genes that are not expressed in females would be unopposed by another allele in males, who have only one copy of that gene, and they are therefore expressed. According to the laws of Mendelian genetics, the diseases inherited due to abnormal alleles are classified as autosomal dominant or recessive, or sex-linked autosomal or recessive, depending on the location of the abnormal allele and whether it is dominant or recessive and present as unicate or in duplicate. The X and Y chromosomes share some alleles, but the longer X chromosome has some genes that are not found on the Y chromosome.

AUTOSOMAL DOMINANT DISORDERS

Autosomal dominant disorders are transmitted by a single gene that is dominant in relationship to the gene on its other allele. The gene is expressed fully in heterozygotes, and because it has a 50% chance of being found in one of the gametes, it is transmitted to 50% of the sons and daughters of an affected person. The trait is evident in every generation. The diseases transmitted as autosomal dominant traits may affect the entire body, as in Marfan's syndrome, osteogenesis imperfecta, or Ehlers-Danlos syndrome; the bones, as in achondroplasia; the hematopoietic system, as in hereditary spherocytosis; the kidneys, as in adult polycystic kidney disease; the central nervous system, as in Huntington's disease; or lipid metabolism, as in familial hypercholesterolemia. They may also be present as hereditary tumor syndromes, such as in familiar forms of retinoblastoma, Wilms' tumor, familial adenomatous polyposis coli, and neurofibromatosis.

Marfan's syndrome is a multisystemic disease caused by a mutation in the gene that encodes an intercellular protein called ***fibrillin***. Fibrillin acts as a glue and without it the connective tissues of many organs are loosely structured. People affected by Marfan's syndrome are typically tall, suffer from loose joints that are prone to luxations, and have cardiovascular symptoms related to loosely structured mitral and tricuspid valves ("floppy valve syndrome") and aneurysmal dilatation of the aorta, and eye problems, such as cataracts, luxation of lens, and detachment of retina.

Osteogenesis imperfecta includes several variants, all of which are related to a defect in the genes encoding collagen type I. Mutation of this gene affects many tissues because collagen type I is the major structural protein of the human body and it is found in essentially all tissues. Affected persons have friable bones prone to fractures. The most severe form of osteogenesis imperfecta is lethal *in utero,* whereas the milder form presents with only minor skeletal deformities and blue sclerae.

Ehlers-Danlos syndrome (EDS) includes several diseases characterized by hyperelasticity of skin, hypermobility of joints, and fragility of blood vessels resulting in frequent bleeding. The disease is heterogeneous and is related to mutations of genes encoding several collagens (*e.g.,* collagen type III in EDS IV, or collagen type I in EDS VII).

Achondroplasia is a defect in endochondral ossification that is essential for normal growth of long bones. Affected persons are dwarfed because they have short limbs. The head, which is formed mostly by intramembranous ossification, is of normal size (*e.g.,* it is disproportionally large in comparison to the arms and legs).

Hereditary spherocytosis is a hemolytic anemia resulting from an intracorpuscular defect of red blood cells. It is caused by a mutation of the gene for ***spectrin,*** a structural cytoskeletal protein of red blood cells. Because of a deficiency of spectrin, the red blood cells assume a rounded shape and are less pliable. These abnormal red blood cells are destroyed at an increased rate during their passage through the spleen, which results in chronic hemolytic anemia.

Adult polycystic kidney disease is related to a gene on chromosome 16 whose function is not fully understood. The genetic defect leads to progressive changes in renal tubules, which undergo cystic dilatation and become afunctional. Renal failure develops in the third or fourth decade.

Huntington's disease is related to an expanded cytosine-adenine-guanine (CAG) trinucleotide repeat on chromosome 4, encoding a gene whose function is not known. The disease presents at midlife as progressive dementia, associated with chorea (involuntary movements), and affective outbursts.

Familial hypercholesterolemia is related to mutation of a gene that encodes the cell surface receptor for the low-density lipoprotein (LDL). Because LDL cannot be removed efficiently from the circulation, hyperlipidemia results, leading to accelerated atherosclerosis and deposition of cholesterol in tissues. Cholesterol-laden macrophages form small yellow subcutaneous nodules known as xanthomas.

AUTOSOMAL RECESSIVE DISORDERS

Autosomal recessive disorders are clinically evident only if both alleles are present (*e.g.,* the person is a homozygote). By definition, both parents must be asymptomatic carriers of the abnormal allele. Numerous diseases are classified as autosomal recessive disorders, and many of the genes causing them have been identified. The most important among these diseases are cystic fibrosis; various lysosomal storage diseases; various forms of hemolytic anemia, such as sickle cell anemia and thalassemia; disorders of glycogen metabolism, such as von Gierke's disease and other glycogenoses; disorders of amino acid metabolism, such as phenylketonuria; hereditary hemochromatosis; Wilson's disease; and alpha-1 antitrypsin deficiency.

Cystic fibrosis is the most common lethal autosomal recessive disorder of humans, affecting 1 in 2500 newborn white babies. The disease was traced to the mutation of a gene on chromosome 7, which encodes the cystic fibrosis transmembrane conductance regulator (CFTR). CFTR regulates the transport of chloride across the cell membrane and is essential for facilitating cellular secretion. Cystic fibrosis affects most notably the pancreas and bronchial glands and the gastrointestinal system. Viscous secretions accumulate in the lumen of these organs, blocking the flow of mucus and enzymes. Cystic dilatation of pancreatic ducts distended with inspissated mucus leads to pancreatic fibrosis, which impairs pancreatic function and causes malabsorption of nutrients. Bronchial obstruction with mucus leads to bronchiectasis and recurrent bouts of pneumonia, which ultimately cause the demise of these patients. Obstruction of the intestines and bile ducts leads to malabsorption and nutritional disturbances, and to hepatic cirrhosis. In neonates, cystic fibrosis may even cause complete obstruction of the intestine (meconium ileus) followed by intestinal rupture. Cystic fibrosis is an incurable disease and most patients die in the third decade of their life.

Lysosomal storage diseases result from storage of intermediate metabolites or undegraded products of metabolism in the lysosomes. These diseases are related to mutations of genes that encode enzymes critical in the intermediate metabolism of lipids, carbohydrates, and proteins. For example, *Tay-Sachs disease* is a deficiency of hexosaminidase-A which results in the accumulation of ganglioside GM_2 in neurons and retinal cells, with subsequent mental deterioration and blindness. *Gaucher's disease* is a deficiency of glucocerebrosidase, resulting in the accumulation of glucosylceramide in macrophages and fixed phagocytic cells of the spleen and the liver. *Mucopolysaccharidoses*, a group of diseases each of which is related to a deficiency of a particular enzyme, result in the accumulation of mucopolysaccharides in lysosomes and consequent development of skeletal, cardiovascular, and neurologic abnormalities.

Disorders of intermediate metabolism of carbohydrates, lipids, and amino acids are often caused by single gene mutations. There are at least twelve distinct forms of *glycogenoses*, each of which is based on a deficiency of a specific enzyme in the intermediate metabolism of carbohydrates. Glycogen accumulates most often in the liver or the muscles, heart, and, to a lesser extent, other organs. The most important of these is von Gierke's disease, a deficiency of glucose-6-phosphatase, which leads to accumulation of glycogen in the liver and the kidneys and high mortality in infancy. Glycogen accumulates in the hyaloplasm except in glycogenosis type II, Pompe's disease, or acid maltase deficiency, which is characterized by lysosomal accumulation. Examples of disorders of amino acid metabolism are *albinism*, a defect in the synthesis of melanin, and *phenylketonuria*, a systemic disorder caused by a deficiency of phenylalanine hydroxylase and accumulation of phenylketones in the body.

X-LINKED RECESSIVE DISORDERS

X-linked recessive disorders are related to mutations of recessive X-chromosome-linked genes, which are not found on the Y chromosome. Accordingly, such genes are expressed only in males, even though they are inherited from the mother. The daughters that inherit the same defective gene from the mother are not affected, although they are asymptomatic carriers and can transmit the disease to their own male offspring. The most important diseases inherited as X-linked recessive traits are Duchenne's muscular dystrophy, hemophilia A and B, and fragile X syndrome. *Duchenne's muscular dystrophy* is caused by a mutation or partial deletion of a very large gene that encodes a structural protein called ***dystrophin***. Without dystrophin, the muscle cells degenerate and most affected patients die by the age of 20 years due to respiratory insufficiency caused by changes in the diaphragm and thoracic muscles. *Hemophilia A* and *B* are severe bleeding disorders caused by a defect in the gene encoding the coagulation factor VIII or IX respectively. *Fragile X syndrome* is a form of mental deficiency, related to a fragile site on the X chromosome that contains abnormally amplified repeats of CGG nucleotide triplets.

Multifactorial Inheritance

In contrast to single gene disorders, which are inherited according to the laws of Mendelian genetics, most human diseases that have a hereditary base are mediated by more than one gene and are thus polygenic. Such polygenic diseases evolve at different rates in different individuals and may be influenced by age, sex, race, and social and environmental factors. These multifactorial diseases, which reflect the balance between nature and nurture, include some of the most important human diseases, such as atherosclerosis, hypertension, diabetes, allergies, congenital heart disease, dysraphic abnormalities of the central nervous system (anencephaly, meningomyelocele), cleft lip, and cleft palate.

NEONATAL DISEASES

Diseases of the neonatal period reflect various disturbances of prenatal development, infections acquired transplacentally or during delivery, or disease acquired immediately after birth. All of these diseases are more common in infants born to diseased mothers, or in infants that have been born before term (*e.g.*, before 38 to 40 weeks of pregnancy).

Prematurely born infants weigh less than normal (normal at 40 weeks is from 2700 to 4000 g). All major organs of such premature infants are functionally immature. Most clinical symptoms result, however, from immaturity of the lungs, which cannot maintain normal respiration. Type II pneumocytes of such infants do not secrete the adult type of pulmonary alveolar surfactant, and therefore their alveoli cannot remain open. A telectasis of the alveoli is typically associated with exudation of fibrin into the alveolar sacs and respiratory bronchioli, and the development of ***hyaline membranes***. Hyaline membrane disease is an acute respiratory distress syndrome of the newborn resulting from pulmonary immaturity; it requires treatment, and without ventilation assistance such infants do not survive. Complications include pulmonary dysplasia, which develops as a result of incomplete healing of severely damaged lungs, intraventricular hemorrhage, and hemorrhagic intestinal necrosis.

Birth injury is relatively common, although most infants injured during delivery recover and have only minimal residual impairment. The most common is *cephalohematoma* or bleeding underneath the periosteum of calvarial bones, which heals without any consequences. Intracranial hemorrhages are a complication of forceps delivery or prolonged birth through a very narrow birth canal. ***Peripheral nerve injuries or avulsions,*** which most often involve the brachial plexus, are rare but may result in permanent paralysis of the extremities.

IMMUNOPATHOLOGY

The normal immune response and the principles of immunity are discussed in the chapter 5 on microbiology and immunity. The following section will focus on general disorders and specific diseases of the immune system. These are included under the following categories:

- hypersensitivity reactions
- autoimmune diseases
- immunologic deficiency syndromes
- amyloidosis

Hypersensitivity Reactions

It is customary to divide hypersensitivity reactions into four types, I through IV.

Type I hypersensitivity (anaphylaxis) occurs as a rapidly developing, local or systemic, immunologic reaction. It evolves within minutes after the combination of an antigen with an antibody is bound to ***mast cells or basophils*** in individuals previously sensitized to the antigen. Systemic reactions produce shock and may lead to death. Local reactions are characterized by cutaneous swellings, nasal and/or conjunctival discharge (hay fever), bronchial asthma, or gastroenteritis (food allergy). Central to these reactions are mast cells and basophils, the contents of which are released by a variety of physical stimuli (*e.g.*, cold, heat), chemical stimuli (*e.g.*, C3a, C5a, IL-8), and some drug stimuli. In humans, the reaction is mediated by ***IgE antibodies***. The mediators responsible for vasodilation and increased permeability include histamine, platelet activating factor (PAF), leukotrienes C_4, D_4, and E_4, neutral proteases that activate complement, and the kinin system and prostaglandin D_4. Those producing muscle spasm include leukotrienes C_4, D_4, and E_4, histamine, prostaglandins, and PAF. Finally, those responsible for cellular infiltration include leukotriene B_4, eosinophil chemotactic factor of anaphylaxis, neutrophil chemotactic factor of anaphylaxis, PAF, and cytokines (*e.g.*, TNF). Conditions precipitating systemic anaphylaxis include the administration of heterologous proteins (*e.g.*, antisera, hormones, enzymes, polysaccharides, and some drugs, such as penicillin). Those conditions precipitating local anaphylaxis include inhalation or ingestion of allergens such as pollen, house dust, and animal dander. Urticaria, angioedema, allergic rhinitis, and at best some forms of asthma are examples of localized anaphylaxis.

Type II hypersensitivity is mediated by antibodies directed toward antigens on cell and/or tissue surfaces. The antigens may be endogenous to the membrane or exogenous and adsorbed to the membrane. The mechanisms by which this occurs may be complement dependent (*e.g.*, transfusion reactions, erythroblastosis fetalis, autoimmune hemolytic anemia, agranulocytosis, and thrombocytopenia); antibody-dependent, cell-mediated cytotoxicity (*e.g.*, parasites, tumor cells); or antibody-mediated cellular dysfunction (*e.g.*, antibodies against acetylcholine in myasthenia gravis).

Type III hypersensitivity (immune complex mediated) is induced by antigen–antibody complexes that produce damage in tissues because of their ability to activate a number of mediators, especially the complement system. Antigens may be exogenous (*e.g.*, foreign proteins, viruses, bacteria) or endogenous (*e.g.*, cell or tissue components). The pathogenesis consists of three phases: (a) the formation of the complex; (b) deposition of the complex in tissues, such as renal glomeruli, joints, skin, heart, serosal surfaces, and small blood vessels; and (c) initiation of an inflammatory reaction. The last step results from the activation of complement and ultimate release of vasoactive and chemotactic mediators. A common morphologic feature seen with the light microscope on hematoxylin-eosin-stained secretions is a smudgy eosinophilic change in the walls of blood vessels. It is caused by the presence of immunoglobulins, complement, and fibrinogen and is called fibrinoid necrosis or fibrinoid change. The latter is a more appropriate term, because this change does not meet the criteria for the definition of necrosis. Serum sickness, poststreptococcal glomerulonephritis, and systemic lupus erythematosus are examples of systemic diseases produced by type III hypersensitivity reactions. The Arthus reaction is an example of a localized disease induced by this mechanism.

Type IV hypersensitivity (cell mediated) is initiated by specifically sensitized T lymphocytes. In these reactions, CD4+ T cells initiate a delayed-typed hypersensitivity reaction with cytotoxicity mediated via CD8+ T cells. Classic examples of this type of hypersensitivity include the tuberculin reaction, contact dermatitis, and graft rejections.

TRANSPLANT REJECTION

The recognition of graft as foreign is mediated via the histocompatibility antigens, which are primarily human leukocyte group A (HLA) antigens. The ensuing process of rejection is complex and involves both cell-mediated and humoral immunity. ***T-cell-mediated reactions*** are characterized by activation of CD8+ cytotoxic lymphocytes, as well as CD4+ T lymphocytes, which initiate delayed-type hypersensitivity reactions. These events are triggered when recipient lymphocytes contact donor HLA antigens. The CD4+ helper lymphocytes recognize class II specific sites, and CD8+ cytotoxic lymphocytes recognize class I determinants. The latter lyse the grafted tissue, while lymphokine-secreting CD4+ lymphocytes cause increased vascular permeability and attract macrophages and lymphocytes to the region, where they accumulate.

Antibody-mediated reactions can take two forms:

1. Hyperacute rejection occurs when pre-formed antibodies against the donor are present in the recipient's circulation (*e.g.*, a recipient who has already rejected a kidney transplant or had prior blood transfusions from donors, or a multiparous woman with anti-HLA antibodies against grafts from husband or children). The rejection occurs immediately. Antibodies rapidly deposit in the graft's vascular endothelium, complement is fixed, and an Arthus reaction is evoked.
2. Exposure of recipients to class I and II HLA antigens from the donor may produce antibodies against the graft. These antibodies can evoke injury by complement-dependent cytotoxicity, antibody-dependent cell-mediated immunity, and/or the deposition of immune complexes. The graft vasculature appears to be the prime target, leading to vasculitis.

Graft rejections are classified as ***hyperacute, acute***, and ***chronic***. Morphologically, as seen in the kidney, ***hyperacute rejections*** occur within minutes to hours after transplantation. The kidney becomes cyanotic and mottled. Histologically, there are neutrophils in arterioles, the glomerular capillaries, and the peritubular capillaries as a result of antigen–antibody complex and complement deposition. Thrombosis ensues, leading to cortical infarction. ***Acute rejection*** may occur within days of the transplantation, or months to years later if immunosuppression is terminated. Acute cellular rejection is characterized by interstitial infiltrates of mononuclear cells, primarily lymphocytes, that are also seen in glomerular and peritubular capillaries. The latter may invade tubules, causing necrosis. If vasculitis is not present, these patients respond to immunosuppression therapy. ***Acute rejection vasculitis*** is seen most commonly in the first few months after transplantation. Histologically, there is necrotizing vasculitis with infiltration by neutrophils, and the deposition of immunoglobulins, complement, and fibrin. Thrombosis ensues and may lead to cortical infarction.

More commonly, a ***subacute vasculitis*** is observed in the first few months after transplantation. This is characterized by marked intimal thickening caused by proliferating fibroblasts, myocytes, and macrophages. The vessel walls often contain immunoglobulins and complement. They become stenotic and may become obliterated.

Chronic rejection is recognized by progressive elevation of creatinine levels over 4 to 6 months. The primary lesions are vascular. Histologically, there is intimal fibrosis primarily in the cortical arteries that lead to ischemia. There is also a mononuclear infiltrate in the interstitium.

Hematopoietic cells are transplanted as a form of therapy for hematologic malignancies, aplastic anemias, and immunodeficiency states. In general, recipients are immunodeficient because of irradiation prior to transplantation, performed either as therapy for their malignancy or to prepare the graft site, or because of their malignancy. This background sets the scene for ***graft-versus-host*** (GVH) disease, a condition in which immunologically competent cells or their precursors are transplanted into immunologically deficient recipients. The donor T lymphocytes recognize recipient HLA antigens and react against them. Thus CD4+ and CD8+ lymphocytes are generated that react against the recipient. ***Acute GVH*** disease occurs within days or weeks of transplantation with allogenic bone marrow. The ensuing clinical manifestations include severe immunosuppression, cutaneous rash, destruction of bile ducts leading to jaundice, and intestinal mucosal ulcers leading to bloody diarrhea. ***Chronic GVH*** disease occurs subsequent to the acute form, or surreptitiously. All of the lesions for the acute form are present, but they are much more severe. Fibrosis of the dermis resembles systemic sclerosis. In addition, esophageal strictures may be present, and recurrent infections are experienced frequently. The GVH response can also be seen in grafts of solid organs that have a lymphoid component (e.g., liver). Finally, bone marrow transplants can also be rejected.

Autoimmunity

Autoimmune diseases are defined by the presence of an immune reaction in diseases where there is no known definable cause and where evidence supports the autoimmune reaction as being a primary cause of the disease and not secondary to tissue destruction. The autoantibodies can be directed to a single organ or tissue or to multiple organs or tissues. Diseases usually associated with the former include Hashimoto's thyroiditis, autoimmune hemolytic anemia, autoimmune atrophic gastritis of pernicious anemia, autoimmune encephalomyelitis, autoimmune orchitis, Goodpasture's syndrome, autoimmune thrombocytopenia, insulin-dependent diabetes mellitus, myasthenia gravis, and Graves' disease. These diseases, generally associated with multiple organs or systems, include systemic lupus erythematosus, rheumatoid arthritis, Sjögren's syndrome, and Reiter's syndrome. The pathogenesis of autoimmunity is complex and appears to involve immunologic, genetic, and viral mechanisms; immunologic tolerance to certain self antigens must be altered for autoimmunity to occur.

Systemic lupus erythematosus (SLE) is a multisystem disease of autoimmune origin. Although every organ in the body can be affected, the skin, kidneys, joints, and serosal membranes are most frequently involved. A vast array of autoantibodies have been identified, particularly antinuclear antibodies (ANAs). These are useful for diagnosis and are also implicated in the pathogenesis of the disease (*e.g.,* immune-complex-mediated glomerulonephritis). Antibodies to double-stranded DNA (ssDNA) and particularly to Smith (Sm) antigen are virtually diagnostic for SLE. The pathogenesis appears to include the interaction of genetic, environmental, and hormonal factors that activate helper T cells and B cells to produce a broad spectrum of autoantibodies. These antibodies are then responsible for producing the clinical manifestations. Nephritis is very common and is manifested in a variety of patterns, including mesangial glomerulonephritis, and focal proliferative, diffuse proliferative, and membranous glomerulonephritis. All of these are associated with the deposition of immune complexes in the glomeruli. Skin lesions are characterized by erythematous regions over the nose and cheeks (''butterfly rash''). Urticaria, bullae, maculopapular rashes, and ulcerations are also observed.

Histologic features include degeneration of the epidermal basal layer, edema of the dermis, perivascular mononuclear infiltrates, and vasculitis with fibrinoid necrosis. Involvement of joints is common. The lesions are characterized by synovitis, neutrophils, and fibrin in the early stages, and little resultant joint deformity. There is also fibrinous pericarditis and pleuritis, and nonbacterial verrucous endocarditis can occur. In addition, the cardiovascular system, spleen, lungs, and a variety of other organs can be involved.

Clinically, the disease is particularly common in young women who, in addition to presenting with the skin rash and arthralgia, are febrile and complain of pleuritic chest pain and photosensitivity. Other forms of lupus are recognized, including a chronic discoid form, a subacute cutaneous form, and a form that is drug induced.

Sjögren's syndrome is characterized by dry eyes and mouth ***(keratoconjunctivitis sicca*** and ***xerostomia).*** It can be primary, but it is most often found in conjunction with other autoimmune diseases, such as rheumatoid arthritis, SLE, and polymyositis. Histologically, periductal and perivascular lymphocytic infiltrates are noted in the salivary glands and lacrimal glands. Other organs are involved to a lesser degree. Clinically, approximately 90% of patients are women between 40 and 60 years of age. They present with signs referable to keratoconjunctivitis and xerostomia. Diagnosis is made clinically and serologically. Approximately 90% of patients have antibodies directed against ribonucleoprotein antigens SS-A (Ro) and SS-B (La).

Systemic sclerosis (scleroderma) is characterized by excessive fibrosis throughout the body, including the skin (the predominant site), gastrointestinal tract, kidneys, heart, muscles, and lung. Two forms of the disease are recognized: (a) ***diffuse scleroderma***, which has initial widespread skin involvement and rapidly progresses to visceral involvement, and (b) ***localized scleroderma***, which has initial localized skin involvement with visceral involvement much later. The localized form is called the ***CREST*** form because of the frequency of calcinosis, Raynaud's phenomenon, esophageal dysfunction, sclerodactyly, and telangiectasia. The etiology is undetermined, but it is proposed that immunologic mechanisms lead to the hallmark fibrosis and microvascular disease by releasing cytokines that stimulate fibrosis and/or cause direct endothelial damage. Histologically, fibrosis is preceded by edema and atrophy. Blood vessels demonstrate endothelial cell damage and hyaline thickening of their walls. In the kidneys, there is fibrinoid necrosis of the walls of small vessels.

Clinically, systemic sclerosis is observed most frequently in women, with the highest incidence noted in the 50- to 60-year old range. It must be differentiated from SLE, polymyositis, and rheumatoid arthritis. Raynaud's phenomenon is often the presenting sign. This is followed by esophageal dysfunction. Abdominal pain dyspnea and/or signs referable to the kidney, from mild proteinuria to malignant hypertension may be present. Numerous ANAs are found with this disease. A rather unusual antibody against DNA topoisomerase I and an anticentromere antibody can be helpful in making a diagnosis.

Inflammatory myopathies consist of three variants, the etiologies of which are unknown, but the pathogenesis of each appears to be immunologically mediated. *Dermatomyositis* appears to result from capillary injury that gives rise to muscle fiber necrosis, regeneration, and fibrosis. Clinically, children or adults can be affected. There is a lilac or heliotrope discoloration on the eyelids, and periorbital edema. Muscle weakness initially affects proximal muscles. Fine movements are affected later. Women with this condition have a slightly higher risk of developing ovarian, lung, and stomach cancer. *Polymyositis* is similar to dermatomyositis, but it does not involve skin. Myofibers are directly injured by CD8+ T lymphocytes. It is a disease of adults and there is a slight increased risk of developing visceral cancers. *Inclusion-body myositis* is mediated by direct injury to myofibers by CD8+ T lymphocytes. Histologically, rimmed vacuoles with basophilic granules are observed in frozen sections of myocytes. Distal muscles are involved initially. The diagnosis of inflammatory myositis is based on clinical signs, electromyography, elevations of muscle-related enzymes in serum, and biopsy. In addition, autoantibodies to tRNA synthetases such as anti-Jo-1 appear to be specific for inflammatory myopathies.

Mixed connective tissue disease (MCTD) is characterized by concomitant clinical features of SLE, polymyositis, and systemic sclerosis. In addition, patients have elevated titers to a complex containing ribonucleoprotein (RNP) and U1 small nuclear RNAs.

Polyarteritis nodosa is part of a group of necrotizing vascular diseases that are not associated with infectious causes. They are thought to be immunologically mediated. Medium sized arteries are most often affected but any size or type of vessel can be involved.

Immunologic Deficiency Syndrome

Immunologic deficiency syndromes are classified as primary or secondary.

PRIMARY IMMUNE DEFICIENCIES (GENETICALLY DETERMINED)

This group of diseases includes several syndromes.

X-linked agammaglobulinemia of Bruton is one of the most common primary immunodeficiencies. It is found exclusively in males and is characterized by an almost total absence of serum immunoglobulins and a virtual absence of B lymphocytes in the blood. Histologically, lymph nodes and spleen have germinal centers and no plasma cells are observed in any tissues. T-lymphocyte populations are normal. Clinically, beginning at 8 to 9 months of age, infants experience severe recurrent bacterial infections, such as conjunctivitis, pharyngitis, and bronchitis. Viral and fungal infections are handled normally.

Common variable immunodeficiency (CVI) is relatively common, may be congenital or acquired, and affects both genders equally. It is characterized by hypogammaglobulinemia, most often affecting all classes of antibody, but sometimes only IgG. In addition, normal numbers of lymphocytes are in the blood, but they cannot differentiate into plasma cells. Histologically, there is hyperplasia of B-cell regions in lymphoid tissue. Clinically, recurrent bacterial infections are the norm. In addition, patients are prone to enteroviral infections, herpes zoster, and *Giardia lamblia*. Finally, these patients have a high incidence of autoimmune diseases, and the risk of lymphoid malignancies is increased.

Isolated IgA deficiency is very common in the United States. It is familial or acquired. The latter is often associated with toxoplasmosis, measles, or other viruses. It is characterized by very low levels of circulating and secretory IgA. The basic defect is in the differentiation of IgA B lymphocytes. Clinically, patients present with infections of the respiratory, gastrointestinal, and/or urogenital systems. There is also a high frequency of respiratory allergies and autoimmune diseases.

DiGeorge's syndrome (thymic aplasia) results from a failure of the third and fourth pharyngeal pouches to develop. There is a T-lymphocyte deficiency that leads to a total lack of cell-mediated immunity. In addition, tetany results due to lack of the parathyroid gland. Finally, there are heart and great vessel defects. Histologically, the thymic-dependent regions of the lymphoid organs are depleted. B-cell-dependent regions are normal, as are serum immunoglobulin levels. Clinically, these patients are susceptible to viral and fungal infections.

Severe combined immunodeficiency diseases (SCID) are characterized by T- and B-lymphocyte deficiencies. The causes are diverse defects in the development of the immune system. Some of these diseases have an X-linked inheritance pattern. Histologically, two forms predominate: in one form, there is a lack of an adenosine deaminase (ADA), the thymus is small, lymphoid cells are depleted, and remnants of Hassall's corpuscles are observed. The other is an X-linked recessive form, in which the thymus contains undifferentiated epithelial cells. Lymphoid tissues in all cases are hypoplastic and there is depletion of T and/or B cells. Clinically, infants are susceptible to severe recurrent bacterial, viral, fungal, and/or protozoal infections. There may be graft-versus-host reactions and in some instances bone marrow transplants are required for survival.

Immunodeficiency with thrombocytopenia and eczema (Wiskott-Aldrich syndrome) is an X-linked recessive disease characterized by depletion of circulating T lymphocytes and those in the thymic-dependent portion of lymphoid tissue. The thymus appears normal in the initial stages. Immunoglobulin levels are variable. IgM may be low, but IgG is normal. IgA and IgE may be elevated. Clinically, patients present with susceptibility to recurrent infections, thrombocytopenia, and eczema, which ends in early death.

Genetic deficiencies of the complement system can give rise to susceptibility to recurrent infections, increased risk of immune-complex diseases, or hereditary angioedema, depending on which of the factors is deficient.

SECONDARY IMMUNE DEFICIENCY (ACQUIRED)

Acquired immunodeficiency syndrome (AIDS) is presently the most significant of the secondary immunodeficiency diseases. It is caused by infection with human immunodeficiency virus (HIV). It is characterized by severe immunosuppression, and it is associated with infections by opportunistic organisms, secondary neoplasms, and neurologic manifestations. The three major routes of transmission are sexual contact, parenteral inoculation, and passage of the virus from infected mothers to newborns. Epidemiologically, five at-risk groups have been designated, based on percentages of recorded cases. In descending order: (a) homosexual or bisexual males including a small percentage of intravenous drug users account for the largest percentage of cases in the United States, (b) intravenous drug users other than those previously described; (c) hemophiliacs, particularly those receiving large amounts of concentrated factor VIII prior to 1985; (d) recipients of blood or blood components who are not hemophiliacs; and (e) heterosexuals contacting members of other high-risk groups. About 2% of AIDS victims are children, the vast majority having contracted the virus *in utero,* during delivery, or by ingesting breast milk. The others are hemophiliacs or nonhemophiliacs who received blood or blood products. Globally, heterosexual transmission is the most common means of HIV transmission. This mode of transmission is now beginning to surpass all others in the United States as well. The HIV virus targets CD4+ T lymphocytes, monocytes, macrophages, and follicular dendritic cells. After lengthy incubations, the CD4+ cells are lysed, leading to profound immunosuppression. Monocytes and macrophages are more resistant to lysis and are thought to act as safe havens for virus replication and storage, and as transporters of the virus, particularly to the brain. The natural history of the disease can be divided into three phases. First, the early, acute phase, in which viral replication, viremia, and viral seeding of lymphoid tissues occurs. This phase is characterized clinically by mild nonspecific symptoms, such as sore throat, fever, and rash. Second, the middle, chronic phase is represented by smoldering, low-level virus replication in lymphoid tissue for several years. Patients are asymptomatic or develop generalized lymphadenopathy. Third, the final crisis phase is represented by marked viral replication, suppression of immunity, and clinical disease (*e.g.*, secondary neoplasms and opportunistic infections). AIDS-defining opportunistic infections include *Pneumocystis carinii* pneumonia, toxoplasmosis, candidiasis, cryptococcosis infections in the central nervous system, mycobacteriosis, and infections with other unusual organisms. Kaposi's sarcoma, non-Hodgkin's lymphomas (*e.g.*, Burkitt's, immunoblastic, primary lymphoma in the brain, and invasive cancer of the uterine cervix) are associated neoplasms. The numbers of CD4+ T lymphocytes in the blood are good measures of prognosis. A CD4+ count above 500/μl suggests a lower probability of progression, whereas a count below 200/μl or a rapidly falling count is indicative of disease progression.

Amyloidosis

Amyloidosis comprises a group of diseases that are characterized by the deposition of fibrillar proteinaceous material between cells in various tissues and organs in a variety of clinical settings. There are several biochemical forms, but morphologically they appear similar: all have a green birefringence when stained with Congo red and examined under polarized light, which differentiates the fibrillar proteinaceous material from collagen and fibrin. Amyloid is classified as systemic or localized. Systemic amyloid is further classified into primary when it is associated with monoclonal B-cell proliferations, such as multiple myeloma, or secondary when it is associated with chronic inflammatory processes. Localized amyloid is seen in Alzheimer's disease, in medullary carcinomas of the thyroid, and in the islets of Langerhans with type II diabetes mellitus. Histologically, amyloid is amorphous, eosinophilic, hyalinized, and extracellular. Systemic amyloidosis most often involves the kidneys, liver, spleen, lymph nodes, adrenals, and thyroid. Immunocyte-associated amyloidosis also involves the heart, gastrointestinal tract, peripheral nerves, skin, and tongue. Clinical symptoms are referable to the organ system. Kidney disease manifested by proteinuria leading to the nephrotic syndrome is a predominant presentation. Prognosis for patients with the generalized form is poor.

NEOPLASIA

The uncontrolled growth of cells that results in a mass (tumor) is the process known as neoplasia (new tissue, new growth). Neoplasms can be ***benign***, in which case they remain localized, or ***malignant***, which allows them to invade surrounding tissue and spread to distant sites. Malignant neoplasms are referred to as ***cancer***, a term that probably derives from their crab-like extension into surrounding structures.

Cancer is the number two killer, behind heart diseases, in the United States. There are more than 1 million new cases, and over 500,000 deaths from cancer annually. Yet the prevalence of cancer is even higher because it does not kill immediately, and because the prognosis for many tumors has been steadily improving.

Although the distinction between benign and malignant neoplasias seems clear, in fact it is not always obvious. Both benign and malignant neoplasms result from accumulation of cells as a result of proliferation that exceeds cellular destruction. This proliferation is outside normal growth controls and unlike hyperplasia, which in some cases appears to predispose to the development of neoplasia, the proliferation persists after the stimulus that evoked it no longer exists. The proliferation is continuous, but it need not be excessively rapid, even in malignant disease. Whereas benign tumors are usually confined to the area in which they arose, they can arise in multiple sites. In general, benign tumors are encapsulated by a layer of connective tissue, which either is a true capsule laid down around the tumor, or is produced by compression of the surrounding supporting stroma *(pseudocapsule)*. Malignancies, too, can produce a pseudocapsule, and some cancers, like basal cell carcinomas, may invade adjacent tissue aggressively but do not spread to distant sites. Whereas benign tumors can be expected to closely resemble their cell or tissue of origin, and they may form products such as hormones that are normally secreted by cells of their type, even malignant tumors can be highly differentiated, forming glands that closely resemble the normal (*e.g.*, follicular carcinoma of the thyroid) and hormones which are appropriate [although sometimes not appropriate (paraneoplastic syndromes)] for their tissue or cell of origin. The single feature of malignancy that most reliably separates it from a benign process is its spread *(metastasis)*.

Much evidence, from both classic circumstantial observation and more recent molecular biological studies, suggests that neoplasms arise by a multistep process *(carcinogenesis)* involving genetic alterations *(mutations)* that are initiated in most instances by environmental factors (carcinogens: chemicals, irradiation, viruses). The classic observations of Percival Pott pointed to accumulation of coal tar on the skin of chimney sweeps as a cause of scrotal cancer and led to the enactment of legislation (not in England, but in Sweden) that required them to bathe, which largely solved the problem.

Neoplasms are classified into several groups according generally to their supposed cell of origin. Thus, epithelial malignancies are called ***carcinomas***, mesenchymal neoplasms are ***sarcomas***, and tumors with more than one component are ***teratomas*** or ***teratocarcinomas***. A ***hamartoma*** is a benign process composed of aberrant components usually found in the area where the overgrowth occurs. They are considered developmental anomalies rather than true neoplasms.

Carcinomas are further classified by cell type into squamous (squamous cell carcinoma), glandular (adenocarcinoma), and transitional (transitional cell carcinoma) types. Similarly, sarcomas that arise from fibrous tissue are ***fibrosarcomas***, those from smooth muscle are ***leiomyosarcomas***, those from skeletal muscle are ***rhabdomyosarcomas***, and so on. The only known cell type that appears not to give rise to a malignant counterpart is the adult neuron. This is probably because it is terminally differentiated. However, embryonic neurons appear capable of malignant transformation (***neuroblastoma***). In general, benign tumors are given the suffix ***-oma*** (***adenoma***) or a descriptive term to indicate their mode of growth (***papilloma, polyp,*** or ***adenomatous polyp***). Time-honored terms, however, like *melanoma* or *lymphoma* are deviations from this rule, in that they indicate malignant growths of pigmented cells or lymphoid cells. Then, too, there are some tumors that have eponymic designations, such as ***Wilms' tumor*** and ***Ewing's sarcoma***.

The degree to which the cells that make up a neoplasm resemble an adult cell type is useful in another way. Cells that have an immature nucleus in a maturing cytoplasm are often said to be atypical or *dysplastic*. Those whose characteristics are more like primitive stem cells exhibit *anaplasia*. The degree of anaplasia can be used to ***grade*** a malignant neoplasm. Those that resemble adult cells that are well differentiated are *low grade*; those that exhibit features that are like stem cells are highly anaplastic, or *high grade*. Sometimes the percentage of anaplastic cells is used to group tumors in a numerical category (1 to 3, or 1 to 4) such as that used in the *Broder's classification*. In addition to the histologic grade, another useful concept in predicting tumor prognosis is the ***stage***. Staging is an attempt to classify the extent of the tumor at the time of diagnosis. Localized tumors do better than those that have spread to adjacent structures, or to regional or distant lymph nodes. Those that have spread to solid organs do particularly poorly. Useful staging systems may use a combination of local involvement and distant spread. The Dukes classification and its modifications for colon cancer use depth of penetration and lymph node involvement (A, B, C), and spread to solid organs (D). The TNM system stages the tumor in terms of the size of the primary tumor (T), the presence of lymph node involvement (N), and whether it has spread (metastasized) to a distant site (M) to gauge the likelihood of cure or progression.

Many factors affect who gets cancer and what type of cancer they get. The incidence of cancer is highest in the very young and the elderly. Many studies indicate that the environment plays a major role. The incidence of stomach cancer, which was at one time the major cancer killer in males in the United States, has decreased significantly in this country but remains very high in Japan. Japanese who emigrate to the United States have fewer gastric cancers than their counterparts in Japan. However, certain types of cancer, such as nasopharyngeal carcinomas, are more prevalent in the Asian population regardless of where they reside. There are many heredity/familial cancer syndromes. Childhood retinoblastoma cases are familial over 40% of the time, and carriers of the gene have a 10,000 times greater probability of developing the tumor, often in both eyes. Therefore, although environmental factors rank high, and certainly occupational exposure to carcinogens such as asbestos can result in tumorigenesis, other factors, such as age, race, sex, and heredity, play a modulating role.

Carcinogenesis

Important causes of cancer include chemical, physical, and viral agents. The process of cancer induction is probably best understood with chemical agents, though the role of viruses in carcinogenesis is rapidly being elucidated. In the classic studies of cancer induction, it appears that there are multiple steps that a cell goes through in transforming from a normal to a benign neoplastic and finally to a malignant cell. The first of these steps is ***initiation***, in which a genetic change, such as gene deletion or mutation, permanently alters the genetic make-up of the cell. At least one cell division is required to fix the mutation.

The next step is ***promotion***, in which the altered cell population expands by clonal growth. Finally, one or more additional events induce ***progression*** of the altered cells toward a more malignant behavior. The study of familial polyposis in the colon has revealed that this sequence might occur at the genetic level. Mutation or deletion of a putative tumor suppressor gene (APC, named for adenomatous polyposis coli) has been mapped to chromosome 5q21. Colon neoplasms appear to lose methyl groups in their DNA (hypomethylation), and there appears to be activation or mutation of the *ras* oncogene in benign adenomas. Subsequent deletions of an allele of chromosome 18q (DCC gene) and 17p (p53, tumor suppressor) appear to be necessary for progression from adenoma to adenocarcinoma.

X-irradiation and ultraviolet irradiation have also been useful in elucidating the sequence of cancer development. However, most research is now focused on viruses as a cause for cancer, because their genetic make-up is easier to elucidate. Two gene types have been identified as most significant: oncogenes and tumor suppressor genes. Studies of transforming retroviruses revealed viral gene sequences (v-*oncs*) that were identical to normal cellular growth-promoting genes *(proto-oncogenes)*. The cancer-causing oncogenes are derived from these proto-oncogenes. The proteins coded by the proto-oncogene include growth factors, growth factor receptors, signal transducing proteins such as GTP-binding proteins, and nuclear regulatory proteins. An example is the *ras* gene, which is the most frequently mutated gene in human cancers. This gene codes for GTP-binding proteins; when it is continuously activated by a mutation in *ras*, control of cellular proliferation is lost. Gene amplification can also supply excessive growth stimuli.

The anti-oncogenic or growth-suppressing activity of *tumor suppressor* genes may be lost through mutation or deletion. An example of this is the ***retinoblastoma gene*** (Rb). Certain families inherit one copy of the gene that is already mutated. If a second mutation occurs that results in a deletion of the intact copy that resides on chromosome 13q14, retinoblastomas develop in one or both eyes. Other tumors occur with increased frequency in these individuals.

It is now suspected that a third factor, control of cell death by ***apoptosis***, may also play a role in tumorigenesis. Thus, continuous proliferation as a result of growth stimuli, and failure of cells to undergo senescence and death, appear to be important mechanisms by which cells accumulate in tumor masses.

Mechanisms of Invasion and Metastasis

The essence of malignant behavior is the invasion of adjacent structures and the spread to distant sites. If these can be controlled, the lethal effects of malignant cell growth can be neutralized. Therefore, the process is being extensively studied, and the essential elements are increasingly understood. Although tumors are thought to arise from a single cell, it is clear that during repeated cell divisions, subclones begin to emerge. Some of these are more aggressive (progression) and are able to loosen themselves from one another, migrate through the extracellular matrix, and enter vascular spaces. Once within the blood vessels, they must still be able to survive, attach to the vessel wall in a distant site, and emerge from the vascular system to produce a secondary tumor nodule. Each of these steps requires specific enzymes and/or membrane receptors and the capability to move. Probably only a very few of those cells that start the journey end up successfully establishing a metastatic focus. Tumors must be capable of inducing their own blood supply *(angiogenesis)* to be able to grow beyond a minimal size and to gain access to the bloodstream. The central area of many tumors becomes necrotic, but this may *not* be the result of outgrowing their vascular systems as was formerly thought, because most are richly supplied by new vessels of all sizes *(neovascularization)*.

To invade and metastasize, tumor cells must first break their attachment to adjacent cells, attach to matrix components such as laminin and collagen, break down the matrix, and be able to move through it to the blood supply. They must then invade the blood vessels and move through the bloodstream to a suitable organ site, where they establish a satellite growth by emigrating from a small vessel and then proliferating again. Cells are held together by a variety of ***adhesion*** molecules, some of which, such as ***cadherens***, appear to be susceptible to digestion by enzymes released by tumor cells. Similarly, carcinomas are known to elaborate enzymes that digest type IV collagen (basal lamina), and other collagenases appear to be important in establishing channels through which the tumor cells can proceed. The tumor cells appear to have specific ***receptors for laminin***, and they can express ***integrins*** that act as receptors for such matrix components as fibronectin and vitronectin as well as various types of collagen. They also elaborate proteases such as ***cathepsin B***. The latter has been shown to correlate with metastatic potential in breast cancer. Once they gain access to the vascular system, it has been shown that tumor cells that are successful in establishing metastases can elaborate specific adhesion molecules that allow them to attach to endothelial cells in specific target organs. Some of these organs may express chemoattractants that guide the tumor cells to an accommodating target site. Not all sites are equally welcoming. Whereas the liver and lung are particularly frequent sites of metastasis, the spleen is rarely involved.

Spontaneous Regression and Tumor Immunity

One would think that, with the myriad cells and the abundance of carcinogens, everyone would ultimately develop one or more malignancies. On the contrary, establishment and growth of a malignant tumor is a relatively rare event, considering the opportunity. It is therefore evident that there are multiple control elements, the bulk of which probably work to eliminate transformed cells before they begin to proliferate. Nonetheless, it is apparent that some successfully transformed cells are eliminated by the body's immune mechanisms. Altered cells apparently are recognized as foreign and cellular mechanisms such as natural killer cells are goaded into action. Many tumors have a lymphoid infiltrate and some of these are well known to behave in a less aggressive fashion. In addition to immunity, there are clearly other factors that limit tumor proliferation and spread. There are well-established cases in which tumors such as melanoma, renal cell carcinoma, and neuroblastomas have "spontaneously" regressed after having established metastatic growth. It is these spontaneous cures that continue to stimulate us to search for the hormones, immune responses, and growth factors that could control neoplastic diseases.

DISEASES OF BLOOD VESSELS

The vascular system is formed early in embryonic life through a process of hollowing-out of islands and tubules of vasculogenic cells. Similar ***angiogenesis*** occurs in adult life in various pathologic processes such as tumors, wound healing *(granulation tissue)*, and various forms of chronic inflammation. Tumor growth can be sustained only because it is able to induce blood vessel development of various types (capillaries, veins, and arteries). Vascular growth in the retina is a primary factor in blindness as a result of diabetes, and the organization of an inflamed area such as an ulcer regularly depends on the formation of vascular channels (granulation tissue).

The blood vascular system of the adult consists of vessels of different calibers with somewhat different functions and substantially different anatomic features. The ***arterial system*** begins with the ***large elastic vessels*** (the aorta and its major branches) whose walls consist of an endothelial layer supported by a small amount of connective tissue (tunica intima) resting on an elastic membrane (internal elastica) that can be penetrated by smooth muscle cells from the medial coat. The smooth muscle cells are interwoven by elastic fibers and there is a well-developed external elastica that separates the media from the adventitia. The adventitia contains fibroblasts and collagen and has blood vessels of its own, the vasa vasorum, that penetrate and provide nutrition for the media. The ***large musculo-elastic arteries*** are similar to the elastic vessels with the progressive loss of elastic fibers in the media and the loss of an external elastic membrane as they reach the size of the muscular arteries and arterioles. The ***small arteries*** and ***arterioles*** are the resistance vessels, and the arterioles, defined as vessels between 20 microns and 100 microns in diameter, regulate the blood flow to the capillaries. ***Capillaries*** are essentially endothelium-lined tubes that can be ***continuous***, ***fenestrated***, or ***discontinuous*** (sinusoids).

The ***endothelium***, which was once thought to be merely a barrier to free diffusion of the luminal contents to the extravascular compartment, is now recognized to be an extremely complex regulatory system. It has surface proteoglycans (heparin-like), which inhibit clotting, and vasodilator and vasoconstrictor substances, which can regulate local blood flow. Endothelial stimulation produces a rapid response (in minutes) that is independent of protein synthesis, and endothelial activation is dependent on new or changed protein synthesis and requires hours to occur. Stimulation results from vasoactive substances such as histamine, and activation follows exposure to substances such as inflammatory cytokines. Vascular ***smooth muscle cells*** (SMCs) are also very responsive cells that can proliferate and migrate in response to appropriate stimuli. They elaborate elastin, various types of collagen, proteoglycans, cytokines, and growth factors. Excessive production of these can be seen in acute and chronic responses of SMCs to injury.

The ***venular end*** of the capillary is apparently a specific site that is important in the attachment of inflammatory cells. ***Veins*** are similar to arteries, except that they have less elastic tissue and smooth muscle, and they have luminal valves that resist backflow (when they are competent). ***Lymphatic vessels*** are similar to veins and capillaries.

Vascular Diseases

Vascular diseases are very common, and the most important, atherosclerosis, accounts for about half of the annual mortality in the United States. The diseases fall into two categories: degenerative or reactive diseases called ***vasculopathy***, and inflammatory diseases referred to as ***vasculitis***. In each there are a number of subcategories.

Congenital anomalies, such as anomalous origin of arteries, are common, and although they may be important for radiologists or surgeons, they are usually clinically inconsequential. Among the rare clinically important anomalies are ***arteriovenus fistulas*** and ***berry aneurysms.*** The latter are found in the ***circle of Willis,*** particularly at branch points, and result from a deficiency of the muscle coat.

VASCULOPATHY

Among the degenerative diseases of blood vessels, the most significant are those characterized by "hardening" (sclerosis) of the vessels encompassed under the term ***arteriosclerosis***. This includes three major variants: ***atherosclerosis***, a disease of major elastic and musculoelastic arteries characterized by lipid-containing intimal plaques; ***Mönkeberg's medial calcific sclerosis***, characteristically involving large muscular arteries with calcium deposits in a thickened media, but minimal luminal compromise; and ***arterial*** and ***arteriolosclerosis***, which involve small arteries and arterioles in a process that produces thickening and fibrosis of the media, narrowing of the lumina with subendothelial fibroplasia, and hyaline change of the vessel wall due to excessive basal lamina (mostly type IV collagen) and plasma proteins.

Atherosclerosis is the most frequent and most devastating of these vascular changes. Luminal narrowing or even complete occlusion by atherosclerosis results in its most frequent complications: ischemic heart disease (IHD, or myocardial infarct), brain infarcts (stroke), and others, such as sudden cardiac death, gangrene of the extremities, and mesenteric artery thrombosis. Over 50% of the annual death rate in the United States is accounted for by atherosclerosis. Predisposing elements include four principal risk factors: (a) hyperlipidemia (hypercholesterolemia, hypertriglyceridemia), (b) hypertension, (c) diabetes, and (d) cigarette smoking. Minor factors include increasing age, obesity, being male, lack of physical activity, and high "stress." Increasing evidence supports the "response to injury" hypothesis in the pathogenesis of the lesions. Injury to endothelial cells causes release of growth factors, proliferation of SMCs, and deposition of lipids that are taken up by circulating monocytes, which are transformed to macrophages. The ***atheroma*** or ***atheromatous plaque*** that is the hallmark of the lesion consists of a raised fibrous cap underneath which there is grumous fatty material which is both extracellular or contained in SMCs and foamy macrophages. Crystals of cholesterol and scattered lymphocytes are also present and the lesion is covered by endothelial cells and lies entirely within the intima. The media may become thinned and hyalinized beneath a plaque, and this weakening may lead to bulging ***(aneurysm formation)***. There are recognized stages in the evolution of atheroma: the ***fatty streak***, which may or may not be a direct stage; the fatty and ***fibrofatty plaque***, which is the characteristic manifestation; and then the complicated lesions that show ***calcification***, ***ulceration***, and ***thrombus*** formation. Hemorrhage into a plaque and rupture of a plaque may also occur.

Of the three types of arteriosclerosis, ***Mönkeberg's arteriosclerosis*** is the least frequent and the least serious. Found principally in large muscular arteries such as those of the upper and lower extremities, the lesion consists of masses of calcium in the media. It is apparently an age-related phenomenon and is rarely found in people under the age of 50 years. It is of little clinical significance because the lumen is rarely compromised.

Arterial and arteriolar sclerosis is the small vessel disease that is principally found in diabetics and hypertensives. Sustained arterial pressure of 90 mm diastolic and 140 mm systolic are accepted levels of the upper limits of normal blood pressure, above which vascular lesions appear to be more frequent. The vascular lesion consists of *hyaline arteriolosclerosis*, which also is frequently encountered in the elderly and in diabetics, and *hyperplastic arteriolosclerosis,* which is usually seen in hypertensives with acute severe hypertension (malignant hypertension). In addition to the hyperplastic lesion, these individuals may show *fibrinoid necrosis* of the arterioles. Hyaline arteriolosclerosis consists of pink smudging and thickening of the media of arterioles. This hyalinization appears to result from the leakage of plasma proteins into the media and the overproduction of basal lamina (type IV collagen) by SMCs. This thickening produces luminal compromise and can result in ischemia. The hyperplastic type has an "onion skin" appearance, which is the result of edema of the wall and proliferation of cells that are probably medial smooth muscle cells. The *fibrinoid* necrosis that usually accompanies this change is often eccentric, may result in focal hemorrhages ("flea bites"), and is often found in parenchymal organs, principally the kidney.

ARTERITIS AND ARTERIOLITIS

Although significantly less frequent than the vascular changes detailed above, inflammatory diseases of the blood vessels encompass a number of well-known and well-defined entities. Although serious inflammation is usually localized to arteries, veins and capillaries may also be involved, giving rise to terms such as ***vasculitis*** and ***angiitis***. These terms are often used as if they were equivalent to arteritis, but they are broader in meaning. The vasculitides can be classified on the basis of their pathogenesis, which includes infectious, immunologic, and unknown etiologies, or the size of the vessel they affect: large, medium, and small. We shall follow the latter approach.

Large Vessel Vasculitis. Two entities included in this category are ***giant cell*** or ***temporal arteritis***, and ***Takayasu's arteritis.*** Both affect the aorta and its major branches and both are a granulomatous type of inflammation.

Giant cell arteritis is characteristically found in adults over 50, and the temporal artery is a frequent site. Although it usually affects medium-sized vessels, it may be found in the aortic arch as well. Biopsy is usually required for diagnosis, but it is negative in a third or more of the patients because of the focal nature of the inflammatory process. Headache and visual symptoms are prominent, and there may be the sudden onset of blindness because of involvement of the ophthalmic artery.

Takayasu's arteritis produces visual disturbances and weak pulses in the upper extremities ***(pulseless disease)***. Of unknown etiology, it affects women predominantly, between the ages of about 15 and 40 and rarely after age 50. Originally described in Asia, it has now been seen worldwide. There is irregular thickening of the aorta, with granulomatous inflammation and fibrosis, and although it is classically found in the aortic arch, it may be found throughout the aorta or only in the descending thoracic and abdominal aorta. There is an early mononuclear adventitial inflammatory infiltrate that also surrounds the vasa vasorum. Later, the media is involved by mononuclear cells and some giant cells.

Medium Vessel Vasculitis. The two principal diseases in this category are polyarteritis nodosa and its variants, and Kawasaki disease.

Polyarteritis nodosa (PAN) is a systemic disease that in its classic form is a necrotizing arteritis that affects medium-sized vessels, typically renal, hepatic, coronary, and mesenteric arteries. This involvement is often eccentric and shows acute, subacute, and healed lesions. In the acute stage, there is a polymorphous infiltrate that includes polymorphonuclear leukocytes, eosinophils, and mononuclear cells. The weakened area of the vessel wall, often at branching points, may form aneurysms that are visible grossly (macroscopic form). It is a disease principally of young adults, although it also may afflict children. About 30% of the patients have hepatitis B antibodies, and there is an association with cytoplasmic antineutrophil antibodies *(C-ANCA)* of the perinuclear type *(P-ANCA)*.

Kawasaki syndrome is also known as ***mucocutaneous lymph node syndrome***. Although it sometimes involves the aorta, it is usually found in medium-sized and small arteries (frequently the coronary arteries). When it affects infants and young children, it is associated with the mucocutaneous lymph node syndrome. In the acute phase, there is fever, oral, and conjunctival reddening and erosion, edema of hands and feet, rash, and lymph node involvement. Aneurysms of the coronary artery may develop as sequelae in up to 20% of patients. The specific etiology is unknown, but an infectious etiology is suspected from the epidemiology of the disorder.

Small Vessel Vasculitis. This includes a number of (fortunately) uncommon syndromes: Wegener's granulomatosis, Churg-Strauss syndrome, microscopic polyangiitis (polyarteritis), Henoch-Schönlein purpura, essential cryoglobulinemic vasculitis, and cutaneous leukocytoclastic angiitis.

Wegener's granulomatosis is a granulomatous inflammatory process that produces a systemic illness that, if untreated, is usually fatal. Immunosuppressive therapy induces an improvement in over 90% of patients. The granulomas are most frequent in the respiratory tract, and ANCA, particularly the C-ANCA (cytoplasmic) is a good marker for the disease. The kidneys, the sinuses, and the nasopharynx are frequently involved. The vasculitis affects mostly small arteries and veins, although the glomerular capillaries may also be affected.

Churg-Strauss syndrome also affects the lungs. Vasulitis is similar to changes seen in PAN but it usually contains numerous eosinophils.

Buerger's disease (thromboangiitis obliterans) is a classic disorder that is particularly frequent in Jewish males. It involves intermediate and small arteries sequentially. Characteristically, veins and nerves are involved as well. Hypersensitivity to cigarettes (tobacco) appears to be the etiologic agent, but the mechanism is not entirely understood. There are microabscesses in the thrombosed vessels that can lead to gangrene. This condition is usually found in young adults (under 35) in contradistinction to atherosclerosis.

INFECTIOUS ARTERITIS

A number of infectious agents can lead to arterial inflammation. Syphilis is a well-known cause of inflammation of the vasa vasora, which leads to fusiform aneurysms of the thoracic aorta. ***Mycotic*** aneurysms result from direct bacterial involvement of the wall of the artery.

ANEURYSMS

The commonest cause of the bulges that occur in arterial walls, termed aneurysms, is atherosclerosis or atherosclerosis in concert with another disease, such as syphilis. These abnormal dilations can be found in many sites, and in vessels of virtually any size, but they are most frequent in the abdominal aorta. Aneurysms can be classified by their shape *(berry, saccular, fusiform)*, their location *(thoracic, abdominal, aortic)*, or their etiology *(atherosclerotic, congenital, dissecting, syphilitic)*. ***True*** aneurysms are surrounded by all or at least part of the vessel wall, whereas ***false*** aneurysms result from a rupture of the vessel wall and are for the most part surrounded by clot (hematoma). Important types of aneurysms include:

Atherosclerotic aneurysms are saccular or fusiform, most common in abdominal aorta but are found in large musculoelastic vessels, too.

Syphilitic aneurysms are usually found in thoracic aorta. They result from inflammation in vasa vasorum and are associated with ''tree bark'' appearance of atherosclerosis and medial fibrosis.

Dissecting aneurysms are really aortic dissections, not true aneurysms; they result from a burrowing of blood (hematoma) along the wall between the inner and middle third. Cystic medial degeneration (''necrosis'') is usually present, as is clinical hypertension. In addition, there is an association with Marfan's syndrome. Type A dissection involves the ascending aorta, or the ascending and descending, whereas type B involves only the descending aorta.

Berry aneurysms occur at the circle of Willis, usually at branch points, as a result of congenital thinning of the media.

Mycotic aneurysms result from focal bacterial infection of the arterial wall.

False aneurysms result from a ruptured vessel with organized hematoma.

AV aneurysms are arteriovenous malformations with bulging; they may be congenital or acquired, such as a AV fistula made for dialysis.

Complications of all aneurysms include rupture, thrombosis, and embolism. Mural thrombosis can propagate and result in occlusion or dissection; blood going into or behind a mural thrombus can result in rupture. Portions of thrombi may dislodge, resulting in embolization. Emboli may also contain atheromatous material.

VENOUS DISEASES

Varicose veins. Veins contain valves that segment the column of blood returning to the heart. When these become incompetent, the full weight of the blood under the force of gravity is exerted on the wall of the vein. Obstruction to flow of any kind will augment this effect and cause dilation of the vein, which in turn leads to incompetency of the valves. Thus, ***phlebectasia*** often precedes ***phlebosclerosis***. The two together are seen in the dilated tortuous veins, particularly of the lower extremities, known as varicose veins.

Thrombophlebitis and phlebothrombosis. If an inflammatory process involves a vein wall, it can become secondarily thrombosed, leading to thrombophlebitis. Phlebothrombosis is simply a clot in a vein that is not inflamed, but because long-standing clots inevitably lead to some inflammation, the two are in fact virtually one entity. Local edema results from the venous obstruction, but pulmonary embolism is the most significant complication. Because the lower extremities are the commonest site of thrombophlebitis/phlebothrombosis, predisposing causes include heart failure, pregnancy, neoplasms, and such prolonged immobilization among others.

Tumors

Hemangiomas, benign tumors, and tumor-like lesions of blood vessels are very common, especially on the skin. There are also lesions of intermediate aggressiveness. Benign tumors include hemangiomas, classified into several subtypes, such as capillary, cavernous, and epithelial. Tumors of low grade malignancy are classified as hemangioendotheliomas. The aggressive malignant tumors are ***angiosarcomas***, ***hemangiopericytomas***, and ***Kaposi's sarcoma.*** The latter is common in AIDS patients.

THE HEART

The most important heart diseases, which account for 85% to 90% of cardiac deaths, include

- ischemic heart disease
- hypertensive heart disease and pulmonary hypertensive disease (cor pulmonale)
- valvular diseases
- congenital heart diseases

These may, in some instances, be related. For example, calcific aortic valve stenosis may impair coronary artery filling, leading to ischemic heart disease. Hypertensive heart disease may evolve to ischemic heart disease because hypertension is a risk factor for atherosclerosis.

Ischemic Heart Disease

Ischemic heart disease includes a spectrum of cardiac disorders stemming from an imbalance between the blood being supplied to the heart and the demand by the heart for that blood. This imbalance gives rise to ischemia, which not only results in hypoxia or anoxia, but also reduces the availability of nutrients and slows the removal of metabolites.

In ischemia, the flow of blood being supplied to the heart through the coronary arteries is often restricted because of stenosis or occlusion by atherosclerotic plaques with or without thrombi. Based on the rate of development of the stenosis, its extent, and the manner in which the myocardium responds to these events, four distinct clinical syndromes have been recognized: (a) angina pectoris, (b) myocardial infarcts, (c) chronic ischemic heart disease, and (d) sudden cardiac death.

ANGINA PECTORIS

Angina pectoris is characterized by intermittent attacks of substernal or precordial chest discomfort caused by transient myocardial ischemia that is not sufficient to cause necrosis. There are three variant forms of angina: (a) stable, (b) variant (Prinzmetal's), and (c) unstable (crescendo).

Stable angina is the most common form, and it generally occurs during exercise. It is associated with depression of the electrocardiographic ST segment, which results from ischemia in the subendocardium. The condition is relieved by rest and vasodilators such as nitroglycerin. The pathogenesis is thought to result from reduction of coronary perfusion by coronary artery atherosclerosis.

Variant angina occurs at rest. There is elevation of the electrocardiographic ST segment, indicating transmural ischemia. It results from vasospasm and is relieved by vasodilators.

Unstable angina is induced in most patients by fissuring, ulceration, or rupture of atherosclerotic plaques with superimposed thrombosis. There may be embolization and/or vasospasm. Microinfarcts may occur. Platelet activation and aggregation are responsible for the widespread thrombosis and vasospasm of small arteries.

MYOCARDIAL INFARCTION

Myocardial infarction is the most important form of ischemic heart disease and the leading cause of death in the United States. There are two types of myocardial infarctions, transmural and subendocardial.

Transmural infarcts are the most common and are characterized by coagulation necrosis that involves from more than half up to the full thickness of the ventricular wall in the distribution of a single coronary artery. They are generally the result of coronary atherosclerotic plaques that are ruptured with superimposed thrombi. These are occlusive in about 90% of cases.

Subendocardial myocardial infarcts are defined as regions of coagulation necrosis involving the inner third to half of the ventricular wall, and they often extend beyond the perfusion zone of a single coronary artery. They are most often associated with diffuse coronary artery stenosis.

Transmural infarcts are most often found (40% to 50%) in the distribution of the left anterior descending branch of the left main coronary artery, the anterior wall of the left ventricle near the apex, and the anterior two thirds of the interventricular septum. Occlusion of the right coronary artery is next in frequency (30% to 40%), and this gives rise to infarctions in the posterior wall of the left ventricle, the posterior one third of the interventricular septum, and, on some occasions, the posterior right ventricular wall. The left circumflex coronary artery is occluded in approximately 15% to 20% of cases, and this causes infarctions in the lateral wall of the left ventricle. The right ventricle is rarely infarcted.

The diagnosis of myocardial infarction is based on the following:

1. Symptoms, including severe substernal or precordial pain, that may radiate to the left shoulder, arm, or jaw. In addition, there may be sweating, vomiting, nausea, or dyspnea.
2. Electrocardiographic changes that are manifested by new Q waves.
3. Elevation levels of serum creatine kinase (CK) and lactic dehydrogenase (LDH). These levels are sensitive indicators of myocardial infarction. The CK rises above baseline levels between 4 and 8 hours postinfarction and returns to normal in approximately 4 days. The LDH level begins to rise at around 24 hours, peaks in 3 to 6 days, and may not return to normal until after 2 weeks. Elevation of the isoenzymes of CK (CK-MB) and LDH (LDH_1) are more specific for diagnosing myocardial infarction.

Complications of myocardial infarction include arrhythmias, left ventricular failure leading to pulmonary edema, cardiogenic shock, rupture of the left ventricular free wall, interventricular septum and/or papillary muscles, left ventricular aneurysm, and mural thrombi that may give rise to thromboemboli.

CHRONIC ISCHEMIC HEART DISEASE

Chronic ischemic heart disease is found in patients who develop congestive heart failure as a result of ischemic myocardial damage. The patients are often, but not always, elderly and usually have a history of angina or previous myocardial infarctions. Most cases are a result of postinfarction cardiac decompensation.

SUDDEN CARDIAC DEATH

Sudden cardiac death is defined as unexpected death from cardiac causes early after the onset of symptoms or without symptoms. The cause is multifactorial but usually associated with myocardial ischemia due to acute changes in coronary artery flow superimposed on long-standing atherosclerosis. Arrhythmias arise in the ischemic myocardium or less frequently in the conduction system.

Hypertensive Heart Disease

Hypertensive heart disease is the second most common cause of heart disease. It results from the increased demands of systemic (above 140/90 mmHg) or pulmonary hypertension. It is diagnosed on the basis of a history of hypertension and left ventricular hypertrophy without other cardiac pathology that might have induced these changes.

Systemic hypertension induces pressure overload in the left ventricle, resulting in concentric hypertrophy. This increases the ratio of the wall thickness to the radius of the ventricular chamber and the weight of the heart. In addition, the increased thickness of the wall imparts stiffness to the wall and impairs ventricular filling. The signs of decompensated hypertensive heart disease include dilatation of the ventricular chamber, thinning of the wall, and enlargement of the external dimensions of the heart. Microscopically, there is enlargement of myocytes. With time, there is variation in cell size and shape, loss of myofibrils, and increased interstitial fibrosis.

Depending on the severity of the hypertension, patients may die of unrelated causes, may develop ischemic heart disease because of the potentiating effects of hypertension on coronary atherosclerosis, or may suffer progressive renal damage, cerebral vascular disease, congestive heart failure, or sudden cardiac death.

RIGHT-SIDED HYPERTENSIVE HEART DISEASE—COR PULMONALE

Pulmonary hypertensive heart disease is right ventricular enlargement resulting from pulmonary hypertension caused by diseases of the lung or pulmonary vessels, disorders affecting chest movement, and conditions causing arteriolar constriction.

Acute cor pulmonale refers to dilatation of the right ventricle after massive pulmonary embolism. *Chronic cor pulmonale* is right ventricular hypertrophy with late-stage dilatation. It is secondary to obstruction of pulmonary arteries or arterioles (*e.g.*, embolism or compression and/or obliteration of septal capillaries, such as chronic obstructive pulmonary disease).

Valvular Heart Disease

Diseases of heart valves cause valvular insufficiency (reverse flow) and/or stenosis (impeding forward flow), the latter resulting from the valve failing to open completely and the former resulting from the valve failing to close completely. Abnormalities in flow around the diseased valves produce murmurs (abnormal heart sounds).

Valvular heart disease can be congenital or acquired. Valvular insufficiency can result from diseases intrinsic to the valve cusps and/or damage/distortion of the aorta, mitral annulus, papillary muscles, chordae tendineae, or ventricular free wall. It may arise acutely or chronically. Stenosis is always associated with abnormalities of the cusp and is generally the result of a chronic process. The mitral and/or aortic valves are most often affected.

Degenerative calcific aortic valve stenosis is the most common valve abnormality. It can be congenital (when obstruction is present at birth) or acquired. The latter is most often associated with age-related degeneration, with lesions due to rheumatic heart disease being relatively rare (10%). Morphologically, these valves have calcified masses within the aortic cusps that eventually make their way into the sinus of Valsalva, preventing opening of the cusp. Most cases are detected clinically in the eighth or ninth decade. In approximately 1% to 2% of the population, aortic valves are congenitally bicuspid and are not abnormal at birth; however, they are predisposed to degenerative calcification in later life. These most often become symptomatic in the sixth to seventh decade.

Mitral valve prolapse (floppy valve) is a condition in which one or both mitral leaflets balloon back into the left atrium during systole. This is a very common condition (*e.g.*, in 5% to 10% of the U.S. population) and is most often found in young women. It is characterized most often by a midsystolic "click" on auscultation. Histologically, the fibrosus layer of the valve is thinned and there is thickening of the spongiousa layer with frequent myxomatous changes in the chordae tendineae. The cause is unknown, but developmental defects in collagen are suspected. It is seen in patients with Marfan's disease. Complications are rare, approximately 3%, but include infective endocarditis, mitral insufficiency, stroke, systemic infarcts, and arrhythmias.

Rheumatic fever is an acute, often recurrent inflammatory disease of children, most often between the ages of 5 and 15 years. Younger and older age groups are susceptible, however. It is characterized by fever, arthralgia, and a group of clinical findings that are categorized as major and minor manifestations. The major manifestations include

- migratory polyarthritis of large joints
- carditis
- subcutaneous nodules
- erythema marginatum of the skin
- Sydenham's chorea

Minor manifestations include: (a) fever, (b) arthralgia, (c) elevated acute phase reactants, and (d) leukocytosis. Diagnosis is made based on the Jones criteria, which include evidence of a preceding group A streptococcal infection (beta-hemolytic) and either two major manifestations or one major and two minor manifestations. The disease is considered to be a postinfectious immunologic disease that arises from immune responses to streptococcal antigens that produce antibodies that cross-react with human tissue antigens, or a form of autoimmune reaction elicited by the infectious agents. Rheumatic fever causes a pancarditis that is characterized by foci of fibrinoid necrosis surrounded by lymphocytes, macrophages, and histiocytes called Anitschkow or Aschoff cells. This pattern of inflammation is called an Aschoff body and is pathognomonic for rheumatic fever. During the acute disease, Aschoff bodies can be found in any layer of the heart. In the pericardium, they are found concomitant with either a serofibrinous or fibrinous exudate. In the myocardium, they are located in interstitial tissue, often perivascular. The endocardium, in particular but not exclusively, and the mitral and aortic valves characteristically have regions of fibrinoid necrosis along the valvular cusps (line of closure) that are 1 to 2 mm in diameter and are called verrucae. They are not Aschoff bodies. These often resolve or give rise to minimal fibrosis.

The chronic disease produces deformity primarily of the mitral and/or aortic valves due to fibrosis. Leaflet thickening, commissural fission, and shortening, thickening, and fusion of the chordae tendineae are most observed.

The incidence of acute arthritis increases with age. The skin lesions are characterized by subcutaneous nodules and erythema marginatum.

The symptoms of acute carditis stem primarily from myocarditis, which may cause arrhythmias, in particular atrial fibrillation. Myocarditis can give rise to thrombi with subsequent thromboembolism to distal sites, such as brain or other internal organs. In addition, myocarditis may cause cardiac dilatation leading to mitral insufficiency and ultimately cardiac failure. The latter is a significant cause of death in these cases. The chronic form of the disease manifests itself most frequently as mitral valve stenosis and less frequently as combined mitral and aortic valve stenosis. Mitral stenosis leads to dilatation of the left atrium with possible thrombus formation and pulmonary congestion. The latter over time leads to right ventricular hypertrophy.

INFECTION OF CARDIAC VALVES

Infective endocarditis is characterized by colonization or invasion of heart valves and/or endocardium by microorganisms, which leads to the formation of friable, bulky vegetations containing organisms. The condition has been divided into acute and subacute forms that describe a spectrum of clinicopathologic findings. These are generally determined by the virulence of the organism and by previous valvular disease. The ***acute form*** is described as being highly destructive, imposed on previously normal valves, and caused by highly virulent organisms, and it is frequently fatal. The ***subacute*** form is imposed on previously injured valves by low virulence organisms; it commences insidiously and has a protracted course. The *Streptococcus viridans* group is the most common cause of the subacute form, and *Staphylococcus aureus* is the most common cause of the acute form. Other bacteria and fungi have been incriminated as well. The mitral and aortic valves are most commonly affected in most cases; however, in intravenous drug abusers, right-sided valves are also involved. The most common conditions that predispose to infectious endocarditis include congenital heart disease, rheumatic fever, myxomatous mitral valve, and degenerative calcific aortic stenosis. Complications include those confined to (a) the heart (e.g., valvular stenosis or insufficiency), (b) embolic complication (*e.g.,* infarcts or metastatic infection), and (c) renal complications, which include infarcts, focal glomerulonephritis due to microemboli, and immune complex glomerulonephritis.

NONBACTERIAL ENDOCARDITIS

Nonbacterial thrombotic endocarditis (marantic endocarditis) is found in debilitated patients. It is characterized by the deposition of small, sterile fibrin thrombi on previously normal valves on either side of the heart. It is thought to result from activation of blood coagulation by underlying disease states (*e.g.,* sepsis or cancer).

Endocarditis of systemic lupus erythematosus

(Libman-Sacks disease) results from valvulitis of the mitral and tricuspid valve. It is characterized by small, sterile vegetations on the undersurface of the mitral and tricuspid valves, chordae tendineae, and mural endocardium of atria or ventricles.

Carcinoid heart disease is caused by bioactive products produced by intestinal carcinoid tumors that have typically metastasized to the liver. This heart disease is characterized by fibrous intimal thickenings of the endocardium of the right ventricle and/or tricuspid and pulmonic valves.

Prosthetic valves, used to replace damaged valves, are either mechanical or bioprosthetic. The most frequent complications of using these valves include thromboembolism, partial dehiscence, infective endocarditis, structural deterioration, and nonstructural dysfunction (*e.g.*, hemolytic anemia).

Congenital Heart Disease

Congenital heart disease is a general term used to describe abnormalities of the heart or great vessels that are present from birth. These disorders arise from faulty embryogenesis during gestational weeks 3 through 8 when cardiovascular structures undergo development. Most are associated with live births. More than 85% of the estimated 25,000 infants born annually with congenital malformations of the heart are likely to reach adulthood.

Congenital heart disease is the most common type of heart disease among children, with reported incidences of 6 to 8 per 1000 live, full-term births. Although the cause of congenital heart disease is unknown in more than 90% of patients, chromosomal defects, viruses, chemicals, and radiation are suspected. Siblings of an affected child have a two- to tenfold increase in congenital heart disease, pointing to genetic influences. In addition, maternal rubella infection in the first trimester of pregnancy has also been incriminated.

Congenital defects fall primarily into two major categories: shunts or obstructions. A ***shunt*** is an abnormal communication between chambers or blood vessels (or both). When blood from the right side of the heart enters the left side *(right-to-left shunt)*, the skin and mucous membranes become cyanotic as a result of poorly oxygenated blood entering the systemic circulation. This type of shunt is called cyanotic congenital heart disease, with examples being *tetralogy of Fallot*, *transposition of the great arteries (TGA)*, *persistent truncus arteriosus*, *tricuspid atresia*, and *total anomalous pulmonary venous connection*. The consequence of these abnormal communications is that septic emboli arising in peripheral veins can bypass the normal filtration of the lungs and enter the systemic circulation. These are called paradoxical emboli.

LEFT-TO-RIGHT SHUNTS

Left-to-right shunts are not associated with cyanosis but can result in progressive pulmonary hypertension and right ventricular overload with hypertrophy. The presence of the shunt may expose the pulmonary circulation to increased volume or pressure in congenital heart disease. These shunts include ***atrial septal defects (ASD)*** and shunts associated with both increased pulmonary blood flow and pressure, including ***ventricular septal defects (VSD)*** and ***patent ductus arteriosus (PDA)***. The pressure on the right side of the heart can rise to exceed that on the left, eventually reversing the shunt to right to left and creating what is called late cyanotic congenital heart disease or Eisenmenger's syndrome. This phenomenon is seen in VSD, ASD, atrioventricular septal defects, and PDA. Once significant irreversible pulmonary hypertension develops, the structural defects of congenital heart disease are considered irreparable.

Clinical findings frequently associated with severe long-standing cyanosis include clubbing of the tips of the fingers and toes (hypertrophic osteoarthropathy), and polycythemia. Cerebral thrombosis is also seen on occasion.

Some developmental anomalies of the heart produce obstructions to flow because of abnormal narrowing of the chambers, valves, or blood vessels. These include valvular stenosis or atresias and are called obstructive congenital heart disease. Coarctation of the aorta, aortic valvular stenosis, and pulmonary valvular stenosis are examples of obstructive diseases. Altered hemodynamics in congenital heart disease often causes cardiac dilatation and/or hypertrophy. A decrease in the volume and muscle mass of the cardiac chamber is called hypoplasia if it occurs before birth and atrophy if it develops after birth.

Left-to-right shunts (late cyanosis) include the following diseases:

1. ***Atrial septal defects*** are abnormal openings in the atrial septum that allow free communication of the blood between the right and left atria. They are the most common congenital cardiac anomalies that may first come to attention in adults. There are three major types of ASDs, depending on their location in the septum. The secundum-type ASD represents approximately 90% of all ASDs. It results from a deficiency or fenestration of the embryonic septum primum, deficiency of septum secundum, or both. The second type of anomaly is found in the septum primum and represents about 5% of ASDs. It occurs low in the atrial septum and is seen especially in Down syndrome patients. Finally, sinus venosus defect is located high in the atrial septum, posterior to the fossa ovalis, near the entrance of the superior vena cava. It accounts for about 5% of ASDs and is commonly accompanied

by anomalous connections of right pulmonary veins to superior vena cava or right atrium.

Atrial septal defects result in left-to-right shunts. In general, ASDs are well tolerated if small (*e.g.*, less than 1 cm in diameter). Even larger defects do not usually constitute serious problems during the first decades of life when flow is from left to right. As this continues, volume hypertrophy of the right atrium and right ventricle develop. A right-to-left shunt may develop later and cause cyanosis. Pulmonary hypertension as well as right ventricular and atrial hypertrophy can develop. Surgical closure is the mode of treatment.

2. ***Ventricular septal defects*** are abnormal openings in the ventricular septum that allow free communication between right and left ventricles. They are the most common congenital cardiac anomaly, often associated with other structural defects such as tetralogy, transposition, and truncus arteriosus. In addition, PDA, ASD, and aortic coarctation are sometimes associated. VSDs are classified according to size and may range from a few millimeters to sufficiently large to create virtually a common ventricle. The functional significance of the VSD depends on the size and the presence or absence of pulmonary stenosis. Approximately 50% close spontaneously and the remainder are generally well tolerated for years. They produce loud holosystolic murmurs. Complications include aortic insufficiency, right ventricular hypertrophy, and pulmonary hypertension. The latter two are present from birth. Ultimately, irreversible pulmonary vascular disease develops in all patients with large unoperated VSDs, leading to shunt reversal, cyanosis, clubbing, and polycythemia. Patients with these lesions are predisposed to infectious endocarditis when lesions are small to moderate size, because of the production of endocardial jet lesions. These defects can close spontaneously, but surgical correction is indicated in children who are older and who have large defects, before pulmonary hypertension and obstructive pulmonary vascular disease develops.

3. ***Patent ductus arteriosus*** results when the ductus arteriosus remains open after birth. The ductus usually closes functionally within the first day or two of life. A patent ductus gives rise to a continuous heart murmur that is described as a "machinery-like" murmur. Obstructive pulmonary vascular disease eventually ensues with reversal of flow, and ultimately cyanosis, clubbing, polycythemia, and right ventricular failure can occur. At this point, lesions are inoperable. In addition to surgical treatment, pharmacologic closure appears to be promising (e.g., indomethacin to suppress prostaglandin D synthesis).

4. ***Atrial ventricular septal defects*** result from abnormal development of the embryologic AV canal in which the superior and inferior endocardial cushions fail to fuse adequately, resulting in incomplete closure of the AV septum and inadequate formation of the septal tricuspid and anterior mitral leaflets. Four potential lesions are possible. The two most common combinations are partial AV septal defect and complete AV septal defect. More than one third of all patients with complete AV septal defect have Down syndrome. Treatment is surgical.

RIGHT-TO-LEFT SHUNTS

Right-to-left shunts (early cyanosis) include the following diseases:

1. ***Tetralogy of Fallot***, the most common form of cyanotic congenital heart disease, is characterized by (a) ventricular septal defect, (b) obstruction to the right ventricular outflow track (subpulmonary stenosis), (c) an aorta that overrides the ventricular septal defect, and (d) right ventricular hypertrophy. Untreated patients often survive into adult life. The severity of obstruction to right ventricular outflow determines the direction of blood flow. The shunt may be left to right if the subpulmonary stenosis is mild. As the obstruction increases, right-to-left shunting predominates and cyanosis ensues. Most infants with this tetralogy are cyanotic from birth or soon thereafter. Surgical repair is possible for classic tetralogy of Fallot.
2. ***Transposition of great arteries*** is characterized by the aorta arising from the right ventricle, and the pulmonary artery arising from the left ventricle. The essential defect is that the aorta, arising from the right ventricle, lies anterior and to the right of the pulmonary artery, in contrast to the positions in the normal heart. The resulting separation of the systemic and pulmonary circulations is incompatible with postnatal life without a shunt. This malformation, common in the offspring of diabetic mothers, causes cyanosis from birth. Patients with transposition and a VSD (35%) have a stable shunt. Those with only a patent foramen ovale or PDA (65%) have an unstable shunt that tends to close and requires surgical intervention to open a right-to-left communication. The right ventricle hypertrophies and the left ventricle becomes atrophic. Without surgery, most patients die within the first few months of life.
3. ***Truncus arteriosus*** arises from a developmental failure of separation of the embryologic truncus arteriosus into the aorta and pulmonary artery. This results in a single great artery that receives blood from both ventricles, accompanied by an underlying VSD that gives rise to the systemic, pulmonary, and coronary circulations. This condition is associated with a large number of concomitant defects. There is early systemic cyanosis as well as increased pulmonary

blood flow. Surgical correction is usually attempted at an early age and is often successful.

4. ***Tricuspid atresia*** is characterized by complete occlusion of the tricuspid valve orifice. It results from unequal division of the AV canal and is almost always associated with a hypoplastic right ventricle. Circulation is maintained by a right-to-left shunt through an ASD or patent foramen ovale. A VSD is also present and allows communication between the left ventricle and the great artery that arises from the hypoplastic right ventricle. Cyanosis is present virtually from birth and there is a high mortality in the first weeks or months of life. Surgical correction is possible.
5. ***Total anomalous pulmonary venous connection*** is characterized by a condition in which no pulmonary veins directly join the left atrium because the common pulmonary vein fails to develop or becomes atretic, causing primitive systemic venous channels from the lungs to remain patent. Venous blood from these anomalies may drain into the right atrium or a variety of other veins. A patent foramen ovale or ASD is always present, allowing pulmonary venous blood to enter the left atrium. Consequences include volume and pressure hypertrophy of the right atrium and right ventricle leading to dilatation. Cyanosis may be present.

OBSTRUCTIVE CONGENITAL ANOMALIES

Obstructive congenital anomalies include the following diseases:

1. ***Coarctation of the aorta*** is one of the more frequent structural anomalies. Males are affected three to four times more frequently than females, although it is common in females with Turner's syndrome. There are two classic forms: (a) the infantile form, a tubular hyperplasia of the aortic arch proximal to a patent ductus that is often symptomatic in early childhood, and (b) an adult postductal form in which there is discrete infolding of the aorta just opposite the closed ductus arteriosus. Clinical manifestations depend almost entirely on the severity of the narrowing and the patency of the ductus arteriosus. Coarctation is often associated with other defects (*e.g.,* bicuspid aortic valve, congenital aortic stenosis, ASD, VSD, mitral regurgitation, and berry aneurysms).

Preductal coarctation leads to clinical manifestations in early life, and many infants do not survive the neonatal period. Right ventricular failure may appear very early. Delivery of unsaturated blood through the ductus arteriosus produces cyanosis in the lower half of the body, whereas the head and arms are unaffected because their blood supply derives from vessels having origins proximal to the ductus.

Children with postductal coarctation are asymptomatic and the disease may go unrecognized. Typically, there is hypertension in the upper extremities, but there are weak pulses and lower blood pressure in the lower extremities, associated with signs of arterial insufficiency (*e.g.,* claudication and coldness).

With uncomplicated coarctation, surgical resection and subsequent end-to-end anastomoses or prosthetic grafts are successful treatment modalities.

2. ***Pulmonary stenosis or atresia with intact ventricular septum*** is a relatively common anomaly that may occur isolated or concomitant with other defects. When the valve is entirely atretic, the anomaly is commonly associated with a hypoplastic right ventricle and an ASD. With atresia, there is no communication between the right ventricle and the lungs, so blood flow bypasses the right ventricle through an ASD and enters the lungs through a PDA. Right ventricular hypertrophy often develops. Mild stenosis may be asymptomatic and compatible with long life. Cyanosis is most severe and appears early with smaller valvular orifices. The isolated valvular stenosis can be corrected surgically.

Miscellaneous Cardiac Diseases

Cardiac transplantation is now frequently performed for severe and intractable heart failure most commonly due to ischemic heart disease and dilated cardiomyopathy. Allograft rejection is a major postoperative problem and endomyocardial biopsy is the only reliable means of diagnosing acute cardiac rejection. Rejection is characterized by interstitial lymphocytic inflammation that, in its more advanced stages, damages adjacent myocytes. More severe stages of rejection are accompanied by extensive myocyte necrosis and frequently inflammatory injury to the vasculature that may lead to edema and hemorrhage. Infections are another significant problem. In addition, lymphomas related to Epstein-Barr virus have been observed. Finally, the major current limitation to long-term success has to do with progressive, diffuse, stenosing, intimal proliferation of the coronary arteries (graft arteriosclerosis). This may lead to myocardial infarction in patients that, because the hearts are denervated, may not experience chest pain.

Neoplasms of the heart are rare. The most common primary tumor of the heart in adults is the *myxoma*, which is located in the atria in about 90% of cases, but can be found in all four chambers. The major clinical manifestation of this neoplasm results from a "ball-valve" obstruction of valves, embolization, or clinical manifestations of fever and malaise. Although not a common site, the heart is the recipient of *metastatic neoplasms*. The most common are those stemming from the lung and breast. In addition, *melanomas, leukemias,* and *lymphomas* may involve the heart.

Diseases of the Pericardium

Pericardial lesions are almost always associated with disease in other portions of the heart or surrounding structures, or they are secondary to systemic disorders.

Pericarditis is usually secondary to a variety of cardiac diseases, to systemic disorders, or to metastasis from neoplasms arising in remote sites. Pericarditis can be caused by infectious agents such as viruses, pyogenic bacteria, tuberculosis, fungi, and other parasites. In addition, a variety of other disease conditions can cause pericarditis, including rheumatic fever, systemic lupus erythematosus, scleroderma, and heart surgery. Finally, miscellaneous conditions can give rise to pericarditis, such as myocardial infarction, uremia, trauma, and radiation.

Chronic or healed pericarditis is characterized by fibrous adhesions extending from the epicardium to the pericardial sac. These vary from being thin and delicate, to a fibrotic process that can completely obliterate the pericardial sac. In the latter instance, the fibrous adhesions can interfere with and restrict cardiac action *(constrictive pericarditis).*

Finally, suppurative or caseous pericarditis, previous cardiac surgery, or radiation to the mediastinum can give rise to adhesive ***mediastinal pericarditis***. In these cases, the pericardial sac is obliterated and adherence of the external aspect of the parietal layer to surrounding structures produces a great strain on cardiac function. The increased workload causes hypertrophy and dilatation mimicking dilated cardiomyopathy.

When excess fluid, usually blood, fills the pericardial sac, there is severe restriction of heart function, which can lead to death. This is called ***cardiac tamponade***.

Heart Failure

Congestive heart failure occurs either because of a decreased myocardial capacity to contract or because of an inability to fill the cardiac chambers with blood. Most instances of heart failure are the consequences of progressive deterioration of myocardial contractile function *(systolic dysfunction).* As often occurs with ischemic injury, pressure or volume overload leads to dilated cardiomyopathy. In some instances, there is inability of the heart chambers to expand sufficiently during diastole to accommodate an adequate ventricular blood volume *(diastolic dysfunction)* as occurs with massive left ventricular hypertrophy, myocardial fibrosis, deposition of amyloid, or restrictive pericarditis. In either instance, there is diminished cardiac output *(forward failure)* or damming back of blood in the venous system *(backward failure)*, or both.

Central to congestive heart failure is cardiac hypertrophy. This is a compensatory response of the myocardium to an increased workload. In pressure-overloaded ventricles resulting from hypertension or aortic stenosis, the hypertrophic change is concentric. In volume-overloaded ventricles, such as in mitral regurgitation, the hypertrophy is associated with dilatation of the free wall, giving rise to eccentric hypertrophy. With an increasing workload, cardiac dilatation progresses beyond the point at which adequate myocardial tension can be generated. Stroke volume and cardiac output are diminished and death often ensues.

Although heart failure is often treated as either a left-sided or a right-sided disease, because the vascular system is a closed circuit, failure of one side cannot exist for long without eventually producing excessive strain on the other side, terminating in total heart failure.

Left-sided heart failure is most often caused by ischemic heart disease, hypertension, aortic and mitral valvular diseases, and myocardial diseases. The left ventricle is usually hypertrophied and often dilated. Enlargement of the left atrium is frequently present. Hydrostatic pressure in pulmonary veins mounts and impacts on capillaries, resulting in pulmonary congestion and edema. In long-standing cases, hemoglobin from extravasated intra-alveolar erythrocytes is phagocytized by macrophages and converted to hemosiderin. These hemosiderin-containing macrophages are called *heart failure cells.* The clinical manifestations of these conditions are dyspnea, orthopnea, and paroxysmal nocturnal dyspnea.

Left-sided heart failure decreases cardiac output, which causes reduction in renal perfusion, activating the renin–angiotensin–aldosterone system, which induces retention of salt and water with consequent expansion of the interstitial fluid and blood volumes. This contributes to pulmonary edema. There is also acute tubular necrosis due to the ischemia caused by renal hypoperfusion.

Hypoxic encephalopathy gives rise to irritability, reduced attention span, and restlessness, which may progress to stupor and coma.

Right-sided heart failure occurs in its pure form in cor pulmonale. Usually, however, it is a result of left-sided heart failure. With right-sided heart failure, the liver is slightly increased in size and weight, and on cut section it displays the prominent "nutmeg" pattern of chronic passive congestion. This is composed of congested red centers of liver lobules surrounded by paler and sometimes fatty peripheral lesions. Central lobular necrosis with sinusoidal congestion can also be observed. There is also congestion of the kidneys, leading to greater fluid retention, peripheral edema, and more pronounced azotemia than with left-sided failure.

Right-sided heart failure leads to elevated pressure in the portal vein. Splenic congestion is observed. Peripheral edema of subcutaneous tissues is seen, especially over the ankles. Also, pleural and pericardial effusions are observed, particularly in the right thoracic cavity; symptoms in the brain due to venous congestion and hypoxia are essentially the same as in patients with left-sided heart failure.

Cardiomyopathies

Cardiomyopathies may be idiopathic or acquired. There are three functional patterns: (a) dilated, (b) hypertrophic, and (c) restrictive.

Dilated cardiomyopathy is a systolic disorder characterized by the gradual development of cardiac failure due to hypertrophy and dilatation of all four chambers of the heart. Acquired dilated cardiomyopathy is seen with infective myocarditis, hemochromatosis, chronic anemia, alcohol abuse, adriamycin treatment, and sarcoidosis.

Hypertrophic cardiomyopathy is characterized as a diastolic disorder caused by massive myocardial hypertrophy which, classically, has a disproportionate thickening of the ventricular septum as compared to the left ventricular free wall *(asymmetric septal hypertrophy).* The left ventricular outflow track can be narrowed during systole when the septum is markedly thickened at the level of the mitral valve. Histologically, muscle fibers are markedly enlarged, there is haphazard disarray of myocytes, and there is interstitial fibrosis. Acquired hypertrophic cardiomyopathy is seen in Friedreich's ataxia, glycogen storage disease, and infants of diabetic mothers.

Restrictive cardiomyopathy is a diastolic disease in which there is impedance of diastolic relaxation and left ventricular filling without an effect on ventricular contraction. The ventricles are normal to slightly enlarged, the cavities are not dilated, and the myocardium is firm. Both atria are often dilated. Histologically, diffuse interstitial fibrosis is noted. Acquired restrictive cardiomyopathy is observed in amyloidosis, radiation fibrosis, endomyocardial fibrosis, and Loeffler's endomyocarditis.

Myocarditis

Myocarditis is inflammation of heart muscle resulting in necrosis of muscle fibers and a leukocytic infiltrate. Most cases are of viral origin. Coxsackieviruses A and B, ECHO (enteric cytopathogenic human orphan) virus, and influenza viruses A and B are mostly commonly implicated.

ANEMIAS

Anemia, in most instances, is defined as a reduction in red blood cell mass below normal limits. This is measured by quantitating the number of red blood cells, the volume of packed red blood cells (hematocrit), or the reduction in hemoglobin concentration. In some instances, such as carbon monoxide poisoning, anemia may result from a reduction in the oxygen-carrying capacity of red blood cells. Anemias can be classified according to their etiology; to whether the red cells are normocytic, microcytic, or macrocytic; or to the mechanism by which the anemia occurs, which lumps a variety of etiologies together. Whatever the cause, there are certain clinical signs and symptoms that are characteristic of anemia. Included are pale skin that is often thin and inelastic, weakness, fatigue, brittle nails (particularly in iron deficiency anemia), and atrophic glossitis, found in iron deficiency anemia and megaloblastic anemias. Fatty change and coagulation necrosis are frequent histologic findings in the myocardium, liver, kidney, and central nervous system.

Anemias Resulting from Blood Loss

Acute blood loss (hemorrhage) results in hypovolemia, which may lead to shock and sometimes death. The hypovolemia results in shifts of interstitial water to the vascular compartment, leading to hemodilution and a lowering of the hematocrit. The peripheral blood morphology remains unchanged early, but erythropoietin production, stimulated by the reduced oxygen, leads to bone marrow hyperplasia, increasing reticulocyte (polychromatophilic macrocytes) counts, which peak at around 7 days. Iron deficiency may result if hemorrhage is severe and external.

Chronic blood loss leads to anemia when the blood loss exceeds the bone marrow's ability to replace the lost red blood cells. Blood loss is the most frequent cause of anemia. Conditions in which this is found include hemorrhage from the gastrointestinal tract and menstrual bleeding. In addition, conditions leading to iron deficiency, such as malnutrition, malabsorption, and increased demands for iron (as in pregnancy), can lead to anemias identical to that of chronic blood loss.

Hemolytic Anemias

Hemolytic anemias are caused by inherited or acquired intracorpuscular or acquired extracorpuscular abnormalities. They are characterized by premature destruction of red blood cells, accumulation of hemoglobin catabolism products, and bone marrow hyperplasia leading to reticulocytosis. If the destruction of red blood cells is intravascular, *hemoglobinemia, hemoglobinuria, methemalbuminemia, jaundice, hemosiderinuria*, and a decrease in plasma *haptoglobin* levels are observed. If the destruction is extravascular, there is no hemoglobinemia or hemoglobinuria; however, jaundice and lower plasma levels of haptoglobin are observed. In addition, because of erythrophagocytosis, there may be *hepatomegaly* and *splenomegaly*. Plasma levels of lactic dehydrogenase (LDH) are elevated in either case.

INHERITED INTRACORPUSCULAR ABNORMALITIES OF RED CELLS

Hereditary spherocytosis is an autosomal dominant condition caused by a defect in the cytoskeleton (*spectrin deficiency* is most common) of red blood cells. This defect makes the red cells spheroidal (because of a loss of membrane), less deformable, and subject to splenic phagocytosis and sequestration. Clinically, patients may have hemolytic crises or aplastic crises, either of which is often triggered by infection. Diagnosis is based on family history, the presence of spherocytes in the peripheral blood, and osmotic fragility of the red cells.

Glucose 6-phosphate dehydrogenase deficiency is a sex-linked inherited condition in which red blood cells cannot protect themselves from oxidative injury due to diminished or deficient enzyme function. The hemolytic crises are triggered by certain drugs, such as primaquine, sulfonamides, and nitrofurans. Infections can also induce crises. Only older red cells are affected.

Sickle cell disease is an inherited hemoglobinopathy in which structurally abnormal hemoglobin is produced (HbS). In the heterozygote (approximately 8% of African Americans), approximately 40% of the hemoglobin is HbS, whereas in the homozygote, 100% is HbS. When the HbS is deoxygenated, it becomes aggregated and polymerizes, leading to distortion of the red cell. Initially, with oxygenation, the red cell subsequently resume their normal shape; however, with repeated bouts, membrane damage occurs, so that the sickle shape remains. Irreversibly sickled cells are sequestered in the spleen, and intravascular hemolysis also occurs. In addition, microvascular occlusions occur, leading to thrombosis. Morphologically, in addition to the classic signs and symptoms of anemia, bone marrow hyperplasia may lead to bone resorption with formation of new bone. Extramedullary hematopoiesis is common in the liver and spleen. Histologically, there is congestion of red pulp, with thrombosis and infarction. Continued scarring leads to autosplenectomy. Infarctions are also seen in the bones, brain, kidney, liver, and retina. Diagnosis is made by clinical findings and by observing sickle cells on peripheral blood smears. It is confirmed by mixing blood with oxygen-consuming reagents such as metabisulfite to induce sickling. This condition is life-shortening and many patients die of overwhelming infections within the first years of life. Those escaping early death live until the fourth or fifth decade.

ACQUIRED INTRACORPUSCULAR ABNORMALITIES OF RED CELLS

Paroxysmal nocturnal hemoglobinuria is an acquired condition in which a somatic mutation in the pluripotential stem cell renders the red cells deficient in proteins anchored to the cell membrane by glycosyl-phosphatidylinositol (GPI). Some of these GPI-linked proteins inactivate complement, and their absence renders the cells vulnerable to lysis by endogenous complement. Most patients have chronic hemolysis, which may lead to iron deficiency over time. Approximately 25% of patients have intravascular hemolysis that is nocturnal and paroxysmal. Other clinical manifestations include venous thrombosis in the hepatic, portal, and cerebral veins, and infections resulting from granulocytopenia.

EXTRINSIC ABNORMALITIES OF RED BLOOD CELLS

These conditions may be mediated by antibodies, mechanical injury, infections, or toxins. The antibody-mediated are most commonly classified in accordance with the nature of the antibody involved. Diagnosis of these anemias is based on the Coombs' antiglobulin test and the temperature dependence of the antibodies. The *warm antibody types* are seen in neoplastic diseases such as lymphomas and leukemias, with treatment using drugs such as penicillin, phenacetin, and α-methyldopa, and in autoimmune disorders, especially systemic lupus erythematosus. The antibodies are IgG, usually do not fix complement, and are active at 37°C. *Cold agglutinin type* antibodies are seen with acute *mycoplasma* infections, some lymphomas, infectious mononucleosis, and some idiopathic conditions. The antibodies are IgM, which is most active at 0° to 4°C. They fix complement at warmer temperatures. Finally, *cold hemolysins* are IgG antibodies that bind to red cells, fix complement, and cause hemolysis when the temperature is raised to 30°C. These are associated with cold-hemolysin hemolytic anemia, which is characterized by acute intermittent massive hemolysis, often with hemoglobinuria in patients exposed to cold. Other antibody-mediated hemolytic anemias include transfusion reactions and *erythroblastosis fetalis*. In addition, extrinsic abnormalities leading to hemolytic anemia can be induced by mechanical means such as in *microangiopathic hemolytic anemia, thrombotic thrombocytopenic purpura*, and *disseminated intravascular coagulation* (DIC). Finally, infections such as malaria and bartonellosis or chemical toxins such as lead are also causes.

Impaired Red Cell Production

These anemias are produced by conditions that either interfere with the proliferation or differentiation of stem cells, or disturb the proliferation and maturation of erythroblasts. They are exemplified by *aplastic anemias*, *megaloblastic anemias*, *thalassemias*, *iron deficiency*, and *myelophthisic anemias*.

APLASTIC ANEMIAS

Aplastic anemias are actually pancytopenias that result from failure or suppression of multipotent myeloid stem cells, resulting in diminished production and release of differentiated cell lines (red cells, granulocytes, and/or thrombocytes). These can be inherited (Fanconi's anemia) or acquired. The latter are often idiopathic. In addition, however, chemicals such as alkylating agents, antimetabolites, chloramphenicol, and organic arsenicals; physical agents such radiation; and viral infections such as hepatitis C, cytomegalic virus, Epstein-Barr virus, and herpes varicella-zoster can cause aplastic anemias. Histologically, the bone marrow is hypocellular: fat cells, fibrous stroma, and a few lymphocytes and plasma cells populate the empty marrow spaces. Few to no megakaryocytes are observed. Clinically, these conditions can occur at any age and in either gender. Signs and symptoms vary, depending on what cell lines are affected. For example, infections are prevalent with agranulocytosis, and bleeding tendencies are observed with thrombocytopenia in addition to the pallor and weakness associated with anemia. Splenomegaly does not occur with aplastic anemia. Red cells are normocytic and normochromic, and there is no reticulocytosis. Diagnosis is based on examining the peripheral blood and bone marrow. The pancytopenia associated with aplastic anemia must be differentiated from that caused by aleukemic leukemias and myelodysplastic syndromes.

MEGALOBLASTIC ANEMIAS

Megaloblastic anemias are characterized by impaired DNA synthesis and distinctive morphologic changes in the bone marrow and peripheral blood. They are caused by deficiencies in either vitamin B_{12} or folate, which are coenzymes in the synthetic pathway of DNA. The synthesis of RNA and proteins is unaffected by these deficiencies. Thus there is cytoplasmic enlargement of red blood cell precursors without concomitant mitotic division (asynchronous cytoplasmic and nuclear maturation). In the peripheral blood, there is marked red cell *anisocytosis*. They are normochromic, but many are macrocytic with mean corpuscular volumes above 100 μm^3. Neutrophils and megakaryocytes are larger than normal and the neutrophils are hypersegmented. The bone marrow is hypercellular and the erythroid-to-myeloid ratio is 1 : 1 (normal is 1 : 3). The bone marrow yields too few mature red cells and there is premature destruction of normoblasts by phagocytosis and hemolysis (ineffective erythropoiesis). Premature destruction of granulocytes and platelet precursors also occurs, leading to leukopenia and thrombocytopenia. Deficiencies of vitamin B_{12} and folate result from inadequate intake in the diet, increased requirement (as in pregnancy), or conditions rendering patients unresponsive to therapy because of treatment with mercaptopurines or fluorouracil. Pernicious anemia is caused by malabsorption of vitamin B_{12} resulting from a lack of intrinsic factor (IF) production caused by atrophic gastritis, characterized by a marked loss of parietal cells. It is believed to result from immunologically mediated destruction of gastric mucosa. Three types of autoantibodies have been recognized: 75% of patients have an antibody that blocks vitamin B_{12}-IF binding; approximately 50% of patients have an antibody that reacts with both IF and the B_{12}–IF complex; and 85% to 90% of patients have an antibody that is directed against the alpha and beta subunits of the gastric proton pump. On the other hand, some evidence supports a cell-mediated immune response as being responsible for the gastric injury. Principal lesions of pernicious anemia include atrophic glossitis, chronic gastritis with atrophy of the fundic glands with loss of both chief and parietal cells, metaplasia of the glandular lining epithelium (intestinalization), and myelin degeneration of the dorsal and lateral tracts of the spinal cord. Complications include increased risk of gastric cancer and cardiac failure caused by hypoxia. Folate deficiency produces an identical clinical presentation.

THALASSEMIA

Thalassemia syndromes are characterized by a lack or decreased synthesis of either the alpha- or beta-chain of hemoglobin A. β-Thalassemia is characterized by reduced or absent synthesis of the beta-globin chain in the presence of normal alpha chain synthesis. The abnormalities in synthesis are a result of point mutations. ***Thalassemia major*** is found in patients who have homozygous genotypes. The incidence is highest in Mediterranean countries and parts of Africa and Southeast Asia. In the United States, immigrants from these regions have the highest incidence. Peripheral blood smears demonstrate microcytic, hypochromic cells with marked anisocytosis. Target cells are common and the reticulocyte count is elevated, but it is not as high as would be expected because of ineffective erythropoiesis. The bone marrow is hyperplastic and there is thinning of the bony cortex concomitant with new bone formation. Splenomegaly and hepatomegaly result from erythrophagocytosis and extramedullary hematopoiesis. Hemosiderosis and hemochromatosis may be present late in the course of the disease as a result of numerous transfusions and possibly tissue hypoxia, leading to enhanced iron absorption. ***Thalas-***

semia minor is more common than thalassemia major and the clinical manifestations are milder. The α-thalassemias are a heterogeneous group of conditions, the severities of which are highly variable.

IRON DEFICIENCY ANEMIA

Iron is required for hemoglobin synthesis. Iron deficiency anemia is considered to be the most common nutritional disorder in the world. Those most often affected are menstruating women, the elderly, children, the poor, and infants. In addition, however, iron deficiency can occur as a result of impaired absorption (such as in sprue), as a result of increased requirement (as in growing children and pregnant women), or as a result of chronic blood loss (as is seen in peptic ulcers, cancers of the gastrointestinal tract, or genitourinary diseases). Morphologically, the bone marrow is characterized by increased numbers of normoblasts and little stainable iron. The peripheral blood contains microcytic, hypochromic red cells. Clinically, the anemia may be diagnosed secondary to the cause of the iron deficiency. However, laboratory studies are required for definitive diagnosis. These include determining serum iron and ferritin levels (low), total plasma iron-binding capacity (high), and transferrin saturation of below 15%.

MYELOPHTHISIC ANEMIAS

Myelophthisic anemias are a result of space-occupying lesions of the bone marrow resulting in marrow failure. They are caused by metastatic cancers from the breast, lung, or prostate; multiple myeloma; leukemias; or myeloproliferative diseases. Other causes of anemias resulting in bone marrow failure include diffuse liver disease and chronic renal failure.

Bleeding Disorders

Bleeding disorders can be caused by abnormalities of vessel walls (nonthrombocytopenic purpuras), decreased numbers or impaired function of platelets, or abnormalities in clotting factors.

Bleeding disorders caused by ***abnormalities of vessel walls*** have varied causes. ***Septicemia*** and ***rickettsioses*** are infectious causes that damage vessel walls directly, thus causing disseminated intravascular coagulation (DIC). ***Scurvy*** and ***Ehlers-Danlos*** syndrome are examples of bleeding disorders caused by impaired collagen formation. ***Henoch-Schönlein*** is a systemic hypersensitivity disease characterized by deposition of immune complexes within vessels throughout the body. Clinically, purpuric rash, colicky abdominal pain, polyarthralgia, and acute glomerulonephritis are manifestations.

Thrombocytopenia is an important cause of generalized bleeding. ***Idiopathic thrombocytopenic purpura*** (ITP) is a chronic autoimmune disorder in which platelets are destroyed by antibodies. Morphologically, the spleen is normal in size, but there is congestion of sinusoids and enlargement of follicles with prominent germinal centers. Megakaryocytes may be seen. The bone marrow appears normal, but there are increased numbers of megakaryocytes, some immature. It occurs most often in adults, particularly women of child-bearing age. Presentations vary from a history of easy bruising, nosebleeds, or melena, to a sudden shower of petechial hemorrhages. Diagnosis is based on thrombocytopenia with normal or increased megakaryocytes in the bone marrow. The bleeding time is prolonged, but clotting tests are normal. All other causes of thrombocytopenia must be ruled out. ***Thrombotic thrombocytopenic purpura*** (TTP) and ***hemolytic-uremic syndrome*** (HUS) are termed thrombotic microangiopathies. Classically, TTP is found in adult women who present with fever, thrombocytopenia, microangiopathic hemolytic anemia, transient neurologic deficits, and renal failure. Although microangiopathic hemolytic anemia and thrombocytopenia are also found in HUS, there are no neurologic signs, renal failure is dominant, and the disease is predominantly found in children.

Bleeding resulting from ***defective platelet function*** is inherited or acquired. Congenital diseases are the result of defects in adhesion or aggregation, or disorders of platelet secretion. Of the acquired diseases, the ingestion of aspirin and other nonsteroidal anti-inflammatory drugs is clinically important. Aspirin inhibits cyclooxygenase which suppresses the synthesis of thromboxane A_2, a potent aggregator of platelets.

Abnormalities in ***clotting factors*** are manifested by the development of large ecchymoses or hematomas after an injury. In addition, they may manifest as prolonged bleeding after laceration or surgery. Deficiencies in factor VIII (***hemophilia A***) is the most common hereditary disease. This is an X-linked recessive trait, and thus it occurs in males. There is a tendency toward massive hemorrhage, although clinical presentation can be variable. These patients have normal bleeding times, normal platelet counts, and prolonged partial thromboplastin times. Factor VIII assays are required for diagnosis. ***von Willebrand's disease*** (vWD) is one of the more common inherited bleeding disorders in humans. Usually it is transmitted as an autosomal dominant disease, but autosomal recessive forms have been recognized. Clinically, spontaneous bleeding from mucous membranes, excessive bleeding from wounds, menorrhagia, and prolonged bleeding time in the presence of a normal platelet count are recognized. This condition is characterized by defects in platelet function and the coagulation pathway. ***Disseminated intravascular coagulation*** (DIC) can be acute, subacute, or chronic. It is characterized by activation of the coagulation cascade, leading to thrombi in the microcirculation. The thrombotic diathesis leads to platelet consumption as well as consumption of fibrin and coagulation factors. In addition, there is activation of fibrinolytic pathways. It is initiated by release of tissue factor or thromboplastic substances into the circulation and by widespread endothelial cell injury. These result from a wide variety of causes, including obstetric complications, infections, neoplasms, massive tissue injury, and other nonspecific causes like snake bite and heat stroke. Morphologically, thrombi are found most often in the brain, followed by the heart, lungs, kidneys, and other organs. Microinfarcts may be seen. Clinically, onset may be acute or chronic. Presentations vary from respiratory signs, to neurologic manifestations, to circulatory collapse. In general, acute DIC presents as a bleeding diathesis whereas the chronic forms present with thrombotic complications.

DISEASES OF WHITE BLOOD CELLS, INCLUDING LYMPH NODES

The white blood cells include the granulocytic and monocytic series. Among the granulocytes are cells that are neutrophilic, eosinophilic, and basophilic. The monocytic series includes lymphocytes that circulate in the blood and those that populate the lymph nodes, and, similarly, monocytes that circulate or contribute to the tissue macrophage pool. Only the most important diseases of each of these will be considered below.

Leukopenia

The predominant circulating cell in the adult is the neutrophil, so that most instances of decreased circulating white cells are a result of ***neutropenia*** (agranulocytosis). ***Lymphopenia*** can occur, much less frequently, in association with conditions such as Hodgkin's disease, immunodeficiencies, and some chronic diseases. Agranulocytosis occurs most frequently as a result of bone marrow depression by drugs (such as antimetabolites, sulfonamides, and chloramphenicol).

The total white cell count is usually under 1000 per μl^3. Symptoms usually relate to superimposed bacterial infection.

Leukocytosis

Increases in white blood cells, often to fairly impressive levels, are relatively common in clinical practice. The reactive disorders of elevated white cell counts must always be distinguished from neoplastic proliferation. Correlation between the peripheral blood counts and morphology and the appearance of the bone marrow or lymph nodes may be essential at times in making this distinction. Varieties of leukocytosis include the following.

Granulocytosis, an increased number of circulating *polymorphonuclear leukocytes* (PMNs), is most often seen in response to bacterial infection. Tissue necrosis after a myocardial infarct or extensive trauma or burns may also cause marked elevations in circulating polys.

In addition to raised levels of circulating neutrophils, ***eosinophilia*** *(eosinophilic leukocytosis)* may be seen in response to *bronchial asthma*, skin diseases such as *eczema* and *pemphigus*, and *parasitic* infestations. ***Basophilia*** is quite uncommon. ***Lymphocytosis*** and ***monocytosis*** can be seen in a variety of chronic infectious diseases *(brucellosis, tuberculosis)* as well as *autoimmune vascular* diseases and others. Lymphocytosis is characteristic of viral diseases as well.

Lymphadenitis

Lymph node enlargement is quite common and can be nonspecific (acute or chronic). Lymphoid hyperplasia with large germinal centers *(follicular hyperplasia)* is seen in conditions such as chronic infection that activates B cells. The paracortical areas are activated by stimulation of T cells *(paracortical hyperplasia)* and the sinuses may be filled with macrophages *(sinus histocytosis)* in lymph nodes draining an area involved by a foreign body or such things as breast cancer.

Leukocyte Neoplasms

For the most part, the neoplastic diseases of white blood cells are, or have the potential to become, malignant. The proliferative disorders of leukocytes fall into two broad categories: *leukemias* and *lymphomas*. As a whole, these are the most important diseases of white cells and they will be discussed in the following categories: the leukemias and myeloproliferative disorders, malignant lymphomas, plasma cell dyscrasias, and histocytoses.

LEUKEMIAS AND MYELOPROLIFERATIVE DISORDERS

Leukemias can be defined as malignancies arising from *stem cells* that overgrow the bone marrow. These cells largely replace the normal marrow elements leading to decreased red cell and platelet production, and then they enter the bloodstream where they can disseminate to solid organs including the spleen, liver, kidney, and lymph nodes.

The classification of leukemias is based on the cell of origin, wherever it can be determined. Some leukemias follow a rapid course, whereas others proceed more slowly, leading to the broad categories of *acute* and *chronic* leukemia. These categories are reflected in the morphology of the cells, at least initially, with acute leukemias being composed of less differentiated cells including *blasts* and chronic leukemias being composed of more mature cells, initially; later in the course of chronic leukemias, blasts may appear in the marrow and the peripheral blood, too.

Acute Leukemias. ***Acute lymphoblastic leukemia*** (ALL) is the commonest form of leukemia in children (80%), with over 2500 new cases yearly. Boys are more often affected than girls, and whites more often than nonwhites. Like most acute leukemias, the onset is often explosive, symptoms are due to replacement of normal marrow *(anemia, bleeding, infection)*, and there is often pain and organ enlargement resulting from leukemic infiltration.

ALL has various subtypes that can be defined by *morphologic* and *immunologic* criteria. The French-American-British system of classification (FAB) recognizes type L1, L2, and L3 variants. Over 80% of ALL cases express *B-cell* markers, and over 90% have karyotypic changes consisting of structural or numerical changes in chromosomes. *Terminal deoxynuceotidyl transferase* (Tdt) is a useful marker that helps distinguish ALL from acute myeloblastic leukemia. Without question, ALL therapy represents one of the signal achievements of modern chemotherapy: over 90% of cases now achieve a remission, and over 60% can be cured.

Acute myeloblastic leukemia (AML) is the principal form of *acute leukemia in adults*. Over 80% of cases occur in patients in their late teens to late thirties. Transformed cells may arise from the myeloid and erythroid stem cells or myelocytic and monocytic lines giving rise to *myelomonocytic leukemia*. Up to eight distinct subtypes are recognized in the FAB classification (M0 to M7). Usually, it is possible to distinguish AML from ALL by a simple Wright or Wright-Giemsa stain, but *myeloperoxidase* staining may be helpful. The presence of a red body called an *Auer rod* in the cytoplasm is also helpful. Up to 90% of patients show chromosomal abnormalities if special banding techniques are used. Prognosis is not as good for AML as for ALL, and less than a third of patients are free of disease after 5 years.

Myelodysplastic Syndromes. The term *myelodysplasia* refers to altered differentiation of stem cells. Erythroid, myeloid, and platelet precursors *(megakaryocytes)* may be affected. Patients are at high risk of developing AML. The condition affects mostly patients in the seventh or eighth decades of life. Almost half of the patients are asymptomatic at the time of diagnosis, but life expectancy is 1 to 3 years in most cases.

Chronic Leukemia. ***Chronic myeloid leukemia*** (CML) accounts for about 20% of all leukemia cases and occurs in adults with a wide range of ages, with a peak in the 30- to 40-year period. Although all cell lines (myeloid, erythroid, megakaryocyte, and B lymphocyte) of the bone marrow are affected, the leukemia principally involves the granulocytes.

There is a distinctive chromosomal abnormality in over 90% of CML cases, usually involving a 9:22 translocation, called the Philadelphia (Ph) chromosome. The *bcr-c-abl* gene is involved, and the presence of bcr-c-abl protein and mRNA are considered diagnostic of CML.

Clinically, CML is slowly progressive. The white count is usually very high, in the 100,000/mm^3 range, and there is marked splenomegaly. Constitutional symptoms include weakness, easy fatigability, anorexia, and weight loss. Mean survival even without treatment is in the range of 3 or more years.

Chronic Lymphocytic Leukemia (CLL). Chronic lymphocytic leukemia (CLL) principally affects males over 50 years old; this form accounts for as much as a quarter of all leukemia cases. It is the least aggressive of the leukemias and shares many features of *lymphocytic lymphoma*. The transformed cells are B cells and express pan-B-cell markers, such as CD19 and CD20, and they may have immunoglobulins on the surface (IgM and IgD). Chromosomal abnormalities are present in up to 50% of cases, with trisomy 12 being most common.

Many patients are asymptomatic, and most often the symptoms are nonspecific. Median survival in the range of 4 to 6 years is recorded, which is not unreasonable in view of the age of the patients who are principally affected.

Hairy cell leukemia is a rare manifestation of chronic B cell leukemia with a distinctive cell population that exhibits a tartrate-resistant acid phosphatase *(TRAP)* histochemically. It is found in older men and may respond to interferon treatment.

Brief mention of ***myeloproliferative*** disorders should also be made. These include ***polycythemia vera***, which, in addition to proliferation of erythroid elements, includes overproduction of granulocytes and platelets, ***CML*** (already described), *myeloid metaplasia*, and essential thrombocythemia. Polycythemia may result in *sludging* caused by the high viscosity of the blood and increased platelets, leading to *thrombosis*. It often evolves into a phase of ***myeloid metaplasia with myelofibrosis***, with bone marrow depression.

LYMPHOMAS

Although the designation ***lymphoma*** would appear to imply a benign neoplasm, almost all neoplasms arising in lymph nodes or lymphoid tissue, such as that of the gastrointestinal tract, are malignant. There are two broad categories: ***Hodgkin's disease*** with its subtypes, and all the others, classified as ***non-Hodgkin's lymphomas***

(NHL). The latter can arise from both T and B lymphocytes *(lymphocytic)* as well as histiocytes *(histiocytic)* and the precursors of both lines *(lymphoblastic and histoblastic)* of differentiation. The classification of these tumors has gone through a number of evolutionary steps in the past several years, especially as *immunocytochemical markers* have come into widespread use. Although the classification of Hodgkin's has become reasonably uniform, classification of NHL remains a problem, with several schemes in current use in the United States and in Europe. This will be discussed further.

Hodgkin's Disease. Hodgkin's disease is a disorder of lymph nodes that arises in a *single node* or in a *contiguous group* of nodes, and then spreads more widely and can even, rarely, involve solid organs. It is separated from NHL because of several distinctive features, not the least of which is that it involves a unique cell, the ***Reed-Sternberg cell (RS)***. In addition, there are both clinical and pathologic features, suggesting an inflammatory process: there is a mixed inflammatory infiltrate consisting of lymphocytes, eosinophils, and plasma cells, and a rather characteristic pattern of fever. Although it is not very common (there are fewer than 8000 new cases each year constituting less than 1% of all neoplastic diseases), it is most frequent in young adults, a population somewhat less frequently affected by malignant neoplasia. It is also an increasingly curable malignancy and proper classification and staging of the neoplastic process is highly predictive of the response to therapy.

The *Rye classification*, which is widely accepted, recognizes four subtypes: ***nodular sclerosis***, ***lymphocyte predominance***, ***mixed cellularity***, and ***lymphocyte depletion***. The diagnosis of Hodgkin's disease rests on the identification of the RS, a giant cell which usually has two *(mirror image)* nuclei which are large and indented and include a very prominent ***macronucleolus*** with a clear halo around it which imparts an "owl-eyed" appearance to these cells. There are mononuclear and multinuclear variants. The classification is based in part on the abundance of RS cells, as well as on other components. Although RS cells are required for the diagnosis of Hodgkin's disease, they can occasionally be found in other disorders, some which are benign. Nodular sclerosis, the most common form of the disease, has another distinctive cell, the *lacunar* cell, and bands of collagen that separate the node into nodules encased in fibrous tissue. This variant is more common in women (the others are all more frequent in men) and has an excellent prognosis if found early. *Lymphocyte predominance* is uncommon and represents fewer than 10% of Hodgkin's disease cases. There are few RS cells and many mature lymphocytes and histiocytes and a cell termed a "popcorn" cell because of its multilobed nucleus. Prognosis is very good with proper treatment. *Mixed cellularity* is the second most frequent form: it has lots of RS cells and a background rich in inflammatory cells such as lymphocytes, eosinophils, and histiocytes. The disease is usually widespread at the time of diagnosis and the patients are usually symptomatic. *Lymphocyte depletion* is the least common form of the disease. There are numerous RS cells and few lymphocytes. It affects older men and has an aggressive course.

The origin of the RS cell is still debated, but much evidence points to a B cell lineage. Staging (I to IV) has important prognostic significance. Stages I and II have limited involvement and are unlikely to have systemic manifestations, whereas patients with stages III and IV have disseminated disease and symptoms such as fever, pruritus, weight loss, and anemia.

Non-Hodgkin's Lymphoma. Non-Hodgkin's lymphomas (NHL) begin usually as localized or widespread lymph node enlargement. In the late stages, they may involve spleen, liver, and bone marrow and enter into the bloodstream producing a leukemia-like picture. Whereas Hodgkin's is unlikely to arise in extranodal lymphoid tissue, NHL arises as a primary tumor in areas such as the gastrointestinal tract in up to a third of cases.

As mentioned previously, there are multiple classifications. *Immunophenotyping*, *DNA hybridization*, *T and B cell receptor rearrangement*, and other techniques are essential adjuncts to histologic assessment in rendering a proper diagnosis and prognosis. A consensus classification called the *Working Formulation for Clinical Usage* is receiving widespread application. It divides NHL into three groups: those of *low grade*, *intermediate grade*, and *high grade malignant potential*. This is based on the 10-year survival, which is about 45% for individuals with low grade tumors, 26% with intermediate grade, and 23% with high grade lymphomas. Histologically, one of the most reliable features for classification is whether the lymphocytes form *nodules* or *follicles*, or whether they obliterate the normal nodal architecture by a *diffuse* involvement. Staging is not as important in NHL as in Hodgkin's disease in predicting the outcome of the disease.

Low Grade Lymphoma. The low grade lymphomas include three types: *small lymphocytic lymphomas*; *follicular, predominantly small cleaved cell lymphomas*; and *mixed small cleaved and large cell lymphomas*. The ***small lymphocytic lymphoma*** (SLL) does not have a follicular pattern, constitutes less than 5% of NHL, and may end up as chronic lymphocytic leukemia in over 50% of cases. It affects older people. The cells are B cells, but they have a T cell marker, CD-5, in addition.

Follicular lymphomas are made up of two types: *small cleaved* and *mixed*. The small cleaved cell type is the most frequent form of follicular lymphomas. The cells are B cells and over 80% have a 14:18 chromosomal translocation. These tumors become leukemic less frequently than SLL, but they also affect older individuals (50 to 60 years of age), and men and women are equally likely to develop the disease. Patients with follicular lymphomas do not respond to treatment very much and do about as well if left untreated. They run a slow but inexorable course.

Intermediate Grade Lymphomas. There are four NHLs in this category: *follicular, predominantly large cell*; *diffuse, small cleaved cell*; *diffuse, mixed small and large cell*; and *diffuse, large cell.*

The most common of these is the diffuse large cell variant. Large noncleaved cells are as much as four times larger than the small cleaved cells. These tumors are phenotypically B cells.

High Grade Lymphomas. The high grade lymphomas have subtypes including *large cell immunoblastic*, *lymphoblastic*, and *small noncleaved lymphomas. Burkitt's lymphoma* falls into the last group.

Large cell immunoblastic lymphomas can be grouped with the *diffuse large cell* and mixed cell lymphomas (intermediate grade) with which they share features that separate them from follicular lymphomas as a group. The large cell tumors make up about 50% of the adult NHL. They show a male predominance, often present as an enlarging mass, and have a wide age range at the time of discovery. Most express B cell markers, but some have T cell indicators. Only infrequently are they composed of cells with macrophage characteristics. They are highly associated with a history of immunologically associated diseases, such as Sjögren's syndrome, thyroiditis, and AIDS or other immunosuppression.

Small noncleaved cell lymphomas include Burkitt's and non-Burkitt's types. Burkitt's, first described in Africa, has a characteristic presentation in children who develop a large mass in the jaw. These tumors are related to the ***Epstein-Barr virus*** (EBV) and histologically show a uniform small cell appearance punctuated by macrophages that stand out like stars *(starry-sky appearance)*. They are B cell tumors.

Lymphoblastic lymphoma characteristically affects adolescents and is a close cousin of T cell acute lymphoblastic leukemia. It shows a 2:1 male preference and although it represents only 5% of all NHLs, it causes more than a third of all childhood lymphomas.

In addition to the above, there are other rare lymphomas such as ***mycosis fungoides*** and ***Sézary syndrome***, which are T cell neoplasms that involve the skin. The ***adult*** form of ***T cell leukemia***, which also presents as a lymphoma, is associated with the human T-cell leukemia virus HTLV-1.

PLASMA CELL DYSCRASIAS

Important among the plasma cell diseases are ***multiple myeloma***, solitary myeloma (***plasmacytoma***) and ***Waldenströms's macroglobulinemia***. There are also extremely rare diseases involving monoclonal gammopathies, such as ***alpha-chain disease***.

Multiple myeloma is a plasma cell tumor arising in the bone marrow, which produces bony involvement in many sites; usually vertebrae and skull are involved. In addition to lytic lesions of bone leading to pathologic fractures, light chains of the immunoglobulin molecule appear in the urine as *Bence-Jones* protein, and these may be deposited in kidney tubules, producing *myeloma nephrosis* along with amyloidosis of the renal glomeruli. Hypercalcemia is frequently present.

Isolated ***plasmacytomas*** can also produce monoclonal gammopathies and are likely to progress to multiple myeloma.

Waldenström's macroglobulinemia accounts for up to 5% of monoclonal gammopathies and derives from invasion of the bone marrow by lymphocytes and plasma cells that produce a monoclonal IgM.

HISTIOCYTOSIS

There are several related diseases that owe their origin to proliferation of a special type of histiocyte, the Langerhans' cell. The older description of these disorders distinguishes different diseases, usually in children, involving characteristic involvement of bone and bone marrow and designated ***Letter-Siwe*** syndrome, ***Hand-Schüller-Christian*** disease, and ***eosinophilic*** granuloma. Later, these were grouped together as ***histiocytosis X***. It is now established that they are derived from histiocytes in the bone marrow that have a characteristic cytoplasmic granule, *Birbeck granules* or *Hx granules*. Electron microscopically, these are racket-shaped and have a tubular "handle" with regular periodicity. The skull is frequently involved with lytic lesions in these disorders which are usually classified as ***unifocal and multifocal Langerhans' cell histiocytosis*** today. The association of diabetes insipidus, lesions in the skull, and exophthalmus is the *Hand-Schüller-Christian triad*. Liver, lymph node, and splenic involvement also occur. Sometimes there is spontaneous remission, and chemotherapy may be curative.

THE LUNGS

The major diseases of the lungs include the following categories of disorders:

- congenital
- mechanical
- vascular
- obstruction
- restrictive
- inflammatory
- neoplastic

In addition to these intrinsic diseases, the lungs, because of their intimate relationship to the cardiovascular system, are subject to vascular diseases that result from heart pathology (*e.g.*, congestive heart failure or valvular disease) and vascular disease (*e.g.*, deep vein thrombosis, which may promote pulmonary emboli). Finally, the lungs, like the liver, are favored targets for tumor metastasis.

Congenital Anomalies

Congenital anomalies can be found in the tracheobronchial tree, lung parenchyma, or vessels.

The more common include the following:

1. ***Agenesis or hypoplasia*** of the lungs or portions of the lungs. Hypoplasia is the most common congenital anomaly of the lung.
2. ***Tracheoesophageal fistula***. This connection between the trachea and the esophagus is most commonly found in the middle of the esophagus. These infants cannot swallow because the esophagus ends in a blind pouch. Instead the food enters the lungs through the fistula, causing aspiration pneumonia.

Mechanical Obstruction

Atelectasis is the major mechanically produced lesion of the lung. It is defined as either incomplete expansion of the lungs or collapse of previously inflated lungs leading to regions of lung parenchyma that are airless. Regions of atelectasis are prone to infection and oxygenation is reduced. Generally, these areas can be reinflated, and thus atelectasis is reversible. There are three causes of atelectasis in adults:

1. *Obstructive atelectasis* results from complete obstruction of an airway, with subsequent absorption of air from that segment. Blood flow remains normal. This is caused by conditions (*e.g.*, asthma, chronic bronchitis, and foreign bodies) that cause excess secretions or exudates in smaller bronchi. The mediastinum shifts toward the atelectasis.
2. *Compressive atelectasis* occurs as a result of the thoracic cavity being filled with fluid, exudates, tumors, blood, or air (pneumothorax), to the point that lung function is compromised. Extrathoracic conditions associated with this condition include congestive heart failure and inflammatory conditions of the peritoneal cavity that elevate the diaphragm. The mediastinum shifts away from the atelectasis.
3. *Patchy atelectasis* is seen in the adult and neonatal respiratory distress syndromes. It is caused by a loss of pulmonary surfactant.

Vascular Disorders

Pulmonary Congestion and Edema

There are three mechanisms by which pulmonary congestion and edema can occur: there are hemodynamic causes, microvascular injury, and idiopathic causes.

- *Hemodynamic causes* include conditions producing increased hydrostatic pressure (left-sided heart diseases), decreased oncotic pressure (liver disease), and lymphatic obstruction (neoplasms, scarring).
- *Microvascular injury* may occur from physical sources (radiation), chemical sources (inhaled gases or liquids, parenteral drugs), biological agents (bacteria, viruses), or systemic disease (sepsis, acute pancreatitis, diabetic ketoacidosis).
- *Idiopathic causes* include high altitude and neurogenic conditions. Hemodynamic pulmonary edema is characterized by heavy, wet lungs that, microscopically, have markedly hyperemic capillaries and a pink fluid filling the alveolar spaces. Free red blood cells are also seen, and in long-standing cases, macrophages bearing hemosiderin pigment (heart failure cells) are observed and the lungs become firm and brown.

Adult respiratory distress syndrome (ARDS; shock lung) is a syndrome characterized by rapid onset of severe dyspnea, cyanosis, and arterial hypoxemia that is refractory to oxygen, and it often leads to multisystem organ failure. It results from a variety of underlying causes including pulmonary infections, shocklike conditions, inhalation of irritant gases, and aspiration. It is characterized by diffuse capillary damage stemming from injury to endothelial or epithelial cells, and leading to severe congestive edema and inflammation with hyaline membranes. In most instances, the lesions do not resolve and scarring ensues. Mortality is high.

Respiratory distress syndrome in the newborn (hyaline membrane disease) is a common, life-threatening condition of (usually) pre-term newborn infants. The idiopathic form is most important. It is characterized by severe progressive dyspnea and cyanosis at birth, which becomes refractory to oxygen therapy. The frequency is dependent on gestational age. The vast majority of cases occur at less than 28 weeks of gestation, and the incidence decreases considerably by 37 weeks of gestation. The primary cause is a deficiency of surfactant, which promotes atelectasis leading to hypoxemia and CO_2 retention. Subsequent acidosis leads to vasoconstriction and then hypoxia, which ultimately causes capillary endothelial and alveolar epithelial damage. The lungs are edematous and microscopically are characterized by poorly developed alveoli, many of which are atelectatic. Necrotic cellular debris is found in terminal bronchioles and alveolar ducts. Hyaline membranes are observed in respiratory bronchioles, alveolar ducts, and alveoli. These are composed of fibrin, and cellular debris.

Pulmonary embolism (PE) is the most frequent cause of vascular occlusions in the lung, and up to 95% are from thrombi in the deep veins of the legs. These account for approximately 10% of acute hospital deaths in adults in the United States. Pulmonary emboli are generally complications in patients who have cardiac disease, cancer, or inherited or acquired hypercoagulable states. Most pulmonary emboli are asymptomatic, particularly if they are small and if there is no underlying cardiovascular disease. Embolic obstruction of small arteries results in alveolar hemorrhage because of influx of blood from bronchial circulation. Large emboli or multiple, simultaneous small emboli that obstruct more than 60% of the pulmonary vasculature cause sudden death due to acute cor pulmonale with ''electromechanical dissociation'' or generalized circulatory collapse. Clinical presentations can vary from minor to severe chest pain, dyspnea, cough, and, in severe cases, shock. Pulmonary angiography is the definitive procedure for establishing a diagnosis. Chest radiographs disclose infarcts 12 to 36 hours after occlusion. Finally, ventilation–perfusion scans are also of value in making a diagnosis. Elevation of LDH is seen with large PEs. Nonfatal acute emboli can resolve via fibrinolysis. Others that are unresolved, if extensive enough, can lead to pulmonary hypertension or chronic cor pulmonale.

Pulmonary hypertension can be primary (idiopathic) or secondary to chronic obstructive (*e.g.,* emphysema) or interstitial diseases (*e.g.,* interstitial fibrosis) of the lung. In addition, recurrent pulmonary emboli, congenital heart diseases (*e.g.,* left to right shunts), truncus arteriosus, and left-sided acquired heart disease cause pulmonary hypertension. The pathogenesis of both primary and secondary forms revolves around physically or functionally disabled pulmonary endothelial cells. Arterioles and small arteries have medial hypertrophy and intimal fibrosis in primary and secondary forms, but they are manifested best in the primary form. The primary form is most common in 20- to 40-year-old women. The clinical presentation is dyspnea, fatigue, and, to a lesser degree, angina-like chest pain. With time, the dyspnea becomes more severe, there is cyanosis and cor pulmonale, resulting in heart failure. Thromboembolism in pneumonia is also a common complication.

Obstructive Diseases

Obstructive diseases are defined as diffuse pulmonary diseases that produce increased resistance in air flow due to partial or complete obstruction anywhere in the tracheobronchial tree. The major obstructive diseases include emphysema, asthma, chronic bronchitis, and bronchiectasis. Neoplasms and foreign bodies can also be obstructive.

Emphysema is characterized by abnormal, permanent enlargement of the air spaces distal to the terminal bronchioles, with destruction of their walls and without fibrosis. The most severe form is found in male smokers in their fifth to eighth decades. Clinically, it is characterized by progressive dyspnea accompanied by prolonged expiration. When severe, patients overventilate and remain well oxygenated, giving rise to the term ''pink puffers.'' There are four types of emphysema. *Centriacinar emphysema* involves the respiratory bronchioles, sparing the alveoli. It is most common in the upper lobes and most often associated with smoking. Smoke particles are believed to establish a nidus of inflammation leading to increased elastase levels from neutrophils. This inflammatory response is generally in the face of decreased alpha-1-antitrypsin levels. *Panacinar emphysema* involves the entire acinus, including the respiratory bronchiole, alveolar duct, and alveolus. It occurs in the lower lobes and is most severe at the bases. It is associated with alpha-1-antitrypsin deficiency. *Paraseptal emphysema* is usually found adjacent to regions of fibrosis or scarring and may be responsible for some cases of spontaneous pneumothorax in young adults. *Irregular emphysema* is most often associated with scarring. Complications of emphysema include respiratory acidosis and coma, right heart failure, and pneumothorax.

Chronic bronchitis is defined clinically as any patient who has persistent cough with sputum production for at least 3 months in at least 2 consecutive years. Any age group and both genders can be affected, but it is generally seen in middle-aged men who are habitual smokers. In addition, it is frequently found in individuals who live in cities with high smog levels. Airway obstruction is caused by the hypersecretion of mucus throughout the tracheobronchial tree. Histologically, there is hypertrophy of mucous-secreting glands in the trachea and bronchi, which increases the ratio of the gland layer to the thickness of the wall (Reid index). In addition, there is bronchiolar narrowing due to goblet cell metaplasia, mucous plugging, inflammation, and fibrosis. Complications include cor pulmonale with heart failure, concomitant emphysema, and superimposed bacterial infections leading to further diminution of the respiratory function (cyanosis), leading to the designation of ''blue-bloaters.''

Bronchial asthma is defined as a condition characterized by hyperactive airways leading to episodic, reversible bronchoconstriction, owing to increased responsiveness of the tracheobronchial tree to various stimuli. There are two types of asthma: *extrinsic,* which is a type I hypersensitivity reaction to specific allergens, chemicals, or antigenic spores (*e.g.,* aspergillosis), and intrinsic, which is induced by nonimmune mechanisms as diverse as cold, respiratory viral infections, and aspirin. Autopsy lesions associated with asthma include overinflated lungs and occlusion of bronchi and bronchioles with thick mucous plugs. Histologically, the mucous contains shed epithelial cells (Curschmann's spirals), eosinophils, and eosinophil membrane protein (Charcot-Leyden crystals). Other characteristic changes include thickening of bronchioepithelial basement membrane, inflammation (primarily eosinophils), edema of the bronchial walls, and hypertrophy of submucosal glands and muscles of the bronchial walls. Complications include emphysema, chronic bronchitis, bronchiectasis, and pneumonia. Cor pulmonale, with resulting heart failure, can also occur.

Bronchiectasis is abnormal, irreversible dilatation of the bronchi and bronchioles in the presence of chronic, necrotizing infection. It results from bronchial obstruction caused by tumors, foreign bodies, chronic bronchitis, asthma, cystic fibrosis, or necrotizing pneumonia. Clinically, bronchiectasis is characterized by severe, persistent cough, foul-smelling sputum that may contain blood, and dyspnea. It usually infects the lower lobes of the lungs bilaterally. Histologically, fully developed cases reveal acute and chronic inflammation, declamation, and also ulceration of bronchial epithelium, and necrosis that may destroy the bronchial walls. Fibrosis is observed in chronic cases. Complications include marked dyspnea and cyanosis. Cor pulmonale, metastatic brain abscesses, and amyloidosis are observed less frequently.

Restrictive Diseases

These diseases are characterized by decreased total lung capacity resulting from reduced expansion of lung parenchyma. They are most often characterized by diffuse, chronic involvement of pulmonary connective tissue, particularly the interstitium of the alveolar wall. The causes are diverse and include coal dust, silicosis, asbestosis, oxygen toxicity, bleomycin, paraquat, gold, viruses, bacteria, fungi, and *Pneumocystis carinii*. In addition, there are many unknown causes. The most frequent causes in descending order are environmental diseases, sarcoidosis, idiopathic pulmonary fibrosis, and collagen vascular diseases.

Pneumoconioses include diseases of the lung resulting from inhalation of mineral dust, organic dusts that induce hypersensitivity pneumonitis, organic dusts that induce asthma, and chemical fumes and vapors. *Coal worker's pneumoconiosis* is a spectrum of conditions that include: (a) asymptomatic anthracosis, in which coal dust pigment accumulates with no cellular reaction; (b) accumulations of macrophages with minimal to no respiratory compromise; and (c) progressive massive fibrosis that leads to pulmonary dysfunction. Complications include pulmonary hypertension and cor pulmonale. There is also an increase in the incidence of tuberculosis.

Silicosis is caused by the inhalation of crystalline silicon dioxide. The initial lesions localize in the upper lung lobes and are characterized by interaction of the particles with epithelial cells and macrophages, which ultimately become fibrotic nodules. Progressive massive fibrosis may occur as a result of coalescing nodules. Pulmonary function is generally normal or may be moderately compromised unless progressive massive fibrosis ensues. In the latter case, the lungs are compromised considerably.

Asbestosis results from the inhalation of asbestos fibers, particularly the amphibole geometric type. It is characterized by diffuse interstitial fibrosis in the lower lung lobes that commences around respiratory bronchioles and alveolar sacs. Subpleural lesions are also noted. Asbestos bodies, fibers coated with iron-containing protein, are observed microscopically, as are "ferruginous bodies." The latter are iron-containing complexes without asbestos-fiber cores. Dyspnea is the presenting symptom. It occurs 10 to 20 years after exposure and is progressive. Cough with sputum production is common as the disease progresses. Complications include pleural effusions, bronchogenic carcinoma, mesothelioma, and laryngeal carcinoma. Concomitant cigarette smoking increases the risk of bronchogenic carcinoma.

Sarcoidosis is an idiopathic disease characterized by noncaseous granulomas in the lungs, lymph nodes, spleen, liver, bone marrow, skin, eye, and, to a lesser degree, other organs. Hilar lymphadenopathy, which is bilateral, or lung lesions are observed on chest x-rays in the majority of cases. It is more frequent in women than men, and in the majority of cases, the presenting clinical symptoms include shortness of breath, cough, chest pain, and hemoptysis. In addition, fever, fatigue, weight loss, anorexia, and night sweats are frequently reported. Histologically, the noncaseating granulomas are characterized by the presence of laminated concretions known as Schaumann's bodies, and stellate inclusions in giant cells called asteroid bodies. There is approximately a 10% mortality; the majority of deaths result from progressive pulmonary fibrosis and cor pulmonale.

Idiopathic pulmonary fibrosis (Hamman-Rich syndrome, chronic interstitial pneumonitis) is a condition characterized by diffuse interstitial inflammation and fibrosis. It is histologically similar to the pneumoconiosis and other conditions causing interstitial fibrosis, but no cause can be determined in these cases. The initial lesions apparently arise in response to type I pneumocyte injury. This leads to pulmonary edema, intra-alveolar exudate, hyalin membranes, alveolar septae infiltration by mononuclear inflammatory cells, and type II pneumocyte hyperplasia. The exudate ultimately organizes and fibrosis results in the alveoli as well as in the alveolar septae. Ultimately, the lung is composed of fibrous tissue separating spaces lined by cuboidal or columnar epithelium *(honeycomb lung)*. Hypoxemia and cyanosis are common in advanced cases. Complications include pulmonary hypertension and cor pulmonale that progresses to cardiac failure.

Pulmonary lesions associated with collagen vascular diseases are discussed in the chapter on Immunopathology.

Pulmonary Infections

Bacterial pneumonias are classified according to etiology, type of host response, or anatomic distribution.

Bronchopneumonia (lobular pneumonia) is characterized by a patchy distribution of consolidated areas that represent an extension of bronchitis and/or bronchiolitis. It is most frequently found in infants or the elderly. Common etiologic agents include staphylococci, streptococci, pneumococci, *Haemophilus influenzae*, *Pseudomonas aeruginosa*, and coliforms. Lesions are frequently bilateral and basal. Histologically, bronchi, bronchioles, and adjacent alveoli contain a purulent exudate with large numbers of neutrophils. Complications include local abscesses, empyema, and bacteremia, which can result in metastatic abscesses, endocarditis, meningitis, and arthritis.

Lobar pneumonia is characterized by consolidation of a large portion of a lobe, or an entire lobe. The vast majority of cases are caused by *Streptococcus pneumoniae*, most commonly types I, III (the most virulent), II, and XII. On occasion, *Klebsiella pneumoniae*, staphylococci, streptococci, *H. influenzae*, and some gram-negative organisms such as *P. aeruginosa* and *Proteus vulgaris* may cause the same changes. The extent of the lesion is dependent on the virulence of the organism and the host's ability or inability to respond. Thus, healthy or immunocompromised adults may be susceptible. Infection is established via the tracheobronchial tree, and it spreads through the alveoli via the pores of Kohn. Classically, four stages are recognized: (a) congestion, in which the lungs are heavy and wet due to hyperemia, alveolar fluid, neutrophils, and large numbers of bacteria; (b) red hepatization, in which the alveoli contain large numbers of red blood cells and a fibrinopurulent exudate; (c) gray hepatization, the third stage, is characterized by lysis of red blood cells and maintenance of the fibrinopurulent exudate; and (d) resolution, the stage in which the exudate undergoes enzymatic digestion and is either reabsorbed, phagocytized by macrophages, or expectorated, returning the lung to normal. With antibiotic treatment, the four stages may be modified considerably. Finally, pleuritis, stemming from the underlying inflammatory response, may resolve or, more often, leads to residual fibrous adhesions. Clinically, patients present with a productive cough, malaise, fever, and pleuritic pain and friction rubs if pleuritis is present. Complications are similar to those of bronchopneumonia.

Primary atypical pneumonia is caused by *Mycoplasma pneumoniae*, a number of viruses, *Chlamydia psittaci*, and *Coxiella burnetii*. It is characterized by multifocal to diffuse inflammatory regions that may be bilateral or unilateral. Histologically, the lesions are characterized by a mononuclear inflammatory cell infiltrate in the interstitium. The alveoli may be free of exudate or they may contain pink proteinaceous material on hyalin membranes. The clinical presentation is varied. Cough may or may not be present. In some cases, the constitutional signs of fever, headache, muscle aches, and leg pain may be the only signs. Elevated cold agglutinins are found in those cases caused by *M. pneumoniae* and in about 20% of those caused by adenovirus. These help distinguish these causative organisms from other viruses. Complications include superimposed bacterial infection.

Pneumocystis pneumonia is caused by *Pneumocystis carinii*. This organism is an opportunist and causes severe pneumonia in HIV-infected patients and is the major cause of death in AIDS. The pneumonia is diffuse or patchy. The alveoli are filled with proliferating organisms and cellular debris. The latter resembles edema fluid. There may be widening of the interstitium because of a mononuclear cell infiltrate. In addition, fibrin exudation, extravasation of red blood cells, and hyaline membranes may be present. Diagnosis is based on identifying the organisms in bronchioalveolar lavage fluid, sputum, or transbronchial biopsy specimens by staining with silver, Giemsa, or toluidine blue.

Lung abscesses are defined as local suppurative processes within the lung characterized by necrosis of lung tissue. They are generally caused by bacteria, including streptococci, *Staphylococcus aureus*, and a variety of gram-negative organisms. In addition, anaerobic organisms, generally found in the oral cavity, can also be isolated from these lesions. The organisms are introduced by (a) aspiration of infected material (*e.g.*, of gastric contents because of acute alcoholism or coma); (b) antecedent primary bacterial infections as a result of pneumonias; (c) septic embolism from thrombophlebitis or bacterial endocarditis; (d) neoplasms that are secondarily infected; and (e) miscellaneous routes, such as direct traumatic penetration and spread of infection from adjacent organs. There are cases in which the cause of the abscess cannot be identified. These are called *"primary cryptogenic" lung abscesses*. The region in which the abscess is located is dependent on the organisms route of entry. Consequently, they may be solitary and right-sided if aspiration is the predisposing cause, or multiple and scattered in cases of septic emboli. Histologically, the lesions are characterized as being well circumscribed with a central area of suppuration and cavitation. Chronic cases are characterized by a fibrous capsule. The clinical presentation is characterized by cough, fever, and copious amounts of foul-smelling purulent or blood-stained sputum. Chest pain and weight loss are also common. Diagnosis is confirmed by chest x-ray and bronchoscopy. Complications include extension of the infection into the pleural cavity, hemorrhage, and the development of brain abscesses or meningitis due to septic emboli. Underlying carcinomas are present in 10% to 15% of cases.

Pulmonary tuberculosis is still the major cause of tuberculosis morbidity and mortality. Lungs are the usual location of primary infections. The Ghon complex, the initial focus of infection, consists of a subpleural lesion between the upper and lower lobes, closely associated with the interlobar fissure. In addition, the lymph nodes draining the parenchymal focus are enlarged and contain caseous lesions. Bacilli from the primary infection can disseminate to regions of high oxygen tension such as the apical parts of the lungs. During this dissemination, individuals are asymptomatic. Reactivation of the disease occurs in the areas where the organisms have established themselves. This reactivated (secondary tuberculosis) is more damaging than the primary disease. Most frequently, the reactivated form commences as a focus of consolidation within the lung apicis. The hylus can also be involved. Regional lymph nodes develop foci of inflammation as well. Histologically, the lungs contain granulomas that often coalesce. These granulomas generally have caseous centers that are surrounded by epithelioid cells. These in turn are surrounded by fibroblasts, lymphocytes, and Langhans giant cells. Larger areas of consolidation are formed as the disease progresses, as a result of the coalescence of granulomas (tubercles). These ultimately become either totally scarred or surrounded by a thick wall of connective tissue. These regions of scar often contain calcium deposits. Diagnosis is confirmed by culturing for acid-fast organisms and staining histologic specimens and smears with acid-fast stains. If the disease progresses, three relatively distinct clinical pathologic conditions ensue. *Cavitary fibrocaseous tuberculosis* is characterized by erosion into a bronchiole, which allows drainage of the caseous focus into that region, transforming the lesion into a cavity. The tubercle bacilli grow favorably in this increased oxygen-tension environment. This allows for spread of the organisms to other sites in the lung, pleura, or upper respiratory tract. *Miliary tuberculosis* is a result of spread of the organisms via lymphatics or blood. The lesions may be confined to the lungs or involve other organs (*e.g.*, bone marrow, liver, or spleen). The individual lesions consist of granulomas varying from one to several millimeters in diameter. *Tuberculous bronchopneumonia* generally occurs in highly sensitized individuals. The pneumonia is diffuse bronchopneumonia, or it can be lobar in distribution.

Bronchogenic Carcinoma

Approximately 90% to 95% of primary tumors in the lungs are bronchogenic carcinomas. It is the most common visceral malignancy in men and accounts for approximately one third of all cancer deaths in men. The incidence is increasing in women, and lung cancer has passed breast carcinomas as a cause of cancer death in women. It is the most frequent fatal malignancy. There is a positive relationship between tobacco smoking and lung cancer, and there are positive links with radiation, uranium, asbestos, and other industrial hazards. The role of genetic factors in the cause and pathogenesis of bronchogenic carcinoma is not clear. There are four major categories of bronchogenic carcinoma.

Squamous cell carcinoma is most commonly found in men who smoke. It originates in the larger, central bronchi and spreads locally. It grows rapidly at its site of origin but metastasizes later than other pulmonary neoplasms. Histologically, well-differentiated neoplasms produce keratin, and intercellular bridges are observed. Undifferentiated neoplasms are also noted that have an appearance similar to that of large cell carcinomas.

Adenocarcinoma is the most common type of lung cancer in nonsmokers. It is usually in peripheral locations and is sometimes associated with scars. Histologically, the well-differentiated neoplasms form glandular elements. Some form papillary lesions, and the more undifferentiated neoplasms form solid masses. The differentiated neoplasms produce mucin. Adenocarcinomas grow more slowly than squamous cell carcinomas.

Small cell carcinoma is a highly malignant tumor of a distinctive cell type. The cells have a lymphocyte-like appearance and are often called ''oat cells.'' Histologically, the cells grow in clusters and neurosecretory granules are found in the cytoplasm by electron microscopy. These neoplasms are associated with paraneoplastic syndromes. This neoplasm is strongly correlated with cigarette smoking. It is generally found at the hilus or central in the lung, and it is the most aggressive of lung tumors. It metastasizes widely and is thus not amenable to surgical excision.

Large cell carcinoma is an anaplastic carcinoma that probably represents undifferentiated squamous cell carcinomas or adenocarcinomas.

Bronchogenic carcinomas metastasize by both lymphatic and hematogenous routes. They metastasize widely and in many instances early in the disease course. In some instances, metastatic lesions are the initial presentation. Favored sites for metastasis are the adrenal glands in more than 50% of the cases. In addition, the liver, brain, and bone are also commonly affected. Within the lung, bronchogenic carcinomas can compress and infiltrate lung parenchyma as well as eroding into the tracheobronchial tree. Additional complications include partial to complete obstruction of bronchi leading to emphysema or atelectasis. Severe purulent and ulcerative bronchitis or bronchiectasis is also observed. Pulmonary abscesses can be found within the neoplasms and they can extend into the pericardial and pleural sacs, giving rise to pericarditis or pleuritis. Finally, they can impinge on the superior vena cava, giving rise to a host of circulatory disturbances. The major presentations of pulmonary neoplasms are cough, weight loss, chest pain, and dyspnea in descending order. Diagnosis can be made by cytologic examination of sputum, bronchial washings, or brushings, or cytologic examination of fine-needle aspirates. The overall 5-year survival rate is around 9%, with adenocarcinomas and squamous cell carcinoma patterns having a slightly better prognosis than the other patterns.

Bronchial alveolar carcinomas, a form of adenocarcinoma, occur in the regions of the terminal bronchi and alveoli as single nodules or more commonly as diffuse nodules that coalesce, sometimes producing consolidation. Histologically, the tumor is composed of tall columnar to cuboidal epithelial cells that line the alveolar septae and project into the alveolar spaces as papilliferous projections. These cells often produce great quantities of mucin. These neoplasms occur from the third decade on. There is equal gender distribution. The presenting signs are similar to those of the other bronchogenic carcinomas. Single lesions can be resected surgically, and in these cases, there is a 50% to 75% 5-year survival rate. The overall survival rate is 25%. Metastasis, which is observed in 45% of cases, occurs late in the course of the disease and is not widely disseminated.

Bronchial carcinoids are low grade malignant tumors that occur typically in individuals younger than 40 and with equal distribution between genders. Histologically, they are composed of nests, cords, or masses of cells separated by fibrous stroma. On electron microscopy, they exhibit dense core granules that are characteristic of neuroendocrine tumors. These granules contain serotonin and a variety of other biologically active mediators. Clinical presentation is characterized by persistent cough, hemoptysis, and other signs of obstructive processes (*e.g.*, bronchiectasis, emphysema, and atelectasis) because of their intraluminal growth. Some of these neoplasms are functional and can produce the carcinoid syndrome. The 5- to 10-year survival rate is 50% to 95%.

Metastatic tumors are the most common malignancy in the lung. They come from a variety of sources, via both the lymphatics and hematogenous routes. Carcinomas include those arising in breast, colon, stomach, kidneys, ovaries, and uterus. Sarcomas include leiomyosarcoma, osteosarcomas, and others. Malignant melanomas also metastasize to the lungs. Finally, esophageal carcinomas and mediastinal lymphomas may be found in the lungs as a result of contiguous growth.

Malignant mesotheliomas are uncommon, but an increased incidence has been observed in individuals with heavy asbestos exposure. There does not appear to be an increase in the incidence of mesotheliomas in asbestos workers who smoke, contrasted to the risk with bronchogenic carcinomas. These neoplasms spread widely in the pleural space and are generally associated with marked pleural effusion. They often invade thoracic structures. Histologically, these neoplasms consist of two cell types with either one predominating in individual cases. Mesothelial cells develop as either mesenchymal stromal cells or epithelial lining cells. Consequently, the tumors may be composed of either a spindle cell sarcoma or a papillary type carcinoma. Special stains, immunohistochemistry, or electron microscopy is often necessary to differentiate these neoplasms from adenocarcinomas. The clinical presentation includes chest pain, dyspnea, and recurrent pleural effusion. The lung is invaded directly and there is often metastatic spread to hilar lymph nodes and other distant organs including the liver. Half of the individuals with pleural disease die within 12 months of diagnosis and very few survive beyond 2 years.

THE MOUTH

In addition to localized conditions, the mouth also manifests systemic diseases.

Inflammatory Diseases

Primary stomatitis is most often caused by infectious agents. ***Herpes simplex virus type I*** produces localized vesicles that upon rupturing produce red-rimmed ulcerations (''cold sores''). Less commonly, a diffuse disease is seen in children 2 to 4 years of age. Histologically, there is inter- and intracellular edema (acantholysis) that leads to vesicle formation. The virus is transported via nerves and ultimately resides in regional ganglia (*e.g.*, the trigeminal) from which it can be reactivated. The lesions in uncomplicated cases resolve in 3 to 4 weeks.

Aphthous ulcers (canker sores) are shallow ulcerations of the oral cavity of unknown etiology. They are painful, recurrent, and most frequently observed in the first and second decades of life. They may be single or multiple. Histologically, the initial inflammatory response is mononuclear, but secondary bacterial infection leads to a neutrophilic response. The lesions persist one to many weeks.

Oral candidiasis (thrush) is characterized by a white to gray, superficial inflammatory membranc that can be scraped off an underlying erythematous region. The membrane is composed of organisms, fibrin, and admixtures of neutrophils and mononuclear inflammatory cells. This condition is generally found in patients who are diabetic, immunologically compromised (*e.g.,* AIDS), or neutropenic, or who have xeroderma or alterations in oral flora as a result of antibiotic therapy.

The term ***glossitis*** is used to describe frank unlcerations of the tongue caused by physical and chemical trauma (*e.g.,* ill-fitting dentures, burns, or caustics). It also is used to describe the atrophic lesions, with or without inflammation, that are caused by deficiencies in the B vitamins and iron.

There are some ***systemic diseases with oral manifestations.*** These include infections (*e.g.,* scarlet fever, measles, infections mononucleosis, diphtheria, and AIDS); dermatologic conditions (*e.g.,* lichen planus, pemphigus, bullous pemphigoid, and erythema multiform); hematologic disorder (*e.g.,* agranulocytosis, aplastic anemia, leukemia, monocytic leukemia); and other conditions, such as melanotic pigmentation (*e.g.,* Addison's disease), phenytoin (Dilantin) ingestion, pregnancy, and Rendu-Osler-Weber syndrome.

Proliferative Diseases

There are two reactive proliferations that must be differentiated from neoplasms. ***Irritation fibromas*** are fibrous nodules that protrude usually from the gingiva–dental margin. They result from chronic irritation. They are common in pregnancy. ***Giant cell granulomas*** (epulis) generally protrude from the site of chronic gingivitis. They are well circumscribed and may be ulcerated. Histologically, they are characterized by foreign body giant cells in a fibrovascular stroma. They must be differentiated from true giant cell tumors.

There are two precancerous lesions of the oral mucosa. ***Leukoplakia*** is a white plaque on the mucous membranes that cannot be scraped off. It is most often associated with the use of tobacco products, particularly smokeless tobacco products. The use of alcohol, ill-fitting dentures, and exposure to persistent irritants (hot foods or beverages) also potentiate it. It appears as solitary or multiple white patches anywhere in the oral cavity. Histologically, it presents as a range of epithelial lesions, from hyperkeratosis or acanthotic epithelium, to dysplastic epithelium, to carcinoma *in situ.* These lesions predominate in males in the 40- to 70-year-old range. ***Erythroplakia*** is less common than leukoplakia, but it is associated with the same potentiating conditions and the same male predominance and age group. It presents as a red, possibly eroded, region in the oral cavity and is level or sometimes depressed below the adjacent mucosa. Histologically, the lesions are eroded and dysplastic; carcinoma *in situ* or adjacent carcinoma is observed. Intense mononuclear inflammation is observed subjacent to the epithelium admixed with dilated, hyperemic blood vessels.

Neoplastic Diseases

Squamous papillomas and ***condyloma acuminatum*** are benign lesions found in the oral cavity. ***Squamous cell carcinomas*** account for approximately 95% of all oral cancer. They are more common in men than women and are usually diagnosed between 50 and 70 years of age. Predisposing conditions giving rise to these neoplasms include the use of alcohol and tobacco products, particularly smokeless tobacco. These neoplasms occur anywhere in the oral cavity, but the floor of the mouth, tongue, hard palate, and tongue base are most frequent. The lesions are raised and present as plaques or verrucose areas. Histologically, they begin *in situ* and extend beyond that site, ranging from well-differentiated to anaplastic lesions. Initially, they infiltrate locally, and they metastasize later to mediastinal lymph nodes, lungs, liver, and bone. Prognosis is best for lip lesions and poorest for lesions at the tongue base and floor of the mouth.

Teeth

Dental caries result from bacteria, the most common of which is *Streptococcus mutans*, that can colonize on the teeth, metabolize carbohydrates, and produce sufficient acid, interacting with a high intake of carbohydrates, to demineralize enamel. Adequate saliva, high-roughage and low-carbohydrate diets, and fluoridation of the drinking water help reduce this incidence of caries. Caries lead to acute or chronic pulpitis, which in turn can lead to apical or periapical granulomas, cysts, abscesses, or osteomyelitis. Chronic periodontal disease is the primary cause of tooth loss in adults. It is caused by bacteria accumulating in the periodontal pocket under the gingiva. These bacteria form masses upon mineralizing calculus (tartar). The initial lesion is marginal gingivitis which can, if untreated, lead to chronic periodontitis. This, in turn, leads to destruction of the periodontium; as a result, there is loosening and ultimate loss of teeth.

Salivary Glands

Inflammation of the salivary glands, ***sialadenitis***, may be caused by viruses, bacteria, or autoimmune disorders. The most common type is mumps. ***Sialolithiasis*** may engender sialadenitis. The origin of the stones is often unknown, but they may be related to impacted food or edema resulting from trauma.

Salivary gland tumors are uncommon. The vast majority arise in the parotid gland (65% to 80%), with approximately 10% arising in the submandibular gland. The majority of malignant tumors are found in the latter gland. Most tumors occur in adults, with benign tumors appearing in the fifth and seventh decades and the malignant tumors appearing later. ***Pleomorphic adenomas (mixed tumors)*** comprise approximately 60% of tumors in the parotid gland and are less common in the other glands. Histologically, these neoplasms are encapsulated and composed of epithelial cells and myoepithelial cells arranged in a myxoid tissue that often has foci of cartilage or, rarely, bone. These neoplasms may recur, and a small percentage of them engender malignancies that are highly aggressive. ***Warthin's tumor (papillary cystadenoma lymphomatosum)*** is the second most common salivary tumor and it almost always arises in the parotid gland. It is predominantly found in men in the fifth and seventh decades. Histologically, narrow mucus-filled cysts or clefts are lined by a double layer of epithelial cells that lie on a stroma densely packed with lymphocytes and some lymphoid follicles. These tumors are benign. ***Mucoepidermoid carcinomas*** account for approximately 10% to 15% of salivary gland tumors. Approximately 70% are in the parotid gland. Histologically, squamous mucus or intermediate cells are arranged in cords, sheets, or cysts. They are classified as low-grade (mostly mucus cells), intermediate grade, and high grade (mostly squamous cells). High grade neoplasms are invasive, recur with some frequency, and are more likely to metastasize than the lower grades.

THE GASTROINTESTINAL SYSTEM

From mouth to anus, the gastrointestinal (GI) tract is exposed to the external environment in a unique way; among the systems of the body, only the skin may have comparable exposure. Add to this the pressure and mechanical trauma, the chemical exposure of the digestive enzymes, and the numerous bacteria that normally populate the gut, and it is clear why it is the principal source of symptoms that generate a visit to a physician. There are common themes that recur in the GI system at every level: diverticula, inflammation, herniation, hemorrhage, ulceration, and neoplasia. As a whole, the GI system is the commonest site of neoplasms in the body.

Esophagus

The esophagus is not just a connecting conduit but an active participant in transferring the food from the mouth to the stomach. In its upper portion, there is skeletal muscle in the wall, and the upper esophageal sphincter is made up of the cricopharyngeus muscle which is under voluntary control. The lower esophageal sphincter is not well defined anatomically, but it is extremely important physiologically as a barrier to the reflux of acidic pepsin-containing gastric contents into the lower esophagus. Normally, the esophagus is lined by squamous epithelium from its origin from the hypopharynx until it joins the cardiac portion of the stomach in the peritoneal cavity.

Diverticula: Diverticula occur at all levels. The upper ones are really in the posterior hypopharynx above the upper sphincter. Termed ***Zenker's*** diverticula, they are most frequent in the elderly. In the middle third, they have been termed ***traction*** diverticula because they were thought to arise from pulling out by inflammatory processes such as tuberculosis of the mediastinum, which was often associated. The esophagus lacks a true serosa. The usual cause of diverticula is pulsion, and this type is found in the lower third above the diaphragm, hence an ***epiphrenic*** diverticulum.

Esophagitis: Inflammation of the lower third of the esophagus is extremely common, usually self-limited, and most often the consequence of ***reflux***. It is usually the result of stimuli such as alcohol that relax the lower esophageal sphincter (LES). Prolonged reflux is associated with histologic changes consisting of papillomatosis and eosinophilic infiltrate, and they may be associated with columnar metaplasia to a ***Barrett's*** type of epithelium. The latter can resemble gastric cardiac or fundic epithelium or intestinal epithelium with goblet cells and villi. The latter appears to be predisposed to malignant transformation. Hiatus hernia is also frequently found in association with reflux esophagitis. Other causes of esophagitis include *Candida* and herpes viruses. These are more likely in immunocompromised hosts.

Hernias: Enlargement of the esophageal hiatus of the diaphragm may or may not be associated with herniation. If the gastroesophageal junction is translocated from its normal subdiaphragmatic location upwards into the thorax, it is called an hiatus hernia. The ***sliding type*** of hiatus hernia occurs where the esophagus joins the stomach in the chest. The less common ***rolling*** type (paraesophageal) occurs where the stomach lies adjacent to the esophagus.

Ulceration: Severe esophagitis can lead to ulceration. Acid and peptic digestion play a major role. Barrett's epithelium can also ulcerate.

Hemorrhage: The esophagus can be a source of major upper GI bleeding. Forceful vomiting can lead to lacerations of the lower esophagus and upper gastric mucosa, with ***hematemesis*** in the so-called ***Mallory-Weiss*** syndrome. ***Esophageal varices*** can lead to massive upper GI bleeding, which is frequently fatal with the first episode.

Varices are in the submucosa, usually of the distal esophagus and cardiac portion of the stomach, because they are the result of portal hypertension, usually caused by cirrhosis of the liver.

Neoplasia: Benign neoplasms are rare in the esophagus, with leiomyomas being the most frequent. Esophageal cancer represents 10% to 11% of GI neoplasms and about 4% of all neoplasms. Squamous cell cancers predominate, but adenocarcinoma is increasing in incidence. About 20% of malignancies arise in the upper third, and 40% to 50% in the middle third. These are almost entirely squamous cell carcinomas. Of the 30% to 40% of the esophageal malignancies arising in the distal third, nearly half are new adenocarcinomas, almost always in association with ***Barrett's*** change, usually of the intestinal type.

Stomach

The stomach has three muscle layers: circular, longitudinal, and transverse. The parietal cells are in the fundus and the body, and the gastrin-secreting cells are in the antrum.

Diverticula are distinctly uncommon in the stomach because of the thick muscle wall. ***Inflammation*** is extremely common but usually mild and self-limited. ***Acute gastritis*** runs a gamut from slight ***hyperemia*** and reddening of the mucosa with engorgement of the rich submucosal blood supply, to intense hyperemia and hemorrhage in the mucosa and even acute gastric ulceration. Red blood cells are prominent, but acute inflammatory cells are rather scanty. Acid, pepsin, and mucosal ischemia play a role with dietary stimuli, such as alcohol, and drugs, such as NSAIDS, probably evoking the response.

Chronic gastritis is a wastebasket term, and uniform classification is lacking. Localized chronic inflammation, usually with some mucosal atrophy, can affect primarily the antrum (type B), primarily the body and fundus (type A), or both (type AB). Antral gastritis is highly associated with *Helicobacter pylori*, and atrophic gastritis of the body and fundus is associated with antibodies to parietal cells or intrinsic factor. With high titers of the latter, gastric acid may be entirely lacking, intrinsic factor may disappear and vitamin B_{12} absorption may be lost with the development of pernicious anemia. Atrophic gastritis may predispose to malignant change.

Rarely, there is hyperplasia of the mucosa, which is better termed ***hypertrophic gastropathy*** than gastritis. One form in which there is excessive gastric fluid secretion and protracted vomiting is termed *Ménétrièr's disease*. The mucosa shows hyperplastic polyps.

Herniation of the stomach can occur as detailed above, or sometimes through a diaphragmatic opening that is congenital or acquired as the result of trauma. Such ***diaphragmatic hernias*** are more likely to result in ***incarceration*** or ***strangulation*** than are ***hiatus hernias***.

Ulceration: Acute gastric ulceration can be considered the severest form of acute gastritis. The ulcers are superficial and tend to be multiple. They are distributed more in the body and fundus than in the antrum, the favored sites for chronic peptic gastric ulcers. "Stress" and mucosal ischemia are important pathogenetic factors. Altered gastric mucosal barrier, including possible loss of prostaglandins, may play a role. Principal associated conditions include shock (of any origin), sepsis, previous surgery, multiple trauma, extensive burns (Curling's ulcer), and raised intracranial pressure (Cushing's ulcer). Severe, even life-threatening bleeding can occur.

Chronic peptic gastric ulcer and chronic peptic ***duodenal*** ulcers are extremely frequent disorders. Duodenal ulcers are more frequent than gastric and are more frequent in men than women. Typically, these ulcers appear within 2 cm of either side of the pyloric sphincter (antrum or proximal duodenum). Gastric ulcers classically involve the lesser curvature, are solitary, and appear scooped out with a regular, clean outline. There are radiating gastric folds that surround the ulcer. Duodenal ulcers often are also present, though if there are multiple duodenal ulcers, the Zollinger-Ellison (*e.g.*, hypergastrinemia syndrome caused by gastrinoma) syndrome must be considered. There is usually chronic gastritis in the antrum surrounding a peptic ulcer, and *H. pylori* infection is highly correlated with both gastric and duodenal ulcers. NSAIDS may be the other principal cause of gastric ulcers. Complications include ***penetration*** into the submucosa, which is almost always present; ***hemorrhage***, which is very frequent and potentially serious; ***perforation***, which is more likely from ulcer on the anterior wall; and ***pyloric obstruction*** as a result of scarring. ***Acquired pyloric stenosis*** affects adults, whereas in childhood, ***congenital hypertrophic pyloric stenosis*** can affect children, usually males, with vomiting that begins at about 4 to 6 weeks of age.

Hemorrhage: The stomach is a particularly frequent site of origin of GI hemorrhage. Causes include gastritis, gastric mucosal tears, gastric varices, acute and chronic ulcers, and gastric neoplasia. Vomited blood is usually red (hematemesis) but may be flecked with black; characteristically upper GI bleeding produces black tarry stools termed ***melena***, as a result of acid action on the blood to produce acid ***hematin***.

Neoplasia: Both benign and malignant neoplasms are still a significant problem in the stomach, more often for men than women. Benign tumors are usually epithelial in origin and project into the lumen as ***polyps***. Hyperplastic (non-neoplastic) polyps are quite frequent; adenomatous polyps, including both tubular and villous varieties, also occur. Hamartomatous polyps occur in the stomach in association with the ***Peutz-Jeghers*** syndrome. Stromal tumors, mostly of smooth muscle origin, are not uncommon. These are sometimes difficult to classify in the stomach as well as other locations and are grouped as gastrointestinal stromal tumors (GIST). ***Leiomyoblastoma*** is a lesion of intermediate malignant potential. Gastric carcinomas are almost always adenocarcinomas. The incidence has been falling in the United States for many years, where they once represented the number one malignancy in men. They are still prevalent in Japan and Scandinavia. Histologic variants include the *intestinal variety*, which resembles colonic glands, and the more aggressive *diffuse* type, which tends to infiltrate the wall with gastric-type mucus-containing cells. The depth of penetration (stage) is a good predictor of outcome. Superficial mucosal involvement predicts a relatively good prognosis. Diffuse wall involvement *(linitis plastica)* has a particularly bad outlook. Five-year survival for superficial cancers is in the 90% range, whereas advanced gastric cancer at diagnosis leaves fewer than 10% of its victims alive at 5 years. Primary intestinal lymphomas and carcinoids also arise in the stomach.

Small Intestine

For all of its length, the small intestine seems to be relatively less frequently involved by serious diseases, particularly neoplasia. Because its principal function is to absorb nutrients, the malabsorption syndrome is one of the more important manifestations of small intestinal disease.

Diverticula: They occur most frequently at the proximal and distal ends. Duodenal diverticula are usually acquired and may arise close to the insertion of the common duct. Meckel's diverticula occur in 2% of the population, are usually 2 inches or less in length, and occur within 2 feet of the termination of the ileum into the caecum (mnemonic: three × 2 !). They represent true diverticula because they have all three coats, and they are remnants of the vitelline (omphalomesenteric) duct. Acquired (false) diverticula occur along the mesenteric border of the small intestine at the insertion of the vessels, but they are less common than false diverticula of the colon.

Inflammation: The most common inflammatory diseases of the small intestine are bacterial infections. On a worldwide basis, they represent a huge problem of morbidity and contribute significantly to mortality in developing countries. *Vibrio cholerae*, *Salmonella*, and *Shigella* are rampant in some parts of the world. Parasites such as *Giardia lamblia* are now prevalent in the natural water supplies all over the United States. AIDS has also made cases of less common organisms such as *Microsporidia* much more frequent than in the past.

The principal noninfectious inflammatory disease that affects primarily the small intestine is ***Crohn's disease***. The distal ileum is involved in up to 85% of cases. The colon and ileum are involved in 35% to 40% of cases, and the esophagus, stomach, and other parts of the small intestine are involved in a small percentage. It is a systemic disease with manifestations in the eye (uveitis), the skin *(pyoderma gangrenosum, erythema nodosum)*, and the bones *(spondylitis)*. Renal calculi and gallstones may be associated. Crohn's and ulcerative colitis are grouped together as idiopathic inflammatory bowel disease and may be indistinguishable in up to 10% of cases. They have a similar epidemiology, affecting young adults most frequently with a smaller secondary peak in the fifth and sixth decade of life. Jews are affected more frequently than non-Jews, females slightly more often than males, and family members may have either ulcerative colitis or Crohn's disease. Pathologically, there are distinct differences. Crohn's is a transmural disease with chronic inflammation. Lymphoid nodules are often present and noncaseating granulomas are found in up to 50% of cases. The mucosal involvement tends to be linear serpiginous ulcers. It may skip areas with normal intervening mucosa. Loops of bowel may adhere to one another and fistulas may develop between loops of bowel, particularly in the anal region. There is an approximately twofold increase in colon cancer in association with Crohn's disease.

Herniation: Small bowel can herniate within the abdominal cavity or externally, as into an ***inguinal*** hernia or an ***umbilical*** hernia. Because its on a long mesentery, the small intestine can kink on itself *(volvulus)* or sometimes an upper segment is carried into a lower segment by peristalsis *(intussusception)*. Either of these can lead to vascular compromise and ischemia *(infarction)*. Fibrous adhesions from previous surgery are often contributors to these processes.

Ulceration: Small intestinal ulcers related to toxicity, such as those associated with potassium supplementation, are well known, and ulcers associated with specific infections such as tuberculosis and typhoid fever (salmonellosis) are also familiar. The ulcers of Crohn's disease and duodenal peptic ulcers represent noninfectious causes of small intestinal ulceration. Ectopic gastric epithelium in a Meckel's diverticulum may ulcerate.

Hemorrhage: The small intestine is a less frequent site of hemorrhage except when it is infarcted or when there is an ulcer in association with a Meckel's diverticulum or Crohn's disease. Bright red bloody diarrhea, ***hematochezia***, is the result of small intestinal as well as large intestinal bleeding.

Malabsorption: Because the major function of the small intestine is to absorb nutrients, malabsorption can generate a syndrome characterized by *weight loss* and *malnutrition*, *diarrhea*, and *steatorrhea* (fatty stools). Various endocrine abnormalities (such as amenorrhea in women), anemia, and other clinical manifestations may also accompany the major symptoms. There are multiple causes, the commonest being gluten sensitivity termed celiac disease, celiac sprue, or nontropical sprue. ***Tropical sprue*** is probably an infectious cause of malabsorption and ***Whipple's disease*** has now been shown to be caused by an actinomycete *Tropheryma whippelii*. Other causes of malabsorption include *short bowel, bacterial overgrowth (blind loop syndrome)*, and *maldigestion* that results from deficiency of pancreatic enzymes.

Neoplasia: Fewer than 1000 malignant neoplasms are identified as arising from the small intestine in the United States yearly, making it the least common site of primary neoplasia in the GI tract. Benign tumors such as adenomatous polyps, lipomas, and leiomyomas are also infrequent. Of the malignancies, although adenocarcinomas are most common in most series, primary non-Hodgkin's lymphoma and carcinoid tumors are almost as frequent. The lymphoid tissue of the intestines [mucosa-associated (MALT)] is abundant, and therefore it is not surprising that primary lymphoid neoplasms are found. The ***Mediterranean*** type and the Western type or maltoma are recognized variants. The small intestine is also richly endowed with neuroendocrine cells that secrete a variety of substances. These can give rise to carcinoids. Ileal carcinoids are more aggressive than those arising in the appendix and can give rise to the ***carcinoid syndrome*** when they spread to the liver.

Large Intestine

The large intestine (colon and rectum) is only about 3½ to four feet in length and parts of it are fixed and retroperitoneal, whereas others, such as the sigmoid and the transverse colon, are on mesenteries. The outer longitudinal muscle is discontinuous and represented by strips known as taenia coli. The blood supply to the proximal third is from the superior mesenteric artery, and that to the distal colon and rectum is from the inferior mesenteric and the hemorrhoidal arteries.

Diverticula: The false diverticula that arise between the discontinuous folds of outer longitudinal muscle at points of vascular insertion are increasingly frequent with advancing age and affect up to 80% of the population after the ninth decade. They may be single or multiple and arise earliest in the sigmoid. Complications include bleeding, inflammation, and perforation. ***Diverticular disease*** is a term that encompasses the older terms of ***diverticulosis*** and ***diverticulitis***.

Inflammation: Many of the infectious diseases that affect the small intestine also infect the large bowel. The bowel normally contains a rich bacterial flora and under appropriate circumstances even relatively innocuous common organisms can become pathogenic. Certain strains of *Escherichia coli* can cause diarrhea and ***hemolytic uremic syndrome***. ***Necrotizing enterocolitis*** in the newborn nursery is probably multifactorial but can be life threatening. Travelers are familiar with the diarrhea that results probably from re-population of the gut with new strains of familiar organisms. Viruses are frequent causes of infectious diarrhea and parasites including ***amebae*** are a huge problem worldwide. Probably 40% or more of our population is affected with diarrhea and/or vomiting yearly. Fortunately, most of it is self-limited. However, therapy can contribute to the development of more serious inflammatory disease such as ***pseudomembranous colitis***, which is often the result of broad-spectrum antibiotic therapy. The pseudomembranes consist of mucus discharged in a volcano-like manner onto the surface of the mucosa and mixed with fibrin and inflammatory cells. *Clostridium difficile* toxin is one of the important causes, but there are others, including ischemia.

The colon is the exclusive target of ***ulcerative colitis*** (UC). This form of inflammatory bowel disease, which shares so many epidemiologic and extraintestinal features (such as uveitis, spondylitis, pyoderma, and gangrenosum) with Crohn's disease, has a distinctive pathologic presentation. It most often begins in the rectum and sigmoid colon and proceeds proximally to involve the entire colon in continuity. It is a mucosal disease that rarely extends below the submucosa. Acute inflammation of the crypts creates cryptitis and crypt abscesses, and denuding of the mucosa results in exuberant granulation tissue. The mucosa is stripped off and regenerates to form pseudopolyps. Complications include ***toxic megacolon***, and prolonged UC increases the risk of cancer significantly more than does Crohn's disease.

Herniation: Because much of the colon is fixed, it is less likely to undergo herniation or torsion, except in the sigmoid or transverse portions. The transverse colon may herniate into the chest, and the sigmoid may undergo *volvulus*.

Ulceration: Aside from the ulcers seen in UC and stercoral ulcers, seen mostly in the rectum and anal canal, ulceration is not particularly common in the colon and rectum.

Hemorrhage: Bleeding in the colon is associated with diverticula or may be a sign of neoplastic transformation. In the past several years, an entity that results from abnormal plexuses of mucosal and submucosal vessels, usually in the right colon in elderly individuals, has been recognized and designated ***angiodysplasia***.

Neoplasia: Benign and malignant neoplasms of the colon and rectum are a major and very frequent problem in the Western world. Lung cancer and breast cancer kill more women and lung cancer and prostate cancer kill more men, but colon cancer is the number two killer of *both* men and women, with more than 150,000 new cases yearly and 55- to 60,000 deaths. Much evidence points to benign polyps as the major precursor, and the sequence of genetic changes leading to malignancy in both polypoid and nonpolypoid epithelium is generally being delineated. Much of this genetic evidence is being derived from familial adenomatous polyposis (FAP) syndrome.

Among the benign lesions, there are a few non-neoplastic and some neoplastic types that require emphasis. Most people over 50 years old develop one or a number of ***hyperplastic*** or ***serrated polyps*** that are considered to have little or no potential to become malignant. In the early decades, polyps may be found in the colon and other sites in the GI tract; these are considered to be hamartomatous and are termed ***juvenile polyps***. Multiple, virtually identical polyps are found at various levels in association with melanosis of the oral and anal mucosa in the familial polyposis syndrome called ***Peutz-Jeghers syndrome*** (P-J). There is little or no propensity for these to become malignant, but P-J patients may also have multiple adenomatous polyps of the tubular type, and these do have malignant potential. The truly neoplastic polyps include tubular adenomas and villus adenomas. The former have about a 3% ± 2% tendency to become malignant, whereas malignancy develops in up to 35% to 40% of villus adenomas. The genetic changes in the adenoma-to-carcinoma sequence have best been delineated in the FAP syndrome, in which there are literally hundreds of tubular adenomas, and the similar multiple polyposis syndrome, ***Gardner's syndrome,*** in which, in addition to tubular adenomas, there are osteomas, epidermal cysts, and fibromatosis. A putative tumor-suppressor gene termed APC (for adenomatous polyposis coli), mapping to the fifth chromosome (5q21), appears to be involved in a process requiring activation of the *ras* oncogene and deletions of chromosomes 17 and 18 before malignancy develops. Flat epithelium apparently can, rarely, also transform. Another multiple polyposis syndrome, ***Turcott's syndrome,*** in which brain tumors, gliomas, and meningiomas are also seen, is less well understood, but it also frequently leads to colonic malignancy.

Carcinomas of the colon are mostly well- or moderately differentiated adenocarcinomas that arise more frequently on the left side (sigmoid and rectum), where polyps are also more frequent. However, in recent years, more right-sided lesions seem to be appearing. In the rectum, carcinomas seem to grow circumferentially and constrict, producing symptoms of obstruction, whereas in the cecum, they are bulky and bleed.

Appendix

The most significant disease of the appendix is appendicitis. The pathogenesis appears to involve impaction of a fecalith with mucosal ischemia and subsequent bacterial invasion with suppression and sometimes perforation. Mucocele of the appendix can be caused by overproduction of mucus by benign or malignant cells. The principal tumor of the appendix is a carcinoid; this can spread, but it usually remains confined to the appendix.

Anal Canal

A principal cause of pain in the anus is ulceration of the hemorrhoidal veins, which, if they are above the squamocolumnar junction, are termed internal hemorrhoids, as opposed to the more frequent external hemorrhoids that are more likely to protrude and cause bleeding after a bowel movement. Fistula-in-ano may be a feature of Crohn's disease.

THE LIVER AND THE BILIARY TRACT

The liver is the largest gland in the body and it weighs about 1500 g on average. It is divided into a large right and a smaller left lobe, with two indefinite smaller lobes clustered around the hilum, which receives the portal vein and hepatic artery. The major bile ducts exit at the hilum and converge to form the common bile duct, which empties into the duodenum at the ampulla of Vater. The cystic duct joins the common hepatic duct after it exits from the gallbladder.

The functional hepatic unit is the classic lobule, which is described as a central hepatic vein around which the cords of hepatic parenchymal cells and sinusoids radiate like spokes of a wheel. In the periphery, the small triangular portal tracts, which contain one or more bile ducts, portal veins, and hepatic arteries, are arranged in a roughly hexagonal pattern. The more physiological concept of the functional unit is the acinar concept, in which the confluence of the hepatic artery and portal vein and the draining bile duct are the center, and the mass of liver cells are grouped in zones surrounding the stem and extending to the draining hepatic venule (zones 1, 2, and 3). Acini are described as simple (one), complex (three associated acini), and agglomerate (three complex acini), draining into a single biliary system. Most pathologic processes are described in terms of the lobule and the change is assigned to periportal, pericentral, and mid-zonal portions of the lobule. Because lobules are visible grossly as about 0.1-cm dots and can more easily be delineated microscopically, we shall use the lobular concept in our subsequent discussion, even though the pathophysiology of liver disease is more easily explained by the acinar model.

Patterns of Liver Cell Injury

The liver is a major metabolic organ that receives virtually everything that is taken in through the digestive system. The highest concentration of a given substance reaches the liver cells adjacent to the portal tract and subsequently the midzonal and pericentral areas. The liver cells next to the portal tract are the most active metabolically and contain enzymes such as the P450 system and others utilized in detoxification. The liver also produces the serum proteins, repackages the fat attached to carrier proteins, produces the bile acids, and metabolizes bilirubin. For these reasons, it is particularly vulnerable, but at the same time it has the capacity to withstand a variety of injurious stimuli. Until about 80% of it is destroyed, it can maintain homeostasis. The lobular arrangement and metabolic gradient explain many of the patterns seen in acute liver cell injury. The liver has an amazing capacity for regeneration. If two thirds of the liver is removed, the remaining liver can restore the lost mass within a matter of weeks. However, nonparenchymal cells can also regenerate, and therefore scarring can distort the pattern of regeneration.

The single most important determinant of the outcome of liver injury is the extent and the pattern of liver cell ***necrosis***. Usually, before they die, or even if they are sublethally injured, the hepatocytes swell (hydropic change). This is evident in ballooning degeneration in viral hepatitis and feathery degeneration in biliary obstruction. Necrotic cells can be condensed as acidophilic bodies (Councilman-like bodies, apoptosis) or they may disappear (drop-out). In addition to acute inflammation (polys), which tends to accompany toxic liver cell injury, mononuclear cells, including lymphocytes, plasma cells, and macrophages such as the Kupffer cells, participate in the inflammatory response, particularly to viral agents. Cytoplasmic hyaline, composed of cytokeratin filaments, is found in liver cells after long or intense exposure to alcohol (alcoholic hyaline or Mallory's hyaline). Fatty change is also a frequent indicator of sublethal injury to hepatocytes. Although hepatocytes constitute 60% of the liver cells and almost 80% of the mass of the liver, the stroma is very important in the overall response to injury, and fibrous scarring probably reflects activity of perisinusoidal cells (Ito cells) as well as periportal and pericentral fibroblasts.

The patterns of cell death are often reflective of the nature of the insult. Massive or submassive necrosis can wipe out whole lobules or several adjacent lobules, whereas zonal necrosis can involve specific hepatocyte populations such as pericentral *(alcohol, carbon tetrachloride)*, midzonal *(yellow fever)*, or periportal *(phosphorus, poisoning, pregnancy)* cells.

Acute Liver Cell Injury

Acute liver cell damage can last for up to 6 months before it is considered chronic. Depending on the extent of the injury, the patient may manifest liver failure (fulminant hepatitis) or only mild malaise with no detectable elevation of bilirubin and only subtle elevation of serum enzymes such as alanine aminotransferase (ALT), aspartate aminotransferase (AST), and lactic dehydrogenase (LDH), indicative of liver cell death. In fact, the majority of individuals with hepatitis go undiagnosed during the initial illness, and only later are they found to have antibodies to a specific virus.

VIRAL HEPATITIS

There are many viruses which affect the liver, but the principal hepatotropic viruses are discussed below:

1. ***Hepatitis A***. Single-stranded RNA, belongs to *picornaviruses*; fecal–oral transmission; incubation period 2 to 6 weeks; virus disappears at onset of clinical illness; fulminant hepatitis in less than 1%; no known carrier state or chronic hepatitis. IgM antibodies develop during illness and disappear; IgG antibodies persist, present in up to 50% of U.S. citizens over 50.
2. ***Hepatitis B***. Double-stranded DNA defines a class of *hepadna viruses*; spread by parenteral routes and intimate contact; incubation period 4 weeks to 6 months; virus not detected after onset of illness; fulminant hepatitis in up to 4%; chronic hepatitis (5%) and asymptomatic carriers (5% to 10%); cirrhosis- and cancer-associated; surface antibodies (HBsAb) indicate immunity and recovery. About 300,000 new infections yearly in the United States.
3. ***Hepatitis C***. Small single-stranded RNA, *Flavivirus*; many strains: antigenicity changes so reinfection possible; mild acute infection, recurrent elevation in transaminases; almost always leads to chronic state; parenteral transmission: leading cause of post-transfusion hepatitis; 80% of non-A, non-B hepatitis; 150,000 to 200,000 new cases yearly; cirrhosis and liver cancer are important complications.
4. ***Hepatitis D***. Defective single-stranded RNA virus, unknown class; requires HBsAg encapsulation to replicate; infects only as *co-infection* or *superinfection* with HBV; co-infection less severe: 3% fulminant hepatitis, 90% recovery; superinfection of HBV carrier: 10% fulminant hepatitis, 80% chronic HBV/HDV; spread by parenteral route, addicts and hemophiliacs at high risk; cirrhosis very frequent in superinfected patients.
5. ***Hepatitis E***. Nonenveloped, single-stranded RNA; water-borne-enteral transmission; no carrier state or chronicity, but high mortality in pregnant women (up to 20%).
6. ***Other viruses***. Epstein-Barr, yellow fever viruses, and others produce hepatitis. Newly discovered viruses F and like hepatitis F and G are on the horizon to account for remainder of "non-A, non-B" hepatitis.

Clinical and pathologic features of viral hepatitis: For the most part, the viral hepatitis diseasses are similar regardless of the infective agent, both from the clinical and the pathologic standpoint. The majority of cases are a mild flu-like illness with fever, malaise, loss of appetite, aches, and pains. Jaundice is present in a minority of patients, so most go undetected in the acute phase. Pathologic features include cell swelling *(ballooning)*, loss of orientation *(disarray)*, single cell necrosis *(drop-out*, or *apoptosis)*, and mild periportal chronic inflammation. Fulminant hepatitis is accompanied by massive or submassive necrosis termed *acute yellow atrophy*; fatty change is more prominent with hepatitis C. Most of the viruses damage the liver through immunologic mechanisms rather than cytotoxicity, but precise mechanisms remain to be elucidated.

TOXIC HEPATITIS

Because everything that is ingested ends up in the liver, the list of hepatotoxins is long. Some agents show a predictable, dose-dependent toxicity. Others are unpredictable and affect only some individuals who are hypersensitive. Some agents are directly toxic, whereas others are activated by detoxifying mechanisms to toxic intermediates. Thus, toxic liver disease can be difficult to predict, and anything can be toxic under the proper circumstances.

Clinically and pathologically, toxic hepatitis is similar to viral hepatitis, especially in the chronic stages. Illness may appear immediately after ingestion/administration of some agents, or it may be delayed. The principal pathologic patterns are necrosis, which can be focal or massive; steatosis *(fatty change)*; and *cholestasis*. Bile accumulation is usually in the canaliculi rather than in the large ducts, but bile plugs are sometimes seen. Inflammation is scattered and most likely to involve acute inflammatory cells (polys) and eosinophils.

Alcoholic liver disease: Alcohol is toxic to the liver. Everyone who ingests alcohol shows at least some fat accumulation in the liver. Liver enlargement *(hepatomegaly)* and fatty liver are very common in alcoholics. Alcohol interferes with fat metabolism in several ways. Fat can accumulate in the liver if there is increased ingestion or mobilization from stores, decreased utilization by decreased oxidation, increased synthesis particularly of triglyceride, and decreased transport by failure to synthesize the necessary carrier proteins. Alcohol interferes with all of these, principally the carrier protein synthesis. Fatty change appears to be entirely reversible. A second pattern is ***alcoholic hepatitis***, with drop-out necrosis. Changes occur in the pericentral region (zone 3) first. Hyaline change is prominent in scattered cells (alcoholic hyaline, Mallory's hyaline). There is fatty change and there are acute inflammatory cells in areas of necrosis, mostly pericentrally. The third pattern is cirrhosis (see later).

Metabolic liver disease: The liver is particularly vulnerable in many systemic illnesses, inborn or acquired, that interfere with carbohydrate protein or fat metabolism. Examples include glycogen accumulation (in several of the glycogen storage diseases), fat accumulation and increased susceptibility to develop cirrhosis (in diabetes mellitus), and cirrhosis (in protein malnutrition, ***kwashiorkor***). Ceruloplasmin deficiency leads to copper accumulation in the liver in ***Wilson's disease***, and affected individuals develop chronic hepatitis and cirrhosis. Iron accumulates in the liver and pancreas in ***hemachromatosis***, which is associated with cirrhosis, diabetes, and hyperpigmentation of the skin. Iron is found mainly in Kupffer cells in transfusional *hemosiderosis*. ***Alpha***$_1$-***antitrypsin deficiency*** is associated with cirrhosis in which characteristic PAS-positive inclusions, composed of the enzyme, are found in many liver cells.

Chronic Liver Injury

Chronic hepatitis: Both viral hepatitis and toxic hepatitis can enter a chronic phase in which inflammation and necrosis predominate, and which appears to be the pathway to cirrhosis in which fibrosis and regeneration become dominant pathologically. Viruses that cause chronic hepatitis and are suspected to cause cirrhosis and hepatocellular cancer are B, C, and D and a new non-A, non-B virus called G. A and E virus do not cause chronic hepatitis. A characteristic of toxic hepatitis is that, if the agent can be found, it is usually possible to get significant recovery of the liver if further exposure is prevented.

The morphologic classification of chronic hepatitis is changing. It was formerly felt that if inflammation was confined to the portal tracts, the prognosis was good, and this change, called ***persistent hepatitis***, ultimately resolved. On the other hand, if the chronic inflammation extended into the lobule and destroyed the limiting plate of cells around the portal tract in a process dubbed *piecemeal* necrosis, and if there were bridges formed between classic lobular landmarks (portal to portal, central to central, portal to central) that consisted of inflammation, necrosis, or fibrosis, the outlook was bad and the patient could die of liver failure as a result of ***chronic active hepatitis***, or progress to ***cirrhosis***. With the delineation of hepatitis C, it is now recognized that even persistent hepatitis C can progress. Thus, we are now switching to an *etiologic diagnosis*, and a system of *grading* and *staging*. However, during this transition the criteria for persistent and chronic active hepatitis remain, and they may be valid in hepatitis B.

Cirrhosis: The best definition of cirrhosis is generalized distortion of the liver architecture by nodules of liver cells as a result of hepatocyte regeneration. The nodules are circumferentially encased in fibrous connective tissue bands, in which are found the afferent and efferent blood supply and the draining bile ducts. The nodules can be big (macronodular) (e.g., more than a lobule in diameter) or small (micronodular). Although there are multiple causes of cirrhosis, alcoholic liver disease accounts for 80% or more in the United States. Cirrhosis is the fifth leading cause of death in men in the fifth or sixth decade of life. Other causes of cirrhosis include certain viruses (posthepatitic or postnecrotic cirrhosis), hemachromatosis, α_1-antitrypsin deficiency, Wilson's disease, primary biliary cirrhosis, and cirrhosis secondary to biliary obstruction. A large number of cases remain ***cryptogenic***.

The major complications of cirrhosis include liver failure with hepatic coma, bleeding from esophageal varices, and other consequences of portal hypertension such as ascites. Men with cirrhosis develop gynecomastia and spider angiomas because the liver fails to metabolize estrogen. Testicular atrophy also occurs.

Hepatic neoplasia: Worldwide primary cancer of the liver is one of the commonest neoplasms. In certain populations, such as male Bantus in South Africa, it is the leading cause of death from cancer. In the United States, almost 90% of hepatocellular cancers arise in a previously cirrhotic liver. The trabecular variant is most frequent, with other variants having a mixed *hepatocellular* and *cholangiocellular* appearance; less common tumors include ***cholangiocarcinoma*** and ***fibrolamellar liver cell carcinoma***. Benign neoplasms and hyperplasia are increasingly frequent. ***Hepatocellular adenomas*** are found in women of childbearing age, particularly those taking contraceptives; ***focal nodular hyperplasia*** is also more frequent in women, but not clearly associated with ''the pill.'' A raised *alpha-fetoprotein* level is a useful serologic marker for hepatic malignancy.

Biliary Tract Disease

Bile and bilirubin: Bile consists of a mixture of ions and salts of bile acids that are essential for the absorption of fat, and bilirubin, a breakdown product of hemoglobin with no known function. Bile acids are synthesized by the hepatocytes, secreted at the canalicular border, and then reabsorbed in the distal ileum. Without reabsorption, insufficient bile salts are available for fat absorption because synthesis cannot keep up with demand. Bilirubin is found in the reticuloendothelial system when the iron is removed from hemoglobin and the tetrapyrole ring is opened, forming biliverdin. The biliverdin is transported to the liver bound to albumin, transferred to the intracellular compartment by a protein called ligandin, and then conjugated to two molecules of glucuronic acid. The mono- or diglucuronide is then secreted again at the canalicular border, and it travels to the gut where it is acted upon by bacteria to form urobilinogens that are partially reabsorbed. Conjugated bilirubin and urobilinogen are water soluble and can appear in the urine. Unconjugated bilirubin is not water soluble. In general, substances that cause excessive breakdown of red blood cells *(hemolytic anemia)* produce an unconjugated hyperbilirubinemia; those that block the biliary system produce a conjugated hyperbilirubinemia.

Cholestasis and jaundice. Normal bilirubin concentration is about 1.2 mg/dL, most of which is (conjugated). Above about 2.5 mg/dL, clinical jaundice is apparent, with yellowish discoloration of the sclera as an early manifestation because of the high elastic tissue content in the eyeball to which bilirubin binds avidly. Usually above about 5 mg/dL, both conjugated and unconjugated bilirubin rise, making it harder to distinguish between obstruction and excess breakdown of rbcs. A mixed hyperbilirubinemia is also indicative of intrahepatic causes of jaundice, such as an intrinsic liver disease. Some causes of predominantly ***unconjugated*** hyperbilirubinemia include excess production by breakdown of rbcs (thalassemia, pernicious anemia), reduced uptake of bilirubin by the liver (drugs), impaired conjugation (genetics, intrinsic liver disease). Conjugated hyperbilirubinemia is seen in genetic abnormalities of transport, such as Dubin-Johnson and Rotor's syndromes; drug-induced impairment of secretion (oral contraceptives); hepatocellular damage (hepatitis); and extrahepatic biliary obstruction (stones, tumors).

Intrahepatic Biliary Tract Diseases

In addition to viral and toxic hepatitis, which can produce canalicular obstruction, there are some distinctive diseases that produce destruction of intrahepatic bile ducts. ***Primary biliary cirrhosis*** is a disease of unknown cause, perhaps involving autoimmunity, with progressive destruction of intrahepatic bile ducts (also called nonsuppurative destructive cholangitis). Affecting women 5 to 6 times more frequently than men, it is found most frequently in the fourth and fifth decades of life. There often is intense itching at the onset, probably resulting from an accumulation of bile salts, followed by jaundice. Xanthelasma and xanthomas (cholesterol deposits) are seen. The disease runs a slowly progressive course that has four stages histologically. Increased levels of antibodies to mitochondria are present in over 80% of cases. The early stage includes bile duct destruction with lymphocytes involved, and there is granulomatous inflammation in over 50%; gradually, the bile ducts disappear and there is progressive fibrosis leading to cirrhosis in the final stage.

Another, probably autoimmune, disease associated

with inflammatory bowel disease (most often ulcerative colitis) is ***primary sclerosing cholangitis***. Again, there is progressive destruction of bile ducts, which become encased in fibrous tissue. The extrahepatic biliary system may frequently be involved too. Ascending inflammation (cholangitis), usually from enteric organisms, can also occur.

Extrahepatic biliary obstruction: The two most frequent causes of extrahepatic obstruction are calculi and tumors. Gallstones almost always form in the gallbladder and are usually a mixture of cholesterol, bilirubin, and calcium salts. Pure stones are most frequently cholesterol, whereas bilirubin stones are found in association with hemolytic anemia. Large stones are less of a problem because they cannot pass through the cystic duct. Small stones can pass into the major ducts (choledocholithiasis) and produce obstruction at various levels. Common duct obstruction over time can produce a micronodular portal cirrhosis, ***secondary biliary cirrhosis***. Obstruction can also be caused by tumors. Malignancies principally affect the gallbladder and, second in frequency, the major bile ducts at the ampulla of Vater. Ductal malignancies arise most often from the large ducts, although intrahepatic malignancies (cholangiocarcinoma) can also be found.

The Gallbladder

The principal disease of the gallbladder is stone formation (cholelithiasis), which affects millions of people in the United States yearly. Bile is stored and concentrated in the gallbladder for secretion in response to a meal. It is an unstable mixture of cholesterol, phospholipids (lecithin), and bilirubin. Lecithin and bile salts tend to keep the mixture soluble, whereas cholesterol and calcium favor precipitation. Stones form when a *nidus* for crystallization develops, which may be a role for focal infection. Stones come in all sizes and shapes, and most (90%) are mixtures, as mentioned previously. Women in midlife who are obese, are fair skinned, and have had several pregnancies are particularly at risk of cholelithiasis (''fat, fair, forty, and fertile'').

Complications of cholelithiasis include obstruction of the cystic duct, in which case ***hydrops*** of the gallbladder, or even calcification (porcelain gallbladder) or mucus accumulation may appear (mucocele). Acute and chronic inflammation (acute cholecystitis; chronic cholecystitis) are strongly associated with calculi. Enteric organisms are most frequently involved as an ascending infection in acute cholecystitis that can lead to a medical emergency termed ***gangrene*** of the gallbladder. Acalculous cholecystitis can also develop.

Gallstones are also highly associated with tumors of the gallbladder. Benign polyps include adenomas, which are similar to those in other parts of the intestinal tract (tubular, villus or papillary, and tubulopapillary). They may be precursors of malignancy that arise principally from the epithelium. ***Carcinoma of the gallbladder*** is the fifth most frequent GI malignancy. It remains silent for some time and often has spread to regional lymph nodes or invaded the liver before it is discovered, so finding it conveys a particularly ominous prognosis.

Miscellaneous Diseases of the Liver

Additional conditions that deserve brief mention include the following:

1. Congenital or hereditary disease of the liver and biliary tree. These include anomalies such as ***biliary atresia***, choledochal cysts (*e.g.*, ***Carole's disease***), and ***cystic disease*** of the liver in conjunction with renal polycystic disease. Hereditary hyperbilirubinemias include benign forms such as the common ***Gilbert's disease***, and ***Dubin-Johnson*** and ***Rotor's syndromes***; and the fatal forms, ***Crigler-Najjar types I and II***.
2. Microvesicular fatty change. Usually large drops of fat are found in hepatocytes, but tiny fatty droplets are characteristic of the fatty liver of *pregnancy*, *Reye's syndrome* (which is generally associated with aspirin intake), and intravenous administration of tetracycline. Other conditions can produce microvesicular fat, but these are the most common.
3. Circulatory disturbances are less frequent in the liver because of its dual blood supply. Nonetheless, infarction does occur in relation to shock, usually in a subcapsular location. So-called ***infarcts of Zahn*** are really hemorrhagic and congested areas that extend to Glisson's capsule and result from portal vein obstruction. Portal vein thrombosis is seen in association with cirrhosis, and hepatic vein thrombosis leads to the ***Budd-Chiari*** syndrome. The commonest cause of hepatic congestion is heart failure, which can lead to acute passive hyperemia or chronic congestion termed nutmeg liver. Pericentral fibrosis can be extensive in long-standing hepatic congestion, which is designated ***cardiac sclerosis*** because regenerative nodules and true cirrhosis are rarely if ever present.

THE EXOCRINE AND ENDOCRINE PANCREAS

The pancreas arises from embryonic buds (dorsal and ventral) of the duodenum, which fuse to form the head, body, and tail of the adult organ. The final pancreatic duct of Wirsung empties into the common bile duct in the majority of individuals before it empties into the ampulla of Vater. In histologic sections, it is made up of two distinct components: the acinar or exocrine component, which drains through a series of ducts into the main pancreatic duct, and the islets or endocrine pancreas. The latter makes up about 1% to 2% of the mass of 100 ± 30 g of pancreatic tissue.

Diseases of Exocrine Pancreas

A variety of inherited and acquired diseases affect the exocrine pancreas, whose principal function is to secrete digestive enzymes including lipases, amylases, and peptidases into the small intestine.

Congenital conditions include hypoplasia and ectopia, which occur in up to 2% of individuals; the stomach, duodenum, and Meckel's diverticula of the ileum are favored sites.

Inherited disease of the pancreas is represented principally by ***mucoviscidosis***, or ***cystic fibrosis*** (CF). CF is the most common lethal genetic disease, occurring in about 1 in 500 Caucasians, and it is the result of a defect in epithelial chloride transport that results in abnormally tenacious mucous secretion. A variety of organs, such as salivary glands and sweat glands, are affected, and at birth it can present as impacted bowel (***meconium ileus)***. Over time, affected individuals develop pulmonary problems, cirrhosis of the liver, and pancreatic insufficiency manifested as ***maldigestion*** with steatorrhea and malnutrition. Pancreatic ducts become plugged with mucus, and the acinar pancreas undergoes atrophy and fibrous replacement.

Pancreatitis is the result of intrapancreatic release of enzymes with consequent acinar injury. Often, the endocrine pancreas is spared until late in the disease. ***Acute pancreatitis*** can be an explosive condition, often with severe necrosis and hemorrhage (acute hemorrhagic pancreatitis). Clinically, pain is a prominent symptom and there is release of enzymes, such as amylase and lipases, into the bloodstream. Various etiologic agents have been identified, with alcohol abuse and impacted gallstones being implicated most frequently. Viruses such as mumps and parasites such as *Clonorchis sinensis* can cause pancreatitis. Interstitial inflammation, proteolysis with necrosis of acinar cells and fat necrosis resulting from lipase release are prominent pathologic features. Plugs of mucus are frequently present in small ducts in cases resulting from diverse etiology, including metabolic causes (uremia, diabetes), ischemia, and alcohol. Hemorrhaging is more prominent than acute inflammation, which is usually minimal. Liquefactive necrosis may produce cystic spaces termed ***pancreatic pseudocysts***.

Chronic pancreatitis: This appears to be the result of repeated episodes of acute pancreatitis with recovery and relapse (chronic relapsing pancreatitis). Therefore, the etiology of chronic pancreatitis is similar to that of acute pancreatitis, with alcoholism and cholecystitis heading the list. Clinically, the patients show pain, weight loss, and malnutrition. They may have associated biliary tract symptoms and develop a pancreatic pseudocyst and focal pancreatic calcification. Diabetes may develop, usually late in the disease, because the acini are preferentially destroyed. Pathologically, the acinar pancreas is replaced by fibrous tissue, and only the ducts and islets remain. Focal calcification, cystic structures, and ductal abnormalities such as squamous metaplasia and ductal plugging are also seen.

Neoplasia: Tumors of the exocrine pancreas arise almost exclusively from the ducts. There are non-neoplastic cystic structures in the pancreas and benign neoplastic cysts. ***Congenital polycystic*** disease may involve the pancreas, but most non-neoplastic cysts are acquired as a result of acute or chronic inflammation (pseudocyst). Pancreatic cysts associated with angiomas of brain and eye are seen in von Hippel-Lindau disease.

Benign cystic tumors include mucinous cystic tumor and mucinous cystadenoma; a microcystic adenoma and a solid-cystic or papillary cystic tumor are most frequent in adolescent girls and young women.

Carcinoma of the pancreas is the sixth most frequent lethal human malignancy and it is increasing in incidence. Fewer than 1% are derived from acinar elements (***acinar carcinoma)***. ***Ductal carcinomas*** are most frequent in the head (60%); about 15% are found in the body and 5% in the tail, and the gland is diffusely involved in up to 20%. The cancer is usually far advanced when it is discovered and thus mortality is very high. There are about 28,000 new cases and 26,000 deaths annually, accounting for about 5% of all cancer deaths.

Symptoms include painless jaundice and an enlarged gallbladder (Courvoisier sign). Migratory thrombophlebitis (Trousseau's sign) is also associated. Histologically, the tumors are usually poorly differentiated adenocarcinomas, and adenosquamous and giant cell and sarcomatoid patterns are seen, but rarely. Acinar cell carcinoma, which is the common form in experimental animals, is uncommon in humans.

Presumptive etiologic factors include multiple dietary factors and cigarette smoking. Partial gastrectomy also has been associated with an increase in pancreatic cancer.

The Endocrine Pancreas

The endocrine pancreas is composed of the islets of Langerhans, which constitute about 1 million separate glomeruloid bodies spread throughout the pancreas, and in aggregate they weigh between 1 and 2 g (1% of the pancreatic weight). They are more frequent in the tail and are composed principally (70%) of beta cells, which secrete insulin. The alpha cells, which secrete glucagon, make up 20% of the islet cell mass, whereas the delta cells (somatostatin) make up about 10%, and the PP cells (pancreatic polypeptide) make up about 1%. There are also scattered enterochromaffin cells, which secrete substances such as vasoactive intestinal polypeptide (VIP) and serotonin.

Diabetes mellitus: The principal disease associated with the endocrine pancreas, diabetes mellitus (DM), results from an absolute lack or a relative lack of insulin. The primary form of diabetes, as opposed to diabetes that is secondary to problems such as chronic pancreatitis or pancreatic resection, has two principal forms: insulin-dependent DM, also known as juvenile onset or type I, and non-insulin dependent (type II, maturity onset). There are other minor forms such as maturity-onset diabetes of the young (MODY).

The symptoms of diabetes include polyphagia, polydipsia, and polyuria. Weight loss may lead to wasting and, particularly, breakdown of adipose tissue. In the absence of insulin, the diabetic will develop ketosis (acetone, acetoacetate, betahydroxybutyrate) and metabolic acidosis.

Of the 15 million or more diabetics in the United States (5% to 6% of the population), nearly half are undiagnosed, and 80% are type II. Although, by definition, all type I diabetics must be treated with insulin, 50% of the type II diabetics could be treated by diet alone. Thus, the bulk of type II diabetics are obese and only a minority are classified as non-obese.

There are some similarities and distinct differences between the two types. Type I diabetes usually has its onset before the age of 20, requires insulin-replacement therapy, and is likely to involve ketoacidosis. There is a familial tendency, with up to 50% concordance in identical twins. There is mounting evidence of an autoimmune origin, with perhaps a triggering event such as an antecedent viral illness. There is an HLA association, and, early in the disease, lymphocytic infiltration if the islets *(insulitis)* is seen. Overt diabetes involves approximately 80% or more destruction of the beta-cell mass, and late in the disease there is atrophy and fibrosis of the islets. The precise antigen is still a matter of debate. Beta-cell antibodies and insulin antibodies are also found, but the latter may be a response to therapy. Type II diabetes characteristically affects obese individuals in the fifth to sixth decade of life. There is a definite genetic predisposition, with both identical twins developing the disease in over 90% of the cases. The pathogenesis is more complex, and absolute lack of insulin and beta-cell destruction may not be present. Type II diabetics are unable to respond appropriately to a glucose load and insulin secretion rises only gradually instead of showing an immediate response. Fasting insulin levels may be normal or even raised. The principal abnormalities include inappropriate insulin release, *decreased hepatic glucose uptake*, increased hepatic glucose ***release***, and decreased insulin response in muscle and adipose tissue, which are the principal insulin-dependent tissues. This *insulin resistance* is probably due to *decreased insulin receptors* in most instances. Diet with weight loss, and exercise can improve the insulin resistance. Antibodies are generally lacking. Pathologically, up to 70% of type II diabetics show some amyloid deposition in the islets, but loss of beta-cell mass is not always documented. The amyloid appears to be the result of deposition of a polypeptide that is capable of assuming the beta-pleated configuration, known as amylin or IAPP. It is co-secreted with insulin, is 37 amino acids long, and has sequence homology, in part, with the calcitonin-releasing gene product. By inference, it is a neuropeptide, but its exact function is debated. Whether it is the cause of insulin resistance remains to be established in humans.

Complications of diabetes are similar in the two types and take about 10 years or more to develop. Although only type I diabetics usually become ketotic, type II diabetics can develop hyperosmolar coma, which is highly lethal. Renal failure is one of the principal causes of death, and diabetes is the principal cause of renal failure in adults. Vascular complications such as stroke, coronary artery occlusion, myocardial infarction, and gangrene of the extremities are all-too-familiar complications of diabetes. Proliferation of retinal vessels leads to diabetic retinopathy, a leading cause of blindness. Increasing evidence indicates that the complications of diabetes are largely a result of the raised blood sugar. This leads to the formation of advanced glycosylation end products (AGE), which cross-link various proteins such as collagen. Hypertension and hyperlipidemia are contributing factors. Insulin excess may account for some of the changes, such as diabetic retinopathy.

Although macrovascular disease (atherosclerosis) does develop, it is probably the microvessel disease *(microangiopathy)* that is the most serious pathologic change. Arteriosclerosis in the small arteries and arterioles of the kidney may trigger hypertension. Mesangial deposits and thickening of the glomerular capillaries lead to the glomerulosclerosis (Kimmelstiel-Wilson) that is responsible for renal failure. Peripheral neuropathy is probably also of vascular origin. With better means of monitoring the blood sugar, such as home monitoring devices and glycosylated hemoglobin (HbA_1) determination, as well as better types of insulin (human) and ways of administering it, complications can probably be avoided by strict adherence to diet, exercise, and insulin requirements. In patients with renal failure and other complications, transplantation of a pancreas along with kidneys is now almost routine. Islet transplantation and other approaches show significant promise.

Islet Cell Neoplasms

The only other disease of real significance in the endocrine pancreas is neoplasm. Most neoplasms behave as benign growths, but they have the potential to disseminate widely.

Insulinoma (beta-cell tumor): This is the commonest type. Symptoms include hypoglycemia, mental confusion brought on by exercise or not eating, and relief of attacks by eating. Most (70%) are single adenomas, but about 10% are multiple and about 10% are diffuse resembling hyperplasia. Up to 10% metastasize and thus are true carcinomas. Diffuse hyperplasia may be seen occasionally, and in infants of diabetic mothers, islet cell enlargement is seen.

Gastrinoma: The occurrence of recurring and/or multiple peptic ulcer(s), gastric hypersecretion, and gastrin-secreting pancreatic islet cell tumor is known as the Zollinger-Ellison syndrome. About 10% of gastrinomas are in the duodenum. Over 50% of gastrinomas are malignant.

Other less common benign neoplasms include ***glucagonomas*** (alpha-cell tumors) and ***somatostatinomas*** (delta-cell tumors). Both of these are associated with mild DM clinically; cholelithiasic is frequently associated with the latter, and a necrotizing red skin rash is associated with the former. Vipoma produces diarrhea.

THE RENAL–URINARY SYSTEM

The Kidneys

The kidneys are paired organs lying in the retroperitoneal area immediately below the diaphragm. They usually each receive a single main renal artery which is a major branch of the aorta. This bifurcates into an anterior or posterior branch before it enters the kidney, and it gives off successively segmental, interlobar, arcuate, and interlobular branches. The afferent arterioles supply the glomerular tuft of capillaries, and the efferent arteriole gives rise to the peritubular capillaries. The venous drainage follows the arterial supply. The renal vessels are said to be an end arterial system, because they do not anastomose with each other. The functional unit is the nephron, which consists of a glomerulus and its associated tubular system, including proximal tubules, Henle's loop (thin and thick limbs), and distal tubules. The collecting ducts drain one or more nephrons into larger and larger ducts, which empty at the renal papilla into the calyceal system. From there, the renal pelvis drains into the ureter, then to the urinary bladder, and ultimately to the urethra, which completes the urinary tract.

The adult kidney weighs about 150 to 200 g and is oval or bean shaped. It measures about $11 \times 5 \times 5$ cm in the adult, and approximately one third of the parenchymal width (10 cm) is cortex, two thirds is medulla, and the rest is pelvis. Renal diseases are most easily discussed in terms of the affected portion of the renal anatomy. Therefore, the following discussion will first cover congenital anomalies as a group, and then the glomerular, tubular, interstitial, and vascular diseases. Then the pelvis, ureter, and urinary bladder will be discussed.

CONGENITAL DISEASES OF THE KIDNEY

The renal–urinary system is one of the most frequently affected systems from the standpoint of congenital anomalies. Nearly 10% of the population has an inherited or, more often, an acquired renal anomaly, most of which are trivial but they may predispose to infection or calculi. ***Polycystic renal disease*** accounts for nearly 10% of chronic renal failure.

Agenesis may be unilateral or bilateral. In the latter case, it is usually found in stillborns. The ureter may not exist, and failure of the nephrogenic mesoderm is responsible. Hypertrophy of the normal kidney may be compatible with normal life.

Congenital hypoplasia involves not only reduction in size, but also the number of calyceal systems is reduced to fewer than five. In acquired hypoplasia, usually from chronic infection, there are the normal complement of 9 to 12 separate calyces.

Ectopic kidneys are usually found in the pelvis because of the embryonic development of the metanephros.

Cystic diseases of the kidney represent a group of anomalies of varying prognoses. Cysts may occur in the cortex or medulla; they may be present in infancy or develop progressively in adulthood. Important types include: adult polycystic disease, which is an autosomal dominant with high penetrance resulting from the APKD1 gene on chromosome 16 in 90% of cases; childhood polycystic disease, an autosomal recessive with several forms, usually fatal in infancy; ***medullary sponge kidney*** of unknown origin; and uremic medullary cystic disease (UMCD), which has its onset in childhood. ***Acquired cysts*** may be single or multiple and usually result from a localized inflammatory or obstructive event that seals off one or more kidney tubules.

GLOMERULAR DISEASES

Glomerular diseases are the most prevalent form of renal disease in young children and young adults. Clinically, they produce various syndromes, including nephritic, nephrotic, and uremic, as well as asymptomatic hematuria or proteinuria. The majority are the result of immunologic mechanisms, with specific diseases developing, for example, from circulating antigen–antibody complexes, and direct antibodies to basement membrane. In later life, degenerative changes predominate, with the laying down of various types of collagen in relationship to hypertension and diabetes.

Patterns of glomerular injury vary from disease to disease, and they are important to remember: if only some glomeruli are affected, the disease is said to be *focal*; if only *part* of the glomerulus is affected, it is termed *segmental*; if all glomeruli are affected, it is *generalized* or *widespread*; and if all of the glomerular tuft is involved, it is *diffuse*.

Nephritic syndrome includes hematuria, azotemia, and proteinuria, and it may include oliguria, hypertension, and edema. The causes of nephritic syndrome include various types of ***acute, rapidly progressive***, and (some forms of) ***chronic glomerulonephritis***. ***Acute*** forms of glomerulonephritis are for the most part immunologically mediated. Among them are the following:

Acute diffuse proliferative glomerulonephritis. The majority of these occur 1 to 4 weeks after group A beta-hemolytic streptococcal infection (types 12, 4, and 1). The exact antigen is unknown, but the disease results from trapping of antigen–antibody complexes to produce a "lumpy-bumpy" fluorescence pattern and subepithelial deposits that can be seen with electron microscopy. Glomeruli are diffusely hypercellular, with mesangial cells and endothelial cells proliferating most, and some increase in epithelial cells and leukocytes. IgG, IgM, and C_3 are present in deposits. More than 90% recover completely. Acute glomerulonephritis can less frequently follow other bacterial infections such as *Staphylococcus, Streptococcus pneumoniae*, and others, and viral infections. Persistence of hypertension, prolonged proteinuria, and low complement are bad prognostic indicators.

Rapidly progressive glomerulonephritis (RPGN) can occur under three circumstances: as an extension of an acute poststreptococcal glomerulonephritis; accompanying systemic diseases such as lupus erythematosus (SLE); and in cases of unknown etiology (idiopathic). Clinically, there is the nephritic syndrome. The hallmark pathologically is *epithelial crescent formation* in Bowman's capsule (crescentic GN is an alternative designation). This appears to be involved in response to fibrin leaking into Bowman's space. Some cases show *linear deposits* of IgG antibodies to glomerular basement membrane and pulmonary hemorrhages, which constitutes Goodpasture's syndrome. More than 50% are idiopathic. In ***SLE***, the disease can begin as a segmental glomerulonephritis with *subendothelial* deposits and progress to crescentic GN. Progression to chronic renal failure is quite common.

Nephrotic syndrome is characterized by edema and massive (more than 3.5 g daily) proteinuria. In addition, there is ***hyperlipidemia*** (cholesterol) and ***hypoalbuminemia***. There is selective loss of albumin in the urine. In childhood, the common cause is lipoid nephrosis or so-called minimal-change disease because with light microscopy the glomeruli are normal. Electron microscopy shows only fusion of foot processes, and deposits are usually absent. Most of these respond promptly to steroids. In cases of recurrence, glomeruli may show ***focal/segmented sclerosis***, which has a less benign course. In adults, ***membranous glomerulonephritis*** (MGN) is a common cause. There are intramembranous deposits that start on the epithelial side and are incorporated into the membrane and then resolve (stages I to IV). Spikes of basement membrane appear between the deposits on silver stain. Associated diseases include neoplasia (particularly of lung, colon, and melanoma), hepatitis B, and a number of other systemic diseases. Another pattern of glomerular injury leading to nephrotic syndrome is ***membranoproliferative glomerulonephritis*** (MPGN), in which there is proliferation mostly of mesangial cells (mesangiocapillary GN). Lobular appearance of the glomerular tuft is accentuated, and dense deposits are mostly subendothelial. Two types (I and II) can be distinguished. Two thirds of cases are type I; type II is distinguished by dense deposits of unknown material (dense-deposit disease).

Other causes of nephrotic syndrome include diabetes (nodular glomerulosclerosis, Kimmelstiel-Wilson disease) and renal vein thrombosis (associated with membranous nephritis).

Other glomerular diseases that may be accompanied by hematuria include ***IgA nephropathy*** (Berger's disease), Henoch-Schönlein purpura, and idiopathic focal GN, in which there may be focal and segmental involvement of glomeruli with necrosis and/or proliferation.

Chronic glomerulonephritis is commonly associated with hypertension and azotemia or uremia. Most of the diseases already described can lead to chronic glomerulonephritis, although frequently the underlying cause remains a mystery. The kidney is shrunken and atrophic, and the glomeruli are usually hyalinized and replaced by collagen.

Glomerular Diseases Associated with Systemic Diseases. Several have already been described, such as DM and SLE. Hereditary disease such as Alport's syndrome, in which there is thinning of the glomerular basement membrane, and amyloidosis, in which typical amyloid is deposited in the glomerulus, should also be mentioned. ***Goodpasture's syndrome*** and ***Wegener's granulomatosis*** are also associated with the acute, the rapidly progressive, and the chronic glomerular diseases.

DISEASES OF TUBULES

The nephron is a unit, so diseases that primarily affect one part will secondarily cause damage to others. Protein filtered through the glomerulus is reabsorbed proximally for the most part, or it may appear as tubular ***casts*** in the urine. Sclerosis of the glomerulus will affect the blood supply to the peritubular capillaries and secondarily cause tubular atrophy. For this reason, it is often difficult to establish the primary cause of ***end-stage*** renal disease.

Acute tubular necrosis (ATN) is one disorder in which tubules are usually affected selectively. In shock from various causes, the blood may be shunted away from the kidneys, resulting in ischemia. The straight portions of the proximal tubules are particularly sensitive, but actual necrosis is usually spotty and not as severe as reversible swelling. Clinically, there is an *initial phase* in which oliguria may progress to complete anuria, followed by a *maintenance phase,* during which fluid and electrolyte balance must be carefully monitored, usually followed in 7 to 10 days by a *recovery phase*. Complete recovery is the usual course, but some patients, such as those with severe bleeding accompanying placental separation, may develop massive ***cortical necrosis*** with widespread necrosis of the kidney cortex bilaterally.

There is a group of diseases referred to as ***tubulointerstitial nephritis*** (TIN), in which the tubules and the interstitium, as well as the blood vessels, may show change. Acute and chronic bacterial infections, *drugs* such as analgesics, *heavy metals* including lead and arsenic, *metabolic* diseases including gout *(urates)*, hyperparathyroidism *(calcium)*, and others, and neoplasms such as *multiple myeloma* may produce this pathologic picture.

INTERSTITIAL DISEASE

The commonest cause of interstitial disease is gram-negative organisms such as *E. coli*, which can ascend to the kidneys in the periureteral lymphatics. ***Acute pyelonephritis*** begins in the interstitial tissue and secondarily involves the tubules. The pelvis and medulla are almost always involved in the acute inflammatory process. An associated bladder infection (cystitis) is usually present and women are much more commonly affected than men, presumably because their short urethras offer access to the lower urinary tract. Flank pain and pyuria with white blood cell casts are helpful in distinguishing acute pyelonephritis from simple cystitis.

Chronic pyelonephritis is thought to be the result of recurrent acute pyelonephritis or failure to completely eradicate the bacteria. Pathogenesis remains a matter of debate, but associated conditions include recurrent lower urinary tract infections, female sex, multiple pregnancies, and urinary tract obstruction from calculi or other causes. Vesicoureteral reflux is another factor. The kidney may undergo severe atrophy and there is interstitial scarring, chronic inflammation that involves the medulla and the cortex, and perivascular and periglomerular fibrosis. Protein casts in the tubules give the appearance of thyroid follicles (thyroidization).

A host of other diseases can affect the renal interstitium. Analgesic abuse, Balkan nephropathy, and nephrosclerosis from renal vascular disease should be mentioned. ***Acute papillary necrosis*** can be seen in diabetics and in people who use analgesics excessively, and the renal medulla may undergo severe atrophy in association with sickle cell anemia.

RENAL VASCULAR DISEASE

All of the angiopathies may affect the renal blood vessels, but arterial and arteriolar sclerosis in association with primary (essential) hypertension is the commonest cause of renal failure in adults in the United States. Over 90% of individuals with long-standing essential hypertension show vascular changes in the kidney, and most show atrophy and fibrosis severe enough to be called ***nephrosclerosis***. In ***benign essential hypertension***, the larger vessels show dilation and thinning of the media with hyaline change, and variable fibrosis of the intima. Small arteries and arterioles show intense hyaline change of the media with some thickening. In rapidly accelerating ***malignant hypertension***, larger vessels show concentric medial and intimal change called "onion-skinning," and small arteries and arterioles show fibrinoid necrosis with eccentric deposits of fibrin and plasma proteins but little inflammation in the wall. Grossly, the kidney may be smooth with focal cortical hemorrhages (flea-bitten kidney).

The role of the renin–angiotensin system in essential hypertension is a matter of debate, but clearly the kidney is involved because of its role in volume regulation at least. The kidney is a principal site of production of renin, an enzyme that cleaves angiotensinogen produced by the liver to form *angiotensin I*, a decapeptide, which is then converted to angiotensin II, a potent vasoconstrictor, by the *converting enzyme,* which cleaves two more amino acids. *Angiotensin II* also stimulates the adrenal cortex to release aldosterone. Although the role of the renin–angiotensin system is still being defined in essential hypertension, it does appear to participate in the *malignant phase* of hypertension and in *renovascular hypertension*. The latter is the result of the narrowing of one or both main renal arteries, usually by ***atherosclerosis*** in adults, or by *fibromuscular dysplasia* in children.

RENAL PELVIS, URETERS, AND URINARY BLADDER

The papillae insert into the minor calyces, which in turn form the major calyces and the renal pelvis. These structures are lined by transitional epithelium (urothelium) and convey the urine without further modification to the urinary bladder for storage. As indicated previously, the principal diseases of the urothelium generally result from ascending bacterial infection (pyelonephritis, ureteritis, cystitis) and obstruction (hydronephrosis, hydroureter). The causes of obstruction include ***renal calculi*** (most of which consist of calcium and are of unknown cause), tumors, congenital anomalies, or acquired stricture. The bladder too can be infected (cystitis) acutely or chronically. Most bladder infections affect the epithelial lining and may produce more hemorrhaging than pus (hemorrhagic cystitis). Women are more frequently affected. Elderly men are susceptible as a result of prostatic enlargement with obstruction. The bladder wall may undergo hypertrophy with trabeculations and the epithelium may undergo metaplasia to a squamous or glandular type (cystitis glandularis). Interstitial cystitis may be of autoimmune origin. A condition called ***malacoplakia***, characterized as infiltration by large macrophages, is seen in transplant recipients.

The urothelium can develop both benign and malignant neoplasms. Benign papillary tumors ***(papilloma)*** of the urothelium may arise in the renal pelvis, ureter, or, most often, in the bladder. ***Transitional cell carcinomas*** constitute 95% of the nearly 50,000 new cases of bladder cancer yearly. They are graded I to III based on their differentiation or degree of anaplasia. ***Squamous cell tumors*** may also arise in the bladder, as can occasional adenocarcinomas.

MISCELLANEOUS RENAL DISEASES

The effect of sickle cell anemia with medullary atrophy has been mentioned. The kidney is frequently the site of thromboemboli, including atheromatous emboli, and these may result in wedge-shaped infarcts. Infarcts are usually evident only at autopsy. Adults and children may develop the so-called ***hemolytic–uremic syndrome***. In children, it often follows diarrheal illness, usually that caused by verocytotoxin-producing *E. coli*. In adults, it may be seen in the malignant phase of hypertension, after complications of pregnancy, or after an infection. There is an inherited form.

RENAL NEOPLASMS

Benign cortical adenomas arise from tubular epithelium, and benign papillomas arise from transitional epithelium. Tubular adenomas can be solid, usually composed of clear cells, or papillary. Sometimes it is difficult to distinguish a clear cell adenoma from an adenocarcinoma, and an arbitrary decision is made on the basis of size (*e.g.*, less than 2 cm in diameter). ***Renal fibroma*** or ***hamartoma***, ***angiolipoma***, and tumors composed of large eosinophilic cells, ***oncocytoma***, constitute the remainder of benign tumors.

Renal cell carcinomas are responsible for up to 3% of all malignancies in adults and constitute more than 80% of renal malignant tumors. They are usually well circumscribed and composed of polygonal cells that are clear or contain liquid droplets, giving them a resemblance to adrenal cells *(hypernephroma)*. Central hemorrhagic necrosis is common. Vascular invasion or extension outside the renal capsule are ominous signs. These carcinomas tend to metastasize widely before they are recognized: painless hematuria is a frequent presenting sign. They are associated with a variety of paraneoplastic syndromes, including polycythemia, hypercalcemia, and either fenestration or masculinization. Urothelial tumors are far less common.

An important tumor of childhood is the ***Wilms' tumor***. This is composed of elements resembling embryonic kidney, and it appears to be the result of specific genetic defects of WT-1 (Wilms tumor) gene on chromosome 11p13.

MALE GENITAL SYSTEM

Testis and Epididymis

The most important developmental anomaly of the testis is ***cryptorchidism***, or undescended testis, which is found in 0.5% of males. Bilateral cryptorchidism is associated with infertility. The undescended testes are at a 10 to 20 times higher risk than normal testes for developing malignant germ cell tumors.

Orchitis (inflammation of the testis) and ***epididymitis*** (inflammation of the epididymis) often occur simultaneously ***(epididymo-orchitis)***. In young and middle-aged men, it is secondary to an ascending spread of sexually acquired pathogens such as *N. gonorrhoeae* or *T. pallidum*. In older men, epididymo-orchitis is secondary to urinary tract infections related to prostatic hyperplasia. These infections are caused by *E. coli* and other uropathogens. Hematogenous epididymo-orchitis is rare, but it may occur in bacteremia. Mumps virus, which typically affects the salivary glands, may disseminate hematogenously and cause orchitis. Bilateral epididymo-orchitis may cause infertility.

Testicular tumors account for 1% of all tumors in men. The peak incidence of these tumors is in the 25 to 40 age group. Germ cell tumors, most of which are malignant, account for 95% of all neoplasms, whereas the remaining 5% represent tumors of sex-cord cells (Sertoli cell tumors and Leydig cell tumors) or lymphomas and metastatic malignancies from abdominal organs. The germ cell tumors occur in several histologic forms, but for clinical purposes it is convenient to subdivide them into two major groups: seminomas and nonseminomatous germ cell tumors (NSGCTs). ***Seminomas*** are composed of slow growing cells resembling undifferentiated germ cells. These tumors do not secrete any tumor markers into the blood and they have an excellent prognosis (5-year survival, >90%,) if treated by surgery and radiotherapy. ***NSGCTs*** are histologically heterogeneous and can be subclassified into *embryonal carcinoma, teratocarcinoma, choriocarcinoma,* and *yolk sac carcinoma*. Mixed forms predominate. Most NSGCTs secrete human chorionic alpha fetoprotein (AFP) and gonadotropin (hCG) into the bloodstream, which serve as reliable markers for these tumors. NSGCTs formerly had a high lethality (35% 5-year survival), but today most patients (90%) can be cured by orchiectomy (removal of the tumorous testis), dissection of the abdominal lymph nodes containing metastatic cancer, and multidrug combination chemotherapy based on platinum compounds.

Prostate

The most important diseases of the prostate are benign prostatic hyperplasia (BPH) and prostatic carcinoma, both of which typically occur in older men.

BPH is a disease of unknown etiology. Some degree of prostatic hyperplasia is found in almost all men above the age of 60 years. BPH develops presumably under the influence of steroid sex hormones, which act on both the glands and the fibromuscular stroma of the prostate. The hyperplastic glands and stromal cells form nodules, which are most prominent in the periurethral zone. These nodules of the lateral lobes may compress the urethra, whereas the hyperplastic median lobe may protrude into the urinary bladder and obstruct the internal urethral orifice. Typical symptoms include urinary retention, dysuria, or frequent urgency to urinate. Retention of urine predisposes to infection of the bladder *(chronic cystitis)*. BPH is treated surgically by transurethral resection or suprapubic prostatectomy.

Carcinoma of the prostate is one of the most common malignant tumors occurring in men. Like BPH, the incidence of cancer increases with age, although the two conditions appear to be independent of one another. Carcinoma usually originates in the posterior lobe and is most often subcapsular in location. Many tumors are present for a long time without being suspected. Histologically, tumors are adenocarcinomas, usually of the desmoplastic type. When such carcinomas metastasize to bones, they form osteoblastic lesions, which appear dense on x-rays. Metastases are most often found in the regional lymph nodes, pelvic bones, and the spine. Prostate-specific antigen (PSA) and prostatic acid phosphatase levels in the serum are often increased. Tumors restricted to the prostate can be resected surgically, but those that have spread outside the prostate are incurable. Grading (Glisson) by the two most frequent patterns of neoplastic glands has prognostic significance.

Penis

Congenital anomalies of the formation of the penis are common in hermaphrodites and pseudohermaphrodites. In genetic males, the anomalies usually involve the penile urethra. In ***hypospadias***, the urethral opening of the urethra is on the lower surface of the penis, whereas in ***epispadias***, which is rare, the opening of the urethra is on the dorsal side. ***Phimosis*** is a narrowing of the prepuce so that it cannot be retracted over the glans.

Infections of the glans penis and the surrounding prepuce is called ***balanoposthitis***. Nonspecific balanoposthitis caused by poor hygiene is more common in men who are not circumcised. Most other infections of the penis are acquired by sexual intercourse. Gonorrhea is characterized by a purulent urethral discharge, syphilis by ulcers on the glans penis, and herpes by vesicles on the glans or the skin of the shaft. Condyloma acuminatum is a wart caused by human papilloma virus (HPV), typically found on the glans or the terminal urethra.

Carcinoma of the penis is uncommon in the United States but prevalent in many underdeveloped countries of South America and Africa. Histologically, these tumors are squamous cell carcinomas. Clinically, such tumors are recognized as persistent ulcerations, indurations, or exophytic verrucous lesions. The prognosis depends on the stage of the tumor at the time of diagnosis, but, overall, 60% of men survive 5 years after diagnosis.

FEMALE GENITAL SYSTEM

Diseases of the female genital system are very common. The most important diseases are infections, hormonally induced changes, tumors, and conditions related to pregnancy.

Infections

Infections of the female genital system may be localized, such as vulvitis, vaginitis, cervicitis, endometritis, and salpingitis, but often the infection involves more than one anatomic site. Infection of the entire internal genital system is called ***pelvic inflammatory disease*** (PID). Most of these infections are acquired through sexual contact. Hematogenous infections are less common.

Common inflammatory lesions of the ***vulva*** include nonspecific bacterial vulvitis (caused by gram-positive or gram-negative bacteria from the environment), genital herpes (which presents in the form of small confluent vesicles), and genital ulcers (such as those of syphilis or lymphogranuloma venereum). Condyloma acuminatum or giant genital warts are papillomas caused by HPV. The ***vagina*** is relatively resistant to invasive pathogens. Most infections are caused by pathogens that grow in the vaginal lumen. Bacterial vaginosis is caused by *Gardnerella vaginalis*. Other common causes of vaginitis are the protozoan *Trichomonas vaginalis* and the fungus *Candida albicans*. These infections present with vaginal discharge, itching, dyspareunia, and even pain. The pathogens may be identified microscopically in Pap smears or by bacteriologic cultures, and if treated appropriately with antibiotics, or antiparasitic or antifungal drugs, they are readily eradicated. ***Cervicitis*** presents most often as a nonspecific infection of the endocervical glands. Gonorrhea also presents as endocervicitis. HPV infection of the exocervix typically leads to formation of flat papillomas or histologic epithelial changes indistinguishable from preinvasive carcinoma. In some instances, these HPV lesions progress to carcinoma.

Pelvic inflammatory disease is a chronic infection involving the uterus, fallopian tubes, and the pelvic peritoneum. In most cases it is a consequence of repeated, polymicrobial, ascending, sexually transmitted infections. Most common pathogens are *Neisseria gonorrhoeae, E. coli, Mycoplasma*, and *Chlamydia*. Pathologic lesions include chronic endometritis or pyometra, chronic salpingitis or pyosalpinx, tubo-ovarian abscess, pelvic peritonitis, and peritoneal adhesions between internal genital organs and the intestines or the urinary bladder. Clinically, PID presents with low grade fever, abdominal pain, and vaginal discharge. Infertility is common. In those women who conceive, the pregnancy may be ectopic due to the implantation of the fertilized egg in the deformed fallopian tubes. Infertility is common. Other complications include intestinal adhesions and obstructions, diffuse peritonitis and bacteremia. Mild PID responds well to antibiotic treatment. Advanced lesions are resistant to medical treatment and a total hysterosalpingo-oophorectomy must be performed to eliminate the persistent source of infection.

Hormonal Lesions

Hormonally induced lesions are most often seen in the uterus and the ovaries. ***Endometrial hyperplasia*** represents thickening of the endometrium caused by excessive proliferation of endometrial glands and stroma in response to estrogenic stimulation. Three histologic forms of endometrial hyperplasia are recognized: (a) simple hyperplasia characterized by cystic dilatation of glands resembling the holes in Swiss cheese, (b) complex hyperplasia without atypia, composed of crowded, hyperplastic glands lined by regular epithelium, and (c) complex hyperplasia with atypia in which the glands show cytologic atypia and architectural abnormalities suggestive of a neoplastic process. All forms of endometrial hyperplasia are associated with abnormal bleeding, which is best treated by endometrial curettage. Complex hyperplasia, especially if associated with atypia, may progress to adenocarcinoma and should be considered a potentially premalignant lesion.

Polyps are localized hyperplastic lesions of endocervical or endometrial mucosa. The pathogenesis of polyps is not known. It is thought that polyps develop as a result of inflammation, or hormonal stimulation accompanied by a localized proliferative tissue response. Histologically, the polyps are composed of hyperplastic or cystically dilated glands and loose stroma infiltrated with chronic inflammatory cells. Polyps may cause menstrual irregularities or bleeding, usually in the form of ''spotting.'' Polypectomy is the treatment of choice.

Ovarian cysts are hormonally induced solitary or multiple lesions. Solitary cysts typically originate from the graafian follicle and are histologically classified as follicular or theca-lutein cysts. Corpus luteum cysts are derived from the corpus luteum.

Polycystic ovary syndrome (POS) presents with bilateral enlargement of the ovaries, which contain multiple follicular cysts. POS is considered to be a disturbance of the hypothalamic–pituitary–ovarian–adrenal hormonal axis. Polycystic ovaries reflect the inability of these women to ovulate in response to hypothalamic stimulation. Hyperestrinism and an excess of androgens are typical. Amenorrhea or menstrual irregularities, infertility, and signs of virilization (*e.g.*, hirsutism) are the most common clinical findings. The treatment is hormonal.

Endometriosis, the appearance of endometrial tissue outside the uterus, is a disease that in some form, usually mild, affects about 20% of women of reproductive age. The pathogenesis of the disease is not understood, but it is thought that it develops most likely from the endometrial tissue shed during the menstrual bleeding period. Because of the reflux of menstrual blood, the endometrial glands and stroma floating in it enter through the fallopian tubes into the pelvis, where they implant on the surface of the ovary and the peritoneum. Foci of endometriosis respond to hormonal stimuli. Like the normal endometrium, these foci enlarge during the proliferative phase and are permeated with blood at the time of menstrual bleeding, because the blood cannot be discharged into the vagina. Endometriosis is associated with periodic pelvic pain, and the larger lesions, especially those on the ovary, may produce nodular masses filled with blood (*endometrioma*, or ''chocolate cysts''). Endometriosis is an important cause of infertility. The treatment includes hormonal suppression of cyclic changes with oral contraceptives or weak androgens, and laparoscopic coagulation of small hemorrhagic foci with a laser beam. Endometriosis is not considered to be a preneoplastic condition and most lesions regress after menopause.

Tumors

Tumors of the female genital organs account for 10% of all neoplasms in women. The most common are tumors of the uterus, followed by tumors of the cervix, ovary, and vulva. Tumors of the vagina and the fallopian tubes are uncommon.

The ***vulva*** is covered by squamous epithelium, which gives rise to squamous cell carcinomas similar to those on other parts of the skin. These tumors typically occur in older women. Histologically, such squamous cell carcinomas may occur in a preinvasive form [called vulvar intraepithelial neoplasia (VIN), or Bowen disease] or an invasive form. Clinically, carcinoma presents as leukoplakia (white plaques), erythroplakia (red plaques), ulcers, or papillary exophytic lesions (verrucous carcinoma). Metastases occur in the inguinal and internal pelvic lymph nodes and then spread to other sites. The prognosis depends on the clinical stage of the tumor, but overall 60% of women survive 5 years after diagnosis. Carcinoma of the vulva must be distinguished from benign lesions that may present as leukoplakia. The most important among these are vulvar dystrophies, which are classified as atrophic (also known as lichen sclerosus et atrophicus), hyperplastic, or mixed atrophic and hyperplastic. Condyloma acuminatum, HPV-induced genital warts, must be distinguished from verrucous carcinoma, which also contains HPV virions. Extramammary Paget's disease, an intraepithelial malignancy composed of mucin-rich cells, may present as an erythroplakia on the inside of the labia majora.

The ***vagina*** is a relatively rare site of neoplasia, accounting for 1% to 2% of all genital cancers. Almost all tumors are squamous cell carcinomas, typically found in older women. Rare adenocarcinomas have been found in young women who were exposed during intrauterine life to diethylstilbestrol (DES). Prenatal exposure to DES leads to formation of vaginal adenosis, a benign lesion that can occasionally undergo malignant transformation and give rise to adenocarcinoma. Botryoid sarcoma is a rare vaginal tumor of children. Histologically, it is a rhabdomyosarcoma, which forms a polypoid grapelike mass protruding from the vaginal orifice.

The ***cervix of the uterus*** is a common site of neoplasia. Carcinoma of the cervix was the leading cause of cancer death up to the mid century but has been partially brought under control by early detection with Pap smears. It still ranks as the sixth major cause of cancer-related death among women. The risk factors for carcinoma of the cervix include early onset of sexual activity, multiparity, promiscuity, low socioeconomic status, and sexually transmitted disease, most notably infections with HPV and herpes simplex virus. The disease begins as an intraepithelial dysplasia and it gradually progresses to carcinoma *in situ* and invasive squamous carcinoma. Intraepithelial dysplasia, graded as mild moderate or severe and carcinoma *in situ* represent stages of the same disease and are collectively called cervical intraepithelial neoplasia (CIN) and graded on a scale from I to III, or low grade or high grade (Bethesda system). Histologic changes correspond to cytologic changes in the Pap smear. Prognosis depends on the stage of tumor at the time of diagnosis. CIN, stage 0 carcinoma, has a 100% cure. Stage I cancer has a 85% to 90% 5-year survival, which drops to 10% to 15% in cancer stage IV. Therapy is based on surgical removal of the tumor or radiation therapy. Chemotherapy is reserved for advanced lesions.

Uterine tumors originate either from the endometrium or myometrium. Myometrial lesions are usually benign (leiomyomas), whereas the endometrial lesions are usually malignant (adenocarcinoma). ***Leiomyomas*** are benign tumors composed of smooth muscle cells. These tumors arise during reproductive age and are almost nonexistent before puberty; they undergo shrinkage and involution after menopause. Leiomyomas may be solitary or multiple. The symptoms depend on the size and the location of tumors. The subendometrial tumors cause bleeding and menstrual irregularities, and they may interfere with implantation of the fertilized ovum, thus causing infertility. Intramural and subperitoneal tumors present as pelvic masses, compressing the rectum and urinary bladder. The treatment of leiomyomas is surgical. *Leiomyosarcomas*, the malignant smooth muscle cell tumors, are rare. They never originate from preexisting leiomyomas but arise *de novo* from the myometrium. Leiomyosarcomas have a poor prognosis.

Adenocarcinoma of the endometrium is the most common malignant tumor of the female genital organs. It has a peak incidence in the postmenopausal period. Endogenous or exogenous estrogens increase the risk of endometrial adenocarcinoma. Other risk factors are obesity, diabetes, hypertension, and infertility. Preexistent endometrial hyperplasia, which is often associated with hyperestrinism, is an important preneoplastic condition. Clinical symptoms include vaginal bleeding and discharge, uterine enlargement, and, in advanced cases, metastatic lesions in various locations. The diagnosis is made by uterine curettage. The prognosis depends on the stage of the tumor at the time of diagnosis. Stage I carcinoma, which is limited to the endometrium, has an excellent prognosis and 85% of women survive 5 years or are cured entirely by hysterectomy. Stage II to IV tumors have a less favorable prognosis.

Ovarian tumors originate from one of the three anatomic compartments of the ovary: (a) surface epithelium (also called germinal or celomic epithelium), which gives rise to 75% of all ovarian tumors and 95% of all malignant tumors; (b) germ cells, which give rise to 15% of all ovarian tumors and 95% of tumors in women under the age of 25 years; and (c) sex cord stromal cells, which give rise to 10% of all ovarian tumors and 95% of all hormonally active ovarian tumors.

Surface epithelial tumors occur in several histologic forms and may be either benign or malignant. These tumors are often cystic and classified as serous cystadenoma and cystadenocarcinoma, or mucinous cystadenoma and cystadenocarcinoma. Most solid tumors are malignant and classified as either endometrioid adenocarcinoma or clear cell carcinoma. Benign cystic tumors are readily curable by surgery. Malignant surface epithelial tumors have a less favorable prognosis that depends on the stage of tumor. These malignant tumors tend to spread by peritoneal seeding and are typically associated with malignant ascites.

Germ cell tumors of the ovary include teratoma, dysgerminoma, embryonal carcinoma, teratocarcinoma, yolk sac carcinoma, and choriocarcinoma. Dysgerminoma corresponds to seminoma of the testis, and all the other tumors are equivalent to testicular tumors of the same name. The most common germ cell tumor is the teratoma, which presents as a cystic lesion lined by skin (dermoid cyst). It typically occurs in the early postpubertal period. Other germ cell tumors are malignant but respond well to chemotherapy.

Sex cord cell stromal tumors include granulosa cell tumors, theca cell tumors, Sertoli-Leydig cell tumors, and fibromas. Granulosa cell tumors are composed of neoplastic granulosa cells capable of estrogen production. They are considered to be low grade malignancies, which tend to recur and metastasize many years after the diagnosis. Theca cell tumors are composed of spindle-shaped, lipid-laden, estrogen-producing cells equivalent to theca interna and externa cells. Theca cell tumors are always benign and hormonally active. Sertoli-Leydig cell tumors are benign or low grade malignant tumors capable of androgen secretion, typically associated with virilization. Fibroma is the most common stromal tumor of the ovary. It does not produce hormonal symptoms. Fibromas may be bilateral and are occasionally, for unknown reasons, associated with pleural effusion (Meigs' syndrome).

Metastatic tumors to the ovary most often originate in primary carcinomas of the gastrointestinal tract and the breast. Bilaterally enlarged ovaries infiltrated with metastatic mucin-producing adenocarcinoma of the stomach are known as Krukenberg tumors.

Placenta and Pregnancy

Pathology of pregnancy and placenta encompasses (a) abnormalities of placentation, (b) abnormal development of placental villi, including neoplastic development of placental cells, and (c) abnormalities of maternoplacental interaction and abnormal placental function, including the effects of the placenta on the maternal organism.

Abnormal placentation is most often a consequence of abnormal implantation of the fertilized ovum, which results in ***ectopic pregnancy***. Ectopic pregnancy occurs most often in the fallopian tubes, but it may also occur on the ovaries or anywhere else on the perineum of the abdominal cavity. Tubal pregnancies occur most often in women who have suffered from PID. The developing placenta penetrates through the thin wall of the fallopian tube, causing abdominal bleeding, which may even be lethal if not adequately treated.

The placenta normally has one disc, but occasionally it may be subdivided into two parts, as *bipartite placenta*. Occasionally, the placenta may have a discrete additional lobe and is called *placenta succenturiata*. In twin pregnancies, the twins are enclosed in a single cavity and have a common placental disc amnion and chorion, or they are enclosed each in a separate cavity. These placenta and membranes are classified accordingly as monochorionic monoamniotic, monochorionic diamniotic, or dichorionic diamniotic. All twins with a monochorionic placenta are monozygotic. Dichorionic placentation may result from either dizygous or monozygous twinning.

Abnormal development of placental villi results in the formation of ***hydatidiform mole*** (HM). In this condition, the placental villi lack the normal vascular core and transform into edematous, afunctional vesicles. The entire placenta transforms into a structure resembling a bunch of grapes. HM cannot support the normal development of the embryo. If parts of a nonviable embryo are included in the mole, it is called *partial* HM. If there is no evidence of the embryo, the HM is considered to be *complete*.

On chromosomal analysis, partial HM shows trisomy (three sets of 23 chromosomes, or 69 chromosomes), whereas the complete HM is always 46, XX (*e.g.*, it contains a normal number of chromosomes). However, all these chromosomes are of paternal origin, indicating that the complete HM is a product of androgenesis, an abnormal fertilization in which the maternal chromosomes are lost.

Hydatidiform mole results in spontaneous abortion, but if it does not occur, the uterus must be evacuated surgically. Such a uterus is usually larger than one would expect by the calculated duration of pregnancy, and the serum contains large amounts of hCG. In most instances, HM has no long-term consequences, although occasionally it may give rise to choriocarcinoma.

Choriocarcinoma is a malignant tumor composed of neoplastic trophoblastic cells: mononuclear cytotrophoblastic cells and multinucleated, hCG secreting syncytiotrophoblastic cells. Approximately 50% of tumors develop from a preexisting hydatidiform mole, whereas the others arise from normal-term placenta, or placental remnants after an abortion. Choriocarcinoma is a highly invasive tumor and 90% of all patients already have pulmonary metastases at the time of diagnosis. With modern chemotherapy based on methotrexate and alkylating agents, excellent results have been achieved in all patients except those who have brain metastases. Overall survival is 70%.

Abnormal maternoplacental interaction may take place in several forms. The most common are various infections that cross the maternoplacental barrier, infecting either the placenta and the membranes or the fetus. ***Placental infection*** is caused by viruses [such as parvovirus, herpesvirus, cytomegalovirus (CMV)], bacteria (such as *Treponema pallidum* and *Listeria monocytogenes,* and various gram-positive and gram-negative bacteria), and protozoa (such as *Toxoplasma gondii*).

Abnormal maternoplacental interaction may result in complex changes known as *preeclampsia* or *eclampsia*. ***Preeclampsia*** presents as a triad of edema, hypertension, and proteinuria. Multiple intravascular thrombi may be found in the renal glomeruli and small blood vessels of other organs. Preeclampsia responds favorably to treatment with magnesium sulfate. If untreated, it may progress to eclampsia, which is characterized by convulsions and significant mortality. In eclampsia, there are hemorrhagic infarctions in major organs, including the brain. The pathogenesis of eclampsia is not understood, but apparently it represents a form of disseminated intravascular coagulation triggered by substances released from the placenta.

Breast

The most important disease of the breasts is carcinoma, which represents, with lung cancer, the foremost cause of cancer-related mortality in women. Infections of the breasts, hormonally induced changes, and benign tumors are other diseases that merit mention.

Mastitis, the infection of breasts, is uncommon in adult women except during the postpartum period of lactation. Lactating breasts are prone to bacterial infections, which usually develop through the nipple. Fissures of the nipple skin caused by the suckling baby and the stagnation of milk that has not been completely evacuated during breast feeding predispose to infection. Mastitis is usually acute and associated with redness, pain, and swelling of the affected tissue. It responds well to antibiotics and proper evacuation of the infected breast. Abscesses require surgical intervention.

Fibrocystic change is the most common hormonally caused alteration of breast tissue. More than 50% of women of reproductive age have some signs of fibrocystic change, but in most instances the symptoms are mild and do not require any treatment. It is thought that fibrocystic change represents an uncoordinated response of the breast epithelium and stroma to the hormonal fluctuations that normally occur during the menstrual cycle. Histologically, the hallmarks of fibrocystic change are *fibrosis* of the intralobular stroma, which merges with the normally denser interlobular connective tissue, *cystic dilatation* of the ducts, and *epithelial proliferation* from the terminal ducts. About 10% of women show *sclerosing adenosis*, marked by intralobular proliferation of small ducts and fibrosis. These histologic features of fibrocystic change are not preneoplastic. However, in a minority of cases, the breasts show intraductal proliferative lesions known as *intraductal papillomatosis* or *intraductal atypical epithelial hyperplasia*, which carry a higher risk for malignant transformation.

Fibroadenoma is the most common benign tumor of the breasts, typically affecting women in the 20 to 35 age group. It presents as a solitary, 3- to 7-cm encapsulated mobile mass distinct from the remainder of the breast. Histologically it is composed of proliferating ducts and stromal cells. Large, rapidly enlarging tumors showing similar features, but characterized by histologically atypical stromal cells, are called ***cystosarcoma phyllodes***. Clinically, phyllodes tumors may be benign or malignant.

Breast carcinoma affects one in 14 women in the United States, which means that every year there are approximately 180,000 new cases diagnosed. Approximately 20% of all cancer deaths are attributed to breast cancer.

Breast carcinoma is rare in young women but its incidence increases after the age of 40 years, reaching a peak in the 50 to 65 age period. The risk factors include family history, nulliparity, long reproductive life (early menarche, late menopause), endogenous or exogenous excess of estrogens, preexisting atypical epithelial intraductal hyperplasia and intraductal papillomatosis of the breast, and preexisting carcinoma of the uterus and ovaries. Two cancer genes, BRCA-1 and BRCA-2, have been found in many affected women and are especially common in familial cases of breast cancer. BRCA-1 appears to be more common in some ethnic groups, such as Askenazi Jews. Several oncogenes have been found to be amplified in breast cancer cells, such as the *erb*-B2/*neu*, c-*ras*, and c-*myc* genes but their exact role in the cancerization of breast tissue remains unclear. The human equivalent of the mouse mammary tumor virus (MMV), a well-known cause of breast cancer in mice, has not been identified yet. Hormonal factors play a crucial role, as evidenced by the fact that breast cancer rarely develops in men: only one male breast cancer is found for every 100 affected women. Thus it appears that both genetic and environmental factors play a role in the pathogenesis of breast cancer.

Breast carcinomas originate from epithelial cells lining the ducts (ductal carcinoma) or lobules (lobular carcinoma). Approximately 50% of cancers are located in the upper outer quadrant, and 20% in the subareolar central area, whereas other quadrants are less often involved. Tumors metastasize preferentially to the axillary lymph nodes. Distant metastases are found in most major organs, most notably the lungs, liver, bones, brain, and adrenals.

Histologically, breast cancers are classified into two major groups: noninvasive (intraductal carcinomas or intralobular carcinoma) and invasive carcinoma. The infiltrating carcinomas are most often classified as infiltrating ductal carcinoma, which accounts for 70% of all malignant tumors. Colloid carcinoma composed of mucinous cells surrounded by pools of extracellular mucus, medullary carcinoma composed of solid nests of tumor cells and scant stroma, Paget's disease characterized by invasion of overlying skin of the nipple, and other less common variants account for the remainder of tumors. Lobular carcinoma is less common and accounts for approximately 5% of both invasive and noninvasive cancer. Clinically, most breast carcinomas are discovered as small nodules on self palpation, by doctors performing routine breast examinations, or by mammography. Cancer may also cause discharge from the nipple and in the case of Paget's disease (intraductal carcinoma with nipple involvement), eczema-like changes on the nipple. A few women present with distant metastases. Noninvasive carcinomas have an excellent prognosis and are curable if diagnosed before they become invasive. Invasive carcinoma has a less favorable prognosis that depends primarily on the stage of the tumor at the time of diagnosis, but also to a minor extent on the histologic type of tumor. Women with stage I lesions (lymph node negative cancer) have an 80% 5-year survival rate, but if the nodes contain metastases, the prognosis deteriorates to 50%. In women with widespread metastases, the disease is incurable.

Besides the size of the primary tumor and the presence or absence of metastases, the prognosis depends to some extent on other factors. Some histologic types, such as medullary carcinoma and colloid carcinoma, carry a better prognosis. Tumors that express estrogen receptors respond favorably to antiestrogenic therapy and oophorectomy.

Male Breast

Enlargement of the male breast, which may be unilateral or bilateral, is called gynecomastia. Histologically, gynecomastia is characterized by proliferation and elongation of ducts that are surrounded by loose, edematous stroma. In most instances, gynecomastia is caused by an excess of estrogen. In cirrhosis of the liver, hyperestrinism reflects the inability of the liver to catabolize endogenous estrogens. In patients with testicular Leydig cell tumors, or adrenal adenomas and carcinomas, estrogen is derived from hormonally active tumor cells. The causes of gynecomastia of puberty, which may be unilateral or bilateral, are not understood.

Carcinoma of the breast is 100 times less common in men than in women. Histologically, it is most often of the infiltrating duct type.

THE ENDOCRINE SYSTEM

The endocrine system, in conjunction with the nervous system, particularly the hypothalamus, is responsible for regulating cellular homeostasis. Hormones produced in the endocrine system regulate cells via receptors (a) on the cell surface, (b) in the cytoplasm, or (c) in the nucleus. Endocrine glands are controlled either by hormones produced in the hypothalamus (*e.g.*, pituitary) or by feedback loops with the pituitary (*e.g.*, peripheral endocrine glands).

Pituitary Gland

The pituitary gland is located at the base of the brain in the sella turcica. It is composed of two major lobes, the anterior and posterior, and the vestigial intermediate lobe. The anterior lobe is derived from the oral canal, Rathke's pouch, and is composed of secretory epithelium. It has six cell types which secrete six major hormones: somatotrophs secrete growth hormone; mammotrophs secrete prolactin; corticotrophs secrete adenocorticotropic hormone (ACTH), melanocyte-stimulating hormone (MSH), endorphins, and lipotropin; thyrotrophs secrete thyroid-stimulating hormone (TSH); and gonadotrophs secrete follicle-stimulating hormone (FSH) and luteinizing hormone (LH). The posterior lobe (neurohypophysis) is derived from outpouchings of the third ventricle. It is connected to the hypothalamus via the pituitary stalk and is composed of unmyelinated nerve fibers that contain granules of stored antidiuretic hormone (ADH) and oxytocin. The hypothalamus regulates the secretion of these hormones by releasing stimulatory or inhibitory factors.

The diseases of the pituitary present as hyperpituitarism and hypopituitarism.

Hyperpituitarism is most commonly produced by adenomas. Carcinomas or hyperfunction of the hypothalamus are rare causes of this disorder. Adenomas can be classified into microadenomas (less than 10 mm) or macroadenomas (greater than 10 mm). The latter may be confined to a portion of the anterior lobe or, by expansile growth, obliterate the anterior lobe, the anterior and posterior lobe or erode through the bone and impinge on adjacent structures.

Somatotrophic adenomas lead to acromegaly or gigantism and account for approximately 14% of pituitary adenomas. Acromegaly is characterized by enlargement of the head, hands, feet, jutting jaw, large tongue, and soft-tissue enlargement. This condition occurs in adults with excess growth hormone. A juvenile form, gigantism, has become very rare. ***Prolactinomas*** are the most common functional pituitary adenomas, accounting for approximately 27%. These neoplasms lead to hypogonadism in both men and women and galactorrhea and amenorrhea in women. Hyperprolactinemia is also produced in hypothalamic lesions, after treatment with serotonin or methyldopa, or after estrogen therapy. ***Corticotroph tumors*** account for approximately 8% of pituitary adenomas. They secrete ACTH, which stimulates the production of cortisol by the adrenal cortex with ensuing Cushing's disease (discussed under the adrenal cortex). ***Gonadotroph adenomas*** account for 6% of pituitary adenomas. They secrete FSH and LH in men, leading to hypogonadism, headaches, and visual disturbances. The hypogonadism results from FSH secretion. It is thought that the LH secreted may not be functional.

Hypopituitarism results from hypothalamic lesions or lesions in the anterior pituitary. The vast majority (90%) of cases are associated with destructive lesions in the anterior pituitary. For hypopituitarism to be manifested, approximately 75% of the anterior lobe must be destroyed. Hypofunction of the thyroid and adrenal glands, as well as gonadal insufficiency, must be differentiated in terms of conditions primary to the organs versus conditions causing hypopituitarism. The major causes of hypopituitarism include

- nonsecretory chromophobe pituitary adenomas
- Sheehan's syndrome
- empty sella syndrome

Nonsecretory chromophobe pituitary adenomas account for 25% to 30% of pituitary tumors. Patients present with clinical signs referable to local effects such as visual field abnormalities, headaches and/or hypofunction of target organs (*e.g.*, thyroid adrenal or gonads). Histologically, these tumors either have small numbers of secretory granules or none.

Sheehan's syndrome (postpartum pituitary necrosis) is defined as acute anterior lobe infarction, generally resulting from obstetric hemorrhage or shock. The pituitary enlarges considerably during pregnancy and compresses adjacent vessels. Anything leading to acute hypotension produces vasospasm, which in turn causes infarction of the anterior lobe but sparing of the posterior lobe. Other causes of pituitary infarction in nonpregnant women and in men include DIC, sickle cell anemia, thrombi in the cavernous sinus, temporal arteritis, and vascular trauma. Clinically, the condition may be symptomatic, or it may manifest as gonadotrophic deficiency or deficiencies of TSH or ACTH. The infarcted region can be pale or hemorrhagic, and ultimately it is replaced by scar tissue. ***Empty sella syndrome*** is an uncommon condition produced by a herniation of the arachnoid through the diaphragma sellae. The pressure of the cerebrospinal fluid (CSF) ultimately causes atrophy of the gland. Infarction of the pituitary (*e.g.*, Sheehan's syndrome) can also cause this condition. Most cases are asymptomatic, with a few manifesting trophic hormone deficiencies. Hypothalamic suprasellar tumors are uncommon lesions that may produce hyper- or hypofunction of the anterior pituitary and/or diabetes insipidus. Gliomas (discussed in the central nervous system chapter) and craniopharyngiomas are most commonly implicated. Craniopharyngiomas arise from remnants of Rathke's pouch or the sella. Histologically, they are characterized by nests of stratified squamous or columnar cells in a loose fibrous connective tissue stroma. The majority contain foci of calcification, which can be seen on radiographs. These tumors are generally seen in children and young adults (5- to 20-year-olds) who usually complain of visual loss, headaches, vomiting, obesity, delayed pubescence, and increased urination (diabetes insipidus). Disorders of the posterior pituitary gland are rare. The majority are caused by injury to the hypothalamohypophysial axis, inflammation, neoplasms (hypothalamic suprasellar), or physical injury.

Diabetes insipidus is the major clinical manifestation of posterior pituitary disorders and is due to a deficiency of ADH. Patients present with excessive thirst, polydipsia, and polyuria. ***Inappropriate ADH secretion*** is usually a result of paraneoplastic secretion of ADH by tumors. It is seen most commonly, but is not limited to, small cell bronchogenic carcinomas of the lung. Secretion is persistent and not governed by plasma osmolality. Because of excess water reabsorption by renal tubules, the extracellular fluid volume is increased, there is hemodilution and hyponatremia, and the urine is concentrated.

Thyroid Gland

The principal diseases of the thyroid gland are

- hyperthyroidism
- thyrotoxicosis
- hypothyroidism
- focal or diffuse enlargement (goiter)

HYPERTHYROIDISM

Graves' disease, toxic multinodular goiter, and toxic adenoma account for approximately 99% of cases of hyperthyroidism. ***Graves' disease*** is responsible for 85% of cases in patients less than 40 years old. It is characterized by a diffuse, hyperplastic goiter that is hyperfunctional. Infiltrative dermatopathy and ophthalmopathy may be present. It is thought to be an autoimmune disease that originates as a result of IgG antibodies interacting with specific domains on the TSH receptor. These antibodies (thyroid-stimulating antibody and thyrotropin-binding inhibitor immunoglobulins) are stimulatory. The gland is uniformly hyperplastic but not considerably enlarged. Histologically, the follicular lining is hyperplastic and tends to become columnar. Papillae project into the lumen of the follicle. There are no lymphocytic infiltrates but lymphoid follicles are common. Clinically, the disease is found predominantly in women and is associated with a moderately enlarged thyroid gland. In addition, patients present with exophthalmos, nervousness, heat intolerance, and fatigue. Diagnosis is based on increased radioactive iodine uptake, decreased levels of TSH, and increased levels of free T_3 and T_4. Hyperthyroidism can also be seen associated with acute or subacute thyroiditis, hyperfunctioning thyroid carcinomas, choriocarcinoma, hydatidiform mole, TSH-secreting pituitary adenoma, and struma ovarii. In addition, it can be induced by iodide or thyroid medication, and it can occur in neonates of women with Graves' disease.

HYPOTHYROIDISM

Hypothyroidism manifests itself as a hypometabolic state that is caused by structural or functional changes that reduce or impair the output of thyroid hormone. The most common cause in the United States is primary idiopathic hypothyroidism *(atrophic autoimmune thyroiditis)*. It is reported that this condition causes anywhere from 15% to 60% of the cases. It is thought that this condition is caused by blocking autoantibodies to TSH receptors. The vast majority of the remaining cases are caused by surgically induced or radiation-induced thyroidal ablation. These are usually performed as treatments for hyperthyroidism or primary neoplasms of the gland. Additional causes of hypothyroidism include developmental defects and Hashimoto's thyroiditis, which reduce the amount of thyroid parenchyma. In addition, heritable biosynthetic defects, iodine deficiency, and certain drugs (*e.g.*, lithium and iodides) as well as Hashimoto's thyroiditis, may interfere with thyroid hormone synthesis. Finally, pituitary lesions reducing TSH secretion and hypothalamic lesions reducing TSH delivery are also incriminated.

Clinically, there are two manifestations of hypothyroidism. When present during infancy and development, ***cretinism*** is observed. This condition can be endemic in areas where there are dietary deficiencies of iodine or it can be sporadic in the face of congenital developmental defects or biosynthetic defects. It is associated with physical and mental retardation. Individuals have dry, rough skin; widely set eyes; periorbital puffiness; a flattened, broad nose; and an overlying large protuberant tongue. When hypothyroidism appears in older children or adults, it is referred to as ***myxedema***. Initially, it is characterized by fatigue, lethargy, cold intolerance, and generalized listlessness and apathy. As it progresses, speech and intellectual functions are slowed. Eventually, the tongue is enlarged and peripheral edema characterized by doughlike thickening of the skin, which is resistant to pitting, it observed. This results from accumulation of hydrophilic mucopolysaccharides in connective tissue.

Diffuse and multinodular goiters result from hypertrophy and hyperplasia of follicular epithelium secondary to conditions that impair thyroid hormone output with concomitant increases in levels of TSH. Over time, these conditions result in hypothyroidism, euthyroidism, or hyperthyroidism. In most cases, the euthyroid state is achieved. ***Diffuse nontoxic simple goiter*** involves the entire gland and is generally associated with hyper- or hypofunction. This condition is also called colloid goiter. The primary cause is an inadequate intake of iodine. This, in turn, leads to decreased synthesis of thyroid hormone with increased production of TSH, leading to follicular cell hypertrophy and hyperplasia. The decreased intake of iodine can occur as a result of iodine deficiencies in certain endemic areas or certain dietary substances that interfere with iodine metabolism. Examples include calcium and fluorides in water supplies, and cabbage, cauliflower, and brussels sprouts. Nonendemic or sporadic simple goiter is less common than the endemic variety. This disease is most common in women, and the cause, most often, is unclear. Histologically, diffuse nontoxic goiter is characterized by a hyperplastic stage in which the follicular epithelium is columnar and the new follicles are small and have little colloid. In addition, there is a stage of colloid involution in which colloid accumulates, enlarging the follicles and flattening the epithelium. The gland is enlarged at this point. Clinically, sporadic goiter due to congenital defects in biosynthesis may induce cretinism. The adult form, however, more often than not, achieves a state of euthyroidism. Multinodular goiters generally stem from simple goiters. They may be euthyroid or hyperthyroid. They are most common in women and cause marked enlargements. They are characterized by irregular nodules that are created by islands of follicles that are either hyperplastic or filled with colloid. In addition, there are multifocal areas of scarring, as well as focal hemorrhages with hemosiderin, calcification in the scars, and microcysts. Clinically, because of their size, they may impinge on the trachea and esophagus. In addition, they may cause hyperthyroidism. They must be differentiated from neoplasms. Scintiscan, ultrasonography, computed tomography (CT) and magnetic resonance imaging (MRI) are techniques used to make the differentiation.

THYROIDITIS

Thyroiditis is most often immune mediated and only rarely results from bacteria or fungal infections.

Hashimoto's disease is an autoimmune disease that causes hypothyroidism. It is characterized by either a goiterous or atrophic thyroid. Autoantibodies to thyroid peroxidases are considered most important in its pathogenesis, but others to thyroglobulin and TSH are also recognized. Histologically, the goiterous form is characterized by a marked lymphocyte, plasma cell, immunoblast, and macrophage infiltrate; sometimes with lymphoid follicles. The atrophic form has abundant fibrosis with a less dense cellular infiltrate. The disease is found predominantly in women and the incidence increases with age. The typical clinical presentation is in a hypothyroid middle-aged woman with goiterous enlargement of the thyroid. Serum levels of TSH are high and T_3 and T_4 levels are low. The condition can be treated effectively with thyroid hormone replacement therapy.

Riedel's fibrous thyroiditis (Riedel's struma) is an idiopathic condition characterized by thyroid atrophy and fibrosis with adhesions to adjacent structures. Hypothyroidism ensues.

Subacute granulomatous (de Quervain's or giant cell) thyroiditis is a distinct form of thyroiditis associated with a granulomatous inflammatory response. It is thought to be of viral etiology, often being associated with previous infections such as mumps, measles, and the influenza virus. Histologically, the characteristic features include free colloid surrounded by macrophages and/or follicular cells admixed with giant cells. With time, chronic inflammatory cells and fibrosis ensue. Clinically, the condition is predominately observed in women in their second through fifth decades. It can present as an acute, febrile illness, with sudden painful enlargement of the thyroid gland, and/or transient hyperthyroidism with less painful enlargement. T_3 and T_4 levels are increased and radioactive iodine uptake is low. The disease is self-limiting.

Chronic lymphocytic (painless) thyroiditis is a common but usually asymptomatic disease. It is predominantly seen in women and is of unknown etiology.

TUMORS

Benign Tumors. Adenomas present as discrete, solitary masses. There is little risk of their becoming malignant; rarely, they are functional and cause hyperthyroidism. Clinically, they need to be differentiated from malignancies, especially if they do not take up radioactive iodine (''cold nodules''). In addition, as they increase in size, they can put pressure on the neck or, because of sudden enlargement, become painful.

Malignant Tumors. Malignant tumors of the thyroid gland are rare. They mainly affect women and the majority are carcinomas. Lymphomas and sarcomas are rare. There is an increased risk of thyroid carcinoma in individuals with a history of irradiation to the head and neck in the first two decades of life. In addition, there may be an increased risk with nontoxic nodular goiter. Finally, there is an increased risk of lymphoma and, to a lesser degree, carcinoma stemming from Hashimoto's disease.

Papillary carcinoma accounts for approximately 75% to 85% of thyroid carcinomas. They are found most often in women in their third to fifth decades. They are rarely encapsulated, they invade lymphatics, and often they are multilobular. Regional lymph node metastasis is common, but not distant spread. Histologically, they range from predominantly papillary to combinations of papillary and follicular patterns. Characteristic findings include hypochromatic ''empty'' nuclei (''Orphan Annie's eyes''), nuclear grooves, invaginations of cytoplasm into the nucleus causing eosinophilic, intranuclear inclusions, and psammoma bodies. In spite of lymph node metastasis, the prognosis is favorable.

Follicular carcinomas account for 10% to 20% of thyroid malignancies. They are most often diagnosed in women in their fifth and sixth decades. Multinodular goiters may be predisposing lesions. These tumors are most often encapsulated. Histologically, there is marked variation in patterns, but most often they have a microfollicular pattern ***without*** psammoma bodies or the nuclear features of papillary carcinomas. Invasion of capsules and blood vessels, but not lymphatics, yields a high frequency of distant metastases in bone, lungs, and liver. Regional lymph nodes are rarely involved. Clinically, follicular carcinomas present as slow-growing, painless thyroid nodules. Prognosis depends on the size of the primary tumor, the presence of metastases or its potential (evidence of capsular and/or vascular invasion), and cellular differentiation. The prognosis is not as good as with papillary carcinomas.

Anaplastic carcinomas account for 5% of thyroid malignancies. They occur most frequently in elderly individuals from areas endemic for goiters. Histologically, there are three patterns: spindle cell carcinomas, giant cell tumors, and a rare small cell carcinoma. They all present clinically as large, rapidly growing lesions. They metastasize widely, but death is often caused by local invasion. Medullary thyroid carcinomas are neuroendocrine neoplasms arising from parafollicular (C) cells. Most secrete calcitonin, although they may secrete a variety of other active substances; many have an amyloid stroma and about 20% to 25% are associated with multiple endocrine neoplasia (MEN) syndromes (to be discussed later). Sporadic tumors occur in the fifth and six decades of life, but those associated with MEN syndromes occur in the third or fourth. A more uncommon familial form is observed in the elderly. The sporadic tumors are usually confined to one lobe, whereas the familial tumors are multicentric. Histologically, polygonal or spindle cells are arranged in nests separated by varying amounts of fibrovascular stroma. Amyloid bands are observed in approximately one half of cases. Clinically, the sporadic tumors present as a thyroid mass or infrequently as paraneoplastic syndromes. Metastasis is via lymphatics and hematogenous routes, with regional lymph nodes, lungs, liver, and bone being frequent sites.

Parathyroid Glands

Disease of the parathyroid glands present as hyperparathyroidism or hypoparathyroidism.

HYPERPARATHYROIDISM

Hyperparathyroidism can be classified as primary or secondary.

Primary hyperthyroidism results from excess parathormone (PTH) produced by abnormal parathyroid glands. It presents with increased bone resorption and calcium mobilization from bones, increased renal tubular resorption and retention of calcium, and increased gastrointestinal resorption of calcium resulting from increased renal synthesis of 1,25-$(OH)_2D_3$. There are three causes: (a) adenomas, (b) hyperplasia, and (c) carcinomas of the parathyroid glands. ***Adenomas*** account for 75% to 80% of the cases. They are generally solitary and involve the inferior glands. Histologically, they are encapsulated and have stromal fat. Most are predominantly composed of chief cells. ***Hyperplasia*** accounts for 10% to 15% of cases. It may occur spontaneously or in the MEN syndrome I and IIA. Classically, all four glands are involved. Histologically, the hyperplasia may be diffuse or nodular. Chief cells predominate and the amount of fat is reduced. Carcinomas comprise less than 5% of cases. They usually involve one gland and may cause enlargement. Histologically, well-differentiated parathyroid cells are arranged in nodular or trabecular patterns. Local invasion and metastasis are the only reliable diagnoses of malignancy. Clinically, women are affected 3 times more frequently than men, and most cases occur the sixth decade and beyond. Classically, nephrolithiasis, osteitis fibrosis cystica, pancreatitis, peptic ulceration, generalized weakness, headaches, seizures, and depression can be observed. Up to half the cases may be asymptomatic, and the diagnosis is based on the presence of hypercalcemia and hypophosphatemia.

Secondary hyperparathyroidism is most often seen in patients with renal failure and, to a lesser degree, vitamin D deficiency or osteomalacia. The mechanism(s) by which it occurs in renal failure is based on the retention of phosphate and hypocalcemia, stimulating increased synthesis of PTH. In addition, there may be a reduction in the synthesis of 1,25-$(OH)_2D_3$, which leads to diminished calcium absorption by the small intestines. The increased synthesis of PTH is a result of diffuse or nodular hyperplasia, primarily of chief cells. Histologically, there is also a concomitant reduction of stromal fat. Clinically, osteitis fibrosa cystica and osteomalacia are common findings.

HYPOPARATHYROIDISM

Hypoparathyroidism results from surgical removal, congenital absence, or destruction of the parathyroid glands by autoimmune diseases, resulting in hypocalcemia. Clinically, a number of symptoms are observed including (a) increased neuromuscular excitability, (b) a range of mental status changes, including irritability and depression, (c) intracranial changes, such as calcification of basal ganglia, and elevations in CSF pressure, (d) calcification of the lens, and (e) cardiac conduction abnormalities. Diagnosis is based on low to undetectable levels of serum PTH in the presence of hypocalcemia.

Adrenal Gland

The adrenal glands are divided into the cortex and medulla. These are functionally distinct units, with the cortex producing steroids and the medulla producing catecholamines.

There are three distinct conditions of the adrenal cortex presenting as hyperadrenalism:

- Cushing's syndrome (excess cortisol)
- hyperaldosteronism (excess aldosterone)
- adrenogenital syndromes (excess androgens)

CUSHING'S SYNDROME

Cushing's syndrome is characterized by hypercortisolism caused by prolonged therapeutic use of corticosteroids; pituitary hypersecretion of ACTH (Cushing's disease); functional adrenal adenomas or carcinomas; hyperplasia; or ectopic ACTH secretion by nonpituitary tumors. ***Pituitary hypersecretion of ACTH*** is responsible for the vast majority (60% to 70%) of endogenous cases. Pituitary adenomas are found in 85% of these cases. The remainder of cases demonstrate corticotroph hyperplasia in the pituitary. The adrenals are bilaterally hyperplastic and serum ACTH levels are elevated. The condition is most common in women. ***Adrenal adenomas***, ***carcinomas***, and ***hyperplasia*** account for approximately 20% to 25% of endogenous cases. The adrenal lesions are solely responsible for the hypersecretion of cortisol in these cases and there is suppression of ACTH secretion. Cortical carcinomas and adenomas are most common in adults and carcinomas are most common in children. Autonomous hyperplasia is uncommon. Hypercortisolism is most severe when it stems from carcinomas. The uninvolved portions of the adrenal glands, and the contralateral gland, when there is unilateral involvement, atrophy because of the ACTH suppression. ***Ectopic ACTH secretion by nonpituitary tumors*** is responsible for approximately 10% to 15% of endogenous cases. The tumors most often associated with this condition include small cell carcinomas of the lung, carcinoids of the bronchus or pancreas, malignant thymomas, pheochromocytomas, thyroid medullary carcinomas, and gastrinomas. This condition is most common in men in their fifth and sixth decades. Cushing's syndrome is characterized by central obesity (trunk and upper back), moon facies, weakness, fatigue, hirsutism, hypertension, plethora, glucose intolerance, osteoporosis, neuropsychiatric abnormalities, menstrual irregularities, and skin striae. Diagnosis is made based on elevated plasma levels of cortisol metabolites (17-hydroxycorticoid). Differentiating the cause of the condition entails using the dexamethasone suppression test to suppress levels of ACTH, and CT of the pituitary and adrenals, and ultrasound of the adrenals.

PRIMARY HYPERALDOSTERONISM

This condition is characterized by prolonged, excessive aldosterone secretion that is primarily independent of the renin–angiotensin system. It is characterized by suppression of plasma renin activity, hypokalemia, sodium retention, and hypertension. Approximately 65% of cases are caused by a solitary aldosterone-secreting adenoma (Conn's syndrome). Approximately 30% of cases are caused by bilateral hyperplasia of the adrenals (idiopathic). There are other less common causes as well. Clinically, the condition is characterized by hypertension that is accompanied by hypokalemia resulting from renal potassium wasting. In addition, muscle weakness, paresthesias, and visual disturbances are observed. Sodium retention expands the extracellular fluid volume, which impacts on the hypertension. Diagnosis of primary hyperaldosteronism is confirmed by demonstrating elevated plasma levels of aldosterone concomitant with depressed levels of renin. Adenomas are treated surgically and idiopathic bilateral hyperplasia is treated medically.

CONGENITAL ADRENAL HYPERPLASIA

These disorders are uncommon and have a variety of forms. The ***adrenogenital syndrome*** (adrenal virilism) can be caused by an androgen-secreting carcinoma or by a group of inborn errors in metabolism which, through deficiencies of particular enzymes associated with the biosynthesis of cortical steroids, lead to increased productions of androgens. The most common of these is a deficiency of 21-hydroxylase, which manifests as three distinct syndromes: (a) salt-wasting adrenogenitalism, (b) simple virilizing adrenogenitalism, and (c) nonclassic adrenogenitalism.

HYPOFUNCTION OF THE ADRENAL CORTEX (HYPOADRENALISM)

Hypoadrenalism may occur as a result of ACTH deficiency, or structural or functional conditions in the cortex that impair the production or synthesis of corticosteroids. There are three distinct patterns of adrenocortical insufficiency:

- primary acute adrenocortical insufficiency (adrenal crisis)
- primary chronic adrenocortical insufficiency (Addison's disease)
- secondary adrenocortical insufficiency

Primary Acute Adrenocortical Insufficiency. This condition is uncommon but can occur as follows: (a) with a crisis in patients with chronic adrenocortical insufficiency that is caused by any form of stress; (b) from too rapid a withdrawal of steroids in patients who have been treated with long-term steroid administration; or (c) from massive destruction of adrenals as is seen in prolonged and difficult deliveries, postsurgical patients with disseminated intravascular coagulation, or massive adrenal hemorrhage as a complication of bacteremic infections (Waterhouse-Friderichsen syndrome).

Primary Chronic Adrenocortical Insufficiency (Addison's Disease). Addison's disease is rare and can be caused by any chronic process that destroys the adrenal cortex. Approximately 90% of all cases are caused by autoimmune adrenalitis, tuberculosis, or metastatic cancer. By itself, ***autoimmune adrenalitis*** is responsible for approximately 60% to 70% of cases. In about half of those, the adrenal is the sole target, and in the other half, other endocrine glands are affected. ***Tuberculous adrenalitis*** accounts for approximately 10% to 15% of cases. Metastatic cancer is uncommon. Those neoplasms that most commonly metastasize to the adrenal are bronchogenic, gastric, and breast carcinomas. In addition, malignant melanomas and lymphomas are also found in the adrenal cortex. Clinically, the disease has an insidious onset and is most often found in adults. The disease is manifested only after approximately 90% or more of the functioning cortical cells are destroyed. It is more common in whites and predominates in women. Its clinical manifestations are referable to low levels of circulating glucocorticoids and mineralocorticoids. These manifestations include weakness, fatigue, weight loss, hypotension, hyperpigmentation in the skin, anorexia, nausea, and vomiting. Plasma levels of cortisol and its metabolites are low. In addition, serum levels of sodium, chloride, bicarbonate, and glucose are also low. Serum levels of potassium are generally elevated. Finally, circulating ACTH levels are also elevated. For the most part, the condition is easily treated with steroids.

Secondary Adrenocortical Insufficiency. Lesions of the hypothalamus and/or pituitary lead to adrenocortical insufficiency by reducing the output of ACTH. Some of the more common conditions leading to this include metastatic cancer, infection, infarction, and irradiation. In addition, however, long-term use of steroids can also reduce the levels of circulating ACTH. Because of the pituitary lesions, secondary adrenocortical insufficiency does not manifest hyperpigmentation. In addition, there is deficiency of cortisol and androgens, but not mineralocorticoids. Consequently, hyponatremia and hyperkalemia are not observed.

Adrenal Medulla

The adrenal medulla is the source of catecholamines including epinephrine, norepinephrine, and dopamine. From a clinical point of view, lesions of the adrenal medulla are not as important as those of the cortex. The most significant of the adrenal medulla disorders are neoplasms and of those, pheochromocytomas, neuroblastomas, and ganglion neuromas are of significance.

PHEOCHROMOCYTOMA

These neoplasms are rare. Their clinical significance is that they are functional and thus produce catecholamine-induced hypertension. Approximately 90% of pheochromocytomas occur sporadically, and the remaining 10% occur in familial syndromes. Approximately 85% of pheochromocytomas arise in the medulla of the adrenal, and the remainder arise in extra-adrenal paraganglia. The extra-adrenal tumors have a higher incidence of malignancy than those found in the adrenal. The malignant neoplasms metastasize, and the most common sites are lymph nodes, liver, lungs, and bones. Clinically, the sporadic neoplasms occur in adults between 40 and 60 years of age. The tumors of familial syndromes, however, arise in childhood and are found predominantly in males, whereas the sporadic tumors have a slight female predominance. The most predominant clinical feature is hypertension. Diagnosis is confirmed by measuring urinary catecholamines and their metabolites, especially metanephrine and vanillylmandelic acid (VMA). The localization of the tumor can usually be defined by CT or MRI scan or ultrasound.

NEUROBLASTOMA AND GANGLIONEUROMA

Neuroblastoma accounts for approximately 15% of childhood cancer deaths and is one of the most common solid neoplasms outside the cranial wall. Approximately 25% to 35% arise in the adrenal medulla. The remainder occur anywhere in the sympathetic chain, but particularly in the paravertebral region of the posterior mediastinum. Histologically, the neoplasms are composed of small primitive cells with dark nuclei and little cytoplasm. Characteristically, the cells are arranged in rosettes (Homer-Wright pseudorosettes). These are characterized by tumor cells arranged around a central space that is filled with fibrillar extensions of the cells. Tumors that are composed of well-differentiated cells resembling sympathetic neurons in a fibrous stroma are called ***ganglioneuromas***. Those with intermediate differentiation are designated ***ganglioneuroblastomas***. Ganglioneuromas are found in young adults, while ganglioneuroblastomas are more frequent in pre-adolescents. Clinically, neoplasms are found primarily in children under 2 years of age and present as large abdominal masses. In addition, fever and possible weight loss are observed. In older children, they may not be diagnosed. In older children, clinical symptoms may not result until metastasis has occurred. In these cases, bone pain, respiratory symptoms, or gastrointestinal complaints may be presenting features.

Thymus

Changes in the thymus can be classified into three major categories:

- developmental disorders
- thymic hyperplasia
- thymomas

Developmental disorders include hypoplasia or aplasia. This malady is seen in DiGeorge syndrome which is characterized by total lack or severe reduction in cell-mediated immune responses. Thymic cysts, another developmental disorder, are also observed. They are usually without clinical significance.

Thymic hyperplasia refers to the formation of lymphoid follicles within the thymus. This is sometimes referred to as thymic follicular hyperplasia. The lymphoid follicles are similar, if not identical, to those encountered in lymph nodes. They occur in conjunction with a number of systemic diseases including myasthenia gravis, Graves' disease, systemic lupus erythematosus, systemic sclerosis, and rheumatoid arthritis.

Thymomas refer to neoplasms arising from thymic epithelial cells. They are classified into benign thymomas and two types of malignant thymomas. Type I include those neoplasms that are morphologically benign but behaviorally capable of local invasion and, in some instances, distant metastasis. Type II have histologic characteristics of malignancy as well as malignant behavioral characteristics. Clinically, thymomas are equally distributed between genders and are usually found in individuals older than 40 years of age. Approximately half of these neoplasms are associated with myasthenia gravis. An additional 40% present as thymic masses that are discovered because they are putting pressure on local structures or by imaging techniques. The remaining 10% are associated with perineoplastic syndromes.

Multiple Endocrine Neoplasia

There are three autosomal dominant multiple endocrine neoplasia (MEN) syndromes. They are characterized by either hyperplasia or tumors of several endocrine glands occurring concomitantly. ***MEN I*** is characterized by adenomas of the pituitary, parathyroid, and pancreatic islets. In addition, there is hyperplasia of the parathyroids, pancreatic islets, and adrenal cortex, and C-cell hyperplasia in the thyroid. Finally, carcinomas can be found in the pancreatic islets.

MEN II or ***IIA*** consists of hyperplasia of the parathyroid and to a lesser degree, adenomas and pheochromocytomas of the adrenal, and most commonly, medullary carcinomas of the thyroid. ***MEN IIB*** or ***III*** is composed of parathyroid hyperplasia, pheochromocytomas in the adrenal, medullary carcinomas of the thyroid, and, mucocutaneous neuromas and ganglioneuromas and a morfanoid habitus.

SKIN

Diseases of the skin are caused by exposure to exogenous physical and chemical agents, by infections, by immune disorders, and by metabolic disturbances within the body. They also include tumors and a number of disorders of unknown etiology. Morphologically, skin diseases present in several forms and can be classified as follows: (a) ***macule***, a flat lesion presenting as a localized discoloration of the skin; (b) ***papule***, a slightly elevated lesion, called a plaque if larger than 5 mm; (c) ***nodule*** or tumor that appears as intradermal but also as a protruding mass; (d) ***vesicles*** and ***bullae***, which are filled with fluid; (e) ***pustules***, which contain pus (polys); (f) ***ulcers***, which present as epidermal defects; (g) ***crusts*** formed of coagulated plasma or blood; and (h) ***scales*** and ***squames***, which are composed of layers of keratin that can be removed by scratching. Histologic terms used to describe these lesions include the usual terms of general pathology, such as necrosis, abscess, and ulcers, but also include specific dermatopathologic terms: ***acanthosis*** (thickening of the epidermis), ***hyperkeratosis*** (thickening of superficial keratin layer composed of squames devoid of nuclei), and ***parakeratosis*** (thickening of stratum corneum with retention of nuclei). ***Acantholysis*** denotes loss of contact between keratinocytes that leads to formation of intradermal vesicles. ***Spongiosis*** is separation by intercellular edema, with the cells stretched apart but remaining attached by desmosomes.

Chronic Dermatitis

Chronic dermatitis, also known as ***eczema***, may develop as a result of obvious exogenous causes, but often it may be an expression of internal diseases, hypersensitivity reactions, or unknown reasons. Exogenous eczema is classified as *irritant contact dermatitis*, usually caused by exposure to soil, dust, or chemicals in the workplace, or *allergic contact dermatitis*, which develops after sensitization to specific allergens, such as gold rings or rubber gloves. Examples of endogenous chronic dermatitis include *atopic dermatitis*, thought to be of allergic origin and related to adverse IgE-mediated reaction to food and environmental allergens; *seborrheic dermatitis*, a disease of unknown origin presenting with excessive dandruff, redness, scaling, and itching of the hairy skin of the chest and intertriginous areas; *dry skin (asteatotic) chronic dermatitis* that develops during winter, especially in the elderly. Chronic dermatitis can be treated successfully if the cause is known. If the cause cannot be identified, the treatment is symptomatic and includes emollient creams and mild topical steroid ointments.

Erythematous Scaly Eruptions

Eczema can be distinguished from several defined clinicopathologic entities that can be identified on the basis of typical clinical and histologic features evident in skin biopsies. These diseases do not have a known cause and are classified as idiopathic. The most common among them are psoriasis and lichen planus.

Psoriasis is a chronic disease of unknown etiology that presents with recurrent eruptions of erythematous, silvery plaques, and scales. It affects approximately 2% of the total population. The lesions, which are thought to originate because of the abnormally rapid proliferation of basal epidermal cells, appear most often on elbows, knees, the lower back, and the scalp. Nails may be involved, and some patients suffer from psoriatic arthritis. Eruptions appear usually without any obvious reason, but occasionally the exacerbation of the symptoms is related to trauma, emotional crisis, infections, and certain drugs, such as lithium and beta-blockers. Treatment modalities, most of which give only partial or temporary relief, include application of tar or steroid ointments and exposure to ultraviolet light or sunshine.

Lichen planus presents with highly pruritic red papules on the flexor sides of the extremities, genital organs, and mucous membranes, especially the mouth. Histologically, the lesions consist of infiltrates of T lymphocytes in the upper dermis invading the epidermis and causing destruction and death of cells in the basal layer. These histologic findings suggest a possible immune mechanism. Occasionally the eruptions are linked to an intake of certain drugs or exposure to chemicals such as film developers. The lesions of lichen planus last for a short period and then heal spontaneously.

Infectious Skin Diseases

Infections of the skin are most often caused by bacteria, viruses, fungi, protozoa, and insects.

Bacterial infections of the skin are extremely common. Such infections occur in all age groups and are caused by a wide variety of pathogens. *Impetigo* is a superficial skin infection typically caused by streptococci or staphylococci; it presents as superficial pustules and yellow crusts. It is most common on the face and arms of children who tend to transmit the disease to other children by close contact or hands. *Furuncles* are abscesses within hair follicles usually caused by *Staphylococcus aureus.* Confluent furuncles are called *carbuncles (boils).*

Erysipelas presents as redness of the skin overlying an infection of the upper subcutis, usually caused by streptococci, which spread through the lymphatics. *Cellulitis* is an infection of the deep subcutis that extends into the adjacent soft tissues. Chronic bacterial infections such as leprosy or tuberculosis are rare in the United States. These diseases present as induration of the skin, often with destruction of underlying tissue and disfigurement.

Acne vulgaris is an inflammatory disease related to the obstruction of the pilosebaceous units. Acne predominantly affects teenagers, but in about 5% of women and some men, the disease may persist into adult life. Most often the lesions appear on the face, upper chest, and back. Pathogenetically it is related to anaerobic *Propionibacterium acnes*, which thrives in stagnant sebum. Hormonal influences, genetic predisposition, and all drugs that stimulate the production of sebum promote the development of lesions. Clinically, acne presents as ***seborrhea*** (greasy skin) reflecting hypersecretion of sebum, and ***comedos***, which represent stagnant sebum in hair follicles. Comedos are classified as open ("blackheads") or closed ("whiteheads"). Infection superimposed on seborrhea and comedos leads to formation of pustules, which may become confluent *(acne conglobata).* Deep infection may result in scarring. Treatment with systemic or local antibiotics usually controls the eruptions. In severe cases, retinoic acid creams and hormonal treatment may be indicated.

Viral infections of the skin may cause acute or chronic lesions. *Measles* cause a maculopapular rash, *varicella* presents with disseminated vesicles. The vesicles caused by *herpesvirus* infection are localized to defined anatomic sites: herpes simplex virus type 1 causes vesicles on the lips, herpes simplex type 2 causes genital vesicles, and herpes zoster causes eruptions of vesicles along specific somatic nerves ("shingles"). *Human papilloma viruses* (HPV) cause warts, which occur in several variants: ***filiform*** common wart or ***verruca vulgaris***, flat ***plantar warts***, or large genital warts ***(condyloma acuminatum).***

Fungal infections of the skin are most often caused by *dermatophytes* (such as *Trichophyton, Epidermophyton*, or *Microsporum* species) which live in the scales of the superficial epidermis. Typical infections are called ***tinea capitis*** if found on the head, ***tinea cruris*** if found in the groin, ***tinea corporis*** (also known as ringworm), or ***tinea pedis*** (also known as athlete's foot). Deep fungal infections, caused by *Blastomyces, Madurella,* and similar pathogens typically occur in the tropics and are rare in the United States.

Insect-related skin diseases are most often caused by insect stings or bites. Mosquitoes, ticks, chiggers, fleas, and lice all cause papulomacular, often indurated skin lesions, which are of a transient nature and rarely leave any consequences unless infected during scratching. Many insects, however, transmit systemic diseases that may appear weeks or even months after the insect bites. *Scabies*, a chronic skin infection caused by *Sarcoptes scabiei*, capable of invading the deep epidermis, is characterized by migratory maculopapular rashes.

Autoimmune Diseases of the Skin

Skin can be affected with all four types of hypersensitivity reactions. *Atopic dermatitis* is an example of a ***type I*** hypersensitivity reaction, mediated by IgE attached to mast cells. Binding of antigen to IgE triggers a release of histamine from mast cells, which causes local increased permeability of the blood vessels, edema, and itching. The best example of ***type II*** or ***cytotoxic hypersensitivity*** reaction is *pemphigus vulgaris*, a blistering disease caused by cytotoxic antibodies binding to the surface of keratinocytes in the epidermis. Antibodies disrupt the cell-to-cell contact junction, which leads to formation of intraepidermal vesicles and bullae. *Discoid lupus erythematosus* and *systemic lupus erythematosus* are examples of ***type III*** hypersensitivity reaction. In these diseases, the circulating immune complexes are deposited along the basement membrane at the epidermal–dermal junction. Deposition of immune complexes activates the complement cascade, which incites a dermal and epidermal inflammation. Skin lesions are most prominent on the face and other areas exposed to sunshine. ***Type IV***, or ***cell-mediated hypersensitivity*** reaction, mediated by T lymphocytes, is typically the underlying cause of skin lesions in ***sarcoidosis***, a systemic disease that often presents with subcutaneous nodules. Histologically, these lesions are noncaseating granulomas. Most forms of contact dermatitis and poison ivy reactions represent also a cell-mediated, type IV hypersensitivity reaction. Graft-versus-host reaction in patients who have received bone marrow transplants is also mediated by T lymphocytes derived from the donor.

Skin Lesions Resulting from Internal Disease

Many internal diseases present with skin lesions. Liver disease presents with spider nevi and palmar erythema. ***Acanthosis nigricans*** is a pigmentation of the skin on the neck and intertriginous areas; it is found as a paraneoplastic syndrome in patients who have carcinoma of the gastrointestinal tract. Porphyria cutanea tarda may present with skin vesicles. Rheumatoid arthritis may present with subcutaneous rheumatoid nodules. Skin pigmentation is a feature of Addison's disease. Hyperthyroidism presents with sweating, warm, moist skin (hyperhidrosis), whereas in hypothyroidism, the skin is doughlike, soft, and pliable (myxedema).

Tumors and Related Lesions

Skin tumors originate from epithelial cells of the epidermis, pigmented cells (melanocytes), neuroendocrine cells (Merkel cells), dermal connective tissue cells, and migratory cells, such as blood-derived white blood cell precursors. Epithelial tumors and melanomas are thought to be induced in many cases by ultraviolet light and occur with greater frequency among people exposed to sunshine (e.g., farmers, sailors) and those of light complexion. ***Epithelial tumors*** may be benign or malignant. The most common benign epithelial tumor is *seborrheic keratosis*, also known as basal cell epithelioma, which presents as wartlike, mildly pigmented, brown lesions on the skin of older people. The most common malignant tumor of the skin is *basal cell carcinoma*, a locally invasive neoplasm of low malignant potential. Most basal cell carcinomas are located on the sun-exposed skin of the face. Histologically, these tumors are composed of cells resembling those in the basal layer of the epidermis. The cells are arranged into nests and strands, and although the tumor is usually locally invasive, distant metastases almost never occur. Excellent results are obtained by surgical resection; the entire tumor must be removed to prevent local recurrence. *Squamous cell carcinoma* differs from basal cell carcinoma in that it is both locally invasive and prone to metastasis. Squamous cell carcinoma also occurs on sun-exposed skin and is often preceded by preinvasive, intraepithelial, neoplastic changes known as *senile* or *actinic keratosis*. Actinic keratosis may present as an atrophy of the skin or in the form of locally hyperkeratotic lesions. Transition to squamous cell carcinoma is characterized by induration of the skin resulting from tumor invasion and accompanied by a desmoplastic dermal reaction, or by exophytic outgrowth leading to formation of nodules and surface ulceration.

Pigmented lesions are classified as benign or malignant. Most benign lesions are not true tumors but rather hamartomas, composed of normal pigmented cells showing abnormal distributions. ***Freckles*** (ephelis) are pigmented macules composed of melanocytes that become more pigmented when exposed to sunlight. ***Lentigo*** is also composed of melanocytes but lentigines do not become darker under the influence of UV light. A ***nevus*** consists of groups of melanocytic cells. Nevi are classified as congenital if present from birth, or acquired if first noticed in adult life. Histologically, nevi are classified depending on the location of the pigmented cells: dermal if the cells are in the dermis, junctional if located at the dermal–epidermal junction, or compound if the lesions shows both junctional activity and dermal location. Most nevi are benign, but in some cases they show histologic atypia and are classified as dysplastic. Dysplastic nevi, which may occur at an increased rate in some families, must be watched carefully because they tend to progress to invasive malignant melanoma. ***Malignant melanomas*** are invasive malignant neoplasms arising from melanocytes residing in normal skin or arranged into nevi. Histologically, melanomas are classified as ***superficial spreading***, ***nodular***, or ***acrolentiginous***. Melanomas are most often located on sun-exposed skin, except the acrolentiginous melanomas, which typically occur on distal parts or extremities and are often subungual. Melanomas are more common in the southern United States but are rare among blacks and other dark-skinned people.

Neuroendocrine tumors of the skin are rare but rather malignant. They originate from Merkel cells and are therefore called ***Merkel cell carcinomas***. ***Connective tissue tumors*** of the dermis are common, but they are usually benign and usually histologically classified as dermatofibromas. Malignant dermal tumors are less common. *Kaposi sarcoma* is a malignant tumor of small blood vessels, which occurs most often in people affected with AIDS. Infiltrates of myelogenous leukemia cells in the dermis may present as yellow-green nodules known as *chloroma*. Both B cell and T cell lymphoma cells may infiltrate the skin. Low grade malignant lymphoma composed of mature T cells that show remarkable dermatotropism is called *mycosis fungoides*. *Urticaria pigmentosa* is a disease of children and young adults in which the skin is infiltrated with mast cells. Urticaria pigmentosa usually heals spontaneously by the time of puberty, and it is debatable whether it represents a neoplasm at all. *Metastatic tumors* to the skin may originate from any internal organ.

BONE AND JOINT

The most important diseases of the skeletal system are metabolic, infectious, autoimmune, and neoplastic.

Metabolic Disorders

Osteoporosis

This condition is characterized by increased porosity of the bone leading to reduction in skeletal mass. It can be localized (as in disuse atrophy) or generalized (as in metabolic diseases). The primary form is associated with senility or postmenopausal changes. Secondary forms can result from (a) endocrine disturbances such as hyperparathyroidism, hyperthyroidism, Cushing's disease, and hypogonadism; (b) neoplasms such as multiple myeloma; (c) gastrointestinal disorders such as malabsorption; (d) rheumatologic diseases; (e) drugs such as corticosteroids or chemotherapeutic agents; and (f) miscellaneous conditions like immobilization or pulmonary disease. The cause of age-related osteoporosis is multifactorial and includes decreased replication of osteoblast precursors and decreased activity of resident osteoblasts. In addition, there is decreased activity of matrix-bound growth factors and reduced physical activity. There is decreased serum estrogen and increased IL-1 leading to increased osteoclastic activity in postmenopausal osteoporosis. Morphologically, the entire skeleton is involved, but the vertebral bodies are most severely involved in the postmenopausal form.

Histologically, trabeculae are thin and lose connections, leading to fractures. There is also enlargement of haversian canals. Clinically, fractures of thoracic and lumbar vertebrae are common. They, in turn, lead to reduction in height, kyphoscoliosis, and lordosis.

RICKETS AND OSTEOMALACIA

Rickets, a disease of children, and osteomalacia, a disease of adults, result from dietary vitamin D deficiency, inadequate vitamin D absorption or metabolism, and disorders in calcium and/or phosphorus metabolism. The resulting defects in bone metabolism result from delayed and/or inadequate mineralization leading to excess unmineralized matrix (osteoid). In rickets, there is the addition of deranged endochondral bone growth resulting from inadequate mineralization of epiphyseal cartilage. Histologically, there is overgrowth of inadequately mineralized epiphyseal cartilage, which is irregular and projects into the marrow cavity. Osteoid is deposited on the cartilage and there is increased osteoblast and osteoclast activity. Finally, there is an overgrowth of capillaries in the region and fibrosis of the marrow. All of this leads to deformation of bones because of a lack of rigidity. This can give rise in children to bowing of the legs, lumbar lordosis, frontal bossing, "rachitic rosary" of the costochondral junction, and anterior protrusion of the sternum (pigeon-breast deformity). Osteomalacia in the adult is not as dramatic and is characterized by osteopenia caused by the inadequate mineralization. Skeletal deformities do not appear, but radiographic evidence of cortical thinning and loss of bone density is observed. Osteomalacia must be differentiated from other osteopenic conditions such as osteoporosis, osteitis fibrosa, and some stages of Paget's disease.

PAGET'S DISEASE (OSTEITIS DEFORMANS)

This condition is characterized by osteoclastic bone resorption followed by a combination of osteoclastic and osteoblastic activity, with the latter predominating. The end stage is quiescent and osteosclerotic. It is thought that a paramyxovirus may be the cause, but this is not proven. Histologically, there is a mosaic pattern to the lamellar bone giving the appearance of a "jigsaw puzzle." Ultimately, the bone has coarsely thickened trabeculae. Clinically, it is seen slightly more frequently in men than women with a peak in the fifth decade. The axial skeleton and proximal femur are involved most frequently. Very often it is asymptomatic. However, pain resulting from microfractures may be present in addition to various postural deformities. High-output heart failure and benign and malignant neoplasms are complications.

OSTEITIS FIBROSA CYSTICA (VON RECKLINGHAUSEN'S DISEASE OF BONE)

This condition results from primary or secondary hyperparathyroidism. It is characterized by marked osteoclastic resorption of bone, particularly in cortical bone. This produces thin corticis. Concomitant osteoblastic activity fills the marrow spaces with fibrovascular tissue. ''Brown tumors'' result from microfractures with resultant hemorrhage, leading to infiltrates by macrophages and fibrous connective tissue. Complications include fractures, deformities, and dysfunction. Control of the hyperparathyroidism leads to significant regression or resolution of the bony lesions.

Infections of Bone

Osteomyelitis is inflammation of the bone and bone marrow. It is generally caused by bacterial infection with *Staphylococcus aureus*, which is responsible for 80% to 90% of cases of pyogenic forms from which positive cultures are obtained. The organisms reach the bone via the hematogenous route (most frequent), extension from an adjacent site, or direct implantation. The infections involve long bones. The regions most commonly involved are the metaphysis and/or epiphysis in neonates, metaphysis in children, and epiphysis and subchondral regions in adults. Histologically, there is acute inflammation and ischemic necrotic bone fragments (sequestra) are noted. Subperiosteal abscesses may lead to draining sinuses. Chronic inflammation, bone resorption, fibrosis, and deposition of reactive bone on the periphery occur with time. Clinically, hematogenous osteomyelitis presents as an acute systemic illness, with marked pain over the involved area. Treatment includes antibiotics and surgical drainage. Complications include suppurative arthritis, usually in infants. Chronic osteomyelitis may give rise to pathologic fractures, secondary amyloidosis, endocarditis, sepsis, squamous cell carcinomas in the sinus tracts, and, rarely, sarcomas in the bone.

Tuberculous osteomyelitis arises from blood-borne organisms that stem from active disease in viscera. Direct extension or lymphatic spread may also occur. The spine (thoracic and lumbar) is the most common site. The lesions are generally focal, but they may be multiple in AIDS patients. The spinal disease (Pott's disease) may involve multiple vertebrae and adjacent soft tissue. Clinically, patients present with pain on motion, fever, chills, and weight loss, as well as localized tenderness. Complications include abscesses of the psoas muscles, vertebral compression fractures, leading to scoliosis or kyphosis, arthritis, sinus tracts, and amyloidosis.

Bone Tumors

Tumors of bone are rare. They can be benign or malignant.

Osteoid osteoma and osteoblastoma: These neoplasms have identical histological features. By definition, osteoid osteomas are less than 2 cm in greatest dimension, and osteoblastomas are larger. Histologically, the lesions are well circumscribed and characterized by trabeculae of bone that are surrounded by osteoblasts and connected randomly. A loose fibrovascular stroma surrounds them. Osteoid osteomas are often surrounded by reactive bone. Clinically, both are found in the second and third decade, with men out-numbering women two to one. Osteoid osteomas are most often found in the appendicular skeleton and are quite painful because of excessive prostaglandin E_2 production. Osteoblastomas occur in the same age group and gender distribution. They are much less painful and most often involve the spine. Both are readily treated and malignant transformation is rare except when treated with radiation. Radiation appears to promote malignant transformation.

Giant cell tumors: These tumors generally arise in the distal femur and proximal tibia but can arise elsewhere. Most are solitary. Histologically, they are characterized by uniform mononuclear cells with indistinct cytoplasm growing in syncytia and having frequent mitoses. Osteoclast-type giant cells are admixed. Necrosis, hemorrhage, hemosiderin deposition, and reactive bone formation are also observed. These tumors arise in the third to fifth decade. They are histologically benign, but they may frequently recur if treated by curettage. A low percentage may metastasize to the lung.

Osteosarcomas: These are malignant mesenchymal neoplasms that produce bone matrix. They account for approximately 20% of primary bone malignancies. The vast majority arise in the metaphysis of long bones. The favored sites in descending order include distal femur, proximal tibia, proximal humerus, and proximal tibia. Mutations have been associated with both inherited and noninherited forms. Histologically, the formation of neoplastic bone by anaplastic cells characterizes these neoplasms. It is coarse and formed in sheets or trabeculae. Vascular invasion is frequent. Clinically, they occur of any age, but the majority occur in patients less than 20 years of age. A significant percentage also occur in the elderly. Males are at higher risk than females. Osteosarcomas present as painful, enlarging masses that may fracture. Metastasis to lungs, bones, and brain is via the hematogenous route.

Chondrosarcoma: These are malignant mesenchymal neoplasms that produce neoplastic cartilage. They are the second most common matrix-producing malignant tumors of bone. They are most commonly found in the pelvis, shoulder, and ribs. Histologically, they are characterized by malignant cartilage infiltrating marrow spaces and surrounding bone trabeculae. Cellularity varies, depending on the grade. Clinically, they are found twice as often in men than in women. Their highest incidence is in the fourth decade or older. They present as painful, progressively enlarging masses. Lower grades are more prevalent and are relatively indolent. Higher grades metastasize to the lungs and skeleton.

Joints

The most important diseases of the joints are classified as:

- degenerative
- infectious
- immunologically mediated
- metabolic

OSTEOARTHRITIS

Osteoarthritis is a degenerative joint disease characterized by erosion of articular cartilage. It can be primary, idiopathic, or secondary to some underlying cause, such as traumatic injury, congenital malformation, or diabetes. The primary form appears to result from intrinsic alterations in cartilage resulting in breakdown. Morphologically, there is erosion of articular cartilage with thickening of underlying bone. Dislodged cartilage and bone migrate into the joint (''joint mice'') and osteophytes develop at the margins of the articular surface. Clinically, primary osteoarthritis is a disease of the sixth decade and beyond. It presents as deep, aching pain, morning stiffness, crepitus, and limitation of movement. Commonly involved joints include hips, knees, lower lumbar and cervical vertebrae, distal interphalangeal joints of the fingers, first carpometacarpal joints, and first tarsometatarsal joints of the feet.

INFECTIOUS ARTHRITIS

The hematogenous route is the most common means by which microorganisms reach joints. Suppurative arthritis is most commonly caused by *Staphylococcus, Streptococcus,* Gonococcus, *Haemophilus influenzae* (in children), and gram-negative bacilli. The large joints are most frequently involved. Clinical presentation includes hot, swollen joints with fever, leukocytosis, and an elevated sedimentation rate. An accompanying synovitis that extends to the articular cartilage may occur as a complication. Arthritis is also observed in tuberculosis and Lyme disease.

RHEUMATOID ARTHRITIS

Rheumatoid arthritis (RA) is a chronic systemic inflammatory disorder that may affect many tissues and organs but mainly affects joints. It is characterized by a nonsuppurative, proliferative synovitis. The cause is unknown, but there is much evidence that incriminates Epstein-Barr virus infections as initiating the condition. The pathogenesis involves a complex interaction of genetic susceptibility, a primary exogenous inducing agent such as a microbial agent, an autoimmune reaction such as IgM autoantibodies against autologous IgG (rheumatoid factors), and mediators of joint damage such as cytokines. Morphologically, the synovium becomes edematous, hyperplastic, and infiltrated by lymphocytes (CD4+), plasma cells, and macrophages. Inflamed, hyperemic synovium (pannus) migrates over the articular cartilage, causing erosion. This, in turn, leads to fibrous or bony ankylosis. Rheumatoid nodules are noted in the skin and rheumatoid vasculitis of small arteries, vasa vasorum, may lead to endarteritis. Clinically, the disease peaks in the third and fifth decades and women are 3 to 5 times more susceptible than men. Involved joints are hot, swollen, and stiff. Initially, small joints such as the metacarpophalangeal and proximal interphalangeal are involved, and, later, larger joints. Diagnosis is based on morning stiffness, arthritis in three or more joints, arthritis of hand joints, symmetric arthritis, rheumatoid nodules (fibrinoid necrosis surrounded by epithelioid cells), serum rheumatoid factor, and typical radiographic findings. Complications include systemic amyloidosis, gastrointestinal bleeding resulting from chronic aspirin use, and infectionsresulting from use of steroids.

GOUTY ARTHRITIS

Gout results from hyperuricemia. It is characterized by transient acute arthritis that eventually leads to chronic arthritis and the deposition of urate masses (tophi) in the joints and other sites, most often including the kidney. Primary gout accounts for approximately 90% of cases. The enzyme defect responsible for it is unknown. Virtually all gout results from conditions causing hyperuricemia. There are numerous predisposing factors including age, duration of hyperuricemia, and genetic predisposition. Once monosodium urate crystals are in the joints, neutrophils and monocytes play a central role in perpetuating the arthritis by releasing mediators and enzymes. Tophi are found not only in the joint space, but also in ligaments, tendons, and soft tissues, such as the earlobes and kidneys. Clinically, gout has four stages: (a) asymptomatic uricemia, (b) acute gouty arthritis, (c) intercritical gout, and (d) chronic tophaceous gout. It rarely appears before 20 to 30 years of hyperuricemia. The initial attacks are most often in the metatarsophalangeal joints and then, in descending order, the insteps, ankles, heels, knees, wrists, fingers, and elbows. Attacks present as excruciating pain with sudden onset, hyperemia, warmth, and severe tenderness. Numerous drugs are available to abort or prevent initial attacks or solubilize the tophi.

EYE

Diseases of the eye are caused by a broad range of conditions that can be categorized as:

- inflammatory
- neoplastic
- miscellaneous

They may be localized or part of a systemic disease process. Many eye diseases reduce visual acuity and may cause blindness.

Inflammatory Diseases

Infections of the external layers of the eye are common and may be caused by bacteria, viruses, or parasites. *H. influenzae* and *Chlamydia trachomatis* cause conjunctivitis. The former is an acute purulent disease in children (''pink eye''). The latter is a disease of infants born to infected mothers, characterized by edema and hyperemia. *Herpes simplex virus I* causes stromal keratitis, which is the major infectious cause of corneal blindness in the United States, secondary to stromal conjunctivitis. Finally, punctate keratitis, caused by inflammation elicited against microfilaria of *Onchocerca volvulus*, causes sclerosing keratitis, iridocyclitis, and retinitis. All these can lead to blindness.

NONINFECTIOUS INFLAMMATORY DISEASES

Sarcoidosis produces a granulomatis iritis or iridocyclitis in about 20% of cases. This is either unilateral or bilateral and leads to glaucoma and/or corneal opacities. Inflammation of the lacrimal gland is a frequent complication. ***Graves' disease*** has an associated exophthalmus of autoimmune origin. It is characterized by lymphocytic infiltrates in the extraocular eye muscles and retro-orbital fat. These areas become edematous and there is increased deposition of mucopolysaccharides and fibrosis. Contractures lead to eye movement incoordination, diplopia, and/or ophthalmoplegia.

Neoplasms

The major neoplasms of the eye include (a) melanomas and (b) retinoblastoma.

Melanomas of the eye arise from melanocytes of the uvea. There are two histologic types. The *spindle cell* type, whose cells are cohesive and have cytoplasm that may have pigment granules, and the *epithelioid cell* type, composed of noncohesive cells with abundant, sometimes pigmented cytoplasm. The former are slow growing and tend to metastasize late. ***Retinoblastomas*** are the most common malignant eye tumors of children from newborn to 15 years of age. They can be sporadic or familial. Histologically, they are composed of small, round, hyperchromatic nuclei with little cytoplasm. In more differentiated tumors, the cells are arranged in rosettes (Flexner-Wintersteiner). Clinically, they present most commonly at 2 years of age with poor vision, strabismus, pain, tenderness, and a white hue to the pupil being the most common symptoms. They are fatal without treatment. Patients with this tumor are at risk of developing other tissue tumors or osteogenic sarcomas.

Miscellaneous Eye Diseases

Refractory disorders, such as ***myopia*** (short sightedness), are so common that they are barely considered diseases. ***Presbyopia*** (far sightedness) is a regular event that accompanies aging. These changes can be easily corrected with eye glasses. ***Glaucoma*** is an eye disease characterized by increased intraocular pressure sufficient to cause degeneration of the optic disc and nerve fibers. Obstruction to the outflow of aqueous humor from the anterior chamber is most common. If not treated, it can lead to blindness. ***Cataracts*** is a disease characterized by clouding (opacification) of the lens. It occurs in the elderly, but it may also be seen, rarely, in the young as a result of rubella infection (congenital) or resulting from metabolic diseases, particularly diabetes mellitus.

SKELETAL MUSCLES

Skeletal muscles vary in size and shape depending on their anatomic location and function, but all of them share certain common features: (a) all muscles are composed of muscle fibers, large multinucleated cells rich in contractile proteins arranged into cytoplasmic functional units; (b) all muscles are composed of two types of fibers intermixed in a haphazard manner: type I fibers (slow fibers), which contain numerous mitochondria and are specialized for long, sustained effort, and type II fibers (fast fibers), which are rich in glycogen and are capable of fast, albeit short-lived, contractions; (c) all muscle fibers are individually innervated by axons extending peripherally from the spinal cord motor neurons, with which they form functional motor units; (d) all muscle fibers are composed of terminally differentiated muscle cells that cannot divide or regenerate. The replacement of lost mature muscle fibers can occur to a limited extent from muscle reserve cells, but this regeneration is of no practical value.

The response of skeletal muscles to injury includes a limited number of reactions. *Atrophy* is caused by immobilization of muscles (*e.g.*, by a cast after bone fractures), malnutrition, aging, chronic disease, or denervation (*e.g.*, by spinal cord trauma). Prolonged strain or exercise (e.g., weight lifting) results in *hypertrophy,* mostly because of an increased size of type II muscle fibers. *Rhabdomyolysis* following a marathon race is a form of focal necrosis of muscle fibers accompanied by pain and a release of creatine kinase (CK) into the circulation. Muscle cell necrosis evokes an inflammatory response that is characterized by an influx of macrophages. Inflammation of muscle (myositis), which usually affects several muscle groups and is therefore called *polymyositis,* occurs in response to muscle cell necrosis; this is a feature of viral infections and autoimmune diseases involving the muscles. All these diseases are accompanied by elevation of blood CK levels.

Overall, the muscle diseases fall into two categories: (a) ***neurogenic muscle disease*** secondary to nerve degeneration that results in atrophy, and (b) primary muscle disease, characterized by destruction and loss of muscle cells and designated ***myopathy***. Myopathies include (a) ***muscular dystrophies***, several genetic disorders involving structural proteins of muscle fibers, (b) ***congenital myopathies***, genetic disorders of enzymes involved in the intermediate metabolism of glycogen, lipids, or proteins, and (c) ***inflammatory myopathies***, which are caused by infections or autoimmune disorders. Myasthenia gravis, a disease involving the neuromuscular junction, is an important muscle disease that cannot be classified into one of the above categories.

Neurogenic Atrophy

Denervation atrophy of skeletal muscles may involve the entire muscle or large muscle fascicles, as in spinal cord injury, or individual muscle fibers, as in ischemic neuropathies characterized by a loss of small axonal branches. Single cell atrophy is common in diabetic neuropathy, which is probably the most common cause of this type of atrophy in clinical practice. Atrophy represents a reversible change and muscle fibers resume their normal size if reinnervated. Reinnervated muscles can be best recognized by immunohistochemistry. Instead of the typical haphazard arrangement of type I and type II muscle fibers in a ''checkerboard'' pattern, the reinnervated muscles show grouping of type I and type II fibers.

Muscular Dystrophy

The term *muscular dystrophy* includes several hereditary diseases, all of which are characterized by progressive destruction and loss of muscle fibers resulting from a genetically determined abnormality of integral components of muscle fibers. Necrosis of muscle fibers is accompanied by an elevation of CK in blood, muscle wasting, and weakness. The most important dystrophies are ***Duchenne's*** dystrophy, ***Becker*** dystrophy, ***facioscapulohumeral*** dystrophy, and ***myotonic*** dystrophy.

Duchenne's dystrophy and *Becker dystrophy* are caused by mutations of the gene encoding ***dystrophin***, a structural protein of the muscle. The dystrophin gene is on the X-chromosome, and its mutations are transmitted in an X-linked recessive manner, so only the male offspring of female carriers are affected. Duchenne's dystrophy presents clinically in early childhood. The symptoms of muscle weakness progress relentlessly, and by school age most children are confined to wheelchairs, and by the age of 20 years most patients have died. Becker dystrophy, also caused by a mutation of the dystrophin gene, is a milder form of the disease. Symptoms begin in puberty or early adult life, and the severe incapacitation does not occur until the age of 40 to 50 years.

Myotonic dystrophy, the second most common dystrophy, is inherited as an autosomal dominant trait causally linked to a gene that shows triple repeats of CGG on chromosome 19. The disease begins between 20 and 30 years of age and is characterized by progressive muscle wasting accompanied by myotonia [*e.g.*, spasm of muscles that cannot relax after contraction (e.g., persistent clasp after a handshake)]. Affected persons also show signs of mental retardation and endocrine disorders, such as diabetes and gonadal atrophy.

Metabolic Myopathies

Congenital metabolic myopathies are rare and occur as part of a generalized metabolic disturbance. The best examples are various glycogenoses, most of which are characterized by muscle symptoms. In ***Pompe*** disease (glycogenosis type II, caused by acid maltase deficiency), muscle weakness is associated with cardiomyopathy. In ***McArdle's*** disease (glycogenosis type IV, muscle phosphorylase deficiency), muscle weakness is the predominant symptom.

Acquired metabolic myopathies are typical of several endocrine disorders, such as diabetes mellitus, Cushing's syndrome, Addison's disease, hypothyroidism, and hyperthyroidism. Hormones are essential for muscle metabolism, and a hormonal imbalance usually affects muscles adversely, causing weakness, easy fatigability, and other functional disturbances. In diabetes, muscle may also show signs of neurogenic atrophy. However, in most other metabolic myopathies, no pathologic changes are apparent in muscle biopsy specimens.

Myositis

Inflammation of the muscles is found in the course of many infectious or autoimmune disease. Infectious diseases are most often systemic and the symptoms of muscle disease are typically overshadowed by other, more serious, ailments. Infectious myositis may be caused by viruses (*e.g.*, Coxsackievirus B) or bacteria such as streptococci, and the muscle cell injury is often mediated by toxins released from such pathogens. The best known toxin-induced myopathy is tetanus, which is characterized by spastic contractions of the muscles. *Trichinella spiralis*, which has a tendency to encyst in the striated muscles, causes an isolated myositis.

Polymyositis is an autoimmune disease affecting the muscles. Histologically, it is characterized by foci of inflammation in which macrophages predominate. Clinically, it is characterized by muscle pain and weakness, elevated CK in blood, and positive serologic tests typical of autoimmunity disorders. Polymyositis may be associated with skin disease (***dermatomyositis***), or with other autoimmune disorders such as systemic lupus erythematosus, but also it may be a paraneoplastic syndrome.

Myasthenia Gravis

Myasthenia gravis is an autoimmune disease characterized by the presence of autoantibodies to acetylcholine receptors at the neuromuscular junction. The binding of antibodies to the receptor prevents the transmission of neural impulses, which impairs the contraction of skeletal muscles. Histologically, the muscle shows no pathologic changes. The disease has a progressive course. Many patients, especially those that are young and female, have thymic lesions such as thymic hyperplasia or thymoma. Removal or surgical resection of such an enlarged thymus could cure the disease. In older patients, medical treatment with inhibitors of cholinesterase or plasmapheresis to remove the harmful antibodies from circulation may give temporary relief.

Tumors of skeletal muscle are rare. These tumors, which are clinically grouped with other *soft tissue tumors*, may be benign or malignant. Most tumors are of connective tissue origin and are classified as *fibroma, myxoma*, or *lipoma* if benign, or *fibrosarcoma, malignant fibrous histiocytoma*, or *liposarcoma* if malignant. Rhabdomyosarcoma is a tumor originating from the striated muscle reserve cells; this typically occurs on the arms and legs of children. *Rhabdomyosarcomas* of adults are less common, and typically they originate from smaller muscles, such as the retro-orbital muscles of the external eye. Surgical resection is the treatment of choice. The prognosis of malignant tumors depends on their size and location, but overall the treatment results are not good.

NERVOUS SYSTEM

The nervous system consists of the central nervous system (CNS), peripheral nerves, and the autonomic nervous system. The nervous system is involved by diseases of many other organ systems, but those will not be discussed here. No mention will be made of important common diseases such as migraine, schizophrenia, or epilepsy, which have a seat in the CNS but are not related to recognizable anatomic changes.

Developmental Malformation

Anencephaly, a congenital defect involving the brain, cerebral meninges, and the calvaria, occurs at a rate of 1 to 2 per 1000 newborns. It reflects an abnormality in the fusion of the neural tube (dysraphic anomaly) that occurs during early stages of pregnancy. Supplementation of maternal diet with folic acid may reduce the risk of this malformation, which is not compatible with normal life. Other dysraphic anomalies that affect both brain and the spinal cord include ***craniorachischisis*** and ***meningoencephalocele***. Incomplete fusion of the spinal cord and posterior vertebrae include ***spina bifida***, ***spina bifida with meningocele***, or ***spina bifida with meningomyelocele***. All these defects are associated with high mortality. Minor defects can be repaired partially but motor defects caused by them remain permanently. ***Spina bifida occulta***, often with a skin dimple or tract (pilonidal sinus) may or may not be associated with identifiable symptoms.

Arnold-Chiari malformation involves downward displacement of the cerebellum and elongation of the medulla oblongata and the fourth ventricle, resulting in hydrocephalus resulting from obstruction of normal CSF circulation. ***Dandy-Walker*** malformation is a hydrocephalus caused by occlusion of the foramina of Luschka and Magendie related to abnormal development of the vermis of the cerebellum.

Phakomatoses are a group of heterogeneous, developmental disorders, unrelated one to another, characterized by distinct pathologic changes in the brain. Some of these disorders have been traced to abnormal genes, but the others remain poorly understood. The most important phakomatoses are listed here.

Tuberous sclerosis presents with aggregates of glial cells, neurons, and large cells intermediate between glia and neurons, forming grossly visible nodules (''tubers'') and subependymal hamartomas that may give rise to astrocytomas. These brain lesions are associated with mental retardation and epileptic seizures. In addition, the patients have facial nodules (nevus sebaceus), skin patches (shagreen patches), areas of hypopigmentation, subungual fibromas, and hamartomatous nodules and cysts in internal organs.

Von Hipple-Lindau disease presents with ***capillary hemangioblastoma*** of the cerebellum and cysts in the liver, kidney, and pancreas, and a tendency to develop renal cell carcinoma. A mutation in the VHL gene on chromosome 3, which acts as a tumor-suppressor gene, accounts for the various neoplasms in this syndrome.

Neurofibromatosis type I (von Recklinghausen disease) is an autosomal dominant disease characterized by multiple cutaneous neurofibromas, pigmented lesions of skin (''café au lait'' lesions), pigmented foci of the iris (Lisch nodules), and, less often, meningiomas, optic gliomas, and acoustic schwannomas. It is associated with a mutation or deletion of the NF tumor-suppressor gene on chromosome 17q. Neurofibromatosis type II is another autosomal dominant disorder characterized by bilateral acoustic schwannomas and, less commonly, meningiomas, related to mutations of a gene on chromosome 22.

Congenital hydrocephalus is usually caused by an obstruction in the flow of CSF resulting from an obstruction at the level of the fourth ventricle or the sylvian aqueduct. Aqueductal stenosis or atresia may result from intrauterine infections caused by viruses (e.g., rubella, CMV, herpesvirus) or toxoplasma, and it is often associated with calcifications that can be recognized by x-rays. The obstruction of the flow of the CSF leads to the dilatation of the lateral ventricles and atrophy of the brain. Because the cranial sutures are not fused during the first few postnatal months, the head expands, resulting in macrocephaly with bulging fontanelles.

Cerebral palsy is a clinical term applied to a heterogeneous group of congenital CNS disorders presumably related to intrauterine brain injury. It affects 2 per 1000 newborns. The symptoms, usually a combination of movement abnormalities, spastic paralysis, speech impairment, and intellectual deficits may be apparent at birth but more often the first symptoms appear during infancy and early childhood. Clinical pathologic correlation is usually poor, because the severity of brain lesions does not reflect the extent of functional impairment. The etiology of the disease remains unknown, but it probably represents a multifactorial prenatal brain injury. Intrauterine anoxia, toxicity, deficiencies, and, to a lesser extent, mechanical brain trauma have been implicated, albeit without any final conclusive evidence.

Trauma to the Central Nervous System

Trauma to the CNS can occur in several forms; it is often associated with fracture of the skull or vertebra, and with various forms of bleeding.

Concussion is a traumatic lesion of the brain that presents with temporary loss of consciousness and reflexes, depression of vital functions (e.g., apnea), but it is not associated with anatomic changes in the brain. The functional changes are reversible even though most patients develop amnesia about the events that preceded or followed the trauma.

Contusion or bruise is a more severe form of brain injury, typically associated with foci of brain necrosis and hemorrhage. Contusion is typically bipolar and includes the *coup lesion* at the site of impact and the *contrecoup lesion* at the opposite side of the skull. It may result in permanent neurologic impairment depending on the site of injury.

Epidural hematoma results from skull fracture lacerating the middle meningeal artery and causing a relentlessly progressive accumulation of blood between the dura and the skull bone. Typically, it is located over the lateral convexity of the cerebral hemispheres. Unless stopped and evacuated, epidural hematoma is usually lethal.

Subdural hematoma results from repeated bleedings from ruptured bridging veins crossing the subdural space between the cerebral hemispheres and the dural venous sinuses. Because the blood accumulates over time, which allows it to clot and become partially organized by the ingrown blood vessels of the arachnoid, it usually appears as a brown-red firm layer between the dura and the arachnoid. Subdural hematomas are typically found in boxers, alcoholics, and old, demented or psychotic persons prone to repeated falls or head injuries.

Intracerebral hematoma is typically found after bullet wounds or other severe trauma to the head, and it is typically associated with marked brain destruction or ***laceration***. Hypertension or aneurysms can also cause intracerebral bleeding (see later).

Spinal cord injury is typically caused by anterior or posterior displacement of the vertebral bodies, resulting in compression or transection of the spinal cord. If the impact hits the chin from below, an overextension injury of the anterior part of the spinal cord and compression of the posterior part result. Trauma to the occiput, flexing the face downward, causes the reverse (*e.g.*, compression of the anterior part of the cervical spine and overextension of the posterior part). These forms of trauma are often lethal, but if the patient survives, complete quadriplegia is the norm. Transection of the spinal cord in the thoracic or lumbar part results in paralysis of the lower extremities and loss of autonomic functions, such as urination, defecation, and erection.

Circulatory Disorders

Cerebrovascular diseases are caused by ischemia or hemorrhage, which are often combined. Pathogenetically, these events are related to (a) atherosclerosis of cerebral vessels, (b) arterial hypertension, and (c) congenital malformations of cerebral vasculature.

Congenital malformations of cerebral vasculature may be asymptomatic but typically they cause hemorrhages. The most common intraparenchymal lesion is the ***arteriovenous malformation***, composed of convoluted or abnormal, usually dilated, and interconnected veins and arteries. Small saccular aneurysms, called ***berry aneurysms***, are typically found in the circle of Willis at the base of the brain, and most often they are located at the site of bifurcation or junction of the major arteries. In about 20% of cases, these aneurysms are multiple. Rupture of berry aneurysms results in subarachnoid hemorrhage, which is often lethal.

Atherosclerosis of cerebral arteries may present in several forms. The symptoms depend on the extent of the disease; whether it involves the major or minor arteries and their branches; and whether it is associated with systemic circulatory disturbances or hypertension.

Cerebral infarcts result from the occlusion of major cerebral arteries. The occlusion is most often caused by a thrombus, originating over a ruptured atheroma. Most common locations of thrombus formation are the carotid artery and its major branches, and the basilar artery. Infarcts can also be caused by thromboemboli originating in the left heart or major thoracic arteries. Cerebral emboli are typically a complication of myocardial infarcts, atrial fibrillation, and valvular heart disease, all of which are accompanied by thrombus formation in the left heart. Thromboemboli carried by arterial circulation tend to lodge preferentially in the middle cerebral artery, but they may occlude any other cerebral vessel as well. Infarcts caused by either thrombi or emboli are initially pale and characterized by liquefactive necrosis of the affected brain region. Because of the dual blood supply of most brain regions, the embolic infarcts are usually reperfused from collateral circulation, and therefore they tend to become hemorrhagic within the first 48 hours. Necrotic brain tissue elicits a glial reaction and an influx of macrophages, but no repair occurs. Ultimately, the necrotic tissue is resorbed and the infarct transforms into a cyst filled with fluid that is clear or yellow (xanthochromic) in previously hemorrhagic lesions.

Hypotensive cerebral infarcts typical of hypotensive vascular episodes (*e.g.*, myocardial infarct or shock) occur without complete occlusion of a major cerebral artery. Vascular collapse results in hypoperfusion of the brain, which affects mostly the border zone between the vascular supply regions of major arteries (watershed). This results in multiple ***watershed zone infarcts*** and laminar necrosis of deeper layers of the cerebral cortex. The most vulnerable area is the marginal zone between the supply region of the anterior and middle cerebral artery, Sommer's sector of the hippocampus, and Purkinje cells of the cerebellum.

Acute cerebral ischemia results in a clinical picture known as ***stroke***. Stroke is typically characterized by a complete or partial loss of consciousness, and abnormal sensory and motor functions. Despite high mortality, most patients recover to some extent, remaining dysfunctional or bed-ridden for many years. Motor deficits are typical.

Ischemic encephalopathy results from widespread ***global ischemia*** of the brain resulting from atherosclerosis of the branches of the cerebral arteries. Atherosclerotic narrowing and occlusion of small blood vessels causes ischemic necrosis of neurons or multiple microinfarcts. This results in transient ischemic attacks (TIAs) and ultimately may impair mental functions of the affected person severely (microinfarct dementia).

Hypertensive cerebrovascular disease may occur in an acute form, as cerebral hemorrhage, or in a chronic form. Hypertension may cause massive cerebral hemorrhage, usually associated with high mortality. Most often, these hypertensive hematomas are located in the basal ganglia–hypothalamic region (65%), pons (15%), or cerebellum (10%), but they may occur in other parts of the brain and they may be multiple. Patients dying of *acute hypertensive encephalopathy*, characterized by a sudden onset of headache, vomiting, blurry vision, or convulsions and coma, may not have any major hemorrhage. Instead, in such patients, the brain shows marked edema, and minor hemorrhages from necrotic arterioles. Arterioles often show ***lipohyalinosis*** (*e.g.*, accumulation of lipid in hyalinized vessel wall) and formation of ***Charcot-Bouchard aneurysms***, prone to rupture and produce intraparenchymal hemorrhage.

Chronic hypertensive encephalopathy is characterized by multiple small cystic infarcts known as lacunae. Lacunar infarcts are most prominent in the basal ganglia, thalamus, internal capsule, and pons. Clinically, it may be characterized by nonspecific neurologic symptoms.

Brain edema is characterized by an accumulation of fluid in the brain parenchyma. Edema may result from other circulatory disturbances, but also it may be provoked by trauma, inflammation, tumors, and metabolic and toxic injuries to the brain. Pathogenetically, there are two types of edema: (a) vasogenic edema, caused by increased vascular permeability and characterized by an increased amount of fluid in interstitial spaces of the white matter; and (b) cytotoxic edema characterized by intracellular accumulation of fluid, predominantly affecting the gray matter. Vasogenic edema is more common and clinically more important because it can be treated more efficiently. Typically, it leads to widening of the white matter, narrowing of the sulci, and widening of the gyri and compression of ventricles. The expanded brain causes herniations, which are typically found in three places: (a) ***subfalcine*** translocation of the gyrus cinguli of the cerebral hemisphere, (b) ***uncal herniation*** underneath the tentorium cerebelli, and (c) herniation of the ***cerebellar tonsils*** into the foramen magnum with compression of the medulla oblongata. The latter herniation is the most common cause of death in patients suffering from brain edema, because it results in compression of the vital medullary centers.

Hydrocephalus

Hydrocephalus is an accumulation of fluid under pressure in the ventricles. It occurs in two forms: ***noncommunicating hydrocephalus*** and ***communicating hydrocephalus***. In noncommunicating hydrocephalus, the obstruction of the CSF fluid occurs at the level of the aqueduct, third ventricle, or the foramina of Luschka and Magendie. In communicating hydrocephalus, the obstruction is in the arachnoid, preventing the reabsorption of CSF into the venous space. Hydrocephalus may be caused by infections, tumors, trauma, or hemorrhage. Such changes must be distinguished from normal pressure hydrocephalus, so-called *hydrocephalus ex vacuo*, in which the accumulation of CSF is related to brain atrophy and consequent dilatation of the ventricles. Hydrocephalus *ex vacuo* is typically found in the elderly and is most prominent in patients with Alzheimer disease.

Infectious Diseases

The infections of the CNS may present in several forms, which include ***meningitis***, ***encephalitis***, ***brain abscess***, and ***myelitis***, all of which may occur in an isolated form, but more often in combination with one another (e.g., meningoencephalomyelitis). The most important pathogens include: (a) *viruses* (e.g., HIV, herpesvirus, rabies virus, and various neurotropic arboviruses, such as St. Louis encephalitis virus), (b) *bacteria* (e.g., *N. meningitidis, E. coli, S. pneumoniae, H. influenzae*), (c) *fungi* (e.g., *Cryptococcus*, *Aspergillus*), and (d) *protozoa* (e.g., *Toxoplasma*).

Main routes of infection of the CNS are: (a) hematogenous from a distant site of infection in the body; (b) local extension from infections of the ear, nose, and nasal sinuses; (c) neurogenic along the axons, as commonly seen in herpes virus infection and rabies; and (d) by direct inoculation, as from trauma.

MENINGITIS

Meningitis typically involves the arachnoid and is therefore also called ***leptomeningitis***, in contrast to ***pachymeningitis***, which involves the dura. Most often it is caused by viruses. Such viral meningitis, which occurs typically during systemic viremia, is usually mild and it is rarely documented. Clinically, it is evidenced by somnolence, or mild mental obtundation, rigidity of the neck or a positive Kernig sign (pain in the knee upon flexing of the hip) and various nonspecific neurologic symptoms. Spontaneous recovery is the norm.

Bacterial meningitis is a more serious disease. In newborns it is most often caused by *E. coli*. In infants, *H. influenzae* predominates, whereas in adults, the disease is most often caused by *Streptococcus pneumoniae* and *Neisseria meningitidis*. Bacterial infection leads to an exudation of neutrophils into the CSF. Signs of infection include fever, leukocytosis, and general malaise. There is severe headache, stiffness of the neck, and the Kernig and Brudzinski signs can be readily elicited. The CSF is under increased pressure, and the lumbar puncture will typically recover purulent fluid that contains an increased level of protein and usually low levels of glucose. The causative bacteria can be seen in smears stained with the Gram stain or in bacteriologic cultures. Antibiotic treatment gives good results, but if the disease is not recognized or if it is associated with Waterhouse-Friderichsen syndrome (as occasionally seen in *N. meningitidis* infection), it may have high mortality.

Chronic meningitis was common before but is rare today except in patients with AIDS. Previously, chronic meningitis was most often caused by *Mycobacterium tuberculosis*, which is still an important pathogen in underdeveloped countries. Tuberculous meningitis preferentially affects the meninges on the basal side of the brain, which are cloudy, overlying the cisterns filled with gelatinous material. Histologically, the meninges contain an exudate composed of incompletely formed granulomas with giant cells and numerous lymphocytes extending into the sulci and encasing the cranial nerves.

Neurosyphilis presents most often as chronic meningitis with prominent plasmacellular infiltrates around the meningeal blood vessels, and obliterative endovasculitis (meningovascular syphilis). Constriction of the posterior nerve roots of the spinal cord by the fibrotic granulation tissue and scars results in compression atrophy of the posterior columns of the spinal cord and loss of sensory proprioceptive and pain-conducting tracts *(tabes dorsalis)*. A loss of cortical neurons, partly because of meningeal vascular changes and in part because of spread of syphilis into the brain parenchyma, leads to *general paresis of the insane*, a form of syphilitic dementia accompanied by a variety of motor and sensory deficits.

BRAIN ABSCESS

Bacterial infection of the brain parenchyma (cerebritis) typically leads to localized suppuration and abscess formation. Such an abscess presents as an expansile space-occupying lesion, showing central liquefactive necrosis and formation of a cavity that is enclosed by a glial capsule. The infection may spread into the surrounding brain tissue with a formation of satellite abscesses. The extension into the meningeal spaces may cause suppurative meningitis. Rupture of the abscess into the ventricles leads to the formation of ***pyocephalus***.

Encephalitis is a term reserved for nonbacterial infections of the brain. Most often, encephalitis is caused by viruses (such as arthropod-born neurotropic viruses, Eastern or Western equine encephalitis, and St. Louis encephalitis), show no predilection for specific anatomic parts of the brain, and therefore produce a diffuse encephalitis. All these viral infections cause lymphocytic exudates around the cerebral blood vessels (Virchow-Robin spaces).

Herpes simplex virus, the most common pathogen in the United States, has a tendency to infect the temporal lobes. Rabies virus localizes preferentially in the brainstem, hippocampus, and the cerebellum. Poliomyelitis virus affects preferentially the motor neuron cells of the anterior horn of the spinal cord and the bulbar motor nuclei. Cytomegalovirus (CMV) affects the periventricular white matter of fetuses and infants. ***Progressive multifocal leukoencephalopathy (PML),*** a disease caused by the JC virus (a papovavirus) in immunocompromised hosts, affects the corticomedullary junction of the cerebral hemispheres. Many of these viruses can be recognized as intranuclear or cytoplasmic inclusions. ***Rabies*** produces typical cytoplasmic inclusions, Negri bodies. Other causes of encephalitis are protozoa, such as malaria, toxoplasma, and rickettsia, and some metazoa, such as cysticercus.

AIDS-related encephalopathy is a common complication of HIV infection, which may cross the blood–brain barrier and infect the microglial cells of the brain. HIV causes an aseptic meningitis, typically early in the course of the disease; HIV encephalopathy, characterized by progressive loss of mental capacity and deterioration of motor and autonomic functions, develops in the later stages of AIDS. Vacuolar myelopathy (involving the posterior columns of the spinal cord), peripheral neuropathy, and myopathy are also features of AIDS. Immunosuppression caused by HIV infection predisposes the patients to a variety of infections that are not normally seen in people who are not immunocompromised. The most important are viral infections (herpes simplex virus, CMV, varicella-zoster virus), fungi such as *Cryptococcus*, and protozoa such as toxoplasma.

SPONGIFORM ENCEPHALOPATHIES

This term includes several infectious diseases such as ***Creutzfeldt-Jakob*** disease, ***kuru***, and ***chronic spongiform encephalopathies*** encountered in sheep and goats. All these diseases are caused by minute infectious particles, ***prions*** (previously known as ''slow viruses'') composed of protein, encoded by the host's gene. The pathologic hallmark of these diseases is formation of small vacuoles in the gray matter and the basal ganglia, imparting a spongelike appearance (''spongiform degeneration'') to the brain. Clinically, spongiform encephalopathies present with progressive dementia, cerebellar symptoms such as ataxia, and corticospinal tract motor symptoms. These diseases are incurable.

Demyelinating Diseases

Diseases characterized by a loss of myelin sheaths of cerebral axons belong to three pathogenetic groups: (a) ***inborn errors of metabolism*** affecting myelin sheaths, also known as *dysmyelinating disorders*, such as ***adrenoleukodystrophy*** and ***Krabbe disease***. These diseases are characterized by defective synthesis of myelin which tends therefore to decompose spontaneously. In Krabbe disease, myelin accumulates in macrophages, which assume the appearance of so-called globoid cells; (b) ***inflammatory diseases*** such as ***progressive multifocal leukoencephalopathy*** (PML), in which the entry of papovavirus JC into oligodendroglia cells (*e.g.*, glial cells that produce the myelin sheaths) impairs the metabolism of myelin, causing demyelination; (c) diseases caused by presumably ***immunological demyelination,*** as in ***multiple sclerosis***, ***acute disseminated encephalomyelitis*** (ADEM), or ***acute hemorrhagic leukoencephalitis*** (AHL). Multiple sclerosis is the most important of these diseases and it affects about 1 per 1000 people yearly. ADEM is a rare complication of acute viral infections or antiviral immunization characterized by multifocal perivenous demyelination and an acute onset of neurologic deficits or coma. AHL has a more fulminant course and is characterized by widespread hemorrhagic necrosis of the white and gray matter. Both of these conditions are thought to represent a hypersensitivity reaction or an autoimmune response against myelin.

MULTIPLE SCLEROSIS

Multiple sclerosis is a chronic recurrent progressive demyelinating disease of unknown etiology. It affects the white matter of the brain, causing multifocal demyelination of cerebral axons. The demyelinated foci, most prominent around the ventricles, in the optic nerve, and in the spinal cord, are called plaques. They can be seen by computerized axial tomography (CAT) scanning and have been found to enlarge as the disease progresses. Histologically, the plaques consist initially of lymphocytes and macrophages, which destroy the myelin, leaving behind denuded axons. Demyelination is accompanied by a loss of motor function, visual problems, and ultimately sensory symptoms and a loss of coordinated neuromuscular action. The disease has an inexorably progressive course, leading to complete incapacitation, usually over a period of 15 to 30 years. There is no effective treatment.

SUBACUTE COMBINED DEGENERATION

A condition called subacute combined degeneration in which there is demyelination of the ascending posterior columns and descending lateral columns is caused by lack of vitamin B_{12}. This is usually seen in association with absence of gastrin intrinsic factor, required for B_{12} absorption, and pernicious anemia.

NEURODEGENERATIVE DISEASES

The term *neurodegenerative diseases* is used to denote a group of unrelated disorders of unknown etiology, which are characterized by degeneration of parts of the CNS, causing defined clinical symptoms. The most important among these diseases are ***Alzheimer*** disease, ***Parkinson*** disease, ***amyotrophic lateral sclerosis***, and ***Huntington*** disease.

Alzheimer disease is a dementia (loss of mental function) that typically occurs in the elderly. The etiology of this disease is not known, albeit there are some familial cases, suggesting a genetic predisposition. Pathologically, it is characterized by atrophy of the brain evidenced as narrowing of the gyri and widening of the sulci and a hydrocephalus *ex vacuo*. Histologic hallmarks of Alzheimer disease include ***neuritic*** (senile) ***plaques*** composed of amyloid and filaments that can be impregnated with silver, neurofibrillary tangles in the cytoplasm of neurons, granulovacuolar degeneration of neurons, and deposition of amyloid in the small cerebral arteries. The first evidence of the disease is a loss of recent memory, but as the dementia evolves, all mental functions deteriorate and the patient becomes completely mentally incapacitated.

Parkinson disease is characterized by a loss of pigmented neurons in the substantia nigra and locus ceruleus. The remaining neurons often contain cytoplasmic Lewy bodies. Clinically, extrapyramidal symptoms dominate. Typically, the muscle movements are slow and lack fine coordination. There is rigidity and tremor at rest, and the face is expressionless (''masklike face''). The patient is stooped and has a shuffling gait. Loss of mental functions and depression occur in advanced cases.

Amyotrophic lateral sclerosis, also known as Lou Gehrig disease (after the baseball player who suffered from it), is characterized by a progressive loss of motor neurons from the anterior horn of the spinal cord, the brainstem, and ultimately the cerebral cortex. Loss of motor neurons is accompanied by demyelination of the lateral corticospinal tracts in the spinal cord and progressive atrophy of skeletal muscles. Loss of muscle fibers presents clinically with fasciculation and progressive weakness, leading ultimately to immobility, slurred speech, and loss of coordination most prominently evident in eye muscles. The mental capacity is, however, preserved.

Huntington disease is an autosomal dominant hereditary disorder that presents at midlife with progressive dementia, movement disorders, and emotional disbalance. It is related to an expansion of trinucleotide CAG repeats on chromosome 4. Persons whose fathers were affected tend to develop symptoms earlier than those whose mothers are the carriers of the abnormal gene. Pathologically, the brain shows cortical atrophy and dilatation of the lateral ventricles, which appear as squares on cross sectioning (*e.g.*, ''box like'') because of the loss of the lateral indentation of the caudate nuclei.

Tumors of the Central Nervous System

Tumors of the CNS are rare, representing only 2% of all human neoplasms. These tumors occur in all age groups. In children and young adults (*e.g.*, age groups in which neoplasms are not common), CNS tumors account for 10% of cancer-related death, being second only to leukemia. Most primary tumors of adults are supratentorial (*e.g.*, in the cerebrum), whereas in children, subtentorial tumors of the cerebellum predominate. In older adults and the elderly, the primary tumors account for approximately one third of all intracranial neoplasms, whereas all others are metastases. The most common primary malignancies metastasizing to the brain are carcinomas of the lungs, breast, gastrointestinal tract, kidneys, and melanomas.

The primary tumors of the CNS originate from glia cells, neuronal cell precursors, cranial nerves, and meninges. *Glial cell tumors* are the most common, accounting for approximately one half of all primary tumors. The most important glial tumors are astrocytoma, glioblastoma multiforme, oligodendroglioma, and ependymoma. All glial tumors are malignant, although some, such as glioblastoma multiforme, are more malignant than others. *Neuronal tumors* develop mostly from precursors of neurons (neuroblasts) and are typically found in children. The most important tumors in this group are medulloblastoma and neuroblastoma. *Cranial nerve tumors,* schwannomas, originate most often from the acoustic nerve in patients affected by neurofibromatosis. Meningeal tumors are called meningiomas.

Astrocytomas are low grade malignant tumors. In children, they are most often cystic and located in the cerebellum, whereas in adults they are usually in the cerebrum. ***Glioblastoma multiforme***, the most common primary malignant CNS tumor, occurs most often in the cerebral hemispheres of adults, but it may also occur in other parts of the brain and spinal cord. It is a rapidly growing, highly malignant tumor, which was named multiforme because on gross examination it has a variegated appearance imparted by broad areas of necrosis and hemorrhage, and histologically it is pleomorphic. ***Oligodendrogliomas*** are slow-growing malignant tumors of the cerebral hemispheres of adults, composed of oligodendroglial cells, commonly speckled with foci of calcification. ***Ependymomas*** originate from the ependymal lining of the cerebral ventricles, central canal of the spinal cord, or the cauda equina. These rare tumors occur mostly in children and young adults, and they are characterized by slow but relentless growth. ***Medulloblastomas*** are tumors of the cerebellum of children. These tumors are composed of primitive undifferentiated cells resembling primitive fetal cells in the neural tube. Because of their location close to vital centers and their rapid growth, these tumors have a dismal prognosis, despite the fact that they are sensitive to radiation and chemotherapy. ***Schwannomas*** of the eighth nerve are slow-growing benign tumors, often bilateral, and usually associated with other stigmata of neurofibromatosis. These tumors are located in the cerebellopontine angle, compressing the cerebellum and the vital centers of the pons. They also cause deafness and vertigo because of the destruction of the eighth nerve.

Meningiomas are well-circumscribed, benign tumors derived from the meninges. They are typically attached to the dura, compressing the brain from the outside. Histologically, meningiomas are composed of elongated meningothelial cells, usually forming interlacing whorls, with occasional calcifications (''psammoma bodies''). There is even a malignant variant, but overall most meningiomas are benign. These tumors can be surgically removed without any residual consequences.

Peripheral Nerves

Trauma. Peripheral nerves are prone to traumatic injury, such as avulsion, transection, or compression. After transection, the distal part of the axon undergoes *wallerian degeneration* and disintegrates. However, if the perikaryon of the nerve cell is intact, new axons will sprout and reestablish peripheral innervation.

Neuropathy. Peripheral nerves may be injured by a number of toxic substances, such as industrial toxins, heavy metals (lead), or drugs. Metabolic injury is found in systemic diseases such as uremia, porphyria, or diabetes. *Diabetic neuropathy*, one of the most common forms of peripheral nerve injury, is only partially induced by metabolic disturbances of diabetes; it is to a large extent secondary to diabetic microangiopathy, which impedes the blood supply to nerves, thus causing axonal atrophy and degeneration. *Nutritional neuropathies* are often caused by deficiency of vitamins such as thiamine (''beriberi neuropathy''), B_{12}, pyridoxine, or niacin. *Viral infections*, such as herpes zoster (''shingles'') and AIDS, and *bacterial infections*, such as leprosy, also affect peripheral nerves. The peripheral nerves can also be affected by demyelinating diseases, the most important of which is the *Guillain-Barré syndrome*. In this syndrome, which develops usually after a viral disease or after an immunization, the nerves are infiltrated with lymphocytes, causing focal demyelination. Although the disease may present with extensive motor defects and even extensive paralysis, most patients recover completely within a few weeks.

Peripheral sensorimotor neuropathy characterized by axonal degeneration and occasional focal demyelination is found in some patients with cancer as a form of *paraneoplastic neuropathy*.

Tumors of the peripheral nerves are usually benign and are histologically classified as ***neurofibromas*** or ***schwannomas***. Malignant peripheral nerve tumors, ***neurofibrosarcomas***, are rare and are most often encountered in patients with preexisting neurofibromatosis.

QUESTIONS IN PATHOLOGY

Multiple-Choice Questions

Choose the one best answer or completion in the following multiple-choice questions. The answers are at the end of the chapter.

1. The type of necrosis that occurs in peripancreatic tissue in acute pancreatitis is:
   (a) Liquefaction
   (b) Fat
   (c) Coagulation
   (d) Gummatous
   (e) Fibrinoid
2. Change of columnar epithelium of the bronchi into mature squamous epithelium is called:
   (a) Metaplasia
   (b) Dysplasia
   (c) Hyperplasia
   (d) Neoplasia
   (e) Hypertrophy

3. The cavity of an abscess contains:
   (a) Caseous necrosis
   (b) Hyalin
   (c) Giant cells
   (d) Pus
   (e) Granulation tissue
4. Prostaglandins are formed from arachidonic acid through the action of which enzyme pathway?
   (a) Cyclooxygenase
   (b) Lipoxygenase
   (c) Myeloperoxidase
   (d) Phospholipase A
   (e) Glutathione reductase
5. All of the following are characterized by granulomatous inflammation *except*:
   (a) Sarcoidosis
   (b) Tuberculosis
   (c) Histoplasmosis
   (d) Diphtheria
   (e) Leprosy
6. An example of a tissue or organ composed of permanent parenchymal cells is:
   (a) Liver
   (b) Bone marrow
   (c) Small intestinal mucosa
   (d) Heart
   (e) Renal tubules
7. The most characteristic feature of granulation tissue is the:
   (a) Resemblance to a granuloma
   (b) Growth of fibroblasts and new capillaries
   (c) Infiltration with neutrophils
   (d) Hemorrhage
   (e) Presence of plasma cells
8. All the following are associated with increased coagulability of blood and a tendency to form thrombi *except*:
   (a) Carcinoma of the pancreas
   (b) Cirrhosis of the liver
   (c) Pregnancy
   (d) Oral contraceptive intake
   (e) Postoperative state
9. Which of the following neoplasms has been linked to a deletion of a tumor suppressor gene?
   (a) Medulloblastoma
   (b) Chondrosarcoma
   (c) Lymphocytic leukemia
   (d) Neuroblastoma
   (e) Retinoblastoma
10. The most common malignant neoplasm in women between the ages of 30 and 55 years is carcinoma of the:
    (a) Breast
    (b) Colon
    (c) Lung
    (d) Cervix
    (e) Ovary
11. Which of the following tumors causes the greatest mortality from cancer in the United States?
    (a) Carcinoma of lung
    (b) Carcinoma of large intestine
    (c) Carcinoma of stomach
    (d) Carcinoma of thyroid
    (e) Carcinoma of kidney
12. Carcinoembryonic antigen is most likely to be significantly elevated in the serum of patients with:
    (a) Colorectal carcinoma
    (b) Carcinoma of the prostate
    (c) Osteosarcoma
    (d) Hepatocellular carcinoma
    (e) Choriocarcinoma
13. Which immunoglobulin mediating the release of histamine in hay fever is bound to mast cells in the nasal mucosa?
    (a) IgA
    (b) IgD
    (c) IgE
    (d) IgG
    (e) IgM
14. Reduced plasma oncotic pressure is the most important cause of generalized edema in:
    (a) Congestive heart failure
    (b) Lung cancer
    (c) Constrictive pericarditis
    (d) Head trauma
    (e) Nephrotic syndrome
15. Which of the following proteins acts as a fibrinolytic factor?
    (a) Bradykinin
    (b) Plasmin
    (c) von Willebrand factor
    (d) Thrombin
    (e) Platelet-activating factor (PAF)
16. Chronic intake of alcohol will always induce which of the following in the liver:
    (a) Fatty change
    (b) Fibrosis of portal tracts
    (c) Cirrhosis
    (d) Liver cell necrosis
    (e) Acute inflammation
17. Portal hypertension is most commonly caused by:
    (a) Cirrhosis
    (b) Portal vein thrombosis
    (c) Pylephlebitis
    (d) Hepatic vein thrombosis
    (e) Tumorous compression of the portal vein

18. Autopsy of a 42-year-old white man found dead and suspected of suicide demonstrated numerous ulcerations of the mucosa of the stomach and ascending colon, along with marked coagulation necrosis of renal tubules. The most likely diagnosis is poisoning with:
    (a) Bismuth
    (b) Mercury
    (c) Arsenic
    (d) Phosphorus
    (e) Inorganic acid or alkali
19. Skin redness and swelling of the arm caused by *Streptococcus pyogenes* is typical of:
    (a) Erysipelas
    (b) Scarlet fever
    (c) Toxic shock syndrome
    (d) Gas gangrene
    (e) Caries
20. Lyme disease is caused by infection with:
    (a) *Leptospira interrogans*
    (b) *Brucella melitensis*
    (c) *Listeria monocytogenes*
    (d) *Streptobacillus moniliformis*
    (e) *Borrelia burgdorferi*
21. Chronic salpingitis is considered to predispose to:
    (a) Ectopic pregnancy
    (b) Carcinoma of the cervix
    (c) Endometriosis
    (d) Cystic hyperplasia of the endometrium
    (e) Choriocarcinoma
22. The most common tumor of major salivary glands is:
    (a) Acinic cell tumor
    (b) Pleomorphic adenoma (mixed tumor)
    (c) Adenolymphoma
    (d) Mucoepidermoid carcinoma
    (e) Adenoid cystic carcinoma
23. All of the following statements regarding viral hepatitis are true *except*:
    (a) Most cases of hepatitis A virus infection are unapparent and clinically not recognized
    (b) Hepatitis B virus infection may progress to chronic hepatitis
    (c) Hepatitis C virus infection may progress to cirrhosis
    (d) Hepatitis D virus infection has the highest mortality of all viral hepatitides
    (e) Hepatitis E virus infection is most often waterborne
24. In the majority of cases of viral hepatitis A, 1 year after recovery the liver most often would appear:
    (a) Coarsely nodular
    (b) Finely nodular
    (c) With residual fibrosis in the portal areas
    (d) With only minimal pseudolobule formation and increased fibrous tissue in portal areas
    (e) Histologically normal
25. In Rocky Mountain spotted fever, rickettsiae tend to invade:
    (a) Endothelial cells
    (b) Nerve cells
    (c) Renal tubular cells
    (d) Hepatocytes
    (e) Fibroblasts
26. Most of the tissue damage evoked by fungi result from:
    (a) Exotoxins
    (b) Their ability to modify the metabolic and reproductive activity of the cells of the host
    (c) Progressive development of sensitization to the fungal antigens
    (d) Endotoxins
    (e) Obstruction of ducts, blood vessels, or lymphatics
27. In patients with AIDS, which organ system is most severely affected by *Cryptococcus neoformans* and *Toxoplasma gondii*?
    (a) Central nervous system
    (b) Genitourinary system
    (c) Alimentary tract
    (d) Respiratory system
    (e) Cardiovascular system
28. The majority of congenital heart disorders are due to:
    (a) Viral infection
    (b) Teratogenic drugs
    (c) Chromosomal defects
    (d) Single gene abnormalities
    (e) Unknown causes
29. Occlusion of the right coronary artery near its origin by a thrombus would most likely result in:
    (a) Infarction of the wall of the left atrium
    (b) Infarction of the anterior left ventricle
    (c) Infarction of the lateral wall of the left ventricle
    (d) Infarction of the posterior left ventricular wall and the posterior septum
    (e) Infarction of the anterior septum
30. All of the following conditions are likely to be complicated by fibrinous pericarditis *except*:
    (a) Bacterial endocarditis
    (b) Uremia
    (c) Myocardial infarct
    (d) Lupus erythematosus
    (e) Rheumatic heart disease
31. The pathognomonic feature of rheumatic heart disease is the presence of:
    (a) Aschoff bodies

(b) Mitral stenosis
(c) Fibrinous pericarditis
(d) Shortening, thickening, and fusion of chordae tendineae
(e) Verrucae along the lines of closure of the valve leaflets

32. Hypochromic microcytic anemia in a 25-year-old woman is most likely caused by a deficiency of:
(a) Folic acid
(b) Vitamin B_{12}
(c) Iron
(d) Cobalt
(e) Copper

33. Which is the most common type of Hodgkin's disease?
(a) Nodular sclerosis
(b) Mixed cellularity
(c) Reticular
(d) Lymphocyte depletion
(e) Lymphocyte predominant

34. Infarction of the spleen is usually due to:
(a) Hypersplenism
(b) Congestion
(c) Arterial embolism
(d) Deposition of connective tissue and pigment
(e) Venous thrombosis

35. Which of the following is the most typical complication of asbestosis?
(a) Asthma
(b) Carcinoma of trachea
(c) Mesothelioma
(d) Tuberculosis
(e) Carcinoid

36. The most common site of carcinoma of the colon is:
(a) Cecum
(b) Ascending colon
(c) Transverse colon
(d) Splenic flexure
(e) Rectosigmoid

37. Most cases of acute poststreptococcal glomerulonephritis:
(a) Progress to chronic glomerulonephritis
(b) Progress to membranous glomerulonephritis
(c) Transform into lobular glomerulonephritis
(d) Progress to crescentic glomerulonephritis
(e) Completely recover

38. Nodular hyperplasia of the prostate involves principally the:
(a) Anterior lobe
(b) Lateral lobes
(c) Posterior lobes
(d) Verumontanum
(e) Prostatic utricle

39. Eczema-like oozing from a nonhealing lesion of the nipple in a 45-year-old woman without a palpable breast mass is most compatible with the diagnosis of:
(a) Fibroadenoma
(b) Sclerosing adenosis
(c) Paget's disease
(d) Fat necrosis
(e) Medullary carcinoma

40. Which of the following pathogens or diseases is most closely causally associated to carcinoma of the cervix?
(a) Herpes simplex virus
(b) Human papilloma virus
(c) Chlamydia
(d) Gonorrhea
(e) Syphilis

41. Intracranial hemorrhage caused by hypertension is most likely located in the:
(a) Frontal cortex
(b) Occipital cortex
(c) Basal ganglia
(d) Lateral ventricles
(e) Medulla oblongata

42. Parkinson disease most often affects the:
(a) Amygdala
(b) Hypothalamus
(c) Internal capsule
(d) Corpus callosum
(e) Substantia nigra

43. Epidural hematomas are characterized by:
(a) Laceration of middle meningeal artery
(b) Rupture of bridging veins
(c) Rupture of berry aneurysm
(d) Preexistent hypertension
(e) Obstructive hydrocephalus

44. Increased number of eosinophils in the circulating blood is most likely found in patients infected with:
(a) *E. coli*
(b) *Streptococcus pneumoniae*
(c) *Pseudomonas aeruginosa*
(d) *Trichinella spiralis*
(e) *Mycoplasma pneumoniae*

45. Renal cell carcinoma:
(a) Rarely metastasizes
(b) Frequently occurs in siblings
(c) Is causally associated to alcoholism
(d) Contains abundant uric acid crystals
(e) Tends to invade renal veins

46. Rapidly progressive glomerulonephritis is characterized by:
(a) Increased mesangial and endothelial cells in capillary loops

(b) Fusion of foot processes by electron microscopy
(c) Crescents in Bowman's space
(d) Thickened glomerular basement membranes
(e) Deposits of IgA in mesangial areas

47. Which of the following is caused by *Treponema pallidum*?
(a) Chancroid
(b) Purulent urethritis
(c) Granuloma inguinale
(d) Lymphogranuloma venereum
(e) Condyloma latum

48. Periventricular plaques of demyelination in the cerebral hemispheres are typical of:
(a) Amyotrophic lateral sclerosis
(b) Syringomyelia
(c) Multiple sclerosis
(d) Huntington disease
(e) Alzheimer disease

49. Circulating immune complexes are typical of:
(a) Myasthenia gravis
(b) Systemic lupus erythematosus
(c) Bronchial asthma
(d) Hay fever
(e) Sarcoidosis

50. Which of the following carcinomas rarely, if ever, metastasizes?
(a) Basal cell carcinoma of the skin
(b) Squamous cell carcinoma of the tongue
(c) Melanoma
(d) Renal cell carcinoma
(e) Seminoma

51. The gallbladder from a 26-year-old white woman was found to contain a solitary, round, firm, yellow stone. This stone was composed of:
(a) Cholesterol
(b) Calcium bilirubinate
(c) Calcium carbonate
(d) Cysteine
(e) Calcium soaps

52. A likely cause of these stones is:
(a) Chronic hemolytic processes
(b) Hypercholesterolemia
(c) Stasis of bile
(d) Infection of the gallbladder
(e) Typhoid fever

Questions 53–55 pertain to the following clinical history:

A 28-year-old man was admitted to the hospital because of severe shortness of breath and cyanosis. He was diagnosed with a heart disease at the age of 2 years, but the left to right shunt, accompanied by a systolic murmur, was never repaired.

53. He was told he had "the most common clinically diagnosed congenital heart defect." The diagnosis is:
(a) Atrial septal defect, ostium primum type
(b) Atrial septal defect, ostium secundum type
(c) Patent ductus ovale
(d) Ventricular septal defect
(e) Persistent ductus arteriosus

54. Cyanosis developed because of:
(a) Left heart failure
(b) Right heart failure
(c) Obliteration of the defect
(d) Endocarditis
(e) Reversal of thc lcft-to-right shunt to a right-to-left shunt

55. At autopsy, one could expect all the following findings *except*:
(a) Right ventricular hypertrophy
(b) Left ventricular hypertrophy
(c) Septal defect
(d) Pulmonary vascular changes of hypertension
(e) Coarctation of aorta

Questions 56–58 pertain to the following clinical history:

A 45-year-old white man, a known alcoholic, was admitted with hematemesis in a shock-like state. He had a history of melena for 1 week prior to admission. He expired soon after admission. An autopsy was performed.

56. The liver was large, nodular, and yellowish brown, divided into small uniform nodules on the cut surface. The most likely diagnosis is:
(a) Cirrhosis
(b) Alcoholic hepatitis
(c) Cardiac cirrhosis
(d) Biliary cirrhosis
(e) Budd-Chiari syndrome

57. Which of the following microscopic changes would you *not* expect to see in his liver?
(a) Fatty change of parenchymal cells
(b) Acute cholangitis
(c) Mallory hyalin in parenchymal cells
(d) Pseudolobule formation
(e) Connective tissue around nodules of liver cells

58. Esophageal varices in this case are most likely the result of:
(a) Generalized hypervolemia
(b) Right-sided heart failure
(c) Decreased albumin in blood
(d) Thrombosis of portal vein
(e) Portal hypertension

59. Which of the following tissues is highly sensitive to ionizing radiation?
(a) Brain
(b) Intestinal mucosa

(c) Liver
(d) Heart
(e) Kidney

60. All of the following lesions are commonly found in diabetes mellitus *except:*
(a) Thickening of capillary basement membranes
(b) Atherosclerosis
(c) Hyaline arteriolosclerosis
(d) Polyarteritis nodosa
(e) Glomerulosclerosis

61. All the following cause disseminated infections in the fetus *except:*
(a) Cytomegalovirus
(b) Herpes simplex virus
(c) *Toxoplasma gondii*
(d) *Treponema pallidum*
(e) *Pneumocystis carinii*

62. Tumors that may produce hormones or commonly cause hormonal paraneoplastic syndromes include all the following *except:*
(a) Oat cell carcinoma of the bronchus
(b) Medullary thyroid carcinoma
(c) Granulosa cell tumor of the ovary
(d) Leydig cell tumor of testis
(e) Oligodendroglioma

63. Patients with α_1-antitrypsin deficiency develop:
(a) Cirrhosis and emphysema
(b) Bronchiectasis and infertility
(c) Chronic lung disease and pancreatic insufficiency
(d) Meconium peritonitis
(e) Atrophic gastritis

64. Which of the following is a cyanotic congenital heart disease?
(a) Tetralogy of Fallot
(b) Patent foramen ovale
(c) Coarctation of the aorta
(d) Patent ductus arteriosus
(e) Ebstein anomaly

65. Hereditary spherocytosis is characterized by:
(a) Decreased osmotic fragility of erythrocytes
(b) Autosomal recessive inheritance pattern
(c) A small contracted spleen
(d) A cell membrane defect involving spectrin
(e) Aplastic bone marrow and heterotopic hematopoiesis in the spleen

66. Features of ulcerative colitis include all *except:*
(a) Superficial mucosal ulcers
(b) Crypt abscesses
(c) Pseudopolyps
(d) Marked thickening of the gut wall
(e) Diffuse involvement of the colon without skip areas

67. Hypertension may result from all the following *except*:
(a) Adrenal medullary tumor
(b) Cushing's syndrome
(c) Adrenal cortical tumor
(d) Amyloidosis of adrenal gland
(e) Chronic renal disease

68. All of the following are true about leiomyomata of the uterus *except*:
(a) Frequently undergo sarcomatous change
(b) Are sharply circumscribed
(c) Composed of smooth muscle cells
(d) Rarely arise after the menopause
(e) Represent the most common benign tumor of the uterus

69. Serous cystadenocarcinoma of the ovary is a:
(a) Benign cystic tumor
(b) Malignant solid tumor
(c) Tumor derived from germ cells
(d) Tumor prone to peritoneal seeding and ascites formation
(e) Tumor characterized by hormonal activity

70. Neuropathologic changes typical of Alzheimer disease include all the following *except*:
(a) Amyloidosis of blood vessels
(b) Abundant senile plaques
(c) Multiple cortical microinfarcts
(d) Neurofibrillary tangles in neurons
(e) Atrophy of the brain

71. Which of the following organisms is the most common cause of meningitis in the newborn period?
(a) *Streptococcus pneumoniae*
(b) *Neisseria meningitidis*
(c) *Escherichia coli*
(d) *Klebsiella*
(e) *Neisseria gonorrhoeae*

72. Characteristics of osteoarthritis include all the following *except*:
(a) Pannus formation
(b) Degeneration of articular cartilage
(c) Osteosclerosis of adjacent bone
(d) Involvement of weight-bearing joints
(e) Osteophytes

73. Epithelioid cells and Langerhans giant cells in granulomas are derived from:
(a) Neutrophiles
(b) Eosinophils
(c) Mast cells
(d) Macrophages
(e) Lymphocytes

74. A fever and leukocytosis in which most leukocytes were neutrophils is typical of:
(a) Acute bacterial infection
(b) Acute viral infection

(c) Chronic viral infection
(d) Parasitemia
(e) Foreign body giant cell reaction

75. Jaundice and diarrhea and desquamation of the skin are typically found complicating transplantation of:
(a) Heart
(b) Lungs
(c) Liver
(d) Kidney
(e) Bone marrow

76. Which of the following neoplastic diseases is typically associated with Epstein-Barr virus infection?
(a) Liver cell carcinoma
(b) Burkitt's lymphoma
(c) Sézary syndrome
(d) Hodgkin's disease
(e) Glioblastoma multiforme

77. Infertility and short stature in a woman with a 45,X karyotype are typical of:
(a) Klinefelter's syndrome
(b) Turner's syndrome
(c) Down syndrome
(d) Achondroplastic dwarfism
(e) Cystic fibrosis

78. Hyperviscosity of blood is a typical feature of:
(a) Megaloblastic anemia
(b) Thrombocytopenia
(c) Polycythemia vera
(d) Hodgkin's disease
(e) Burkitt's lymphoma

79. Demyelination of the posterior and lateral columns of the spinal cord is a feature of deficiency of vitamin:
(a) A
(b) B_1
(c) B_{12}
(d) C
(e) D

80. *Pneumocystis carinii* infection is typically found in:
(a) Neonates with TORCH syndrome
(b) Epidemic pneumonia among recruits
(c) Pregnant women
(d) Debilitated elderly men
(c) AIDS patients

81. Hepatitis A virus is transmitted by:
(a) Blood transfusion
(b) Contaminated needles and syringes
(c) Oral route
(d) Inhalation
(e) Transdermally from contaminated water

82. Bladder cancer is common in men infected with:
(a) *Schistosoma hematobium*
(b) *Clonorchis sinensis*
(c) *Strongyloides stercoralis*
(d) *Ascaris lumbricoides*
(e) *Trichuris trichiura*

83. Cholera infection primarily affects the:
(a) Stomach
(b) Small intestine
(c) Cecum
(d) Transverse colon and sigmoid
(e) Rectum

84. All the following represent localized brown pigmented skin lesions *except*:
(a) Ephelis
(b) Malignant melanoma
(c) Leucoplakia
(d) Junctional nevus
(e) Lentigo

85. Poison-ivy-induced bullous lesions of the skin represent:
(a) Type I hypersensitivity reaction
(b) Type II hypersensitivity reaction
(c) Type III hypersensitivity reaction
(d) Type IV hypersensitivity reaction
(e) Graft-versus-host reaction

86. Brown hyperpigmentation of the skin is typical of:
(a) Graves' disease
(b) Cushing's syndrome
(c) Addison's disease
(d) Pernicious anemia
(e) Wilson's disease

87. Which of the following is most typical of systemic lupus erythematosus?
(a) Skin lesions on sun-exposed areas
(b) Myxedema
(c) Dental decay
(d) Osteoporosis
(e) Ovarian cysts

88. Fibrinoid necrosis of renal arterioles is a feature of:
(a) Poststreptococcal glomerulonephritis
(b) Goodpasture's syndrome
(c) Malignant hypertension
(d) Diabetes
(e) Gout

89. Necrotizing arteritis associated with foci of pulmonary thrombosis and infarction, and upper respiratory lesions associated with renal lesions are typical of:
(a) Buerger's disease
(b) Wegener's granulomatosis
(c) Kawasaki disease
(d) Raynaud's disease
(e) Giant cell arteritis

90. Dissecting aneurysms of the aorta are typical of:
(a) Cystic fibrosis
(b) Osteogenesis imperfecta

(c) Marfan's syndrome
(d) Neurofibromatosis type I
(e) Tyrosinosis

91. The most common cause of death during the first 3 hours after a myocardial infarct is:
(a) Arrhythmia
(b) Cardiac rupture
(c) Acute aortic stenosis
(d) Acute mitral insufficiency
(e) Acute pericarditis and compression of the heart

92. All of the following conditions predispose to bacterial endocarditis *except*:
(a) Congenital heart disease
(b) Rheumatic heart disease
(c) Marantic endocarditis
(d) Cardiac valvular surgery
(e) Mitral valve prolapse resulting from floppy valves

93. All the following hormones can be produced from gastrointestinal carcinoid tumors *except*:
(a) Serotonin
(b) Gastrin
(c) Cholecystokinin
(d) Glucagon
(e) Cortisol

94. Meconium ileus is typical of:
(a) Cholelithiasis
(b) Cholangitis
(c) Cystic fibrosis
(d) Acute pancreatitis
(e) Celiac sprue

95. Amyloid of multiple myeloma is derived from:
(a) Serum amyloid precursor protein secreted by the liver
(b) Lambda chain of immunoglobulin
(c) Antigen linked into immune complexes
(d) Complement attached to immune complexes
(e) Calcium released from punched-out bone lesions

96. Rotation of the loops of sigmoid colon caused by twisting of the mesentery is called:
(a) Intussusception
(b) Volvulus
(c) Hernia
(d) Incarceration
(e) Toxic megacolon

97. All of the following conditions are accompanied by thrombocytopenia *except*:
(a) Aplastic anemia
(b) Myelofibrosis
(c) Leukemia
(d) Hypersplenism
(e) Hemophilia

98. Hypoparathyroidism caused by surgical removal of parathyroid glands during thyroid cancer surgery is characterized by:
(a) Hypocalcemia
(b) Hypermagnesemia
(c) Hypophosphatemia
(d) Hypernatremia
(e) Osteitis fibrosa cystica

99. The most common malignant tumor of the thyroid is:
(a) Papillary carcinoma
(b) Follicular carcinoma
(c) Medullary carcinoma
(d) Insular carcinoma
(e) Sarcoma

100. Creutzfeldt-Jakob disease is caused by:
(a) *Neisseria meningitidis*
(b) Measles virus
(c) Epstein-Barr virus
(d) Fungi
(e) Prions

101. Which of the following diseases is a cause of dementia?
(a) Amyotrophic lateral sclerosis
(b) Neurofibromatosis
(c) Guillain-Barré syndrome
(d) Huntington disease
(e) Tabes dorsalis

102. Which of the following symptoms is most typical of craniopharyngioma?
(a) Polyuria and polydipsia
(b) Hypercalcemia
(c) Hypocalcemia
(d) Hypophosphatemia
(e) Hyperphosphatemia

103. Membranous nephropathy presents with:
(a) Proteinuria
(b) Polyuria
(c) Hematuria
(d) Oliguria
(e) Red blood cell casts in the urine

104. The most prominent feature of Legionnaires' disease is:
(a) Encephalitis
(b) Myocarditis
(c) Pneumonia
(d) Liver abscesses
(e) Peritonitis

105. A tophus in the subcutaneous tissue is typical of:
(a) Rheumatic fever
(b) Gout
(c) Diabetes mellitus
(d) Diabetes insipidus
(e) Pellagra

ANSWERS TO MULTIPLE-CHOICE QUESTIONS

1. b
2. a
3. d
4. a
5. d
6. d
7. b
8. b
9. e
10. a
11. a
12. a
13. c
14. e
15. b
16. a
17. a
18. b
19. a
20. e
21. a
22. b
23. d
24. e
25. a
26. c
27. a
28. e
29. d or a
30. a
31. a
32. c
33. b
34. c
35. c
36. e
37. e
38. b
39. c
40. b
41. c
42. e
43. a
44. d
45. e
46. c
47. e
48. c
49. b
50. a
51. a
52. b
53. d
54. e
55. e
56. a
57. b
58. e
59. b
60. d
61. e
62. e
63. a
64. a
65. d
66. d
67. d
68. a
69. d
70. c
71. c
72. a
73. d
74. a
75. e
76. b
77. b
78. c
79. c
80. e
81. c
82. a
83. b
84. c
85. d
86. c
87. a
88. c
89. b
90. c
91. a
92. e
93. e
94. c
95. b
96. b
97. e
98. a
99. a
100. e
101. d
102. a
103. a
104. c
105. b

Rypins' Basic Sciences Review, 17th Edition,
edited by Edward D. Frohlich. Lippincott–Raven Publishers,
Philadelphia © 1997.

7

Pharmacology

Margaret A. Reilly, Ph.D.
Adjunct Assistant Professor
Department of Pharmacology
New York Medical College
Valhalla, New York

Adjunct Assistant Professor of Pharmacology
Concordia College
Bronxville, New York

Instructor in Pharmacology
Phillips–Beth Israel School of Nursing
New York, New York

INTRODUCTION

Pharmacology is the study of the interactions of drugs with living systems. Drugs are substances that have the ability to influence the physiological or biochemical activity of cells. Included are substances used in the diagnosis, prevention, and treatment of disease, as well as substances used for nonmedical or ''recreational'' purposes, such as alcohol, heroin, and cocaine. Interactions of drugs with living systems are often complex, resulting not only in desired or therapeutic actions but also in unwanted and occasionally life-threatening effects. A full understanding of these actions requires a strong foundation in the principles of anatomy, physiology, and biochemistry.

Drug Names

Every drug is a chemical substance and thus will have a name that describes exactly its molecular structure. Chemical names are rarely encountered in clinical pharmacology; their major importance is in the area of drug development and production.

When a drug is ready for clinical testing, a generic or nonproprietary name will be selected after discussion by committees or representatives of the American Medical Association, the Food and Drug Administration (FDA), the United States Pharmacopeia, the World Health Organization (WHO), the National Formulary, and the commercial sponsor of the drug. Since 1961, the names finally selected have been known as United States Adopted Names (USAN), and they are intended to provide the features of brevity, easy recall, and some syllable or stem that indicates the group to which the drug belongs. International recognition of the USAN reduces the occasion for worldwide multiplicity of names.

Proprietary or trademark names are the property of the commercial developer of the drug. Trademarked drugs must always be identified by their generic names also. Exclusive manufacturing and distributing rights may be held under patent for 17 years.

Administration of Drugs

Drugs are given for a wide variety of purposes under many clinical situations. All drugs possess the potential to induce serious adverse reactions. To administer drugs safely and effectively, the physician must have extensive knowledge of pharmacology. This chapter serves merely as a review of some of that body of knowledge, and focuses mainly on drugs currently in frequent use. Other more comprehensive sources must be consulted before drugs are prescribed. One valuable publication is ***AMA** Drug Evaluations,* prepared by committees and consultants of the American Medical Association. It is particularly useful to determine available preparations and currently accepted therapeutic practices. The ubiquitous *Physicians' Desk Reference (PDR)* is a compilation of extensive drug information supplied by pharmaceutical manufacturers, much of it in the form of official package inserts that are in compliance with FDA regulations pertaining to drug labelling. Newly released drugs, newly recognized adverse effects, and other items of importance to the practicing physician are presented in publications such as the *FDA Drug Bulletin* and *The Medical Letter on Drugs and Therapeutics.*

Regulatory Control of Drugs

The Food and Drug Administration is charged with protection of the public interest insofar as it is affected by the sale and the distribution of drug products. This agency was founded in 1906 but had little authority until 1938, when the Food, Drug and Cosmetic Act empowered the FDA to require demonstrations of reasonable safety at recommended drug doses, and, in 1962 (the Kefauver-Harris Amendment), to require proof of efficacy. In both instances, legislation followed disastrous incidents: in one case, the "elixir of sulfanilamide" tragedy, which cost over 100 lives because of unexpected toxicity of diethylene glycol, the solvent; in the other, the thalidomide experience, in which teratogenic effects of an apparently harmless sedative occurred in several thousand cases, almost all of them outside the United States. The U.S. Pharmacopeia (USP) and the National Formulary (NF), now combined in a single publication, specify the standards for manufacture of drugs in the United States.

In 1971, the FDA, in collaboration with the National Academy of Sciences and National Research Council, began rating the efficacy of drug products already on the market. The efficacy ratings are commonly referred to as drug efficacy study implementation (DESI) ratings, and include "effective," "effective with restrictions or qualifications," "probably effective," "possibly effective," and "ineffective."

In 1952, the Durham-Humphrey Amendment to the Food, Drug and Cosmetic Act established specific regulations in regard to prescription practices. Distinction was made between drugs that may be dispensed on prescription only ("legend" drugs) and those that may be sold "over the counter." The first category bears the prescription legend "Caution: Federal law prohibits dispensing without prescription." Among the prescription-legend drugs, certain ones can be refilled for the time specified by the prescriber, as indicated by the "refill" instructions; however, it should be noted that such instructions as "refill prn" or "refill ad lib," or other notations that place no limit on the length of time in which the prescription may be refilled are not recognized by the FDA as valid refill authorizations. Persons receiving prescription drugs should be under continuous medical supervision, to detect changes in their clinical conditions or development of adverse effects.

The Comprehensive Drug Abuse Prevention and Control Act (Controlled Substances Act) of 1970 limits the prescribing and refilling of certain depressant, stimulant, and hallucinogenic drugs in five different "schedules." Those drugs that have no legal use (such as heroin and LSD) are all placed in schedule I. Those drugs in the remaining schedules (II through V) are rated according to their decreasing potential for addiction or habituation. Prescriptions for drugs in schedule II (morphine, cocaine, and methamphetamine, for example) cannot be refilled. Prescriptions for drugs in schedules III and IV may be refilled, if the prescriber authorizes, not more than five times nor for longer than 6 months after the prescription is issued. Small quantities of schedule V drugs may be obtained from a pharmacist without a prescription.

When prescribing controlled substances, the prescriber must include the full name and address of the patient, must sign the prescription in ink, and must show his or her own address and Drug Enforcement Administration (DEA) registration number. It is illegal for a pharmacist to fill a prescription for a controlled substance unless all these requirements are met.

The Drug Regulation Reform Act of 1979 is a major revision of the way in which new drugs are brought onto the market and includes provisions for their surveillance after marketing. The Orphan Drug Act of 1983 was intended to foster development of agents useful in rare diseases. Economic incentives are provided to compensate for drug research that holds little potential for monetary return.

The Drug Price Competition and Patent Term Restoration Act passed in 1984 has simplified the requirements for approval of generic forms. The result has been a greatly increased number of such agents on the market. Although few serious bioequivalence discrepancies have been reported, transfer of patients from one drug form to another always requires careful observation for variations in therapeutic response.

In addition to federal legislation, states, municipalities, institutions, and agencies often have regulations that will govern the dispensing and use of drugs.

Drug-Receptor Interactions

Many drugs appear to exert their effects by combining with structural components (or receptors) on cell membranes or within cells. Endogenous substances such as neurotransmitters and hormones also act by combining with these receptors. The kinetics of attachment and release are regulated by such chemical forces as covalent electron sharing, electrostatic charge, hydrogen bonding, and van der Waal bonding. Some attachments of drugs to receptors are stable and long-lasting, while others are relatively weak and easily reversible.

In interacting with receptors, some substances elicit physiological or biochemical responses from cells. These substances are called ***agonists*** and are said to have both affinity (the ability to bind to a receptor type) and intrinsic activity (the ability to provoke a cellular response). For example, the β-adrenergic agonists isoproterenol and epinephrine activate adenylate cyclase when they bind to beta receptors. The ensuing increase in intracellular levels of cyclic AMP (the "second messenger") sets into motion biochemical responses that are ultimately expressed as alterations in physiological activity of those cells that possess beta receptors.

Other substances bind to receptors but do not initiate cellular responses, that is, these substances have affinity but not intrinsic activity. Drugs called ***antagonists*** act in this manner, blocking the effects of endogenous substances as well as of other drugs by preventing their access to receptors. For example, the β-adrenergic antagonist propranolol can decrease the intensity of those physiological responses attributable to stimulation of (or agonist activity at) β-receptors.

STRUCTURE–ACTIVITY RELATIONSHIPS

Drug-receptor interactions are specific or selective. Certain structural or spatial relationships must be present in a drug's molecular makeup in order for it to act as an agonist or antagonist at a receptor. Small molecular modifications can produce agonists or antagonists of varying potency, or convert agonist activity to antagonism. The pharmaceutical industry has utilized these structure–activity relationships in its efforts to develop drugs that will have greater therapeutic efficacy or lower incidence of adverse effects than prototype drugs. Narcotic antagonists and histamine H_2-receptor blockers were developed in this manner, as well as drugs with increased oral efficacy (*e.g.*, the antidysrhythmic tocainide) and decreased susceptibility to hepatic or renal inactivation (*e.g.*, the β-blocker nadolol). Drugs with more selective actions have been discovered (*e.g.*, β-agonists and antagonists selective for β_1 or β_2 receptors). Completely new classes of drugs have evolved, for example, the sulfonylurea oral hypoglycemic drugs from the sulfonamide antiinfective agents. However, some agents thus developed do not represent major differences from related compounds, and merely contribute to the vast number of available drugs.

DOSE–RESPONSE CURVES

Physiological responses to drugs are usually related to the dose administered, up to a maximal limit. The dose–response curve (characteristically S-shaped or sigmoid) is a graphic representation of this observation. Greater potency will shift the dose–response curve to the left, that is, lower doses will produce the same effect as larger amounts of less potent analogues. Efficacy refers to the maximal limit of the response produced; the height of the dose–response curve is greater for drugs with increased efficacy.

Interactions between drugs also yield characteristic dose–response curves. Competitive or reversible inhibition results in a parallel shift of the curve to the right, with no change in height (or efficacy). This type of inhibitory effect can be overcome by administration of increasing amounts of agonist. A noncompetitive antagonist, or one that is not reversible by increasing dosages of agonist, will produce a dose–response curve in which the maximal height is diminished.

Pharmacokinetics

Pharmacokinetics describes the fate of a drug after it has been administered. Many factors influence absorption, distribution, biotransformation, and elimination of drugs. The onset, duration, and intensity of a drug's actions are in turn modified by these interactions with physiological and biochemical functions.

The movement of a drug through the human body depends upon its lipid solubility, which enables it to cross biological membranes with ease. Most drugs are, to some degree, lipid soluble. A solution of a drug that is a weak acid or a weak base will contain both nonionized (lipid soluble) and ionized (water soluble) molecules. Alterations in the pH of the solution will change the ratio of nonionized to ionized molecules. Alkalinization will enhance ionization of acids and reduce that of bases; acidification has the opposite influence. The pKa of a drug is that pH at which equal amounts of the molecules in solution are nonionized and ionized.

Absorption refers to the entry of drug molecules into the circulatory system. Drugs administered for systemic effects must be transported from the site of administration to the site of action. Intravenous administration places the drug directly into the circulatory system. Other routes, however, depend upon the ability of molecules to gain access to the blood by crossing biological membranes. Most drugs are passively absorbed down a concentration gradient. Lipid-soluble molecules are most readily absorbed, although capillary walls in many tissues are quite permeable to both lipid- and water-soluble molecules. The rate of blood flow through the site of administration affects the concentration gradient. Normal perfusion rapidly carries drug away and enhances entry of more molecules into the circulatory system. Sluggish flow, as might be encountered in shock or heart failure, will impede absorption from peripheral sites. Bioavailability refers to the fraction of an administered drug dose that reaches the circulatory system and thus becomes available for distribution to sites of action.

Distribution occurs when drug molecules leave the circulatory system and enter body tissues where sites of action, storage, or inactivation are located. Again, the importance of the ability of molecules to cross membranes is apparent. Drugs have relatively uniform access to most tissues, with the exception of brain. There, the blood–brain barrier formed by the tight junctions of capillary cells tends to exclude ionized, lipid-insoluble molecules.

Distribution of drug can be delayed by the binding of molecules to plasma proteins such as albumin and alpha-acid glycoprotein. These macromolecules normally are restricted to the circulatory system, and only the unbound portion of a drug dose will be distributed to body tissues. The binding of drug to plasma protein is reversible, and as molecules leave the circulatory system additional drug will dissociate from its binding sites. Drugs that bind extensively to plasma proteins will have prolonged plasma half-lives and durations of action. Physiological and pathological states (*e.g.*, very young or old age, or hepatic or renal disease) that induce changes in the amounts of plasma protein can influence characteristic patterns of protein binding.

Other tissues also will bind and accumulate certain drugs. For example, adipose tissue can sequester significant amounts of lipid-soluble drugs. Perfusion of this tissue is low, thus drugs will accumulate and subsequently be released slowly.

Biotransformation, frequently accomplished by hepatic enzymes, involves the conversion of drugs to other substances. The action of many lipid-soluble drugs is terminated by transformation to molecules that are less lipid soluble and thus more readily excreted by the kidneys. Drug metabolites also are usually less pharmacologically active than the parent drug. However, some agents (*e.g.*, diazepam and procainamide) yield active metabolites that prolong the duration of pharmacological action. A few drugs are administered in inactive or prodrug form, and are biotransformed to active substances. Impairment of hepatic function (*e.g.*, in elderly persons or in the presence of hepatic disease) will reduce the effectiveness of biotransformation. Induction or enhancement of hepatic enzyme activity will increase the rate of drug metabolism. Some drugs are extensively extracted from the portal circulation by the liver. This ''first-pass effect'' greatly diminishes the effectiveness of drugs such as propranolol, and precludes the oral administration of drugs such as nitroglycerin and lidocaine.

The final factor in pharmacokinetics is excretion, which removes drugs and their metabolites from the body. The kidneys accomplish most excretion, although some drugs are eliminated by the lungs, in perspiration, or by secretion into bile and feces. Some drugs that are carried by bile into the gastrointestinal tract are reabsorbed in the intestine. This enterohepatic circulation contributes to the prolonged action of drugs such as the neuroleptics and digitoxin. Water-soluble drugs can be filtered by the kidneys and excreted as unmetabolized molecules. Changes in urinary *p*H will influence the ionization of drug molecules and alter rates of excretion. Some agents (*e.g.*, penicillins) are actively secreted by the nephron. Renal impairment can markedly prolong the plasma half-life of drugs eliminated by renal excretion.

The rate of drug excretion is expressed as the biological half-life, which is the time interval required for the amount of drug in the body to decrease by one half. This is usually measured in clinical pharmacology as the plasma half-life, which can be influenced by many of the previously discussed pharmacokinetic factors. The total amount of drug in the body is difficult to ascertain, except immediately following an initial IV bolus. Drugs vary in distribution to and sequestration in body compartments. The volume of distribution (V_d), estimated by comparing the total amount of drug present to the concentration in plasma, indicates the ability of the drug to diffuse from the circulatory system and enter tissues and cells.

SPECIAL CONSIDERATIONS

Pharmacokinetic factors differ considerably among persons, allowing much interindividual variation in therapeutic responsiveness. Age, sex, nutrition, hydration, genetic traits, and pathological status all influence the fate of drugs in the human body. Special precautions are thus required when drugs are administered to certain groups of persons.

Geriatric Pharmacology. The elderly population (*i.e.*, those over 65 years of age) consumes a disproportionately large percentage of the drugs sold annually in the United States. Many elderly persons have multiple illnesses and are often receiving several drugs simultaneously. This age group is at greater risk of experiencing adverse drug reactions and interactions.

Alterations in certain pharmacokinetic factors predispose elderly persons to greater responsiveness to drugs.

Physiological functions, such as hepatic and renal activity, become less efficient. Drugs that are hepatically biotransformed (*e.g.*, sedatives and narcotic analgesics) or inactivated by renal excretion (*e.g.*, antibiotics) can have prolonged and intensified action in the elderly.

Changes in patterns of blood flow may delay absorption and distribution of drugs and can also hinder their delivery to the liver and kidney for inactivation. An increase in the proportion of adipose tissue enhances the sequestration of lipid-soluble drugs.

Dehydration, occurring frequently in the elderly as renal water-conserving efficacy is lost, results in higher plasma levels of drugs, particularly those that are water soluble.

In addition to factors that affect many drugs in general, some physiological changes in the elderly will have an impact, particularly on individual types of drugs. For example, anticoagulants can be especially hazardous for several reasons. The elderly have fragile skin and blood vessels that increase the risk of hemorrhage following injury. In addition, decreased hepatic function will hinder the inactivation of these drugs, and also result in depletion of hepatically synthesized clotting factors and of plasma proteins to which these drugs avidly bind. Drugs that induce orthostatic hypotension can cause severe blood pressure fluctuations, since the vascular response to changes in position is reduced in the elderly. Drug-induced hypotension is believed to be a major cause of falls in older persons, who often have fragile bones (osteoporosis) that are easily fractured. Alterations in receptor sensitivity may occur at advanced age: this appears to underlie in part the increased responsiveness to benzodiazepines such as diazepam.

Despite the physiological changes that occur with age, many precautions can be taken to make drug administration safe and effective in the elderly. Only those drugs that are absolutely necessary should be given. Initial prescriptions should be written for smaller than normal amounts, and careful observation will reveal whether dosage adjustments are needed. Information can be provided to patients about anticipated adverse effects, in particular those that can warn of impending drug toxicity (*e.g.*, anorexia caused by digitalis glycosides) and those that endanger personal safety (*e.g.*, drowsiness or orthostatic hypotension). Attention can also be paid to possible drug interactions, especially those involving foods, alcohol, or over-the-counter preparations. If the patient's clinical condition deteriorates, or new symptoms appear, consider the very real possibility that these effects may be drug related.

Pediatric Pharmacology. Very young persons respond to drugs differently than adults. Most drugs are not specifically studied for their safety and efficacy in children. Instead, retrospective observation provides a body of knowledge that skilled physicians can use to administer drugs appropriately to pediatric patients. Several mathematical formulas, based on age, body weight, and surface area, can be used to proportion adult doses to suitable amounts for children. Drug prescriptions may also be based on body weight (*e.g.*, mg/kg) to provide for a child's smaller size.

Several physiological factors can alter drug pharmacokinetics in children. Neonates, in particular those born prematurely, are most at risk of heightened drug effects. Their hepatic enzyme systems that inactivate drugs are immature. Suboptimal renal blood flow and function result in inefficient excretion of drugs and metabolites. The blood–brain barrier is not fully developed, allowing entry of water-soluble drugs into the central nervous system. Levels of plasma proteins are reduced and are frequently bound with endogenous substances such as bilirubin. The neonate has higher body water volume and a lower proportion of adipose tissue than older infants, thus distribution of drugs may be altered. Many substances are easily absorbed across the neonate's permeable skin. Differences in gastrointestinal *p*H, motility, and bacterial population can affect absorption of drugs following oral administration.

Physiological systems gradually attain the maturity found in adults. However, development occurs at varying rates, and drug responses may be quite different among children of the same age and size. Close observation and careful adjustment of doses can help to make pediatric drug administration safe and effective.

Drugs During Pregnancy. Drugs administered during pregnancy gain access to the fetus via the placental circulation. Lipophilic drugs cross the placenta most readily, but it must be considered that almost any chronically administered drug can reach the fetus. Drugs can exert a variety of adverse effects on the developing fetus, which, like the neonate, has little ability to inactivate these substances. During the first trimester, some drugs interfere with the early establishment of organs and systems. At birth, the infant may have major anatomical malformations. Called teratogens, these drugs include the sedative thalidomide, several antineoplastic agents, and alcohol.

In later pregnancy, drugs can retard mental and physical development of the fetus, or can produce effects identical to those observed in the mother. For example, β-adrenergic antagonists can markedly depress fetal cardiac function, and oral anticoagulants can induce severe fetal or neonatal hemorrhage even though the mother's prothrombin time is within acceptable limits. Women who are physiologically dependent on drugs such as opiates and barbiturates during their pregnancy will often give birth to an "addicted" infant who will exhibit abstinence signs during the first hours or days of life. Smoking of cigarettes during pregnancy results in fetal damage and low birth weight. Drugs administered during labor and delivery (*e.g.*, anesthetic and analgesic agents) can evoke respiratory depression in the neonate.

Pregnancy must be considered a contraindication to the administration of all drugs. However, maternal diabetes, hypertension, convulsive disorders, or preeclampsia must be controlled for the safety of both mother and infant. Required drugs should be administered in the lowest possible doses, and under close medical supervision. Breast-feeding is also a contraindication for drug administration, although there is controversy regarding which agents reach sufficient levels in breast milk to be harmful to the nursing infant.

DRUG INTERACTIONS

Drugs administered concurrently or sequentially can enhance or diminish each others' actions. Some drug interactions are beneficial, such as the potassium-retaining effects of angiotensin converting enzyme inhibitors offsetting the potassium-losing effects of thiazides. Enhancement of effect can be due to simple addition of the similar actions of two drugs, for example, severe suppression of the cholinergic nervous system when two drugs with anticholinergic efficacy are given simultaneously. ***Potentiation*** (occasionally referred to as synergism) refers to the marked intensification of a drug's action by another, so that the combined effect is greater than the sum of the two drugs acting independently. For example, very small amounts of alcohol and benzodiazepines combined can produce central nervous system depression of greater severity than anticipated.

Drug interactions can be pharmacokinetic or pharmacodynamic. ***Pharmacokinetic interactions*** involve alterations in drug absorption, distribution, biotransformation, or excretion. Bile acid sequestrants will bind many orally administered drugs, including digoxin and warfarin, in the gastrointestinal tract and impede their absorption. Probenecid prolongs the action of the penicillins by inhibiting their renal secretion. Tricyclic antidepressants reduce the efficacy of guanethidine by hindering its entry into presynaptic nerve terminals. ***Pharmacodynamic interactions*** generally occur at the site of drug action. The dopamine-blocking action of neuroleptic drugs will antagonize dopamine agonists such as levodopa and bromocriptine, used in the treatment of Parkinson's disease.

Chemical or physical interactions can occur *in vitro*. Combining sodium bicarbonate and epinephrine in the same solution will inactivate the latter. Diazepam is precipitated from solution by several drugs and solvents. Many such incompatibilities exist and will preclude the combination of drugs in one syringe or infusion.

In addition to its interaction with central nervous system depressants, alcohol can react adversely with many other drugs. It will enhance gastric irritation of salicylates and other nonsteroidal anti-inflammatory drugs. It potentiates the hepatotoxicity of methotrexate and acetaminophen. Severe vasodilatation and hypotension can occur when alcohol and antianginal nitrates are concurrently administered. Because of the widespread use of alcohol, patients should always be advised when its consumption may be hazardous.

Drugs can also interact with components of foods. Wines, cheeses, and other foods containing tyramine can provoke hypertensive emergencies in persons receiving monoamine oxidase inhibitors. Pyridoxine (vitamin B_6) is a cofactor for the decarboxylase that inactivates levodopa, and will reduce the efficacy of this antiparkinsonian agent. Bile acid resins such as cholestyramine will bind fat-soluble vitamins and prevent their intestinal absorption.

Beneficial interactions have prompted the use of drug combinations to treat some diseases. For example, hypertension is frequently managed with two or three agents that provide a good therapeutic response in patients refractory to single drugs. Cancer also is often treated with carefully selected combinations of drugs.

The incidence of undesirable drug interactions can be decreased by health care personnel who are familiar with the pharmacology and the recognized interactions of the drugs they administer. A thorough medical history will reveal other drugs (including over-the-counter) that the patient is taking, and any clinical condition that might enhance interactions. Patients can be given information regarding potential drug or food interactions.

AUTONOMIC DRUGS

The autonomic nervous system, consisting of sympathetic (adrenergic) and parasympathetic (cholinergic) branches, modulates a vast variety of physiological activities. Thus it is not surprising that drugs that either stimulate (agonists) or inhibit (antagonists) these systems are frequently used in the management of many disorders. Some agonists have a direct effect on receptors, while others enhance the release of neurotransmitters or block their enzymatic degradation. Norepinephrine, the neurotransmitter or "chemical messenger" in the sympathetic system, acts upon both α- and β-adrenergic receptors. Acetylcholine stimulates muscarinic receptors at the autonomic effector sites, and also nicotinic receptors in the autonomic ganglia and at the neuromuscular junctions of the somatic nervous system. Both of these acetylcholine receptor types appear to be present in the central nervous system. Antagonists of the effects of the autonomic nervous system are relatively selective for only one type of receptor. Because of the diffuse distribution of the autonomic nervous system, and its considerable influence on physiological activity, drugs that alter its activity will have many side effects that occasionally limit their usefulness.

TABLE 7-1. Cholinergic Drugs

GENERIC NAME	TRADE NAME
Direct-Acting Stimulants	
Bethanechol	Urecholine
Carbechol	Carbacel
Pilocarpine	Pilocar
Anticholinesterases	
Ambenonium	Mytelase
Echothiophate	Phospholine iodide
Edrophonium	Tensilon
Neostigmine	Prostigmin
Physostigmine	Eserine, Antilirium
Pyridostigmine	Mestinon

Parasympathomimetic Drugs

Acetylcholine is synthesized in the nerve terminal by the enzyme choline acetyltransferase and is stored in synaptic vesicles for release subsequent to action potentials transmitted along the neuron. Acetylcholine is inactivated in the synaptic cleft by the enzyme acetylcholinesterase, and choline is transported back into the terminal for resynthesis to acetylcholine. Among the numerous autonomic effects of this neurotransmitter are miosis, ciliary muscle spasm, salivation, lacrimation, sweating, negative chronotropy, peripheral vasodilation, and stimulation of smooth muscle contraction and secretion in the respiratory, gastrointestinal, and urinary tracts.

Acetylcholine itself is not a useful pharmacologic agent because it is too rapidly metabolized and not orally active. Several synthetic analogues that directly stimulate muscarinic receptors have proved to be effective (Table 7-1). These drugs can be given subcutaneously (SC) or orally (PO) but should not be administered IV or IM since subsequent extreme bradycardia, bronchospasm, and bronchial secretion may be fatal. Fortunately, the toxic effects of these cholinergic agonists can be reversed by atropinelike drugs (see below). ***Bethanechol*** stimulates in particular the urinary and gastrointestinal smooth muscle, thus is administered to alleviate neurogenic, postsurgical, and postpartum nonobstructive urinary retention, bladder atony, and abdominal distention. It has a prolonged duration and relatively little influence on cardiovascular activity. Carbachol and pilocarpine are used mainly as topical agents to reduce intraocular pressure in glaucoma and to induce miosis during ocular surgery. ***Pilocarpine*** may be administered systemically (PO, SC) to restore flow of saliva. ***Methacholine*** is seldom used, although it will terminate paroxysmal atrial tachycardia, and its stimulation of catecholamine release can be diagnostic in pheochromocytoma.

Side effects of the acetylcholine agonists in general include gastrointestinal distress, involuntary urination and defecation, salivation, marked bradycardia, postural hypotension, syncope, and dyspnea. These drugs are contraindicated in patients with peptic ulcer, asthma, obstruction or weakness of the gastrointestinal or urinary tract, pregnancy, and many cardiovascular disorders. Hypertensive patients may experience a profound reduction in blood pressure.

Muscarine is a cholinergic agonist of toxicologic importance, since it is the substance in *Amanita muscaria* responsible for poisoning when this mushroom is ingested.

ANTICHOLINESTERASES

Some parasympathomimetics are reversible inhibitors of the enzyme acetylcholinesterase. By slowing inactivation of endogenous acetylcholine, these anticholinesterases (see Table 7-1) increase the intensity and duration of cholinergic actions. In contrast to direct-acting cholinergic agents, these drugs can affect ganglionic and neuromuscular junction transmission because they will inhibit acetylcholine degradation at these sites also. The anticholinesterases have been especially useful in the management of glaucoma and myasthenia gravis.

Physostigmine (Antilirium) is a naturally occurring alkaloid with a relatively short duration of action. It is frequently used to reverse both central and peripheral effects of anticholinergic drug overdose. Children are especially sensitive to this drug; thus its pediatric use is limited to life threatening episodes of anticholinergic poisoning.

The longer acting agents ***neostigmine*** (Prostigmin), ***pyridostigmine*** (Mestinon), and ***ambenonium*** (Mytelase) are used in the management of myasthenia gravis. This neuromuscular deficit in acetylcholine transmission causes extreme skeletal muscle weakness. In addition to cholinesterase inhibition, neostigmine appears to have a direct effect on nicotinic receptors. Although usually given orally, these drugs can be administered parenterally in myasthenic crisis or to patients who cannot swallow. ***Edrophonium*** (Tensilon) has a very short duration of action, making it especially useful in the diagnosis of myasthenia gravis and in differentiating myasthenic from cholinergic crises. Both of these emergencies are characterized by extreme muscular weakness that can lead to respiratory failure. However, while anticholinesterases alleviate myasthenic crisis, they will exacerbate cholinergic crisis.

The anticholinesterases are also used to reverse muscle paralysis induced by nondepolarizing neuromuscular junction blockers such as curare derivatives and gallamine. However, they will intensify the effects of the depolarizing muscle relaxant succinylcholine.

The adverse effects of the anticholinesterases include all the symptoms of excessive parasympathetic action:

increased gastrointestinal and respiratory secretion, intestinal and urinary tract hypermotility, bronchoconstriction, convulsions, bradycardia, and hypotension. In addition, nicotinic symptoms such as fasciculations, weakness, and respiratory paralysis can occur. Atropine will reverse the muscarinic actions of these drugs but will not alter neuromuscular effects. Drug tolerance, or "anticholinesterase insensitivity," may develop with chronic use. Drugs must then be withheld and patients provided with respiratory assistance as needed until cholinergic responsiveness returns.

Irreversible inhibition of cholinesterases is achieved by the use of several organophosphates. Topical preparations containing demecarium (Humorsol), isoflurophate (Floropryl), and echothiophate (Phospholine) are used in the management of glaucoma and strabismus. Diisopropyl fluorophosphate (DFP) and parathion are contained in commercial insecticides. The nerve gases of biological warfare, sarin and tabun, for example, are organophosphate compounds. Organophosphates phosphorylate the cholinesterase enzyme, rendering it incapable of hydrolyzing acetylcholine. Recovery of neurotransmitter inactivation may take up to 3 months, since new cholinesterase molecules must be synthesized.

The highly lipid-soluble insecticides can be absorbed through the skin as well as by inhalation and ingestion. Poisoning provokes both peripheral and central manifestations of excessive acetylcholine levels. Bronchoconstriction, bradycardia, and hypotension are autonomic in origin, while somatic nicotinic activity causes fasciculations and weakness of skeletal and respiratory muscles. Central nervous system symptoms include restlessness, tremors, convulsions, respiratory depression and paralysis, and circulatory collapse. Atropine will ameliorate central and peripheral muscarinic effects, but mechanical ventilation may be required to sustain respiration. Diazepam will alleviate convulsions induced by organophosphate toxicity. Measurement of plasma cholinesterase levels can indicate the extent of insecticide poisoning. Pretreatment with the anticholinesterase pyridostigmine can block the action of the nerve gases soman and tabun.

Pralidoxime (Protopam) reverses organophosphate toxicity by reactivating the cholinesterases. Its greatest effect is upon skeletal and respiratory muscle paralysis; it does not enter the central nervous system. Usually given IV, pralidoxime is relatively short-lived and can be readministered if needed. However, it has some cholinergic depolarizing action and can induce muscular weakness, vision disturbances, and hyperventilation. The action of atropine may be accelerated, and barbiturates are potentiated by pralidoxime.

Tacrine (Cognex) is a lipid-soluble, reversible cholinesterase inhibitor that may slow the deterioration of cognitive function and activities of daily living in Alzheimer's disease. This drug is almost completely metabolized in the liver, and there is first-pass extraction that may decrease with larger doses. Adverse effects are nausea, vomiting, diarrhea, ataxia, headache, myalgia, and changes in liver function, which are reversible when drug is terminated. The inactivation of theophylline, and possibly of other drugs metabolized by the cytochrome P450 system, is inhibited by tacrine. Absorption of tacrine is decreased by food in the gastrointestinal tract.

TABLE 7-2. Anticholinergic Drugs

GENERIC NAME	TRADE NAME
Antimuscarinics	
Atropine	Atropisol, Dey-Dose, others
Hyoscyamine	Levsin, Bellaspaz, others
Scopolamine	Transderm-Scōp, others
Antispasmodics	
Clidinium	Quarzan
Dicyclomine	Bentyl
Glycopyrrolate	Robinul
Oxybutynin	Ditropan
Propantheline	ProBanthine
Antiparkinsonism Agents	
Benztropine	Cogentin
Biperiden	Akineton
Ethopropazine	Parsidol
Procyclidine	Kemadrin
Trihexyphenidyl	Artane

CHOLINERGIC ANTAGONISTS

Drugs that reverse the effects of acetylcholine are relatively specific for the autonomic nervous system, for ganglionic transmission, or for the neuromuscular junction. This selectivity becomes somewhat obscured at high drug doses. The first type of drug is considered in this section; the latter two are discussed subsequently.

Atropine, a belladonna derivative that competitively blocks the postganglionic effects of parasympathetic stimulation, is the prototype anticholinergic drug. (In large doses, atropine has some nicotinic blocking action also.) There are naturally occurring and synthetic analogues (Table 7-2) that have much the same characteristics and uses as atropine. Some are quaternary rather than tertiary amines, thus having less central nervous system activity but greater potential to alter ganglionic transmission. Atropine will reverse all the effects of parasympathetic stimulation. Low doses inhibit perspiration and salivation; gradually higher doses will exert cardiac actions and suppression of gastrointestinal and urinary smooth muscle. Quite large amounts are required to reduce gastric secretion.

The anticholinergics are used in the treatment of spastic

and inflammatory bowel and biliary disorders, and as adjunctive peptic ulcer therapy to reduce gastric acidity. As presurgical medication (atropine and scopolamine in particular), these agents reduce respiratory tract secretions and prevent bradycardia, bronchospasm, and laryngospasm. Asthmatic bronchoconstriction can be alleviated, as can urinary tract irritability. ***Ipratropium*** (Atrovent) is administered by inhalation to alleviate chronic obstructive respiratory difficulty. Cold medications may contain an anticholinergic to reduce nasal secretions. Some anticholinergics are used to alleviate symptoms of parkinsonism and are discussed under that topic. ***Scopolamine*** in transdermal patches (Transderm Scōp) has provided a new route of administration for a time-honored remedy for motion sickness. Atropine will reverse digitalis suppression of atrioventricular conduction and vagally induced bradycardias such as those encountered in acute myocardial infarction. (However, it must be noted that low doses of this drug can further slow heart rate, and high doses can induce tachydysrhythmias and postural hypotension.) Scopolamine combined with a narcotic analgesic such as morphine or meperidine produces a particular kind of analgesia called "twilight sleep" that was once used frequently in obstetrics. Anticholinergics are included in some over-the-counter sleeping aids, and brief-acting agents, such as ***homatropine*** and ***eucatropine***, are topical mydriatics and cycloplegics that facilitate ocular examination. Anticholinergic drugs are also used to manage overdose or exaggerated response to parasympathomimetic agents.

Because the anticholinergics have a wide variety of effects, those actions that are therapeutic in some instances can become unwanted side effects in others. For example, the increase in heart rate that is beneficial when bradycardia accompanies acute myocardial infarction may be undesirable when anticholinergics are used as gastrointestinal antispasmodics. Additional side effects include dry mouth, constipation, urinary retention, blurred vision, elevated intracranial pressure, intestinal paralysis, suppression of perspiration, nervousness, and insomnia. In hot environments, normal doses of anticholinergics may induce fatal hyperthermia. Low doses of anticholinergics can depress central nervous system activity, while higher doses cause stimulation. Elderly persons, who are especially sensitive to anticholinergics, may experience marked mental confusion or excitation.

Anticholinergic overdose induces cutaneous vasodilation and flushing (hot, dry skin), hyperthermia, respiratory stimulation followed by depression, tachycardia, dilated pupils, changes in blood pressure, muscular incoordination, confusion, delirium, and coma. The anticholinesterase physostigmine is the drug of choice to control anticholinergic overdose; benzodiazepines may also be given to reduce central nervous system stimulation. Pressor agents such as norepinephrine or metaraminol will alleviate hypotension.

Anticholinergics are contraindicated in glaucoma, prostatic hypertrophy, some types of cardiovascular disease, gastrointestinal atony or obstruction, ulcerative colitis, and myasthenia gravis. Caution must be used in patients with renal or hepatic disease or hyperthyroidism. In addition to the elderly, young children also are especially sensitive to anticholinergic effects. Many types of drugs (*e.g.,* tricyclic antidepressants, neuroleptics, antihistamines) can significantly suppress cholinergic function; thus, they are subject to all the precautions and contraindications relevant to anticholinergics.

Concomitant administration of two drugs that reduce parasympathetic activity requires great caution to ensure that excessive suppression does not occur. Monoamine oxidase inhibitors block the hepatic biotransformation of cholinergic antagonists, thus intensifying their effects. Anticholinergics administered IV to persons receiving cyclopropane anesthesia can precipitate ventricular dysrhythmias. Absorption of orally administered drugs can be enhanced by the prolonged gastrointestinal transit time induced by cholinergic antagonists.

Sympathomimetic Drugs

There are at least four distinct receptor types in the adrenergic nervous system. Alpha$_1$ receptors, found postsynaptically, mediate in particular contraction of blood vessels, gastrointestinal and urinary sphincters, and the radial muscle of the eye. Presynaptic α_2 receptors, so-called "autoreceptors," exert negative feedback inhibition of norepinephrine release. Postsynaptic α_2 binding sites appear to influence intestinal secretion and glucose-induced insulin release. Lipolysis and cardio-stimulant actions of the adrenergic system are mediated through β_1 receptors, while β_2 receptor stimulation induces relaxation of smooth muscle resulting in vasodilation, uterine relaxation, decreased gastrointestinal motility, and bronchodilation. Muscle glycogenolysis is also a β_2 function.

Adrenergic drugs have varying degrees of selectivity for receptors. Norepinephrine, the adrenergic neurotransmitter, stimulates α_1 and α_2 as well as β_1 (but little at β_2) receptors. Epinephrine, released from the adrenal medulla in response to various stressors, stimulates all four of the adrenergic receptors.

The synthetic β-agonists ***isoproterenol***, ***albuterol***, and ***terbutaline*** are especially useful as bronchodilators. Isoproterenol in addition is a powerful β_1 receptor stimulant. Beta antagonists may block both β_1 and β_2 receptors (*e.g.,* ***propranolol***) or may be somewhat selective (*e.g.,* metoprolol and atenolol) for the cardiac β_1 sites, except at higher doses where β_2 activity also becomes apparent (*e.g.,* ***metoprolol***). ***Clonidine***, a centrally acting antihypertensive, is an α_2 agonist that reduces sympathetic stimulation apparently by inhibition of norepinephrine release.

Some sympathomimetics work by direct stimulation of receptors (*e.g.*, isoproterenol) while others act indirectly by releasing endogenous catecholamines (*e.g.*, amphetamines). Still others have both direct and indirect effects (*e.g.*, ***metaraminol***). Tachyphylaxis can develop to the effects of indirect acting agents, as norepinephrine is depleted from nerve terminals.

The catecholamines (norepinephrine, epinephrine, dopamine, and isoproterenol) must be administered parenterally. All are rapidly inactivated, norepinephrine and epinephrine by presynaptic reuptake as well as by the catechol-o-methyltransferase and monoamine oxidase enzyme systems. 3-Methoxy-4-hydroxy mandelic acid, the final metabolite, is occasionally measured as an indicator of catecholamine synthesis and turnover.

Norepinephrine, in the form of the synthetically prepared levo isomer levarterenol bitartrate (Levophed), is used in the management of acute hypotensive states (*e.g.*, those accompanying spinal anesthesia or cord damage). Blood volume deficits must be replaced before or concurrently with pressor amine administration. Norepinephrine returns blood pressure toward normal levels by vasoconstriction (mediated by α_1 receptors) and cardiac stimulation (mediated by β_1 receptors). Cardiac irritability and force of contraction as well as myocardial oxygen consumption will be increased. Cardiac output and venous return increase, and systemic blood flow and coronary artery perfusion improve. Heart rate, often reflexly increased in hypotension, will slow as blood pressure rises.

Administered intravenously, the rate of infusion of norepinephrine must be carefully and constantly adjusted to the patient's response. Severe hypertension and reflex bradycardia can develop; cardiac output can fall as a result of extreme elevations in total peripheral resistance. Headache can be a symptom of elevated blood pressure due to excessive α stimulation. A large vein in the upper body should be selected as the infusion site, which must be constantly observed for signs of extravasation. The intense vasoconstrictor action of norepinephrine will deprive subcutaneous tissue of its blood supply, and cause necrosis and sloughing. If extravasation occurs, infiltration of the α-antagonist phentolamine can help to limit subcutaneous tissue damage. Termination of drug administration should be accomplished gradually, with frequent monitoring of blood pressure. Norepinephrine administration requires caution in persons with vascular disease or heart failure.

Epinephrine's actions differ somewhat from those of norepinephrine. Vascular beds possessing β-receptors (*e.g.*, skeletal muscle and coronary artery) will dilate in response to low doses of epinephrine. Epinephrine, acting on extracardiac β-receptors, induces glycogenolysis and release of fatty acids from adipose tissue. Blood glucose and lactic acid concentrations increase. By its action on pulmonary β_2 receptors, epinephrine is a powerful bronchodilator.

Solutions of epinephrine ranging from 1 mg/ml to 0.01 mg/ml are available for IV, IM, or SC administration. Direct intracardiac injection may be used to restore heart beat in cardiac arrest. Epinephrine can also be administered by endotracheal tube in an aerosol. Epinephrine is the drug of choice in anaphylaxis and other life-threatening allergic reactions; it rapidly alleviates shock and asthmatic bronchoconstriction. It is available as a spray for nasal decongestion, and also as an ophthalmic vasoconstrictor and mydriatic. Epinephrine is frequently combined with local or intraspinal anesthetics to induce vasoconstriction and retard systemic absorption. Inadvertent IV administration can cause marked central nervous system and cardiovascular stimulation.

Isoproterenol (Isuprel) is a synthetic, purely β-adrenergic agonist. It is administered IV, sublingually (although absorption is inconsistent), by rectal suppository, and by inhalation. It may reverse atrioventricular heart block and can assist in the reversal of cardiac arrest. It is contraindicated in tachydysrhythmias, except for those dysrhythmias that may be ameliorated by its marked action on the sinoatrial node. Isoproterenol is a highly effective bronchodilator. However, it has caused sudden death (often attributable to excessive use); propellants contained in aerosol forms may sensitize myocardial cells to the dysrhythmogenic action of the catecholamines. Isoproterenol can increase myocardial oxygen consumption and may exacerbate situations in which coronary perfusion is compromised (*e.g.*, acute myocardial infarction).

Dopamine (Intropin), the precursor of epinephrine and norepinephrine, is used in the treatment of shock subsequent to myocardial infarction, congestive heart failure, renal failure, septicemia, and trauma. In low doses (2 to 5 μg/kg/min) dopamine acts at dopaminergic receptors to dilate renal and splanchnic blood vessels. Glomerular filtration rate and sodium excretion are increased. Doses in the range of 5 to 10 μg/kg/min stimulate cardiac β receptors and also release norepinephrine from sympathetic nerve terminals, thus improving myocardial function. Alpha receptors are responsive at higher doses (10 to 20 μg/kg/min) of dopamine, and vasoconstriction will occur. Dopamine can exert significant positive inotropy with less increase in myocardial oxygen requirement than isoproterenol. Dopamine is administered only by IV infusion, carefully adjusted to the patient's response. Urinary output should be monitored. Extravasation should be avoided. Dopamine is also a central nervous system neurotransmitter.

Dobutamine (Dobutrex), similar in structure to dopamine, is indicated in the short-term management of cardiac decompensation subsequent to cardiac surgery or refractory heart failure. Its main action is direct β_1 receptor stimulation, producing a marked increase in contractile force with less effect on heart rate and myocardial oxygen demand. In contrast to norepinephrine's vasoconstrictive effects, renal and splanchnic vessels are dilated by dobutamine. It has a short plasma half-life and is administered by IV infusion.

Many of the responses to adrenergic β stimulation have been linked to activation of adenylate cyclase. Catecholamines and other sympathomimetics are considered "first messengers," which activate this enzyme that catalyzes the conversion of ATP to cyclic AMP. The latter "second messenger" then activates other enzyme systems that alter cellular activity and produce characteristic adrenergic actions.

Among the many adverse effects of catecholamines and other adrenergic agonists are anxiety (epinephrine in particular induces apprehension), restlessness, tremor, convulsions, vertigo, headache, nausea, urinary retention, palpitations, severe changes in blood pressure, dysrhythmias, anginal pain, and cardiac or respiratory arrest. Sympathomimetics are contraindicated in severe hypertension, certain cardiovascular disorders, hyperthyroidism, narrow angle glaucoma, and in persons receiving monoamine oxidase inhibitors or anesthesia with halothane or cyclopropane. The effects of direct-acting agents can be potentiated by tricyclic antidepressants, while those of indirect-acting amines that require entry into presynaptic terminals is reduced. Reserpine also will reduce the effectiveness of indirect acting agents since this drug depletes synaptic stores of norepinephrine. Risk of arrhythmias is increased by concomitant administration of digitalis or thyroid hormones.

Amphetamines (Table 7-3) appear to act indirectly by releasing endogenous catecholamines. They are powerful central nervous system stimulants (see discussion under that topic), and also possess vasoconstrictor and cardiac stimulant properties. Because of their euphoriant and energizing actions, the amphetamines are subject to abuse. Both psychological and physiological dependence can develop to these schedule II controlled substances. Amphetamines have a brief anorexient action (2 to 3 weeks) that has occasioned their use in initiating weight reduction or intermittently sustaining such programs. They should be used only when other dietary and nondrug measures have failed. A large number of anorexients (Table 7-4) are available, but are generally subject to rapidly developing tolerance and drug dependence. ***Phenylpropanolamine*** (PPA) is available over the counter, but marked cardiovascular stimulation is a not infrequent adverse effect of this drug.

Amphetamines also have some value in the management of childhood attention-deficit disorders (minimal brain dysfunction), and narcolepsy. ***Methylphenidate*** (Ritalin) is used similarly to amphetamines in attention-deficit disorders, and as an antidepressant: elderly women with refractory depression can be especially responsive to this latter action.

The α-receptor agonists ***metaraminol*** (Aramine) and ***methoxamine*** (Vasoxyl), will alleviate hypotensive states. By producing reflex bradycardia, these agents can terminate paroxysmal atrial tachycardia. These drugs are administered parenterally and have a longer duration of action than the catecholamines. Many α-adrenergic drugs are utilized as nasal decongestants (Table 7-5; see also Respiratory Pharmacology).

Ephedrine is an indirect-acting sympathomimetic that can be administered orally. It has a relatively long duration of action, and is an effective bronchodilator, mydriatic, and decongestant. Significant central nervous system stimulation induced by ephedrine can be reversed by concomitant administration of a barbiturate.

The β-agonists ***metaproterenol*** (Alupent), ***terbutaline*** (Bricanyl, Brethine), and ***albuterol*** (Ventolin, Proventil) can be administered orally, SC, or by inhalation to prevent

TABLE 7-3. Amphetamines

GENERIC NAME	TRADE NAME
Amphetamine	—
Benzphetamine	Didrex
Dextroamphetamine	Dexedrine
Methamphetamine	Desoxyn

TABLE 7-4. Anorexients

GENERIC NAME	TRADE NAME
Fenfluramine	Pondomin
Mazindol	Mazanor, Sanorex
Phendimetrazine	Bontril
Phenmetrazine	Preludin
Phenylpropanolamine	Acutrim, Dexatrim

TABLE 7-5. Adrenergic Decongestants

GENERIC NAME	TRADE NAME
Ephedrine	Efedron
Epinephrine	—
Naphazoline	Privine
Oxymetazoline	Dristan
Phenylephrine	Neo-Synephrine
Propylhexedrine	Benzedrex
Tetrahydrozoline	Tyzine
Xylometazoline	Otrivin

or alleviate bronchoconstriction (see Respiratory Pharmacology).

Ritodrine (Yutopar) is a β-agonist that relaxes uterine smooth muscle and will reverse premature labor that occurs *after the 20th week of pregnancy.* Intravenous infusion can terminate acute episodes, then oral administration is instituted to prevent recurrence. This drug is not used when postponement of delivery may threaten the survival of either the mother or the fetus (*e.g.,* in the presence of uncontrolled maternal diabetes mellitus, eclampsia, or intrauterine fetal death). Because of its β-stimulating properties, ritodrine is also contraindicated by tachydysrhythmias and hypertension. Intravenous administration can elevate serum free fatty acid, glucose, and insulin levels, and decrease potassium levels. Diabetic patients and those receiving diuretics that promote potassium loss require close observation. Adverse effects that occur most frequently following IV infusion include alterations in heart rate (both maternal and fetal) and blood pressure, pulmonary edema, palpitations, nausea, tremor, and anxiety. Sudden significant changes in maternal or fetal heart rate or blood pressure, or signs of circulatory overload, require that IV infusion of ritodrine be slowed or terminated. In the neonate, hypoglycemia, hypocalcemia, hypotension, and paralytic ileus may be present.

ADRENERGIC ANTAGONISTS

Adrenergic blocking agents are generally selective for either α- or β-receptors. Most are competitive antagonists at postsynaptic sites. Alpha antagonists, which reduce sympathetically induced vasoconstriction, are administered in vasospastic diseases such as Reynaud's syndrome, and in the management of pheochromocytoma. They are investigational in the treatment of shock, since a marked vasoconstrictive component may occur before the final vasodilatory response characteristic of circulatory failure.

α-Adrenergic Blocking Agents ***Phenoxybenzamine*** (Dibenzyline) binds to both α_1 and α_2 receptors. It produces a gradually developing (4 to 6 hours) but long-lasting (1 to 4 days) ''nonequilibrium'' blockade by forming with the receptor a stable complex that is reversible only in the early stages of interaction. This drug is administered orally in the management of pheochromocytoma. Because of its slow onset, doses must be increased cautiously. Phenoxybenzamine is hazardous in the presence of marked cerebral or coronary arteriosclerosis, when a fall in blood pressure can further compromise perfusion of vital organs. Nasal congestion, reflex tachycardia, miosis, and postural hypotension can occur. Severe hypotension may follow concomitant administration of β-adrenergic agonists, which will induce unopposed vasodilation.

Phentolamine (Regitine) has a more rapid onset and shorter duration of action than phenoxybenzamine. Administered either orally or parenterally, it also blocks both types of α receptors and also has a direct vasodilatory action. Phentolamine will control hypertensive episodes before and during surgical removal of pheochromocytoma, and has been used in hypertensive emergencies induced by abrupt termination of antihypertensive medication and by drug interactions with monoamine oxidase (MAO) inhibitors. Vasoconstriction and tissue damage resulting from extravasation of norepinephrine or dopamine can be minimized by local infiltration with phentolamine. Contraindicated in coronary artery disease, this drug can cause coronary and cerebral artery occlusion following IV administration. Its side effects are similar to those of phenoxybenzamine. Reflex tachycardia can be alleviated with a β-antagonist, and excessive hypotension can be treated with norepinephrine or a purely α agonist to reverse the competitive alpha blockade. Epinephrine is contraindicated in the presence of an α-blocker; the beta vasodilatory action of epinephrine predominates and will further decrease blood pressure. This effect has been termed ''epinephrine reversal.''

Tolazoline (Priscoline) is similar to phentolamine, and has the ability to stimulate the myocardium, gastric secretion, and gastrointestinal motility. It is ''possibly effective'' in the management of peripheral vascular disease, and is used investigationally to reduce elevated pulmonary vascular resistance in infants.

In contrast to phenoxybenzamine and phentolamine, which can enhance norepinephrine release by their blockade of presynaptic α_2 receptors, ***prazosin*** (Minipress) and ***terazosin*** (Hytrin) are selective antagonists at postsynaptic α_1 receptors. These drugs do not potentiate sympathetic stimulation of cardiac β-receptors, and are effective antihypertensive agents (see discussion under that topic).

β-Adrenergic Blocking Agents. Indications for the ''β-blockers,'' such as ***propranolol*** (Inderal), include many cardiovascular disorders that are alleviated by reduction of β-receptor-mediated positive inotropic (contractile force) and chronotropic (heart rate) effects. These drugs alleviate symptoms of angina pectoris and hypertrophic subaortic stenosis and can control dysrhythmias induced by excessive β receptor activation; propranolol's membrane-stabilizing or local anesthetic effect enhances its antidysrhythmic efficacy. β-blockers may be administered prophylactically to patients who experience frequent and severe migraine headaches. Propranolol appears to prevent the vasodilatory initiation of this disorder but will not reverse acute migraine attacks. β-blockers are effective in preventing recurrence of myocardial infarction and sudden death. Once considered contraindicated in congestive heart failure, these drugs may be cautiously administered to reduce excessive sympathetic stimulation that has become detrimental to cardiac activity.

Perhaps the most common indication for β-blockers is in the management of hypertension. These drugs appear to have both central (reduction of sympathetic outflow from the central nervous system) and peripheral (decreased inotropy and chronotropy, and suppression of renin release) hypotensive actions, and will also block reflex tachycardia induced by many other antihypertensive agents such as diuretics and vasodilators. The β-blockers are discussed further under such topics as Antihypertensive Agents and Pharmacotherapy of Angina Pectoris.

The clinically available β-receptor blockers (Table 7-6) have many similarities, although some possess special characteristics. While most are inactivated hepatically, ***atenolol*** and ***nadolol*** are excreted renally. These two agents have a longer duration of action, which allows for once-daily oral administration. Because of their lower lipid solubility, they are less able to cross the blood–brain barrier. Some "cardioselective" agents (*e.g.*, ***metoprolol*** and ***atenolol***) are more selective for β_1 receptors and can be administered cautiously to persons with asthma. However, these drugs may cause β_2 mediated bronchoconstriction at higher doses or in sensitive individuals.

Acebutolol (Sectral), ***pindolol*** (Visken), ***carteolol*** (Cartrol), and ***penbutolol*** (Levatol) have some intrinsic activity at β-adrenergic receptors, and may cause less reduction in heart rate and cardiac output than other β-blockers. However, this action has not been demonstrated to be of significant advantage in any of the indications for these drugs. Acebutolol yields a pharmacologically active metabolite with a long plasma half-life. This may be of possible benefit in some indications, although once-daily dosing with any of the beta blockers often appears to be effective in the treatment of hypertension. ***Labetalol*** (Normodyne, Trandate) blocks both α- and β-receptors, and is reported to produce a greater incidence of orthostatic hypotension and sexual dysfunction. This agent can be effective in hypertensive emergencies (see discussion under that topic).

Timolol (Timoptic), ***levobunolol*** (Betagan), and ***betaxolol*** (Betoptic) are used topically on the conjunctivae to decrease intraocular pressure in chronic open angle glaucoma. In contrast to the cholinergic agonists, β-blockers cause little vision disturbance. Sufficient amounts of drug can be absorbed to produce characteristic systemic adverse reactions; thus these agents are subject to all the usual precautions for β-blockers (see below). ***Betaxolol*** is a selective β_1 receptor antagonist, while ***timolol*** and ***levobunolol*** are nonselective.

Esmolol (Brevibloc), administered only by IV infusion, is a cardioselective agent with rapid onset and brief duration of action. Extensively inactivated by an esterase found in erythrocytes, it is used for rapid short-term control of supraventricular tachycardias.

Since the β-blockers will suppress all physiological functions mediated by β-receptors, they have numerous side effects. Bradycardia, atrioventricular heart block, hypotension, heart failure, pulmonary edema, sexual dysfunction, fatigue, and cold hands and feet may develop. Caution is required in the presence of congestive heart failure, in which a high degree of β stimulation can be essential to maintaining circulation. Beta-blockers, except for those that are cardioselective, are contraindicated in persons susceptible to asthma since bronchoconstriction can occur. In persons with diabetes, β-blockers will suppress the signs and symptoms (tachycardia, tremor) of hypoglycemia. Agents that block β_2 receptors can enhance insulin-induced hypoglycemia and inhibit insulin release in response to hyperglycemia. Blockade of cardiac β-receptors can exacerbate bradycardia or atrioventricular (AV) heart block. The manifestations of thyrotoxicosis may be suppressed. Abrupt discontinuance of β-blockers can precipitate dysrhythmias, angina pectoris, rebound hypertension, and myocardial infarction. β-blockers can induce mental depression and may be contraindicated in persons with a history of this disorder. β-blockers are also contraindicated in peripheral vascular disease.

Beta-blockers interact with several types of drugs. Additional suppression of AV conduction occurs with digitalis, and of cardiac activity with catecholamine depletors (*e.g.*, reserpine), calcium channel blockers (*e.g.*, nifedipine), and other cardiac depressants. The actions of β-

TABLE 7-6. β-Adrenergic Antagonists

GENERIC NAME	TRADE NAME
Nonselective	
Nadolol	Corgard
Propranolol	Inderal
Timolol	Blocadren
Cardioselective	
Acebutolol	Sectral
Atenolol	Tenormin
Betanolol	Kerlone
Bisoprolol	Zebeta
Esmolol	Brevibloc
Metoprolol	Lopressor
Intrinsic Activity	
Carteolol	Cartrol
Penbutolol	Levatol
Pindolol	Visken
α Blockade	
Labetalol	Normodyne, Trandate
Ophthalmic	
Betaxolol	Betoptic
Levobunolol	Betagan
Timolol	Timoptic

agonists are blocked. Administration of MAO inhibitors (MAOI) must be terminated 2 weeks before β-antagonist therapy. Hepatic enzyme induction shortens the half-life of lipid soluble β-blockers, while cimetidine (Tagamet) prolongs their action.

Ganglionic Antagonists

Although ganglionic blocking agents will interrupt transmission through both parasympathetic and sympathetic ganglia, they are used most frequently to reduce blood pressure by suppressing the sympathetic branch of the autonomic nervous system. ***Mecamylamine*** (Inversine) is occasionally administered orally in the management of severe hypertension. ***Trimethaphan*** is a short-acting agent infused IV to produce controlled hypotension during surgery or to alleviate hypertensive emergencies. Blood pressure must be monitored, and drug administration is reduced gradually to prevent rebound hypertension. Preexisting cardiovascular disorders, especially those exacerbated by decreased tissue perfusion, mandate the use of caution when ganglionic blockers are used. Orthostatic hypotension is a prominent side effect; others are manifestations of parasympathetic blockade: decreased gastrointestinal and urinary tract tone, pupillary dilation, dry mouth, and exacerbation of glaucoma. Trimethaphan releases histamine from tissue storage sites such as mast cells. Mecamylamine crosses the blood–brain barrier and may induce hallucinations, tremor, and convulsions through central nervous system stimulation. Renal impairment increases mecamylamine toxicity. The hypotensive action of the ganglionic blockers is enhanced by concomitant administration of other drugs that cause a fall in blood pressure. Vasopressor agents such as the α-adrenergic agonists phenylephrine and mephenteramine can reverse excessive hypotension.

Other ganglionic blockers include ***pempidine*** (Perolysen), ***pentolinium*** (Ansolysen), and ***chlorisondamine*** (Ecolid). Nicotine will stimulate and then block ganglionic nicotinic receptors.

DRUGS AFFECTING SKELETAL MUSCLE

Neuromuscular Junction Blockers

Neuromuscular junction (NMJ, Table 7-7) blockers interact with nicotinic receptors to interrupt the flow of impulses from the somatic nervous system to the motor end plate of skeletal and respiratory muscle. Two types of blockers are available. Nondepolarizing or competitive blockers can be reversed by agents that increase or mimic acetylcholine at the receptors. Depolarizing blockers produce sustained nonresponsiveness of muscle fibers that is intensified by acetylcholine or its analogues. Both types of agents produce flaccid paralysis and can cause respiratory arrest. Facial muscles are affected at low doses of drug, then the extremities, and, finally, at high doses, the diaphragm ceases to function.

TABLE 7-7. Neuromuscular Junction Blockers

GENERIC NAME	TRADE NAME
Nondepolarizing	
Atracurium	Tracrium
Doxacurium	Nuromax
Gallamine	Flaxedil
Mivacurium	Mivacron
Pancuronium	Pavulon
Pipecuronium	Arduan
Rocuronium	Zemuron
Tubocurarine	Tubocuraine
Vecuronium	Norcuron
Depolarizing	
Succinylcholine	Anectine

d-Tubocurarine and dimethyl tubocurarine (***metocurine***, Metubine) are nondepolarizing analogues of the alkaloid curare. Metocurine has a shorter onset and greater effect than *d*-tubocurarine. These agents have some blocking action at the ganglionic nicotinic receptors, and also cause histamine release that will result in bronchoconstriction and hypotension. ***Pancuronium*** (Pavulon) is more potent than the alkaloid derivatives, has a more rapid onset of action, and is relatively free of histamine-releasing properties. Its vagolytic actions may result in significant tachycardia and hypertension. ***Pipecuronium*** (Arduan) and ***doxacurium*** (Nuromax) are long-acting nondepolarizing NMJ blockers reported to have minimal cardiovascular effects. ***Gallamine*** (Flaxedil) also does not release histamine, and has a shorter duration of action. It also has vagolytic effects and can induce tachycardia that may be hazardous in cardiovascular disorders. ***Vecuronium*** (Norcuron) and ***atracurium*** (Tracrium) are relatively short acting blockers with low incidence of side effects. ***Mivacurium*** (Mivacron) has a short duration, can release histamine, and is inactivated by plasma cholinesterase. At high doses, ***rocuronium*** (Zemuron) has the most rapid onset of the nondepolarizing NMJ blockers, but also has a long duration of action.

Succinylcholine (Anectine) is the most frequently used depolarizing NMJ blocker. Initial depolarization of the motor end plate will cause fasciculations. Subsequent nonresponsiveness of the receptors yields irreversible paralysis. Despite its potentially more dangerous adverse effects (*e.g.*, hyperkalemia, malignant hyperthermia, and cardiac arrest), succinylcholine has the advantages of faster onset and shorter duration, compared with the nondepolarizing blockers.

NMJ blockers are used during surgery to provide deep muscle relaxation to accompany those general anesthetics that do not have this capability. Short-acting NMJ paralysis facilitates endotracheal intubation, and will protect patients from injury during electroconvulsive shock therapy. These agents may also be used in the management of patients on mechanical ventilation. Administration is usually by the IV route, although IM injection can be used if it is more appropriate.

Except for atracurium and mivacurium, which are inactivated in plasma, the nondepolarizing agents are excreted renally and thus will have a prolonged plasma half-life in the presence of kidney dysfunction. Succinylcholine is usually rapidly inactivated by a plasma cholinesterase that is genetically defective in some persons, who will experience intense and persistent muscle paralysis. Dehydration and electrolyte imbalance (*e.g.*, potassium depletion, acidosis) can alter responsiveness to NMJ blockers. These drugs are usually contraindicated in patients with myasthenia gravis and respiratory depression. The intensity of NMJ blockade is enhanced by calcium, magnesium, general anesthetics, antibiotics (*e.g.*, aminoglycosides, polymixins, tetracyclines) that depress myoneuronal transmission, and drugs having a membrane-stabilizing or local anesthetic effect. Preadministration of nondepolarizing blockers will prevent the effects of succinylcholine, probably by blocking its interaction with receptors. On the other hand, nondepolarizing blockers given after succinylcholine will intensify paralysis. Patients who have received NMJ blockers can be completely paralyzed and unable to communicate yet may be fully aware of their surroundings. Means for mechanical respiration must be immediately available when these drugs are used. Succinylcholine may cause malignant hyperthermia that can usually be controlled with dantrolene (Dantrium). Succinylcholine is contraindicated in open-eye injuries and glaucoma. Administration during labor and delivery may cause apnea and muscle flaccidity in the neonate.

Skeletal Muscle Relaxants

Skeletal muscle relaxants will alleviate painful spasm induced by injury and by musculoskeletal disorders such as cerebral palsy, multiple sclerosis, and inflammation. These agents are often used in conjunction with rest, heat, physical therapy, and analgesics. Some have sedative and anxiolytic properties that possibly contribute to reduction in muscle tension. A placebo effect may also be involved.

Baclofen (Lioresal) is an analog of ***gamma aminobutyric acid*** *(GABA),* an inhibitory neurotransmitter in the central nervous system. Although its mechanism of action is uncertain, it crosses the blood–brain barrier and appears to reduce reflex efferent motor stimuli. It is well absorbed from the oral route and is excreted renally largely as unchanged drug. Baclofen administered intrathecally is especially useful in alleviating the spasticity of multiple sclerosis and spinal cord injury. The gradual diffusion of the drug in the cerebrospinal fluid results in a slow onset of action. Respiratory support may be required. Malfunction of the pump can result in overdose or abrupt termination of drug, the latter leading to increased spasticity, seizures, and hallucinations. The seizure threshold in persons with convulsive disorders may be lowered. Side effects that can be minimized by cautious drug administration include drowsiness, confusion, mood alterations, hypotension, and nausea.

Chlorzoxazone (Paraflex), and ***carisoprodal*** (Rela, Soma), which is structurally related to the antianxiety drug meprobamate, may induce muscle relaxation due to their sedative actions. Drug dependence can develop to carisoprodal, which has also been reported to induce an idiosyncratic reaction characterized by extreme muscle weakness, confusion, and ataxia. Chlorzoxazone can be hepatotoxic, and both drugs may provoke allergic responses.

Benzodiazepines such as diazepam, chlordiazepoxide, and clonazepam are used as skeletal muscle relaxants. These agents are sedative and anxiolytic, and also appear to inhibit polysynaptic reflexes in the spinal cord. The pharmacology of these drugs is discussed in the section Antianxiety Agents.

Dantrolene (Dantrium) is a peripherally acting skeletal muscle relaxant that blocks calcium availability and utilization and thus ''uncouples'' muscle contraction from stimulation. Intravenous administration of dantrolene is an important adjunct to supportive measures in malignant hyperthermia induced by neuroleptic or general anesthetic agents, and can be given orally to prevent this medical emergency in susceptible persons. It is hepatotoxic and thus contraindicated in persons with liver disorders. Drowsiness, weakness, and diarrhea that can be severe are frequent adverse effects. Respiratory impairment can be exacerbated. Dantrolene has a long (up to 9 hours) plasma half-life, binds to plasma proteins, and is metabolized hepatically.

Administration of central nervous system depressants, including alcohol, concurrently with the skeletal muscle relaxants is generally contraindicated. Caution is also advised in patients who are dependent upon some degree of muscle rigidity to walk or perform other daily activities.

Interferon beta-1b given SC can decrease the number and severity of attacks in mild-to-moderate relapsing-remitting multiple sclerosis. A flu-like syndrome and reactions at the injection site are the most common adverse effects.

PSYCHOTHERAPEUTIC AGENTS

Major psychiatric disturbances are categorized into psychotic (*e.g.*, schizophrenic) and effective (*e.g.*, depressive) disorders. A significant number of psychiatric patients will respond to neuroleptic and antidepressant drugs, although many require long-term treatment to keep symptoms under control. The causes of psychiatric disorders are not fully understood. The observation that specific central nervous system neurotransmitter systems are altered by psychotherapeutic agents has generated biochemical theories for the evolution of these disorders. Many drugs induce mental changes and must be ruled out as possible causes when psychiatric disturbances are diagnosed.

Antidepressants

Although the selective serotonin reuptake inhibitors (SSRI) have become widely used for mild-to-moderate depression, the tricyclic antidepressants (TCA) continue to be clinically important antidepressant drugs, especially for severe depression. Suppressed inactivation of central nervous system neurotransmitters, norepinephrine and serotonin in particular, appears to play a role in the mechanism of action of these agents. The original ''amine hypothesis'' of depression proposed that a deficit in these neurotransmitters resulted in depressed mood. However, the inhibition of transmitter inactivation occurs rapidly, while clinical effects develop over several weeks. More recent studies have indicated that most if not all antidepressant agents, including electroconvulsive therapy, cause a slowly evolving decrease or down-regulation in β-adrenergic receptor density that may be related to their therapeutic efficacy.

TRICYCLIC ANTIDEPRESSANTS

The TCA (Table 7-8) inhibit presynaptic reuptake of norepinephrine or serotonin, or both. The onset of therapeutic effectiveness is delayed for 3 weeks or longer, and patients may need encouragement to continue taking a drug when they are experiencing no apparent benefit. Severely depressed patients may require hospitalization during this time, and electroconvulsive therapy can provide a more rapid antidepressant effect. If necessary, drug doses can be gradually increased, with time allowed for a therapeutic response. Studies have suggested that treatment of depression is often abandoned before adequate dosages and time intervals are achieved.

The therapeutic usefulness of the TCA is limited at times by their adverse effects. The intensity of anticholinergic activity varies among these agents. Most can cause the characteristic side effects discussed earlier in this chapter, and are subject to the usual precautions and contraindications for anticholinergic drugs. High drug doses can induce central nervous system symptoms such as confusion, convulsions, delirium, and coma. The anticholinesterase physostigmine will reverse many of these effects, and diazepam can be given IV to terminate convulsions. Elderly persons in particular are at risk of TCA-induced anticholinergic toxicity.

The α-adrenergic blocking action of the TCA probably accounts for their ability to cause orthostatic hypotension and nasal congestion. Sedation is a prominent adverse effect, although the degree of drowsiness produced differs among the TCA. Since these drugs have a long duration of action (up to 72 hours), this effect can often be minimized or used to advantage by giving most or all of the daily dose at bedtime.

Cardiac toxicity is most likely to appear after TCA overdose or in persons with preexisting cardiovascular disease. TCA depress cardiac conduction in a manner similar to the antidysrhythmic agent quinidine. A widening of the QRS interval is characteristic of TCA toxicity. Severe bradycardia or tachycardia as well as cardiac failure can develop. Lidocaine or propranolol may control rhythm disturbances. Small doses of TCA can induce lethal cardiotoxicity in children.

Therapeutic doses of TCA can provoke seizures, especially in persons with convulsive disorders. Other central

TABLE 7-8. Antidepressant Drugs

GENERIC NAME	TRADE NAME
Tricyclic Antidepressants	
Amitriptyline	Elavil
Desipramine	Norpramine, Pertofrane
Doxepin	Adapin, Sinequan
Imipramine	Tofranil
Nortriptyline	Aventyl, Pamelor
Protriptyline	Vivactil
Trimipramine	Surmontil
Clomipramine	Anafranil
Second-Generation Antidepressants	
Amoxapine	Asendin
Bupropion	Wellbutrin
Maprotiline	Ludiomil
Venlafaxine	Effexor
Trazodone	Desyrel
Nefazodone	Serzone
Monoamine Oxidase Inhibitors	
Isocarboxazid	Marplan
Pheneizine	Nardil
Tranylcypromine	Parnate
Selective Serotonin Reuptake Inhibitors	
Fluoxetine	Prozac
Sertraline	Zoloft
Paroxetine	Paxil
Fluvoxamine	Luvox

nervous system effects include panic reactions, mania, hostility, insomnia, and exacerbation of psychosis. Extrapyramidal disorders such as parkinsonism and tardive dyskinesia can develop. Increased appetite and weight gain, endocrine changes, sexual dysfunction, and gastrointestinal discomfort are additional adverse effects.

The TCA are hepatically biotransformed, some to metabolites that also possess antidepressant activity. Extensive binding to plasma proteins occurs.

Drug interactions are numerous. Central nervous system depressants, including alcohol, will enhance the sedative action of TCA. Other anticholinergic drugs will add to the suppression of the parasympathetic nervous system. Sympathomimetic amines that are transported by the presynaptic reuptake mechanism will be potentiated, while peripherally acting antihypertensive agents such as guanethidine and guanadrel will be less effective. Elevated serum levels of thyroid hormones (either endogenous or exogenous) can increase the risk of cardiac dysrhythmias. Although the combination of TCA and monoamine oxidase inhibitors (MAOI) can be hazardous, skillful concomitant administration of these two types of antidepressants is often effective in persons with refractory illness. Both drugs may be instituted simultaneously, although greater safety is probably ensured if the TCA is begun first, followed by careful administration of an MAOI. Cardiovascular responses must be monitored, and dietary restrictions relative to MAOI therapy (see below) must be observed. Abrupt termination of TCA may cause headache, gastrointestinal disturbance, and other withdrawal effects.

The so-called "second-generation" antidepressants (see Table 7-8), although related to the TCA, do differ in some important aspects. ***Trazodone*** interacts with serotonin receptors, causes less cardiotoxic and anticholinergic action, and can be combined with other antidepressants. ***Nefazodone***, related to trazodone, decreases reuptake of and blocks receptors for serotonin and norepinephrine and blocks α-adrenergic receptors. Extensive first-pass hepatic metabolism produces three active metabolites. Taking nefazodone with food can decrease the bioavailability of this drug. Trazodone and nefazodone cause sedation, headache, dizziness, nausea, dry mouth, blurred vision, hypotension, and sexual dysfunction (priapism also is reported, especially with trazodone). Nefazodone inhibits inactivation of some benzodiazepines and of terfenadine and astemizole; the latter two drugs are antihistamines occasionally associated with potentially lethal ventricular dysrhythmias. ***Maprotiline*** has a marked tendency to provoke seizures. ***Clomipramine*** (Anafranil) is used to manage obsessive-compulsive disorder. Bupropion has a lower incidence of anticholinergic and cardiovascular effects and sexual dysfunction than does TCA. ***Venlafaxine*** is chemically related to bupropion, inhibits norepinephrine and serotonin reuptake, and has adverse effects similar to the SSRI. It has less anticholinergic action, but can cause dry mouth and constipation. Sustained diastolic blood pressure elevation is reported, especially with high doses. Drugs that inhibit cytochrome P450 may decrease venlafaxine biotransformation. ***Amoxapine***, structurally related to the neuroleptic loxapine, has antipsychotic efficacy and may be especially useful when agitation or psychosis coexists with depression. It can, however, cause characteristic neuroleptic effects such as malignant hyperthermia and extrapyramidal disturbances.

SELECTIVE SEROTONIN REUPTAKE INHIBITORS

Fluoxetine (Prozac), the first of the SSRI (see Table 7-8), rapidly became the most frequently prescribed antidepressant in the United States. The side-effect profile of these agents differs from that of other antidepressants. Nervousness, insomnia, nausea, headache, and weight loss are characteristic, while orthostatic hypotension, cardiac toxicity, and anticholinergic effects are less. Seizures, sexual dysfunction, and extrapyramidal effects may occur; reports of increased incidence of violent behavior have appeared. Fluoxetine and its active metabolite have long plasma half-lives; care must be taken when it is administered in the presence of decreased hepatic function. Like tricyclics, the onset of action can be several weeks. Several drug interactions have been reported. The toxicity of digoxin, warfarin, and tricyclics can be increased. Concomitant lithium, haloperidol, or carbamazepine may cause adverse neurological responses. Monoamine oxidase (MAO) inhibitors must be avoided, as hyperpyrexia, convulsions, coma, and death may result. Because of its side effect of weight loss, fluoxetine may be of brief benefit in weight-reduction programs. ***Sertraline*** (Zoloft) has a shorter half-life than fluoxetine and its active metabolite. Taking it with food will increase the bioavailability of sertraline, which is extensively bound to plasma proteins. Unlike fluoxetine, sertraline has little effect on the cytochrome P450 enzymes and thus fewer interactions with other drugs. ***Paroxetine*** (Paxil) undergoes extensive first-pass biotransformation, generally to inactive metabolites. It inhibits cytochrome P450 and thus has a greater risk of drug interactions than sertraline. Paroxetine enters breast milk in large quantity. ***Fluvoxamine*** (Luvox), like fluoxetine and clomipramine, ameliorates obsessive-compulsive behavior. Drug interactions are similar to those of fluoxetine: plasma levels of many drugs are elevated.

Of special note is the "serotonin syndrome," which can occur when serotonergic drugs and MAOI interact. Autonomic instability, confusion, delirium, hyperpyrexia, convulsions, coma, and death can occur. MAOI

TABLE 7-9. Foods Contraindicated by Administration of Monoamine Oxidase Inhibitors

Aged cheese
Beer
Wines (*e.g.*, Chianti)
Chicken liver
Bananas
Avocados
Broad beans
Soy products
Preserved meats
Protein supplements and extracts
Meat tenderizers
Chocolate
Caffeine (in excess)

require a two-week washout interval; two weeks is also needed for sertraline and paroxetine; two to three weeks is needed for fluvoxamine; and five weeks is needed for fluoxetine.

MONOAMINE OXIDASE INHIBITORS

Although the MAOI are effective antidepressants, they have been consigned to second-line status by their characteristic potential for provoking hypertensive episodes when certain foods or drugs are ingested concurrently. The MAOI irreversibly inhibit the enzymatic deamination of many amines, including the catecholamines. Thus they, like the TCA, enhance the availability of norepinephrine and serotonin at the synapse. Because new enzyme synthesis is required to overcome the action of MAOI, their effects can persist up to 14 days.

Common adverse effects include orthostatic hypotension, confusion, insomnia, dry mouth, blurred vision, sexual dysfunction, mania, and alterations in cardiac rhythm. Severe hepatotoxicity can occur. The MAOI are usually not administered in the presence of hypertension, cerebrovascular disorders, or renal or hepatic dysfunction. Abrupt discontinuation of MAOI may cause tachycardia, insomnia, nightmares, and psychotic reactions. Drug overdose can induce muscular hyperexcitability, hyperthermia, convulsions, marked changes in blood pressure and heart rate, and cardiovascular collapse.

Ingestion of pressor amines when MAO is inhibited can result in hypertensive crisis. Many over-the-counter cold remedies and appetite suppressants contain α-adrenergic stimulants, and many foods (Table 7-9) contain tyramine. Catecholamines or their precursors, or substances that release these agents or sensitize the myocardium to their effects can be hazardous, as are any drugs that affect inactivation pathways for neurotransmitters such as norepinephrine and serotonin. Many such drugs, (*e.g.*, other antidepressants) have long durations of action that must be considered when drug regimens are changed. Meperidine (Demerol) is contraindicated, since it may trigger potentially fatal hyperpyrexic reactions in the presence of MAOI. Dosages of other narcotic analgesics should be reduced, since MAOI potentiate their actions. MAOI are hepatically inactivated and will interfere with the metabolism of many drugs. Concomitant use of hypotensive agents such as diuretics and spinal anesthesia may induce a marked fall in blood pressure.

ADDITIONAL AGENTS

Lithium carbonate is effective in preventing and ameliorating the manic aspects of bipolar affective disorder. It is also reported to have antidepressant action and to enhance the efficacy of TCA and MAOI. The mechanism of lithium's action appears to be linked to an ability to decrease phosphoinositide turnover, which is an important biochemical pathway involved in transmembrane signaling by neurotransmitter receptors.

Lithium is excreted renally, in direct proportion to levels of filtered sodium. Thus, sodium depletion (*e.g.*, that induced by chronic diuretic administration) will promote retention of lithium. The plasma half-life of lithium is also prolonged in the elderly and in persons with renal dysfunction. Large amounts of lithium may be required to control manic behavior. Dosages should then be reduced to maintenance levels. Onset of action of lithium is slow (2–4 weeks), thus acute mania may be treated initially with antipsychotics or benzodiazepines.

Lithium has a low therapeutic index. Plasma concentrations must be monitored; the range of 0.6 to 1.0 mEg/liter is generally effective with acceptable risk for adverse effects. Elderly persons in particular may experience toxicity at levels as low as 0.4 mEq/liter. Adverse effects include nausea, severe diarrhea, weakness, tremor, ataxia, confusion, weight gain, fatigue, thirst, frequent urination (polyuria), nephrogenic diabetes insipidus, cardiac dysrhythmias, circulatory failure, seizures, changes in thyroid function leukocytosis, and teratogenicity (cardiac abnormalities). Lithium may increase the central nervous system toxicity of neuroleptics, including haloperidol, fluphenazine, thioridazine, and clozapine. Nonsteroidal antiinflammatory drugs (NSAID) can impede renal excretion of lithium. The anticonvulsants ***carbamazepine*** (Tegretol) and valproic acid (Depakene, Depakote) can alleviate severe refractory manic episodes.

Neuroleptics

Antipsychotic or neuroleptic agents will alleviate symptoms of schizophrenic disorders, and will calm aggressive and agitated behavior. Generally, the so-called positive

TABLE 7-10. Neuroleptic Drugs

GENERIC NAME	TRADE NAME
Phenothiazines	
Acetophenazine	Tindal
Carphenazine	Proketazine
Chlorpromazine	Thorazine
Fluphenazine	Permitil, Prolixin
Mesoridazine	Serentil
Perphenazine	Trilafon
Prochlorperazine	Compazine
Promazine	Sparine
Thioridazine	Mellaril
Trifluorperazine	Stelazine
Triflupromazine	Vesprin
Thioxanthenes	
Chlorprothixene	Taractan
Thiothixene	Navane
Butyrophenone	
Haloperidol	Haldol
Additional Agents	
Clozapine	Clozaril
Loxapine	Loxitane
Molindone	Moban
Pimozide	Orap
Risperidone	Risperdol

symptoms are more responsive to standard neuroleptics than are "negative" symptoms. Although these drugs do not cure psychoses, they often reduce the need for institutional care and enable patients to maintain relatively stable lives. The observation that clinically effective neuroleptics are dopamine receptor antagonists has yielded the hypothesis that enhanced dopaminergic activity in the central nervous system underlies schizophrenic behavior. Amphetamines, which stimulate dopamine receptors, can induce psychotic behavior that closely resembles schizophrenia.

Neuroleptics are classified mainly into three chemical groups (Table 7-10). Antipsychotic activity was first recognized in the phenothiazines; chlorpromazine is the prototype drug against which other neuroleptic agents are compared. The exact site of antipsychotic action is not known. However, the limbic system of the central nervous system has been proposed as the site of action because of its participation in emotional responsiveness and its rich dopaminergic innervation. Chronic administration of neuroleptics is often required to prevent recurrence of symptoms.

Side effects of the ***phenothiazines*** are numerous. Marked sedation is characteristic of many agents in this group, although tolerance can develop to this effect. Their anticholinergic action makes the neuroleptics subject to all the precautions and contraindications that pertain to drugs with parasympatholytic action. Blockade of α-adrenergic receptors induces nasal congestion and orthostatic hypotension. Severe reduction in blood pressure can occur in elderly or debilitated persons. Tachycardia, bradycardia, electrocardiographic (ECG) changes, and cardiac arrest have been reported.

The phenothiazines exert an antiemetic effect via suppression of the central chemoreceptor trigger zone. They are used in particular to suppress vomiting induced by antineoplastic and general anesthetic agents. Paradoxically, they do not suppress vestibular emesis (*e.g.*, motion sickness) despite their antihistaminic action.

Extrapyramidal disturbances believed to result from dopamine receptor blockade or subsequent hypersensitivity occur frequently with neuroleptics. Parkinsonism, acute dystonias, and motor restlessness (akathisia) may develop early in treatment and can usually be controlled by reduction or termination of neuroleptic, or by administration of antiparkinson drugs or the antihistamine diphenhydramine. Beta-blockers and benzodiazepines have also been used to alleviate akathisia. The most troublesome extrapyramidal response is tardive dyskinesia: choreiform movements usually involving facial muscles. Characteristic of chronic administration of neuroleptics, this syndrome is usually irreversible and does not respond to antiparkinsonism drugs. Tardive dyskinesia may not appear until drug administration is terminated, and can be precipitated or exacerbated by abrupt discontinuance of a neuroleptic. Simultaneous administration of antiparkinson drugs may mask the early symptoms that should prompt gradual drug withdrawal. To decrease the risk for tardive dyskinesia, the lowest effective dose of neuroleptic should be given.

The ability of neuroleptics to alter temperature regulatory control can be especially hazardous in elderly persons. Fatal hyperthermia (neuroleptic malignant syndrome) has been reported at normal and elevated ambient temperatures. Hypothermia also can occur. Bone marrow depression, lowering of seizure threshold, weight gain, obstructive jaundice, hyperprolactinemia, and other endocrine changes are additional adverse effects. Neuroleptic agents can add to the effects of anticholinergic and central nervous system depressant drugs. Because they are dopamine receptor antagonists, neuroleptics counteract antiparkinsonism agents and are contraindicated in this neurological disorder. Neuroleptics administered simultaneously with drugs such as lithium and digitalis may mask the nausea that warns of impending toxicity. The major site of neuroleptic inactivation is the liver, where several enzymatic pathways produce water-soluble metabolites.

The ***thioxanthenes*** are quite similar in structure and have much the same pharmacology as the phenothiazines. The butyrophenone ***haloperidol*** does not differ markedly, although sedation and adrenergic and cholinergic antagonism may be less than that occurring with other neuroleptics. ***Haloperidol*** will suppress the manifestations of Tourette's syndrome. ***Molindone*** and ***loxapine*** are additional agents used in the treatment of schizophrenia; their actions are quite similar to other neuroleptics. Loxapine appears to pose considerable risk for convulsive episodes.

Clozapine (Clozaril) has less risk for extrapyramidal effects but can cause fatal agranulocytosis. Its use is restricted to persons who are refractory to or cannot tolerate standard neuroleptics. White cell counts must be monitored closely throughout treatment with this drug. If the total leukocyte count is below $3{,}000/mm^2$ or the granulocyte count is below $1{,}500/mm^2$, drug administration should be interrupted until counts recover. Counts below $2{,}000/mm^2$ or $1{,}000/mm^2$, respectively, suggest that clozapine be permanently terminated. Granulocyte colony-stimulating factor may alleviate clozapine-induced agranulocytosis. Other adverse effects include seizures, anticholinergic action, weight gain, dizziness, sedation, hypotension (orthostatic in particular), tachycardia, and transient hyperthermia. Pancreatitis and priapism may occur. Cimetidine taken concurrently can decrease the rate of biotransformation of clozapine. Lithium combined with clozapine has caused involuntary movement, tremor, confusion, poor concentration, and memory deficit. Simultaneous administration of carbamazepine and clozapine may increase the risk for neuroleptic malignant syndrome; simultaneous benzodiazepines may cause respiratory arrest.

Risperidone (Risperdol) binds to serotonin 5-HT_2, dopamine D_2, histamine H_1, and α-adrenergic receptors. This drug may have a more rapid (one-week) onset of action than other neuroleptics (*e.g.,* haloperidol) and appears to be more effective in alleviating negative symptoms such as apathy, blunted affect, and social withdrawal. The risk for extrapyramidal toxicity may be lower with risperidone. This drug is extensively biotransformed by the hepatic cytochrome P450 system to the active metabolite 9-hydroxyrisperidone. Side effects include sedation, poor concentration, orthostatic hypotension, weakness, weight gain, increased serum prolactin, and sexual dysfunction.

Antianxiety Agents

Benzodiazepines (Table 7-11) are frequently prescribed to alleviate emotional and somatic symptoms of overwhelming anxieties. They are best utilized only for brief periods of time, since chronic administration of high doses can lead to psychological and physiological dependence, and tolerance develops to their effects. (Benzodiazepines are Schedule IV controlled substances.) Patients should be encouraged to resolve anxiety provoking situations, or to investigate nondrug modalities for coping with those that cannot be eliminated. Prior to the development of the benzodiazepines, the barbiturates were used as antianxiety agents and daytime sedatives, but frequently produced an unacceptable degree of drowsiness. The benzodiazepines have a more favorable therapeutic index, producing less general central nervous system depression when used in recommended doses and not combined with other depressants. Benzodiazepines are also used clinically as skeletal muscle relaxants, hypnotics, anticonvulsants, and as presurgical sedatives. The benzodiazepine mechanism of action may involve the ability to enhance the affinity of GABA for its central nervous system binding sites. This inhibitory neurotransmitter increases the influx of chloride ions through cell membrane channels and thus inhibits membrane depolarization.

TABLE 7-11. Benzodiazepines

GENERIC NAME	TRADE NAME
Antianxiety Agents	
Alprazolam	Xanax
Chlorazepate	Tranxene
Chlordiazepoxide	Librium
Diazepam	Valium
Halazepam	Paxipam
Lorazepam	Ativan
Oxazepam	Serax
Prazepam	Centrax
Sedatives	
Estazolam	ProSom
Flurazepam	Dalmane
Midazolam	Versed
Quazepam	Doral
Temazepam	Restoril
Triazolam	Halcion
Zolpidem	Ambien

Benzodiazepines are well absorbed from the gastrointestinal tract but less so from IM sites. The onset of therapeutic action is gradual; several days may be required to attain good anxiolytic effect. Some benzodiazepines (*e.g.,* ***diazepam***, ***lorazepam***, and ***chlordiazepoxide***) are available in IV form. Changes in blood pressure, respiration, and heart rate may occur when this route is used. Respiratory and cardiac arrest have been reported following IV diazepam. Extensive hepatic metabolism converts benzodiazepines to a variety of metabolites including *n*-desalkylated and hydroxylated compounds and glucuronide conjugates. Several of these metabolites are pharmacologically active and serve to prolong the duration of action. In persons with decreased hepatic function (*e.g.,* the elderly) drugs such as diazepam and ***halazepam*** will produce extended periods of sedation.

Benzodiazepines appear to exert their greatest depressant action in the limbic system. However, these agents can elicit a significant degree of sedation, especially at the initiation of therapy. Driving a car or operating machinery can be hazardous activities for persons taking benzodiazepines. Anterograde impairment of memory has been reported with benzodiazepines. Concomitant use of other central nervous system depressants, including alcohol, can markedly potentiate central nervous system suppression to produce coma, respiratory failure, and death. Preexisting respiratory impairment greatly increases the risk of severe respiratory depression. Cross-tolerance in the mechanism of physiological dependence to alcohol and benzodiazepines enables the latter drugs to alleviate symptoms of the alcohol withdrawal syndrome. Long-acting agents such as diazepam and ***chlordiazepoxide*** are most useful in this context. Paradoxically, benzodiazepines have occasionally caused central nervous system stimulation resulting in confusion, delirium, and aggressive behavior. Abrupt termination of benzodiazepines can result in withdrawal characterized by anxiety, irritability, insomnia, nausea, muscle cramps, delirium, and occasional seizures. ***Estazolam, triazolam,*** and ***alprazolam*** appear to have greater toxicity and to produce more difficult withdrawal.

Some benzodiazepines are valuable for the alleviation of insomnia (see Table 7-11). These drugs prolong sleep stages 1 and 2 and shorten stages 3 and 4 and REM sleep. Agitation and aggressive behavior can result from REM deprivation. ***Flurazepam*** rapidly induces sleep but can cause persistent daytime drowsiness. ***Temazepam*** has a slower onset and a longer duration, making it advantageous for persons who have difficulty maintaining adequate sleep time. ***Triazolam*** has a short duration and is especially useful in patients whose difficulty is in falling asleep. However, early morning awakening can occur. Abrupt discontinuance of these hypnotics may occasionally induce "rebound" REM sleep, nightmares, and anxiety.

Zolpidem (Ambien) is structurally different from the benzodiazepines but binds to the benzodiazepine receptors. Lacking significant anxiolytic or anticonvulsant action, it is used only for induction and maintenance of sleep. It does not decrease stages 3 and 4 or REM sleep. Metabolized in the liver, its half-life of 2.5 hours is prolonged in persons with impaired hepatic function, including the elderly who are especially vulnerable to confusion and falls following high doses. Other adverse effects are nausea, diarrhea, headache, dizziness, persistent daytime sedation, and occasional anterograde amnesia. Termination of drug administration may cause mild rebound insomnia. Although zolpidem has little abuse potential, this drug is a Schedule IV controlled substance. Central nervous system depressants combined with zolpidem can be lethal. The benzodiazepine antagonist flumazenil reverses zolpidem's effects.

Midazolam is a rapid-acting parenteral benzodiazepine that provides sedation for brief diagnostic procedures and before surgery, and induction for general anesthesia. It can be mixed in solution with perioperative opiates and anticholinergics. (Diazepam is incompatible with most drugs.) Respiratory depression and occasional failure can occur. Hypotension can be especially severe when the opiate fentanyl (Sublimaze) is administered concurrently.

Alprazolam is unique among benzodiazepines in its reported antidepressant action and it may be effective in panic disorder. Other benzodiazepines are not recommended for patients with notable depression or psychosis, which may be exacerbated.

Flumazenil (Mazicon), a selective benzodiazepine receptor antagonist, is used to reverse sedation following clinical administration or overdose of benzodiazepines. Flumazenil is rapidly metabolized in the liver (its half-life is one hour), and significant resedation may occur, especially following administration of longer-acting benzodiazepines (*e.g.*, diazepam). Patients should be monitored, and flumazenil readministered if necessary. Flumazenil may be less effective in reversing benzodiazepine-induced respiratory depression. It has no effect on central nervous system depression induced by drugs other than benzodiazepines, except when these drugs are taken in combination with benzodiazepines. In such instances, the benzodiazepine component, which intensifies central nervous system depression, is reduced. Treatment of tricyclic antidepressant plus benzodiazepine overdose with flumazenil may result in seizures as the anticonvulsant action of the benzodiazepine is reversed and the seizure-inducing action of the tricyclic becomes predominant. Adverse effects of flumazenil include headache, dizziness, nausea, blurred vision, anxiety, and possibly cardiac arrhythmias. Persons physically dependent on benzodiazepines or with epilepsy controlled with benzodiazepine administration may develop seizures if flumazenil is given.

Meprobamate (Equanil, Miltown), introduced as a skeletal muscle relaxant, was the first of the "modern" antianxiety agents but has subsequently been largely replaced by the benzodiazepines. This drug causes drowsiness, hypotension, and occasional hematological disturbances. REM sleep is suppressed. Tolerance and physical dependence can develop. Drug overdose produces respiratory depression, shock, and pulmonary edema.

Buspirone (BuSpar), a nonbenzodiazepine anxiolytic, has a long (up to 4 weeks) onset of action. Sedation and impairment of motor skills are not induced by this drug, nor is the depressant action of alcohol enhanced. Dizziness, headache, restlessness, and dysphoria have been reported. Buspirone interacts with serotonin and dopamine receptors in the central nervous system. Persons who have used benzodiazepines may not respond to buspirone: its lack of sedative action may serve to dissuade patients of its benefit. Buspirone is rapidly extracted from the portal circulation and inactivated hepatically. It binds extensively to plasma proteins and may displace digoxin.

SEDATIVES AND HYPNOTICS

Insomnia, or difficulty in falling asleep or maintaining adequate sleep, is a not uncommon disorder that can severely compromise physiological and psychological well-being. Attempts must be made to determine the cause(s) for sleep disturbance, and to alleviate problems through nonpharmacological measures. Drugs should be used only when other means are unsuccessful, and only for brief periods of time. Tolerance rapidly develops to the sleep-inducing action of sedatives and hypnotics, and chronic use may lead to psychological and physiological drug dependence.

A variety of drugs are used for promoting sleep. Ideally, such drugs should have a rapid onset of action, a duration of 7 to 8 hours (to sustain a full night's sleep), and no adverse effects that persist into the following day. Unfortunately, no single agent possesses all of these characteristics. Many sedatives produce a daytime lethargy or "hangover." As central nervous system depressants, these drugs interact with other depressants including alcohol, and many can induce marked respiratory depression and cardiovascular insufficiency when used at high doses. When taken in overdose, either by accident or with suicidal intent, many of these agents are lethal. The benzodiazepines are the exception to this: overdoses can produce marked lethargy and somnolence, but are not reported to be fatal unless a second central nervous system depressant has been ingested concomitantly. For this reason, the benzodiazepines have largely replaced other hypnotic agents.

The "short to intermediate acting" barbiturates (*e.g.*, ***pentobarbital***, Nembutal; ***secobarbital***, Seconal; ***butabarbital***, Butisol; ***talbutal***, Lotusate) are still available for the management of insomnia. In contrast to the benzodiazepines, which appear to suppress discrete brain areas selectively, the barbiturates are general central nervous system depressants. However, the reticular activating system is particularly sensitive to the latter group of drugs. Both classes of sedatives appear to exert their effects through interaction with the inhibitory neurotransmitter GABA.

The ***barbiturates*** are controlled substances; their continual use induces psychological and physiological drug dependence similar to that of alcohol. Withdrawal can be severe; symptoms include delirium, hyperthermia, convulsions, hypotension, and cardiovascular failure. Deaths have been reported to occur during uncontrolled barbiturate withdrawal. Detoxification of dependent persons can be most safely accomplished by substituting gradually diminishing doses of a long-acting barbiturate such as phenobarbital. This is usually done in hospital under close observation. The dose of barbiturate can be increased slightly if withdrawal symptoms appear, and seizures can be controlled with IV diazepam.

The barbiturates, like many other hypnotic agents, suppress REM sleep. Although the exact physiological function of this aspect of sleep in which dreams take place has not been determined, REM deprivation results in sleep that is not restful, and in rebound REM once use of the suppressive agent is discontinued. Consequent unpleasant dreams or nightmares may cause patients to resume drug use.

The barbiturates have many additional adverse effects. Paradoxical excitation, confusion, and anxiety may occur, especially in children and the elderly. Gastrointestinal disturbances and suppression of respiration and cardiovascular function develop. Hypersensitivity reactions, in particular skin rashes that may be severe, are likely to occur in persons with allergies. Rarely, hematological abnormalities appear. Barbiturates can heighten the awareness of pain, although in combination with analgesics they ameliorate the apprehension provoked by pain and help to promote rest. Barbiturates are teratogenic, and can cause neonatal hemorrhage. Habitual use during later pregnancy results in neonatal drug dependency with an abstinence syndrome appearing shortly after birth. Administration of barbiturates during labor can suppress uterine contractions and lead to central nervous system and respiratory depression in the neonate. Nursing mothers who use barbiturates may find their infants excessively lethargic.

Overdose of barbiturates causes severe respiratory depression; supportive measures must be instituted rapidly to prevent fatalities. Symptoms include markedly depressed respiration, Cheyne-Stokes syndrome, hypotension, tachycardia, hypothermia, renal failure, and loss of consciousness. Maintenance of respiration with supplemental oxygen may minimize hypoxic tissue damage. Attempts should be made to retrieve any unabsorbed drug from the stomach. Intravenous fluids may ameliorate hypotension and shock. Mannitol diuresis or alkalinization of the urine will promote barbiturate excretion, unless renal failure has developed. Hemodialysis can assist in the removal of drug. Patients who survive intentional overdose of barbiturates (or other substances) must be offered psychological as well as physiological assistance. The abuse of these drugs is further discussed under that topic.

The barbiturates are metabolized in the liver, and are capable of inducing enzyme activity. This is the basis for the decreased effectiveness of many drugs (*e.g.*, oral anticoagulants, digitoxin, corticosteroids, tricyclic antidepressants, and estrogens including those contained in oral contraceptives) administered concurrently. When barbiturates are discontinued, patients receiving other hepatically inactivated drugs must be observed for signs of overdose. The MAOI enhance barbiturate action by delaying their biotransformation. Barbiturate effects are also potentiated by concomitant administration of other respiratory or central nervous system depressant; respiratory arrest can occur. Administration of narcotics should be well-spaced between doses of barbiturates if both types of drugs are required.

Porphyria, severe hepatic dysfunction, or previous drug dependence contraindicates the use of barbiturates. Extreme caution is required in patients with respiratory depression or renal impairment. Abrupt termination of barbiturate administration may provoke status epilepticus or other severe withdrawal symptoms. Injectable solutions of barbiturates are usually prepared at alkaline *p*H to promote ionization and water solubility of the drugs. Given IM or SC, these preparations can produce considerable local irritation, occasionally with abscess formation. Sodium phenobarbital is the least irritating of these agents.

Several drugs with pharmacological action similar to the barbiturates have been used as sedatives and hypnotics; these also are now largely replaced by the benzodiazepines. ***Glutethimide*** (Doriglute) has marked anticholinergic activity in addition to its barbiturate-like central nervous system depression and suppression of REM sleep. ***Ethchlorvynol*** (Placidyl) may interact with tricyclic antidepressants to induce delirium. These agents, along with methyprylon and ethinamate, are controlled substances, capable of producing psychological and physiological drug dependence. Methaqualone (Quaalude) became so widely abused that it was taken off the market in the United States.

Relatively little respiratory depression is caused by ***chloral hydrate*** and triclofos, both of which are metabolized to the pharmacologically active trichloroethanol. Used as sleeping aids and for presurgical sedation, these agents are gastric irritants. Dysrhythmias may develop, particularly in persons with cardiac disease. ***Paraldehyde*** (Paral) is a liquid with unpleasant taste and odor. It can be administered enterally or parenterally in the emergency management of convulsions (*e.g.,* in eclampsia, status epilepticus, and intoxication with central nervous system stimulants) and of hyperexcitable psychiatric episodes. The use of paraldehyde has been largely replaced by benzodiazepines, chlordiazepoxide in particular. Drug inactivation is largely by way of hepatic enzymes although up to 20% of a dose is eliminated from the pulmonary capillaries. Impairment of either of these systems can delay paraldehyde removal. Intramuscular injections are usually painful, and sites traversed by major nerve trunks must be avoided since paraldehyde can damage nerves. Intravenous injection, used only in extreme emergencies, can induce coughing. ***Disulfiram*** (Antabuse) interferes with paraldehyde metabolism, resulting in the characteristic reaction observed when alcohol and this aldehyde dehydrogenase inhibitor are ingested concurrently. Overdose of paraldehyde, although rare because of its disagreeable physical properties, can elicit respiratory and cardiovascular depression, hypotension, pulmonary edema, metabolic acidosis, renal failure, and prolonged coma.

Central Nervous System Stimulants

Central nervous system stimulants vary considerably in their pattern of effects, some acting most intensely at the cerebrum, others in the pons-medulla or the spinal cord. All have the potential to cause seizures, and many are also cardiovascular stimulants. These drugs have few clinical indications, since other supportive measures are generally more effective and more easily titrated to the patient's response.

Doxapram (Dopram) and ***nikethamide*** (Coramine), which act in the brain stem, are occasionally administered to stimulate respiration (see Respiratory Pharmacology). ***Pentylenetetrazol*** (Metrazol) may be used in the diagnosis of seizure disorders. These analeptic agents appear to interact with GABA-mediated movement of chloride ions in the central nervous system. The possible occurrence of convulsions and severe cardiovascular and respiratory stimulation makes their administration hazardous. Barbiturates can terminate such seizures but will also produce return of respiratory depression.

Amphetamines and related agents (discussed under Autonomic Drugs) are psychomotor stimulants that interact with sympathetic transmission. Amphetamines and ***methylphenidate*** (Ritalin) reverse the central nervous system depression that induces the sleep and cataplexy characteristic of narcolepsy. Methylphenidate, amphetamines, and ***pemoline*** (Cylert) alleviate the symptoms of childhood attention-deficit disorder (ADD, hyperkinetic syndrome). Suppression of nutrition and growth, and interference with sleep are adverse effects. The α_2-adrenergic agonist clonidine and some antidepressants are administered to some children having ADD. These drugs should be used only when clear benefit is derived. Amphetamines have very limited use as anorexients, since tolerance and drug dependence (both physiological and psychological) develop rapidly.

Xanthines (discussed under Respiratory Pharmacology) produce varying degrees of central nervous system stimulation. Caffeine, found in coffee, tea, chocolate, and cola, produces wakefulness and mild euphoria. This substance is available in combination with sodium benzoate to alleviate alcohol- and drug-induced respiratory depression, and in over-the-counter preparations to ward off drowsiness. The latter use is hazardous, since profound fatigue can develop. Excessive caffeine consumption induces insomnia, nervousness, palpitations, and other symptoms of central nervous system and cardiovascular hyperactivity. A mild form of dependence can develop, so that abrupt discontinuance of consumption causes headache and fatigue. Caffeine is combined with aspirin or ergot alkaloids, as it may be somewhat effective in ameliorating headaches.

Many drugs produce unwanted central nervous system stimulation, as do many illegal abused substances. The latter are discussed under Drug Abuse.

ANTICONVULSANTS

Seizures arise from aberrant electrical activity in the central nervous system that is manifested in involuntary motor activity and changes in level of consciousness. Generalized seizures include general convulsions and absence seizures as well as akinetic and atonic episodes in which muscle tone is reduced. In partial seizures, limited areas of the body are affected, and consciousness may be lost. Convulsions have many causes, including epilepsy, brain tumors, head injury, hypoglycemia, eclampsia, childhood fever, drug overdose, and withdrawal from drug dependence. Astute diagnosis is required before chronic drug therapy is instituted.

Several drugs (Table 7-12) are available for the management of seizure disorders. Although these drugs represent several classes of chemical compounds, similarities are conferred by various combinations of five- and six-membered ring structures. Most anticonvulsants are effective for either generalized convulsions or absence seizures, and may exacerbate the type of seizure that they do not control. Termination of any anticonvulsant medication must be accomplished by a gradual reduction in dosage, since abrupt termination can precipitate seizures. Some patients respond inadequately to drugs; trials of several single agents should precede a decision to use multiple-drug regimens. Many complex interactions occur among the various anticonvulsant drugs.

TABLE 7-12. Anticonvulsants

GENERIC NAME	TRADE NAME
Barbiturates and Related Agents	
Phenobarbital	Luminal
Mephobarbital	Mebaral
Primidone	Mysoline
Hydantoins	
Phenytoin	Dilantin
Mephenytoin	Mesantoin
Succinimides	
Ethosuximide	Zarontin
Methsuximide	Celontin
Oxazolidinediones	
Trimethadione	Tridione
Paramethadione	Mysoline
Benzodiazepines	
Clonazepam	Klonopin
Diazepam	Valium
Additional Agents	
Carbamazepine	Tegretol
Valproic acid	Depakene
Acetazolamide	Diamox
Phenacemide	Phenurone
Felbamate	Felbatol
Gabapentin	Neurontin
Lamotrigine	Lamictal

The use of ***phenobarbital*** in the control of generalized convulsions and partial seizures has declined as other anticonvulsants have become available. The mechanism of action of this long-acting barbiturate may include potentiation of the inhibitory action of the neurotransmitter GABA. The most frequent adverse effect of this barbiturate is sedation. Tolerance may develop, although some patients continue to report an unacceptable level of daytime drowsiness. Ataxia, teratogenicity, bleeding in the neonate, behavior disturbances, poor concentration, depression, and allergic rashes can occur.

Phenobarbital is biotransformed by the hepatic enzymes that are also induced by the presence of this drug. An initial reduction in the inactivation of concurrently administered drugs will often progress to more rapid metabolism and decreased efficacy. Drug doses that have been increased to compensate for this interaction must subsequently be reduced when use of phenobarbital is terminated. The coumarin anticoagulants in particular have been involved in this type of interaction. Phenobarbital can enhance the action of central nervous system depressants.

Phenobarbital is also excreted renally as unchanged drug; up to 25% may be inactivated by this mechanism. Alkalinization of the urine promotes drug ionization and enhanced excretion. ***Primidone***, partially metabolized to phenobarbital, has pharmacology and toxicology similar to this barbiturate.

Phenytoin, or diphenylhydantoin, is used extensively in the treatment of general and partial seizures. By decreasing intracellular sodium and calcium, phenytoin appears to suppress the spread of abnormal electrical activity in the central nervous system. A major advantage of phenytoin is its lack of sedative action, although it may interfere with cognitive function. Numerous other adverse effects can limit the use of this drug. Ataxia, visual disturbances, nystagmus, hepatitis, nephritis, rashes (can be severe), hematologic disturbances (including bleeding in infants exposed in utero), dizziness, behavioral changes, gingival hyperplasia, teratogenicity, and hirsutism are characteristic reactions. Chronic administration of phenytoin can induce vitamin D metabolism and deplete serum levels of folic acid, thyroxine, and vitamin K. Since phenytoin is a myocardial depressant, IV administration can induce cardiovascular collapse. This drug has some use in the management of cardiac dysrhythmias, in particular, those induced by cardiac glycosides.

Many drugs affect the hepatic metabolism of phenytoin. Inhibition of hepatic inactivation of phenytoin occurs with concomitant use of diazepam, cimetidine, dicoumarol, and disulfiram. Inactivation is accelerated by carbamazepine and valproic acid. Phenobarbital and alcohol may either increase or decrease the hepatic metabolism of phenytoin.

Carbamazepine may be more effective than phenytoin in the treatment of generalized convulsions and partial seizures; it is often the drug of choice. Although these agents appear to work by similar mechanisms, they can have additive effects that provide control of seizures that are refractory to each drug alone. Carbamazepine is metabolized hepatically and induces enzyme activity. Its biological half-life can extend to 60 hours. Common adverse effects include drowsiness, headache, and gastrointestinal and vision disturbances. More serious reactions such as hepatitis, teratogenicity (neural tube defects), hematological disturbances, hallucinations, hypotension, congestive heart failure, and rashes progressing to Stevens-Johnson syndrome are reported. Carbamazepine can exacerbate myoclonic and absence seizures. Inadequate bioavailability of both trade and generic forms of this drug can result in poor response.

Valproic acid is effective in absence seizures, occasionally in cases that are refractory to other drugs. This agent will also suppress generalized convulsions and partial seizures. Valproate potentiates the inhibitory action of GABA in the central nervous system. It is well absorbed following oral administration, and is highly bound to plasma proteins. Adverse effects include teratogenicity, endocrine disturbances in women, hair loss (alopecia), headache, drowsiness or insomnia, weight gain or loss, and suppression of platelet function. Valproate can produce potentially fatal hepatotoxicity. Nausea and vomiting induced by valproate can be decreased with enteric coated forms or by taking with food.

Valproic acid can elevate plasma levels of phenobarbital and primidone, and reduce those of phenytoin. Close observation is required whenever anticonvulsant agents are combined, and adjustment of dosages may be necessary. Valproic acid can enhance the effects of central nervous system depressants.

Ethosuximide is a succinimide used very effectively in the management of absence seizures. Other drugs in this chemical group are methsuximide and phensuximide. Ethosuximide has a long plasma half-life; it is both metabolized hepatically and excreted as unchanged drug. Hepatic and renal function should be monitored in patients receiving these agents. Gastrointestinal disturbances occur frequently. Psychological aberrations, hematological disorders, a lupuslike reaction, and skin rashes including Stevens-Johnson syndrome may develop. The succinimides can induce generalized seizures in susceptible patients; they may be administered concurrently with other anticonvulsants to persons who experience other types of seizures in addition to absence seizures. Methsuximide is occasionally effective in refractory patients.

Some benzodiazepines are used as anticonvulsants. ***Diazepam*** or ***lorazepam*** administered IV are especially effective in terminating status epilepticus. ***Clonazepam*** can reduce the incidence of atonic and akinetic seizures. Central nervous system depression and drug dependence are adverse effects of the benzodiazepines, which are discussed under Antianxiety Agents. Intravenous phenobarbital and phenytoin are alternative drugs for treatment of status epilepticus.

Severe aplastic anemia and acute liver failure have restricted the use of ***felbamate*** (Felbatol). Effective in partial seizures with or without secondary generalization, felbamate can also be used in children with Lennox-Gastaut syndrome, which can produce intractable seizures. Partly metabolized in the liver, it has a half-life of almost 24 hours. Among the adverse effects of felbamate are gastrointestinal disturbances, headache, fatigue, insomnia or sedation, and rashes. Felbamate can be combined with other anticonvulsants, but interactions can be numerous. Felbamate inhibits and induces the cytochrome P450 enzyme system. Plasma carbamazepine is decreased, but its active metabolite increases, as do levels of phenytoin and valproic acid. Phenytoin and carbamazepine induce the metabolism of felbamate. Felbamate in combination with other drugs occasionally causes hematologic dyscrasias.

Gabapentin (Neurontin) is an analogue of the inhibitory neurotransmitter gamma amino butyric acid (GABA) but does not work through any known aspect of GABAergic neurotransmission. It is rapidly absorbed following oral administration, possibly through a saturable intestinal transport system. Gabapentin differs from most anticonvulsants in that it is inactivated almost entirely by renal excretion. Doses must be decreased in persons with renal impairment or on hemodialysis. Adverse effects are nystagmus, fatigue, dizziness, ataxia, and drowsiness. Extremely high doses of gabapentin induced pancreatic adenocarcinomas in male rats. Usually combined with other drugs, this agent does not alter their hepatic biotransformation. Antacids administered concurrently can decrease the absorption of gabapentin.

Lamotrigine (Lamictal) is approved for add-on treatment of partial seizures in adults. Similarly to carbamazepine and phenytoin, lamotrigine blocks voltage-dependent sodium channels and decreases the release of the excitatory neurotransmitters glutamic and aspartic acids. Well absorbed from the gastrointestinal tract, lamotrigine is inactived by hepatic glucuronidation and has a half-life of approximately 24 hours. Lamotrigine can cause severe rashes, sedation, headache, nausea, dizziness, ataxia, and visual disturbances. Disseminated intravascular coagulation may occur. Carbamazepine, phenytoin, phenobarbital, and primidone all induce the hepatic biotransformation of lamotrigine. In contrast, valproate slows the rate of inactivation of lamotrigine. Lamotrigine does not affect the cytochrome P450 system.

Phenacemide is used to treat refractory cases of partial seizures, especially those originating in the temporal lobe. Phenacemide has a high incidence of adverse effects such as psychosis, depression and other behavioral changes, hepatotoxicity, leukopenia, anemia, and nephritis. Treatment with phenacemide should be initiated in the hospital to allow for close observation.

Magnesium is occasionally administered parenterally to control convulsions in eclampsia, glomerulonephritis, and hypothyroidism, conditions in which hypomagnesemia may contribute to seizure activity. Adequate renal function is required, since this ion is inactivated solely by renal excretion. Magnesium is a uterine relaxant that can inhibit labor. Marked depression of the central nervous system and of cardiac and respiratory function can occur. Calcium salts (chloride or gluconate) administered IV can reverse the toxic effects of magnesium.

A characteristic shared by many of the anticonvulsants is their potential teratogenic action. These agents should be administered with caution in women of childbearing age. However, therapy must be continued during pregnancy; the possible adverse effects must be weighed against the benefit of preventing seizures and possible fetal hypoxia. Phenobarbital and phenytoin in later pregnancy may cause a neonatal coagulation deficit.

While anticonvulsants do not ''cure'' seizure disorders, medication can occasionally be withdrawn from persons who have been seizure-free for a considerable time interval. Careful reduction of dosage with close observation is required.

Pharmacotherapy of Parkinson's Disease

Degeneration of dopaminergic neurons traveling from the substantia nigra to the basal ganglia (caudate nucleus, pallidus, and putamen) underlies the gradually developing tremor, rigidity, and bradykinesia characteristic of Parkinson's disease. This disorder can be induced by exposure to manganese, carbon monoxide, and other neurotoxins such as 1-methyl-4-phenyl-1,2,5,6-tetrahydropyridine (MPTP). Arteriosclerosis, and some forms of encephalitis, may also be causative factors in some forms of parkinsonism. In most instances, however, the cause of this movement disorder is not known. Reversible states of ''parkinsonism'' can be induced by administration of dopamine receptor antagonist drugs such as the neuroleptics.

Levodopa was the first effective drug available for Parkinson's disease. In modern practice, its use is often delayed until resistance to other therapies has occurred. Levodopa (L-dopa) is the precursor of dopamine but differs from the latter substance in its ability to cross the blood–brain barrier. Once in the central nervous system, levodopa enters dopaminergic neurons, is metabolized to dopamine, and released in the same manner as endogenous neurotransmitter. L-Aromatic amino acid decarboxylase, the enzyme that converts L-dopa to dopamine, is found in tissues outside the central nervous system, most notably the gastrointestinal tract, liver, and kidneys. To prevent breakdown of levodopa before it reaches the brain, a decarboxylase inhibitor is frequently administered concurrently. Agents such as ***carbidopa*** do not cross the blood–brain barrier, thus will selectively block peripheral decarboxylation. Lower doses of levodopa become effective, and side effects due to peripheral actions of dopamine can be alleviated. ***Sinemet*** combines levodopa and carbidopa, although the inhibitor alone is also available as ***Lodosyn*** to facilitate dosage adjustment for each drug.

Levodopa can effect marked improvement in parkinsonian symptoms, with tremor more slowly and incompletely resolved than rigidity and bradykinesia. However, levodopa often gradually loses its effectiveness, apparently as the loss of nigrostriatal neurons progresses. Rapid variations in effectiveness may develop during treatment with levodopa. Fluctuations in the plasma level of drug may be related to this ''on-off'' phenomenon, which is occasionally relieved by more frequent administration of levodopa or by the addition of bromocriptine. Also, Sinemet is available in controlled-release form to provide more sustained plasma levels of levodopa.

Adverse effects attributable to levodopa include nausea and vomiting, orthostatic hypotension, dyskinesias, psychoses, and cardiac dysrhythmias. Many of these will respond to reduction in dosage, and tolerance will develop to some. Nausea may be alleviated by taking the drug with meals, although food can delay the absorption of levodopa, and amino acids derived from dietary proteins can compete with levodopa for transport into the central nervous system. Levodopa should not be discontinued abruptly, as rigidity and fever similar to neuroleptic malignant syndrome can develop.

Levodopa is contraindicated in persons with narrow-angle glaucoma or with a risk or history of melanoma. Extreme caution is required in the presence of asthma, peptic ulcer, or cardiovascular disease. Levodopa is not administered concurrently with monoamine oxidase inhibitors. Cautious use of tricyclic agents may alleviate the depression that often accompanies parkinsonism. The anticholinergic action of the latter drugs can be beneficial to parkinsonian symptoms, but may also exacerbate orthostatic hypotension induced by levodopa or the disease itself. Levodopa can potentiate the actions of adrenergic agonists. Neuroleptics and other agents that block dopamine receptors are contraindicated in parkinsonian patients regardless of drug treatment, since antagonism will further aggravate the striatal dopamine deficit. Pyridoxine (vitamin B_6), a cofactor for the decarboxylase enzyme, will enhance peripheral conversion of L-dopa to dopamine. This action of pyridoxine is suppressed in the presence of decarboxylase inhibition.

Bromocriptine (Parlodel) and ***pergolide*** (Permax) are dopamine receptor agonists that work in much the same manner as dopamine. Adverse effects, attributable to receptor activation, are similar to those of levodopa. Bromocriptine augments the action of levodopa, and can be effective when levodopa's usefulness is waning or unstable. Since dopamine exerts inhibitory influence over prolactin release, these agonists will suppress hyperprolactinemia and postpartum lactation. Chronic administration occasionally induces pleural effusion and pulmonary infiltrates.

Amantidine (Symmetrel) is a moderately effective agent that can enhance the action of levodopa. Its mechanism may involve release of dopamine from striatal nerve terminals, thus its action would be expected to decrease as neuronal degeneration progresses. Tolerance does develop to the beneficial effects but can often be reversed by interrupting therapy. Adverse effects similar to those of levodopa can occur. Congestive heart failure and a lowering of seizure threshold also are reported. Characteristic is livedo reticularis, a bluish discoloration of the skin, particularly at the ankles where edema may also develop. Abrupt termination of amantidine may exacerbate parkinsonian symptoms.

Selegiline (Eldepryl) inhibits the MAO-B enzyme that metabolizes dopamine in the CNS. It can enhance the effectiveness of levodopa, although selegiline itself loses efficacy within 1 to 2 years. In higher doses (*e.g.*, above 10 mg per day), MAO-A inhibition occurs and presents the risk of hypertensive crisis with certain foods and other medications, including meperidine and fluoxetine. Selegiline causes nausea, insomnia, and orthostatic hypotension.

The efficacy of anticholinergic agents (see Table 7-2) in alleviating symptoms of parkinsonism appears to arise from a reciprocal inhibitory relationship between dopamine and acetylcholine in the striatum. As dopaminergic influence wanes, that of acetylcholine increases. Anticholinergics are especially effective in alleviating tremor early in the course of disease, and like other drugs, can add to the effectiveness of levodopa. Histamine H_1 receptor blockers that possess anticholinergic activity are also used; diphenhydramine is the most notable among these.

ANESTHETICS

General Anesthetics

The basic mechanisms by which drugs depress the central nervous system to produce general anesthesia are not clear. Theories based on alterations in membrane permeability, depression of cellular respiration, and formation of crystal hydrates have been proposed to explain the effects of these agents, which represent several diverse chemical groups. The Meyer-Overton correlation relates their oil-water partition coefficient to their ability to act, or to reach their sites of action. The most potent anesthetics are those with the greatest lipid solubility. Agents with low blood solubility but high lipophilicity will rapidly leave the circulatory system and cross the blood–brain barrier. Drugs with a higher capacity to remain in the vascular compartment will require greater plasma concentrations to attain equilibrium and reach anesthetic levels in the central nervous system. However, there are many substances with comparable oil–water partition coefficients that do not induce general anesthesia.

The major site of action of general anesthetics is thought to be the reticular activating system of the brain stem. This multisynaptic pathway has been shown to be primarily responsible for the control of sleep and waking patterns, as well as the integration of prolonged behavioral response to sensory perception. Anesthetic action at this level serves the dual purpose of producing sleep and decreasing sensory perception by reducing neural transmission to the cortex.

The objectives of general anesthesia are to produce unconsciousness, analgesia, amnesia, and muscular relaxation. Ether is virtually the only agent that can induce all of these responses. Other anesthetics must be combined with each other or with nonanesthetic drugs to achieve an adequate response. This is referred to as balanced anesthesia.

STAGES OF ANESTHESIA

The classic stages of anesthesia are most apparent when ether is utilized. Because this agent is quite soluble in blood and body tissues, effective concentrations are slowly achieved in the central nervous system and characteristic changes in levels of consciousness and involuntary activity are prominent. While many general anesthetics produce a somewhat similar sequence of events, some stages are minimized. Simultaneous administration of other drugs (*e.g.*, in balanced anesthesia) can obscure these classic hallmarks that indicate the level of anesthesia.

Stage I, or induction of anesthesia, begins with drug administration and ends when consciousness is lost. If analgesia is provided, minor surgical procedures can be performed in this state.

Stage II, reduced with the use of many modern anesthetics, begins with loss of consciousness, and is characterized by central nervous system excitation, rapid, possibly irregular respiration, dilated but reactive pupils, and delirium. Involuntary movement and vocalization may occur; patients should be restrained to prevent injury. Salivation and vomiting present the risk of aspiration; thus general anesthesia is best preceded by several hours of restricted oral intake. Myocardial stimulation, evidenced by increases in heart rate and blood pressure that occur during this stage, can seriously compromise the safety of persons with cardiovascular disease.

Stage III begins with the return of rhythmic respiration, and is divided into four planes of deepening surgical anesthesia and muscular relaxation. In plane 1, the swallowing and pharyngeal (gag) reflexes disappear, as do spontaneous and reflex eyelid closure. The eyes are generally wandering and off-center. When the eyes become centrally fixed, plane 2 has begun. Most surgery is performed at this level, which is characterized by marked skeletal muscle relaxation when ether is the anesthetizing agent. Other anesthetics frequently must be supplemented with skeletal muscle relaxants to prevent reflex responses to painful stimuli. Increasing suppression of intercostal muscles, and greater diaphragmatic maintenance of respiration signal the beginning of plane 3. Skeletal muscle becomes profoundly relaxed, and certain types of surgery may require this degree of anesthesia. However, respiration can be seriously impaired. Paralysis of intercostal muscle activity marks plane 4, which is dangerously close to stage IV and complete diaphragmatic and respiratory arrest. Obviously, heroic measures must be rapidly instituted to prevent cardiovascular failure and death. Plane 4 and stage IV should be avoided, through careful administration of the anesthetic agent and close observation of patient response.

When drug administration is terminated, the patient will go through the stages of anesthesia in reverse order. Those agents that produce a characteristically slow induction will have a prolonged recovery period. Vomiting may again occur, and patients should not be left unattended until they have emerged from the delirium stage.

General anesthetics (Table 7-13) include both inhalation and intravenous agents, all having characteristic advantages and hazards. The choice of agent (or combinations of agents) is based upon many factors, including the physiological condition of the patient and the type of surgery to be performed.

TABLE 7-13. General Anesthetics

GENERIC NAME	TRADE NAME
Halogenated Inhalation Anesthetics	
Desflurane	Suprane
Enflurane	Enthrane
Halothane	Fluothane
Isoflurane	Forane
Methoxyflurane	Penthrane
Sevoflurane	Ultane
Barbiturates	
Methohexital	Brevital
Thiamylal	Surital
Thiopental	Pentothal
Other Agents	
Alfentanil	Alfenta
Droperidol + fentanyl	Innovar
Etomidate	Amidate, Hypnomidate
Fentanyl	Sublimaze
Ketamine	Ketaject, Ketalar
Nitrous oxide	—
Propofol	Diprivan
Sufentanil	Sufenta

INHALATION ANESTHETICS

Inhalation anesthetics include gases and volatile liquids that are absorbed from the alveoli. Their lipid solubility enables these agents to cross biological membranes, including the blood–brain barrier, and partial pressure gradients govern their pharmacokinetics to a large extent. Anesthetics are drawn into the lungs by either spontaneous or assisted respiration. Inspired gases contain a high concentration of the anesthetic, which will travel across the alveolar wall and into the pulmonary capillaries. A large fraction of cardiac output is delivered to the brain; thus, this tissue is exposed to a high concentration (or partial pressure) of anesthetic. Those agents that are less water soluble (*e.g.*, nitrous oxide) will leave the systemic circulation rapidly, entering the central nervous system as well as other tissues. Anesthetics with greater water solubility (*e.g.*, ether) will remain longer in the vascular compartment and have an extended onset of action. These agents are also sequestered in adipose tissue, although accumulation of drug occurs gradually because of the low rate of perfusion of this tissue. When anesthesia is terminated, the partial pressure of the agent in inspired gases is low, and promotes the removal of drug from the circulatory system and body tissues. Anesthetic in adipose tissue is gradually released, and can contribute to slow emergence from anesthesia.

Inhalation anesthetics are generally administered with

"anesthesia machines." Completely open systems, in which liquids were dropped onto gauze or cloth face coverings, are obsolete. Current practice utilizes semiclosed and closed systems of administration. In both types of systems, anesthetic gas or vapor (the latter from heated volatile liquids) is mixed with oxygen and administered through a close-fitting face mask. Respiration may be spontaneous or assisted with a rebreathing bag. In a semiclosed system, exhaled gases are released to the environment. In a closed system, gases are circulated through a chamber that adsorbs carbon dioxide, and are remixed with oxygen and additional anesthetic and readministered to the patient. The latter system greatly reduces the exposure of operating room personnel to anesthetic, but does not allow precise control over the amount of drug in the inspired mixture.

The most frequently used inhalation anesthetics are the halogenated volatile liquids such as halothane, isoflurane, enflurane, desflurane, and methoxyflurane. Although these agents are similar in structure, their individual properties give them characteristic advantages and disadvantages. Because these drugs are nonflammable, they have largely replaced the use of ether and cyclopropane.

Halothane (Fluothane), relatively insoluble in blood, provides a rapid onset and termination of action. Because anesthesia is accomplished rapidly, close observation is necessary to prevent lethal overdose. Respiration is significantly depressed by halothane; ventilatory assistance is often required, especially at deeper levels of anesthesia. Hypotension, due in part to vasodilation, and myocardial depression occur. In the presence of halothane, catecholamines (including those exogenously released) can induce severe cardiac dysrhythmias. The risk of hepatitis and liver necrosis is reported to be increased in halothane administration, although many factors can contribute to this reaction. Biliary surgery and history of hepatic disease may contraindicate use of this anesthetic agent. Several months should be allowed between halothane administrations, since drug-induced hepatitis may represent a hypersensitivity response. Halothane, which produces little analgesia or skeletal muscle relaxation, is usually combined with other agents in balanced anesthesia. Halothane is partially metabolized by hepatic enzymes.

Isoflurane (Forane) is often the choice halogenated anesthetic for its rapid induction and emergence and its low potential for organ toxicity. It produces less myocardial depression and sensitization to catecholamines than halothane. Pressor amines can be coadministered with caution. A greater degree of skeletal muscle relaxation is achieved, thus lower doses of neuromuscular blockers are required. Isoflurane undergoes less biotransformation than halothane, and appears less likely to cause hepatic changes. A major disadvantage of this agent is its unpleasant odor.

Enflurane (Enthrane) shares many characteristics with halothane, including rapid induction and emergence and suppression of cardiovascular and respiratory function. Myocardial sensitization to catecholamines and the incidence of hepatitis are reported to be less pronounced. An increase in respiratory secretions may occur. Compared to halothane, enflurane achieves a greater degree of skeletal muscle relaxation. However, at deeper levels of anesthesia, paradoxical muscle contraction may occur.

Methoxyflurane (Penthrane) produces slow induction and prolonged recovery; the latter may be shortened by discontinuing drug administration approximately 30 minutes before the completion of surgery. Its effects on the cardiovascular and respiratory systems are similar to those of halothane, except that myocardial sensitization is less marked. Methoxyflurane has significant analgesic activity. The use of this agent, however, has been greatly curtailed by its characteristic nephrotoxicity. Hepatic metabolism produces free fluoride ions that irreversibly damage tissue and result in high-output renal failure, hypernatremia, and elevated blood urea nitrogen levels.

Desflurane (Suprane) has the most rapid induction of the halogenated anesthetics. It is a vasodilator and depressant of respiratory and myocardial activity, with a characteristic unpleasant odor. Tachycardia, hypertension, laryngospasm during induction, and nausea and vomiting during emergence may occur. Organ toxicity is not anticipated with this agent. ***Sevoflurane*** (Ultane) also has rapid uptake and excretion, but much lower pungency than desflurane. Nausea and vomiting do occur, and hypotension, nephrotoxicity, hepatotoxicity, and malignant hyperthermia are possible adverse effects.

Ether, once widely used, has generally been discontinued; it is highly explosive and flammable. Induction and emergence are prolonged and characterized by significant risk of emesis.

Nitrous oxide is a widely used anesthetic gas that induces analgesia and loss of consciousness but little skeletal muscle relaxation. It may be used alone for brief procedures, and is often a component of balanced anesthesia since it provides rapid induction and potentiates the effects of other agents. Nitrous oxide is administered in fairly high concentrations and must be mixed with oxygen to prevent hypoxia and subsequent tissue damage. This combination of gases is hazardous as it readily supports combustion. Central nervous system excitation and nausea may occur during nitrous oxide administration. Respiratory and cardiovascular function are relatively unchanged by nitrous oxide. The actions of central nervous system depressants such as barbiturates and opiates may be potentiated. Hypotension caused by halothane may be ameliorated by concomitant administration of nitrous oxide, in part by a reduction in the amount of the halogenated agent required.

Cyclopropane also has generally been discontinued, because of its explosive nature and its sensitization of the myocardium to catecholamine-induced arrhythmias. Induction is rapid, with good skeletal muscle relaxation achieved at levels of surgical anesthesia. Respiration and cardiovascular function are usually well maintained.

INTRAVENOUS ANESTHETICS

Similarly to the inhalation anesthetics, the IV agents are often used as components of balanced anesthesia. These are quite lipid soluble and are rapidly delivered to the central nervous system, quickly inducing loss of consciousness. The inactivation of (or emergence from) IV agents depends upon redistribution of drug to tissues such as skeletal muscle, and ultimately upon hepatic biotransformation. This is in contrast to the inhalation agents, which are relatively rapidly excreted by the lungs once the flow of anesthetic vapors is terminated. Thus the IV agents are not suitable for prolonged administration, since recovery would require an excessive period of time. Intravenous anesthetics generally do not enhance myocardial responsiveness to catecholamines, and they rarely produce emesis during induction and emergence.

The barbiturates include several drugs with varying durations of action that make them suitable for a variety of clinical purposes (*e.g.*, see under Sedatives and Hypnotics and under Anticonvulsants). Those barbiturates that are "ultrashort-acting" can be used as IV anesthetic agents. Rapid loss of consciousness and subsequent amnesia are achieved, but neither analgesia nor skeletal muscle relaxation is provided by the barbiturates.

Thiopental (Pentothal) is frequently used to produce rapid and comfortable induction of anesthesia that is then maintained with inhalation agents. Occasionally, brief procedures are accomplished under thiopental supplemented with nitrous oxide for analgesia. Characteristic of all barbiturates, the ultrashort-acting agents can induce respiratory depression and laryngospasm. Consequent elevation of plasma CO_2 may cause cerebral vasodilation and an increase in intracranial pressure. Myocardial depression and peripheral vasodilation, with subsequent changes in heart rate, can be hazardous in patients with cardiovascular disease or blood volume depletion. Allergic reactions to the barbiturates can occur. Drug-induced changes in hepatic enzyme activity exacerbate acute intermittent porphyria; these agents are contraindicated in persons with this disorder. Hepatic impairment prolongs the actions of barbiturates.

Methohexital (Brevital) has a shorter duration of action (5 to 7 minutes) and is used in a manner similar to thiopental. ***Thiamylal*** (Surital) is reported to cause fewer adverse effects than thiopental; both can be given to obtain control of status epilepticus. Thiopental can be administered by rectal suspension for preanesthetic sedation. These agents are sequestered in adipose tissue, from which gradual release prolongs their plasma half-life. Barbiturates are prepared in alkaline solutions (*p*H 11) and may precipitate in the circulatory system following rapid administration. Since methohexital is more potent, it is administered in smaller doses and is less likely to separate out of solution. Barbiturates should not be added to IV solutions containing acid drugs.

Etomidate (Amidate, Hypnomidate) is a rapid-acting nonbarbiturate used for the induction of anesthesia and to supplement agents such as nitrous oxide for brief surgical procedures. This drug does not provide analgesia. It has less pronounced effects on cardiovascular and respiratory functions than the barbiturates. Pain may occur at the site of injection; this can be reduced by slow administration into a large vein. Involuntary movement of skeletal muscles, and occasional changes in blood pressure and heart rate, are reported. Hypersensitivity reactions occur less frequently than with barbiturates. Etomidate may suppress stress-induced adrenal release of corticosteroids. This agent is not recommended for children under 10 years of age, nor for obstetric patients.

Propofol (Diprivan), with a rapid onset and brief duration, is used in induction and balanced anesthesia. Cardiac and respiratory depression can occur.

Ketamine (Ketaject, Ketalar) produces a dissociative anesthesia in which patients appear to be conscious but do not respond to external stimuli. In contrast to other IV anesthetics, ketamine produces profound analgesia. It can be used alone in subanesthetic doses for brief painful procedures. Cardiovascular and respiratory stimulation commonly occur, although suppression of these systems resulting in bradycardia, hypotension, and apnea are also possible. Persons with cardiovascular insufficiency or blood volume depletion may experience a marked reduction in blood pressure. Skeletal muscle tone increases. Elevations in intracranial and intraocular pressures may occur, making ketamine hazardous in head or eye injury or surgery. Emergence from ketamine anesthesia can be characterized by confusion, hallucinations, vivid unpleasant dreams, delirium, and vomiting. Patients should be kept in a quiet environment under close observation for 24 hours following ketamine administration. Severe reactions can be ameliorated with diazepam. Ketamine can be given IM, and is safe for cautious administration to children. It is inactivated hepatically.

Droperidol (Inapsine), a butyrophenone similar to the neuroleptic haloperidol, and the narcotic analgesic ***fentanyl*** (Sublimaze) are combined in the IV formulation known as ***Innovar*** that induces a state of marked analgesia and reduced motor activity. In this ***neuroleptanalge-***

sia, patients appear somewhat detached from reality but are able to respond to verbal communication. Nitrous oxide may be administered concurrently to provide loss of consciousness. Cardiovascular function is usually not markedly altered, although changes in heart rate and blood pressure can occur. The opiate component can induce respiratory depression and emesis; these effects can be rapidly reversed by narcotic antagonists. Laryngospasm and bronchospasm have been reported, as well as extrapyramidal symptoms. Innovar can be administered also for presurgical sedation.

Opiates such as fentanyl, ***sufentanil*** (Sufenta), ***alfentanil*** (Alfenta), and morphine can be used as sole agents for some types of surgery. Because these drugs have little effect on myocardial activity, they can be especially useful to anesthetize persons with cardiac disorders. The drug doses required to induce anesthesia can severely depress respiration, frequently necessitating mechanical ventilation. Hypotension can occur, particularly with the use of morphine. This effect may be in response to opiate-induced release of histamine, since it can be ameliorated by concomitant administration of H_1- and H_2- receptor antihistamines. Excessive muscle rigidity may require the addition of neuromuscular blocking agents that will further compromise respiration. Close observation of the patient is necessary to ensure that an adequate level of anesthesia is maintained. Once surgery is completed, the effects of the opiate can be rapidly reversed by administration of a narcotic antagonist. Additional doses of antagonist may be required as the opiate is gradually biotransformed and eliminated.

ADJUNCTS TO GENERAL ANESTHESIA

Several types of agents are used in conjunction with general anesthesia to supplement or counteract drug effects. Since apprehension and anxiety can significantly interfere with induction of anesthesia, presurgical medication often includes a phenothiazine or a benzodiazepine. The latter group of drugs also induces amnesia, while the antiemetic action of the neuroleptic agents can suppress nausea during induction and emergence. Anticholinergics may be administered to reduce laryngospasm, bronchospasm, vagally induced bradycardia, or respiratory secretions, although most contemporary anesthetic agents are less irritating to the respiratory tract than ether. To provide skeletal muscle relaxation, neuromuscular blocking agents such as tubocurarine, pancuronium, and vecuronium are given. The action of these drugs is enhanced by nitrous oxide and the halogenated hydrocarbons, and respiratory arrest may occur. Succinylcholine, with its brief duration of action, facilitates endotracheal intubation.

Postsurgically, narcotic analgesics may be administered to alleviate intense pain. Patient-controlled intravenous administration of opiates is reported to provide satisfactory pain reduction with minimal adverse reactions.

TABLE 7-14. Local Anesthetics

GENERIC NAME	TRADE NAME
Benzocaine	Anbesol, Solarcaine, Unguentine, Americaine, others
Butacaine	—
Butamben	Butesin
Bupivacaine	Marcaine
Cocaine	—
Chlorprocaine	Nesacaine
Dibucaine	Nupercainal
Etidocaine	Duranest
Lidocaine	Xylocaine, others
Mepivacaine	Carbocaine, isocaine
Prilocaine	Citanest
Procaine	Novocain
Tetracaine	Pontocaine

Local Anesthetics

A number of agents (Table 7-14) are used to provide local and regional suppression of peripheral nerve function. Sensory nerves, with their smaller fiber size and relatively more surface area for drug action, are paralyzed more rapidly and at lower concentrations than motor nerves. Local anesthetics are thought to work at the neuronal membrane surface, suppressing depolarization and subsequent propagation of the action potential. Temporary stabilization of the membrane, apparently achieved as local anesthetics compete with calcium ions at neuronal membrane sites, prevents the influx of sodium that normally occurs during depolarization. Calcium-binding sites may regulate sodium entry into nerve cells; reinforcement of calcium ion concentrations will reduce the efficacy of local anesthetics.

Two chemical classes, esters and amides, are represented among the local anesthetics. Both types of agents possess a lipophilic and a hydrophilic region. Esters are inactivated by plasma pseudocholinesterase; amides are biotransformed hepatically. Additional differences among these agents include onset and duration of action, local irritation, passage across mucous membranes, and incidence of systemic toxicity.

Cocaine, the oldest of the local anesthetics, currently is limited to topical application. This drug induces vasoconstriction, which tends to slow systemic absorption from skin. Absorption from mucous membranes, particularly of the urinary tract, where its use is contraindicated, can be quite extensive. Cocaine inhibits presynaptic neuronal uptake of norepinephrine, and thus can exert sympathomimetic actions. This drug is discussed further under Drug Abuse.

Procaine (Novocain) is regarded as one of the safest of the local anesthetic agents; it induces serious toxicity much less often than other drugs in this group. The duration of action (usually 1 hour) can be extended by the inclusion of epinephrine in injectable preparations. The vasoconstrictor action of the catecholamine slows systemic absorption of the anesthetic. Although the quantity of epinephrine is small, inadvertent IV administration of this powerful adrenergic stimulant can elicit marked cardiovascular responses. A major limitation of procaine is its inadequate penetration through skin and mucosal surfaces. ***Chloroprocaine*** is similar in action to procaine, although its duration of effect is shorter.

Lidocaine is a widely used agent that is highly effective following injection or topical application. Lidocaine's amide structure is biotransformed hepatically, in part to metabolites that retain pharmacological activity and appear to contribute to this drug's central nervous system toxicity. Epinephrine is frequently combined with lidocaine to intensify its local action. The use of lidocaine as an antidysrhythmic agent is discussed under that topic. ***Mepivacaine***, quite similar to lidocaine, has a longer duration of action.

Tetracaine has a greater potency than procaine or lidocaine; its longer onset of action is coupled with a more prolonged duration. ***Dibucaine*** and ***bupivacaine*** also have greater potency and duration of action. Most of these agents are effective both topically and when given by injection.

Some agents (*e.g.*, ***benzocaine***, ***butamben***) are used only for surface anesthesia to alleviate discomforts of skin or mucous membrane disorders and injuries. Since these drugs are so poorly absorbed, systemic reactions rarely occur when they are used. Their most prominent adverse effects are dermatological in nature.

TOXIC EFFECTS

Topical application or injection of local anesthetics can result in sufficient quantities entering systemic circulation to induce serious side effects. The considerable lipid solubility of many of these agents promotes central nervous system reactions that may be excitatory or depressant. Toxic responses can include characteristics of both types of reactions; stimulation may be followed by depression. Central excitation elicits restlessness, anxiety, tremor, hyperpyrexia, and convulsions. Sedation, coma, and respiratory difficulty and arrest can also occur. Cardiovascular effects of local anesthetics include changes in blood pressure and heart rate, myocardial depression, and cardiac arrest. Upon injection, local anesthetics must not be inadvertently delivered into blood vessels. Means for resuscitation must be immediately available when these agents are used. Vasopressor amines and IV fluids may alleviate drug-induced hypotension; seizures can be controlled with diazepam or a short-acting barbiturate. Persons receiving MAO inhibitors or tricyclic antidepressants may develop severe hypertension following administration of local anesthetic formulations that contain a vasoconstrictor.

ADMINISTRATION

Anesthesia is accomplished by infiltration of a large volume of a weak solution (*e.g.*, procaine 0.5%) into the operative area, or by conduction block or regional block, in which small volumes of a more concentrated solution (procaine 1 to 2%) are injected around nerve trunks supplying the operative area.

Spinal anesthesia is a form of block anesthesia in which the drug is injected into the subdural space. Puncture usually is made just below the level of the second and third lumbar vertebrae, and the anesthetic is directed to the desired level by varying the injected volume, by barbotage, or by the position of the patient. Sensory and sympathetic nerve structures are paralyzed for a longer time and at lower concentrations than are motor nerve roots.

Tetracaine is currently the most frequently used agent for spinal procedures; lidocaine, dibucaine, and procaine are also used in this manner. Formulations that contain preservatives are not intended for spinal or epidural use.

Spinal anesthesia provides good muscular relaxation with a minimum of metabolic disturbances and no pulmonary irritation. Postoperative distention is less than with general anesthetics, since vagal tone is not affected. Disadvantages of this route include postpuncture headache (presumably due to meningeal leakage) and occasional paralysis of bladder function (due chiefly to paralysis of sacral autonomics supplying the detrusor muscle of the bladder).

Deaths from spinal anesthesia rarely are attributed to a rise of anesthetic in the spinal canal, causing corresponding paralysis of nerve structures regulating respiration and circulation. Patients must be closely monitored for indications of cardiovascular or respiratory difficulty, and resuscitative measures must be promptly instituted as necessary.

The disadvantages of meningeal puncture are avoided by the use of epidural or peridural anesthesia, in which the anesthetic is injected into the peridural space to travel out with the nerve trunks through the intervertebral foramina. Since relatively large amounts of anesthetic are needed, there is increased danger of systemic drug absorption.

Continuous caudal anesthesia is a special form of extradural block used chiefly in obstetrics. The anesthesia is delivered incrementally through a needle or a catheter inserted into the caudal canal through the sacral hiatus.

ANALGESICS

Analgesics provide relief from pain. Those used clinically can be classified into narcotic analgesics, which will alleviate severe pain, and nonnarcotic agents, generally effective only for "mild to moderate" pain. Narcotic and nonnarcotic agents are frequently combined, their additive analgesic effect allowing reduced dosage of the opiate. Since pain is symptomatic of an underlying disorder, the cause for persistent pain must be investigated.

Both types of analgesics have other therapeutic indications. Many nonnarcotic agents are also antipyretic and anti-inflammatory. Narcotic or opiate drugs are used as antitussive and antidiarrheal agents and for presurgical sedation and anesthesia.

Nonnarcotic Analgesics

Aspirin (acetylsalicylic acid) is the most effective and widely used salicylate, although others (*e.g.,* sodium salicylate) are available. Diflunisol (Dolobid) is a derivative of salicyclic acid that retains many of the characteristic salicylate effects. Aspirin is analgesic, antipyretic, and anti-inflammatory. Its actions appear to involve both central and peripheral mechanisms. At the hypothalamus, aspirin interferes with the transmission of pain impulses, and restores the heat-dissipating efficacy of the thermoregulatory centers. Aspirin also inhibits the cyclooxygenase pathway of prostaglandin synthesis, the biochemical mediators involved in the production of pain, fever, and inflammation.

Aspirin (up to 325 mg daily) is recommended for the prevention of myocardial infarction in persons with unstable angina pectoris or history of previous myocardial infarction, and also for the prevention of transient ischemic attacks and strokes in men. Suppression of the synthesis of thromboxane A_2, a vasoconstrictor and platelet aggregating factor, appears to be the mechanism by which aspirin exerts its protective action. Aspirin irreversibly blocks platelet aggregation and thus will significantly prolong blood-clotting time. Anemia or spontaneous gastrointestinal bleeding may develop. Salicylates generally are contraindicated after surgery or concomitantly with anticoagulant medications.

Salicylates are gastric irritants that can induce stomach pain, nausea, vomiting, and erosion of the gastric lining. Additive effects of alcohol, corticosteroids and the nonsteroidal anti-inflammatory drugs will increase the risk of peptic ulceration. Other adverse effects, seen particularly in persons maintained on chronic high doses of salicylates, include dizziness, confusion, and tinnitus. Allergic reactions may take the form of rashes, angioedema, asthma, or anaphylaxis. Children who are prone to asthma often are hypersensitive to aspirin; the appearance of bronchospasm shortly after administration of a salicylate suggests that nonsalicylate agents be substituted.

Controversy persists over the relationship of aspirin administration during chicken pox (varicella) and influenza infections and subsequent appearance of Reye's syndrome in children. Many authorities recommend that acetaminophen be used if antipyretic or analgesic action is necessary in the course of these or other diseases in children. Children who must receive salicylates for the chronic management of inflammatory disorders should be inoculated annually against the prevailing strains of influenza.

Salicylates depress tubular secretion of uric acid and in high doses block its reabsorption, exerting a uricosuric effect. The ability of probenecid and sulfinpyrazone to promote uric acid secretion is reduced by salicylates. Aspirin is contraindicated in persons receiving methotrexate since the renal excretion of the latter drug can be suppressed. The toxicity of drugs that bind to plasma proteins (*e.g.,* thyroid hormones, nonsteroidal anti-inflammatory drugs, penicillins, oral anticoagulants) can be enhanced as the salicylates compete for available binding sites.

Salicylates are well absorbed from the acid environment of the stomach. Because they are largely nonionized at normal urinary *p*H, these drugs are reabsorbed from the renal tubules. Alkalinization of the urine promotes ionization and excretion, and can be used to aid in the management of aspirin overdose. Hepatic enzymes biotransform the salicylates to inactive water-soluble metabolites.

Aspirin overdose can be lethal, especially in children. Acid-base imbalances occur as a consequence of respiratory stimulation, renal excretion of bicarbonate ion, uncoupling of oxidative phosphorylation, and accumulation of pyruvic and lactic acid. Hyperthermia, hypoglycemia, convulsions, circulatory collapse, and coma can occur. Extensive supportive measures are required to prevent death.

Diflunisol has a long (8 to 12 hours) duration of action. It is a less effective antipyretic, but its analgesic and anti-inflammatory actions are comparable to aspirin. A lower incidence of platelet dysfunction and gastrointestinal bleeding are reported.

The nonsteroidal anti-inflammatory drugs (NSAID, Table 7-15) are a rapidly expanding group of agents closely related to aspirin and sharing many of its therapeutic and adverse actions. These prostaglandin synthetase inhibitors are useful in the treatment of rheumatoid arthritis and other inflammatory disorders in persons who do not respond to or cannot tolerate the side effects of aspirin. It must be emphasized that while aspirin and NSAID relieve the symptoms of arthritis, they do not prevent progression of the disease. ***Ibuprofen*** (Motrin, Nuprin, Advil) and ***naproxen*** are intermittently adminis-

TABLE 7-15. Nonsteroidal Anti-inflammatory Drugs

GENERIC NAME	TRADE NAME
Diclofenac	Voltaren
Etodolac	Lodine
Fenoprofen	Nalfon
Flurbiprofen	Ansaid
Ibuprofen	Motrin, Advil, Nuprin
Indomethacin	Indocin
Ketoprofen	Orudis
Ketorolac	Toradol
Meclofenamate	Meclomen
Mefenamic acid	Ponstel
Nabumetone	Relafen
Naproxen	Anaprox, Naprosyn
Oxaprozin	Daypro
Phenylbutazone	Butazolidin
Piroxicam	Feldene
Sulindac	Clinoril
Tolmetin	Tolectin

tered for relief of dysmenorrhea; their suppression of prostaglandin synthesis is thought to be the mechanism by which they alleviate menstrual discomfort. ***Indomethacin*** will induce closure of neonatal patent ductus arteriosus. ***Phenylbutazone,*** among the original NSAIDs, is seldom used now because of its potentially severe toxicity that includes hematological disorders. ***Piroxicam*** is reported to have a longer duration of action than other NSAIDs and can be effective in single daily doses. ***Ketorolac*** (Toradol) can be administered parenterally, and may be as effective as opioid analgesics. ***Oxaprozin*** (Daypro) has a half-life of up to 60 hours, making once-daily administration effective. This NSAID may cause greater frequency of adverse gastrointestinal effects then some other drugs in this class, while ***nabumetone*** (Relafen) may be less toxic to the gastric mucosa.

Although reported to be less severe than those induced by aspirin, gastrointestinal disturbances are a frequent effect of NSAIDs. Gastric ulcer and severe hemorrhage can develop; ***misoprostol*** (Cytotec) will reduce this risk. Preexisting peptic ulcer contraindicates the use of NSAIDs, indomethacin in particular. Severe diarrhea induced by mefenamic acid requires dosage reduction or termination.

NSAIDs inhibit synthesis of prostaglandins that are renal vasodilators, thus changes in renal function, including azotemia and anuria, occur. Preexisting renal impairment increases the risk of this adverse action; kidney function should be monitored in persons receiving NSAID. Sodium and fluid retention can exacerbate cardiovascular disorders. Hematological disturbances are reported. Inhibition of platelet aggregation is reversible and less pronounced with NSAID therapy, although these drugs require caution when administered to persons with coagulation abnormalities. Dizziness, anxiety, drowsiness, and confusion may occur. Changes in vision and liver function can develop; monitoring of ophthalmic and hepatic activity may be necessary. Chronic administration of fenoprofen may cause hearing impairment. Persons who are allergic to aspirin are frequently also hypersensitive to NSAIDs. Asthmatic patients may develop bronchospasm and respiratory failure. Several NSAIDs are available as ophthalmic preparations. Diclofenac and flurbiprofen reduce inflammation following cataract surgery, and ketorolac may alleviate itching of allergic conjunctivitis.

These agents bind avidly to plasma proteins and may displace other bound drugs. The effect of anticoagulant agents can be enhanced. Indomethacin and other NSAIDs have been reported to reverse the antihypertensive efficacy of thiazide diuretics and β-adrenergic blockers, and to inhibit renal clearance of lithium.

Acetaminophen (Tylenol and other over-the-counter and prescription preparations) has analgesic and antipyretic efficacy similar to that of aspirin, but has negligible anti-inflammatory action. Its site of action appears to be mainly in the central nervous system. It causes minimal changes in gastrointestinal or platelet function. Cross-allergenicity with aspirin does not occur. Chronic administration can induce methemoglobinemia and hemolytic anemia. Acetaminophen overdose provokes slowly developing irreversible hepatic damage, and has been used by persons intent upon suicide. Administration of sulfhydryl donors such as ***acetylcysteine*** (Mucomyst) within 12 hours (possibly up to 18 hours) following acetaminophen overdose can prevent fatal hepatic damage. Chronic alcohol ingestion potentiates acetaminophen hepatotoxicity.

Additional nonanalgesic agents are used in the management of gout, rheumatoid arthritis, and other painful disorders. While these agents often are beneficial, they require close monitoring to avert serious adverse reactions. ***Colchicine*** appears to reduce migration of neutrophils to areas of uric-acid-induced inflammation. It provides rapid relief and can prevent recurrence of acute attacks. Gastrointestinal disturbances occur in a large portion of patients. Uricosuric drugs such as ***probenecid*** and ***sulfinpyrazone*** inhibit renal tubular reabsorption of uric acid. ***Allopurinol*** inhibits xanthine oxidase, which catalyzes the formation of uric acid from xanthine and hypoxanthine. Since the antineoplastic agents mercaptopurine and azathioprine are inactivated by xanthine oxidase, their toxicity is markedly potentiated by allopurinol.

Gold salts appear to interact with the immune system to prevent or retard the progressive deterioration of function in rheumatoid arthritis. These agents can induce severe toxicity, and are reserved for refractory patients. However, the greatest benefit is derived when gold salts are administered before significant damage to joints has occurred. Other anti-inflammatory agents can be administered concurrently. Gold is retained in body tissues for a prolonged period of time, although its removal can be facilitated with penicillamine or dimercaprol (BAL). Gold salts are administered orally (auranofin, Ridaura) or IM-aurothioglucose (Myochrysine, Solganol).

Penicillamine (Cuprimine) can alleviate the symptoms of arthritis; its onset of action, like that of gold salts, is gradual. Gastrointestinal, renal, and hematological disturbances may necessitate drug termination. ***Antimalarials*** (chloroquine, Aralen; hydrochloroquine, Plaquenil), which interact with several aspects of immune responsiveness, can ameliorate the symptoms of arthritis, as can the corticosteroids. Cytotoxic immunosuppressant agents such as ***azathioprine*** and ***cyclophosphamide***, may be administered in severe degenerative refractory arthritis. Oral, low-dose ***methotrexate*** (Rheumatrex) is reported to be quite effective. Its toxicity may be increased by concomitant NSAIDs.

The anticonvulsants ***phenytoin*** and ***carbamazepine*** can alleviate the discomfort of trigeminal neuralgia, while the tricyclic antidepressants are occasionally effective in diabetic neuropathy.

The alkaloid ***ergotamine*** is effective in aborting impending migraine headaches. However, the potent vasoconstrictor action of this drug can lead to gangrenous fingers and toes. ***Methysergide*** (Sansert), a related substance, is a serotonin receptor antagonist that may prevent migraine. Its chronic use is limited by the development of pulmonary and retroperitoneal fibrosis. Beta-adrenergic blockers also can reduce the incidence of migraine but are not effective in acute attacks.

Sumatriptan (Imitrex) is a serotonin agonist that can relieve migraine. The action of this drug involves constriction of intracerebral blood vessels and reduction of inflammation around sensory nerve fibers. It is given orally or parenterally, and is hepatically inactivated. Oral doses undergo extensive first-pass extraction from the circulatory system. Nausea, chest pressure, and a feeling of heaviness are adverse effects. Because sumatriptan can constrict coronary arteries, it is contraindicated in angina.

Narcotic Analgesics

The narcotic analgesics (Table 7-16) differ from others in their ability to alleviate severe pain, in particular sustained dull visceral pain. In addition, the narcotics are neither antipyretic nor anti-inflammatory. These analgesics work via opiate receptors in specific areas of the central nervous system. Both the perception of pain and the emotional response to pain are altered by the opioid drugs. Endorphins are endogenous substances that interact with opiate receptors and appear to modulate transmission of information relating to pain, emotional behavior, and other physiological processes.

TABLE 7-16. Narcotic Analgesics and Antagonists

GENERIC NAME	TRADE NAME
Pure Agonist Analgesics	
Morphine	Several
Codeine	—
Fentanyl	Sublimaze
Hydromorphone	Dilaudid
Levorphanol	Levo-Dromoran
Meperidine	Demerol
Methadone	Dolophine
Oxycodone	Hycodan
Propoxyphene	Darvon
Tramadol	Ultram
Partial Agonist Analgesics	
Buprenorphine	Buprenex
Butorphanol	Stadol
Dezocine	Dalgan
Nalbuphine	Nubain
Pentazocine	Talwin
Pure Antagonists	
Nalmefene	Revex
Naloxone	Narcan
Naltrexone	Trexan, ReVia

The usefulness of the opiates is limited by their adverse effects. Both drug tolerance and dependence develop to these agents, rendering them unsuitable for the management of chronic pain. Administration for more than a few days is advisable only in instances of severe pain accompanying terminal illness. Should the patient survive, drug dependence can be reversed. Tolerance will develop, thus drug doses should be just sufficient to reduce pain to an acceptable level. The euphoriant effect of these drugs makes pain less noxious; patients will experience pain but its anxiety-provoking aspect is ameliorated.

Opiate analgesics are respiratory depressants at therapeutic doses. Action at the respiratory control centers in the brain stem produces slow, shallow, irregular breathing. These drugs are contraindicated in persons with depressed respiration; they can progress to respiratory failure. Mechanical respiratory assistance must be available when opiates are administered. Because a reduction in pulmonary gas exchange will elevate P_{CO_2} and induce cerebral vasodilation, these agents must not be administered when intracranial pressure is or may become elevated. Furthermore, the central nervous system depression produced by the opiates can obscure the characteristic signs of neurological deterioration.

Although sedation usually results from narcotic administration, restlessness, dysphoria, and excitation may also occur. Loss of mental acuity (''mental clouding'') is characteristic. Diagnostic of opiate use is marked miosis (''pinpoint pupils''), unless cerebral hypoxia and dysfunction have become sufficiently severe to produce pupillary dilation.

Nausea and orthostatic hypotension following narcotic administration can be reduced by encouraging the patient to remain recumbent. Tolerance rapidly develops to nausea, and higher doses have an antiemetic effect. Through their action on opiate receptors within the gastrointestinal tract, the narcotics increase smooth muscle tone, decreasing motility and prolonging transit time through the stomach and intestines. Constipation is a frequent consequence, to which little tolerance develops. Opiates are contraindicated in some gastrointestinal disorders; thus the cause for abdominal pain must be determined before these analgesics are administered.

Biotransformation of the opiates occurs in the liver, and doses must be reduced in the presence of hepatic dysfunction. Opiates potentiate the action of other central nervous system depressants.

Morphine is generally administered parenterally since its rapid hepatic extraction from portal circulation reduces its oral efficacy. It is used particularly to alleviate severe pain of brief duration. Often administered during acute myocardial infarction, it reduces pain and allays the accompanying apprehension that heightens sympathetic stimulation and increases myocardial oxygen demand. The labored breathing resulting from pulmonary edema is converted by morphine to slower, more efficient respiration. Presurgical sedation can include morphine, although low doses of this drug can enhance the emetic action of some general anesthetics. Morphine is antitussive and antidiarrheal; however, oral medications are usually preferred for these indications. Morphine can release histamine that will cause bronchoconstriction. Extreme caution is necessary when this drug is administered to asthmatic persons. Morphine also promotes release of antidiuretic hormone and of epinephrine from the adrenal medulla, which in turn causes mild hyperglycemia.

Codeine, like morphine, is a naturally occurring substance. It is a less potent analgesic but a highly effective antitussive. Codeine, which is orally active, is often combined with nonnarcotic analgesics such as aspirin (*e.g.,* in Emcodeine and Percodan) or acetaminophen (*e.g.,* Percocet, Tylenol with codeine). Adverse effects occasionally observed with codeine include central nervous system stimulation and seizures.

As a result of efforts to develop potent analgesics free of opiate toxicity, many semisynthetic and synthetic narcotic agents have become available. Although they vary in potency and duration of action, their side effects do not differ significantly from each other nor from morphine.

Meperidine (Demerol) is administered orally or parenterally. Its duration of action is shorter than morphine, but it produces less intense spasm of the gastrointestinal tract. The use of this drug is decreasing, due in part to its biotransformation to a toxic metabolite having a long (up to 20 hours) half-life. This metabolite can cause dysphoria, tremors, seizures, and a lethal interaction with monoamine oxidase inhibitors.

Methadone is an orally active analgesic that has a prolonged duration of effect. This opiate is also used in the detoxification and maintenance of persons physiologically dependent upon opiates. Detoxification involves administration of methadone in amounts just sufficient to suppress the abstinence (withdrawal) syndrome; doses are then gradually reduced over several days until the patient is drug-free. Methadone maintenance substitutes this opiate for morphine, heroin, and other opiates. A well-managed methadone program should enable former ''addicts'' to return to a stable life-style although their opiate dependency is maintained. Withdrawal symptoms develop more slowly in methadone dependence because of its prolonged plasma half-life.

Propoxyphene (Darvon) is structurally similar to methadone but its actions bear closer resemblance to those of codeine. It is a moderately effective analgesic frequently combined with aspirin (Darvon with acetylsalicylic acid) and acetaminophen (Wygesic, Darvocet). In large doses, propoxyphene can induce seizures. ***Levorphanol*** (Levo-Dromoran) is effective orally and parenterally and produces less nausea than morphine. ***Dextromethorphan,*** the d-isomer of levorphanol, has considerable antitussive effect but a negligible degree of other characteristic opioid actions. ***Hydromorphone*** (Dilaudid) and ***oxycodone*** (Hycodan) are semisynthetic analgesics with activity similar to morphine and codeine.

Fentanyl (Sublimaze) is a potent short-acting opiate used as a component of balanced anesthesia. Innovar combines fentanyl with droperidol to induce a sedated analgesic state known as neuroleptanalgesia. General anesthesia produced with large doses of opiates such as morphine, fentanyl, and the related ***sufentanil*** (Sufenta) and alfentanil (Alfenta) can be used for surgery in high risk myocardial patients (see discussion under General Anesthetics). A transmucosal fentanyl lozenge (Fentanyl Oralet) is available for preanesthetic sedation in children and adults, and may be useful for painful diagnostic and treatment procedures and for postoperative and cancer pain. Fentanyl in a transdermal patch (Duragesic) has a slow onset (8 to 12 hours) and long duration (48 to 72 hours) of action and can alleviate severe chronic pain refractory to nonnarcotic analgesics. In addition to the characteristic opioid effects, the transdermal preparation can cause localized redness and pruritis.

Natural opium alkaloids are available in several forms (Pantopon, paregoric, opium tincture) that have the indications and adverse effects common to all opiates. Heroin, or diacetylated morphine, has no approved use in the United States, but is used in some countries as a component of Brompton's mixture and for the maintenance of persons dependent upon opiates. All of the opiates are controlled substances.

Tramadol (Ultram) works selectively at opioid μ receptors in the central nervous system to produce analgesia. It is as effective as codeine, and has a 6-hour duration of action. Renal or hepatic impairment can prolong tramadol's half-life. Headache, nausea, constipation, sedation, and dizziness are side effects. Tramadol may potentiate the action of central nervous system depressants, including alcohol, and should not be given concurrently with monoamine oxidase inhibitors. Tramadol is reported to have neglible abuse potential and is not a controlled substance.

Agonist–Antagonist Analgesics

The search for nonaddicting potent analgesics has yielded several agents that have both agonist and antagonist action at opiate receptors. ***Pentazocine*** (Talwin) produces the characteristic analgesia, respiratory depression, and sedation of the opiates, although gastrointestinal effects such as nausea and constipation are milder. In higher doses its euphoriant effect is replaced with dysphoria, and hallucinations can occur. Caution is required in its use during acute myocardial infarction, since pentazocine can elevate heart rate and blood pressure. Parenteral administration can cause subcutaneous tissue damage. Tolerance and physiological opiate dependence develop with chronic administration. Talwin Nx reduces the abuse potential of pentazocine by combining it with naloxone (see Narcotic Antagonists below), which is not absorbed from the gastrointestinal tract and will not interfere with analgesia when tablets are ingested orally. However, if this form of pentazocine is injected, naloxone will block the opiate receptor binding of the agonist. ''Ts and blues'' is a street drug combination of pentazocine and the histamine H_1-antagonist tripelennamine, which frequently induces pulmonary disturbances, vascular obstruction, and seizures. Related to pentazorine, ***dezocine*** (Dalgan) is administered only by the parenteral route.

Nalbuphine (Nubain) is a potent rapidly acting antagonist-analgesic that in high doses produces less dysphoria and respiratory depression than pentazocine. Its abuse potential is reported to be low. ***Butorphanol*** (Stadol) shares characteristics of both pentazocine and nalbuphine and is available as a nasal spray. These analgesics are administered parenterally and have a relatively short duration of action (3 to 4 hours). They can produce sufficient respiratory depression to cause elevations in intracranial pressure. ***Dezocine*** (Dalgan) is an agonist–antagonist analgesic, and ***buprenorphine*** (Buprenex) is a partial agonist.

Because of their weak narcotic antagonist activity, the agonist–antagonist analgesics can precipitate an abstinence syndrome in persons who are physiologically dependent on opiates.

NARCOTIC ANTAGONISTS

Narcotic antagonists are classified as ''mixed'' or ''pure.'' Mixed (or agonist–antagonist) agents exert both stimulating and blocking action at the opiate receptors, and include ***levallorphan*** (Lorphan), ***nalorphine*** (Nalline), and the agonist–antagonist analgesics discussed above. Pure antagonists have no agonist activity; they merely block the access of opiates to the receptors. ***Naloxone*** (Narcan) and ***naltrexone*** (Trexan) are in the latter category.

Narcotic antagonists reverse the effects of the opiates only; the actions of other central nervous system depressants are not ameliorated by these agents. A highly specific interaction of drugs and receptors appears to be the basis for the effects of the opiates and their antagonists. The latter drugs have greater affinity for opiate receptors, and will reverse the effects of agonists by displacing them from cellular binding sites. Thus, antagonists can rapidly reverse the symptoms of opiate overdose, and can just as rapidly induce (or ''precipitate'') the abstinence syndrome in persons who are physiologically dependent upon opiates. This type of withdrawal is not easily reversed by administration of opiates, since their access to the receptors is blocked until the antagonist is inactivated. Observations of the interactions of these opposing drug types led to the first investigations of drug receptors. Subsequent studies suggest that at least four distinct types of opiate receptors mediate various effects of these agents.

The mixed antagonists cause characteristic respiratory depression, although with a lower maximal intensity than that of opiate agonists. For this reason, mixed antagonists are contraindicated in respiratory depression unless it is severe and known to be caused by opiates. Mixed antagonists can exacerbate respiratory depression from other origins. In contrast to the euphoria usually induced by opiate agonists, the response to mixed antagonists can include dysphoria, anxiety, and hallucinations.

The pure antagonist naloxone is the drug of choice for reversing opiate overdose. Intravenous administration rapidly alleviates sedation and respiratory depression. However, this drug has a relatively short half-life, and central nervous system depression can recur if sufficient amounts of opiate remain after the antagonist is metabolized. Patients must be observed for returning signs of overdose, and additional doses of naloxone may be required.

Naltrexone is an orally active analogue of naloxone that has a considerably longer half-life. Chronic alternate-day administration of this antagonist may assist former addicts to remain drug-free, since it will prevent the euphoriant effect of opiates and obviate this positive reinforcing aspect of drug abuse.

Nalmefene (Revex), a parenteral naltrexone analog, has a rapid onset with IV administration, and a half-life of 11 hours. It is hepatically inactivated. It may cause nausea and vomiting, and like all narcotic antagonists, it can precipitate withdrawal in opioid-dependent persons.

CARDIOVASCULAR PHARMACOLOGY

Inotropic Agents

Inotropic agents are used in congestive heart failure (CHF) to improve cardiovascular hemodynamics. CHF is characterized by decreased cardiac contractility resulting in decreased cardiac output and underperfusion of tissues. Peripheral vascular resistance increases reflexly, adding to afterload and further reducing cardiac output. Preload also is increased because of increases in venous return. The diameter of the heart enlarges, and cardiac efficiency declines further. Inadequate renal perfusion mobilizes responses that enhance vasoconstriction and sodium and fluid retention. As hydrostatic pressure builds in capillaries, fluid leaks out of the circulatory system and becomes evident as ascites and pulmonary and peripheral edema. Reflex sympathetic stimulation provokes a rapid but ineffective rate of cardiac contraction.

Inotropic agents are effective in CHF because they increase the contractile force of the heart. Cardiac output increases, renal perfusion improves, sodium and fluid are excreted, sympathetic activity abates, venous return falls, and cardiac dilation is alleviated. Myocardial efficiency improves while oxygen consumption remains the same or decreases.

Originally derived from the foxglove plant, the ***digitalis glycosides*** (Table 7-17) have long been used as inotropic agents. The basic digitalis structure is a steroid nucleus with a lactone ring at C17 (together called the aglycone or genin) and one to four sugar residues attached at C3. Removal of the sugars reduces the potency and duration of action of the drug. Saturating or removing the lactone ring nullifies inotropic activity. All of the digitalis glycosides exhibit the same pharmacology and toxicity. They differ in potency, degree of binding to plasma protein, route of inactivation, gastrointestinal absorption, and plasma half-life.

TABLE 7-17. Digitalis Glycosides

GENERIC NAME	TRADE NAME	ROUTE	INACTIVATION
Deslanoside	Cedilanid-D	IM, IV	Renal
Digitoxin	Crystodigin	IM, IV, PO	Hepatic
Digoxin	Lanoxin	IV, PO	Renal

An important characteristic of the digitalis glycosides is their narrow therapeutic index. The dose required to achieve beneficial effects is close to the dose that can provoke serious cardiac dysrhythmias such as paroxysmal tachycardia with block, premature ventricular contractions, nodal rhythms, bigeminy, multifocal ventricular ectopic tachycardias, and ventricular fibrillation. Persons receiving digitalis must be observed for signs and symptoms of impending drug toxicity: anorexia, nausea and vomiting, visual disturbances, weakness and fatigue, mental confusion and depression (especially in elderly patients), and psychotic behavior.

The toxic cardiac effects, and possibly the therapeutic actions, of digitalis appear to occur through inhibition of myocardial cell membrane sodium-potassium ATPase. This ''sodium pump'' normally extrudes sodium that enters the cell during depolarization, and transports potassium back into the cell. Na^+-K^+ ATPase has been proposed as the ''digitalis receptor site.'' By influencing myocardial electrolyte concentration, digitalis alters cardiac electrophysiology. Increased amounts of free intracellular calcium enhance the force of contraction of the heart. Digitalis also has marked effects on myocardial conduction velocity. Atrioventricular (A-V) node conduction and refractory periods are prolonged, predisposing to varying degrees of heart block. (Thus, digitalis can be effective in managing some atrial dysrhythmias.) A pulse lower than 60 beats/minute (50 beats for some patients) in persons receiving digitalis can be a warning of approaching toxicity. In the ventricles, particularly in Purkinje fibers, digitalis shortens the action potential and decreases the refractory period. Automaticity is enhanced, giving rise to ectopic pacemakers and ventricular escape rhythms. The ability of ventricular cells to assume control of heart rate is enhanced by digitalis-induced A-V block that hinders sinus rhythm.

In addition to its direct effects on the heart, digitalis also exerts cholinergic or ''vagal'' effects on cardiac activity. These actions, which can be reversed by atropine, include slowing of A-V conduction at low digitalis doses, and shortening of the atrial refractory period. The vagal action of digitalis may help to slow cardiac rate in the failing heart, although the improvement in hemodynamics (*i.e.*, increased stroke volume, increased ejection fraction, decreased end-diastolic volume, decreased central venous pressure) and subsequent reduction in sympathetic stimulation also contribute to this effect.

The toxic effects of digitalis on the myocardium are enhanced by hypokalemia, hypomagnesemia, and hypercalcemia. While diuretics such as the thiazides and organic acid (''loop'') agents promote renal excretion of potassium, these drugs are often administered concurrently with digitalis in the management of CHF. Patients' serum electrolyte levels must be monitored and consumption of foods rich in potassium (*e.g.*, fresh orange juice, bananas) should be encouraged. Vomiting and diarrhea, which often occur in digitalis overdose, can exacerbate K^+ loss and further enhance toxicity. Potassium supplements may be required. In persons receiving digitalis, calcium salts (especially when given parenterally) are hazardous and usually contraindicated. Renal insufficiency increases the risk of digoxin toxicity, while hepatic impairment increases that of digitoxin.

Several agents are used in the management of digitalis-induced dysrhythmias. The antidysrhythmics phenytoin and lidocaine can be effective. Use of a beta blocker such as propranolol must be carefully monitored since these drugs can enhance A-V heart block. Potassium salts may alleviate ventricular dysrhythmias only if hypokalemia is present. Elevated levels of potassium also can slow A-V conduction, and the blocking action of digitalis on entry of K^+ into cells will promote hyperkalemia. A specific antidote is now available for toxicity induced by digitoxin and digoxin. ***Digoxin immune fab*** (Digibind) utilizes drug-specific antibodies (similar to those used for radioimmunoassay of blood levels of digitalis) to bind the drug in the circulatory system and promote its removal from body tissues. The agent is usually reserved for severe life-threatening digitalis intoxication that is unresponsive to other therapy.

Additional drug interactions can enhance the toxicity of digitalis. Concurrent administration of quinidine, amiodarone, and calcium channel blockers will elevate serum digoxin levels, apparently through a decrease in renal clearance. Severe bradycardia may develop when digitalis and beta blockers are administered concomitantly. Sympathomimetic agents enhance ventricular responsiveness to digitalis, and anticholinergics, erythromycin, and tetracycline promote its gastrointestinal absorption. On the other hand, the efficacy of digitoxin is reduced by bile sequestrants such as cholestyramine that bind the drug following oral administration, and by hepatic enzyme inducers (*e.g.*, barbiturates) that accelerate its biotransformation. The plasma half-life of digitoxin is prolonged in hepatic impairment, and that of digoxin by renal insufficiency.

In persons who are seriously ill, therapeutic serum levels of digitalis may be achieved rapidly by administering large loading or digitalizing doses of drug. Lower maintenance doses are then substituted. The use of radioimmunoassay to monitor serum drug levels can be helpful in selecting drug doses that are therapeutic but not toxic. However, individual characteristics influence responsiveness to digitalis. Hyperthyroid states, or administration of thyroid hormone, make digitalis less effective while hypothyroidism enhances its actions. Infants, especially premature, and the elderly are sensitive to the actions of digitalis.

In addition to CHF, the therapeutic indications for digitalis include certain atrial dysrhythmias. Through its prolongation of A-V conduction, digitalis will slow the ventricular rate in response to atrial flutter or fibrillation. Digitalis can convert flutter to fibrillation, which may revert to sinus rhythm once drug administration is stopped. In paroxysmal atrial tachycardia, the vagal action of digitalis can help to slow atrial rate.

Drugs that decrease preload and afterload are often useful in congestive heart failure. Angiotensin converting enzyme (ACE) inhibitors such as captopril (discussed under Antihypertensive Agents) promote vasodilation, thus alleviating symptoms and improving exercise tolerance in patients with congestive heart failure. These drugs appear to slow the progression of congestive heart failure and may prolong survival. Vasodilators such as hydralazine, nitroprusside, and nitrates will decrease preload and afterload. ***Flosiquinan*** (Manoplax), chemically related to the fluoroquinolone antibiotics, dilates both arteries and veins and can be useful in persons refractory to ACE inhibitor therapy. Hepatic biotransformation converts this drug to an active metabolite with a long half-life (up to 50 hours in the presence of congestive heart failure), thus once daily dosing provides therapeutic drug levels. Headache, tachycardia, palpitations, dizziness, syncope, and nausea are side effects. Kidney failure may develop in persons with renal artery stenosis. Flosiquinan has been reported to hasten mortality in cardiac patients. Cimetidine inhibits flosiquinan inactivation, flosiquinan augments the action of anticoagulant drugs.

β-adrenergic blockers can decrease the ineffectual reflex sympathetic stimulation that occurs in congestive heart failure. However, these agents must be used with great care, as their negative inotropic and chronotropic action can exacerbate heart failure.

Amrinone (Inocor), a nondigitalis cardiotonic agent, often alleviates CHF refractory to conventional therapy. A phosphodiesterase inhibitor, this drug elevates intracellular cAMP, decreasing Ca^{2+} utilization and inducing vasodilation. Amrinone improves myocardial efficiency with little change in heart rate or blood pressure. However, adverse central nervous system and gastrointestinal reactions limit the use of this agent to short-term IV administration. ***Milrinone*** (Corotrope) may have a more favorable side effect profile.

Antidysrhythmic Drugs

Several types of drugs have the ability to suppress myocardial action and alleviate abnormal patterns of contrac-

TABLE 7-18. Antidysrhythmic Drugs

GENERIC NAME	TRADE NAME
Class Ia	
Procainamide	Pronestyl
Quinidine	Quinaglute, Cardioquin
Disopyramide	Norpace
Class Ib	
Lidocaine	Xylocaine
Mexiletine	Mexitil
Tocainide	Tonocard
Phenytoin	Dilantin
Class Ic	
Encainide	Enkaid
Flecainide	Tambocor
Propafenone	Rythmol
Other Class I	
Moricizine	Ethmozine
Class II*	
Acebutolol	Sectral
Esmolol	Brevibloc
Propranolol	Inderal
Sotalol	Betapace
Class III	
Bretylium	Bretylol
Amiodarone	Cordarone
Class IV	
Verapamil	Calan, Isoptin
Diltiazem	Cardizem
Class V	
Digoxin	Lanoxin
Adenosine	Adenocard

* For additional β-adrenergic blockers, see Table 7-6.

tion. A classification based on electrophysiological effects (Table 7-18) has been established, although some drugs may have multiple antidysrhythmic actions. The class I agents inhibit sodium entry into cells and thus reduce myocardial automaticity and excitability, slow the rate of depolarization, and prolong the effective refractory period. They depress ventricular automaticity to a greater degree than that of the sinoatrial node. Class IB agents have less effect on the rate of depolarization than those in IA, while IC drugs cause a profound slowing of depolarization. Class II antidysrhythmics are β-adrenergic antagonists (''β-blockers'') and will suppress the dysrhythmogenic influence of sympathetic stimulation. Some of these agents (*e.g.*, propranolol) also possess membrane-stabilizing activity. The major action of the class III agents is a prolongation of the myocardial action potential that can reverse refractory ventricular tachycardia and prevent fibrillation. Class IV drugs, the calcium channel antagonists, reduce the entry of calcium into cells during myocardial depolarization and recovery. Activity in the sinus and A-V nodes is most influenced, making these agents especially effective against supraventricular dysrhythmias. Additional antidysrhythmic drugs are digitalis (discussed under Cardiotonic Drugs), magnesium sulfate, which is especially effective in torsade de pointes, and adenosine.

Characteristic of class IA antidysrhythmics, ***quinidine*** depresses activity in atria and ventricles. Its action at the A-V node can be influenced by the dose and by the degree of parasympathetic tone. In small amounts, quinidine is anticholinergic and will enhance A-V conduction and sinus node depolarization rate. In higher doses, the direct depressant effect of the drug will prolong A-V conduction time. Quinidine markedly prolongs the PR, QRS, and QT intervals of the electrocardiogram.

The indications for quinidine include ventricular tachycardias and premature ectopic beats arising in the atria, A-V node, or ventricles. It can convert atrial flutter and fibrillation to normal sinus rhythm, although digitalis is usually administered first to slow A-V conduction and reduce the ventricular response. Reentrant tachydysrhythmias (*e.g.*, Wolff-Parkinson-White syndrome) can be controlled with quinidine. This drug is usually given orally, often to prevent recurrence of dysrhythmias. IV administration is hazardous since the cardiodepressant action of quinidine combined with its direct vasodilatory effect can produce a profound fall in blood pressure. Extensive binding to plasma proteins occurs. Quinidine is inactivated by the liver, although a small amount is also excreted renally. Alkalinization of the urine reduces the degree of ionization of this basic drug and enhances its renal reabsorption. Hepatic dysfunction or congestive heart failure also prolongs its plasma half-life.

Like all antidysrhythmics, quinidine is also dysrhythmogenic. Prolongation of the QT interval facilitates the occurrence of ventricular rhythms such as torsade de pointes. Quinidine can induce or exacerbate A-V heart block and may depress ectopic pacemakers, leading to cardiac arrest. Sudden death due to ventricular tachycardia or fibrillation has occurred in persons taking normal doses and in those on maintenance quinidine (''quinidine syncope''). Quinidine reduces the renal clearance of digoxin, and in higher doses may add to the block of A-V conduction. Additional adverse effects of this drug include gastrointestinal disturbances, blood dyscrasias, and cinchonism.

Procainamide has many characteristics similar to, and is used in much the same way as, quinidine. However, its vasodilatory and cardiosuppressant actions are less intense and thus it is more appropriate for IV administration. Procainamide is both inactivated hepatically and excreted renally. Renal impairment shifts biotransformation to the liver, and also causes increased plasma levels of the *n*-acetyl metabolite that also has antidysrhythmogenic action. Procainamide has a short plasma half-life, making it less suitable than quinidine for chronic prophylactic administration.

Procainamide can elicit hypotension, A-V heart block, and ventricular dysrhythmias, especially following rapid infusion. Chronic administration elevates serum levels of antinuclear antibodies and may induce a lupuslike syndrome that is usually alleviated by discontinuing use of the drug. Cross-allergenicity between procainamide and the local anesthetic procaine occurs frequently.

Because of their cardiodepressant action, both quinidine and procainamide require extreme caution in the presence of impaired A-V node or ventricular conduction. Actions of other cardiosuppressants are additive, and congestive heart failure can be exacerbated. Hyperkalemia enhances responsiveness to these agents while hypokalemia reduces their efficacy. Because of their membrane-stabilizing effect, these drugs are contraindicated in patients with myasthenia gravis.

Disopyramide is administered orally and has a longer duration of action than other class IA agents. Its effects, both direct and via cholinergic antagonism, resemble those of quinidine and procainamide. It is used in particular for ventricular dysrhythmias. Disopyramide is reported to have a lower incidence of adverse effects, although it can induce hypotension, congestive heart failure, and dysrhythmias. Either renal or hepatic impairment may require a reduction in dosage.

Lidocaine has long been the prototype class IB antidysrhythmic. Its major disadvantage is its lack of effectiveness following oral administration, caused by extensive first-pass hepatic extraction that prevents attainment of therapeutic blood levels. Its short plasma half-life necessitates continuous IV infusion (often preceded by a bolus dose) and is lengthened by impairment of hepatic function or perfusion. Lidocaine's greatest effect is on ventricular conduction, with minimal actions in supraventricular areas. The PR, QRS, and QT intervals usually are unaffected. Lidocaine is often the drug of choice to terminate or prevent ventricular dysrhythmias subsequent to acute myocardial infarction or digitalis toxicity. Neurotoxic metabolites of lidocaine can cause drowsiness, disorientation, respiratory depression, and convulsions. Concurrent propranolol or cimetidine administration can prolong lidocaine's action.

Mexiletine and ***tocainide*** are orally active analogues of lidocaine. Their effectiveness and pharmacokinetics are similar to lidocaine, with the exception that hepatic metabolism occurs more slowly and sustained ventricular tachycardia is less responsive. Adverse effects of these agents include gastrointestinal disturbances (foods or antacids may alleviate these symptoms) and central nervous system toxicity. Tocainide can induce agranulocytosis. Changes in urinary *p*H can significantly influence renal clearance.

Phenytoin has electrophysiological actions quite similar to lidocaine. It can be given orally or IV, although rapid administration by the latter route can cause cardiac arrest. Absorption after oral administration is slow; hepatic metabolism of this drug shows great variability among patients. Phenytoin is most effective in ventricular dysrhythmias that result from acute myocardial infarction and digitalis toxicity. Hypotension following phenytoin administration is due partly to its vasodilatory action. Hyperglycemia, hematologic abnormalities, and severe skin rashes may occur. Other characteristics of phenytoin are discussed under Anticonvulsants.

Class IC drugs such as ***flecainide*** and ***encainide*** markedly suppress myocardial conduction and prolong the ventricular refractory period. Ventricular dysrhythmias are especially responsive to these agents, and paroxysmal supraventricular tachycardias may also be controlled. These agents can, however, provoke or intensify rhythm disturbances, and have been linked to increased mortality among postmyocardial infarction patients. Encainide has been removed from the market, although it remains available for some persons who respond well and safely to it. The extent of biotransformation of encainide to a pharmacologically active metabolite varies among individuals. Flecainide should be used only for refractory, life-threatening dysrhythmias. Adverse effects include dizziness and blurred vision. Congestive heart failure or less than 30% ejection fraction contraindicate this drug. Inactivated by both hepatic and renal mechanisms, flecainide has a half-life of 13 to 16 hours, which may be extended in the presence of cardiovascular disease. Concurrent administration of other antidysrhythmics or cardiac suppressants is usually contraindicated. However, digoxin or a β-blocker may be used to prevent an increase in ventricular rate when flecainide is given to slow atrial contraction rate. Amiodarone and quinidine inhibit inactivation of flecainide. ***Propafenone*** (Rythmol) is a third class IC agent, and ***moricizine*** (Ethmozine) has class I characteristics but does not fall into any one of the subclasses.

Those β-blockers with membrane-stabilizing action (*e.g.*, propranolol and acebutolol) are the most effective class II antidysrhythmics. Suppression of sympathetic stimulation also contributes to control of rhythm disturbances but can be hazardous in patients with compensated heart failure sustained by increased adrenergic tone. Beta-blockers suppress activity in all cardiac regions. Sinoatrial node depolarization and A-V node conduction are slowed, atrial excitability and conductivity and ventricular automaticity are reduced. Beta-blockers are especially useful in suppressing dysrhythmias enhanced by prolongation of the QT interval as well as those induced by excessive catecholamine activity, as in thyrotoxicosis and halothane or cyclopropane anesthesia. Treatment with some β-blockers has reduced mortality in postmyocardial infarction patients. Beta-blockers can elicit hypotension, hypoglycemia, and bronchospasm that is resistant to β-agonists. Likewise, congestive heart failure exacerbated or induced by β-blockers can be unresponsive to catecholamines. However, glucagon or amrinone can stimulate cardiac activity in the presence of β-receptor blockade. Other cardiac depressants can add to that effect of the β-blockers. Acebutolol is somewhat β_1 receptor-selective and has less intense metabolic and respiratory effects than propranolol. It also has partial agonist activity and thus causes less slowing of atrial rate. Esmolol given IV for supraventricular dysrhythmias has a rapid onset and brief duration of action. The β-blockers are discussed further under Sympathomimetic Drugs.

The class III antidysrhythmic agents prolong the duration of the myocardial action potential and are especially effective in controlling refractory ventricular tachydysrhythmias and in preventing ventricular fibrillation. ***Bretylium*** is administered IV to patients who have not responded to other first-line antidysrhythmics. An initial release of catecholamines from sympathetic nerve terminals can elicit a brief exacerbation of tachycardia and vasoconstriction. Then a decrease in sympathetic activity ensues due to depletion of norepinephrine stores. Duration of therapy is usually limited to 5 days. Hypotension is the major adverse reaction. Bretylium enhances myocardial responsiveness to electrical defibrillation.

Amiodarone is administered orally to control severe refractory ventricular dysrhythmias. It prolongs the myocardial refractory period and the PR, QRS, and QT intervals. A large percentage of persons treated with this drug experience a variety of adverse effects. Hepatotoxicity, nephrotoxicity, pulmonary alveolitis, congestive heart failure, and exacerbation of dysrhythmias are among the most serious. Nausea, corneal microdeposits, central nervous system dysfunction, changes in thyroid activity, photosensitivity, and skin discoloration also occur. Amiodarone is excreted in the bile and has a remarkably long (from 10 to 50 days) plasma half-life. The inactivation of many drugs, including digoxin, oral anticoagulants, and other antidysrhythmics, is inhibited.

Sotalol (Betapace) combines characteristics of class II and class III antidysrhythmics. It prolongs repolarization and is a β-adrenergic antagonist. Sotalol is renally excreted and has a half-life of 12 hours. Bradycardia and fatigue are adverse effects. Risk of torsade de pointes with sotalol is increased at high doses or with hypokalemia. Tricyclic antidepressants, phenothiazines, and the nonsedating H_1 receptor antihistamines enhance sotalol's dysrhythmogenic potential.

Verapamil is the calcium channel blocker most frequently used for treatment and prevention of supraventricular tachycardias. It causes marked depression of A-V conduction and slowing of sinus node depolarization may occur. Verapamil binds extensively to plasma proteins and is inactivated hepatically. IV administration produces a rapid onset of action. Combination with a β-antagonist can elicit extreme bradycardia, while concurrent disopyramide can precipitate congestive heart failure. Verapamil administered in the presence of Wolff-Parkinson-White syndrome is hazardous. The calcium channel blocker diltiazem also is an effective antidysrhythmic. The calcium channel blockers are used also as antihypertensive and antianginal agents and are discussed under those headings.

Class V includes other agents that have proven effective against some dysrhythmias. Adenosine has a very brief plasma half-life; its major adverse effects are dyspnea and hypotension. Given IV, adenosine has a very rapid onset and a brief half-life and thus generally a short duration of adverse effects such as hypotension and nausea. It depresses A-V conduction and terminates reentrant supraventricular dysrhythmias. Caffeine and theophylline block the action of adenosine.

Digoxin is discussed under Inotropic Agents.

Hypolipemic Agents

The complexes of lipid and protein (lipoproteins) found in the circulatory system are of several types. Chylomicrons are the least dense. They are composed mainly of dietary triglycerides and are present in the greatest amounts shortly after eating. Very-low-density lipoproteins (VLDL) or prebeta lipoproteins carry triglycerides and cholesterol within the circulatory system. Low-density lipoproteins (LDL) contain large amounts of cholesterol; elevated levels of LDL have been found to correlate with increased risk of coronary heart disease (CHD). High-density lipoproteins (HDL) contain triglycerides and cholesterol and appear to transport the latter from body tissues to the liver. Elevated levels of these lipoproteins are associated with reduced risk of CHD.

Hyperlipidemia, or elevated blood levels of lipoproteins, occurs in various forms. Although there is still some controversy over the relationship between elevated serum lipid levels and the development of CHD, attempts are usually made to correct hyperlipidemia. Decreasing serum cholesterol levels appears to slow the progression and may promote regression of atherosclerosis. Dietary changes such as decreased calorie and saturated fat ingestion are used first in the management of elevated lipid levels. If these measures are not effective after a trial of at least 6 months, drugs may have to be administered. Dietary modifications must be continued to enhance the efficacy of pharmacotherapy. Hypolipemic drugs usually

TABLE 7-19. Hypolipemic Drugs

GENERIC NAME	TRADE NAME
Bile Acid Sequestrants	
Cholestyramine	Questran
Colestipol	Colestid
HMG-CoA Reductase Inhibitors	
Fluvastatin	Lescol
Lovastatin	Mevacor
Pravastatin	Pravachol
Simvastatin	Zocor
Other Agents	
Clofibrate	Atromid-S
Gemfibrozil	Lopid
Nicotinic acid	Nicobid, Nicolar, others
Probucol	Lorelco

must be continued indefinitely, because serum cholesterol rises when they are terminated.

Several types of hypolipemic agents are available (Table 7-19). The bile acid-binding resins ***cholestyramine*** (Questran) and ***colestipol*** (Colestid), which bind bile acids in the intestine and promote their excretion in the feces, are used in the management of type II hyperlipidemia. Cholesterol metabolism is increased, while its serum levels and those of LDL are lowered. The resins are suspended in water or juice and are consumed at mealtimes. Gastrointestinal distress is the most frequent adverse effect. Increased ingestion of fiber can ameliorate bloating and constipation. Since fat-soluble vitamins (A, D, and K) also bind to these resins, deficiencies can develop. The gastrointestinal absorption of many drugs (*e.g.*, digoxin, warfarin, antibiotics, and thiazide diuretics) is reduced by concomitant resin administration. Cholestyramine is also used to alleviate pruritus associated with biliary tract obstruction.

Nicotinic acid (niacin) lowers plasma levels of VLDL and LDL and elevates HDL levels. Its administration has been associated with decreased risk of CHD. The prominent side effect of cutaneous flushing can be alleviated with inhibitors of prostaglandin synthesis, such as aspirin. Nicotinic acid is hepatotoxic, can decrease glucose tolerance, and can activate peptic ulcer. Blurred vision, gastrointestinal upset, and hyperuricemia can occur. Because of its relaxant effect on blood vessels, it should not be administered to persons with marked hypotension. It can add to the effects of antihypertensive agents. In the treatment of hyperlipidemia, nicotinic acid used concurrently with bile-acid binding resins is an effective regimen for achieving maximal reductions in LDL cholesterol.

Probucol (Lorelco) reduces plasma levels of both LDL and HDL. Its mechanism of action is not completely understood, and may involve increased LDL catabolism and the biliary excretion of cholesterol. Since this drug is cardiotoxic, it is contraindicated in patients with cardiac dysrhythmias or QT interval prolongation. The most frequent adverse effects are gastrointestinal disturbances and headache. Probucol sequesters in adipose tissue and thus remains in the body for extensive periods of time.

HMG-CoA (3-hydroxy-3-methylglutaryl-coenzyme A) reductase inhibitors such as ***Lovastatin*** (Mevacor) are probably the most effective drugs for lowering total cholesterol and LDL. However, their long-term safety is not established, and other drugs should be tried first. The HMG-CoA reductase enzyme catalyzes the rate-limiting step in the synthesis of cholesterol. Cholesterol is an important constituent of cell membranes, and decreased synthesis *may* promote other causes of mortality. Myositis, a lupus-like syndrome, renal failure, headache, gastrointestinal distress, severe increases in serum creatine phosphokinase, and elevation of serum aminotransferase levels have been reported. Hepatic function should be monitored. HMG-CoA reductase inhibitors may be combined with other antihyperlipidemic drugs, but concurrent niacin or gemfibrozil as well as erythromycin or cyclosporine can increase the risk for myopathy. HMG-CoA reductase inhibitors are most effective when taken in the evening, as most endogenous cholesterol synthesis appears to occur just after midnight.

Pravastatin (Pravachol), ***simvastatin*** (Zocor), and ***fluvastatin*** (Lescol) are additional HMG-CoA reductase inhibitors. Fluvastatin may have less risk of myopathy, but several drug interactions have been reported. Bile acid-binding resins interfere with absorption of fluvastatin, which should be taken at least two hours before or four hours after the resin. Rifampin will increase the inactivation of fluvastatin, while the antiulcer drugs cimetidine, ranitidine, and omeprazole will inhibit its inactivation. Fluvastatin is highly bound to plasma proteins and is subject to extensive first-pass extraction.

Gemfibrozil (Lopid) lowers VLDL and can elevate HDL. Gastrointestinal distress is the most common adverse effect; formation of gallstones may occur. Gemfibrozil can enhance the action of oral anticoagulants. ***Clofibrate*** (Atromid-S) is similar in action to gemfibrozil. Clofibrate may be linked to incidence of fatal malignancies, gallstones, and gastrointestinal disease. It is now recommended as second-line therapy.

The observation that premenopausal women have a low incidence of CHD led to the investigation of female hormones as antilipemic agents. While estrogens lower serum cholesterol levels, they elevate triglyceride levels and have not been proven effective. They produce feminizing side effects, and are contraindicated in the presence of thromboembolic disorders, pregnancy, and estrogen-dependent breast carcinoma.

Omega-3 fatty acids derived from cold-water fish have

modest effects on serum lipids, and may decrease early mortality among myocardial infarction survivors.

Pharmacotherapy of Angina Pectoris

Angina pectoris is chest pain that occurs when the myocardial oxygen supply becomes inadequate. Effort-induced or classic angina (chronic stable angina) develops when atherosclerotic deposits encroach upon the coronary blood supply and compromise the ability of coronary vessels to dilate. An increased cardiac workload fails to elicit an increase in blood flow, and oxygen demands are not satisfied. Variant or Prinzmetal's angina, which appears to result from coronary artery vasospasm, can occur even in the absence of physical or psychological stress. Myocardial infarction can occur if periods of ischemia are prolonged. Drugs that increase coronary perfusion or decrease the myocardial workload can alleviate ischemic pain. Some antianginal drugs exert both effects. Reduction in the incidence and severity of anginal attacks, and increased exercise tolerance, are the goals of antianginal therapy.

Nitroglycerin and related nitrates continue to be the primary drugs used in the prevention and alleviation of angina. Nitroglycerin, the drug of choice for terminating acute anginal attacks, is inactive when given orally but its marked lipid solubility allows rapid absorption and onset of action following sublingual administration. Transdermal, translingual, and transmucosal forms of this nitrate are also available (Table 7-20). Tolerance develops rapidly with continuous use of the transdermal patches, thus intermittent rather than continuous use is recommended. Intravenous nitroglycerin (Tridil, Nitro-Bid IV, Nitrostat IV) can be used to maintain consistent plasma levels of drug. ***Isosorbide dinitrate***, ***isosorbide mononitrate*** (the major active metabolite of the dinitrate), ***erythrityl tetranitrate*** (Peritrate), and ***pentaerythrityl tetranitrate*** are administered orally and sublingually. ***Amyl nitrate*** is inhaled to alleviate anginal pain. Sustained-release forms can prolong the duration of action of these drugs, which are rapidly inactivated in the liver.

TABLE 7-20. Nitrate Vasodilators

GENERIC NAME	TRADE NAME
Amyl nitrate	—
Erythrityl tetranitrate	Cardilate
Isosorbide dinitrate	Isordil, Sorbitrate
Isosorbide mononitrate	Izmo
Nitroglycerin	Nitrostat, Nitrogard, Deponit, Nitrodisc, Transderm-Nitro, Tridil, Nitrostat IV, Nitrospan, Nitrol
Pentaerythrityl tetranitrate	Peritrate, Duotrate, Naptrate, others

The nitrates relax smooth muscle of arteries and veins. Arteriolar dilation decreases the resistance to cardial outflow (afterload), while dilation of veins reduces venous return to the right atrium (preload). Both of these effects reduce myocardial oxygen demand. The nitrates can elicit marked hypotension with reflex tachycardia that may intensify myocardial ischemia. Postural hypotension frequently occurs, and dilation of cerebral vessels can induce headaches, nausea, and syncope. Tolerance may develop to side effects and also to the beneficial effects of the nitrates; this can be minimized by administering doses that are just effective and by providing drug-free intervals each day. When tolerance reaches unacceptable levels, temporary termination of nitrate administration allows reversal of tolerance. Sublingual nitroglycerin tablets should provide rapid relief from pain. Failure of two or three tablets administered 5 minutes apart may indicate acute myocardial infarction. Nitroglycerin tablets must be stored properly to prevent spontaneous decomposition. Termination of nitrate administration must be accomplished gradually to avoid angina recurrence or myocardial infarction. Persons exposed to industrial sources of nitroglycerin may experience these consequences when removed from their work environment. Methemoglobinemia can occur with overdose of nitrates. Individual sensitivity or concomitant alcohol consumption can provoke profound hypotension characterized by nausea, weakness, anxiety, and loss of consciousness.

Beta-adrenergic antagonists, in particular those with no intrinsic activity (*e.g.*, propranolol and nadolol) are also used to prevent the occurrence of angina. By reducing sympathetic stimulation of the heart, these drugs have negative inotropic and chronotropic effects that reduce myocardial oxygen demand. When given with nitrates, the β-antagonists suppress the reflex tachycardia induced by the vasodilators. The pharmacology of these drugs is discussed under Adrenergic Antagonists.

The calcium antagonists (or slow channel calcium entry blockers) are effective in preventing both effort-induced and variant angina. The entry of calcium ions through specialized membrane channels is altered by these agents. Reduced intracellular calcium causes slowing of sinus nodal depolarization and prolonged A-V conduction time. Relaxation of vascular smooth muscle, particularly in the coronary and cerabral vessels, also occurs. The sensitivity of various tissues to the calcium antagonists is not uniform. Cardiac cells are most responsive to ***verapamil*** and ***diltiazem***, while vascular smooth muscle is most affected by the dihydropyridines, such as ***nifedipine***, ***amlodipine***, and ***nicardipine***. Vasodilation can, in turn, provoke reflex increase in sympathetic activity and greater anginal pain.

Calcium antagonists alleviate both stable and variant anginal pain. Nifedipine and diltiazem have slightly greater efficacy than verapamil. These drugs can be combined with nitrates and also with beta antagonists, although the latter combination may precipitate heart failure or A-V conduction block. Concomitant IV administration of a beta blocker and verapamil is contraindicated. Side effects such as dizziness, headaches, and tachycardia that result from vasodilation occur most frequently with the dihydropyridines. Verapamil and diltiazem are most likely to cause negative inotropy and chronotropy, and can induce heart failure when left ventricular function is inadequate. Bradycardia and heart block can occur. These consequences of cardiac depression are more likely to occur when β-adrenergic blockers are coadministered. Verapamil can cause severe constipation. Peripheral edema can occur. The calcium antagonists are inactivated in the liver. ***Bepridil*** (Vascor), a blocker of both slow calcium and fast sodium channels, can be effective in refractory angina. Metabolized in the liver and highly bound to plasma protein, bepridil has a half-life of 30 to 50 hours. Adverse effects include dizziness, gastrointestinal symptoms, headache, tremor, and ECG changes that predispose to serious ventricular dysrhythmias, including torsade de pointes. Bepridil may enhance the action of other antianginal agents. Amlodipine's gradual absorption and long plasma half-life make it effective with once-daily administration.

Antihypertensive Agents

Hypertension (persistent elevation of systolic and diastolic pressure) is broadly defined as essential (primary) or secondary. The latter results from some identifiable disease process such as nephritis, renal artery obstruction, arteriosclerosis, or toxemia of pregnancy. When the underlying cause is corrected, secondary hypertension is resolved.

The cause of essential hypertension, which accounts for 90% of patients with elevated blood pressure, is not known. Hyperactivity of the sympathetic nervous system may contribute to the development of hypertension. Regardless of its origin, chronic high blood pressure produces end-organ damage chiefly of the vasculature of the kidney, heart, and brain, resulting in myocardial infarction, stroke, renal failure, and premature death. Reduction of elevated pressure, through diet (weight loss and decreased sodium intake), reduction in smoking and alcohol use, increased physical activity, or the use of antihypertensive drugs if these measures are ineffective, can prevent potential adverse sequelae. Essential hypertension can remain asymptomatic for many years; thus periodic measurement of blood pressure is important.

A considerable number of drugs have been used in the management of essential hypertension (Table 7-21). Several different mechanisms of action are represented, and persons refractory to one type of agent often respond to another. In addition, combinations of two or three types of drugs are frequently used, with the advantage that low doses can be given, thus reducing the incidence of side effects while maintaining an adequate therapeutic response. "Stepped therapy" for hypertension refers to initiating treatment with a single agent (usually a thiazide, β-blocker, angiotensin-converting enzyme inhibitor, or calcium antagonist), then increasing doses or adding in a stepwise manner additional drug(s) as necessary. Multiple drug regimens are also used to reduce adverse effects

TABLE 7-21. Antihypertensive Drugs

GENERIC NAME	TRADE NAME
Centrally Acting Agents	
Clonidine	Catapres
Methyldopa	Aldomet
Guanabenz	Wytensin
Guanfacine	Tenex
Peripheral Amine Depletors	
Reserpine	several
Guanethidine	Ismelin
Guanadrel	Hylorel
Vasodilators	
Hydralazine	Apresoline
Minoxidil	Loniten
α-Adrenergic Antagonists	
Prazosin	Minipress
Terazosin	Hytrin
Doxazosin	Cardura
Angiotensin-Converting Enzyme Inhibitors	
Captopril	Capoten
Enalapril	Vasotec
Lisinopril	Prinivil, Zestril
Benazepril	Lotensin
Fosinopril	Monopril
Ramipril	Altace
Quinapril	Accupril
Moexipril	Univasc
Angiotensin Receptor Antagonist	
Losartan	Cozaar
Calcium Channel Blockers	
Amlodipine	Norvasc
Diltiazem	Cardizem
Felodipine	Plendil
Nifedipine	Procardia
Verapamil	Calan, Isoptin
Nicardipine	Cardene
Nimodipine	Nimotop
Isradipine	DynaCirc
Diuretics (see Table 7-25)	
β-Adrenergic Antagonists (see Table 7-6)	

of antihypertensive agents. For example, diuretics will reverse the sodium and fluid retention caused by calcium channel blockers, and β-adrenergic antagonists will block the reflex tachycardia of vasodilators.

Essential hypertension will frequently require life-long therapy, although gradual reduction in drug dosage can be attempted when blood pressure has been controlled for a year or more. Compliance with drug regimens can be problematic: annoying side effects experienced by a previously asymptomatic patient may elicit a decision to abandon drug treatment. Patients must be told of the possible severe consequences of untreated hypertension, and must be encouraged to take measures to reduce blood pressure. Often, a different type of drug with more tolerable side effects can be substituted.

The thiazide diuretics (see Table 7-25) are among the most frequently used antihypertensive drugs, both as single agents and as components of combination therapy. Their mechanisms of action include sodium depletion and reduction of plasma volume. In addition, there is evidence that the thiazides have a direct relaxant effect on arteriolar smooth muscle and may reduce vascular responsiveness to endogenous constrictors. Older persons frequently respond well to low doses of thiazides. The "potassium-sparing" diuretics such as spironolactone and triamterene may be combined with the thiazides to minimize potassium loss. Metolazone (Zaroxolyn) and indapamide (Lozol) have actions very similar to the thiazides and can be effective when decreased renal function impairs the action of thiazides. The loop diuretics such as furosemide are occasionally used in treating hypertension, although their greater diuretic action can result in increased incidence and severity of adverse effects. Loop diuretics are generally less effective than thiazides as antihypertensives, except in the presence of impaired renal function. Diuretics can elevate plasma lipid levels. The diuretics are discussed further elsewhere in this chapter.

The β-adrenergic antagonists such as propranolol, atenolol, or metoprolol also are used widely in the management of hypertension, frequently in combination with thiazides and other agents. Their mechanism of antihypertensive efficacy may include reduction in sympathetic outflow from the central nervous system, suppression of response to sympathetic stimulation of cardiac β_1 receptors, and inhibition of renin release. Black and elderly patients may respond poorly to β-blockers. Because β-blockers will reduce many aspects of sympathetic stimulation, they cause a wide range of side effects. Metoprolol (Lopressor), atenolol (Tenormin), acebutolol (Sectral), and betaxolol (Kerlone) are "cardioselective" β-antagonists that preferentially block β_1 receptors in cardiac tissue. However, higher doses will block the β_2 receptors in bronchial and vascular tissues. This selective action confers advantages over β-blockers such as propranolol. For example, there is relatively less danger of provoking undesirable bronchoconstriction in patients with asthma and other forms of chronic obstructive pulmonary disease, and a temporary rise in peripheral resistance at the start of therapy, and sudden pronounced rises in blood pressure after physical exertion and emotional stress, are less likely to occur. The most common adverse reactions of the β-blockers are tiredness and dizziness, depression, diarrhea, impotence, loss of libido, changes in plasma lipid levels, and shortness of breath with bradycardia. There have been reports of exacerbation of angina pectoris and occasional myocardial infarction following abrupt cessation of therapy. Beta-blockers are contraindicated in sinus bradycardia, heart block greater than first degree, and cardiogenic shock. Cardioselective β-blockers are safer in diabetic persons. The β-blockers are discussed further under Adrenergic Antagonists.

Other antihypertensive agents that appear to work by reducing sympathetic outflow from the central nervous system are methyldopa (Aldomet), clonidine (Catapres), guanabenz (Wytensin), and guanfacine (Tenex). Several theories have been proposed to explain the action of ***methyldopa.*** It is now generally accepted that α-methylnorepinephrine, a metabolite of this drug, activates presynaptic α_2 receptors (autoreceptors) that in turn inhibit release of the neurotransmitter norepinephrine. Methyldopa also reduces plasma renin levels. Common adverse effects are sedation, dry mouth, nasal congestion, and postural hypotension. Similarly to β-blockers and vasodilators, methyldopa causes sodium and fluid retention; thus a diuretic is usually given concurrently. Methyldopa can induce autoimmune reactions in the form of elevated antiglobulin antibodies (positive Coombs test), hemolytic anemia, thrombocytopenia, and leukopenia. Fever and hepatitis may develop, making this drug contraindicated in patients with hepatic disease.

Clonidine acts by direct stimulation of central α_2-adrenergic receptors and may also stimulate the baroreceptor reflex pathway, inducing a fall in blood pressure. The greatest effect of clonidine occurs when the patient is in the upright position. The most commonly encountered side effects are drowsiness and dry mouth. Constipation may occur and, rarely, orthostatic hypotension. Administration of clonidine (like propranolol) must not be terminated abruptly, since rapid withdrawal can provoke restlessness, tachycardia, and rebound hypertension. A diuretic is usually given concurrently to enhance hypotensive action. Tricyclic antidepressants can reverse the therapeutic effects of clonidine. Investigational uses for this drug include treatment of migraine and of the symptoms of opiate withdrawal. Clonidine is available in a transdermal form (Catapres TTS) that is applied once weekly. ***Guanabenz*** and ***guanfacine*** work in much the same manner as clonidine to reduce blood pressure. Guanfacine is reported to cause milder side effects than other agents in this class.

Some drugs reduce blood pressure by decreasing sympathetic activity at the peripheral nerve terminals. Because of their wide range of adverse effects, these drugs are used less frequently. ***Reserpine,*** one of the earliest antihypertensive agents, depletes neuronal norepinephrine, dopamine, and serotonin. Numerous adverse effects are reported for this drug. Its suppression of sympathetic activity allows parasympathetic predominance that leads to bradycardia, increased gastrointestinal motility and diarrhea, and exacerbation of peptic ulcer. A most troublesome aspect of reserpine is its ability to elicit profound mental depression; a history of affective disorder contraindicates this drug. The onset of action of reserpine is slow, requiring several days to produce a full antihypertensive effect. Beta-adrenergic blockers add to the sympatholytic action of reserpine; if these drugs are combined, severe hypotension and bradycardia can occur. Patients taking reserpine may experience marked hypotension under general anesthesia. Once used in the management of psychiatric disorders, reserpine has largely been replaced by phenothiazines and other neuroleptics.

Guanethidine (Ismelin) depletes adrenergic neuronal norepinephrine and also inhibits its release in response to sympathetic stimulation. Its onset of action is several days. Guanethidine has a long plasma half-life (5 days) that may be extended in persons with renal impairment. To exert an antihypertensive action, guanethidine must enter the adrenergic nerve terminal. Thus, tricyclic antidepressants and other drugs that inhibit the neuronal membrane uptake system can reverse the actions of this drug. Side effects include diarrhea, bradycardia, retrograde ejaculation, postural hypotension, and sodium and fluid retention that is managed with concurrent diuretic administration. In the presence of pheochromocytoma, guanethidine may elicit hypertension as it suppresses neuronal reuptake of catecholamines. Extreme caution is required when this drug is administered to persons with peptic ulcer, asthma, coronary insufficiency, cerebral vascular disease, severe cardiac failure, or recent myocardial infarction. Use of MAOIs must be terminated at least 1 week prior to guanethidine administration. Drugs or other factors (*e.g.,* warm environment) that cause vasodilation can exacerbate postural hypotension of this agent. Guanadrel (Hylorel) works in a manner similar to guanethidine but has a shorter duration of action. Bretylium also has a similar mechanism but is no longer used extensively for the treatment of hypertension.

Prazosin (Minipress), ***terazosin*** (Hytrin), and ***doxazosin*** (Cardura) block postsynaptic α_1-adrenergic receptors, thus reducing sympathetic vasoconstriction. Dilation of arterioles and veins results in a reduction in both preload and afterload. Because of these effects, prazosin may be used to ameliorate congestive heart failure refractory to digitalis and diuretics. Prazosin rarely causes tachycardia. A ''first-dose phenomenon'' is marked postural hypotension and syncope 30 to 90 minutes after the initial administration or a rapid increment in dose. This may be prevented by instituting treatment with a low dose that is gradually increased as required. Because α-blockade will relax smooth muscle, terazosin can enhance urine flow in persons with prostatic hypertrophy.

Hydralazine (Apresoline) and ***minoxidil*** (Loniten) are direct-acting arteriolar dilators. Hydralazine reduces diastolic pressure more than systolic. A diuretic is usually given concurrently to prevent sodium and fluid retention, and a β-blocker or centrally acting sympathetic inhibitor is given to minimize reflex tachycardia. Chronic administration of doses in excess of 200 mg/day can provoke development of a lupuslike syndrome. Other adverse effects include headache, tachycardia, angina pectoris, nausea, vomiting, and diarrhea. These may be alleviated by reducing the dosage. The presence of cardiovascular disease requires caution in the use of hydralazine. This drug appears to increase renal blood flow, in contrast to many antihypertensives that reduce renal perfusion.

Minoxidil, which can cause marked fluid retention and occasional pericardial effusion that may progress to tamponade, is usually reserved for severe hypertension that is refractory to other drugs. Congestive heart failure can occur; concomitant administration of a diuretic (frequently furosemide) is advised. Tachycardia can be suppressed with a β-blocker or other sympatholytic agent. Guanethidine should not be used concurrently with minoxidil because severe hypotension may occur. Hypertrichosis is a frequent side effect, and topical preparations of minoxidil (Rogaine) are available as a treatment for baldness.

The ***angiotensin converting enzyme (ACE) inhibitors*** captoril (Capoten) and others (see Table 7-21) reduce blood pressure primarily by suppressing the renin-angiotensin-aldosterone system. Angiotensin II is a powerful endogenous vasoconstrictor. Persons with elevated plasma levels of renin (*e.g.,* those with renovascular hypotension or who are volume depleted) are most responsive to these agents and may experience severe hypotension. Proteinuria and hyperkalemia may develop, especially in persons with preexisting renal impairment. However, captopril can slow renal deterioration in diabetic persons. Dry cough, acute renal failure, especially with renal artery stenosis, hematological changes, and altered taste perception are characteristic side effects; myelosuppressive drugs can exacerbate agranulocytosis. ACE inhibitors impair renal excretion of lithium. Because the ACE inhibitors can cause potassium retention, potassium supplements or potassium-sparing diuretics are contraindicated when these drugs are used. Impaired renal function increases the risk for ACE inhibitor–induced hyperkalemia. ACE inhibitor–induced angioedema indicates immediate cessation of drug administration. A diuretic may be given concurrently to enhance the action of the ACE inhibitors. An ACE inhibitor, added to digitalis/diuretic therapy, can be beneficial in refractory congestive heart failure. Nonsteroidal anti-inflammatory drugs decrease the antihypertensive action of many agents including ACE inhibitors, β-blockers, and diuretics. ACE inhibitors should not be used during pregnancy because they increase the risk of fetal death. Quinapril is a prodrug converted to an active ACE inhibitor in the liver and small intestine.

Losartan (Cozaar) is an antagonist of angiotensin II binding at type I angiotensin receptors found in blood vessels as well as other tissues. The diuretic hydrochlorothiazide enhances its antihypertensive effect. Losartan is hepatically biotransformed to an active metabolite with a plasma half-life of 6 to 9 hours. Adverse effects reported thus far for this drug are dizziness and some elevation of serum potassium and aminotransferase. Like the ACE inhibitors, losartan is contraindicated in pregnancy; but, unlike the ACE inhibitors, it is not associated with cough and angioneurotic edema.

The MAOI were among the earliest antihypertensive agents but have largely been replaced by newer drugs. ***Pargyline*** (Eutonyl) is occasionally used in the management of moderate to severe hypertension. Common side effects include gastrointestinal disturbances, dry mouth, fluid retention, and postural hypotension. A major disadvantage of the MAOI is the number of potentially severe drug interactions that can occur. Sympathomimetic amines, or drugs that can release or block uptake of catecholamines, may cause hypertensive crisis in the presence of MAOI. Foods that contain tyramine (*e.g.*, certain wines and cheeses) can provoke the same type of occasionally fatal response (the so-called "cheese reaction"). The hepatic biotransformation of many drugs (*e.g.*, sedatives and opiates) is suppressed. Meperidine (Demerol) is contraindicated in persons receiving MAOI. These drugs can exacerbate parkinsonian symptoms as well as the adverse effects of antiparkinsonism drugs. Diabetic patients may experience severe hypoglycemia. MAOI are used also in the management of depression, and are discussed further under that topic.

The calcium channel blockers (or calcium antagonists) such as verapamil are effective antihypertensive agents. They are discussed under Pharmacotherapy of Angina Pectoris. These drugs reduce the entry of calcium ions into vascular and cardiac muscle, thereby reducing contractility. Vasodilation occurs and blood pressure falls. Nifedipine (capsular formulation) can induce a reflex increase in heart rate, while verapamil and diltiazem prolong A-V conduction time. Verapamil is used as an antidysrhythmic drug. Because of their cardiac suppressant action, the calcium channel blockers can exacerbate congestive heart failure.

MANAGEMENT OF HYPERTENSIVE EMERGENCIES

Hypertensive emergencies occur when extreme risk of vascular or organ damage coexists with markedly elevated blood pressure. Clinical episodes including aortic dissection, excessive adrenergic stimulation, severe hypertension accompanying vascular surgery, intracranial hemorrhage or pulmonary edema, and malignant hypertension with evidence of organ damage require lowering of blood pressure to a safer level in a relatively rapid but carefully controlled manner. Excessive fall in pressure can adversely affect renal, cerebral, or coronary perfusion and function and may induce vomiting. Persons who are elderly or have vascular disorders are especially at risk of such adverse consequences. In some acute hypertensive situations, more gradual (*i.e.*, over several hours) reduction of pressure is appropriate.

Several types of drugs (Table 7-22) are used in the management of hypertensive episodes. Although the choice of drug can be influenced by the cause of the crisis, therapeutic measures often must be instituted before a diagnosis is definitive. Intravenous administration is required in true emergencies; other routes can be effective in less urgent cases.

Nitroprusside is the drug of choice for certain hypertensive emergencies; it dilates veins and arterioles. Its rapid onset is coupled with a brief duration of action that necessitates continuous IV infusion but allows fine control of patients' response. Since a marked reduction in blood pressure may occur rapidly, close observation of patients is required. Elderly and hypertensive persons are especially sensitive to the effects of this and other hypotensive agents. Nausea, headache, psychotic behavior, palpitations, tachycardia, and anxiety can accompany ni-

TABLE 7-22. Drugs Used in the Management of Hypertensive Emergencies

GENERIC NAME	TRADE NAME
Nitroprusside	Nipride
Diazoxide	Hyperstat
Hydralazine	Apresoline
Nitroglycerin	Several
Trimethaphan	Arfonad
Labetalol	Normodyne, Trandate
Verapamil	Calan, Isoptin
Nifedipine	Procardia
Phentolamine	Regitine

troprusside administration. Biotransformation of this drug yields cyanide and thiocyanate. Hepatic and renal impairment, and administration for longer than 24 hours, increase the risk of toxic accumulations of these substances. Metabolic acidosis or tolerance to drug effects often presage this toxicity. Nitroprusside is rapidly decomposed; infusion solutions should be protected from light with aluminum foil wrapping, and darkly discolored solutions should be discarded. A β-blocker such as propranolol may be used to suppress reflex tachycardia and to minimize additional damage in aortic dissection.

The arteriolar vasodilator ***diazoxide,*** administered by IV bolus, has a rapid onset (within minutes) but an extended duration (several hours) of action. Severe prolonged hypotension may be avoided by the use of small doses (miniboluses or pulse injections) and close observation. Diazoxide is contraindicated in patients with aortic dissection, coronary artery disease, and myocardial infarction. Reflex tachycardia can be reduced by concomitant administration of a β-adrenergic antagonist. Diazoxide promotes sodium and fluid retention, and extended use may require the administration of a diuretic. Similarly to the related thiazide diuretics, this drug can induce hyperglycemia that necessitates adjustment in dosage of antidiabetic medication. Phlebitis and myocardial and cerebrel ischemia can occur following diazoxide administration. Since diazoxide relaxes uterine muscle, it can terminate contractions during labor.

Hydralazine, also an arteriolar dilator, is considered by many to be the drug of choice to ameliorate hypertension that accompanies eclampsia. The IM or IV route provides a prompt onset of effect, although patients' responses are variable. Reflex tachycardia and an increase in myocardial oxygen demand can induce angina. Additional adverse effects include those that frequently accompany rapid lowering of blood pressure: nausea, dizziness, and palpitations. Sodium and fluid retention can be avoided by concurrent administration of a diuretic, and β-blockers can reduce excessive cardiac stimulation.

Nitroglycerin, administered by IV infusion, provides a rapid reduction in blood pressure that can be titrated to the patient's response. Dilation of veins and of coronary blood vessels occurs, and at higher drug doses arterioles also are affected. The resultant hemodynamic changes usually will decrease myocardial oxygen demand. Glyceryl trinitrate should be considered for use in hypertensive patients with coronary insufficiency. Adverse effects can include nausea and vomiting, headache, tachycardia, and marked hypotension.

The ganglionic blocker ***trimethaphan***, especially useful in the management of aortic dissection, dilates both veins and arterioles. Elevation of the patient's head potentiates the hypotensive action of trimethaphan, which is administered by continuous IV infusion. Trimethaphan releases histamine from mast cells and thus can be hazardous in persons sensitive to this amine. The development of coronary and cerebral ischemia can be relieved by cautious administration of sympathomimetic pressor agents such as phenylephrine. Respiratory arrest has been reported following rapid infusion rates. Pupillary dilation induced by the anticholinergic action of trimethaphan can hinder detection of cerebral anoxia. Since tolerance develops to this drug, hypertension may recur during administration.

Labetalol is an α- and β-adrenergic antagonist that appears to have additional direct vasodilator action. It will rapidly lower blood pressure while its β-component prevents reflex tachycardia. Severe hypotension may develop. Persons with coronary insufficiency or myocardial infarction often respond favorably to this drug. Continuous IV infusion or intermittent low-dose bolus injections with close monitoring provides the most satisfactory responses. The usual contraindications to β-blockers apply also to labetalol; bradycardia, bronchial asthma, congestive heart failure, or heart block greater than first degree. The α-blocking efficacy of labetalol can induce orthostatic hypotension.

Calcium channel blockers cause vasodilation and provide rapid lowering of elevated blood pressure. Verapamil is available for IV administration; both bolus and infusion are reported useful in hypertensive emergencies. Verapamil's negative inotropic action may exacerbate heart failure, and heart block may develop. Nifedipine capsules can be administered orally or sublingually to elicit a fall in blood pressure within 15 minutes. However, excessive hypotension may be difficult to manage since this drug has prolonged action. Calcium channel blockers can elicit either bradycardia or tachycardia. Concomitant administration of β-blockers, however, can be hazardous since both types of drugs have a depressant effect on cardiac conduction. Preexisting conduction deficits may contraindicate the use of calcium channel blockers.

Phentolamine possesses α-adrenergic blocking efficacy that is particularly advantageous in hypertensive emergencies induced by excessive sympathomimetic activity. Abrupt termination of antihypertensive drugs such as clonidine and propranolol can predispose to "rebound" hypertension. In addition to the usual hypotensive adverse responses, phentolamine can induce severe dysrhythmias or myocardial infarction.

Certain oral antihypertensive agents (see previous section of this chapter) are used to induce more gradual reduction in blood pressure when hypertensive episodes are not so likely to produce immediate life-threatening consequences. Minoxidil will produce prompt reduction in blood pressure. However, marked hypotension and reflex tachycardia can occur. Beta-blockers and diuretics are frequently administered concomitantly.

The angiotensin converting enzyme inhibitor captopril is well absorbed from the gastrointestinal tract and can reduce blood pressure within 30 to 60 minutes. Precipitous hypotension may occur in persons who are receiving diuretics or are otherwise hypovolemic. These agents may be particularly useful in patients with cardiac failure. Enalapril is available for intravenous administration.

Clonidine can lower pressure within 2 to 3 hours, usually without altering cardiac output or rate of contraction or causing severe hypotension.

Precautions and contraindications relevant to each of these drugs must be considered when emergency antihypertensive therapy is selected. Once the hypertensive episode is controlled, steps must be taken to determine its cause and to prevent its recurrence. Transition from IV to oral drug administration must be accomplished carefully to avoid return of hypertension.

DRUGS AFFECTING BLOOD COAGULATION AND COMPOSITION

Anticoagulants

Intravascular coagulation of blood can occur when the endothelial lining of the vessels is damaged and platelets come into contact with the subendothelial surface. Thrombi impede local circulation, and can be the source of emboli that cause ischemia in distant vital organs. The risk of thromboembolism is increased by blood flow stasis. Controversy over use of anticoagulants in management of acute myocardial infarction continues. Some studies suggest that administration of anticoagulants for 2 to 4 weeks following infarction provides significant benefit to certain patients.

Anticoagulants are of two types: heparin, including its low molecular weight forms, which must be given parenterally (SC or IV); and the coumarin-type or orally active agents. The major toxic effect of both is excessive suppression of clotting mechanisms, resulting in severe spontaneous or accidental hemorrhage. Conditions that predispose to risk of bleeding (*e.g.,* thrombocytopenia, gastrointestinal ulceration, severe hypertension, spinal anesthesia) generally preclude the administration of anticoagulants. Caution is required in elderly patients who frequently have fragile skin, blood vessels that are easily damaged, and reduced plasma levels of hepatically synthesized clotting factors.

Heparin sodium USP (Liquaemin), a large, highly charged sulfated polymer of paired units of acetylated glucosamine and glucoronic acid, is inactivated in the gastrointestinal tract and must be administered parenterally. Preparations ranging from 10 to 40,000 units/ml are derived from bovine lung and porcine intestinal mucosa. ''Low-dose'' heparin (5,000 units SC every 8 to 12 hours) is frequently adequate to prevent thrombosis. When there is overt thromboembolism, high doses of up to 30,000 units IV per day may be required. Continuous infusion rather than intermittent bolus injection best maintains consistent therapeutic plasma levels and reduces the danger of severely compromised coagulation. Careful monitoring of the partial thromboplastin time (PTT) will assist in the selection of properly individualized drug doses. The PTT should be maintained at 1.5 to 2.0 times the control value.

Heparin interacts primarily with the ''intrinsic'' pathway of coagulation by inactivating several factors that are essential to the complex process of clot formation. Heparin enhances the action of a required plasma cofactor, antithrombin III, which chiefly inactivates thrombin. Because of its direct interference in clot formation, the onset of heparin's effect is rapid (almost immediate with IV administration; within 2 hours after SC injection). The plasma half-life of this drug is 1 to 2 hours. Inactivation is by both hepatic metabolism and renal excretion of unchanged drug; renal impairment delays its removal from blood. Because of the risk of hematoma, heparin should not be administered IM, and other IM administration should be avoided in persons receiving heparin.

The use of heparin to treat disseminated intravascular coagulation (DIC) is controversial. This condition is characterized by excessive activity in both the fibrinogenic and fibrinolytic systems; thrombi may occlude small vessels at the same time that severe hemorrhage is occurring. Close monitoring of patients is required since many do not respond to heparin. Therapy should be discontinued after 4 to 8 hours if no significant benefit is derived. Indeed, all forms of treatment, including fresh plasma, may be hazardous. Aminocaproic acid may be administered concomitantly.

Intravenous heparin has the ability to produce rapid clearance of dietary lipids from plasma. It appears to release from various tissues a lipase that catalyzes the hydrolysis of triglycerides in chylomicrons. Beta-lipoproteins of high molecular weight and low density are converted into low-molecular-weight, high-density lipids.

In addition to an increased risk of hemorrhage, heparin can suppress aldosterone synthesis, resulting in increased sodium and fluid excretion. Paradoxically, heparin can cause thrombocytopenia by inducing platelet aggregation and thromboembolism (white clot syndrome). Chronic high doses of heparin have caused osteoporosis. Hypersensitivity reactions, often to the animal protein contaminating the drug, have occurred. Other drugs that inhibit coagulation, such as dextran, dipyridamole, aspirin, and other nonsteroidal anti-inflammatory drugs, are usually contraindicated in heparinized patients.

Enoxaparin (Lovenox) and ***dalteparin*** (Fragmin),

TABLE 7-23. Oral Anticoagulants

GENERIC NAME	TRADE NAME
Anisindione	Miradon
Dicumarol	—
Phenprocoumin	Liquamar
Warfarin	Coumadin, Antithrombin-K

fragments of the heparin molecule, inhibit Factor X_a-induced production of thrombin but cause less thrombin inactivation, less platelet inhibition, and less vascular permeability than heparin and thus may lower risk for severe hemorrhage. These agents have longer half-lives than heparin, and bind less extensively to plasma proteins.

Positively charged protamine sulfate, administered by slow IV infusion, binds to negatively charged heparin in the circulating blood and prevents its anticoagulant action. One mg will neutralize approximately 100 units of heparin; the time interval between the last dose of heparin and protamine administration must be considered in estimating the dose of the latter drug. Protamine also is anticoagulant (this effect becomes apparent when protamine is in excess of heparin) and has a longer plasma half-life than heparin. Adverse effects include hypotension, bradycardia, anaphylaxis in previously sensitized subjects, and exacerbation of DIC.

Oral anticoagulant therapy, which has a more prolonged onset of action, may be initiated concomitantly with heparin. The mechanism of action of these drugs (Table 7-23) differs from heparin in that they decrease hepatic synthesis of clotting factors II, VII, IX, and X by preventing utilization of vitamin K. Those factors already present in circulating blood must be depleted (over 3 to 5 days) before the full anticoagulant effect of the oral drugs becomes apparent. ***Warfarin*** is used most frequently because it is well absorbed from the gastrointestinal tract. The action of the oral anticoagulants affects in particular the ''extrinsic'' clotting pathway and is monitored through the prothrombin time (PT). One-stage PT should be maintained at 1.5 to 2.0 times greater than control value. When heparin is administered concurrently, blood for prothrombin testing should be drawn at least 4 to 5 hours after the last IV dose or 12 to 24 hours after SC injection.

As with heparin, the major adverse effect of oral anticoagulant therapy is hemorrhage. Gastrointestinal bleeding, widespread petechiae, prolonged hemorrhage from open wounds, hematuria, and excessive bruising can occur. Adrenal hemorrhage and resultant insufficiency (which can occur also with heparin) may require glucocorticoid replacement therapy.

The hemorrhagic action of oral anticoagulants can be reversed by vitamin K preparations (phytonadione, Mephyton, Konakion) that stimulate hepatic synthesis of clotting factors. Control of hemorrhage can usually be achieved within 3 to 6 hours following parenteral phytonadione, with prothrombin attaining normal levels after 14 hours. Oral phytonadione is effective in 6 to 12 hours, while parenteral menadiol requires 8 to 24 hours. Because of this long onset of action, significant bleeding may necessitate emergency administration of plasma, whole blood, or factor IX complex (Konyne, Proplex). The efficacy of vitamin K is dependent upon functioning hepatocytes. The action of heparin is not reversed by these drugs. Administration of vitamin K can reduce the effectiveness of subsequent doses of oral anticoagulant for several weeks.

Additional adverse reactions observed with the oral anticoagulants include diarrhea, depressed levels of formed elements of blood, hepatitis, renal damage, and dermatological symptoms. Lack of bioequivalence among warfarin preparations from various manufacturers has been reported. Anticoagulant therapy should be interrupted several days before anticipated surgery. Patients should wear or carry medical identification noting their use of anticoagulants and must be observant of signs of hemorrhage.

Many drugs, including over-the-counter preparations, interact with the oral anticoagulants to either enhance or reduce their actions (Table 7-24). The PT must be closely monitored whenever drug doses are increased or decreased, or when drugs are added to or withdrawn from the patient's regimen. The oral anticoagulants are hepatically inactivated and induction of drug-metabolizing enzymes will decrease their effectiveness. Patients should not concomitantly use aspirin, which has its own anticoagulant effect and also displaces the coumarintype drugs from plasma protein binding sites. Alcohol should be

TABLE 7-24. Drug Interactions Affecting Oral Anticoagulant Activity

Drugs That Enhance Anticoagulant Effect
Cimetidine
Clofibrate
Dipyridamole
Gemfibrozil
Quinidine
Salicylates, other nonsteroidal anti-inflammatory drugs
Sulfinpyrazone
Sulfonylureas
Many antibiotics
Drugs That Reduce Anticoagulant Effect
Barbiturates
Bile sequestrants
Carbamazapine
Estrogens
Phenytoin
Vitamin K

avoided, as well as activities that increase the risk of injury. Consumption of large amounts of leafy green vegetables that contain vitamin K can suppress anticoagulant action. Impaired renal or hepatic function can prolong the plasma half-life of these drugs. Discoloration of urine by indandiones may mimic hematuria.

Ticlopidine (Ticlid), an inhibitor of the adenosine diphospate pathway of platelet aggregation, can decrease the risk of recurrent thrombotic stroke and myocardial infarction. Its onset of action is 2 days, reaching a maximum effect in 7 days. Anticoagulant action can continue up to 2 weeks after the drug is terminated. The liver inactivates ticlopidine, thus significant hepatic dysfunction contraindicates its administration. Adverse effects are gastrointestinal upset including diarrhea, rash, severe disruption of white cell and platelet production, aplastic anemia, hepatic dysfunction, and elevated serum cholesterol. Antacids inhibit absorption of ticlopidine, while cimetidine can inhibit its inactivation. Ticlopidine can enhance theophylline's effectiveness and inhibit that of cyclosporine.

Abciximab (ReoPro) is a monoclonal antibody fragment that decreases platelet aggregation by inhibiting the binding of adhesive glycoproteins. It prevents abrupt occlusion of coronary blood vessels following percutaneous transluminal coronary angioplasty. However, it carries the risk of severe hemorrhage.

Thrombolytics

Although anticoagulants prevent additional clot formation, they do not generally dissolve those already present. Thrombolytic or fibrinolytic agents (***streptokinase***, Streptase; ***urokinase***, Abbokinase; ***tissue plasminogen activator [tPA] alteplase***, Activase; ***anistreplase***, Eminase or APSAC) are used for this purpose. Disruption of clots is desirable in the management of thrombosis and pulmonary embolism, and the maintenance of access shunts and intravascular catheters. Several studies have indicated that thrombolytic agents, administered early in the course of evolving myocardial infarction, can restore blood flow through occluded coronary arteries and may limit myocardial damage.

Circulating blood contains a fibrinolytic system that dissolves intravascular fibrin aggregates as they form. Fibrinolysin (or plasmin), the major component of this system, is a proteolytic enzyme that disrupts fibrinogen and fibrin. Plasminogen is the inactive circulating precursor of fibrinolysin. Thrombolytic drugs convert plasminogen to plasmin, thereby setting into motion the fibrinolytic mechanism.

Streptokinase is derived from streptococcal bacteria strains. Its action is suppressed by antistreptococcal antibodies, commonly found in patients' blood in response to prior streptococcal exposure. Large loading doses may be required. Streptokinase itself can induce antibody formation. Readministration of this drug can result in allergic responses or in inadequate thrombolytic action. ***Urokinase*** is derived from human urine or from cultures of human embryonic renal cells. Its actions are similar to those of streptokinase. It is less likely to induce antibody production but is more costly. ***Tissue plasminogen activator*** (alteplase, Activase) is an endogenous activator of the fibrinolytic system. Produced by recombinant DNA technology, ***anistreplase*** has a longer plasma half-life (90 minutes) than other thrombolytics and is more convenient to administer.

Since these drugs may also lyse fibrinogen and other blood-clotting factors, a major disadvantage is the risk of severe hemorrhage. Active internal bleeding, or significant potential for cerebral hemorrhage, contraindicate their use. Streptokinase and urokinase have a more widespread effect on blood clotting throughout the circulatory system. The action of tPA occurs more selectively at the surface of thrombi, although this agent is not completely free of systemic anticoagulant action. However, tPA also has a relatively short plasma half-life (6 to 8 minutes). In the management of acute myocardial infarction, tPA given IV may be more effective than streptokinase unless the latter drug is administered by the hazardous, costly, and time-consuming procedure of intracoronary injection. To be effective in limiting myocardial damage, thrombolytic drugs must be given early (usually within 6 hours) in the course of vessel occlusion. Patients receiving thrombolytic therapy must have some measure of clotting time or fibrinogen content monitored, and must be protected from activities or procedures that may evoke bleeding. Observation for signs of spontaneous bleeding (*e.g.*, nausea, abdominal pain, or change in neurological status) is necessary. Cardiac dysrhythmias often develop as perfusion of myocardial cells is reestablished and may be controlled with lidocaine. Heparin and/or oral anticoagulants may be administered subsequently to reduce the risk of additional thrombosis.

Debriding Agents

Streptokinase-streptodornase (Varidase) is a debriding agent used topically to remove blood clots and purulent material from wounds. Sufficient enzyme may be absorbed to produce systemic anticoagulation. This agent is contraindicated in active hemorrhage. Other enzymatic debriding preparations include ***fibrinolysin*** with ***desoxyribonuclease*** (Elase), ***trypsin*** (Granulen) and ***chymotrypsin, papain*** (Panafil), and ***sutilains*** (Travase). When applied topically, these agents remove necrotic debris and promote healing of dermatological ulcers, severe burns, and other wounds. ***Collagenase*** (Santyl) removes necrotic tissue and attached strands of collagen and may induce more rapid healing. ***Dextranomer*** (Debrisan) hydrophilic beads are applied to draining wounds to remove exudates and bacteria that can hinder tissue repair.

Agents That Restore Plasma Volume

Circulating plasma volume is maintained largely by the oncotic influence of plasma proteins such as albumin. When plasma volume becomes inadequate (*e.g.*, following severe hemorrhage, generalized vasodilation, trauma, or extensive burns) survival may depend upon a rapid replenishment of circulating fluid. Solutions such as dextrose and saline have limited capacity to maintain vascular volume, since their components of relatively small molecular size readily diffuse across capillary walls. Much more effective in restoring plasma volume are the nondiffusable colloids such as ***dextran*** (Gentran, Macrodex) and ***hetastarch*** (Hespan). These substances are relatively stable and inexpensive, and do not present the risk of infection or incompatibility that may be encountered when blood products from natural sources are used. However, colloids can provoke allergic or anaphylactoid reactions, and in persons who are dehydrated they may severely deplete extravascular volume by attracting interstitial fluid into the vascular compartment. The latter hazard can be reduced by concomitant IV infusion of fluids. Observation for circulatory overload and signs of pulmonary edema or congestive heart failure is necessary. Colloidal solutions do not enhance the oxygen-transporting capacity of blood; erythrocyte replacement is required to correct this deficit.

Dextran is a polymer produced by the action of *Leuconostoc mesenteroides* on sucrose solutions. The large, extensively branched colloids are modified by acid hydrolysis to molecular weights averaging 40,000 and 75,000. Preparations containing predominantly one size of molecule are available. The lower-molecular-weight solution (dextran 40) is used as a volume expander, and as a hemodiluent for pump-oxygenators during extracorporeal circulation. Since dextran suppresses platelet agglutination, it is used to prevent venous thromboembolism following orthopedic surgery. Because it can prolong bleeding time, dextran is contraindicated in persons with coagulation deficits including those induced by anticoagulant drugs. Active hemorrhage can be exacerbated as blood volume and perfusion pressure increase. Renal failure, probably due to viscous obstruction of renal tubular flow, has occurred in persons receiving dextran.

Dextran 70, consisting of larger-molecular-weight particles, is more efficient in maintaining plasma volume because it remains longer (24 hours or more) within the vascular compartment. However, it produces a higher incidence of adverse effects including histamine release from mast cells, increased bleeding time, and alteration of erythrocyte sedimentation and aggregation. An osmotic diuretic such as mannitol may be coadministered with dextran to maintain urinary output.

Hetastarch is used as a volume expander, and also in leukapheresis where it improves the recovery of granulocytes. This colloid, prepared by ethylene oxide treatment of waxy sorghum starch, has many of the same properties and adverse effects of dextran. It may be somewhat less allergenic.

Plasma protein fractions (Buminate, Plasminate) are albumin and protein preparations derived from human blood. These are administered to correct volume depletion and are useful adjuncts in the management of hypoproteinemia that may occur in premature infants or consequent to renal or hepatic disease. Because these substances are of human origin, the incidence of adverse effects such as anaphylaxis is low. Changes in blood pressure may occur. The possibility of hepatitis transmission has been obviated by heating these solutions for 10 hours at 60° C, which destroys the virus but does not denature plasma proteins.

Antiplatelet Drugs

Platelet aggregation is a contributing factor to thrombus formation that can result in coronary and cerebral artery occlusion. Platelet interaction with collagen may also enhance the development of arteriosclerotic deposits on blood vessel walls. Drugs that reduce platelet adhesion may prove to be effective inhibitors of these cardiovascular disorders.

Thromboxanes and prostacyclin, synthesized by the cyclo-oxygenase pathway, have been implicated in platelet function. Aspirin, which blocks the action of this enzyme, is reported to reduce the incidence of transient ischemic attacks and the risk of myocardial infarction in men with unstable angina. Low doses (40–325 mg daily) are most effective, possibly because they do not affect vascular endothelial prostacyclin production, which itself has antiplatelet activity.

The coronary vasodilator ***dipyridamole*** (Persantine), occasionally used to alleviate angina pectoris, suppresses *in vitro* platelet interaction with damaged blood vessel endothelium. Inhibition of phosphodiesterase and accumulation of cyclic AMP within platelets may account for the antiplatelet effects of dipyridamole. However, this drug alone has not been shown to reduce recurrence of myocardial infarction. The efficacy of anticoagulants or other antiplatelet agents may be enhanced by dipyridamole; drug combinations are used following cardiac valve implantation. Adverse effects of this drug are generally mild and transient; gastrointestinal disturbances, nausea, and syncope may occur, and angina can be exacerbated.

Sulfinpyrazone (Anturane), usually used as a uricosuric, has a platelet inhibitory action that may be beneficial in persons with coronary artery disease or implanted cardiac valves. Persons receiving this drug may develop hematological deficits; close monitoring of blood counts is required. Sulfinpyrazone can precipitate gout, renal stone formation, and possibly renal failure. Adequate hydration and urinary alkalinization can reduce the precipitation of uric acid in the urinary tract. Aspirin may be given concurrently with sulfinpyrazone to reduce deep venous thrombosis following hip surgery.

Pentoxyfylline (Trental) is a methylxanthine phosphodiesterase inhibitor that decreases serum levels of fibrinogen and reduces aggregation of platelets. Its greatest action, however, appears to be promotion of capillary blood flow by enhancing erythrocyte flexibility. Pentoxyfylline alleviates symptoms of intermittent claudication in some patients. Adverse effects of this drug, which is metabolized by erythrocytes and hepatocytes, include headaches, dizziness, and nausea. Clinical response may require up to 8 weeks of drug administration.

Hemostatic Agents

Local application of a variety of substances will retard bleeding from small vessels such as capillaries. ***Thrombin*** (Thrombostat) helps to control bleeding during surgery or in easily accessible sites, for example, nose and dental socket bleeding, in hemophiliac and other patients. Administration of this substance, which catalyzes the conversion of fibrinogen to fibrin, is limited to body surfaces since its entry into large blood vessels can result in potentially lethal intravascular clotting. ***Oxidized cellulose*** (Oxycel, Surgicel) reacts physically with blood to form a clotlike complex. It can be used to control surgical or mucous membrane bleeding. Epithelialization and bone regeneration are suppressed by prolonged topical application to denuded areas and fracture sites.

Absorbable gelatin hemostatics (Gelfoam, Gelfilm) need not be removed when surgical incisions are closed. The film can be used to ''patch'' dural or pleural injuries. Healing of skin incisions may be inhibited, although leg and decubitus ulcers are treated with these agents. Infection usually contraindicates their use.

Antihemophilic Factor VIII will replace the factor absent in classic hemophilia (type A) and help to control bleeding in persons with this deficit. Administration is by the IV route, and doses are closely individualized to patients' needs. Factor VIII inhibitors can develop. Preparations of this substance derived from human plasma can transmit hepatitis and AIDS. Monoclate and Hemofil M are purified Factor VIII preparations that may carry less risk of blood-borne infections. Recombinate and Kogenate are Factor VIII preparations produced by genetic engineering, and are free of risk for transmitting hepatitis and HIV.

Factor IX complex (Konyne, Proplex), containing several vitamin K-dependent clotting factors, can prevent or alleviate hemorrhagic episodes in Christmas disease (hemophilia B). Risk of hepatitis usually precludes the use of this plasma-derived product in persons with preexisting liver disease. Intravascular coagulation can be exacerbated by administration of Factor IX complex. Rapid infusion rates cause hypotension and tachycardia that necessitate temporary termination of drug administration.

Vitamin K (discussed under Vitamins) is beneficial in deficiencies of vitamin K-dependent factors, provided that hepatocytes are functional.

Aminocaproic acid (Amicar) inhibits fibrinolysis and is useful in bleeding states caused by excessive fibrinolytic activity, such as open heart surgery, bleeding of the urinary tract, neoplastic diseases, hepatic cirrhosis, and abruptio placentae. This amino acid, which is related to lysine, inhibits the conversion of plasminogen to plasmin and also, to a lesser degree, directly inhibits the action of plasmin, the active fibrinolytic enzyme. In severe hemorrhagic emergencies, concomitant administration of fibrinogen and fresh whole blood may be necessary. Aminocaproic acid is contraindicated in DIC, unless heparin is coadministered. Hyperfibrinolysis should be established before this drug is administered.

Tranexamic acid (Cyklokapron), similar to aminocaproic acid, is administered (PO or IV) concomitantly with coagulation factors (VIII or IX) to reduce the risk of hemorrhage following dental extraction in hemophiliac patients. DIC or preexisting hematuria or subarachnoid hemorrhage preclude the use of tranexamic acid. Vision aberrations, including changes in color discrimination, have been reported.

Aprotonin (Trasylol) is a fribrinolysis inhibitor administered IV to decrease bleeding following coronary artery bypass graft. It is usually reserved for patients at high risk for severe blood loss. Allergy to the bovine protein in aprotonin can occur.

Drugs That Correct Hemoglobin Deficits

Iron is required for the synthesis of hemoglobin. Deficiency of this essential element, resulting from malabsorption of dietary iron or excessive blood loss (*e.g.*, menstrual or occult gastrointestinal bleeding) will cause anemia. Iron deficiency attributed to inadequate dietary intake is not unusual in children aged 6 to 24 months, teenagers, and pregnant women.

Several preparations (including many over-the-counter) are available for the reversal of negative iron balance.

Oral administration is preferred, although iron dextran (Imferon) can be given IM or by slow IV infusion to persons with inadequate gastrointestinal absorption or intolerance to the oral route. The ferrous form of iron is most readily absorbed, chiefly in the duodenum. Vitamin C promotes this action. In the circulatory system, iron is bound to a plasma protein (transferrin) that transports it to tissue sites of storage and utilization. Normally, only a small proportion of dietary iron is absorbed. However, when iron stores are depleted, the capacity of the intestinal mucosa to transport iron into the circulatory system increases. Certain malabsorption diseases will interfere with absorption of iron, and loss of blood interrupts the physiological cycle that captures used iron from the spleen and other tissues and transports it back to bone marrow for further use in hemoglobin, or to sites (*e.g.*, the liver) for storage.

Oral administration of iron salts (*e.g.*, ferrous fumarate, gluconate, and sulfate) can cause nausea, diarrhea, constipation, abdominal cramps, and changes in fecal pigmentation. Gastrointestinal symptoms can be reduced by taking these preparations with meals. However, simultaneous ingestion of eggs, milk, antacids, and tetracycline antibiotics suppress the intestinal absorption of iron. Supplements should be used only by persons with true iron deficiency, as excessive amounts of this metal can be hazardous. Acute overdose causes severe gastrointestinal irritation and mucosal injury, which further enhances iron absorption. Lethargy, dyspnea, shock, and metabolic acidosis can develop. Chronic overdose induces iron storage excess (hemosiderosis and hemochromatosis). Parenteral administration of chelating agents such as deferoxamine (Desferal) will promote renal excretion of iron. Dimercaprol should not be administered in cases of iron excess.

Peptic ulcer and inflammatory disorders of the intestines usually contraindicate oral administration of iron. Parenteral administration requires extreme caution. Intramuscular injections may be painful; leakage of iron solutions can discolor the skin; IV infusion can induce phlebitis. Patients must be closely observed for allergic responses including anaphylaxis; a test dose of drug followed by 1 hour of observation may be given initially. The required parenteral dose should be calculated based upon measurement of the patient's hematocrit. Oral and parenteral administration must *not* be used concurrently.

Megaloblastic anemias occur when insufficient amounts of vitamin B_{12} (cyanocobalamin) and folic acid are available for production of formed elements of blood. These substances are discussed under Vitamins. In pernicious anemia, gastric mucosal cells fail to secrete intrinsic factor that is required for vitamin B_{12} absorption. Pernicious anemia may be accompanied by glossitis and specific neurological deficits (loss of vibratory sensation, paresthesias of hands and feet, ataxia) due to degenerative changes in dorsal and lateral columns of the spinal cord.

Hematopoietic Growth Factors

Several endogenous hematopoietic factors have been isolated and produced by recombinant DNA technology. ***Erythropoietin*** (epoetin alfa, Epogen) stimulates production of erythrocytes; it may ameliorate the anemia which accompanies chronic renal failure or that occurs with zidovudine administration to AIDS patients. Hypertension, thrombosis, gastrointestinal and cardiac irregularities, seizures, and fatigue are possible adverse effects.

Granulocyte colony-stimulating factor (G-CSF, filgastrim, Neupogen) and ***granulocyte-macrophage colony-stimulating factor*** (GM-CSF, sargramostim, Leukine, Prokine) stimulate the production of leukocytes and are used following antineoplastic therapy to protect against infection, and also after bone marrow transplant to promote myeloid activity. These agents may be useful in other conditions characterized by leukopenia. Adverse effects include bone pain, enlarged spleen, and with GM-CSF, pleural and pericardial effusion.

DIURETICS

Diuretics are used extensively in the management of cardiovascular disorders such as hypertension and congestive heart failure. Edema accompanying renal dysfunction, hepatic cirrhosis, and administration of drugs such as estrogens and corticosteroids also can be alleviated by diuretics. In addition, some diuretic agents are used for specific conditions: mannitol to relieve cerebral edema, and the carbonic anhydrase inhibitor acetazolamide (Diamox) to reduce elevated intraocular pressure in glaucoma and to alleviate altitude sickness.

The mechanism of action of most diuretics appears to involve reduction of active sodium and/or chloride reabsorption at the basal surface of the tubular epithelial cells. Sodium in the tubular filtrate enters the epithelial cells and is then transported out into the interstitial space through the activity of an ATPase-dependent sodium-potassium exchange. Water is reabsorbed passively along an osmotic gradient in those regions of the nephron that are water permeable, chiefly the collecting ducts.

Several types of drugs (Table 7-25) have the ability to induce diuresis. Their sites of action in the renal tubule vary and can influence the net effect of the drug. The mercurial and organic acid (''loop'') diuretics, such as furosemide, exert their greatest effect in the ascending limb of the loop of Henle, where active transport of sodium and chloride contributes to the countercurrent gradient that promotes passive reabsorption of water in the

TABLE 7-25. Diuretics

GENERIC NAME	TRADE NAME
Thiazides	
Benzthiazide	Hydrex, others
Chlorothiazide	Diuril
Hydrochlorothiazide	Hydrodiuril, others
Trichlormethiazide	Diurese
Carbonic Anhydrase Inhibitors	
Acetazolamide	Diamox
Dichlorphenamide	Daranide
Methazolamide	Neptazane
Organic Acids (Loop Diuretics)	
Bumetanide	Bumex
Ethacrynic acid	Edecrin
Furosemide	Lasix
Torsemide	Demadex
Potassium-Sparing	
Amiloride	Midamor
Spironolactone	Aldactone
Triamterene	Dyrenium
Osmotic Diuretics	
Mannitol	Osmitrol
Urea	Ureaphil
Additional Diuretics	
Chlorthalidone	Hygroton
Metolazone	Zaroxolyn
Indapamide	Lozol

collecting tubules. The carbonic anhydrase inhibitors and the thiazides impede sodium reabsorption in the proximal and distal tubules of the nephron, respectively. Potassium-sparing diuretics reduce the distal tubule exchange of sodium for potassium and hydrogen ions. They may act by inhibiting the action of aldosterone (*i.e.*, spironolactone) or the sodium-for-potassium pump mechanism (*e.g.*, amiloride or triamterene). Osmotic agents, filtered by the glomeruli but not reabsorbed, promote the excretion of an osmotically equivalent amount of water. Drugs such as the xanthines (*e.g.*, theophylline and caffeine) and agents that affect secretion of antidiuretic hormone (ADH) also have a diuretic action.

Although they are a varied group of drugs, causing varied degrees of diuresis and effects on electrolyte excretion, these agents share some noteworthy characteristics. Most have the potential to induce severe electrolyte depletion and imbalance; preexisting electrolyte disturbances should be corrected before diuretics are administered. Diuretics require extreme caution in the elderly, who are already placed at risk for dehydration and electrolyte imbalance by declining renal function. Several diuretics can provoke severe dehydration with attendant hypovolemia, progressing to circulatory collapse and predisposing to thrombosis and embolism. The thiazides appear to reduce vascular responsiveness to the neurotransmitter norepinephrine, which may account in part for their antihypertensive efficacy. Diuretics suppress renal excretion and enhance the toxicity of lithium; thus concomitant administration is usually contraindicated. Corticosteroids enhance the potassium loss that occurs with most diuretics. Although digitalis and diuretics are often given simultaneously, the hypokalemia induced by the latter will enhance the risk of toxicity of the cardiac glycosides. Concurrent administration of potassium salts or potassium-sparing diuretics can ameliorate this interaction. Dopamine, which in small doses will enhance renal perfusion, can increase diuretic effects. Nonsteroidal anti-inflammatory drugs (NSAIDs) decrease renal perfusion and thus can inhibit diuretic action.

Thiazides (Benzothiodiazides)

The thiazide or sulfonamide diuretics are currently among the most widely used drugs in the United States. The onset of action of most thiazides is 2 hours after oral administration, with a duration up to 12 or more hours. ***Chlorthalidone*** and ***indapamide***, closely related diuretics, are effective up to 36 and 72 hours, respectively. The action of the thiazides, unlike carbonic anhydrase inhibitors and organomercurials, is little influenced by variations in *p*H of body fluids. Since thiazides are secreted by the same tubular transport mechanism that excretes uric acid, hyperuricemia and exacerbation of gout are side effects. Hyperglycemia (probably via inhibition of pancreatic insulin release) also may occur, necessitating increased dosage of insulin or oral hypoglycemics for diabetic persons. Thiazide and loop diuretics can elevate plasma levels of cholesterol and triglycerides.

Thiazides are often combined with digitalis in the management of congestive heart failure. Their use as antihypertensives is discussed in that section. Paradoxically, thiazides are used to decrease urine volume in diabetes insipidus, particularly the nephrogenic form. Thiazides affect calcium absorption; their ability to ameliorate hypercalciuria enables them to inhibit formation of calcium stones in the kidneys.

Caution is required when thiazides are administered in the presence of renal impairment because azotemia may occur. In persons with hepatic disease, alterations in fluid or electrolyte balance can precipitate hepatic coma. Thiazides administered during pregnancy can induce neonatal jaundice and aberrant carbohydrate metabolism. However, these drugs are used cautiously in the management of eclampsia.

Like most diuretics, the thiazides promote excessive potassium excretion and increase the risk of digitalis toxicity. Thiazides can reduce the excretion of quinidine (by urinary alkalinization) and may induce hypercalcemia when calcium salts are given concurrently. Thiazides potentiate the action of most antihypertensive agents, and will produce severe postural hypotension in combination with opiates, barbiturates, and alcohol.

Carbonic Anhydrase Inhibitors

Acetazolamide (Diamox) causes diuresis through its inhibition of carbonic anhydrase which catalyzes the reaction of $CO_2 + H_2O$ to yield H^+ and CO_3^-, reduces tubular reabsorption of sodium in exchange for hydrogen ions and results in alkalinization of the urine. Metabolic hyperchloremic acidosis develops and hinders the efficacy of the carbonic anhydrase inhibitors, probably by inhibiting hydrogen-sodium ion exchange. Intermittent drug administration allows normalization of plasma *p*H by facilitating natural correction of the metabolic acidosis.

Carbonic anhydrase inhibitors alleviate elevated intraocular pressure in glaucoma by decreasing the formation of aqueous humor. Their effectiveness in some forms of epilepsy may be due to decreased formation of cerebrospinal fluid with reduction in intracranial pressure. Acetazolamide is used investigationally to ameliorate high-altitude hypoxia. Analogues of acetazolamide include ***dichlorphenamide*** (Daranide) and ***methazolamide*** (Neptazane). These drugs, like the thiazides, are sulfonamide derivatives and are contraindicated in persons allergic to this chemical class.

Organic Acid Diuretics

Furosemide (Lasix), ***ethacrynic acid*** (Edecrin), ***torsemide*** (Demadex) and ***bumetanide*** (Bumex) work primarily in the loop of Henle, thus their designation as "loop" diuretics. This portion of the nephron extends down into the medullary region of the kidney where much of the sodium, chloride, and urea (but not water) are reabsorbed in the thick ascending limb of the loop. Urine entering the distal tubule is hypotonic, while the medullary interstitium is hypertonic. This osmotic gradient (or countercurrent multiplier) becomes important in the collecting ducts that traverse the medullary region and that, under the influence of ADH, are rendered permeable to water. The greater the osmolarity of the medulla the greater the water reabsorption, resulting in a concentrated urine. The loop diuretics reduce medullary osmolarity, and cause intense diuresis with significant excretion of sodium, chloride, and potassium. These drugs have greater efficacy than most other agents including the thiazides, and are often referred to as "high ceiling" diuretics. Refractory edema often will respond to the loop diuretics, which can be given orally or IV and have a rapid onset of action.

These agents are highly bound to plasma proteins, and are secreted into the proximal tubules by the same system that transports thiazides and uric acid. This transport is necessary for their effects, since they work at the luminal side of the nephron.

Because of their intense diuresis, the loop diuretics produce excessive dehydration and marked depletion of electrolytes, including hypokalemia and hypochloremic alkalosis. Elderly persons, in whom renal function usually is less than optimal, are especially at risk and require close observation when these drugs are given. Some physicians recommend that loop diuretics not be administered to the elderly, preferring instead to use thiazides, although the latter can lose their effectiveness as renal functions declines. Loop diuretics can cause hyperuricemia, hearing impairment, and glucose intolerance. Toxicity is enhanced in patients with renal disease, thus doses should be reduced.

Characteristic drug interactions of the loop diuretics include inhibition of salicylate excretion and potentiation of theophylline and succinylcholine. Nonsteroidal anti-inflammatory drugs reduce the efficacy of loop diuretics. The ototoxicity of the aminoglycoside antibiotics may be enhanced.

Potassium-Sparing Agents

The potassium-sparing diuretics are unique in their propensity to cause hyperkalemia rather than potassium depletion. Their site of action is the distal convoluted tubule, where the hormone aldosterone mediates sodium reabsorption in exchange for potassium and hydrogen ions. ***Spironolactone*** (Aldactone) is a specific competitive aldosterone antagonist, while ***triamterene*** (Dyrenium) and ***amiloride*** (Midamor) inhibit sodium entry into the collecting tubular cell. Spironolactone is most effective in the presence of high levels of renin and aldosterone, and is used in the management of hyperaldosteronism.

Most diuretics result in delivery of increased amounts of sodium to the distal tubule. As the nephron exerts a final attempt to reabsorb this ion, much potassium can be lost. The greatest use of the potassium-sparing agents, which alone produce only mild diuresis, is in combination with other diuretics to reduce this potassium wasting. Excessive potassium intake, either dietary (including table salt substitutes containing potassium) or in the form of supplemental salts, must be avoided, particularly in the presence of renal disease, which might produce dangerous elevations of potassium when a potassium-sparing agent is given. Concomitant administration of ACE inhibitors should be avoided.

Osmotic Diuretics

As their name implies, the osmotic diuretics carry fluid through the circulatory system and the renal tubules by elevating oncotic pressure. Administered IV, these substances are restricted to the vascular compartment and attract considerable amounts of extravascular fluid. ***Mannitol*** (Osmitrol), the most frequently used in this class of drugs, is completely filtered at the glomeruli but is neither secreted nor reabsorbed by the nephron. Osmotic diuretics are used to alleviate intracranial edema, to enhance renal excretion of toxic substances, and to prevent renal failure by maintaining urine flow. Refractory elevation of intraocular pressure may respond to osmotic agents. Urinary output must be maintained during administration of these drugs; renal failure or severe dehydration contraindicate their use. Persons with cardiovascular disease may tolerate poorly a sudden increase in intravascular volume produced by the osmotic diuretic agent.

Corticosteroids may be coadministered with mannitol in the management of elevated intracranial pressure. However, both types of drugs promote potassium excretion, and marked hypokalemia may develop.

RESPIRATORY PHARMACOLOGY

Pharmacotherapy of Asthma

Asthma, or difficulty in breathing attributable to reversible airway obstruction, is a frequent component of allergic reactions and may also result from psychological stress, respiratory infections, or exposure to irritant environmental chemicals. Because chronic airway inflammation is perceived as a major factor in asthma, the use of corticosteroids is increasing.

Corticosteroids (Table 7-26) administered orally or by inhalation have a gradual onset but prolonged duration of action and can reduce the required doses of other drugs such as the β-adrenergic agonists. To reduce the occurrence of adverse effects, corticosteroids can be administered on alternate days as a single oral dose taken shortly after awakening. The numerous adverse effects of the corticosteroids are discussed under Adrenocortical Hormones. Asthmatics receiving systemic corticosteroids should not be switched abruptly to inhaled corticosteroids without tapering the systemic dosage to allow recovery from adrenal cortical suppression. Following inhalation, sufficient drug may be systemically absorbed to suppress the hypothalamic–pituitary–adrenal axis and result in severe adrenal deficiency in times of stress, or when drug doses are reduced or terminated. Administration of corticosteroids should be discontinued gradually rather than abruptly. Oral infections with *Monilia* (candidiasis) may occur with inhalation of these drugs. The propellants utilized in some aerosol formulations have been implicated in sudden deaths among asthmatics.

Also used in the management of asthma are the β-adrenergic agonists, which stimulate β_2 receptors in airways to induce bronchodilation. ***Epinephrine*** and ***isoproterenol*** can be administered by injection (SC in particular) or by inhalation. ***Metaproterenol*** is active orally and by inhalation. Although hazardous, isoproterenol can be administered IV to control refractory status asthmaticus, especially in children.

TABLE 7-26. Bronchodilators

GENERIC NAME	TRADE NAME
β-Adrenergic Agonists	
Epinephrine	Bronkaid, Medihaler
Isoproterenol	Isuprel
Metaproterenol	Alupent
Albuterol	Proventil, Ventolin
Bitolterol	Tornalate
Ephedrine	Efedron
Isoetharine	Bronkometer
Salmeterol	Serevent
Terbutaline	Brethine, others
Pirbuterol	Maxair
Methylxanthines	
Theophylline	Theo-Dur, Bronkodyl, Slo-Phyllin, others
Dyphylline	Dylline, Lufyllin
Aminophylline	Amoline, Somophyllin, others
Oxtriphylline	Brondecon, Choledyl
Corticosteroids	
Beclomethasone	Beclovent, Vanceril
Budesonide	Pulmicort
Flunisolide	AeroBid
Triamcinolone	Azmacort
Prednisone	Several
Prednisolone	Several
Anticholinergic	
Ipratropium	Atrovent

Several relatively β_2 receptor-selective agonists (Table 7-26) available in aerosol and oral forms have a longer duration of action than epinephrine and isoproterenol, and cause less cardiac (β_1 receptor) stimulation. ***Terbutaline*** can be administered SC. These agents are used to alleviate acute attacks and also to reduce the recurrence of bronchospasm.

Tremor is a major adverse effect of the sympathomimetic bronchodilators, induced by stimulation of β_2 receptors in skeletal muscle. Anxiety, cardiac dysrhythmias, and pulmonary edema may occur particularly following use of nonselective β-agonists. Beta$_2$-selective agonists can stimulate β_1 receptors in high doses or in sensitive persons. Inhalation of drugs usually provides prompt relief of symptoms with a lower incidence and severity of adverse effects than is observed following systemic routes. Tolerance to the therapeutic actions of β-agonists can develop. Excessive β_2 bronchodilator use has been associated with increased mortality in asthmatic persons. Other characteristics of these agents are discussed under Autonomic Drugs.

Theophylline and ***aminophylline*** are effective bronchodilators that can be administered by slow IV infusion to reverse acute asthma. Several oral and rectal formulations are used in chronic asthma to reduce the incidence and severity of symptoms. Rates of inactivation of theophylline vary extensively among patients and doses must be adjusted to each person's response. Cardiac, hepatic, or pulmonary disease, fever, cigarette smoking, age, and the presence of other drugs will influence hepatic metabolism of theophylline. Concomitant food ingestion has variable effects on absorption of oral preparations. Adverse effects include tachycardia, headache, tremor, restlessness, nausea, and insomnia. The therapeutic index of theophylline is low, and overdose can result in seizures and fatal cardiac dysrhythmias. Plasma concentrations of drug should be monitored; optimal levels range from 10 to 20 μg/ml.

Cromolyn sodium (Intal), an inhaled powder that prevents release of histamine from mast cells, is used prophylactically to reduce inflammation and responsiveness of the airways. It is most effective against exercise- or cold-induced asthma. It is of no use and is contraindicated during asthmatic episodes. Adverse effects are relatively infrequent, although pharyngeal irritation and nausea do occur. ***Nedocromil*** (Tilade) is similar in action and effectiveness to cromolyn. Bronchospasm, headache, unpleasant taste, and nausea are reported adverse effects.

Ipratropium (Atrovent) is available as an inhaled, poorly absorbed, atropinelike bronchodilator with a slower but more prolonged action than the β-agonists. Blood levels are very low and inhalation is usually free of adverse effects. Ipratropium does not cross the blood–brain barrier. It apparently does not increase the viscosity of respiratory secretions or interfere with their expectoration.

Cystic Fibrosis

Pulmozyme is human deoxyribonuclease (DNAse) produced by recombinant DNA technology. Administered as an aerosol mist, this agent hydrolyzes extracellular DNA and decreases sputum viscosity in cystic fibrosis. Pulmonary function improves and the incidence of respiratory infection deceases. Laryngitis, pharyngitis, and chest pain are side effects.

Nasal Decongestants

Several α-adrenergic agonists (***ephedrine, epinephrine, naphazoline, oxymetazoline, phenylephrine, tetrahydrozoline,*** and ***xylomethazoline***) are applied locally in sprays and drops to alleviate nasal ''stuffiness'' that accompanies upper respiratory tract infections and allergic reactions. Otic congestion of middle ear infections may also respond to these drugs. Stimulation of α-receptors constricts blood vessels and reduces capillary leakage that causes swelling and excessive secretion. Adverse effects that can occur if sufficient drug is systemically absorbed include anxiety, psychotic disturbances, dysrhythmias, and changes in blood pressure. These agents are contraindicated in persons with hyperthyroidism, hypertension, and other cardiovascular disorders. Young children and the elderly are particularly sensitive to the effects of α-agonists. Concomitant administration of MAO inhibitors is contraindicated. The effectiveness of some antihypertensive drugs that utilize neuronal amine pump uptake mechanisms may be reduced. Excessive use of decongestants can result in rebound congestion, leading to the need for a further increase in dosage.

For nasal congestion that is refractory to decongestants, topical preparations of corticosteroids (***betamethasone, dexamethasone, beclomethasone, budesonide,*** and ***flunisolide***) are available, and cromolyn may be helpful. Administration of topical corticosteroids should not be continued beyond 3 weeks unless definite symptomatic relief is obtained. Systemic absorption of corticosteroids may alter adrenal function. Local responses include nasal dryness, irritation, epistaxis, sneezing, and infection.

Antitussives

The cough reflex is a protective mechanism that clears obstructive substances from the respiratory tract. A dry, nonproductive cough that interferes with proper rest is ameliorated by antitussives. Opiates and related drugs that suppress the central cough reflex are most effective. ***Codeine*** and ***hydrocodone*** can induce characteristic opiate effects such as respiratory depression and drug dependence. ***Dextromethorphan*** and ***noscapine*** have antitussive but not analgesic activity, and cause relatively few adverse reactions. ***Diphenhydrmine,*** an antihistamine that mildly suppresses the cough center, characteristically causes sedation. ***Benzonatate*** is a nonnarcotic that decreases responsiveness of stretch receptors and central cough mechanisms. Locally acting agents such as glycerin or honey help to alleviate pharyngeal irritation. Expectorants (*e.g.*, ***glyceryl guaiacolate,*** and ***potassium iodide***) may increase fluidity of respiratory secretions so that they may be expectorated more easily. Sufficient hydration and humidified air can ameliorate respiratory irritation and reduce the viscosity of secretions.

Acetylcysteine (Mucomyst) administered by inhalation reduces the viscosity of mucus by depolymerizing mucopolysaccharides, thus enhancing the removal of respiratory secretions.

Respiratory Stimulants

Respiratory stimulants (analeptics) are seldom used, since mechanical ventilatory assistance is generally a more effective and safer mode of supporting respiration. ***Doxapram*** (Dopram) and ***nikethamide*** (Coramine) may alleviate drug-induced respiratory depression (*e.g.*, following general anesthesia) and may enhance ventilation in persons with chronic pulmonary disorders. The major adverse effect of these drugs is central nervous system stimulation including convulsions. Patients must be closely observed for untoward reactions and also to ensure that ventilation is adequate.

The carbonic anhydrase inhibitor acetazolamide is investigational in the treatment of high-altitude hypoxia or "mountain sickness." It induces a mild degree of acidosis that stimulates respiration but also reverses the efficacy of the drug. Intermittent administration, or addition of bicarbonate, can prevent drug tolerance.

Therapeutic Gases

Oxygen, essential to many forms of life including mammalian, normally constitutes 20% of inspired air. This gas is frequently administered in clinical conditions that foster hypoxia (reduction in tissue oxygenation) or anoxia (absence of tissue oxygenation). Oxygen deficit occurs by several mechanisms. In anoxic anoxia, entry of oxygen into the lungs or the pulmonary capillaries is reduced. Such anoxia, frequently encountered in pulmonary disease and general anesthesia, is most amenable to oxygen administration. Stagnant anoxia occurs in disorders such as myocardial infarction, congestive heart failure, and shock, when systemic circulation fails to supply adequate blood flow to tissues including the lungs. An enhanced oxygen supply may be of some benefit in these situations. The value of oxygen administration is lower in anemic anoxia, characterized by a deficient oxygen-transporting capacity of blood, and in histotoxic anoxia, caused by substances that suppress cellular utilization of oxygen.

Oxygen is supplied in tanks, commonly color-coded green in the United States. Several devices, capable of delivering varied amounts of oxygen, are available. The rate of flow of oxygen will determine the final concentrations in inspired air. Nasal cannulae or nasopharyngeal catheters, which allow considerable concomitant inspiration of ambient air, can provide 25% to 50% oxygen. Face masks, dependent upon tightness of fit and type of valve (rebreathing or nonrebreathing) can deliver up to 100% oxygen. When spontaneous respiration is absent, mechanical ventilation is required to achieve movement of gases into and out of the lungs. Arterial blood gases (*i.e.*, oxygen and carbon dioxide) must be monitored to determine the actual extent of pulmonary gas exchange.

Oxygen administration should be limited to as brief a time as possible. Oropharyngeal and pulmonary irritation induce coughing and respiratory difficulty. Prolonged exposure to oxygen alters normal patterns of pulmonary gas exchange by provoking edema, fibrosis, hemorrhage, and formation of a hyaline membrane. This adult respiratory distress syndrome occurs most frequently at high oxygen tension, and may become irreversible. Seizures have been reported to occur with oxygen administration. Premature infants given oxygen are at marked risk of retrolental fibroplasia and blindness. If required, extended periods of oxygen therapy in such infants should utilize oxygen concentrations lower than 40% of inspired air. Commercially prepared oxygen is anhydrous and will dehydrate mucous membranes and cause increased viscosity of respiratory secretions. Since oxygen supports combustion, its use always requires strict precautions to avoid explosion or fire. Smoking, use of open flame, and sparks from electrical appliances must be avoided.

Administration of oxygen is especially hazardous in persons with chronic obstructive pulmonary diseases, as it may aggravate hypoxemia and hypercapnea. Prolonged hypoxia alters the sensitivity of carotid and aortic chemoreceptors, and spontaneous respiration becomes dependent upon low plasma oxygen tension. Increased oxygenation of arterial blood can cause respiratory arrest, necessitating mechanical assistance to breathing. Ventricular dysrhythmias may occur with rapid reduction of chronically elevated arterial carbon dioxide levels.

Hyperbaric chambers can provide an atmosphere of increased oxygen pressure. Their use may be of value in the treatment of obstructive lung disease, gas gangrene, decompression sickness, severe and extensive burns, and carbon monoxide poisoning. The usefulness of oxygen in carbon monoxide poisoning is limited by the impaired oxygen-transport capacity of hemoglobin. Oxygen is somewhat soluble in plasma, and inspiration of 100% oxygen can provide small increases in delivery to tissues via this route. The potential adverse effects of oxygen administration can be decreased by keeping chamber pressures at or below three atmospheres.

Oxygen is added to perfusing fluids for excised organs being readied for transplantation, and is used to oxygenate blood during extracorporeal circulation (*i.e.*, in cardiopulmonary bypass). Carbon dioxide is added to pump oxygenators to maintain optimal gas concentrations. The latter is a powerful stimulant to respiration, but excessive amounts in the circulatory system induce respiratory acidosis. Although carbon dioxide dilates cerebral blood vessels, it has been used with little success to alleviate cerebrovascular insufficiency. Carbon dioxide should not be administered to persons with cerebral edema, head injury, or any other source of increased intracranial pressure.

Histamine and Antagonists

Histamine is endogenous to many mammalian cell types, most notably mast cells in the skin and lungs, parietal cells of the gastric mucosa, and basophils. Histamine is also found in the central nervous system, where it appears to be a neurotransmitter. Secretion of gastric acid is markedly influenced by histamine. Antigen-antibody interactions, as well as several drugs (*e.g.*, morphine, trimethaphan) stimulate release of histamine from mast cells. Allergy symptoms such as urticaria, rhinitis, asthma, and anaphylactic shock are attributable at least in part to this amine.

Histamine exerts its effects by interacting with two distinct types of binding sites, designated H_1 and H_2 histamine receptors. H_1-receptors are most responsible for allergy responses, while H_2-receptors mediate gastric secretion. Both types of receptors are found in brain, and both receptor types probably mediate cardiovascular actions of histamine.

Histamine was administered in the past as a test for gastric secretion when pernicious anemia was suspected. Betazole, a relatively H_2-receptor-specific analogue of histamine, was used in a similar manner. However, side effects that can be life threatening have made this use obsolete. ***Pentagastrin*** (Peptavlon) has replaced histamine as a test for gastric-acid secretory responses. Histamine use as a provocative test in the diagnosis of pheochromocytoma is also obsolete. Histamine stimulation of the cells of the adrenal medulla, coupled with an exaggerated reflex response to histamine-induced hypotension, results in massive release of catecholamines in these individuals. Chemical assays of catecholamines are now used. Administration of histamine can provoke all the symptoms of allergy, including asthma and anaphylactic shock, especially in persons with allergies who are especially responsive to histamine. Additional adverse reactions are headache, dizziness, hypotension, tachycardia, and exacerbation of peptic ulcer symptoms. Betazole causes fewer and less intense side effects.

The conventional or ''classic'' antihistamines are H_1-receptor antagonists (Table 7-27). They are used extensively in the prevention and control of allergic reactions, and several are available without prescription. The most prominent side effect of these drugs is sedation, although recently developed agents such as ***terfenadine*** (Seldane) and astemizole (Hismanol) are reported not to cross the blood-brain barrier. H_1-antihistamines are also anticholinergic and will produce dry mouth, urinary retention, thickening of bronchial secretions, and exacerbation of glaucoma. Over-the-counter sleeping aids and motion sickness preventatives often contain antihistamines. Antihistamines are combined with α-adrenergic agonists such as pseudoephedrine, the latter to alleviate nasal congestion of allergic reactions.

TABLE 7-27. Antihistamines

GENERIC NAME	TRADE NAME
H_1-Receptor Antagonists	
Astemizole*	Hismanal
Azatadine	Optimine
Brompheniramine	Dimetane
Chlorpheniramine	Chlor-Trimeton, others
Clemastine	Tavist
Cyproheptadine	Periactin
Diphenhydramine	Benadryl, others
Loraladine*	Claritin
Terfenadine*	Seldane
Tripelennamine	Pyribenzamine
Triprolidine	Actidil
H_2-Receptor Antagonists	
Cimetidine	Tagamet
Famotidine	Pepcid
Ranitidine	Zantac
Nizatidine	Axid

* Second generation

A second generation of H_1-antihistamines lacks the major sedating and anticholinergic effects of the ''classic'' agents. Terfenadine (Seldane) and astemizole (Hismanal) are hepatically metabolized, and many drugs, including some antifungals and antibacterials, can inhibit that inactivation. An important adverse effect of these antihistamines is ventricular dysrhythmias, which can be lethal and which occur especially at higher plasma concentrations. Hepatic dysfunction and hypokalemia also increase the risk for dysrhythmia. Cholestatic jaundice can occur with both drugs. Terfenadine causes rash and alopecia, while astemizole causes weight gain. ***Loratidine*** (Claritin) induces little drowsiness at recommended doses but becomes sedating at higher doses. Recommended doses also seem not to potentiate the sedative effect of other CNS depressants. Loratidine has not been reported to cause ventricular dysrhythmias. It is hepatically inactivated, and its 8- to 14-hour half-life can extend to 24 hours in older patients and those with hepatic impairment.

H_2-receptor antagonists (see Table 7-27) are used clinically for their ability to suppress both daytime and nocturnal gastric acid secretion in response to a variety of stimuli (*e.g.*, pentagastrin, insulin, histamine, and food ingestion). Treatment and prevention of peptic ulcers, including those that can occur with stress or with Zollinger-Ellison syndrome, are the major indications for these drugs. During clinical development, ***cimetidine*** (Tagamet) appeared remarkably free of adverse effects. However, postmarket surveillance revealed an inhibition of hepatic cytochrome P-450 enzymes that can result in elevated serum levels of such drugs as diazepam, warfarin, theophylline, and propranolol. Other H_2-receptor antagonists have lower potential for such drug interactions. Although the H_2-receptor antagonists do not readily cross the blood–brain barrier, they can cause lethargy, depression, hallucinations, and mental confusion, particularly in patients who are elderly or have impaired renal function. Agranulocytosis and thrombocytopenia can occur. Cimetidine's anti-androgenic action can cause impotence and gynecomastia. Some H_2-antihistamines are now available over the counter.

Prostaglandins

Most tissues can synthesize prostaglandins from free arachidonic acid, which is released from phospholipids by phospholipases. The nonsteroidal antiinflammatory drugs, including aspirin, inhibit the enzyme cyclo-oxygenase, the first step in the formation of prostaglandins. These substances, which have a relatively short biological half-life, exert local actions frequently via activation of adenyl cyclase. Prostaglandins have varied and occasionally opposing action on physiological functions. For example, prostaglandin E_2 (PGE_2) dilates bronchioles while $PGF_{2\alpha}$ is a bronchoconstrictor. PGE_2 and $PGF_{2\alpha}$ both stimulate the pregnant uterus but have opposite effects on the nonpregnant uterus and on blood pressure.

The actions of the prostaglandins have prompted research into possible clinical uses for these substances. Prostaglandins and their analogues have been used as second-trimester abortifacients. Clinical studies on prostaglandin analogues for the alleviation of peptic ulcer and asthma are ongoing. The prostaglandin analogue misoprostol (Cytotec) can decrease the risk of nonsteroidal anti-inflammatory drug-induced ulcers. Prostaglandins are involved in inflammation, dysmenorrhea, patent ductus arteriosus in the neonate, and other disease processes. PGE_2 appears to have an important role in renal function.

Additional members of the prostaglandin family are thromboxane A_2 (TxA_2), a potent vasoconstrictor and platelet-aggregating agent, and prostacyclin (PGI_2), which is a vasodilator and antiaggregant. PGI_2 is synthesized in the vascular endothelium and Tx in platelets. The balance between PGI_2 and TxA_2 contributes to the aggregability of platelets.

Another pathway of arachidonic acid metabolism is via lipoxygenase, which gives rise to the leukotrienes. These products, which constrict airways and most blood vessels, have been implicated in the pathogenesis of allergic reactions. A mixture of leukotrienes including C_4 and D_4 account for the activity of slow-reacting substance of anaphylaxis (SRS-A).

GASTROINTESTINAL PHARMACOLOGY

Treatment of Peptic Ulcer

Mildly alkaline salts are used to relieve gastric discomfort arising from hyperacidity or peptic ulcer. Healing of the latter is promoted by the addition of antacids to other regimens of treatment. Antacids can also be administered to achieve alkalinization of the urine, which can be of value in combatting urinary infections and in preventing precipitation of uric acid and various types of drugs.

Antacids contain aluminum, calcium, magnesium, and sodium ions in varying combinations and concentrations. Aluminum and calcium salts have a constipating effect while magnesium salts cause diarrhea, thus antacids are often combined or alternated to promote normal lower intestinal function. Antacid preparations that contain sodium can be deleterious in persons who must restrict their intake of this ion. Magnesium ion in particular can accumulate to toxic levels in the presence of renal impairment. Antacids consumed for an extended time may induce systemic alkalosis; this occurs especially with the water-soluble sodium bicarbonate. Some antacids contribute to the formation of renal stones. Many antacids are available over-the-counter; persons receiving drugs such as digitalis and tetracyclines must be advised of possible interference with drug absorption.

Sucralfate (Carafate), a complex of aluminum hydroxide and sulfated sucrose, promotes healing of duodenal ulcers apparently by forming a local protective barrier on ulcerated tissue. Constipation is the major adverse effect of this drug, which is poorly absorbed. Aluminum toxicity can occur in persons with chronic renal impairment. Possible interference with gastrointestinal absorption of digoxin, cimetidine, warfarin, phenytoin, lansoprazole, or fluoroquinolone and tetracycline antibiotics can be avoided by administering these drugs at least 2 hours before or after sucralfate.

Omeprazole (Prilosec) and ***lansoprazole*** (Prevacid) inhibit the H^+/K^+ ATPase proton pump that is the final step in gastric secretion of hydrogen ions. These drugs strongly reduce gastric acidity and thus promote healing of ulcers and control of hypersecretory disorders. Adverse effects include abdominal pain, nausea, and diarrhea. Chronic administration to rats induced gastric carcinoid tumors, and long-term safety in humans is not known. Omeprazole can increase plasma levels of digitalis, diazepam, warfarin, and phenytoin.

Omeprazole and lansoprazole have some activity against *Helicobacter pylori* but do not completely eradicate this bacteria, which is associated with peptic ulcer development. Antibacterials such as amoxicillin, tetracycline, clarithromycin, and metronidazole are frequently combined with other anti-ulcer agents. Complete eradication of *H. pylori* greatly decreases recurrence of ulcer.

H_2-histamine receptor antagonists and anticholinergic agents, also used in the management of peptic ulcer and Zollinger-Ellison syndrome, are discussed elsewhere in this chapter.

Emetics

Emetics can be useful in evacuating some toxic substances from the stomach if gastric lavage is unavailable. It must be noted, however, that induction of vomiting is contraindicated following ingestion of corrosive substances that may further damage the esophagus. Guidance from a poison control center can be useful in determining proper treatment of some poisonings. Emetics should not be administered to persons who are lethargic or unconscious. Patients should be monitored until vomiting has ceased.

Drugs that induce vomiting may act through nonspecific gastric irritation, or may stimulate the chemoreceptor trigger zone or the vomiting center in the central nervous system. ***Apomorphine*** has a central site of action, producing vomiting within 15 minutes following SC administration. A single dose only is given. Apomorphine can induce characteristic opiate central nervous system depression and cardiovascular failure.

Ipecac syrup appears to act through local irritation of the gastric mucosa and stimulation of central control areas. This drug is administered orally. If vomiting does not ensue, ipecac *must* be evacuated from the stomach by other means. Systemic absorption of this drug is hazardous because of its marked cardiovascular effects. The more highly concentrated ipecac fluid extract should not be confused with ipecac syrup.

Antiemetics

Suppression of vomiting may be desirable to reduce the risk of malnutrition, dehydration, and electrolyte depletion. Emesis itself is a sign of local or central irritation, and the cause for persistent vomiting must be investigated.

Antihistamines such as dimenhydrinate, hydroxyzine, and meclizine are most effective in alleviating emesis of vestibular origin. Several motion sickness remedies containing these drugs are available over the counter. The anticholinergic ***scopolamine*** is incorporated into a transdermal form (Transderm-Scōp) for this indication. Phenothiazines and other drugs such as ***metoclopramide*** (Reglan), which block central dopaminergic receptors, can be used to alleviate vomiting following general anesthesia, and may be somewhat effective in reducing the severe emesis that often accompanies antineoplastic therapy. ***Diphenidol*** (Vontrol) and ***benzquinamide*** (Emete-Con) can alleviate moderate nausea and vomiting. Caution must be exercised in the use of drugs with antiemetic action because they can suppress this manifestation of drug toxicity or organic disease. Oral tetrahydrocannabinal (***dronabinol,*** Marinol) or its synthetic analogue ***nabilone*** (Cesemet) can be used to treat the vomiting associated with cancer chemotherapy.

Ondansetron (Zofran) is a serotonin antagonist administered IV to decrease nausea and vomiting induced by antineoplastic drugs. Dopamine receptors are not blocked by this drug, thus extrapyramidal effects should not occur. Inactivation occurs in the liver; common side effects are diarrhea or constipation, dizziness, and headache. Coadministration of dexamethasone enhances the antiemetic action of ondansetron.

Granisetron (Kytril), a serotonin 5-HT_3 antagonist, is approved for prevention of nausea and vomiting induced by antineoplastic agents. Metabolized in the liver and excreted in urine and feces, granisetron has a half-life of 9 hours. The recommended dose of 10 μg/kg is administered IV over 5 minutes, no earlier than 30 minutes before the start of chemotherapy. Concomitant dexamethasone (Decadron) may enhance the antiemetic efficacy. Induction or inhibition of hepatic enzymes can decrease or increase the half-life of granisetron. Adverse effects include headache (acetaminophen can be given), somnolence, asthenia, diarrhea, or constipation. Cardiovascular changes including increase or decrease in blood pressure, sinus bradycardia, atrial fibrillation, A-V heart block, and ventricular dysrhythmias may be related to granisetron administration. Long-term high doses induced hepatic tumors in rodents.

Laxatives

Laxatives are used to facilitate evacuation of contents from the lower intestinal tract. The irritant action of laxatives including ***bisacodyl, cascara, castor oil,*** and ***phenolphthalein*** promotes peristalsis. They also affect water content by increasing secretion by PGE_2, cAMP and inhibition of Na^+-K^+-ATPase. Other laxatives add moisture and bulk to fecal material, softening the stool and enhancing passage through the bowel. Nonabsorbed, bulk-forming laxatives include ***methylcellulose*** and ***psyllium.*** Saline or osmotic laxatives (*e.g.,* glycerin, lactulose, magnesium salts, and sodium phosphates) draw fluid into the intestinal tract. Calcium ***polycarbophil*** can act as a bulk-forming laxative, or can alleviate diarrhea by drawing excess water out of loose fecal matter.

Surface-acting or wetting agents such as the docusates do not relieve constipation but will counteract further formation of hard dry feces. Persons with cardiovascular disease or hernia, in whom straining to defecate can be hazardous, benefit from the use of these drugs.

Abdominal pain, nausea, or other indications of gastrointestinal obstruction or acute abdomen contraindicate the administration of laxatives. Persons who experience frequent constipation should be encouraged to increase their intake of fluids and fiber-rich foods. Regular exercise also can promote normal intestinal function. Chronic use of laxatives, many of which are available without prescription, can induce dehydration, electrolyte imbalance, and dependence upon these agents for bowel function. The use of laxatives can reduce the absorption of orally administered drugs by shortening their transit time through the intestine.

Other Gastrointestinal Agents

Ursodiol (Actigall) is available as an alternative to surgery for dissolution of small, radiolucent, noncalcified gallbladder stones. Long-term therapy (up to 2 years) may be required for removal of stones. Ursodiol should not be administered to persons with chronic liver disease or hypersensitivity to bile acids. Concurrent administration of ***chenodiol*** (Chenix) may enhance efficacy.

Mesalamine (***5-aminosalicylic acid***, Rowasa) enema to decrease inflammation in ulcerative colitis is now available in an oral coated form (Asacol), which releases the drug in the lower gastrointestinal tract. ***Olsalazine*** (Dipentum) is a dimer of mesalamine that also prevents upper gastrointestinal absorption of this drug. Adverse effects include headache, gastrointestinal disturbance, and rarely pericarditis, asthma, nephrotoxicity, diabetes insipidus, pancreatitis, and a lupus-like syndrome.

Cisapride (Propulsid) relieves symptoms of gastroesophageal reflux. It appears to work through serotonin receptors, releasing acetylcholine to improve esophageal motility, raise pressure at the lower esophageal sphincter, and hasten gastric emptying. Cisapride is highly bound to plasma proteins and is hepatically metabolized. Nausea, vomiting, diarrhea, and headache can occur, and this drug should not be administered during pregnancy or lactation because of the possibility of fetal or neonatal harm. Because cisapride affects gastrointestinal motility, it can alter the absorption of other drugs given orally.

Bleeding of esophageal varices can be treated with the sclerosing agent ***ethanolamine oleate*** (Ethamolin).

ENDOCRINE PHARMACOLOGY

Anterior Pituitary Hormones

Under the regulation of stimulatory and inhibitory factors released by the hypothalamus, the anterior pituitary synthesizes and releases several hormones that affect growth and development, often through actions on other endocrine organs. Somatostatin, which inhibits release of growth hormone, is found also in the gastrointestinal tract and pancreas, where it reduces secretion of insulin, glucagon, and digestive fluids.

Adrenocorticotropic hormone (ACTH) promotes synthesis and release of hormones such as cortisol from the adrenal cortex and is in turn subject to negative feedback control by plasma levels of these hormones. It is used clinically to differentiate between primary and secondary adrenocortical insufficiency. In persons with functional adrenals, administration of ACTH provokes secretion of corticosteroids that is reflected in elevated plasma and urinary levels of 17-hydroxycorticosteroid and 17-ketosteroid metabolites. ACTH is seldom used to treat adrenal insufficiency, since administration of corticosteroids provides more consistent and reliable hormone replacement. Symptoms of multiple sclerosis, myasthenia gravis, and hypercalcemia resulting from carcinoma may be alleviated with ACTH. This hormone is derived from animal pituitary and must be administered parenterally. Adverse effects are similar to those observed with adrenocortical hyperactivity or administration of corticosteroids. Allergic reactions, some provoked by contaminating porcine protein, can develop. Sustained action forms of ACTH that contain zinc hydroxide and gelatin must not be administered IV. Contraindications to the use of ACTH include osteoporosis, congestive heart failure, and hypertension.

Cosyntropin (Cortrosyn) is a synthetic analogue containing the first 24 amino acids in the ACTH sequence. It is a diagnostic agent for adrenocortical responsiveness, and is less likely than ACTH to provoke allergic reactions.

Metyrapone (Metopirone), an agent diagnostic for anterior pituitary function, inhibits the enzymatic biosynthesis of the corticosteroids. This reduces negative feedback control and increases the release of ACTH if pituitary function is adequate. Subsequent synthesis of corticosteroid precursors will be reflected in elevated urinary levels of 17-hydroxy and 11-deoxy metabolites. Responsiveness of the adrenals should be determined before metyrapone is administered. Phenytoin, cyproheptadine, exogenous estrogen, and pregnancy may alter the results of metyrapone testing.

Thyroid-stimulating hormone (TSH, thyrotropin) induces iodine uptake and hormone synthesis in the thyroid gland. Similarly to ACTH, TSH is used to diagnose primary and secondary hypothyroidism. Because it provokes release of triiodothyronine (T_3) and thyroxine (T_4), inappropriate administration of TSH can elicit symptoms similar to hyperthyroidism and thyrotoxicosis; tachycardia, angina pectoris, and congestive heart failure may develop or be exacerbated. The long onset (up to 8 hours) and duration (24 to 48 hours or more) of action necessitate persistent observation of patients. Secretion of TSH is stimulated by the hypothalamic thyrotropin-releasing hormone (TRH), and is under negative feedback control relative to plasma levels of thyroid hormones.

The gonadotropic hormones of the anterior pituitary promote and maintain sexual development and function. ***Follicle-stimulating hormone*** (FSH) induces maturation of ovarian follicles and secretion of estrogen. ***Luteinizing hormone*** (LH) causes rupture of the follicle (ovulation) and supports secretion of progesterone by the corpus luteum. LH also induces synthesis and release of testosterone from testicular Leydig cells. ***Menotropins*** (human menopausal gonadotropins, Pergonal) are derived from urine of postmenopausal women and contain large amounts of FSH and LH. Anovulatory women with functional ovaries can be given menotropins to induce follicular development, and subsequent administration of ***human chorionic gonadotropin*** (HCG, Follutein, which has pronounced LH-like activity) will elicit ovulation. This treatment for infertility presents the risk of ovarian hyperstimulation resulting in rupture of cysts and severe intraperitonal hemorrhage. The incidence of multiple fetuses is increased, and pregnancies often terminate with the premature birth of high-risk infants. Spermatogenesis also can be stimulated by menotropins, and HCG is used to induce testicular descent in prepubertal boys. ***Urofollitropin*** (Metrodin) is another human gonadotropin preparation used to induce ovulation.

Human growth hormone (HGH, somatotropin, Asellacrin) will stimulate growth and development in children with growth hormone deficiency. Treatment must be given before epiphyseal closure, and concomitant or induced hypothyroidism must be corrected. HGH is diabetogenic and influences protein, fat, and electrolyte metabolism. Fluid retention and intracranial hypertension may occur. Recombinant DNA technology has made available a more abundant supply of HGH (***somatrem***, Protropin; ***somatropin***, Humatrope, Nutropin) free of the risk of transmitting Creutzfeldt-Jakob disease.

Prolactin, normally elevated only during pregnancy and lactation, stimulates the mammary glands to produce milk. Release of this anterior pituitary hormone is under inhibitory control of the neurotransmitter dopamine. The dopamine agonist bromocriptine (Parlodel) is administered to reverse hyperprolactinemia that is not GH-dependent and to suppress unwanted postpartum lactation. Pharmacological agents that deplete dopamine (*e.g.*, alpha methyldopa) or which block dopamine receptors (*e.g.*, the neuroleptics) will promote prolactin release.

Posterior Pituitary Hormones

Vasopressin (antidiuretic hormone, ADH) and ***oxytocin*** are secreted by the posterior pituitary (neurohypophysis). Vasopressin influences renal reabsorption of water by altering membrane permeability in the distal tubule and collecting duct of the nephron. Vasopressin (Pitressin) and the synthetic analogues ***desmopressin*** (DDAVP) and ***lypressin*** (Diapid) will alleviate diabetes insipidus caused by endogenous ADH deficiency. (Nephrogenic diabetes insipidus, characterized by renal unresponsiveness to ADH, is treated with thiazide diuretics.) Fluid intake and output must be monitored, because water intoxication can occur. Like many hormone preparations, vasopressin must be administered parenterally. Desmopressin and lypressin are given intranasally. Vascular constriction caused by vasopressin can induce hypertension, angina pectoris, and myocardial infarction; persons with cardiovascular disease are at greatest risk. Oxytocic-like activity, apparent at high doses, makes this drug hazardous during pregnancy. The synthetic analogues cause less stimulation of vascular and uterine smooth muscle and are, therefore, preferable to ADH in pregnancy. Vasopressin is also used to alleviate postsurgical abdominal distention. Desmopressin induces a temporary increase in plasma levels of clotting factors that can help to control abnormal bleeding in some types of von Willebrand's disease and hemophilia. Desmopressin may also ameliorate nocturnal enuresis in children older than 6 years.

Oxytocin secreted by the posterior pituitary appears to have an important physiological role in parturition and lactation. Responsiveness of the uterine muscle to oxytocin gradually intensifies during pregnancy. Increased amounts of this hormone are released at the time of labor and delivery, possibly in response to dilation of the cervix and vagina.

Exogenous ***oxytocin*** (Pitocin) is occasionally administered to enhance uterine activity in carefully selected patients in whom pregnancy or labor is not progressing normally. It is too hazardous for use in routine deliveries since powerful sustained contractions can result in fetal hypoxia or uterine rupture. Fetal or maternal dysrhythmias and water intoxication (oxytocin has some ADH activity) can be severe. There are many contraindications to the use of oxytocin, such as malpositioning of the fetus, maternal history of cervical or uterine surgery (including cesarean section), placenta previa, and umbilical cord prolapse. Oxytocin is administered by slow IV infusion carefully titrated to produce contraction patterns similar to those of normal labor. Patients must be under continual observation, and drug administration is terminated if fetal distress, uterine hyperactivity, or significant changes in maternal vital signs occur. After the infant and placenta have been delivered, oxytocin can be given to control uterine atony and hemorrhage. The sustained uterine contractions help to seal off bleeding from arterioles. Oxytocin is an abortifacient, especially in later pregnancy (during the first trimester, the uterus is relatively unresponsive to oxytocin). Flow of milk (''milk letdown'') is stimulated by this hormone, which is available in a nasal spray to be used by lactating women. Oxytocin can potentiate the pressor effect of sympathomimetic drugs.

The ergot alkaloids (***ergonovine*** and ***methylergonovine***) are oxytocics that are used to control postpartum atony and hemorrhage of the uterus. Vasoconstriction can occur and occasionally produces severe hypertension or circulatory stasis in the extremities.

Thyroid Hormones

The thyroid gland synthesizes ***thyroxine*** (T_4) as well as small amounts of ***triiodothyronine*** (T_3). Many tissues in the human body convert T_4 to T_3, which is the more active form of thyroid hormone. In the circulatory system, most T_4 and T_3 is bound to thyroid hormone-binding globulin and to albumin.

Thyroid hormone is essential for proper growth and metabolism. Its absence is especially severe in infants and very young children, in whom arrested physical and mental development known as cretinism can occur. Thyroid deficiency is treated with hormone-replacement therapy. Thyroid USP and thyroid extract (Proloid) are prepared from animal thyroid. ***Levothyroxine*** (Synthroid) and ***liothyronine*** (Cytomel) are synthetic sodium salts of T_4 and T_3 that can be administered either orally or intravenously. ***Liotrix*** (Euthyroid, Thyrolar) combines levothyroxine and liothyronine in a 4 : 1 ratio that approximates the endogenous levels of thyroid hormones. Thyroid preparations have a gradual onset and long duration of action due in part to their extensive binding to circulatory proteins. (Levels of thyroid hormone-binding globulin can be decreased by corticosteroid administration and increased in pregnancy.) Thyroid hormones are used clinically to suppress excessive release of TSH.

The replacement dosage of thyroid hormone must be individualized to produce the desired response in each patient. Many drugs (*e.g.*, aspirin, lithium, propranolol, and estrogens) can alter the results of thyroid function tests. Excessive amounts of hormone will produce symptoms similar to those of hyperthyroidism (*e.g.*, tachycardia, angina pectoris, irritability, insomnia, and heat intolerance). Hormone administration is contraindicated in persons with cardiovascular disease unless hypothyroidism coexists. Thyroid hormones appear to increase the number of myocardial β-adrenergic receptors, producing increased responsiveness to catecholamines and to sympathetic stimulation. The action of the oral anticoagulants can be increased by concomitant thyroid hormone administration, while the effectiveness of antidiabetic therapy is decreased.

Hyperactivity of the thyroid can be alleviated by surgical removal of the gland, or by pharmacological treatment. The antithyroid drugs ***propylthiouracil*** (PTU) and ***methimazole*** (Tapazole) inhibit the synthesis of thyroid hormones. They do not block the actions of the hormones, which are occasionally administered concurrently (*e.g.*, during pregnancy) to maintain a desirable level of thyroid influence. Because antithyroid drugs deplete circulating amounts of T_4 and T_3, the negative feedback control of TSH release is reduced. The resulting increase in TSH can induce enlargement and vascularization of the thyroid. Bone marrow suppression, which increases susceptibility to infections and severe hemorrhage, is a major adverse effect of antithyroid agents. Oral anticoagulant activity can be potentiated. Fatal hepatitis can be induced by administration of these drugs. Their use is contraindicated in nursing mothers because of the danger of inducing cretinism in the infant.

High doses of iodides (sodium and potassium iodides, and ''strong iodine'' or Lugol's solution) are given to suppress thyroid hormone synthesis and release. They may be combined with antithyroid drugs in the presurgical treatment of thyroidectomy patients. Intravenous administration is indicated for the management of thyrotoxicosis (thyroid crisis or storm). These agents have a slow onset and prolonged duration of action. Marked sensitivity to iodides may cause laryngeal edema and suffocation. Pretesting for reactivity is advisable, especially if the parenteral route is to be used.

Radioactive iodine (^{131}I), which is concentrated by the thyroid, is used to assess thyroid function and to treat hyperthyroidism and thyroid carcinoma. ^{131}I is contraindicated in pregnancy and lactation, and is rarely administered for hyperthyroidism in persons younger than 30 years of age. Treatment with ^{131}I can cause sore throat, bone marrow suppression, radiation sickness, and eventual hypothyroidism as the gland is destroyed. Antithyroid drugs will hinder uptake of ^{131}I, thus administration of such agents must cease 3 to 4 days before isotope therapy. Radiation safety precautions may be instituted to protect patient, staff, and visitors from injury.

Parathyroid Hormones

Parathyroid hormone (PTH) strongly influences plasma calcium levels by increasing bone resorption, enhancing renal reabsorption of calcium and excretion of phosphate, promoting intestinal uptake of dietary calcium, and stimulating the activation of vitamin D. Secretion of this hormone is regulated by plasma calcium levels. PTH is rarely used in the management of hypocalcemia since it rapidly provokes formation of antibodies. Administration of PTH (teriparatide acetate, human parathyroid hormone 1–34, Parathar) is diagnostic for hypoparathyroidism, provoking an excessive increase in urinary phosphorus and cAMP excretion in persons with hormone deficiency.

Hypocalcemia can be alleviated by administration of vitamin D, which is converted to its active forms, calcitriol and dihydrotachysterol, in the kidneys and liver. Vitamin D promotes intestinal absorption of calcium; thus adequate dietary intake is essential for the efficacy of this treatment. Calcium salts (*e.g.*, chloride, gluconate, and glucepate) can be administered IV to alleviate severe hypocalcemia manifested as tetany or marked prolongation of the myocardial QT interval. Calcium enhances responsiveness to defibrillation, and may help to restore cardiac rhythm. Extreme caution is required in patients receiving digitalis because calcium potentiates both the inotropic and toxic effects of the cardiac glycosides. Sodium bicarbonate will precipitate calcium salts from solution. The use of oral calcium to alleviate osteoporosis in women after menopause is controversial: studies indicate that concomitant estrogen replacement is required for adequate use of this ion.

Excessive amounts of vitamin D can produce hypercalcemia. Symptoms include muscle weakness, nausea, and diarrhea. Significant demineralization of bone can occur, and renal stones and soft-tissue calcium deposits may develop.

Calcitonin, a hormone synthesized by the thyroid, has actions opposite to those of PTH (*i.e.*, inhibition of bone resorption and enhancement of renal excretion of calcium and phosphate). Hypercalcemia induces the release of calcitonin. This hormone is used in the treatment of osteoporosis, hypercalcemia, and Paget's disease, which is characterized by abnormal osteoclastic and osteoblastic activity. Salmon calcitonin (Calcimar) provokes antibody formation and allergic responses. Synthetic hormone (Cibacalcin) identical to human calcitonin is also available.

Etidronate (Didronel), a diphosphatase that suppresses bone formation and resorption, also is used to manage Paget's disease, to reduce aberrant ossification following hip replacement or spinal cord injury and may be effective in decreasing bone loss of osteoporosis. Etidronate is administered only for a limited time (6 months for Paget's disease, 3 months following surgery or injury). The onset of action is gradual, and the dosage should be increased cautiously. Adequate calcium and vitamin D intake must be maintained.

Pamidronate (Aredia) can correct hypercalcemia and alleviate bone pain that frequently accompanies cancers, such as of the breast and prostate. This drug also may prove useful in osteoporosis, Paget's disease, and hyperparathyroidism, all of which are characterized by bone demineralization. Fever, leukopenia, and nausea are adverse effects of pamidronate, which is administered IV.

Adrenocortical Hormones

Adrenocortical hormones are essential for human survival. Addison's disease and other forms of adrenal insufficiency necessitate chronic corticosteroid replacement therapy. Endogenous cortical secretions are of two types: the ***glucocorticoids,*** which serve mainly to regulate carbohydrate and protein metabolism and resistance to stress; and the ***mineralocorticoids,*** which influence sodium and water balance. Synthesis of ***hydrocortisone*** (cortisol), the principal glucocorticoid in humans, is stimulated by ACTH. Plasma levels of glucocorticoids follow a pattern of circadian variation, with highest amounts just after awakening. Administration of exogenous cortisol in a similar pattern (*i.e.*, once daily or on alternate days early in the waking period) often provides a good therapeutic response with lower incidence of adverse effects. An increase in dosage may be necessary in times of increased stress (*e.g.*, illness or surgery).

Secretion of the mineralocorticoids (***desoxycorticosterone*** and ***aldosterone***) is regulated by circulating blood volume. A decrease in volume activates the juxtaglomerular apparatus and the renin–angiotensin system, which in turn stimulates aldosterone release. This hormone acts in the distal tubule of the nephron, promoting sodium reabsorption in exchange for potassium and hydrogen ion. The naturally occurring glucocorticoids possess some mineralocorticoid activity, and some persons with adrenal insufficiency can be maintained solely on hydrocortisone plus adequate dietary sodium chloride. ***Fludrocortisone*** (Florinef) is an orally active synthetic steroid possessing glucocorticoid and mineralocorticoid activities and is useful in patients with Addison's disease who need greater assistance in maintaining water and electrolyte balance. ***Desoxycorticosterone*** (Percorten) can be administered when the parenteral route is preferred. In Addison's disease, response to the mineralocorticoids may be heightened, resulting in edema, hypokalemia, hypertension, and cardiac dysrhythmias. Increased aldosterone secretion can occur in adrenal hyperplasia or malignancy, toxemia of pregnancy, renal hypertension, and hepatic cirrhosis with ascites. The potassium-sparing diuretic spironolactone (Aldactone) is an aldosterone antagonist.

In addition to their use in replacement therapy, the naturally occurring glucocorticoids and their synthetic analogues (Table 7-28) are administered in pharmacologic

TABLE 7-28. Glucocorticoids

GENERIC NAME	TRADE NAME
Cortisone	Cortisan, others
Hydrocortisone	Cortef, Hydrocortone, others
Beclomethasone	Beclovent, Vanceril
Betamethasone	Celestone
Dexamethasone	Decadron, others
Flunisolide	AeroBid
Methylprednisolone	Medrol
Prednisone	Meticorten, others
Prednisolone	Delta-Cortef, Cortalone
Triamcinolone	Aristocort, Azmacort, others

doses in the management of many illnesses including rheumatoid arthritis, rheumatic fever with carditis, acute leukemia, exfoliative dermatitis, pulmonary fibrosis, ulcerative colitis, nephrotic syndrome, systemic lupus erythematosus, and other inflammatory and autoimmune diseases. Cerebral edema and anaphylactic shock are indications for the glucocorticoids. The use of prednisone in particular to suppress immunity aids the survival of organ transplants. High-dose methylprednisolone administered IV within 8 hours of spinal cord injury may enhance neurological recovery but can cause gastrointestinal bleeding and increase the risk of wound infection.

The adverse effects of these drugs are numerous and can be serious, even life-threatening. Suppression of the hypothalamic–pituitary–adrenal axis falls into the latter category. Prolonged administration of glucocorticoids inhibits release of corticotropin (CRF) and ACTH, allowing the adrenal cortex to atrophy. If administration of hormone is abruptly terminated, the individual is left in a state of adrenal insufficiency. For this reason, glucocorticoid dosages must always be tapered gradually, with careful observation for signs of hypoadrenalism. Once daily or alternate-day dosing is reported to affect ACTH release minimally.

Administration of glucocorticoids suppresses immune responsiveness, predisposing to the development or exacerbation of infections. Bone demineralization (osteoporosis), diabetes, weight gain, edema, hypertension, weakening of blood vessel walls, peptic ulcer, electrolyte imbalance, mental changes, cataracts, glaucoma, impaired wound healing, menstrual irregularities, muscle weakness, and protein wasting are a few of the many additional adverse reactions to the glucocorticoids. Administration during pregnancy may cause cleft palate and pituitary-adrenal suppression in the fetus. Glucocorticoids are contraindicated in active tuberculosis, malignant hypertension, uremia, psychoses, active peptic ulcer, and in nursing mothers. Both types of adrenal hormones are biotransformed in the liver to a variety of metabolites such as sulfates and glucoronides, which are renally excreted.

Many of the synthetic corticosteroids (*e.g.*, ***prednisone***, ***prednisolone*** and ***dexamethasone***) have greater anti-inflammatory potency with lower mineralocorticoid activity than cortisone and cortisol. Synthetic glucocorticoids also have a longer duration of action than the natural substances. Prednisone acts for 18 to 36 hours while dexamethasone's effects may persist up to 48 hours.

Because glucocorticoids influence carbohydrate metabolism, they can increase the requirement for insulin or oral hypoglycemics in diabetic patients. Drugs that induce hepatic enzymes can enhance the biotransformation of corticosteroids, while oral contraceptives may inhibit their inactivation. Corticosteroids can alter blood coagulation; concomitant administration of aspirin or coumarin-type drugs requires observation for abnormal bleeding tendencies. Mineralocorticoid-induced potassium loss will add to diuretic-induced hypokalemia, and can enhance digitalis toxicity.

Beclomethasone (Beclovent, Vanceril), ***flunisolide*** (AeroBid), and ***triamcinolone*** (Azmacort) are corticosteroids in aerosolized form used in the management of asthma. Drug amounts absorbed through the lungs can be sufficient to suppress the hypothalamic-pituitary-adrenal axis, yet insufficient to substitute for systemically administered corticosteroids. Any alteration in drug regimen requires close observation for adrenal deficiency.

Nasal aerosols of beclomethasone and dexamethasone will alleviate inflammatory nasal conditions (see Respiratory Pharmacology). A variety of ocular inflammatory disorders are treated with ophthalmic ointments and solutions of dexamethasone and prednisolone. Topical corticosteroid creams and ointments, some available over-the-counter, will relieve pruritic and inflammatory dermatoses such as eczema; poison ivy, oak, or sumac; insect bites; and allergic reactions. ***Betamethasone*** (Diprolene) and ***clobetasol*** (Temovate) are the most potent of these agents, and present the greatest risk of adrenal suppression due to systemic absorption.

Aminoglutethimide (Cytodren) blocks the conversion of cholesterol to pregnenolone, thus reducing adrenal synthesis of steroids. This agent is occasionally used in the control of Cushing's syndrome, and may be palliative in some patients with advanced breast cancer or metastatic carcinoma of the prostate.

Insulin

The pancreas secretes insulin (from β-cells in the islets of Langerhans) and glucagon (from α-cells), both important for proper metabolism. Insulin is essential for the entry of glucose into many human tissues (exceptions to this are brain, liver, red blood cells, β-cells, and kidney tubules). This hormone appears to work by interacting with receptors on cell membranes. Release of insulin is stimulated by elevated blood levels of glucose, and by gastrin, secretin, ketone bodies, and glucagon. Epinephrine and norepinephrine, acting at α-adrenergic receptors, suppress insulin release while β-stimulation increases insulin release. Many of the actions of insulin are opposed by glucagon, which promotes ketogenesis, glycogenolysis and hyperglycemia. Glucagon release is promoted by amino acids and suppressed by glucose, ketones, and free fatty acids.

In diabetes mellitus, insulin is lacking (Type I, insulin-dependent, or juvenile-onset diabetes) or fails to function adequately (Type II, noninsulin-dependent, or maturity-onset diabetes). Failure of the pancreas to synthesize insulin requires that this hormone be administered throughout the lifetime of the patient. Diet and exercise must be properly balanced against insulin intake to maintain blood glucose within relatively safe levels. Persons who have diabetes are at greater than normal risk for cardiovascular disease, renal disease, and degenerative ocular changes. Hyperglycemia can cause brain damage, coma, and death, and can be fetotoxic.

Several forms of insulin are available for the management of diabetes mellitus. Most are derived from animal sources; all must be administered parenterally. Crystalline zinc insulin or ***regular insulin*** is a clear solution that can be administered by either the SC or IV route. It has a rapid onset and short duration (6 to 8 hours) of action. All other forms of insulin can be given only by the SC route.

Ultralente insulin is crystalline insulin with an onset of 4 to 6 hours and a duration of action up to 18 hours. ***Semilente*** or ***amorphous insulin,*** with an onset of 2 to 4 hours and duration of 12 to 16 hours, can be mixed with ultralente to provide an intermediate-acting lente insulin. Protamine insulin suspensions are gradually absorbed from the SC site and provide a long duration of action. ***Neutral protamine Hagedorn*** (NPH) insulin or isophane insulin is a crystalline modification of protamine zinc insulin. Regular insulin can be added to NPH insulin without losing its rapid, intense action. Protamine zinc insulin will retard the absorption of regular insulin.

Insulins can be combined to provide both immediate and sustained control of blood glucose. Three concentrations of insulin are currently available: U100 (or 100 units per ml) is most commonly used, U40 is available for administration of small doses, and U500 is used by persons who have developed insulin resistance and must receive large doses.

Hypersensitivity can develop to contaminants such as glucagon and somatostatin found in insulin. Highly purified insulin preparations (*e.g.,* single-component and purified porcine insulin) are available but are more expensive and limited in supply. Recombinant DNA technology has produced a ***biosynthetic human insulin (Humulin)*** that may be less allergenic than that derived from animals.

Since chronic SC injection of insulin can cause atrophy or hypertrophy of subcutaneous tissue, injection sites should be rotated. Administration of insulin carries the risk of overdose or underdose and subsequent hypoglycemia or hyperglycemia. Changes in exercise or eating habits, or increased physiological or psychological stress, alter insulin requirements. Persons who are diabetic must be aware of all factors that can affect their well-being. Regular testing of the blood for glucose is essential to diabetic control. Patients must also be alert to symptoms of hypoglycemia (hunger, nausea, irritability, tremor, mental confusion, tachycardia, ataxia), which can be alleviated by administration of some source of glucose. Severe hypoglycemia, which can result in convulsions, coma, and irreversible brain damage, can be treated with IV dextrose or SC or IM glucagon. Since β-adrenergic blockers can mask the symptoms of hypoglycemia, these drugs are hazardous in diabetic persons.

TABLE 7-29. Oral Hypoglycemic Drugs

GENERIC NAME	TRADE NAME
First Generation	
Acetohexamide	Dymelor
Chlorpropamide	Diabinese
Tolazamide	Tolinase
Tolbutamide	Orinase
Second Generation	
Glipizide	Glucotrol
Glyburide	Diabeta, Micronase

Persistent hypoinsulinemia leads to elevated plasma levels of glucagon, epinephrine, and growth hormone, which mobilize free fatty acids and eventually produce ketoacidosis or diabetic coma. Administration of insulin will reverse these effects by normalizing glucose utilization. Hydration with normal saline and infusion of dextrose may also be necessary. Marked depletion of body stores of potassium can accompany ketoacidosis, although plasma levels of this electrolyte may be normal. Administration of insulin promotes reentry of potassium into cells with subsequent hypokalemia. However, potassium supplements are given only when plasma levels persistently fail to normalize, and renal function is adequate.

Type II diabetes can often be ameliorated by administration of the sulfonylurea or oral hypoglycemic agents (Table 7-29). These drugs are ineffective in the total absence of endogenous insulin. The exact mechanism of action of the oral hypoglycemics is not known; they may enhance release of insulin from the pancreas or promote the utilization of insulin by body tissues. Control of Type II diabetes should initially be attempted through diet, exercise, and weight loss where appropriate. Patients receiving oral hypoglycemics must balance food intake, physical activity, and stress with their drug regimen. Failure to do so can cause hypoglycemia or hyperglycemia.

Side effects of the oral hypoglycemics include dermatological allergic reactions and gastrointestinal disturbances. Chlorpropamide may cause sodium and fluid retention, while the newer agents, glyburide and glipizide, have a mild diuretic effect. Tolerance can develop to the hypoglycemic action of these drugs. Controversial results of the University Group Diabetes Program study suggested that these drugs may increase the risk of cardiovascular disease.

Some of the oral hypoglycemics, chlorpropamide in

particular, can induce a disulfiramlike reaction following alcohol ingestion. Extensive plasma protein binding of these drugs may alter the actions of other drugs. Many drugs can affect blood glucose levels (*e.g.*, thiazide diuretics and sympathomimetics elevate while β-adrenergic blockers lower glucose levels) and may thus alter insulin or oral hypoglycemic requirements.

Metformin (Glucophage) increases cellular uptake of glucose and decreases hepatic glucose production. It does not have the risk for hypoglycemia presented by other antidiabetic agents. Insulin is required for metformin's action, and oral hypoglycemic agents can be given concurrently. Metformin inhibits the degradation of lactic acid and can cause lactic acidosis. Renal dysfunction, hypoxia (*e.g.*, with shock or heart or hepatic failure) and excessive alcohol ingestion will increase the risk for acidosis. Common adverse effects are gastrointestinal, including anorexia, nausea, diarrhea, metallic taste, and decreased absorption of vitamin B_{12} and folic acid. Although metformin is renally excreted, cimetidine can cause elevated blood levels of this drug.

Female Hormones

Estrogens and ***progesterone*** are endogenous steroid hormones synthesized principally in the ovary and the placenta. In addition, small amounts of these substances are formed in adipose tissue, adrenal cortex, liver, kidney, and other organs; these remain a source of female hormones in postmenopausal women. Naturally occurring estrogens include ***estradiol, estriol,*** and ***estrone.*** Salts and esters of these hormones, as well as synthetic analogues, are available (Table 7-30). In general, the naturally occurring estrogens must be administered parenterally, although ***conjugated estrogens*** (Premarin, sodium salts of sulfate esters) and ***esterified estrogens*** (Amnestrogen) are active when given by the oral route. Many topical preparations, and estradiol in a transdermal system, are also used. Estrogens are extensively metabolized in the liver.

TABLE 7-30. Estrogens and Progestogens

GENERIC NAME	TRADE NAME
Estrogens	
Chlorotrianisene	Tace
Conjugated estrogens	Premarin
Diethylstilbestrol	Stilphostrol
Estradiol	Estrase, Estraderm, others
Estrone	Theelin
Ethinylestradiol	Estinyl
Quinestrol	Estrovis
Progestogens	
Hydroxyprogesterone	Delalutin
Medroxyprogesterone	Depo-Provera
Norethindrone	Norlutin
Norgestrel	Ovrette
Progesterone	Femotrone, Progestaject

The estrogenic substances have many physiologic actions: *e.g.*, the primary effects of stimulation of the development of female reproductive organs, proliferation of the endometrium during the menstrual cycle, and maintenance of pregnancy. Secondary sex characteristics such as skin texture, adipose tissue distribution, and skeletal growth are influenced by estrogens. Adverse effects caused by these hormones include nausea, menstrual changes, headache, depression, sodium and fluid retention, thromboembolism, hypertension, hyperglycemia, and closure of epiphyses when administered before completion of skeletal development. Estrogens may increase the risk of endometrial carcinoma; concomitant administration of progestogens has a protective effect.

A major clinical use for estrogens is in combination with progestogens in oral contraceptives (discussed below). Estrogen can help to slow bone demineralization in osteoporosis; it is most effective when administration is begun before extensive bone loss has occurred. The effectiveness of calcium salts in osteoporosis is greatly enhanced by concomitant estrogen administration. Estrogens will alleviate menopausal symptoms, including urogenital atrophy, and are used as replacement therapy in endogenous hormone deficiency. Treatment of inoperable breast or prostate cancer may include estrogenic substances.

Progesterone is secreted principally by the corpus luteum. This hormone converts endometrial proliferation to the secretory phase of the menstrual cycle, prepares the uterus for ovum implantation, and subsequently maintains pregnancy. Progesterone is not active when taken orally, but several synthetic progestogens (see Table 7-30) are effectively absorbed from the gastrointestinal tract. Inactivation of these substances is accomplished mainly by hepatic enzymes.

Progestogens are widely used in oral contraceptives, for regulation of menstrual abnormalities, and in endometrial and renal carcinoma. Progesterone may occasionally be effective in relieving symptoms of premenstrual syndrome. Progestogens induce many of the same adverse effects attributable to estrogens. Both types of hormones are contraindicated during pregnancy since the risk of subsequent cancer and of fetal damage resulting in congenital defects is considerable.

Many of the oral contraceptives combine an estrogen and a progestogen. The mechanism of action of these preparations is thought to be suppression of ovulation by inhibiting the release of pituitary gonadotropins in a negative feedback manner. However, there is evidence that they are effective in doses lower than those necessary to suppress gonadotropins, and there may also be a direct effect on the ovary or interference with transport of ova or with fertilization or implantation. Oral contraceptives are a unique pharmacological entity, as they are used for substantial intervals of time by large numbers of relatively healthy young women to alter normal physiological functions. Although the incidence of serious side effects is low, the potential for thrombophlebitis, embolism, and hypertension must be recognized. Cigarette smoking greatly increases the risk of serious cardiovascular sequelae, particularly in women older than 35 years. Coexistence of both of these conditions should contraindicate the use of oral contraceptives. More frequent adverse reactions include nausea, sodium and fluid retention, breast tenderness, and breakthrough bleeding. Because of possible adverse effects on the fetus, pregnancy must be absolutely ruled out before oral contraceptive therapy is begun, and drug administration must be terminated if pregnancy is suspected. Cardiovascular disease, including hypertension and thrombotic tendency, and certain types of cancer contraindicate the use of oral contraceptives.

Combination contraceptives consist of 21 daily doses of an estrogen plus a progestogen, followed by 7 drug-free days. (Placebos frequently are substituted for this interval, to maintain the daily pattern of taking one tablet.) ***Ethinyl estradiol*** or ***mestranol*** provides the estrogen component; the progestogen may be ***norgestrel, levonorgestrel, norethindrone, ethynodiol diacetate, desogestrol,*** or ***norgestinate*** (the latter two may be less androgenic than other progestins). Recent formulations contain the lowest effective doses and correspondingly produce minimal adverse effects. A second type of oral contraceptive, the "minipill," which contains progestogen only, has a lower efficacy than combination drugs. Sequential formulations, in which 16 days of estrogen-only administration was followed by 5 days of estrogen plus progestogen have been discontinued because of an apparent risk of endometrial carcinoma. Drugs that induce hepatic enzymes can enhance the inactivation of these hormones and reduce the efficacy of contraception. Norplant is a subdermally implanted system of levonorgestrel that provides contraception of 5 years' duration.

Estrogens given alone postmenopausally can cause endometrial hyperplasia and increased incidence of endometrial cancer and possibly of breast cancer. Prempro and Premphase combine the conjugated estrogen Premarin with medroxyprogesterone to decrease estrogen-induced endometrial growth.

The antiestrogen ***clomiphene*** (Clomid) enhances pituitary release of gonadotropins, which in turn induces ovulation. Used as a fertility agent, this drug frequently results in multiple fetuses. Blurring or other visual disturbances occasionally develop, and can impair the ability to drive or operate machinery.

TABLE 7-31. Androgenic Drugs

GENERIC NAME	TRADE NAME
Androgens	
Testosterone (several forms)	Several
Danazol	Danocrine
Fluoxymesterone	Halotestin
Methyltestosterone	Metandren, others
Testolactone	Teslac
Anabolic Steroids	
Ethylestrenol	Maxibolin
Nandrolone	Anabolin, Durabolin
Oxandrolone	Anavar
Oxymetholone	Androyd
Stanazolol	Winstrol

The antiestrogen ***tamoxifen*** (Nolvadex) is discussed under Chemotherapeutic Drugs.

Male Hormones

Testosterone is the principal endogenous androgen. Like the female hormones, it is metabolized in the liver and is ineffective when given orally. Several synthetic analogues (Table 7-31) can be administered PO. These hormones stimulate the maturation of male reproductive organs and sexual characteristics. Androgens are also potent anabolic substances, promoting skeletal muscle development.

Androgens are administered as replacement therapy when endogenous testosterone is deficient. Several nortestosterone derivatives are used particularly for their anabolic action, which may be of value in severely debilitated or burn patients who are experiencing negative nitrogen balance. The use of such steroids to enhance athletic ability is of questionable efficacy but considerable hazard. Androgens may be administered to suppress unwanted lactation, and to ameliorate endometriosis, fibrocystic breast disease, and advanced breast cancer.

Adverse effects of androgens include hypercalcemia, psychological aberrations, sodium and fluid retention with exacerbation of congestive heart failure, and increased plasma levels of low-density lipoproteins, which may promote coronary artery disease and changes in hepatic function. Negative feedback inhibition of pituitary-gonadotropin release can induce sexual dysfunction. Hypertension, hepatic impairment, hormone-sensitive carcinomas, and pregnancy contraindicate the administration of androgens.

Finasteride (Proscar) blocks the conversion of testosterone to dihydrotestosterone, which promotes prostate enlargement, and thus can reverse prostatic hypertrophy. Several months of administration may be required before reduction of prostate size occurs, and termination of drug allows hypertrophy to recur. Suppression of 5-alpha reductase synthesis of dihydrotestosterone by finasteride may prevent development of prostate cancer. However, finasteride interferes with screening for prostate cancer by decreasing prostate-specific antigen (PSA). Impotence and decreased libido have been reported occasionally. Pregnant women should avoid all contact with this drug, including the semen of men who are taking it, because it can be teratogenic in the male fetus.

CHEMOTHERAPEUTIC DRUGS

Antineoplastic Agents

Antineoplastic drugs have effected cures in some forms of cancer, and can produce remissions and alleviation of symptoms in other forms. Hodgkin's and non-Hodgkin's lymphomas, myelogenous and acute lymphocytic leukemia, testicular, and breast cancers all respond exceptionally well to treatment, particularly when instituted early in the course of neoplasia.

Unfortunately, antineoplastic agents are cytotoxic also to normal cells and can provoke severe, even life-threatening adverse responses. Cells that are rapidly replicating are most affected by these drugs. Suppression of bone marrow synthesis of formed blood elements results in anemia, thrombocytopenia, and leukopenia; severe hemorrhage or infections can prove to be lethal. Another rapidly proliferating tissue that can be severely damaged is the gastrointestinal mucosa; ulceration may develop at any location along that tract, including the oral cavity. Germinal epithelium is suppressed, resulting in amenorrhea and decreased spermatogenesis. Interaction with fetal growth, which involves rapid cell division, can cause fetal damage or death. Perhaps the most innocuous effect in terms of physiological damage is suppression of follicular activity resulting in alopecia (hair loss); however, this response can have marked psychological impact in persons who are already coping with a severe disease. Many antineoplastic agents have additional characteristic organ toxicities that produce damage to the liver, kidneys, lungs, and myocardium. Hyperuricemia, resulting from tumor cell metabolism or destruction, may be alleviated with urinary alkalinization, proper hydration, and the xanthine oxidase inhibitor allopurinol. Anaphylaxis and other allergic symptoms can occur following administration of antineoplastic drugs. ***Gallium*** (Ganite) will reduce hypercalcemia associated with cancer. Adequate hydration must be maintained with this drug.

One of the most prominent adverse reactions characteristic of many antineoplastics is nausea and vomiting. Physiological sequelae include dehydration, malnutrition, and electrolyte imbalance; psychological responses include psychogenic nausea and reluctance or refusal to undergo subsequent courses of drug treatment. The exact mechanism of antineoplastic induction of vomiting is not understood. Stimulation of central mechanisms, formation of toxic products during cell destruction, and direct gastric irritation have all been proposed. A degree of relief is afforded to some persons by the concomitant administration of antiemetic agents such as ***phenothiazines***, ***metoclopramide*** (Reglan), ***ondansetron*** (Zofran), and ***corticosteroids***. ***Nabilone*** (Cesemet) and ***dronabinol*** (Marinol), derivatives of the active marijuana component tetrahydrocannabinol, seem to have some usefulness in young adult patients. The benzodiazepine lorazepam (Ativan) can decrease anticipatory nausea.

A variety of chemotherapeutic agents (Table 7-32) is used. Alkylating agents and antibiotics suppress cell growth by interacting with DNA replication. Antimetabolites, analogues of essential naturally occurring substances, enter into and disrupt cellular metabolic functions. Alkaloids interfere with mitotic spindle integrity. Hormones and the antiestrogen, tamoxifen, are effective in hormone-responsive neoplasms, and some will alleviate the symptoms of other cancers.

Alkylating Agents

Alkylating agents interfere with strand separation of DNA chains. Suppression of this requisite for cell division imparts antineoplastic activity, but also gives these drugs mutagenic and carcinogenic potential. Alkylation of other cell constituents is the probable basis for many of their less specific cytotoxic actions.

Nitrogen mustard (mechlorethamine, Mustargen) was among the earliest antineoplastics. Its current use is relatively limited to the treatment of Hodgkin's disease and other lymphatic cancers, often as a component of the MOPP combination (Table 7-33). Rapid inactivation of mechlorethamine gives it a characteristically brief (approximately 10 minutes) half-life. Adverse reactions include marked myelosuppression, nausea and vomiting, diarrhea, stomatitis, hyperuricemia, and alopecia. Herpes zoster infections may be activated. Concurrent radiation therapy can potentiate bone marrow suppression. Persistent infertility in men and women has followed mechlorethamine therapy. This drug is also reported to be teratogenic.

Because of its vesicant action, thrombophlebitis can be a complication of the IV administration of mechlorethamine. Dilution into a rapidly flowing infusion, and administration into a large vein can reduce the incidence of this effect. Extravasation into subcutaneous tissues can cause marked irritation and sloughing that may be prevented by immediate local infiltration with isotonic sodium thiosulfate. Health care personnel must take precautions to avoid inhalation or skin or eye exposure to mechlorethamine. Accidental contact necessitates immediate irrigation of accessible sites.

TABLE 7-32. Antineoplastic Drugs

GENERIC NAME	TRADE NAME
Alkylating Agents	
Busulfan	Myleran
Mechlorethamine	Mustargen
Chlorambucil	Leukeran
Melphalan	Alkeran
Cyclophosphamide	Cytoxan
Dacarbazine	DTIC
Ifosfamide	Ifex
Nitrosoureas	
Carmustine	BICNU
Lomustine	CeeNU
Semustine	
Antimetabolites	
Methotrexate	Mexate, Folex
Mercaptopurine	Purinethol
Thioguanine	Lanvis
5-Fluorouracil	5-FU, Adrucil
Cytarabine	Cytosar
Fludarabine	Fludara
Pentostatin	Nipent
2-Chlorodeoxyadenosine	Leustatin
Antibiotics	
Doxorubicin	Adriamycin
Daunorubicin	Cerubidine
Dactinomycin	Cosmegen
Bleomycin	Blenoxane
Plicamycin	Mithracin
Mitomycin	Mutamycin
Idarubicin	Idamycin
Mitoxantrone	Novatrone
Vinca Alkaloids	
Vinblastine	Velban
Vincristine	Oncovin
Vinorelbine	Navelbine
Additional Antineoplastics	
Tamoxifen	Nolvadex
Megestrol	Megace
Mitotane	Lysodren
Leuprolide	Lupron
Goserelin	Zoladex
Flutamide	Eulexin
Cisplatin	Platinol
Carboplatin	Paraplatin
Etoposide	VePesid
Teniposide	Vumon
Streptozocin	Zansar
Procarbazine	Matulane
Hydroxyurea	Hydrea
L-asparaginase	Elspar
Pegaspargase	Oncaspar
Paclitoxel	Taxol
Estramustine	Emcyt
α-interferon	Intron, Roferon
Altretamine	Hexalen

Mechlorethamine is given in short courses of IV therapy, allowing for sufficient recovery of bone marrow function before subsequent drug administration. Intracavity instillation may reduce pleural or peritoneal effusion; analgesics may be required to alleviate accompanying discomfort.

Chlorambucil (Leukeran), used in the management of lymphomas, is administered orally and produces less severe adverse reactions than mechlorethamine. Myelosuppression is its prominent toxic effect. Frequent monitoring of formed blood elements is required; radiation therapy generally is not utilized concomitantly. This drug has teratogenic and carcinogenic potential.

Melphalan (Alkeran) is similar to chlorambucil in its route of administration and toxicity. Sustained myelosuppression may occur. Pulmonary toxicity has been reported with both of these drugs.

Cyclophosphamide (Cytoxan) is a nitrogen mustard derivative that is biotransformed hepatically into antineoplastic metabolites. It is administered PO, IM, or IV, and is active against a wider range of cancers than other mustard compounds. Several chemotherapy combinations include cyclophosphamide (see Table 7-33). Renal function should be monitored to forestall toxic accumulations of this drug and its metabolites. Adverse effects include myelosuppression, nausea and vomiting, pulmonary fibrosis, and induction of bladder carcinoma and other secondary cancers. Adequate hydration can reduce the risk of hemorrhagic cystitis, apparently due to bladder irritation, that is characteristic of cyclophosphamide therapy. Early detection of hematuria and termination of drug can minimize urinary tract damage. Cyclophosphamide has additional clinical use as an immunosuppressant agent in severe refractory autoimmune disorders (see Immunosuppressants).

Ifosfamide (Ifex), which is similar to cyclophosphamide, is administered in metastatic germ-cell testicular cancer. ***Mesna*** (Mesnex) is coadministered to detoxify the metabolites of ifosfamide that cause hemorrhagic cystitis.

Dacarbazine has the characteristic actions of alkylating agents, and can cause hepatic necrosis. Extravasation will damage subcutaneous tissue. ***Busulfan*** is relatively selective; it has virtually no pharmacological action other than myelosuppression and is useful in the induction of remission in chronic granulocytic leukemia. ***Thio-tepa***

and ***uracil mustard*** are additional alkylating agents used in the treatment of neoplasms.

The ***nitrosourea*** compounds (***carmustine, lomustine,*** and ***semustine***) are lipid soluble and will cross the blood–brain barrier. They are used in the treatment of brain tumors as well as other types of neoplasms. Their toxicity is similar to that of other alkylating agents. Myelosuppression may be delayed and severe. Sustained courses of treatment can induce pulmonary fibrosis. ***Streptozocin***, a water-soluble nitrosourea, is administered IV or intra-arterially in carcinoid and pancreatic tumors. Release of insulin as malignant pancreatic cells are destroyed may result in marked hypoglycemia. Nausea, vomiting, and nephrotoxicity are frequent. Renal function must be monitored, and the use of other nephrotoxic drugs is to be avoided.

Antimetabolites

FOLIC ACID ANTAGONISTS

Methotrexate is the major folate antimetabolite currently in use. Amelioration and maintenance of remission in choriocarcinoma and childhood leukemia can be achieved with PO or IV administration. The intrathecal route is used in meningeal neoplasia. Methotrexate blocks the enzymatic conversion of folic acid to tetrahydrofolate, an intermediary in the synthesis of DNA, by covalently binding to dihydrofolate reductase. Tumor cells can develop resistance to methotrexate, resulting in termination of remission and unresponsiveness to folic acid analogues.

Methotrexate has numerous adverse effects, some of which can be lethal. Blood counts must be monitored; marked myelosuppression requires that drug administration be stopped. Nausea and vomiting, stomatitis, and gastrointestinal ulceration can occur. Characteristic is renal damage caused by precipitation of drug in the nephrons. Renal function must be monitored, since this is also the route of elimination of this highly toxic drug. Renal dysfunction contraindicates its use. Salicylates and probenecid reduce renal excretion and enhance toxicity, as do drugs that compete for plasma protein binding sites. Hepatic toxicity can occur; alcohol and other hepatotoxic drugs should be avoided. Methotrexate is tetratogenic and abortifacient. Folinic acid (leucovorin or citrovorum factor) can minimize some of the toxic effects of this drug.

The immunosuppressant action of methotrexate has been utilized in the management of severe, refractory psoriasis and rheumatoid arthritis. However, the extremely hazardous nature of this drug must be considered against the relatively nonlethal course of these diseases. Close and persistent monitoring of patients for early indications of toxicity is necessary.

PURINE ANALOGUES

Mercaptopurine, among the earliest effective antineoplastics, is most useful against leukemias. The action of this drug evolves from its ability to disrupt the synthesis of nucleic acid and other substances that contain the purines adenine and guanine. Myelosuppression, stomatitis, gastrointestinal ulceration, nausea, and vomiting are anticipated adverse effects. Leukocyte counts should be monitored. Potentially lethal hepatitis can develop; monitoring of liver function can detect early changes that require termination of drug use.

Allopurinol, which may be concomitantly administered to alleviate hyperuricemia, inhibits the xanthine oxidase enzyme necessary for inactivation of mercaptopurine. To avoid serious toxicity, the dosage of the latter drug should be reduced to one third and often as low as one quarter of the usual dose.

Thioguanine is a guanine analogue that acts in a manner similar to mercaptopurine. Its toxicity is generally less severe than that of mercaptopurine. However, myelosuppression and hyperuricemia can occur. Dosage reduction is not required in concomitant allopurinol administration since thioguanine is not inactivated by xanthine oxidase. This drug is administered orally, although its absorption is slow and incomplete. Cellular resistance to the actions of purine analogues can arise through an acquired reduction in the enzyme (hypoxanthine-guanine phosphoribosyltransferase) necessary for their activation. ***Fludarabine*** (Fludara), ***pentostatin*** (2-deoxycoformin, DCF, Nipent), and ***2-chlorodeoxyadenosine*** (CdA, Leustatin) all interact with adenosine deaminase and thus decrease purine metabolism and DNA synthesis. Fludarabine is approved for refractory chronic lymphocytic leukemia, and pentostatin (and possibly CdA) for the rare hairy-cell form of chronic lymphocytic leukemia. All three may be effective against non-Hodgkin's lymphoma.

Azathioprine is a purine analogue immunosuppressant. It is metabolized to mercaptopurine, thus its actions are potentiated by allopurinol.

PYRIMIDINE ANALOGUES

5-Fluorouracil is a pyrimidine analogue that must be enzymatically activated in order to disrupt DNA synthesis. Intravenous administration achieves the most favorable response from this drug, which undergoes rapid hepatic inactivation. The considerable potential for toxicity with 5-fluorouracil mandates close patient monitoring and termination of drug administration if stomatitis, severe diarrhea or vomiting, or hemorrhage or precipitous changes in formed-blood elements occur. Myelosuppression can be severe. Since this drug crosses the blood–brain barrier, it can produce central nervous system symptoms such as lethargy, weakness, and ataxia. It is catabolized as uracil and is more effective with allopurinol support. Topical preparations of 5-fluorouracil are used in the treatment of keratoses and superficial basal cell carcinoma.

Floxuridine, an analogue of 5-fluorouracil with similar toxicity, is infused intra-arterially in patients with inoperable hepatic metastases.

Cytarabine (cytosine arabinoside), an analogue of the pyrimidine cytidine, is activated by tumor cells and subsequently inhibits DNA synthesis. It is used particularly in the treatment of leukemias. Because it is rapidly metabolized by several body tissues, cytarabine is most effective when administered by continuous IV infusion. This drug crosses the blood–brain barrier, and can be administered directly into the cerebrospinal fluid. Myelosuppression, particularly of white cell production that may continue to fall 2 to 3 weeks after drug therapy is stopped, is a frequent consequence of cytarabine. Drug therapy may be interrupted to allow recovery of leukocyte and platelet counts. Nausea and vomiting can be severe; slow IV infusion rates reduce the incidence of this response. Stomatitis and hyperuricemia also occur.

Antibiotics

Numerous antibiotics are useful cancer chemotherapeutic agents. ***Doxorubicin*** is effective against many types of neoplasms and is a component in many combination chemotherapy regimens (see Table 7-33). It intercalates by hydrogen bonds into the DNA double helical structure, thus suppressing the synthesis of nucleic acids. Cardiotoxicity is characteristic of this drug; preexisting cardiovascular disease may increase the risk of potentially lethal myocardial changes. At total doses greater than 550 mg/m^2, doxorubicin can induce congestive heart failure that is refractory to cardiotonic drugs. Monitoring of ECG and observation for signs of myocardial deterioration may reveal early cardiomyopathy, although severe dysrhythmias can develop rapidly. ***Dexrazoxane*** (Zinecard) may decrease myocardial damage from doxorubicin by chelating intracellular iron and preventing the antineoplastic agent's production of oxygen free radicals. However, dexrazoxane may increase doxorubicin's myelosuppressant action and may decrease its antitumor efficacy. Myelosuppression also occurs with doxorubicin; preexisting bone marrow dysfunction contraindicates initiation of therapy with this drug. Biliary excretion is the major route of inactivation; hepatic insufficiency increases the risk of toxicity. The IV route of administration is utilized, and extravasation can destroy subcutaneous tissue. Infiltration with a corticosteroid may minimize damage. ***Mitoxantrone*** (Novatrone), used in adult acute nonlymphocytic leukemia, can severely depress bone marrow function.

Daunorubicin is structurally and pharmacologically similar to doxorubicin, but its use is limited mainly to treatment of leukemias. It too is myelosuppressant and cardiotoxic, and both drugs can cause red discoloration of the urine that may be mistaken for hematuria. ***Idarubicin*** (Idamycin) is used in the treatment of acute myelogenous leukemia in adults.

Actinomycin D (dactinomycin), useful for a variety of tumors, is a frequent component of drug combinations. On a molar basis, it is one of the most potent antitumor agents. Major adverse effects are nausea and vomiting, myelosuppression, stomatitis, and a synergistic effect with exposure to radiation. Like many antineoplastics, it disrupts DNA function. Its plasma half-life averages 36 hours; unchanged drug is excreted in bile and urine.

Bleomycin appears to damage DNA by liberating free oxygen radicals such as superoxide. The characteristic toxic effects of this drug are pneumonitis and pulmonary fibrosis. Renal impairment enhances the risk of toxicity. An idiosyncratic reaction of fever, hypotension, and wheezing has been reported; volume expansion or pressor amines may be required to support blood pressure.

Plicamycin is used to ameliorate elevated plasma and urine levels of calcium that accompany advanced cancers. It can be severely toxic; patients require close (preferably in-hospital) observation. Life-threatening hemorrhage can occur; platelet counts should be monitored. Preexisting coagulation deficits contraindicate use of this drug. Electrolyte imbalance (depletion of plasma calcium, potassium, and phosphate), nausea and vomiting, and changes in hepatic and renal function should be anticipated. Thrombophlebitis and tissue damage upon extravasation indicate the irritant nature of plicamycin.

Mitomycin is usually a second-line or combination drug for gastric or pancreatic carcinoma. Because myelosuppression frequently occurs, intermittent therapy must allow adequate recovery of thrombocyte and leukocyte counts. Renal and pulmonary toxicity and nausea and vomiting are other adverse effects. Extravasation may damage subcutaneous tissue.

Vinca Alkaloids

Vinblastine and vincristine, alkaloids from the periwinkle plant, interrupt the function of the mitotic spindle. These drugs are useful in the treatment of several types of tumors, including lymphatic cancers. However, they are not identical in either therapeutic or adverse actions. ***Vinblastine*** markedly suppresses bone marrow function; severe leukocyte depletion places patients at considerable risk of secondary infection.

Vincristine is a component of many chemotherapy combinations. The characteristic toxicity is neurological. Muscular weakness, loss of sensation and deep-tendon reflexes, ataxia, and suppression of gastrointestinal and urinary tract function are usually reversible upon termination of drug. Paralytic ileus may lead to upper colon fecal impaction. In contrast to vinblastine, there is little myelosuppression. Both drugs are potent vesicants; extravasation can damage subcutaneous tissue. Infiltration of hyaluronidase may be beneficial.

Vinorelbine (Navelbine) is a semisynthetic vinca alkaloid for IV administration in non-small-cell lung cancer. Hepatically metabolized, vinorelbine has a half-life of 1 to 2 days. Severe neutropenia, venous irritation, and dyspnea can occur. Vinorelbine may cause less peripheral neuropathy than vincristine. It can be combined with cisplatin.

Hormones

Corticosteroids (cortisone, prednisone, and prednisolone) have some antileukemic action, and will alleviate symptoms of these disorders. Dexamethasone, a synthetic glucocorticoid, may reduce the severity or the psychological impact of chemotherapy-induced vomiting.

Estrogen can effect some degree of regression in prostatic carcinoma, probably by suppression of androgen release and subsequent remission of hormone-dependent cellular growth. ***Estramustine*** is a combination of estradiol and nitrogen mustard. Estrogens may alleviate symptoms of breast cancer, but may also promote development of endometrial and mammary carcinoma. Conflicting reports have made this a controversial topic. Bone metastasis of breast cancer is an indication for the administration of androgens, particularly in postmenopausal patients. The characteristics of these hormones are discussed under Endocrine Pharmacology.

Tamoxifen is an antiestrogen useful in breast cancer, particularly in postmenopausal women. Estrogen-sensitive neoplasia, evidenced by the presence of estrogen receptors in tumor tissue, is most responsive to tamoxifen, although some studies have indicated that estrogen-receptor-negative tissue can also be suppressed by this drug. Metastatic cells are responsive; transient bone pain and increase in the size of soft-tissue lesions appear to be indicative of therapeutic drug action.

Tamoxifen is slowly absorbed from the gastrointestinal tract and metabolized in the liver to active metabolites. Excretion into bile and subsequent enterohepatic circulation probably contribute to its long (7 days) plasma half-life. Doses should be evenly spaced 12 hours apart to maintain consistent therapeutic plasma concentrations. Side effects are generally mild: nausea, hot flashes, edema, vaginal discharge or bleeding, and hypercalcemia in patients with significant bone metastases. Long-term administration of high doses has occasionally induced deterioration in vision.

Mitotane is an adrenocortical suppressant that may afford symptomatic relief in inoperable adrenal cortex carcinoma. Adrenal insufficiency can develop, necessitating steroid replacement. Nausea, vomiting, or diarrhea occurs in a large percentage of patients; depression, lethargy, and dizziness also occur frequently. Large doses and long-term administration may be required for clinical response. The appearance of adverse effects should guide the upper limits of dose as long as beneficial effects are apparent, although a 3-month (occasionally longer) interval of drug administration may be necessary to induce the latter.

Leuprolide, an analogue of LHRH, can suppress pituitary release of LH, diminishing hormone synthesis in the ovaries and testes. Amelioration of mammary and prostatic cancers can be obtained. Sexual hypofunction can occur. ***Goserelin*** (Zoladex); similar to leuprolide, is used in palliation of advanced prostate cancer. ***Flutamide*** (Eulexin) is an oral antiandrogen for administration with LHRH analogues.

Additional Antineoplastic Agents

Cisplatin is especially effective both alone and in drug combinations against ovarian, testicular, and bladder tumors, although it is also used in the treatment of various other cancers. Disruption of DNA function appears to be its mechanism of action. Severe vomiting that is often refractory to antiemetics occurs in almost all patients treated with cisplatin. Metoclopramide, ondansetron, granisetron, or dexamethasone may partially alleviate this response. Renal toxicity, also a prominent adverse effect, may be reduced by maintaining sufficient hydration. Intravenous fluids can be initiated 8 hours before and continued throughout drug administration. Mannitol administered concurrently with the drug will promote rapid elimination from the renal tubules. Dehydration subsequent to vomiting may enhance nephrotoxicity. Renal damage is cumulative, and function should return to normal levels before subsequent drug doses are given. Simultaneous use of other nephrotoxic agents is contraindicated. Cisplatin is ototoxic; loop diuretics and aminoglycoside antibiotics should not be given concurrently. Myelosuppression, neurotoxicity, and hyperuricemia are additional adverse reactions. Infusion equipment that contains aluminum will inactivate cisplatin. The related ***carboplatin*** (Paraplatin) may have less severe adverse effects, except for myelosuppression, which is greater.

Etoposide induces bone marrow dysfunction in a large percentage of patients, and causes other adverse effects common to antineoplastics. It is generally used in combination therapy of refractory testicular cancer. Hypotension can occur with rapid IV infusion.

Teniposide (VM26, Vumon) is approved for combination with methotrexate or cytarabine in induction treatment of refractory acute lymphoblastic leukemia (ALL) in children. Like etoposide, this drug inhibits topoisomerase II to prevent resealing of chromosome breaks and thus arrest the cell cycle before mitosis. The average half-life of teniposide is 5 hours, and renal or hepatic impairment or hypoalbuminemia (teniposide binds extensively to plasma proteins) can increase the toxicity of this drug. Severe hypersensitivity reactions (urticaria, angioedema, flushing, chills, fever, bronchospasm, hypotension) following teniposide administration may be due to the drug vehicle of castor oil plus alcohol. Other adverse effects are alopecia, nausea, vomiting, diarrhea, mucositis, myelosuppression (resulting in infection or hemorrhage), and secondary leukemias. Teratogenesis and embryotoxicity were observed in animal studies. Induction of hepatic enzymes may decrease the effectiveness of teniposide. The high alcohol content may increase the central nervous system depressant activity of other drugs. Immediately prior administration of teniposide and etoposide can decrease the action of cytarabine, and teniposide may increase peripheral neuropathy caused by vincristine. Teniposide may be useful in other cancers, and may enhance radiation-induced bone marrow ablation for organ transplant.

Procarbazine is a component of several drug combinations. Myelosuppression, nausea, and vomiting occur frequently. The drug readily enters cerebrospinal fluid and can cause central nervous system symptoms such as depression, anxiety, ataxia, tremors, and confusion. An MAO inhibitor, procarbazine may provoke hypertensive emergencies when drugs or foods containing sympathomimetics are ingested. Effects of other central nervous system depressants and of some antihypertensives can be potentiated. Consumption of alcohol may induce a disulfiramlike reaction.

Hydroxyurea can reduce leukocyte levels in chronic myelocytic leukemia. Preexisting bone marrow depression or renal insufficiency contraindicates use of this drug. Hyperuricemia is a frequent adverse effect.

L-asparaginase, an enzyme that deaminates asparagine, exploits the asparagine-dependent characteristic of certain tumor cells. Its use in acute lymphoblastic leukemia is associated with a significant number of hypersensitivity reactions as well as induction of diabetes mellitus. Depletion of clotting factors can lead to hemorrhage. Renal failure and central nervous system symptoms occur. ***Pegaspargase*** (Oncaspar), a polyethylene glycol conjugate of L-asparaginase, is recommended for persons with acute lymphoblastic leukemia who are allergic to asparaginase. Allergic reactions may still occur with pegaspargase, and this drug, like asparaginase, can cause pancreatitis, hemorrhage, and hepatic impairment.

Interferon Alfa, a biological response modifier, is currently indicated for hairy-cell leukemia and AIDS-related Kaposi's sarcoma. (It may also be effective in chronic viral hepatitis and genital warts.) This naturally occurring component of the immune system can be produced in *E. coli* by recombinant DNA technology. Its proposed mechanism of action is inhibition of DNA and protein synthesis. Fatigue and a flulike syndrome of chills and fever, malaise, and headache are the most common adverse reactions. Antipyretics and analgesics can alleviate patient discomfort. Myelosuppression and cardiovascular and central nervous system disturbances can occur. Extreme caution is recommended in persons with preexisting cardiac, hepatic, or renal disease or with seizure or other central nervous system disorders. Interferon must be administered parenterally (SC, IM).

Paclitaxel (Taxol) is extracted from the bark of the western yew tree. Fungus-derived paclitaxel and a semisynthetic analog (***taxotere***) may supplement the somewhat limited availability of this drug. Paclitaxel inhibits cell replication by inducing formation of stable microtubule bundles, which interfere with late G-2 mitosis of the cell cycle. Intravenous administration of paclitaxel is effective in some patients with refractory ovarian cancer, and may be of use in the management of metastatic breast cancer, malignant melanoma, advanced non-small-cell lung cancer, and head and neck tumors. Paclitaxel is infused over 24 hours every 3 weeks for three to six cycles. The inactivation route of this drug is not fully identified. The drug has a half-life of 1 to 9 hours, appears to be highly protein bound, and does not enter the central nervous system. Granulocytopenia is a major adverse effect, but can be eased by concomitant administration of granulocyte colony-stimulating factor (G-CSF). Severe hypersensitivity reactions (probably due to the castor oil vehicle) such as urticaria, angioedema, hypotension, and dyspneas can be inhibited by pretreatment with dexamethasone and diphenydramine plus cimetidine or ranitidine. Slowing the infusion rate may also decrease hypersensitivity reactions. Other adverse effects are alopecia, nausea, vomiting, diarrhea, mucositis, arthralgia, myalgia, peripheral neuropathy, bradycardia (which generally requires no intervention), occasional heart block, and fatal myocardial infarction. The antifungal agent ketoconazole (Nizoral) may increase paclitaxel toxicity. Polyvinyl chloride (PVC) bottles and tubing must not be used for paclitaxel administration.

Altretamine (Hexalen) is converted to metabolites that are cytotoxic to ovarian cancer cells. Adverse effects resemble those of many antineoplastics: myelosuppression, vomiting, peripheral neuropathy, and CNS symptoms including confusion, dizziness, depression, and seizures. Severe othostasis may occur if MAO inhibitors are given concurrently.

Octreotide (Sandostatin) decreases release of serotonin, vasoactive intestinal peptide, and other vasoactive substances secreted by carcinoid and other tumors, thus alleviating the hypotension that often accompanies these neoplasms.

TABLE 7-33. Frequently Employed Chemotherapy Combinations

NAME	DRUGS	NEOPLASM
ABDV	Doxorubicin, bleomycin, vinblastine, dacarbazine	Hodgkin's disease
BACOP	Bleomycin, doxorubicin, cyclophosphamide, vincristine, prednisone	Diffuse histiocytic lymphoma
BEP	Bleomycin, etoposide, cisplatin	Testicular
BCVPP	Carmustine, cyclophosphamide, vinblastine, procarbazine, prednisone	Hodgkin's disease
CAF	Cyclophosphamide, doxorubicin, 5-Fluorouracil	Breast
CAMP	Cyclophosphamide, doxorubicin, methotrexate, procarbazine	Lung
CAP	Melphalan, cisplatin, doxorubicin	Ovarian
CAV	Cyclophosphamide, doxorubicin, vincristine	Ewing's sarcoma
CHAP	Cyclophosphamide, hexamethylmelamine, doxorubicin, cisplatin	Ovarian
CMFP	Cyclophosphamide, methotrexate, 5-Fluorouracil, prednisone	Breast
COMLA	Cyclophosphamide, vincristine, methotrexate-leucovorin, cytarabine	Diffuse histiocytic lymphoma
CVPP	Chlorambucil, vinblastine, procarbazine, prednisone	Hodgkin's disease
FAM	5-Fluorouracil, doxorubicin, mitomycin	Gastric
M-2 Protocol	Vincristine, carmustine, cyclophosphamide, melphalan, prednisone	Multiple myeloma
M-Bacop	Bleomycin, doxorubicin, cyclophosphamide, vincristine, prednisone, methotrexate-leucovorin	Diffuse histiocytic lymphoma
MOPP	Mechlorethamine, vincristine, procarbazine, prednisone	Hodgkin's disease
POCC	Procarbazine, vincristine, cyclophosphamide, lomustine	Lung
PVB	Cisplatin, vinblastine, bleomycin	Testicular
VP	Vincristine, prednisone	Acute lymphocytic leukemia

Combination Therapies

The use of several antineoplastic drugs simultaneously has been remarkably effective in suppressing some types of cancers. Mechlorethamine, vincristine, procarbazine, and prednisolone (MOPP) and other combined chemotherapies have effected cures of Hodgkin's disease; other frequently used combinations are listed in Table 7-33.

Combinations of drugs must be carefully chosen, using agents that have varied antineoplastic mechanisms and do not duplicate each other's toxicities. Drugs may be administered intermittently for several cycles to achieve complete eradication of malignant cells.

Antineoplastic drugs are also used in conjunction with surgery or radiation therapy. This adjuvant chemotherapy can delay or prevent the recurrence of neoplasia. Since treatment may continue for months or years, drugs with minimal adverse effects are the most appropriate.

RADIOISOTOPIC AGENTS

Radioisotopes are useful in clinical medicine as diagnostic agents because their selective localization to specific body tissues can be easily measured. They are also useful as antineoplastic agents because of their cytotoxicity. Elements commonly used include ^{125}I and ^{131}I, ^{32}P, ^{51}Cr, and ^{14}C-labelled carbohydrates. Generally, small doses are used for diagnostic purposes, while larger amounts of isotope are required to destroy tissue. Doses are often expressed as curies or fractions of this unit, such as the millicurie or microcurie. Energy is emitted in the form of α, β, or γ radiation. A fixed percentage of atoms disintegrate per unit of time; therefore these substances have a predictable radioactive half-life.

Radiolabelled iodine is particularly useful in the diagnosis of thyroid dysfunction or in the management of hyperactivity or carcinoma of this gland. Iodine concentrates within the thyroid; persons with overactivity of the gland will exhibit increased accumulation of isotope in the region of the thyroid, increased serum protein-bound isotope, and slower than normal urinary excretion of radioactive material. The objective of the treatment of hyperthyroidism or carcinoma is destruction of thyroid cells. This can be facilitated by coadministration of thyroid-stimulating hormone, which enhances iodine uptake by the gland. Extensive destruction of thyroid tissue should be anticipated, and clinical manifestations of hypothyroidism may require replacement hormone therapy. Sore throat and transient swelling of the neck may develop. Antithyroid medications and recent administration of iodine in any form can suppress uptake of isotopic iodine. Allergy to iodine or seafood (which contains this element) mandates close observation of patients for anaphylactic or asthmatic reactions. Administration of high doses of this or other isotopes should be accompanied with radiation safety precautions to protect patients, visitors, and health-care personnel from inadvertent injury. Because of their carcinogenic and mutagenic potential, labelled iodine as well as other radioisotopes are usually contraindicated in pregnancy and during lactation.

Albumin with radiolabelled iodine is used to measure plasma volume, and iodohippurate tagged with this isotope can assess renal function.

^{32}P can suppress certain types of leukemia, and may alleviate polycythemia vera. Phosphorus concentrates in rapidly proliferating tissue such as bone marrow. Excessive myelosuppression can result in pancytopenia, and isotope-induced leukemias have been reported. Blood counts must be determined repeatedly before and after isotope therapy.

Radioactive gold (^{198}Au) can be instilled into body cavities (*e.g.*, pleural and peritoneal) to alleviate effusion and ascites that accompany malignancy. Open tumors or wounds contraindicate the use of this isotope. Labelled chromic phosphate can be used in a similar manner.

Strontium-89 (^{89}Sr, Metastron) relieves pain of metastatic bone lesions, which are sequelae to prostate and breast cancer in particular. ^{89}Sr, which decays by beta emission, is extensively taken up by bone, particularly around metastatic regions. The isotope's half-life of 14 days in noncancerous bone is greatly extended in the presence of mestastasis. A single dose given by slow IV injection provides pain relief usually within 7 to 20 days; doses can be repeated at 90-day intervals. A transient increase (36 to 72 hours after administration) in bone pain may be predictive of a subsequent favorable response. ^{89}Sr is myelosuppressant, especially with repeated administration. Rapid IV injection can cause flushing. Teratogenicity and carcinogenicity have been reported in animal studies of ^{89}Sr, which probably enters breast milk.

Indium 111 (^{111}In, a gamma emitter) bound to ***satumomab pendetide*** (a chelating agent conjugated with a monoclonal murine antibody to the tumor-associated glycoprotein TAG 72) (CYT 103) can be of assistance in detecting metastases of colorectal and ovarian adenocarcinomas. Immunoscintigraphy detects localization of the isotope, which also binds to many noncancerous and nonspecific sites. Extensive uptake by the liver prevents this agent's ability to detect hepatic metastasis, which occurs in particular with colorectal cancer. (Computed tomagraphy is much more accurate in diagnosing liver involvement.) In addition, CYT 103 does not distinguish between benign and malignant primary ovarian tumors. Both false-positive and false-negative readings can occur. Administration of this agent can cause fever, chills, changes in blood pressure, nausea, diarrhea, and rash. The development of antimurine antibodies, which can persist longer than 12 months, can interfere with subsequent accuracy of other imaging techniques or *in vitro* diagnostic agents, including detection of carcinoembryonic antigen (CEA) in colorectal cancer and CA125 in ovarian cancer.

Additional uses of isotopes include measurement of cerebral and skeletal-muscle blood flow, bodywater distribution, renal and hepatic function, utilization and storage of iron, and detection of pancreatic carcinoma, bone metastases, and ischemic heart disease.

Radiographic Diagnostic Contrast Media Agents

Radiopaque contrast media are used to visualize blood vessels and the biliary and urinary tracts. Because of their potential for inducing adverse reactions, these agents are administered only by personnel skilled in their use and in facilities equipped to manage life-threatening responses. Iodine atoms attached to a benzene ring confer radiopacity. Some of these agents, such as the ***diatrizoate salts***, are negatively charged in solution. The addition of sodium or methylglucamine as a balancing cation results in a highly hypertonic preparation (2,000 mOsm/kg compared to 300 mOsm/kg for blood). Intravenous administration of these agents induces pain, vomiting, and cardiovascular changes that may be related to their hypertonicity. Other agents such as ***iohexol***, ***iopamidol***, and ***ioxaglate*** have decreased ionic content (below 900 mOsm) and may be safer for persons with cardiovascular or pulmonary disorders.

Hypersensitivity reactions are unrelated to osmolarity and can be lethal. The risk of cardiovascular collapse necessitates close observation of patients during and for at least 1 hour following diagnostic testing. Means for resuscitation must be immediately available. A small test dose of drug may be helpful, although a lack of adverse response does not always ensure safe administration of the full diagnostic dose. Severe myocardial depression and hypotension may occur by mechanisms other than anaphylaxis. Persons with a history of allergy (particularly to iodine) or of previous adverse response to contrast media appear to be at increased risk of shock and cardiac arrest. Pretreatment with antihistamines or corticosteroids may reduce the incidence of life-threatening reactions. Radiopaque media have induced renal toxicity in patients with multiple myeloma, especially if dehydration was coexistent. These agents can exacerbate symptoms of sickle cell anemia and may induce hypertension in the presence of pheochromocytoma. Renal impairment can hinder the excretion of radiopaque materials.

ANTIMICROBIALS

Antibacterials

Drugs that suppress bacterial growth are among the most widely prescribed in the United States. (The hazards of inappropriate use are discussed below.) Many of these agents are naturally occurring substances, synthesized by bacteria and fungi. Molecular modification of these antibiotics has yielded numerous semisynthetic substances, often with broader efficacy than the naturally occurring analogues. For example, acid-stable and penicillinase-resistant penicillins have increased the spectrum of activity of the parent drug, penicillin G (see discussion under Penicillins). Some antibacterial agents such as the sulfonamides are totally synthetic anti-infectives.

The mechanism of action of the antibacterial drugs, indeed of all the antimicrobials, involves interference with some aspect of the physiological function of the microorganism, for example, suppression of cell wall or protein synthesis, or alteration of cellular metabolism. Bacterial cell function frequently differs sufficiently from mammalian cell function, so that some antibacterial agents are not markedly cytotoxic in humans. There is a range of antibacterial activity from bacteriostatic, which slows but does not irreversibly prevent bacterial growth, to bactericidal in which microbes are destroyed. Some agents are bacteriostatic at lower doses and bactericidal in larger amounts. Anti-infective drugs are most useful in persons with competent immune systems that assist in the removal of infectious agents.

Antibacterials vary widely in their spectrum of susceptible organisms. Some are active against a wide variety of pathogens (''broad spectrum'') while others are effective against a limited number of microorganisms (''narrow spectrum''). Viruses are generally impervious to these agents, which are appropriately administered to persons with viral infections *only* when secondary bacterial invasions are present. The sensitivity of specific pathogens to drugs should be determined so that the most appropriate antibacterials can be selected. Some conditions (*e.g.*, meningitis and bacteremia) require immediate institution of antibacterial treatment. The initial choice of agents is based on the probable infecting pathogen, and the drug regimen may be altered once the susceptibility of the specific organisms is identified. Body fluids for sensitivity testing should be obtained before drug therapy is begun.

Several *in vitro* susceptibility tests are available to aid in the identification of specific pathogens. Disk diffusion tests utilize paper filters impregnated with anti-infective drugs placed on the surface of agar inoculated with bacteria isolated from patients' body fluids or tissues. Following a period of incubation, the presence or absence of bacterial growth around each disk will indicate the effectiveness of the various drugs. Methods that test dilutions of anti-infectives against microbial cultures can provide information regarding minimal inhibitory concentrations (MIC) and minimal bactericidal concentrations (MBC), which are particularly important in the management of meningitis and endocarditis. The *in vivo* efficacy of a drug can be predicted by considering achievable serum or cerebrospinal fluid concentrations.

The inappropriate use of antibacterials has caused a number of serious consequences. Among these is the problem of acquired drug resistance: organisms once susceptible to a particular drug develop the ability to survive in the presence of that drug. Spontaneous mutations can occur among bacteria, and excessive administration of anti-infectives can suppress the growth of susceptible bacteria, therefore providing unopposed opportunity for survival of resistant cells. On the other hand, premature termination of antibacterial administration also fosters development of drug resistance, and it is important for patients to complete a full regimen of treatment even though the symptoms of infection have waned. Many nosocomial (hospital-acquired) infections are attributable to drug-resistant organisms.

Superinfections are secondary infections that arise from administration of antibacterials. The gastrointestinal, respiratory, and genitourinary tracts are normally inhabited by a variety of microorganisms that grow together and exert their own inhibitory influence to prevent overabundance of any one organism. Administration of drugs will suppress the growth of susceptible bacteria, and allow nonsusceptible organisms (with either acquired or natural resistance) to increase in numbers and induce infections. The risk of this response is increased when broad-spectrum agents are used, and when administration continues beyond 7 to 10 days. Elderly and seriously ill persons, in whom immune responsiveness may be less than optimal, are most susceptible to the development of superinfections. The best defense against this type of secondary infection is to administer antibacterials only when and as long as absolutely necessary, and to use agents known to be effective against the invading organism.

Prophylactic administration of antibacterials is appropriate in a limited number of clinical situations. Persons with a history of certain cardiovascular diseases, such as valvular heart disease, may be protected against bacterial endocarditis by brief regimens of penicillin or other antibiotics at times of dental or surgical procedures. Routine perioperative administration of antibacterials appears to reduce the occurrence of infection following some types of surgery, such as open heart surgery. Persons with AIDS may require continuous antibacterial therapy to prevent recurrence of opportunistic infections.

A frequent manifestation of superinfection is colitis. Pseudomembranous colitis induced by *Clostridium difficile* causes severe diarrhea and dehydration that can be lethal. Vancomycin or metronidazole may help to suppress this secondary infection. Many antimicrobials cause diarrhea, which if severe may require that drug therapy be terminated.

Allergic reactions are another frequent adverse response to anti-infective drugs. Symptoms can range from skin rashes to asthma and anaphylactic shock. Penicillin-responsive infections that occur in persons with penicillin hypersensitivity have been treated with the antibiotic after desensitization. Very low initial "desensitizing" doses are gradually increased until a favorable antibacterial response is obtained. However, persons thus treated must be closely observed for signs of anaphylaxis and supportive measures must be immediately available. Pretreatment with antihistamines may circumvent possible severe reactions.

Decreases in renal function, including those normally observed in older persons, require a reduction in dosage of antibacterial drugs inactivated by renal excretion. Plasma concentrations of anti-infectives should be monitored to ensure that toxic levels are avoided and therapeutic levels are achieved. Renal capacity should be determined before administration of drug to persons in whom inadequate function is suspected, and periodically during prolonged therapy. Many antibiotics are themselves nephrotoxic; changes in renal function detected during treatment with these agents usually require that drug administration be terminated.

Many antibiotics are well absorbed from the oral route, while others are not and must, therefore, be administered parenterally for the treatment of systemic infections. Oral administration of the latter, however, can be used to eradicate bacteria from the intestinal tract. Most antibiotics do not readily cross the blood–brain barrier; thus large doses must be given to treat central nervous system infections. Inflammation of the meninges can increase the permeability of cerebral capillary walls to drugs.

Carefully selected combinations of antibacterial agents are appropriately utilized for a limited number of clinical indications. Penicillins plus aminoglycosides can facilitate each others' effects against some bacteria. In contrast, some drug combinations result in reduced efficacy. In general, bactericidal and bacteriostatic agents are not administered concurrently. Bactericidal drugs are most effective against microorganisms that are rapidly dividing; this advantage is lost when bacterial replication is slowed by a bacteriostatic drug.

Antibacterial activity may be enhanced by concomitant use of other types of drugs. Probenecid competes for renal tubular secretion, prolonging the plasma half-life of penicillins and cephalosporins. Beta-lactamase inhibitors such as clavulanic acid will broaden the antimicrobial spectrum of activity of agents that are destroyed by these enzymes. The characteristics of microorganisms and their responses to antiinfective agents are further described in Chapter 5, "General Microbiology and Immunology."

PENICILLINS

Penicillin G, a naturally occurring product of the *Penicillium* mold, was the first significantly effective agent developed in this group of drugs. It is, however, quite acid-labile and its characteristic β-lactam structure is rapidly destroyed by β-lactamase ("penicillinase") produced by some types of bacteria (*e.g.*, staphylococci and gonococci). Numerous semisynthetic penicillins (Table 7-34) have been developed; some derivatives are less susceptible to gastric acid degradation (*e.g.*, ***ampicillin*** and ***amoxicillin***) while others are penicillinase-resistant (*e.g.*, ***methicillin, oxacillin,*** and ***nafcillin***). A particularly broad spectrum of antibacterial activity is obtained in ***mezlocillin*** and ***azlocillin.***

TABLE 7-34. Penicillins

GENERIC NAME	TRADE NAME
Naturally Occurring	
Penicillin G	Pentids, Pfizerpen
Penicillin V	Pen-Vee, V-Cillin
Semisynthetic	
Penicillinase-resistant	
Methicillin	Staphcillin
Nafcillin*	Unipen, Nafcil
Oxacillin*	Prostaphlin
Cloxacillin*	Tegopen
Dicloxacillin*	Dynapen
Amdinocillin	Coactin
Extended spectrum	
Ampicillin*	Omnipen, Polycillin
Amoxicillin*	Amoxil, Wymox
Carbenicillin	Geopen
Ticarcillin	Ticar
Mezlocillin	Mezlin
Azlocillin	Azlin
Piperacillin	Pipracil
Pro-ampicillins	
Bacampicillin	Spectrobid
Hetacillin	Versapen

* Acid-stable penicillins.

Penicillins block the action of a transpeptidase that is required for cross-linkage of structural units of the bacterial cell wall. Deprived of their protection against a lower extracellular osmotic pressure, susceptible bacteria are destroyed by the influx of fluid from their environment. Penicillins are bactericidal, and are most effective during phases of rapid pathogen division when cell wall construction is essential to ensure survival.

The penicillins have a considerable range of antibacterial efficacy, and are the drugs of choice for many infections. Penicillin G is especially effective by parenteral routes; oral activity can be enhanced by administering large doses spaced between meals, when gastric acid secretion is relatively low. Penicillin V is a natural derivative with greater acid stability. Penicillin G and V are most effective against facultative gram-positive cocci and rods. Those penicillins resistant to the β-lactamase enzyme will destroy penicillinase-producing staphylococci. Broad-spectrum derivatives have a range of activity that includes several gram-negative rods. Among the infections commonly treated with penicillin are gonorrhea, bacterial endocarditis, syphilis, *Haemophilis influenzae,* and streptococcal invasions, and some urinary tract infections. The acquired ability to synthesize β-lactamase has conferred resistance on many strains of staphylococci that now cause nosocomial infections that are difficult to eradicate. The spectrum of activity can be extended by combining penicillins with β-lactamase inhibitors. ***Clavulanic acid*** is combined with amoxicillin (Augmentin) and ticarcillin (Timentin), ***sulbactam*** with ampicillin (Unasyn), and ***tazobactam*** with piperacillin (Zosyn). The β-lactamase inhibitors do not appear to alter penicillin pharmacokinetics nor to have notable adverse effects. Tetanus, typhoid, and diphtheria, which can be avoided through proper immunization procedures, can be treated with penicillins. Amoxicillin is the preferred drug for Lyme disease in pregnant or lactating women, or children under age 8. ***Amdinocillin,*** which is slightly different from the basic β-lactam structure, is especially effective against gram-negative bacteria.

Penicillin G is rapidly absorbed following IM administration and rapidly extracted from the plasma as unchanged drug by the renal tubules. Probenecid blocks this tubular secretion and can sustain significant plasma levels of drug. Repository forms of penicillin (*e.g.,* procaine and benzathine penicillin G, or ***Bicillin***) provide IM depots that can provide detectable plasma levels of drug for up to 4 weeks. Large doses of penicillins contain significant amounts of sodium, which may result in electrolyte imbalances. Intermittent rather than sustained therapeutic concentrations of penicillins are considered to be effective since microorganisms are sensitive only when replicating. In addition, drug levels are more uniformly maintained in body tissues and lymph, where bacteria are most abundant.

Penicillin allergy, occurring in up to 5% of patients, is one of the most frequent adverse effects of this group of antibiotics. Reactions range from mild transitory rhinitis and urticaria to angioneurotic edema, periarteritis nodosa, fever, and anaphylactic shock. The more severe reactions occur particularly following parenteral administration. Ampicillin has a marked propensity to cause skin rashes. Predetermination of sensitivity may be obtained through intradermal testing with a penicillin-polylysine conjugate. The previously used intradermal testing with penicillin G is no longer recommended, since sensitive persons can respond with a severe anaphylactoid reaction. Persons allergic to one form of penicillin are usually hypersensitive to all others, and may also be allergic to the cephalosporin antibiotics, which have a similar molecular structure. More slowly developing reactions (''accelerated reactions'') may occur 1 to 72 hours following use of penicillin: urticaria is the most common of these. Delayed reactions may develop up to several weeks after administration; skin rashes, hemolytic anemia, and serum sickness characterize these late responses.

Oral administration of penicillins can cause nausea and diarrhea. Superinfections may develop, particularly with prolonged therapy using extended-spectrum drugs. Large doses of penicillins, especially when given IV to persons with meningeal infection or seizure susceptibility, may reach sufficient central nervous system concentrations to induce convulsions. Parenteral injection sites should avoid arteries or nerves. Thrombophlebitis may accompany IV administration, and pain often occurs at the IM site. Nephrotoxicity that can lead to acute renal failure is most characteristic of methicillin. Renal impairment necessitates reduction in dosage of all penicillins except nafcillin, which can be shunted to a hepatic route of inactivation. Penicillinase-resistant penicillins in particular have been linked to myelosuppression, and some penicillins interfere with platelet function.

Additional possible drug interactions include a reported reduced efficacy of oral contraceptives when penicillin V or ampicillin is concurrently administered, and an increased risk of dermatological reactions when ampicillin and allopurinol are present concomitantly. Penicillins should not be combined in solution with aminoglycosides because the latter drugs may be rendered inactive. Sulbactam and clavulanic acid are penicillinase inhibitors that are combined with penicillins to enhance their activity.

CEPHALOSPORINS

The cephalosporins, derived from the *Cephalosporium* mold, (Table 7-35) are similar to the penicillins in both structure (they possess a β-lactam nucleus) and mechanism of antibacterial action. A rapidly expanding and widely utilized group of drugs, the cephalosporins are classified into ''generations'' based upon their spectrum of activity. ''First-generation'' agents are particularly effective against gram-positive organisms that are also susceptible to penicillin. The ''second-generation'' agents are active against many anaerobic organisms, while the ''third generation'' includes gram-negative strains in its extended spectrum.

Many of the cephalosporins are β-lactamase resistant, and are useful in the eradication of penicillinase-producing bacteria including staphylococci, *Neisseria,* and *Haemophilus influenzae.* Most of the cephalosporins have a relatively short plasma half-life, although ***cefonocid*** is reported effective with once-daily dosing. The first-generation agents ***cephalexin, cephradine,*** and ***cefadroxil,*** plus second-generation ***cefaclor, cefuronime,*** and ***cef-***

TABLE 7-35. Cephalosporins

GENERIC NAME	TRADE NAME
First Generation	
Cephaloridine	Loridine
Cephalothin	Keflin
Cefazolin	Ancef, Kefzol
Cephapirin	Cefadyl
Cephalexin*	Keflex
Cephradine*	Velocef, Anspor
Cefadroxil*	Duricef, Ultracef
Second Generation	
Cefamandole	Mandol
Cefonicid	Monocid
Cefoxitin	Mefoxin
Cefuroxime*	Zinacef, Ceftin
Ceforanide	Precef
Cefaclor*	Ceclor
Cefmetazole	Zefazone
Cefprozil*	Cefzil
Third Generation	
Cefotaxime	Claforan
Cefotetan	Cefotan
Ceftizoxime	Catizox
Ceftriaxone	Rocephin
Ceftazidime	Fortaz, Tazidime
Cefoperazone	Cefobid
Cefiximo*	Suprax
Cefpodoxine*	Vantin
Moxalactam	Moxam

* Available in oral formulations.

prozil, and third-generation ***cefpodoxime,*** and ***cefixime*** are resistant to acid degradation, thus are orally active; other cephalosporins are administered parenterally. Since they are quite water soluble, these drugs are for the most part renally excreted (both by filtration and secretion) and do not cross the blood–brain barrier in appreciable amounts. However, some second- and third-generation agents are effective in bacterial meningitis; their entry into the central nervous system is enhanced by meningeal inflammation. Some cephalosporins bind extensively to plasma proteins. ***Cefoperazone*** is hepatically deacylated and secreted into bile.

The cephalosporins are highly effective against many bacterial invasions. Upper and lower respiratory tract as well as urinary tract pathogens are responsive. ***Cephtriaxone*** IV has been useful in treating Lyme disease. Second- and third-generation agents will destroy *H. influenzae, Pseudomonas aeruginosa, Serratia, Proteus,* and *Enterobacter*. Intraabdominal and gastrointestinal infections are often ameliorated by cephalosporins. Their use, however, is occasionally limited by cross-allergenicity with penicillins; extreme caution is necessary if cephalosporins are administered to persons reporting penicillin hypersensitivity.

Side effects can vary among the members of this large family of drugs. Some cause diarrhea, others induce a disulfiramlike reaction following ingestion of alcohol. Renal tubular damage (enhanced by concomitant administration of other nephrotoxic drugs) and superinfections (particularly with extended spectrum agents) can occur. Pain following IM injection and thrombophlebitis after use of the IV route are not uncommon. Several cephalosporins, most notably ***cefamandole, cefoperazone,*** and ***moxalactam,*** disrupt vitamin K metabolism and lead to deficiencies in clotting factors. Severe bleeding that may require transfusion of blood products can develop, especially in persons with renal impairment or poor nutritional status. Vitamin K supplementation can minimize the risk of coagulopathy. Because of the risk for fatal hemorrhage, use of monolactam is not recommended.

Aztreonam (Azactam) is a monobactam antibiotic especially effective against specific gram-negative bacteria and *P. aeruginosa*. It is not susceptible to β-lactamase degradation and is active by oral and parenteral routes.

Loracarbef (Lorabid) is a carbacephem having a β-lactam structure similar to penicillins and cephalosporins. It is well absorbed from the gastrointestinal tract, and has antibacterial activity comparable to cefaclor and cefuroxime. Diarrhea is the most frequent adverse effect, although allergy, including cross-sensitivity with other β-lactams, must be considered.

AMINOGLYCOSIDES

The aminoglycosides (Table 7-36), derived from *Streptomyces* strains of bacteria, are especially effective against gram-negative infections. These bactericidal antibiotics bind intracellularly to microsomal subunits, disrupting protein synthesis. The aminoglycosides are not well absorbed from the gastrointestinal tract; oral administration is used to eradicate microorganisms from the intestinal lumen. Treatment of infections elsewhere in the body requires parenteral administration. Because of their marked

TABLE 7-36. Aminoglycosides

GENERIC NAME	TRADE NAME
Parenteral	
Streptomycin	Generic
Kanamycin	Kantrex
Gentamicin	Gentamycin
Tobramycin	Nebcin
Amikacin	Amikin
Netilmicin	Netromycin
Oral	
Neomycin	Mycifradin
Paromomycin	Humatin
Spectinomycin	Trobicin

water solubility, these agents are generally restricted to extracellular fluid compartments. Penetration into ocular and cerebrospinal fluids is poor, and the presence of ascites can draw large amounts of these drugs out of the circulatory system. Inactivation is by glomerular filtration, with large amounts of drug concentrating in renal tissue. Because of the narrow therapeutic index of these antibiotics, impairment of kidney function requires that dosages be reduced.

The major adverse effects of the aminoglycosides are ototoxicity (deafness and vestibular disturbance) and nephrotoxicity. The risk of toxicity is greatest in persons with renal impairment, in the elderly, and in the presence of dehydration. Tinnitus and ataxia are symptoms of auditory damage that may become irreversible. Audiometric testing before and throughout drug therapy can assist in the early detection of ototoxicity; high-frequency hearing is usually lost earliest. Preexisting hearing deficits preclude the use of these drugs, and concomitant administration of other ototoxic agents (*e.g.*, furosemide) should be avoided. Diuretics can also induce dehydration, which will enhance toxicity. Streptomycin and gentamicin have a greater propensity to affect vestibular function, while the other aminoglycosides most frequently cause hearing loss. Tobramycin affects both of these functions of the cranial nerve VIII.

Adequacy of renal function should be determined before initiation of aminoglycoside therapy. Impairment suggests that alternative drugs be considered. Periodic testing throughout therapy can detect deterioration of function that may require termination of the aminoglycoside. Maintenance of adequate hydration and avoidance of concomitant nephrotoxic agents (*e.g.*, furosemide and cisplatin) decreases the incidence of renal damage.

An additional adverse effect of these antibiotics is suppression of neuromuscular transmission that can be manifested in respiratory depression and muscular weakness. These become most evident in persons with preexisting disorders of transmission, such as myasthenia gravis. Calcium depletion, or concurrent administration of other neuromuscular junction blocking agents, can potentiate this action. Aminoglycosides are therefore hazardous in persons undergoing surgery who may require administration of such drugs as curare and succinylcholine.

The aminoglycosides are reported to cause occasional changes in hepatic and bone marrow activity. Allergic reactions, skin rashes in particular, occur. Many bacterial strains rapidly acquire resistance to these drugs.

The use of ***streptomycin,*** the earliest of the aminoglycosides, has been largely replaced by the newer drugs in this class. Tularemia, brucellosis, and plague are special indications for the use of streptomycin. Gram-negative bacillary infections of the urinary tract can be treated with streptomycin as long as renal function is adequate and the microorganisms have not developed resistance. The use of streptomycin in the management of tuberculosis has declined; isoniazid and other antitubercular agents are discussed under that topic.

Gentamicin has a wide range of activity, including *Enterobacter, Serratia,* and *Staphylococcus aureus.* It can be effective against strains that have acquired resistance to other aminoglycosides. The combination of carbenicillin or ticarcillin plus gentamicin is especially useful in the eradication of *Pseudomonas.* Disruption of cell wall synthesis effected by the penicillin facilitates the action of the aminoglycoside at the intracellular ribosomes. As noted earlier, these drugs should not be combined in the same solution.

A penicillin plus gentamicin or streptomycin can be administered to persons with cardiac valvular abnormalities undergoing surgery or invasive diagnostic procedures. Such patients are particularly at risk of developing bacterial endocarditis. Gentamicin is frequently used in the initial therapy of bacteremia. Intrathecal and subconjunctival routes for gentamicin can make this drug useful in meningeal and ocular infections.

Amikacin, netilmicin, and ***tobramycin*** are used in much the same manner as gentamicin. Netilmicin and tobramycin are reported less ototoxic and nephrotoxic. Tobramycin is more active against *Pseudomonas.* Neomycin is no longer administered systemically.

TETRACYCLINES

The tetracyclines (Table 7-37) are broad-spectrum bacteriostatic antibiotics derived from *Streptomyces* bacterial strains. Semisynthetic analogues have been produced by molecular modification of the tetracycline structure. These agents inhibit protein synthesis by preventing attachment of transfer RNA to the 50 S ribosomal subunit. Gram-positive and gram-negative facultative and obligatory anaerobes are susceptible to the tetracyclines, although many microorganisms have acquired resistance to these antibiotics. Brucellosis, syphilis, gonorrhea, cholera, pelvic inflammatory disease, chlamydia, rickettsia (typhus, Lyme disease, and Rocky Mountain spotted

TABLE 7-37. Tetracyclines

GENERIC NAME	TRADE NAME
Tetracycline	Achromycin
Chlortetracycline	Aureomycin
Oxytetracycline	Terramycin
Demeclocycline	Declomycin
Methacycline	Rondomycin
Doxycycline	Vibramycin
Minocycline	Minocin

fever), and urinary tract infections are among the many clinical indications for tetracyclines, which can be used as alternative antibiotics in persons allergic to the β-lactam agents. Protozoal infections (*e.g., Entamoeba histolytica* and malaria due to *Plasmodium falciparium*) are frequently responsive to this group of drugs. ***Minocycline*** can be effective against *Staphylococci* and *Nocardia* that are resistant to other tetracyclines. Acne may be treated with chronic tetracycline therapy.

The tetracyclines can be administered orally or parenterally. Gastrointestinal absorption is inhibited by the presence of food, and particularly by ions such as calcium, iron, and magnesium. Dairy products and antacids should be ingested not less than 1 hour before or 2 hours after tetracycline dosages. Exceptions to this are ***doxycycline*** and ***minocycline.*** Doxycycline and minocycline are lipid soluble and will cross the blood–brain barrier. These two drugs have a longer plasma half-life than other tetracyclines. They are metabolized hepatically and excreted in bile and feces, being somewhat safer than many other antibiotics in persons with renal impairment. The less lipid-soluble tetracyclines are excreted by glomerular filtration, giving them greater efficacy in urinary tract infections.

Tetracyclines can induce renal dysfunction, and nephrogenic diabetes insipidus is reported to occur with ***demeclocycline***. Hepatotoxicity may develop, in particular following large IV doses. Pregnancy or kidney impairment increases the risk of hepatic damage. Tetracyclines are antianabolic, causing elevated blood urea nitrogen levels. Fanconi's syndrome, consisting of acidosis, proteinuria, glycosuria, and aminoaciduria, is caused by degradation products in outdated tetracycline preparations. Because tetracyclines chelate with calcium ion, they are incorporated into dental enamel and bone. The risk of subsequent staining of teeth and suppression of skeletal development contraindicates the use of these drugs during pregnancy or in children younger than 8 years. Photosensitivity can be especially severe with demeclocycline; minocycline produces a high incidence of vertigo. Chronic administration of tetracyclines frequently induces secondary infection due to nonsusceptible organisms. Nausea and diarrhea can accompany oral administration and allergic reactions can occur. Tetracyclines enhance the actions of digoxin and anticoagulants, and reduce the efficacy of oral contraceptives.

FLUOROQUINOLONES

Fluoroquinolones have a broad spectrum of activity including streptococci, staphylococci, *Haemophilus influenzae, Escherichia coli, Proteus mirabilis* and *vulgaris, Pseudomonas aeruginosa, Salmonella* and *Neisseria gonorrhoeae*. ***Ciprofloxacin*** (Cipro) and ***ofloxacin*** (Floxin) have greater efficacy than ***norfloxacin*** (Noroxin), ***lomefloxacin*** (Maxaquin), and ***enoxacin*** (Penetrex). Fluoroquinolones are well absorbed following oral administration, although gastric acidity will alter their bioavailability. Hepatic and renal routes are involved in inactivation of these drugs. Adverse effects include nausea, diarrhea, abdominal pain, headache, insomnia, dizziness, photosensitivity, and rarely, hypersensitivity reactions, hematologic and hepatic changes, and seizures. Erosion of cartilage in young animals contraindicates the use of these agents in pregnancy, lactation, and children under 18 years of age. Sucralfate and dairy products, antacids, and dietary supplements containing metals such as calcium, aluminum, iron, zinc, or magnesium can inhibit gastrointestinal absorption of fluoroquinolones. Ciprofloxacin and enoxacin can interfere with inactivation of methylxanthines, leading to theophylline toxicity.

CHLORAMPHENICOL

Chloramphenicol (Chloromycetin) is a broad-spectrum antibiotic with a range of activity similar to that of the tetracyclines. Typhoid fever, typhus, and other rickettsial infections are especially responsive. Chloramphenicol penetrates the blood–brain barrier, making it a useful agent in *Haemophilus influenzae* infections in the central nervous system. The mechanism of action of this antibiotic involves inhibition of protein synthesis by disruption of peptide bond formation at the 50 S ribosomal subunit level.

Chloramphenicol is well absorbed from the gastrointestinal tract, thus the oral route of administration is used most frequently. Inactivation is by hepatic glucuronidation and renal clearance by both filtration and secretion.

Myelosuppression is the major toxic effect of chloramphenicol. The risk of potentially lethal anemia, thrombocytopenia, and agranulocytosis limits the use of this drug to serious infections unresponsive to other forms of treatment. Chloramphenicol is hazardous in children, especially neonates, who appear to lack sufficient capacity to metabolize the drug. A cyanotic or "gray baby" syndrome that includes vomiting, abdominal distention, hypothermia, and respiratory and circulatory collapse is often fatal. Slowly developing hematological abnormalities, including leukemia, have been attributed to this antibiotic. Frequent monitoring of bone marrow function can assist in detecting early changes that may be reversed by immediate discontinuation of the drug. Renal and hepatic impairment increase the risk of chloramphenicol toxicity. The effects of dicumarol and the oral hypoglycemics can be increased during concomitant chloramphenicol administration. The efficacy of penicillins and the hematopoietic actions of iron and vitamin B_{12} may be reduced.

MACROLIDES

Erythromycin is a macrolide antibiotic available in several forms for oral, topical, and parenteral administration. The mechanism of its inhibition of protein synthesis is not clear. The spectrum of activity is similar to that of the penicillins but, like that of the tetracyclines, it also includes the psittacosis–lymphogranuloma venereum group of large viruses. Erythromycin is destroyed by gastric acid; the stearate and oleate salts are relatively acid-stable and are preferred for oral administration. Enteric coated forms of this drug also are available. Erythromycin is usually utilized as an alternative to penicillin.

Cholestatic hepatitis can develop over 2 to 3 weeks of therapy with the estolate salt, or may appear rapidly in persons who have previously experienced this reaction. Hepatic impairment precludes administration of this form of erythromycin. Nausea and diarrhea can follow oral administration.

Food ingestion does not affect absorption of ***clarithromycin*** (Biaxin), which is more effective than erythromycin against staphylococci and streptococci. Inactivation occurs by both the hepatic and renal routes; renal impairment may necessitate a reduction in dosage. Blood levels of carbamazepine and theophylline may be elevated by clarithromycin, which binds approximately 70% to plasma proteins. ***Azithromycin*** (Zithromax), which has greater efficacy against *Haemophilus influenzae,* should be taken between meals. Azithromycin has a plasma half-life of about 3 days, with negligible amounts renally excreted as unchanged drug. These two macrolides cause much lower incidence of nausea compared with erythromycin. High doses may cause hearing loss; high doses of clarithromycin in pregnant animals have been fetotoxic. Staphylococci and streptococci resistant to erythromycin also are resistant to these macrolides. ***Dirithromycin*** (Dynabac) concentrates in tissues and has a long (up to 44 hours) half-life, which makes it effective with once-daily dosage. Food does not hinder its gastrointestinal absorption. Adverse gastrointestinal effects are similar to erythromycin. Drug interactions reported for other macrolides, including cardiotoxicity with nonsedating antihistamines, are not anticipated with dirithromycin.

Troleandomycin is a seldom-used orally administered macrolide antibiotic.

SULFONAMIDES

Once widely used, the sulfonamides have been largely replaced with newer antibiotic agents. The action of these synthetic anti-infective drugs involves interference with bacterial utilization of para-aminobenzoic acid (PABA) in the synthesis of folic acid. Since mammalian cells derive folic acid from dietary constituents, their growth is not affected by this action. The efficacy of the sulfonamides will be suppressed by pus or other sources of para-aminobenzoic acid. Low doses of the sulfonamides are bacteriostatic, while larger amounts are bactericidal. Bacteria, in particular gonococci, pneumococci, and streptococci, can acquire resistance to these drugs apparently by developing increased production of PABA or alternative enzymes that incorporate PABA into folic acid. Reduction in bacterial cell wall permeability to sulfonamides may also occur. Many of the organisms that have acquired sulfonamide resistance are susceptible to penicillins.

Sulfonamides can be administered orally or parenterally, according to their water solubility and intended site of action. Biotransformation of systemic sulfonamides is by enzymatic acetylation in the liver. Metabolites as well as unchanged drugs are excreted by the kidney. Crystallization of some sulfonamides in the nephrons can cause renal damage. ***Sulfisoxazole, sulfadimetine,*** and ***sulfacetamide*** are highly soluble in urine at low *p*H, making these drugs useful in the treatment of urinary tract infections.

Topical sulfonamide preparations are available for ocular and vaginal infections. Sulfonamides that are poorly absorbed following oral administration can be used to eliminate intestinal bacteria. ***Sulfasalazine*** is used in the management of ulcerative colitis; the 5-amino salicylate metabolite may account in part for its beneficial effects. ***Silver sulfadiazine cream*** (Silvadene) and ***mafenide*** (Sulfamylon) are used to control infection in burn patients. Absorbed systemically, mafenide can induce metabolic acidosis, particularly when renal excretion of the drug and its metabolites is hampered. Application of these preparations can be severely painful and is often preceded by administration of an analgesic.

Trimethoprim is an antifolate frequently combined with ***sulfamethoxazole*** (Bactrim, Septra). Synergistic antibacterial action occurs since the drugs inhibit different steps in the synthesis of folic acid. This combination is used especially in urinary tract infections, and may help to control *Pneumocystis carinii* in persons with acquired immune deficiency syndrome (AIDS).

Hypersensitivity reactions to the sulfonamides can include severe dermatological responses such as Stevens-Johnson syndrome. Hematological abnormalities can develop; persons deficient in glucose-6-phosphate-dehydrogenase (G6PD) are at significant risk of hemolytic anemia. Photosensitivity can occur. Precipitation of drugs in the kidneys can be nephrotoxic; adequate hydration and urinary alkalinization can help to prevent this adverse effect. Sulfonamides should not be administered in late pregnancy or to neonates since the competition of these agents with bilirubin for plasma protein binding sites can result in hyperbilirubinemia. Megaloblastic anemia due to folic acid deficiency may develop in pregnant or malnourished patients, particularly when trimethroprim is administered concurrently.

Systemic sulfonamides compete with other drugs for plasma protein binding sites. In bacteriostatic doses, these broad-spectrum agents reduce the efficacy of bactericidal antibiotics. Sulfonamides can prolong the plasma half-life of methotrexate, phenytoin, and the oral hypoglycemic agents.

ADDITIONAL AGENTS

Polymixins (colistin and polymixin B), which appear to increase bacterial cell wall permeability, have their greatest efficacy against *P. aeruginosa.* Nephrotoxicity limits the systemic use of these agents. Renal impairment delays the clearance of polymixins, which are extensively bound in many tissues and are slowly eliminated by glomerular filtration. Because they are poorly absorbed after oral administration, these drugs can be used to eradicate susceptible bacteria from the gastrointestinal tract. Several preparations for topical use (dermatological and ophthalmological) contain polymixin B. These drugs can induce respiratory failure in combination with neuromuscular blocking agents or in persons with myasthenia gravis.

Bacitracin interferes with bacterial cell wall formation, and has a spectrum of activity similar to that of the penicillins. It is reserved for topical use, since systemic administration presents a marked risk of renal damage. Ophthalmic and dermatological invasions of streptococci and staphylococci often respond to this agent. However, significant amounts of drug may enter the systemic circulation following application to infected or denuded skin.

Vancomycin, an inhibitor of bacterial cell wall synthesis, is derived from *Streptomyces orientalis.* Its action is directed mainly against streptococci and staphylococci, making it useful in treating methicillin-resistant infections. Parenteral administration is required for systemic efficacy. The oral route is used to eradicate infections, such as those caused by overgrowth of *Clostridium difficile,* within the lumen of the gastrointestinal tract. Vancomycin is ototoxic; hearing deficits contraindicate its use. Like most antibiotics, this drug is inactivated by renal excretion.

Lincomycin and ***clindamycin*** are closely related broad-spectrum antibiotics especially useful in alleviating anaerobic *(Bacteroides)* infections. Both are available as oral and parenteral preparations. These agents bind extensively to plasma proteins and penetrate most tissues except the central nervous system. Since these drugs are inactivated hepatically, impairment of renal function does not appear to enhance their toxicity. The potentially life-threatening pseudomembranous enterocolitis associated with these drugs (as well as occasionally with ampicillin, tetracyclines, and chloramphenicol) appears to be caused by a toxin elaborated by a resistant strain of *C. difficile,* which proliferates inordinately when other gastrointestinal flora are suppressed. Vancomycin administered orally ameliorates this superinfection. Unfortunately, lincomycin and clindamycin also cause a diarrhea that can be difficult to differentiate from colitis.

Nitrofurantoin is active against a variety of urinary infections. It is well absorbed following oral administration (delayed gastric emptying enhances absorption) and is rapidly concentrated in urine by both glomerular filtration and tubular secretion. Additional rapid metabolism of this drug by various tissues contributes to its brief (20- to 30-minute) plasma half-life. Renal impairment markedly prolongs this time interval, and decreases the drug's efficacy within the urinary tract. Low urinary *p*H promotes reabsorption and elevated drug concentrations in renal parenchyma; alkalinization of the urine enhances renal excretion. Persons with G6PD deficiency are at considerable risk of drug-induced hemolytic anemia. Late pregnancy and age of less than 1 month contraindicate the use of this drug. Pulmonary toxicity, occasionally due to hypersensitivity, is reported with nitrofurantoin. Chest pain, pleural effusion, and interstitial fibrosis occur. Patients must be observed for dyspnea, cough, and other indications of respiratory changes since pulmonary damage may become irreversible.

Nitrofurazone, a topical agent related to nitrofurantoin, helps to control infection following severe burns or skin graft. The polyethylene glycol vehicle can be absorbed through damaged skin and attain toxic serum levels in persons with impaired renal function.

Nalidixic acid and ***oxalinic acid*** have been particularly effective in inhibiting growth of gram-negative bacteria in the urinary tract. They appear to act by inhibition of DNA synthesis. Administered orally, these agents are hepatically biotransformed (nalidixic acid to an active metabolite) and renally excreted. Adverse effects include photosensitivity, hypersensitivity, gastrointestinal and visual disturbances, and central nervous system and hematological abnormalities.

Methenamine (Urotropin) in an acid urine is converted to formaldehyde, which is bactericidal, particularly to gram-negative organisms. The drug is administered orally and is partially destroyed in the stomach. Enteric-coated formulations are available. Mandelic or hippuric acid, ammonium chloride, or acid-sodium phosphate often is administered simultaneously to attain a urinary *p*H below 5.5. Irritation of the urinary bladder can occur. Dehydration and renal impairment contraindicate the use of methenamine and its salts.

Phenazopyridine (Pyridium) imparts a local anesthetic action in the urinary tract to relieve pain and discomfort accompanying infections, injury, or diagnostic procedures. Administration by the oral route is usually limited to brief periods of time. Methemoglobinemia, hemolytic anemia, and hepatic and renal failure can occur. Renal dysfunction increases the risk of toxicity. Urine may become discolored; yellow discoloration of the skin or sclera can indicate dangerously elevated plasma levels of phenazopyridine.

Antitubercular Agents

Pulmonary *Mycobacterium* infections are treated with a combination of drugs administered for 6 to 9 months or longer. Because of the emergence of drug-resistant strains, isolates should be tested for specific susceptibility. Test results may not be available for as long as 3 weeks, and initial drug treatment can be based on various risk factors. Persons with no history of prior tuberculosis, no history of HIV infection, and no time spent in areas where resistant tuberculosis strains are known to occur, and older persons infected before the emergence of drug resistance are likely to be infected with fully susceptible mycobacteria. Persons from areas where substantial resistance, especially to isoniazid, is known should initially be presumed to be infected with resistant bacteria. Homeless persons, HIV-infected persons, persons with previous tuberculosis history, and persons probably exposed to resistant strains should be presumed to be infected with multiple-drug–resistant bacteria. In all cases, drug regimens can be changed when susceptibility test results are known.

Immunocompetent persons infected with nonresistant strains of mycobacteria should receive ***isoniazid*** (INH) and ***rifampin*** for at least 6 months, including 3 months after culture conversion. In addition, pyrazinamide is given for the first 2 months. Treatment of infection with possibly resistant organisms should begin with a combination of INH, rifampin, pyrazinamide, and either ethambutol or streptomycin. Organisms resistant only to INH require 12 months' treatment with rifampin and ***ethambutol*** and the possible addition of pyrazinamide. If HIV infection, disseminated tubercular disease, or meningitis are present, drug treatment should continue for 6 months after culture conversion. Pyrazinamide continued throughout treatment may improve drug response in meningitis. Multiple-drug–resistant tuberculosis is treated with at least three drugs to which the strain is not resistant, and drug administration should continue for 12 to 24 months after culture conversion. Because poor compliance leads to treatment failure and contributes to the emergence of resistant bacterial strains, it is often recommended that administration of antitubercular drugs be closely supervised.

Isoniazid, a highly specific inhibitor of mycobacterial cell wall formation, is used in both the prevention and treatment of tuberculosis. It is most effective against actively replicating bacteria. Isoniazid is hepatically acetylated at varying rates dependent upon genetically determined enzyme capacities. Renal impairment slows excretion of the acetylated metabolite.

The major toxicity of isoniazid is potentially fatal hepatitis. Liver function must be monitored when this drug is administered. Up to 20% of patients receiving isoniazid will initially develop elevations in serum aminotransferase levels, although this frequently reverts to normal levels without drug termination. Persistent marked elevations of aminotransferase, a concomitant rise in serum alkaline phosphatase or bilirubin, or other indications of hepatic deterioration require that drug administration be interrupted. Persons over the age of 35 appear to be at greatest risk of hepatic impairment. Chronic consumption of alcohol increases the incidence of this adverse reaction, and the presence of hepatic disease often precludes the use of isoniazid. Persons who have recovered from drug-induced hepatitis may be given a carefully controlled second trial of the drug. Recurrence of hepatic symptoms, however, requires abandonment of therapy with this agent.

Peripheral neuropathy and convulsions can be induced by isoniazid, particularly in malnourished persons. Pyridoxine (vitamin B_6) reduces this risk. Hematological aberrations and allergic reactions are additional adverse effects. Isoniazid slows the biotransformation of phenytoin, benzodiazepines, and carbamazepine, and can act as an MAO inhibitor. Overdoses of isoniazid can result in fatal central nervous system depression and respiratory failure. Convulsions may occur, and can be alleviated with IV barbiturates and pyridoxine. Concomitant metabolic acidosis may require sodium bicarbonate administration.

Prophylaxis with isoniazid may be indicated for close contacts of persons with active tuberculosis and for positive tuberculin reactors, particularly persons under age 35. Immunosuppressive therapy as well as disorders such as diabetes, leukemia, Hodgkin's disease, and AIDS increase the risk of tuberculosis and may justify preventive treatment with isoniazid. Although pregnancy is a relative contraindication, women at significant risk of disease can receive isoniazid. (Persons exposed to INH-resistant strains may be given various drugs and combinations including rifampin, ethambutol, pyrazinamide, ciprofloxacin, and ofloxacin.)

Rifampin, usually coadministered with isoniazid, is active against tuberculosis, leprosy, and a number of other bacterial infections. This drug inhibits RNA synthesis by interacting with DNA-dependent RNA polymerase. Like isoniazid, rifampin enters cerebrospinal fluid and is effective in meningeal disease. Hepatic biotransformation produces an active metabolite. The parent drug is partially secreted into bile and is subject to enterohepatic circulation. The drug should be administered 1 hour before or 2 hours following meals, since food hinders gastrointestinal absorption.

Rifampin induces hepatic enzymes, lowering the efficacy of many drugs. Hepatitis can occur in persons receiving rifampin, particularly in the presence of liver dysfunction or other hepatotoxic drugs. Although synergistic hepatotoxicity from isoniazid combined with rifampin does not seem to occur, persons receiving both drugs must be closely observed. Since microorganisms can develop resistance to rifampin, drug sensitivity should be determined before therapy is begun. The most common adverse reactions include gastrointestinal symptoms, headache, ataxia, rashes, thromobocytopenic purpura, and hematological aberrations. Intermittent administration induces a flulike syndrome. Renal failure has been reported. Urine and other body fluids can acquire a red discoloration in persons receiving rifampin. Soft contact lenses and lens implants may be stained by rifampin. ***Rifabutin*** (Mycobutin, formerly ansamycin) is a related antibacterial agent effective against mycobacterium avium complex in AIDS patients.

Ethambutol is not effective against all strains of *Mycobacterium,* and is administered only as an adjunct to other drugs. Unmetabolized drug is excreted in feces and urine; renal impairment may necessitate dosage adjustment. Optic neuritis is the unique toxicity of this drug, although it rarely occurs if daily doses do not exceed 15 mg/kg. A complete ophthalmological evaluation of the patient should precede institution of drug therapy, and vision should be tested periodically thereafter. Changes in acuity of red-green color discrimination mandate that ethambutol be terminated. Other reactions to this drug include hepatic dysfunction, hyperuricemia, allergy, and gastrointestinal and central nervous system symptoms.

Pyrazinamide combined with other antitubercular drugs can shorten the time required for successful eradication of mycobacterial infections. The drug and its metabolites are excreted renally. Hyperuricemia and hepatotoxicity occur. In contrast to that induced by ethambutol, elevation of serum uric acid levels induced by pyrazinamide is not alleviated by probenecid. Other adverse effects are optic neuritis, arthralgia, and gastrointestinal upset.

The aminoglycoside antibiotics such as ***streptomycin*** and ***kanamycin*** are effective agents for the management of tuberculosis. Because of their ototoxicity and nephrotoxicity, these drugs require caution in the elderly and in persons with auditory or renal impairment. Streptomycin-resistant mycobacteria frequently respond to kanamycin. Microorganism strains that are resistant to both of these drugs may be affected by ***viomycin,*** although the use of this drug is limited by its great incidence of toxicity. These drugs must be administered IM since they are not absorbed from the gastrointestinal tract. Fluoroquinolones such as ***ciprofloxacin*** and ***ofloxacin*** may be of some use against multiple-drug–resistant strains.

Ethionamide (Trecator) and ***cycloserine*** (Seromycin) are less potent antitubercular agents occasionally used as second-line adjunctive agents. Magnesium depletion induced by the latter drug leads to neurological symptoms such as confusion, depression, convulsions, and psychosis. ***Para-aminosalicylic acid*** (PAS) frequently causes gastrointestinal ulceration and has been largely replaced by other drugs. This agent is bacteriostatic, and some mycobacteria are not at all affected by it. However, PAS given concomitantly with other agents appears to suppress the development of drug-resistant strains. Serum levels of isoniazid are elevated by PAS. Hepatotoxicity and hypersensitivity reactions can occur.

Leprosy (Hansen's disease) is relatively rare in the United States and is optimally treated by specialists associated with the Public Health Service. The sulfone ***dapsone*** (Avlosulfon) is the drug of choice for this mycobacterial infection; rifampin may be coadministered. Several years of therapy are usually required to achieve complete eradication of the causative microorganism. Adverse reactions such as nausea, tachycardia, and hematological disturbances occur with relative infrequency and are generally mild. Hemolytic anemia may develop in persons deficient in G6PD. Dapsone-resistant strains of *M. leprae* have appeared.

Clofazimine (Lamprene) is effective against dapsone-resistant organisms. Combined with dapsone, it can hinder the development of drug resistance; rifampin can be added to this regimen. Clofazimine is slowly absorbed following oral administration. It accumulates in adipose tissue and leukocytes and has an elimination half-life of 2 months. An anti-inflammatory action, beneficial in erythema nodosum leprosum, has been reported for this drug. Clofazimine can cause reddish brown discoloration of skin, conjunctivae, and lepromatous lesions. Perspiration and lacrimation may be suppressed by anticholinergic action of clofazimine, and gastrointestinal disturbances are reported, particularly when large doses are given.

Antifungals

Fungal (mycotic) infections can be superficial or internal, thus both topical and systemic forms of antifungal agents are utilized. Microorganisms most commonly invading the human host include *Candida, Blastomyces, Cryptococcus, Histoplasma, coccidioides,* and *Aspergillus.*

Despite its considerable potential for toxicity, ***amphotericin B*** (Fungizone) has activity against all mycotic organisms and is usually the drug of choice for systemic fungal infections. By combining with sterols in the fungal membrane, amphotericin B disrupts the selective permeability of the cell. Since it is poorly absorbed, this drug is usually administered IV. Intraventricular or intrathecal routes can be used for meningeal involvement, and topical forms are available for superficial infections (see below).

Once-daily or alternate-day therapy may extend for several months. Amphotericin B is extensively bound within the body, and gradually excreted in the urine.

Amphotericin B has severe adverse effects. Suppression of renal function may persist for months following therapy; irreversible renal damage can occur. Renal function should be monitored; indications of significant renal failure require dosage reduction or termination of drug therapy. When serum creatinine levels are used to determine function, it must be remembered that in elderly patients this parameter may be low due to a decreased muscle mass. Thrombophlebitis (due to intravenous administration), hypokalemia and bone marrow suppression are additional reactions that can have serious sequelae. Erythropoietin may alleviate resultant anemia.

The initial infusion of amphotericin B characteristically provokes nausea, vomiting, headache, wheezing, hypotension, hypoxemia, fever, and shaking chills. These symptoms may be ameliorated by concurrent administration of steroids, antipyretics, or antihistamines. Although hypersensitivity is uncommon, amphotericin B therapy is often initiated with a test dose of 1 mg in a small volume of 5% dextrose administered over 20 to 30 minutes.

Flucytosine (Ancobon) administered orally can be combined with amphotericin B in the treatment of systemic candidiasis or cryptococcosis. This drug interferes with nucleic acid synthesis; it is fungistatic and microorganisms can develop resistance. Inactivation is by renal excretion, and dosage reduction is required in persons with impaired kidney function. Adverse effects of flucytosine, which include hepatitis, myelosuppression, and diarrhea, can be severe. Blood counts, renal function, and serum levels of drug should be monitored. Amphotericin B may hinder the elimination of flucytosine, thus potentiating its toxicity.

Griseofulvin (Fulvicin), administered orally, is concentrated in the keratin layer of the skin. It is utilized in dermatophytoses that do not respond adequately to topical antifungal drugs. Concomitant ingestion of foods with high fat content promotes gastrointestinal absorption of this drug. Griseofulvin is metabolized hepatically and is excreted in bile. Headache, mental aberrations, gastrointestinal upset, and skin rashes can develop.

Ketoconazole (Nizoral) is effective in the treatment of a variety of fungal invasions. Its effectiveness is enhanced by an active immune response. (Serum concentrations of drug are frequently lower in AIDS patients.) The mechanism of action of ketoconazole is inhibition of synthesis of ergosterol, which is the main sterol in fungal cell membranes. Oral absorption is substantial, although the therapeutic response may be gradual and courses of treatment may extend 6 to 12 months. Ketoconazole is inactivated hepatically and binds extensively to plasma proteins. Gastrointestinal side effects are most common, and may be alleviated by giving the drug with food or before sleep. Drug-induced hepatic changes on rare occasions progress to potentially lethal hepatic necrosis. Ketoconazole suppresses testosterone synthesis, can cause gynecomastia, decreased libido and potency in men, and menstrual dysfunction, and may be of benefit in prostatic cancer. Inhibition of corticosteroid synthesis has also been reported. Ketoconazole interferes with inactivation of cyclosporine, phenytoin, and the H_2 antihistamines astemizole and terfenidine, which are implicated in potentially life-threatening ventricular dysrhythmias.

Itraconazole (Sporanox) an oral antifungal related to ketoconazole, is effective against a variety of mycoses. Administration with food enhances absorption. Severe hepatic impairment requires that plasma concentrations of itraconazole be monitored. Nausea, vomiting, hypokalemia, hypertension, hypoadrenalism, rhabdomyolysis, and hepatic changes that may progress to hepatitis are reported adverse effects. Hepatic enzyme inducers will decrease the effectiveness of itraconazole. Plasma concentrations of many drugs, including phenytoin, cyclosporine, warfarin, oral hypoglycemics, terfenadine, and astemizole, are increased by itraconazole. As with any drug that induces hypokalemia, concomitant administration of other drugs that also decrease plasma potassium demands close observation. Prolonged administration of itraconazole may be required, especially in immunocompromised persons.

Fluconizole (Diflucan) can be given PO or IV in the treatment of cryptococcal meningitis and candidiasis. It is more water soluble than ketoconazole, and excreted unchanged in urine with a half-life of approximately 30 hours. Fluconazole enters CSF. Less toxic than some other antifungal agents, fluconazole can cause gastrointestinal distress, headache, hepatic changes and rash that may progress to Stevens-Johnson syndrome. Liver dysfunction contraindicates its administration. The action of several drugs, including phenytoin, cyclosporine, and warfarin, may be enhanced.

Miconazole (Monistat) administered IV can elicit cardiorespiratory arrest following the initial dose. Close observation and immediately available means for resuscitation are required. A variety of systemic fungal invasions are susceptible to this drug, which disrupts cell wall synthesis. Administration into the urinary bladder or the spinal column is suitable for treatment of refractory localized infections. Thrombophlebitis can occur with IV infusion; thrombocytosis and severe pruritus also may develop. Renal impairment usually does not enhance toxicity. Topical preparations of miconazole are also available.

Several additional agents are applied topically in the treatment of superficial fungal infections. ***Tolnaftate, tioconazole, naftifine*** (Naftin), ***terbinafine*** (Lamisil) and

undecylenic acid and its salts are included in over-the-counter creams, ointments, and powders. ***Clotrimazole*** and ***econazole,*** analogues of miconazole, have a broad spectrum of antifungal activity. ***Ciclopirox*** (Loprox), which disrupts fungal cell energy metabolism, is active against several types of mycotic infections. ***Nystatin*** (Mycostatin), ***clotrimazole, miconazole, terconazole*** (Terazol), ***butoconazol*** (Femstat), and ***tioconazol*** (Vagistat) are used topically in the management of vaginal candidiasis. Some of these products are available over the counter. Localized burning and irritation can develop following the application of many of these drug forms.

Amebicides

Infection with *Entamoeba histolytica* is characterized by fatigue, fever, myalgia, arthralgia, intestinal bleeding, and severe diarrhea. Trophozoites in the lower bowel lumen can enter the circulatory system and infect extraintestinal tissues including lung and liver. Drug therapy for amebiasis is divided broadly into treatment of acute symptoms; treatment of tissue invasion such as intestinal ulceration, hepatitis, and liver, lung, and brain abscesses; prevention of relapse by eradicating all cysts from the gastrointestinal lumen; and elimination of cysts in asymptomatic carriers. Because of differing body locations and chemical susceptibilities of active motile trophozoites as contrasted with encysted microorganisms, no single drug has proved to be curative for both gastrointestinal lumen and tissue infections.

Metronidazole (Flagyl), the best single agent for treatment of amebiasis, is amebicidal at both intestinal and extraintestinal sites, but relapses of luminal infections occur. This drug, which inhibits DNA replication, is active against a broad spectrum of microorganisms. Metronidazole can be administered IV or orally, with good absorption from the gastrointestinal tract. It is inactivated hepatically and excreted via the kidney. Renal impairment does not prolong its usual half-life of approximately 8 hours. Hepatic dysfunction may necessitate dosage reduction. Treatment for 5 to 10 days is required to ameliorate amebiasis. To avoid drug decomposition, reconstitution and use of parenteral metronidazole must follow manufacturers' instructions precisely.

Gastrointestinal distress is the most frequently reported adverse response to metronidazole. Because the drug enters cerebrospinal fluid, central nervous system symptoms such as convulsions, vertigo, insomnia, and mental deterioration can occur. Peripheral neuropathy, leukopenia, changes in renal function, hypersensitivity reactions, and thrombophlebitis (the latter following IV infusion) can develop. Candidiasis may be exacerbated during administration of this drug. Metronidazole in therapeutic doses is carcinogenic for mice and rats but it has not been shown to be mutagenic for cells of other mammalian species. However, concentrations of metronidazole equivalent to those in body fluids of humans receiving therapeutic doses produce mutations in Ames' test salmonella (an *in vitro* mutagen assay system). This drug crosses the placenta and is secreted in breast milk. Teratogenicity and adverse effects in nursing infants have not been demonstrated to date but additional years of follow-up are necessary to rule out such actions. Use of metronidazole during late pregnancy and lactation is warranted only when risks of withholding metronidazole (hepatic amebiasis may be fatal) are greater than the risks of administering this drug.

The efficacy of metronidazole may be reduced by drugs that induce activity of hepatic enzymes. Metronidazle can potentiate the anticoagulant action of coumarin-type drugs, and concurrent alcohol consumption may provoke a disulfiramlike reaction.

Oral metronidazole is used frequently to eradicate vaginal trichomoniasis, as either a single dose or a 7-day course of treatment. Sexual partners, even when asymptomatic, should receive similar treatment to avoid reinfection. In research studies, metronidazole appears to enhance tumor responsiveness to radiation therapy. ***Amacrine*** in topical preparations can help to control this infectious agent.

The antimalarial ***chloroquine*** (Aralen), administered for 2 to 3 weeks, is amebicidal for extraintestinal infections but has little efficacy in alleviating acute symptoms of dysentery or in removing intraintestinal cysts, since it is almost completely absorbed from the upper gastrointestinal tract, and is present in low concentrations in the lower bowel lumen. The hydrochloride is available for IM administration when the oral route is inappropriate. Renal excretion of chloroquine is promoted by an acid urine.

Adverse reactions to chloroquine include alterations in ophthalmic and cardiovascular functions, gastrointestinal distress, headache, and occasional central nervous system stimulation manifested as convulsions or psychotic symptoms. Chronic administration (as in the management of malaria) can induce muscular weakness and exacerbation of psoriasis and porphyria. The occasional hepatotoxicity of chloroquine can be intensified by other hepatotoxic drugs. Chloroquine binds extensively to tissue proteins, particularly in the eye. Daily long-term use (years) for treatment of collagen diseases has caused irreversible retinal damage.

Emetine and ***dehydroemetine*** are toxic alkaloids derived from ipecac. They inhibit protein synthesis and eradicate trophozoites from extraintestinal sites such as liver. Prompt alleviation of symptoms including fever, arthralgia, and myalgia, and reduction in size, tenderness, and abscess of the liver have been obtained. In the past, these agents were usually combined with chloroquine to treat amebic hepatitis. Administered parenterally (IM or SC but not IV) emetine alkaloids are gradually excreted in the urine and may be detected in body tissues for long periods of time. The recommended 10-day course of therapy should not exceed a 650 mg total dose of drug, and a rest period of several weeks (6 or more) should elapse before a second course of treatment is given. Today, metronidazole is the drug of choice for treatment of extraintestinal amebiasis, and has replaced chloroquine and highly cardiotoxic emetine alkaloids for this purpose.

Iodoquinol (diiodohydroxyquin, Yodoxin) is an 8-hydroxyquinoline that will alleviate intestinal amebiasis. Intraluminal trophozoites and cysts are eradicated, but insufficient drug is absorbed for extraintestinal activity. Asymptomatic carriers of *E. histolytica* can be treated with iodoquinol. The usual course of therapy is 20 days; chronic therapy with hydroxyquinolines, particularly clioquinol, can elicit subacute myelo-optic neuropathy (SMON). More common adverse reactions are gastrointestinal and dermatological disturbances. Diarrhea or emesis with subsequent dehydration and electrolyte imbalance can occur, and thyroid function tests may be altered by iodoquinol (because of absorption of released iodine).

Diloxanide (Furamide), available from the Centers for Disease Control and Prevention, is the drug of choice for treatment of asymptomatic cyst passers. The aminoglycoside ***paromomycin*** (Humatin) administered orally remains within the intestinal lumen where it destroys *E. histolytica*. Although a direct amebicidal action cannot be ruled out, the antiamebic efficacy of erythromycin and the tetracyclines is probably accomplished by their suppression of lower bowel flora that synergistically support growth and colonization of *E. histolytica*.

CHEMOTHERAPY OF OTHER PROTOZOAL INFECTIONS

Schistosomiasis is caused by trematodes (blood flukes) that enter the body through the skin or gastrointestinal mucosa and invade the vascular compartment. Malaise, fever, anemia, and hepatic and gastrointestinal symptoms appear within 2 to 3 weeks of exposure to the microorganism, several species of which can induce illness. *Schistosoma japonicum* and *mansoni* produce intestinal disturbance, while *S. haematobium* causes urinary tract symptoms.

Praziquantel (Biltricide) is active against the three species of schistosoma and other helmintic infestations as well. It is well absorbed following oral administration, and is rapidly excreted in the urine. Gastrointestinal disturbances, headache, and dizziness are the most common adverse reactions to praziquantel.

Oxamniquine (Vansil), active against *S. mansoni* infections, can induce headache, dizziness, gastrointestinal disturbance, convulsions, or central nervous system depression. The antischistosomal ***hycanthone*** (Etrenol) is contraindicated in hepatic disease, and may be teratogenic and carcinogenic. Single IM doses can be repeated at 3-month intervals.

Antimalarials

Malaria, caused by four species of plasmodia transmitted by the *Anopheles* mosquito, is endemic in many underdeveloped areas of the world. *Plasmodium falciparum* induces a potentially lethal tertian infection. Early treatment can be effective, although inadequate therapy often results in recurrence of symptoms caused by persistence of parasites in the circulatory system. *Plasmodium vivax* is a much milder malaria of tertian occurrence, although relapses may occur up to 2 years following the initial infection. Much rarer is infection with *Plasmodium ovale;* the course of this malaria is similar to that caused by *P. vivax*. *Plasmodium malariae* is quartan in nature; rarely, relapses can occur for several years. The malarial parasite, which gains entry to the human circulation via the bite of female *Anopheles,* localizes in hepatic cells. During this exoerythrocytic stage of 5 to 16 days' duration, tissue schizonts (primary tissue forms) develop and eventually rupture to release merozoites into the circulatory system. In the subsequent erythrocytic stage of malarial infections, the red blood cell is the site of development of trophozoites that mature into schizonts and cause the disruption of the erythrocyte and the classic malarial symptoms (nausea, headache, chills, and fever that may approach 105° F). Merozoites released in erythrocyte rupture will infect other red blood cells to propagate the cyclical nature (tertian or quartan) of clinical malarial attacks. *P. falciparum* and *P. malariae* leave no residual parasites in hepatic cells, while *P. vivax* and *P. ovale* may persist in dormant forms (secondary tissue forms) that can yield periodic recurrence of symptoms for several months or years. Plasmodial gametocytes also evolve during the erythrocytic stage but develop further only when transmitted back into the female *Anopheles*.

Drugs used in the treatment of malaria act at various points in the life cycle of the parasite. Agents that suppress primary tissue forms of plasmodia will prevent initial malarial attacks; those effective against secondary tissue forms can prevent recurrence of disease. Complete eradication of parasites from the body is referred to as a radical cure. Drugs that affect erythrocytic stages of malaria will achieve a clinical cure, that is, will terminate acute symptoms of disease.

Chloroquine (Aralen) is usually the drug of choice to alleviate symptoms and suppress recurrence of acute malarial attacks. The usual route is oral, although the hydrocholoride salt is available for IM injection in patients with severe disease. Chloroquine is concentrated in infected erythrocytes where it destroys the parasite. *P. falciparum* has no secondary exoerythrocytic phase and can be completely eradicated by chloroquine unless the invading organism has acquired resistance to this drug. (Primaquine must be administered to effect radical cure in other forms of malaria, *i.e.,* to eradicate the secondary exoerythrocytic foci of reinfection.) Chloroquine taken once weekly prevents nonresistant malaria attacks in persons travelling to or residing in endemic areas. Administration is begun 2 weeks before exposure, and one daily dose of primaquine is added during the final 2 weeks of chloroquine prophylaxis to prevent reinfection and obtain a radical cure for *P. vivax* infections. The pharmacology of chloroquine is discussed under Amebicides.

Mefloquine (Lariam) kills *P. falciparum* and *vivax schizonts* in the circulatory system. It is effective against some chloroquine-resistant strains. Gastrointestinal disturbances and CNS toxicity, including dizziness, confusion, psychosis, and seizures, can occur. Mefloquine is teratogenic in animals. Its prolongation of cardiac conduction leads to interactions with other cardiac depressant drugs.

Quinine, an alkaloid derived from cinchona, is currently used mainly to eradicate chloroquine-resistant strains of *P. falciparum.* **Pyrimethamine,** sulfadiazine, and tetracycline may be concomitantly administered. Quinine is well absorbed from the gastrointestinal tract, metabolized in the liver, and rapidly excreted in urine. Urinary alkalinization decreases the ionization and promotes reabsorption of this weak base.

Cinchonism often develops with therapeutic doses of quinine; symptoms include tinnitus, vertigo, gastrointestinal disturbances, and visual changes that usually remit if the drug is promptly discontinued. Hematological deficits and hypersensitivity reactions, particularly skin rashes, occur. Hemolyic anemia of an allergic or idiosyncratic nature can develop. Quinine can potentiate the actions of oral anticoagulants, digitalis glycosides, and neuromuscular blocking drugs.

Quinacrine (Atabrine), which acts by suppressing DNA synthesis, is seldom used for malaria although it is still available as an anthelmintic. This drug binds extensively to plasma and tissue proteins and is slowly excreted in the urine. Common adverse effects include headache, vertigo, nausea, and diarrhea. Psychiatric symptoms, visual changes, severe skin rashes, and anemia can develop, and skin and urine may acquire a yellow discoloration.

Amodiaquin (Camoquin) is a congener of chloroquine and has similar antimalarial actions.

Primaquine is used to prevent relapses by eradicating secondary exoerythrocytic foci of reinfection in liver. It has little direct effect on erythrocytic infection, and other antimalarials such as chloroquine are used to prevent acute attacks or to produce a radical cure of falciparum malaria after the patient leaves the endemic area. Methemoglobinemia and potentially fatal hemolytic anemia can appear in persons whose red cells are deficient in G6PD or other enzymes involved in the reduction of methemo globin. Myelosuppressant drugs may exacerbate the hematological disturbances, including leukopenia, induced by primaquine.

Pyrimethamine (Daraprim) and ***trithioprim*** (Proloprim) block dihydrofolate reductase synthesis of tetrahydrofolate and inhibit the vital capacity of plasmodia to synthesize folic acid. Sulfonamides are PABA antagonists and are usually administered simultaneously with dihydrofolate reductase inhibitors to suppress further folate formation and to reduce development of resistant microorganisms. The slow antimalarial action of both types of antifolates makes them unsuitable for treatment of acute attacks. A single formulation, ***Fansidar***, combines pyrimethamine with sulfadiazine. The considerable toxicity of these drugs limits their use to prophylaxis of chloroquine-resistant *P. falciparum.* Combining a sulfonamide with pyrimethamine increases the risk of severe dermatological reactions such as Stevens-Johnson syndrome. The appearance of a rash requires that drug administration be terminated. Pyrimethamine has a long duration of action, due in part to its ability to bind to tissue protein. Hematological disturbances induced by folic acid deficiency may develop; leucovorin (folinic acid, citrovorum factor) can reverse folate depletion in the human host but not the plasmodial parasite.

Anthelmintics

Anthelmintics are used to eradicate worm infestations. A variety of helminths can reside in the human gastrointestinal tract and induce debilitating, even life-threatening disease (*e.g.,* malnutrition, anemia). Some infections involve migration of microorganisms to additional sites in the body. Anthelmintic drugs take advantage of differing metabolic sensitivities of helminths compared to human cells.

Piperazine (Antepar) is effective against enterobiasis (pinworm) and ascariasis (roundworm) infestations, producing a flaccid paralysis that allows evacuation of worms from the intestine. The drug is available as tablets or syrup, administered for 2 days for roundworm (feces should be examined for expulsion of worm) and 7 days for pinworm. Adverse effects are relatively few, although piperazine is absorbed from the gastrointestinal tract. Gastrointestinal upset and allergic reactions can develop. Central nervous system toxicity, occurring particularly in persons with renal impairment, can include dizziness, tremors, visual disturbances, and seizures. Convulsive disorders contraindicate the use of this drug. Pinworms are easily transmitted; thus family members may also be infected and require drug therapy.

Pyrvinium (Povan) is administered in a single dose to eradicate pinworms; if required, a second dose can be given after 14 to 21 days. Administration with food reduces the incidence of gastrointestinal disturbance. Although this drug is poorly absorbed from the gastrointestinal tract, hypersensitivity reactions and Stevens-Johnson syndrome may occur. Pyrvinium kills worms by inhibition of oxygen and glucose uptake. The drug will color feces and vomitus a bright red; to avoid staining of dental enamel, drug tablets should not be chewed.

Thiabendazole (Mintezol) is useful in a variety of infestations including ascariasis, enterobiasis, strongyloidiasis (threadworm), trichinosis, cutaneous larva migrans, and uncinariasis (hookworm). Absorbed systemically, this drug can cause headache, drowsiness, hepatic changes, cardiovascular and visual symptoms, and hypersensitivity that can include severe dermatological reactions. Gastrointestinal disturbances are the most frequently reported adverse effects, and may be reduced by administering the drug with food. Courses of treatment vary depending upon the type of invading organism. Corticosteroids may be given concurrently to alleviate symptoms of trichinosis.

Mebendazole (Vermox) is effective against several species of helminth. Its mechanism of action—inhibition of glucose uptake—is similar to that of thiabendazole. Fever, hypersensitivity, and gastrointestinal disturbances (particularly when large numbers of worms are expelled) can occur. Little of the drug is absorbed systemically.

The antimalarial quinacrine (Atabrine) in large doses will eradicate several species of tapeworm. Interference in protein synthesis appears to be the mechanism of action. Sodium sulfate or saline is used to purge the gastrointestinal tract before and following drug administration. Feces should be examined for expulsion of worms. Brief courses of drug therapy can induce headache and gastrointestinal disturbances. Seizures and cardiovascular collapse may occur following ingestion of large drug doses.

Pyrantel (Antiminth) in a single oral dose is highly effective in the treatment of enterobiasis and ascariasis, while three consecutive daily doses are administered to remove hookworm. The drug is poorly absorbed from the gastrointestinal tract, although systemic amounts can become sufficient to cause headache, dizziness, and drowsiness. Gastrointestinal disturbances are the most frequently reported adverse effects. Depolarizing neuromuscular paralysis induced in worms accounts for the action of this drug.

Tapeworm infestations can be responsive to ***niclosamide*** (Niclocide), which inhibits mitochondrial oxidative phosphorylation. The dorsal part of the worm is killed, and may be digested in the gastrointestinal tract. *Taenia solium* (pork tapeworm) may release viable eggs that are not affected by niclosamide. Cysticercosis may be prevented by purging the intestine. Patients should be examined for 3 months to ensure the helminth eradication is complete. Little of this drug is absorbed, and gastrointestinal upset is the most frequent adverse reaction.

Diethylcarbamazine (Hetrazan) is effective in filariasis, apparently by promoting hepatic destruction of microorganisms. Fever, lymphadenopathy, leukocytosis, and tachycardia may occur as large numbers of filariae are killed. Drug treatment continues for 2 to 3 weeks.

The aminoglycoside ***paromomycin*** (Humatin), used primarily in intestinal amebiasis, will induce removal of tapeworms. Sufficient drug can be absorbed to cause nephrotoxicity. Paromomycin can decrease the intestinal absorption of methotrexate, and may interfere with vitamin K metabolism to potentiate the action of the oral anticoagulants.

Antiviral Agents

Because viruses invade and replicate within host cells, this type of infection is particularly resistant to drug treatment. Management of viral diseases often consists solely of supportive measures until the natural cycle of the pathogen is over. Anti-infective agents may be used to ameliorate secondary bacterial or other invasions. These drugs generally are not effective against viruses, although they have often been administered inappropriately to persons with "colds" or influenza. This use fosters the development of superinfections and resistant strains of microorganisms, as discussed under Antibacterials. Certain viral diseases (*e.g.*, poliomyelitis, influenza, measles, mumps, hepatitis B) can be prevented by administration of immunostimulant substances. A few virucidal agents, with limited spectra of activity, are available.

Amantadine (Symmetrel) and ***rimantadine*** (Flumadine) appear to block the entry of the influenza A virus into host cells. Although annual inoculation with influenza vaccine is the preferred prophylactic measure, persons at risk of developing this infection can be given one of these drugs in daily oral doses for several weeks. Following known or suspected exposure, vaccine and amantadine or rimantadine may both be utilized, the latter to prevent infection while an immune response is emerging. These drugs are also useful for persons in whom vaccine is contraindicated. Amantadine causes CNS effects ranging from insomnia, confusion, nervousness, lightheadedness, and difficulty concentrating to hallucinations and seizures. Risk of these adverse reactions is increased by advanced age, convulsive or psychiatric disorders, and renal impairment. Rimantadine has relatively low potential for central nervous system effects. Because of their teratogenicity in animals, both of these drugs are contraindicated in pregnancy. Renal impairment necessitates reduced dosage of amantadine, which has an average plasma half-life of 20 hours. Rimantadine is not excreted as unchanged drug.

Acyclovir (Zovirax) is used mainly in the management of herpes and varicella-zoster infections. Initial episodes of genital herpes are most responsive, with a significant reduction in duration of pain and viral shedding. The occurrence and duration of viral reactivation may also be reduced. Oral, IV, and topical routes of administration can be used. Acyclovir can protect immunocompromised patients against local or systemic herpes infections, although viral activity frequently resumes when drug therapy is terminated. This drug has largely replaced vidarabine in the treatment of viral infections.

Acyclovir, itself not active, is phosphorylated by viral thymidine kinase to a substance that inhibits the polymerase required for viral DNA synthesis. Glomerular filtration and tubular secretion inactivate this drug. Frequent dosing, renal impairment, and dehydration enhance the risk of nephrotoxicity attributable to drug precipitation in the renal tubules. Bone marrow and hepatic changes may occur, and PO administration can elicit gastrointestinal disturbances.

Ganciclovir (Cytovene) is administered IV to prevent and to treat cytomegalovirus (CMV) infections in immunocompromised persons such as AIDS patients and transplant recipients. A major adverse effect of ganciclovir is myelosuppression, which may be exacerbated by concomitant administration of ***zidovudine*** (Retrovir, AZT). Ganciclovir is teratogenic, mutagenic, and carcinogenic, and can cause headache, gastrointestinal distress, fever, rash, confusion, changes in liver and kidney function, and psychiatric symptoms.

Famciclovir (Famvir) is given orally to decrease postherpetic neuralgia of shingles (herpes zoster). Famciclovir is hepatically deacetylated to the active drug penciclovir, which like acyclovir inhibits viral DNA polymerase. Penciclovir remains in cells for up to 20 hours and is renally excreted by both glomerular filtration and tubular secretion. Rarely occurring adverse effects include tremor, hallucinations, seizures, and coma. Viral strains that acquire resistance to famciclovir are often susceptible to foscarnet.

Foscarnet (Foscavir) inhibits herpes virus DNA polymerase and HIV reverse transcriptase. Like ganciclovir, it can be given IV for CMV invasion of the retina. This infection is a major cause of blindness in AIDS patients, and prophylactic administration of drug may be necessary. Foscarnet can be effective against CMV strains resistant to ganciclovir and acyclovir. Renal dysfunction prolongs the half-life of this drug, which can sequester in bone for long time intervals. Nephrotoxicity of foscarnet may be prevented by maintaining hydration. Adverse effects include headache, seizures, electrolyte imbalances (divalent cations are chelated), nausea, anemia, fatigue, and genital ulceration. Concomitant IV pentamidine increases the risk for hypocalcemia, and nephrotoxic drugs such as the aminoglycosides increase risk for renal damage.

Interferon-alfa may be effective in chronic hepatitis B and C. Given IM or SC, this drug produces a variety of adverse effects, including a flu-like syndrome, myelosuppression, fatigue, susceptibility to bacterial infection, changes in liver and thyroid function, and psychiatric symptoms.

Idoxuridine and ***trifluridine*** (Viroptic) are available in topical ophthalmic preparations for the alleviation of herpes simplex infections of the eye.

Ribavirin (Virazole) can inhibit both RNA and DNA replication. Administered as an aerosol, it will control lower respiratory syncytial virus infections in infants and young children. Such infections are frequently lethal in children who have cardiac disorders. A small particle aerosol generator intended specifically for drug administration is utilized, and high concentrations of drug are achieved in the respiratory tract. Persons requiring assistance in respiration are not good candidates for this therapy, because drug precipitation in respirator valves and tubing causes mechanical failure. Filters can reduce this danger.

Three inhibitors of the reverse transcriptase needed for replication of HIV are used in the treatment of AIDS. ***Zidovudine*** (Retrovir, originally named azidothymidine [AZT]) can increase CD4 T-cell counts, reduce the occurence of opportunitistic infections, and prolong survival. Unfortunately, this drug has many adverse effects, including confusion, fatigue, nausea, vomiting, headache, myopathy, hepatitis, and severe myelosuppression leading to anemia and neutropenia. In some patients, erythropoietin (Epogen) may enhance red cell production, and colony-stimulating factors G-CSF (Neupogen) and GM-CSF (Leukine, Prokine) can ameliorate the suppression of leukocyte production. Zidovudine seems most effective when administered precisely every 4 hours throughout the day and night. This drug can interact unfavorably with many drugs, including acetaminophen, ribavirin, and acyclovir. ***Didanosine*** (DDI, Videx) is administered to AIDS patients refractory or intolerant to zidovudine. Gastrointestinal distress, pancreatitis, severe peripheral neuropathy, and hepatic failure are side effects. Didanosine inhibits gastrointestinal absorption of ketoconazole and itraconazole. ***Zalcitibine*** (DDC, Hivid) may be given together with zidovudine in advanced HIV infection. Peripheral neuropathy, stomatitis, esophageal ulceration, fever, and rash are side effects of this third reverse transcriptase inhibitor. It bears repeating that to date there is no "cure" for AIDS. Prevention remains the best defense against this devastating disease.

Many antimicrobial agents are utilized for the amelioration of opportunistic infections that develop in AIDS patients (Table 7-38). ***Atovaquone*** (Mepron) and ***pentamidine*** (Pentam 300) may be useful in *Pneumocystis carinii* pneumonia. Trimethoprim-sulfamethoxazole, usually the treatment of choice for this infection, appears to provoke severe reactions in the presence of AIDS. Among the numerous adverse effects reported for pentamidine are nephrotoxicity, hepatic changes, pancreatic damage, and cardiac and hematological abnormalities. IM administration can cause sterile abscess. A promising investigational treatment of *Pneumocystis carinii* pneumonia in AIDS patients involves simultaneous administration of the dihydrofolate reductase inhibitor trimetrexate (Neutrexin) and folinic acid (Leucovorin). Acyclovir (Zovirax) and foscarnet (Foscavir) can ameliorate herpes virus infections. Foscarnet as well as gancyclovir (Cytovene) are effective against cytomegalovirus. Continuous prophylactic administration of anti-infective agents may be required to prevent recurrence of infections in AIDS patients.

Antiseptics

Several chemical preparations are used topically to remove microorganisms from body surfaces. Their actions involve alteration of pathogen protein and cell membrane integrity. Application of these substances to injured skin requires great caution, because toxic quantities may enter the systemic circulation.

Benzalkonium chloride (Zephiran) can be safely applied to skin, body cavities, the eyes (in concentrations less than 1:5,000 or 0.02%) and mucous membranes (concentrations less than 1:3,000 or 0.03%). Many vaginal infections respond to this antiseptic. Benzalkonium can be bacteriostatic or bactericidal, depending upon the concentration used. To avoid inactivation of this cationic antiseptic, substances such as soaps and detergents that are anionic must be completely removed from surfaces to be treated. Ingestion of benzalkonium can induce gastrointestinal irritation; systemic absorption elicits central nervous toxicity such as anxiety, weakness, convulsions, respiratory difficulty, and paralysis. Supportive care and evacuation of gastric contents may be necessary to prevent fatalities.

Hexachlorophene (pHisoHex) is used only on intact skin. Systemic absorption can induce hypotension and neurological symptoms including convulsions. Routine bathing of neonates with this detergent was discontinued following several deaths attributed to transdermal absorption. Application to injured skin or mucous membranes, or use with occlusive dressings, is contraindicated. Eyes should be protected from contact with hexachlorophene. This antiseptic leaves a surface film that is especially

TABLE 7-38. Drugs for Opportunistic Infections of AIDS

	DRUGS USED	
INFECTION	**Generic Name**	**Trade Name**
Pneumocystis carinii	Trimethoprim–sulfamethoxazole	Bactrim Septra
	Pentamidine	Pentam 300, NebuPent
	Trimethoprim	Trimpex
	Dapsone	
	Pyrimethamine	Daraprim
	Atovaquone	Mepron
	Clindamycin + primaquine	Cleocin
	Trimetrexate	Neutrexin
Toxoplasmosis	Pyrimethamine + sulfadiazine or clindamycin	
Cryptosporidiosis	Octreotide	Sandostatin
	Paromomycin	Humatin
	Azithromycin	Zithromax
Candidiasis	Nystatin	Mycostatin
	Clotrimazole	Mycelex
	Ketoconazole	Nizoral
	Fluconazole	Diflucan
Cytomegalovirus	Ganciclovir	Cytovene
	Foscarnet	Foscavir
Herpes simplex and Varicella	Acyclovir	Zovirax
	Foscarnet	Foscavir
Systemic fungal infections	Amphotericin B	Fungizone
	Flucytosine	Ancobon
	Fluconazole	Diflucan
	Itraconazole	Sporanox

effective against many gram-positive bacteria. Irritation, photosensitivity, and dermatitis may develop in areas treated with hexachlorophene.

Chlorhexidine (Hibiclens), applied only to the skin, can be bactericidal to gram-positive and gram-negative bacteria. Eyes and ears should be protected from contact with antiseptic preparations. Adverse effects occur with less frequency than with hexachlorophene.

Iodine preparations including iodophors (water-soluble complexes such as povidone-iodine) release free iodine, which will destroy a broad spectrum of microorganisms. Of the iodine preparations, iodophors are reported to be the least irritating to skin. The most frequent adverse responses are allergic rashes that may be severe.

Mercury, in the form of ***merbromin*** (Mercurochrome) or ***thiomerosal*** (Merthiolate) may provide some antiseptic action when applied to skin or mucous membranes. It appears to act by inhibiting sulfhydryl enzymes and precipitating proteins.

Silver nitrate 1% may be used to prevent neonatal ophthalmic gonorrheal infections. More concentrated solutions treat dermatological disorders; 50% solutions are used in podiatry to remove plantar warts. Irritation of skin and conjunctivae can occur; application to injured skin is hazardous. Prolonged use can result in hyponatremia and hypochloremia as these ions are attracted to silver nitrate dressings. Ingestion of this antiseptic can induce severe gastrointestinal irritation and inflammation that can be lethal. Administration of 1% sodium chloride will precipitate inactive silver chloride. Nitrate ions in the circulatory system can elicit methemoglobinemia.

Ethylene oxide is a flammable gas used for the sterilization of instruments. Four hours of gas exposure at room temperature will effectively eradicate bacteria and viruses. Ten to 12 hours must then be allowed for dissipation of gas, since irritation and burns can result from minute amounts that remain on equipment. Exposure to this gas can cause nausea and neurotoxicity; appropriate safety precautions must be followed.

IMMUNOMODULATORS

Immunostimulants

Protection against many infectious diseases can be gained by exposure to naturally occurring pathogens or by administration of vaccines, toxoids, or immune sera. Vaccines and toxoids contain modified antigens that provoke an active immune response; the resulting production of antibodies and ''memory'' cells maintains prolonged resistance to infection. Immune sera contain antibodies (globulins) derived from humans or other animals and provide passive immunity that is immediate but transient. Both active and passive agents are administered following exposure to such diseases as hepatitis B or rabies; the passive agent provides immediate protection while the active agent stimulates an immune response. Otherwise, administration of these agents is separated by 3 months since antibodies present in passive agents may suppress the response to active agents. Agents for active immunity are most effective in persons with a responsive immune system, and should be withheld in the presence of severe infections.

All of the immunostimulants are biological preparations, derived from natural sources. Allergic reactions, especially to products from nonhuman species, must be anticipated with the availability of adequate means for resuscitation. To avoid drug decomposition, use and storage must comply with manufacturers' instructions.

Many vaccines and toxoids are routinely administered (*e.g.*, DTP, poliovirus vaccine), at an early age when possible, to establish life-long immunity. Other preparations are administered only to persons at risk of or following exposure to infectious materials (*e.g.*, hepatitis B or rabies). These agents are generally safe in most persons, and the benefit of avoiding potentially serious infections usually outweighs the risks incurred. Awareness of these risks can help to reduce the incidence and severity of occasional adverse reactions.

The DTP triple antigen contains pertussis bacteria and diphtheria and tetanus toxoids. Usually administered at age 2, 4, 6, and 18 months, a course of treatment can be given at similar time intervals later in life. Pertussis, however, should not be administered to children over 6 years of age because of an increased risk of adverse reactions. Preparations omitting this component are available. Pertussis has been implicated in rare but serious neurological responses in young children, and is contraindicated by the presence or familial history of neurological disorders or by severe reactions to previous doses of antigen. DTaP (Acel-Imune, Tripedia) is a triple antigen preparation containing an acellular pertussis component and is recommended for the fourth and fifth DTP doses usually administered at 15 to 18 months of age and at entry to school. DTaP produces less local reaction to inoculation and less fever and irritability than standard DTP. Tetramune combines Haemophilus influenzae Type b vaccine with standard DTP vaccine to decrease the number of individual vaccines given to young children. Diphtheria and tetanus immunity should be reinforced every 10 years. Localized reactions are the most frequent adverse effects, although allergic responses including anaphylaxis can occur. The latter contraindicate further administration of any component of the vaccine.

Poliovirus vaccine is available in both oral and parenteral forms. Oral vaccine (TOPV, Orimune), which confers prolonged immunity, is administered in four doses to children as young as 2 months or as old as 18 years, or to adults at significant risk of exposure to the virus. Immunodeficiency in the candidate for vaccination or in others who reside in the same household will contraindicate oral polio vaccine. Viruses are present transiently in the gastrointestinal and upper respiratory tract, and rare cases of paralytic poliomyelitis have occurred. Immunosuppressed persons are at increased risk of infection, and parenteral vaccine is more appropriate in such circumstances. An inactivated injectable polio vaccine may also be safer in all adults, who appear at greater risk for paralytic polio following oral vaccine.

Haemophilis influenzae type B can be prevented by administration of a conjugate vaccine (HibTITER, PedvaxHIB). It is recommended that infants be inoculated on a schedule similar to that for DTP. ProHIBit vaccine is effective in children older than 15 months. Measles, mumps, and rubella vaccines are routinely administered to children at 15 months of age. Some of these preparations are produced in chick embryo cell cultures and are contraindicated by previous severe reaction to ingestion of eggs. Rubella vaccine is absolutely contraindicated in pregnancy because of the fetotoxic nature of this viral infection. (Most vaccines are best avoided during pregnancy, unless the risk of severe disease, *e.g.*, hepatitis B, poliomyelitis, or rabies, is present.)

Hepatitis B vaccination is recommended for all infants and many adolescents as well as persons, including health-care professionals, who are at risk of exposure to this infection. Three preparations are available: Heptavax B, from human plasma, and Recombivax HB and Engerix B, produced by recombinant DNA technology. If exposure has occurred, vaccine and hepatitis immune globulin (H-BIG) can be administered simultaneously. Infants born to carriers of this virus should receive immediate inoculation to prevent infection. Hepatitis A vaccine (Havrix) is prepared in human cell culture and inactivated with formalin. Two doses (three for children 2 to 18 years) spaced 6 to 12 months apart are given. Immunosuppressed persons may require additional doses. Immune globulin can be given concurrently if immediate protection is desired. Adverse effects are local reactions and, rarely, anorexia, nausea, headache, fever, fatigue, and anaphylactic reactions.

A live attenuated varicella vaccine is currently recommended for all persons over age 1 year having no history of varicella. Two doses are given over a 4- to 8-week interval. Local reactions and rash within 1 month are adverse effects. Immunodeficiency, recent large doses of immunosuppressant steroids, and pregnancy (varicella infection during the first and second trimester are implicated in birth defects) contraindicate varicella vaccine. Salicylates should not be given for 6 weeks after varicella vaccine because of the apparent risk for Reye's syndrome.

Annual administration of influenza vaccine is recommended for children with inflammatory disorders that require chronic aspirin therapy (due to the possible relationship between aspirin administration during influenza infection in children and the subsequent development of Reye's syndrome), for elderly persons, and for those with chronic debilitating disorders or immunodeficiency. The antigen content of this vaccine is varied yearly to include prevalent strains or mutations of virus. Localized reactions are the most frequent adverse response; neurological disorders such as Guillain-Barré syndrome are occasionally reported. Anaphylactic hypersensitivity to eggs contraindicates this preparation. Amantadine (Symmetrel) can be administered to prevent or ameliorate influenza (see Antiviral Agents). A pneumococcal vaccine appears effective in decreasing the incidence of this type of pneumonia in elderly persons.

Rabies infections develop slowly and are generally fatal. Vaccines are available for both preexposure administration to persons at risk, and for postexposure administration together with rabies immune globulin, which imparts immediate passive protection. Because of the lethal nature of this disease, there are no contraindications to postexposure inoculation, which should be initiated as soon as possible after contact with the virus.

In addition to hepatitis and rabies immune globulins, several other agents of passive immunity are utilized. Immune serum globulin (gamma globulin) can forestall the development or reduce the intensity of measles, chickenpox (varicella), poliomyelitis, and hepatitis A and B. Although most immunostimulants are not administered IV, gamma globulin may be given intermittently by this route to immunodeficient persons. Intravenous immune globulin is also used in the management of idiopathic thrombocytopenic purpura, Kawasaki disease, and chronic lymphocytic leukemia. Headache, a flulike syndrome, and severe prolonged pain at IM injection sites are common reactions. Agents of active immunity usually are not administered within 3 months of immune globulins.

Rho(D) immune globulin (RhoGam), derived from human plasma, will prevent sensitization to the Rh blood factor. Rh-negative persons are at risk following transfusion of mismatched blood, or pregnancy with an Rh-positive fetus.

Antitoxins to botulism, diphtheria, and tetanus are derived from the blood of horses inoculated with these bacterial toxins. Hypersensitivity to equine proteins can result in anaphylactic shock or serum sickness. However, persons desperately in need of the life-preserving actions of these agents can be administered desensitizing doses accompanied by close observation and immediate availability of means of resuscitation.

Several biological response modifiers, including interleukins, interferons, and hematopoietic growth-stimulating factors, are used as immunostimulants, reproducing the action of these naturally occurring substances.

Immunosuppressants

Immune responsiveness, beneficial when it protects the human body against potentially lethal infections, can be undesirable when it threatens the survival of grafted tissues, or when it aberrantly destroys normal host cells. The development of drugs that suppress the immune system has markedly enhanced the success of organ transplant surgery and may aid in the identification and alleviation of autoimmune diseases. However, the nature of these drugs' beneficial action leaves the recipient at significant risk of developing infections and neoplasms that are themselves a threat to survival. Therefore, these drugs are administered only by personnel well-skilled in their use, and in facilities that are adept at managing the special pharmacotherapeutic problems encountered. In the treatment of autoimmune disorders, which generally are not life-threatening, careful consideration must be given to the risk of potentially lethal consequences of immunosuppressant therapy. Severe disabling disease that is refractory to all other forms of treatment is the most acceptable indication for these drugs.

Cyclosporine (Sandimmune), a fungal derivative, has proven to be a valuable adjunct in kidney, heart, and liver transplantation and can suppress graft-versus-host disease in bone marrow recipients. Since this drug is water insoluble, it is prepared in alcohol and oil (olive oil for oral administration, castor oil for the IV route). Therapy is begun 4 to 12 hours before surgery, and must be maintained daily thereafter to prevent tissue rejection. Although gastrointestinal absorption is slow and incomplete, this is the preferred route; IV administration is utilized only when the oral route cannot be tolerated. The average plasma half-life of cyclosporine is 19 hours; it is metabolized hepatically and excreted in bile. Extensive binding to plasma proteins occurs, and the drug is sequestered in erythrocytes. Measurement of circulating levels will yield substantially higher values for whole blood than plasma.

Cyclosporine has a more selective action on the immune system than most previously available agents. The proliferation of T lymphocytes, in particular T-helper cells, which are important to the mobilization of the immune response, is suppressed by this drug. Thus the risk of opportunistic infections is reduced but not completely abolished. Viral diseases such as Epstein-Barr infection and infectious mononucleosis have been troublesome in persons receiving cyclosporine.

Nephrotoxicity is a major adverse response to cyclosporine. In renal transplant recipients, deterioration of kidney function induced by drug toxicity is difficult to differentiate from that arising from graft rejection. Symptoms occurring soon after surgery suggest the latter, while more slowly developing impairment is characteristic of drug-induced damage. Cyclosporine frequently produces hypertension and fluid retention, of particular concern following heart transplant. Neurotoxicity, hepatotoxicity, diabetes, and hypersensitivity can occur. Embryotoxicity has been found in animal studies.

A corticosteroid such as prednisone is usually coadministered to enhance cyclosporine's effectiveness. Azathioprine may also be given. Most other immunosuppressants, as well as other nephrotoxic agents, including NSAIDs, are avoided. Hepatic enzyme inducers can increase the rate of cyclosporine metabolism, while cimetidine and some antimycotic agents prolong drug action. To control secondary infections, concomitant use of antibiotics is often necessary during immunosuppressant therapy.

Tacrolimus (Prograf, formerly FK506) has action like that of cyclosporine but causes less hypertension and decreases the required amounts of additional immunosuppressant drugs. Other adverse effects of tacrolimus are similar to those of cyclosporine, with a greater risk for neurotoxicity, such as tremor and insomnia. Inhibitors of cytochrome P450 III A may interfere with inactivation of cyclosporine and tacrolimus. Tacrolimus has reversed graft rejection in persons receiving standard immunosuppressant regimens.

Mycophenolate (CellCept) suppresses T- and B-cell proliferation via inhibition of inosine monophosphate dehydrogenase. Administered orally, it is combined with cyclosporine and a corticosteroid. Bioavailability approaches 100%. The liver inactivates mycophenolate, which has a half-life of 18 hours. Diarrhea, leukopenia, gastrointestinal hemorrhage, and CMV infection are adverse effects. Antacids and drugs that disrupt enterohepatic recirculation decrease absorption of mycophenolate.

Azothioprine (Imuran), a derivative of the antineoplastic 6-mercaptopurine, suppresses bone marrow synthesis of the cells involved in immune responsiveness. This drug can be administered PO or IV. Xanthine oxidase is important for drug inactivation, thus the enzyme inhibitor, allopurinol, will markedly prolong the plasma half-life of azathioprine. Low doses of this drug are occasionally administered in severe degenerative rheumatoid arthritis refractory to other treatment. Adverse effects resemble those of antineoplastic agents: myelosuppression, nausea and vomiting, alopecia, hypersensitivity, hepatotoxicity, and carcinogenesis. Pregnancy is a contraindication. Azathioprine may be combined with other immunosuppressants, which increases the risk of infections. Nonsteroidal anti-inflammatory drugs can be added in the management of arthritis.

Oral, low-dose ***methotrexate*** (Rheumatrex) may be used in severe refractory rheumatoid arthritis. Myelosuppression, hepatic and pulmonary toxicity, nausea, and gastrointestinal ulceration are among the adverse reactions. Salicylates and other nonsteroidal anti-inflammatory drugs must be used with great care, since these can inhibit renal excretion of methotrexate. Renal function must be monitored. Pregnancy contraindicates this drug, which is both teratogenic and abortifacient. Concomitant use of nephrotoxic drugs, or alcohol and other hepatotoxic agents, can increase the risk of organ damage.

The antineoplastic ***cyclophosphamide*** (Cytoxan) can be used clinically for its immunosuppressant action. Hemorrhagic cystitis is of special concern with this drug (see Antineoplastic Agents).

Antithymocyte globulin (Atgam), extracted from blood of horses sensitized to human T lymphocytes, blocks the immune reactivity of T cells. It is administered IV in combination with other agents to suppress transplant rejection. Aplastic anemia can also be ameliorated by this drug. Thrombophlebitis, chills and fever, arthralgia, diarrhea, and hypersensitivity (particularly to equine protein) are possible adverse reactions.

Muromonab CD-3 (Orthoclone OKT3) is a monoclonal antibody that suppresses T-cell activity. Patients must be carefully screened for fever, fluid overload, or allergy to murine substances before this drug is administered. Fever and pulmonary edema are among the adverse effects. Therapy is usually limited to less than 14 days; during this time severe infections can develop.

High doses of corticosteroids such as prednisone and prednisolone continue to be useful when immunosuppression is required. The actions of these drugs are discussed under Endocrine Pharmacology.

VITAMINS

Vitamins may be considered a special category of drug. Not only do they influence the actions of many types of cells, but they are also essential to proper physiological function. Vitamin deficiencies occur infrequently in the United States, except among persons who lack access to a well-balanced diet. Deficiencies may also be induced by malabsorption syndromes, extensive surgery, and the use of certain drugs, for example, inadequacy of fat-soluble vitamins when bile sequestrants are administered. Vitamin replacement therapy is highly effective in restoring proper nutrition. Widespread use of vitamins prophylactically and as therapy for actual or presumed subclinical deficiencies has occasionally resulted in ingestion of toxic amounts of these substances. Vitamin deficiency can often be alleviated by improved dietary intake.

Vitamin A is essential for retinal function, bone growth, and skin integrity. This fat-soluble vitamin is available as fish-liver oil with high content of the vitamin, as concentrates from such natural sources, and as manufactured synthetic products. Water-miscible forms can be administered by slow IV infusion; rapid injection can cause fatal anaphylactoid reactions. The recommended daily allowance of this vitamin for adults is 5,000 units. Hypervitaminosis A has occurred in numerous instances of excessive self-medication, causing symptoms such as irritability, headache, arthralgia, drying and cracking of the skin, and hematological deficits. Jaundice and enlargement of the liver may develop, since vitamin A is stored tenaciously in this organ. New bone formation and premature closure of the epiphyses have occurred, with serious alterations of skeletal development. Bone decalcification is also reported. ***Tretinoin*** (Retin-A) is a vitamin A derivative administered topically in the treatment of acne. It may also decrease skin damage induced by exposure to the sun. The drug can be irritating to the skin, and is believed to be teratogenic.

Vitamin D affects calcium and phosphate metabolism, influencing the development and function of tissues that use these essential ions. Endogenous vitamin D formation in the skin is induced by exposure to sunlight. This substance occurs in several forms: vitamin D_2 ***(calciferol)*** and D_3 ***(cholecalciferol)*** appear to have similar activity. ***Dihydrotachysterol*** (Hytakerol) is hepatically transformed to active vitamin; it is used particularly in amelioration of hypoparathyroidism. ***Calcitriol*** (Rocaltrol) has special application in alleviating hypocalcemia in renal dialysis patients. Bile is essential for the absorption of vitamin D from the gastrointestinal tract; persons with inadequate amounts of this digestive secretion often benefit from administration of bile acids.

The recommended daily intake of vitamin D is 400 units. Replacement dosages must be highly individualized. Symptoms of overdose include nausea, diarrhea, weakness, convulsions, polyuria, and metallic taste. Hypercalcemia can induce calcification of blood vessels, renal tubules, and other soft tissues. Serum calcium and phosphatase levels should be monitored; a reduction in the latter can warn of developing calcium excess. Vitamin D is lipid soluble and may be stored in large amounts in body tissues. Hypercalcemia in infants is occasionally reported to be induced by vitamin D administration. Persons receiving digitalis must avoid hypercalcemia, because this electrolyte may elicit cardiac arrhythmias. Hepatic enzyme induction decreases the efficacy of vitamin D.

Vitamin E occurs in several forms known collectively as the tocopherols. The functions of this fat-soluble vitamin appear to include antioxidant and enzyme cofactor. Deficiency seldom occurs, although malnourished infants may exhibit the characteristic hemolysis, muscle necrosis, and creatinuria. Premature infants maintained on formulas high in iron and polyunsaturated fatty acids also are at risk of vitamin E deficiency. Anemia in these patients is corrected by administration of vitamin E. Recommended adult daily intake ranges from 12 to 15 units.

Vitamin K is essential for the hepatic synthesis of several clotting factors including prothrombin. Intestinal bacteria are an important source for this vitamin; administration of certain anti-infective drugs can eradicate these microorganisms and induce coagulation deficits. Absorption of this fat-soluble vitamin is dependent upon the presence of bile in the intestine. Administration of vitamin K will correct vitamin-dependent coagulopathies only if hepatocytes retain their ability to synthesize clotting factors. Oral anticoagulants such as warfarin suppress formation of K-dependent factors; overdose or overresponsiveness to these drugs can be ameliorated by administration of the vitamin. The onset of improved coagulation requires several hours. Emergency measures such as transfusion of blood products may be necessary in severe hemorrhagic episodes.

Several synthetic analogues of vitamin K are available. ***Phytonadione*** (Mephyton) can be administered orally or parenterally, although the IV route is used only with extreme caution since anaphylactic reactions may occur. The efficacy and potency of this substance are nearly identical to those of the naturally occurring vitamin. Phytonadione has a more rapid onset and longer duration of action than other analogues, and appears to be safer and more effective in ameliorating responsive neonatal coagulopathies. ***Menadione*** and ***menadiol*** (Synkavite) do not require the presence of bile for gastrointestinal absorption. These analogues can provoke hemolytic anemia in G6PD-deficient persons or in neonates, and are contraindicated in late pregnancy. Newborn infants also are at risk of vitamin K analogue-induced hyperbilirubinemia. Administration of vitamin K can transiently suppress responsiveness to oral anticoagulants. There is no interaction between this vitamin and heparin.

Vitamin B complex includes several water-soluble substances that are essential for many physiological functions. Since these vitamins are not stored in body tissues to any appreciable extent, deficiencies readily occur if daily intake is inadequate. Usually more than one vitamin in this group will be lacking.

Thiamine (vitamin B_1) is a coenzyme in carbohydrate metabolism. Requirements for this vitamin are increased during pregnancy, febrile diseases, and by high dietary intake of carbohydrates. Thiamine deficiency (beriberi) leads to malfunction of the gastrointestinal, cardiovascular, and nervous systems. Korsakoff syndrome, characteristic of chronic alcohol abuse, is caused by inadequate amounts of this vitamin. Replacement can be given by oral or parenteral routes. Intramuscular injection can be painful; IV administration is hazardous and should be used only when other routes are unacceptable. Intradermal pretesting can help to identify hypersensitive persons.

Riboflavin (vitamin B_2) is an essential component of coenzymes involved in the transfer of hydrogen ions in tissue respiratory systems. Symptoms of riboflavin deficiency include corneal and dermatological changes. Oral and IM routes are used for replenishment of this vitamin.

Pantothenic acid (vitamin B_5) is a component of coenzyme A that takes part in many energy-releasing reactions. Synthesis and utilization of fatty acids and steroid hormones are dependent upon this vitamin. Deficiencies have not been reported, except when induced by administration of an antagonist of pantothenic acid.

Pyridoxine (vitamin B_6) interacts with carbohydrate, protein, and lipid metabolism. Deficiencies may occur in persons receiving isoniazid, oral contraceptives, hydralazine, or penicillamine. Chronic alcoholism, malnutrition, diabetes, and seizure disorders increase the risk of deficiency. Infants also may exhibit deficiency. Abdominal disturbances, convulsions, and peripheral neuritis are prominent A genetic pyridoxine-dependent seizure disorder and pyridoxine-responsive anemia are occasionally reported. Pyridoxine reverses the antiparkinsonism efficacy of levodopa, unless a peripheral decarboxylase inhibitor is given simultaneously.

Cyanocobalamin (vitamin B_{12}) is required for cell replication, hematopoieses and myelin synthesis. Deficits elicit neuropathies such as weakness, paresthesias, ataxia, and loss of bladder and bowel control. Erythrocytes fail to mature, resulting in megaloblastic anemia. Primary vitamin deficiency may respond to oral replacement therapy, although treatment in the presence of abnormal gastrointestinal absorption often requires parenteral forms of vitamin B_{12}. In pernicious anemia, oral administration of vitamin must be accompanied by intrinsic factor in order to effect absorption. Intramuscular and SC injections provide for rapid vitamin replacement. Since this is a water-soluble substance, excess amounts are not retained in body tissues. Adequate amounts of iron, potassium, and folic acid are also needed for the production of erythrocytes. Chloramphenicol and other drugs that suppress bone marrow function can reduce the hematopoietic efficacy of vitamin B_{12}.

Adverse responses to vitamin B_{12} administration include pain at the injection site, diarrhea, thrombosis, pulmonary edema, congestive heart failure, and allergic reactions. An initial intradermal test dose can help to avoid anaphylaxis. Preparations should not be administered IV. Large amounts of vitamin may be required to correct deficiencies, with smaller doses continued at monthly intervals.

Folic acid deficiency usually accompanies states of inadequate vitamin B_{12} and appears to contribute to the incidence of megaloblastic anemia. Both vitamins participate in synthesis of DNA. Folic acid is usually well absorbed following oral administration, and may also be given SC, IM, or IV. Few adverse reactions other than allergy have been reported. Folic acid can reduce the efficacy of phenytoin, leading to loss of seizure control. Phenytoin, primidone, and phenobarbital can accelerate folate metabolism. Several antineoplastic agents (*e.g.*, methotrexate) and antibiotics (*e.g.*, sulfonamides) are also folate antagonists. Oral contraceptives can induce mild folate deficiency.

Nicotinic acid (niacin) and ***nicotinamide*** are utilized in the prevention and treatment of pellagra. Administration of isoniazid may induce deficiency of nicotinamide, which is essential for lipid and carbohydrate metabolism. Nicotinic acid is a component of nicotinamide adenine dinucleotide (coenzyme II). This drug has some value in hyperlipidemia and is discussed under that topic. Peptic ulcer, hepatic impairment, and severe hypotention contraindicate its administration.

Vitamin C (ascorbic acid) is essential for many physiological functions. Deficiency leads to collagen changes (scurvy) and loss of integrity of bone, capillaries, and connective tissue, and inadequate healing of wounds. Fever, infections, extensive burns, chronic illness, and cigarette smoking will increase the daily requirement for vitamin C. This water-soluble substance is not stored in body tissues; its renal excretion can produce significant lowering of urinary *p*H. Formation of oxalate or urate stones in kidneys has occurred with large doses. Excessive amounts of vitamin C can cause diarrhea, and are contraindicated during pregnancy since an increased need for the vitamin may be induced in the neonate.

A variety of drug interactions has been attributed to vitamin C. Alterations in the actions of oral anticoagulants and interference with oral contraception may occur. Urinary acidification can enhance reabsorption of acidic drugs and reduce that of alkaline drugs. The action of disulfiram may be impeded. Vitamin C facilitates intestinal absorption of iron.

TOXICOLOGY

Exposure to ***carbon monoxide,*** a product of most forms of combustion as well as a constituent of artificial fuel gases, is exceptionally common. This gas combines with hemoglobin to form carboxyhemoglobin, which is incapable of transporting oxygen. When approximately 20% of the blood pigment is thus combined, the subject experiences headache and dizziness; with 40% combined, there is collapse; with 60%, coma; higher proportions of carboxyhemoglobin are usually lethal. The dissociation pressures of the remaining oxyhemoglobin are less than normal under these conditions. Carboxyhemoglobin is a red pigment, and cherry-red flushing of the skin can be diagnostic. Large skin blisters may occur. The combination of monoxide and hemoglobin dissociates slowly, since the affinity of monoxide for hemoglobin is 200 to 300 times greater than the affinity of oxygen for hemoglobin. Continuous exposure to a carbon monoxide concentration of 0.1% can be fatal in about 2 hours. Administration of oxygen, occasionally under hyperbaric pressure, promotes dissociation and restoration of hemoglobin; respiratory assistance may be required concomitantly.

Cyanides and ***hydrocyanic acid*** represent a special danger because of their use in industries and fumigation procedures. They are also encountered as poisons used in suicide attempts. Cyanides rapidly and directly inhibit the respiratory mechanism of cells by a highly sensitive inactivation of the cytochrome oxidase system. Histotoxic anoxia in the thoracic chemoreceptors induces pronounced hyperpnea. Convulsions, probably anoxic in character, are followed by respiratory failure. Rapid IV administration of amyl or sodium nitrite and sodium thiosulfate to inactivate cyanide ion can be life-saving. Although less effective, methylene blue may be more readily available in an emergency.

Methemoglobin is formed by the action of certain inorganic substances (chlorates, nitrites), aniline dyes, and drugs such as acetaminophen and sulfanilamide that are aniline derivatives. (The use of acetanilid was discontinued because of its propensity to oxidize hemoglobin.) Methemoglobin, like carboxyhemoglobin, is incapable of transporting oxygen, since the ferrous ionic form is converted to the ferric state. Cyanosis, headache, and respiratory difficulty are symptomatic of methemoglobinemia.

Neonates, particularly premature infants, are at risk of methemoglobinemia. In adults, susceptibility follows genetic trends and is associated with deficiency of enzymes such as G6PD.

Methemoglobin is partially eliminated in the urine and partially reconverted to normal hemoglobin over the course of several hours. Erythrocytes are hemolyzed, and chronic methemoglobinemia leads to anemia. Treatment of acute poisoning consists of administration of oxygen and methylene blue (1 to 2 mg/kg intravenously). Identification and elimination of the causative agent are necessary to prevent recurrence.

Kerosene ingestion often causes pneumonitis due to aspiration. Vomiting should not be induced, and gastric lavage must be carried out with extreme caution. There is evidence also that kerosene produces pulmonary inflammation due to transport through the bloodstream from the alimentary canal. ***Turpentine*** has similar effects, with a more conspicuous degree of renal inflammation.

Methyl alcohol (methanol) is similar to ***ethyl alcohol*** (ethanol) in its central nervous system depressant action.

This organic solvent is especially toxic to retinal cells and the optic nerve; its ingestion can lead to blindness. Methanol is metabolized to formate, which can induce metabolic acidosis. Sodium bicarbonate administered PO or IV will neutralize excess H^+ ions in plasma. Since ethanol slows the oxidation of methanol, its administration may minimize toxic effects.

Isopropyl alcohol is used extensively as a substitute for ethyl alcohol in external medicinal preparations, such as rubbing and disinfecting alcohols. Ingestion can cause marked renal impairment; large amounts of isopropyl alcohol can be lethal.

Boron hydrides such as pentaborane and decaborane have been responsible for acute and chronic toxicities. Mild symptoms resemble those of common respiratory infections and allergies. In more severe cases, muscle spasms, convulsions, disorientation, and coma develop, frequently after a latent period of several hours. Liver tenderness and abnormal liver function tests may continue for some time.

Lead is a commonly used element, found in paints, pottery, and other household items. Toxic effects can develop after ingestion of a few miligrams daily over several weeks. Toxicity occurs most rapidly following inhalation of dusts and of the volatile tetraethyl lead, although poisoning also results from oral ingestion and through absorption of organic compounds through the skin. Signs and symptoms of lead poisoning include stippling of red cells, reticulocytosis, anemia, pallor, lead line on the margin of teeth and gums, muscle weakness, and gastrointestinal distress. Encephalopathy with convulsions and coma can be fatal.

X-ray density at the epiphyseal line is diagnostic in infants who more commonly exhibit cerebral and meningeal symptoms.

The elimination of stored lead is promoted by IV administration of the chelating agent ***calcium disodium ethylenediamine tetraacetic acid*** (EDTA, Versene, Sequestrene). This substance complexes with lead to form a soluble compound that is readily excreted in the urine. ***Dimercaprol*** (BAL) may be administered concurrently to enhance excretion. ***Succimer*** (DMSA; Chemet) is given orally to children to promote lead excretion. The source of lead intake must be identified and eliminated.

Another effective chelating agent is ***penicillamine***, which is capable of removing copper as well as lead. This drug is used in the management of copper excess such as Wilson's disease. It must be remembered, however, that the administration of an antidote carries the risk of drug side effects.

Mercury in soluble ionized form is intensely corrosive, and after absorption it has conspicuous toxic effects in the kidney tubules. Mercuric chloride (corrosive sublimate), metallic mercury (*e.g.*, in thermometers and manometers), and mercury contamination of fish are sources of this poisoning. Toxicity develops in two stages. The first, chemical trauma due to corrosive action, is characterized by immediate burning in the upper gastrointestinal tract, followed by severe vomiting and diarrhea. The second stage, systemic toxicity, becomes apparent within a few days as renal tubular necrosis and azotemia develop.

Treatment consists of stomach lavage, proteins from egg whites and milk to provide local protection, and parenteral fluids. The chelating agents dimercaprol and penicillamine assist in the removal of mercury ion but do not reverse renal damage, which can be lethal.

Arsenic, utilized in pesticides and weed killers, has been a frequent cause of accidental and suicidal poisonings. Acute poisoning may result from ingestion of as little as 100 mg arsenic trioxide (white arsenic). It is characterized by gastrointestinal disturbances, usually with severe vomiting and diarrhea. Arsenic can gain entry into the central nervous system, and will cause convulsions and coma. The chief systemic action is capillary dilation, most marked in the splanchnic area.

Replacement of fluids and electrolytes can be life-saving. Gastric lavage followed by administration of ferric hydroxide or sodium thiosulfate and a sodium sulfate cathartic will evacuate metal from the gastrointestinal tract. Dimercaprol may prevent further systemic action of the arsenic.

Chronic ***beryllium*** poisoning was once of special interest, largely because of its incidence in the early days of the flourescent-lamp industry. Presently it is used in alloys, atomic energy technology, and in ceramics. Skin granulomas may develop following direct contact. Small amounts of inhaled beryllium produce nodular and diffuse granulomas, replacing lung parenchyma. Symptoms of weakness, dyspnea, cough, and weight loss may develop at varying intervals following exposure. Polycythemia has been reported. Administration of prednisone may reduce the toxic effects of beryllium.

Cigarette smoking exposes the smoker to many toxic substances, particularly nicotine, carbon monoxide, tars containing known carcinogenic hydrocarbons, pesticides, and polonium 210 (^{210}Po). Concern over health hazards posed by these toxins has been emphasized by the report of the advisory committee to the Surgeon General of the Public Health Service. Conclusions were that cigarette smoking is causally related to lung cancer, is a significant factor in the incidence of cancer of the larynx, and may be related to cancer of the mouth, esophagus, and urinary bladder. It is considered to be the most frequent cause of chronic bronchitis in the United States and to have a causative relationship to pulmonary emphysema. Deaths attributable to these nonneoplastic conditions are significantly more frequent among cigarette smokers than among nonsmokers. Graded epithelial changes have been observed in the tracheobronchial tree in approximate dose–response relationships to cigarette smoking. These changes include loss of cilia, basal cell hyperplasia, and appearance of atypical cells with hyperchromatic nuclei; bronchial glands also exhibit hyperplastic changes. Smoking during pregnancy increases the risk of abortion, stillbirth, and low birthweight infants. Smoking is also associated with an increased incidence of myocardial infarction, hypertension, and peptic ulcer. Nonsmokers exposed to "sidestream" or "secondhand" smoke appear also to be at risk for adverse consequences.

Radiation exposures to doses of the order of 50,000 rads at high dose rates are followed by immediate injury and death, presumably as the result of damage to the central nervous system; exposure to about 1,000 rad leads to death in several days as gastrointestinal epithelium is lost; total body irradiation with several hundred rads is followed by profound myelosuppression with death in 2 to 4 weeks; smaller doses of 100 rad or less may produce only equivocal acute symptoms followed by slowly developing sequelae such as cataracts, degenerative disease, and neoplasia, long after the initial radiation insult.

The testing of nuclear weapons and more recently the construction of nuclear power plants has fastened interest on radiation effects in exposed populations, with intensive monitoring in various parts of the world. The predominant long-lived nuclide from fusion reactions is tritium; from fission reactions, ^{90}Sr. ^{90}Sr and ^{137}Cs appear in plants through uptake from soil. The fallout behavior of ^{131}I differs because of its short half-life and usually is related to rain and the surface area of plants; transfer of ^{131}I to human occurs principally through milk.

Rodenticides and ***insecticides*** have been made increasingly effective, and their consequent greater use has increased the hazards of public exposure to these agents.

Red Squill is one of the oldest and most common rodenticides. It contains cardiac glycosides (scillaren) and other glycosides. It produces alternating convulsions and paralysis in rats. Household pets and humans usually vomit the poison before a lethal dose is absorbed.

Sodium fluoroacetate (1080) is volatile and stable and can be absorbed through the skin in toxic amounts. It is used only by specially trained commercial exterminators. The mechanism of death is by ventricular fibrillation.

Alpha-naphthol-thiourea (ANTU) stimulates powerfully the flow of lymph and kills by massive pulmonary edema and pleural effusion.

The anticoagulant ***warfarin*** is an effective rodenticide. Vitamin K can reverse the hemorrhagic effects of this drug, although several hours are required for the resynthesis of clotting factors.

Pyrethrum, a mixture of plant esters used as an insecticide, is a central nervous system stimulant. Oral ingestion by humans results in hydrolysis of the esters to inactive compounds, which gives it a wide margin of safety. However, its allergenic properties are marked in comparison with other insecticides.

Rotenone is a neutral crystalline derivative of derris root. It causes death in mammals through convulsions and respiratory depression.

Some chlorinated hydrocarbons are unusually effective against a considerable variety of infestations. Usually they are applied in kerosene solution and, when ingested accidentally, the symptoms of poisoning may be those of kerosene. ***Chlorophenothane*** (DDT) is a central nervous system stimulant and sensitizes the heart to fibrillation. Chronic poisoning is characterized by nervous system symptoms and severe liver damage. ***DDD, TDE,*** and methoxychlor are similar. Some isomers of benzene hexachloride, particularly gammexane or ***lindane,*** are extremely potent central nervous system stimulants, while others are depressant. Chlorinated ***camphene*** (Toxaphene) produces reflex excitability and convulsions that can be ameliorated by barbiturates. ***Chlordane,*** a chlorinated indane derivative, has action similar to DDT; it is more readily absorbed through skin thus has a greater incidence of toxicity. ***Dieldrin*** and ***aldrin*** also are chlorinated hydrocarbons related in action and uses to chlordane and camphene. The chlorinated hydrocarbons accumulate tenaciously in body fat, but their excretion rate increases in proportion to accumulated amounts. The organophosphate insecticides, which are inhibitors of cholinesterase, are discussed under Autonomic Drugs.

DRUG ABUSE

Many drugs are misused or abused for a variety of purposes. This section will focus on those drugs that are used in a nonmedical or "recreational" manner based upon their central nervous system actions. Both stimulants and depressants of central nervous system function are included. The abuse of such drugs can lead to drug dependence that may be psychological or physiological. Psychological dependence, characterized by intense craving for drug, or by feelings of inability to function without drug use, fosters repetitious drug use that in many instances can lead to physiological (or physical) dependence. In the latter, the persistent presence of drug appears to induce poorly understood physiological changes; when the drug is not present, physical symptoms called an abstinence or withdrawal syndrome develop.

Persons dependent upon (or "addicted to") drugs often become totally preoccupied with obtaining drugs, first for their pleasurable aspects, then as physiological dependence develops, for their ability to stave off the discomforts of withdrawal. Drug abuse has become a problem of major proportions in the United States, having economic, social, and moral as well as medical ramifications. Only the latter will be outlined here. However, the physician must be mindful that psychological and social assistance must be offered and encouraged along with medical care if the patient is to overcome his or her dependency.

Tobacco Abuse

Amid controversies over health consequences and addictive properties of nicotine, the proportion of smokers among the United States population has decreased significantly. Some smokers desiring to quit can benefit from transdermal nicotine patches (Habitrol, Nicoderm) that reduce nicotine craving and abstinence symptoms such as headache, irritability, and difficulty concentrating. Although the delivery system is designed to deliver small amounts of nicotine into the circulatory system, nicotine poisoning (characterized by dizziness, nausea, convulsions, and respiratory failure) can develop. Persons who smoke while wearing the patch are especially at risk for drug overdoses. Use of the patch can cause local irritation, nausea, headache, gastrointestinal distress, and sleep disturbances. (See discussion also under ''Toxicology.'')

Alcohol Abuse

Alcohol is a central nervous system depressant that sedates and induces a calm euphoric response in most persons. Chronic consumption of ethyl alcohol severely damages many body tissues. Hepatotoxicity, cardiomyopathy, esophageal varices, gastritis, central nervous system atrophy, nephrotoxicity, and teratogenicity are among the adverse responses attributed to the use of this drug. Large quantities of alcohol can severely, even fatally, depress respiration. Perhaps the greatest toxicity of alcohol is the number of persons killed and injured annually in accidents, automobile and other, caused by people under the influence of this drug.

Alcohol is metabolized hepatically, first to acetaldehyde through the action of alcohol dehydrogenase, then to acetate by aldehyde dehydrogenase. Acetate enters the tricarboxylic acid cycle to be transformed finally to carbon dioxide and water. The early steps of this pathway tend to follow zero-order kinetics, so that the rate of metabolism is not affected by the quantity of alcohol present. Blood levels of alcohol in most persons closely parallel the degree of intoxication, and in most states are accepted as medicolegal evidence of impairment. Emotional instability and motor incoordination occur with 80 to 100 mg/100 ml plasma (0.08 to 0.1%); ''legal'' drunkenness begins at 100 to 150 mg/100 ml; marked central nervous system depression appears at 200 to 400 mg/100 ml; loss of consciousness at 500 mg/100 ml; concentrations above this level can be lethal.

Alcohol provides substantial amounts of calories but virtually no nutritional components. In addition, alcohol appears to impair intestinal absorption of foodstuffs and nutrients. Thus persons who chronically consume quantities of alcohol frequently suffer from malnutrition. Mental aberrations such as Wernicke's encephalitis and Korsakoff's syndrome, frequent among alcoholics, are at least in part amenable to administration of thiamine (vitamin B_1).

Withdrawal from physiological dependence upon alcohol can be especially severe. Nausea, tremors, hyperreflexia, and hallucinations progress to seizures, delirium tremens, and disorientation. In extreme uncontrolled withdrawal, cardiovascular and respiratory failure can occur. Dehydration, electrolyte imbalance, and hypoglycemia can be present. Controlled detoxification from alcohol dependence can be accomplished in-hospital, with the administration of small, gradually reduced doses of a long-acting central nervous system depressant such as chlordiazepoxide, paraldehyde, or phenobarbital to suppress withdrawal symptoms. A marked craving for alcohol usually persists after detoxification, and patients will need a period of psychological support and assistance to avoid relapse into alcoholism.

Disulfiram (Antabuse) can occasionally be of assistance in maintaining abstinence from alcohol use. Disulfiram interferes with inactivation of alcohol, inducing accumulation of a toxic metabolite that is probably acetaldehyde. Alcohol ingestion in the presence of disulfiram elicits an unpleasant and at times hazardous reaction. Nausea, headache, dizziness, cutaneous vasodilation, hypertension, and tachycardia are characteristic. The rationale for such therapy is to provide negative conditioning or a perception that the results of alcohol consumption are not pleasant. Unfortunately, the disulfiram–alcohol interaction can also induce hypotension, coma, and death. Cardiovascular disease and psychiatric disorders contraindicate the use of disulfiram. This drug must be administered only to persons who willingly accept its use and have full knowledge of the potential severity of the consequences of concomitant alcohol consumption.

The opiate antagonist ***naltrexone*** (ReVia, Trexan) can reduce alcohol craving and consumption in abstinent alcohol-dependent persons. If opiate dependence coexists, naltrexone can precipitate withdrawal. Thus, persons should be opiate-free for several days (7 days for short-acting opiates, up to 14 days for those with longer durations of action) before naltrexone is given. Naltrexone should not be combined with disulfiram, as both can be hepatotoxic. Naltrexone may potentiate the central nervous system depressant action of the neuroleptic thioridazine.

Opiate Abuse

The pharmacology of the opiates is discussed under Narcotic Analgesics.

Because these drugs induce an intense euphoria, they are subject to abuse. Tolerance to the pleasurable responses, as well as physiological drug dependence, rapidly develop to drugs such as heroin, morphine, methadone, hydromorphone, meperidine, and other opiates. ''Designer drugs,'' similar in structure to the potent narcotic fentanyl, have the curious situation of being ''legal'' substances simply because their chemical structure is not specified as ''illegal.'' In addition to the usual dangers inherent in substance abuse, these drugs may contain contaminants such as 1-methyl-4-phenyl-1, 2, 3, 6-tetrahydropyridine (MPTP), which has induced parkinsonian destruction of dopaminergic neurons.

Withdrawal from opiate dependence can be unpleasant but is rarely as severe as that from alcohol. Fatigue, anxiety, nausea, drug craving, chills, and fever are characteristic. Detoxification is often accomplished by substituting methadone, which is orally effective and has a long duration of action, for the abused opiate. Stepwise reduction in methadone dosages keeps abstinence symptoms under control while allowing physiological mechanisms to readjust to a drug-free existence. Clonidine also has been used to manage opiate withdrawal symptoms. Clonidine is a centrally active antihypertensive agent whose site of action is at the presynaptic, α_2 adrenoceptor. It suppresses the autonomic symptoms of withdrawal.

Detoxification does not abolish the patient's craving for opiates, and the rate of recidivism among abusers is high. For some persons, methadone maintenance programs offer a more stable life-style. Methadone, itself an opiate, suppresses (or satisfies) drug craving and also blocks the euphoriant action of other opiates. L-alpha-acetyl-methadol (LAAM), a methadone analog, is available for maintenance treatment of opiate-dependent persons. It has much the same pharmacology and toxicology as methadone, but has a longer duration of action (*i.e.*, up to 72 hours compared with an average of 24 hours for methadone). Naltrexone, the orally active opiate antagonist having a long duration of action, also can be used to block the pleasurable aspects of opiate use.

Sedative–Hypnotic Abuse

Dependence upon barbiturates and other sedatives often begins with legitimate use of these agents (see discussion under Sedatives and Hypnotics). Psychological dependence on the calming or sleep-inducing effects fosters prolonged use and the development of physiological dependence. Overdose of hypnotics, not uncommonly with suicidal intent, can result in respiratory depression and failure. Withdrawal from dependence upon these drugs is similar to that from alcohol. Symptoms can be severe, and can be suppressed by gradual withdrawal of central nervous system depressant substances.

Antianxiety Drug Abuse

Benzodiazepines and related antianxiety agents produce both psychological and physiological dependence. In contrast to other central nervous system depressants, overdose of these drugs is not lethal unless other central nervous system depressants are ingested concurrently. Withdrawal symptoms from benzodiazepines such as diazepam and chlordiazepoxide may develop slowly, since these drugs have a long duration of action. Tremor and restlessness, often mistaken for return of anxiety, progress to seizures and delirium. As with other central nervous system depressants, dependence upon benzodiazepines is best managed by gradual reduction in drug dosage.

Psychostimulant Abuse

Central nervous system stimulants induce less pronounced physiological dependence than do the depressants. However, the intense euphoriant and energizing effects of drugs such as the amphetamines and cocaine promote marked and persistent drug craving. Termination of drug use can elicit depression, fatigue, and other subjective symptoms that may constitute a physiological withdrawal syndrome.

Amphetamines are used either orally or intravenously, and have a relatively prolonged duration of action. Intravenous abusers may carry out successive bouts of injection for several days without sleep or food. Restlessness, hyperthermia, increases in blood pressure and heart rate, psychotic episodes, cerebral hemorrhage, and convulsions can occur. Treatment of acute reactions involves supportive measures aimed at normalization of vital signs. An antipsychotic agent such as haloperidol can reduce agitation; urinary acidification promotes excretion of the weakly basic amphetamines.

Cocaine, in particular the free base (''crack''), has become a widely abused drug. The free base can be smoked to produce a rapid and intense but shortlived response that leaves the user craving additional drug. Physiological effects are similar to those of amphetamines: lethal dysrhythmias, myocardial infarction, and seizures can occur. Haloperidol (to control agitation), diazepam (to alleviate seizures), and antidysrhythmics all can be used in the management of cocaine reactions.

Psychotomimetic Abuse

Tetrahydrocannabinol (cannabis, contained in marijuana and hashish) is rapidly absorbed from pulmonary alveoli.

Euphoria; intoxication; drowsiness; alterations in auditory, visual, and time perception; failure of short-term memory; impairment of skilled behavior; hallucinations; and panic reactions are prominent central nervous system responses. Vasodilation, changes in blood pressure, and tachycardia occur. ''Bloodshot'' eyes are a hallmark of marijuana use. An ''amotivational syndrome,'' characterized by apathy and personality changes, has been attributed to this drug. Physiological dependence does not seem to develop, and little tolerance occurs. Controversy has long centered on the relative ''safety'' of marijuana abuse. Possible therapeutic usefulness of tetrahydrocannabinol has fostered development of a synthetic analogue, nabilone (Cesamet), for bronchodilation, antiemesis in antineoplastic therapy, and to decrease intraocular pressure in glaucoma. Tetrahydrocannabinol is available as Dronabinol.

Mescaline, an alkaloid derived from peyote, induces anxiety, tremors, nausea, and disturbed auditory and visual sensations.

Lysergic acid diethylamide (LSD) and an ''alphabet soup'' of related substances (DOM-STP, DMT, DET, MDA, MDMA, as well as psilocin and psilocybin) produce distortions in sensory awareness, hallucinations, euphoria or dysphoria, and panic, the latter often referred to as a ''bad trip.'' These substances are active in extremely small (microgram) amounts. Flashbacks to previous drug experiences commonly occur. Schizophreniform psychoses, transient and more prolonged, can be induced by these hallucinogens. Tolerance to drug effects is rapidly developed and rapidly lost. Physiological dependence does not occur; time intervals between drug experiences may be extensive. Panic and psychotic reactions can be subdued with phenothiazine administration.

Phencyclidine (PCP, angel dust) has been a widely abused drug despite its tendency to produce personality changes and severe toxic psychoses. This substance appears to interact with several central nervous system neurotransmitter systems. Characteristic reactions range from a comatose state to agitated, violent behavior. Convulsions, hyperthermia, anxiety, suicidal ideation, stereotyped activity, hallucinations, and mood alterations are a few of the unpredictable responses elicited by phencyclidine. Irrational behavior may put the drug user or those around him or her in imminent danger of harm. The most appropriate management of severe adverse reactions usually consists of supportive measures administered in an environment relatively free of sensory stimuli. Diazepam can alleviate agitation or seizures. Neuroleptic drugs may suppress psychotic behavior but can also induce marked hypertension. Barbiturates can cause extreme central nervous system depression, and thus should be avoided.

The nutmeg spice contains a hallucinogen thought to be myristicin. Ingestion of large amounts produces euphoria, hallucinations, and psychosis as well as anticholinergic responses such as tachycardia, dry mouth, and apprehension.

Anticholinergics have become drugs of abuse. Excessive ingestion of tricyclic antidepressants and antiparkinson cholinolytics, as well as of belladonna and related plant alkaloids, induces central nervous system responses of disorientation, confusion, and hallucinations. Coma, convulsions, dysrhythmias, and death may ensue. Physostigmine, discussed under Autonomic Drugs, can be used cautiously to reverse anticholinergic overdose.

Numerous volatile substances and gases have been inhaled for their euphoriant actions. Industrial solvents in a variety of preparations ranging from glues to typewriter correction fluid and lighter fluid are often toxic to bone marrow, renal, hepatic, brain, and myocardial cells. Fatal reactions are not uncommon.

In addition to the adverse reactions that can be elicited by abused drugs, further physiological detriment can arise from contaminants that are used to ''cut'' street drugs. Polydrug abuse is often present, together with infections induced by sharing of needles among IV drug users. This latter practice places persons at extreme risk for development of the acquired immune deficiency syndrome (AIDS).

QUESTIONS IN PHARMACOLOGY

Multiple-Choice Questions

ONE-ANSWER TYPE

1. Which of the following symptoms are alleviated by anticholinergic drugs?
   (a) Tardive dyskinesia
   (b) Parkinson symptoms
   (c) Both
   (d) Neither
2. Which of the following is (are) used only as a diagnostic agent in myasthenia gravis?
   (a) Edrophonium
   (b) Pyridostigmine
   (c) Both
   (d) Neither
3. Therapeutic doses of which of the following are associated with decreased heart rate at rest?
   (a) Propranolol
   (b) Pindolol
   (c) Both
   (d) Neither
4. The principal route for succinylcholine inactivation is a:
   (a) Mitochondrial enzyme
   (b) Microsomal enzyme

(c) Plasma enzyme
(d) Cytosolic enzyme
(e) None of the above

5. The principal route for epinephrine methylation is a:
(a) Mitochondrial enzyme
(b) Microsomal enzyme
(c) Plasma enzyme
(d) Cytosolic enzyme
(e) None of the above

6. The principal route for diazepam glucuronidation is a:
(a) Mitochondrial enzyme
(b) Microsomal enzyme
(c) Plasma enzyme
(d) Cytosolic enzyme
(e) None of the above

7. Which of the following is associated with chronic alcohol consumption?
(a) Depressed platelet function
(b) Hypertension
(c) Both
(d) Neither

8. Which of the following is the most serious and dose-limiting adverse effect of morphine?
(a) Extreme sedation
(b) Increased intracranial pressure
(c) Decreased respiration
(d) Decreased myocardial conductivity
(e) Decreased blood pressure

9. Which of the following statements about enflurane is *not* true?
(a) It is a halogenated compound.
(b) It sensitizes the myocardium to catecholamines less than halothane does.
(c) It undergoes more hepatic metabolism than halothane does.
(d) It potentiates nondepolarizing muscle relaxants.

10. Which property of β-blockers is unlikely to increase peripheral resistance?
(a) Selectivity towards β_1-adrenoceptor
(b) Intrinsic β-adrenoceptor stimulating activity
(c) Both
(d) Neither

11. Which property of β-blockers is unlikely to produce respiratory distress?
(a) Selectivity towards β_1-adrenoceptor
(b) Intrinsic β-adrenoceptor stimulating activity
(c) Both
(d) Neither

12. The most commonly used hypnotic agents are from which following class of drugs?
(a) Tricyclic antidepressants
(b) Monoamine oxidase inhibitors
(c) Phenothiazines
(d) Benzodiazepines
(e) Butyrophenones

13. An ideal general anesthetic would have all of the following properties *except:*
(a) Low blood gas solubility
(b) Nonflammable
(c) Primary hepatic elimination
(d) Muscle relaxation

14. Side effects of which of the following may include salivation and sweating?
(a) Physostigmine
(b) Pyridostigmine
(c) Both
(d) Neither

15. Which of the following is used as an antidote in tricyclic antidepressant overdose?
(a) Physostigmine
(b) Pyridostigmine
(c) Both
(d) Neither

16. Select the correct statement about nitrous oxide:
(a) It is an adequate surgical anesthetic by itself.
(b) It does not undergo biotransformation.
(c) It has no analgesic properties.
(d) It is rarely used in modern anesthesia techniques.

17. Injection of a drug *X* into an anesthetized dog increased blood pressure and decreased heart rate. Following bilateral vagotomy drug *X* elicited a pressor response without changes in heart rate. Drug *X* is probably:
(a) A ganglionic stimulant
(b) A sympathomimetic amine acting on α- and β-adrenoceptors
(c) A sympathomimetic amine acting only on α-adrenoceptors
(d) An indirect acting sympathomimetic amine

18. Which of the following is a veterinary anesthetic with hallucinogenic effects?
(a) Cannabis
(b) Cocaine
(c) Phencyclidine
(d) Mescaline
(e) MPTP (methylphenyltetrahydropyridine)

19. Which of the following is a psychedelic phenylethylamine derived from a mushroom?
(a) Cannabis
(b) Cocaine
(c) Phencyclidine
(d) Mescaline
(e) MPTP (methylphenyltetrahydropyridine)

20. Which of the following produces reddening of the conjunctiva and aggravation of angina pectoris?
(a) Cannabis
(b) Cocaine
(c) Phencyclidine
(d) Mescaline
(e) MPTP (methylphenyltetrahydropyridine)
21. Each of the following is an effective antidepressant drug *except:*
(a) Lithium
(b) Imipramine
(c) Phenelzine
(d) Desipramine
(e) Chlorpromazine
22. Which of the following drugs would have the shortest onset of action for its recommended indication?
(a) Diazepam
(b) Imipramine
(c) Amitriptyline
(d) Phenelzine
(e) Desipramine
23. Which of the following causes muscle paralysis by sustained depolarization of the post-junctional membrane?
(a) Pancuronium
(b) Atracurium
(c) Both
(d) Neither
24. Dosage adjustment is not required for the patient with renal dysfunction for which of the following?
(a) Pancuronium
(b) Atracurium
(c) Both
(d) Neither
25. For which of the following drugs are blood levels *routinely* determined for therapeutic purposes?
(a) Phenelzine
(b) Lithium
(c) Chlorpromazine
(d) Diazepam
(e) Flurazepam
26. Which of the following drugs has a short elimination half-life?
(a) Diazepam
(b) Oxazepam
(c) Both
(d) Neither
27. Dosage of which of the following drugs may have to be reduced during concomitant administration of cimetidine?
(a) Diazepam
(b) Oxazepam
(c) Both
(d) Neither
28. Which of the following has a low therapeutic index?
(a) Diazepam
(b) Oxazepam
(c) Both
(d) Neither
29. There is a high incidence of seizures during withdrawal from:
(a) Heroin
(b) Phenobarbital
(c) Both
(d) Neither
30. Tolerance and dependence develop with repeated use of:
(a) Heroin
(b) Phenobarbital
(c) Both
(d) Neither
31. Which of the following drugs has reduced effects in patients who chronically consume alcohol?
(a) Barbiturates
(b) Warfarin
(c) Both
(d) Neither
32. In an emergency room setting, which of the compounds listed below would probably be most useful in treating a drug overdose in a patient exhibiting coma, decreased respiration, and pinpoint pupils but no other remarkable signs?
(a) Amphetamine
(b) Diazepam
(c) Haloperidol
(d) Naloxone
(e) Atropine
33. Which of the following statements about pentazocine is *false?*
(a) It will not precipitate withdrawal in heroin addicts.
(b) It has fair oral bioavailability.
(c) It can cause dysphoria.
(d) It can cause respiratory depression.
(e) It possesses moderate analgesic activity.
34. Which of the following is *not* usually a therapeutic indication for the use of a strong narcotic agonist?
(a) Obstetrical pain
(b) Chronic ''low-back'' pain
(c) Dyspnea of pulmonary edema
(d) Myocardial infarction
(e) Cardiac surgery
35. Cardiac dysrhythmias caused by exogenous catecholamines are most commonly seen during anesthesia with:
(a) Enflurane
(b) Isoflurane

(c) Halothane
(d) Methoxyflurane
(e) Nitrous oxide

36. Diminution or prevention of reflex tachycardia is caused by:
(a) Ganglionic blockade
(b) β-Adrenoceptor blockade
(c) Both
(d) Neither

37. Diminution or prevention of reflex bradycardia is caused by:
(a) Ganglionic blockade
(b) β-Adrenoceptor blockade
(c) Both
(d) Neither

38. Diminution or prevention of norepinephrine pressor response is caused by:
(a) Ganglionic blockade
(b) β-Adrenoceptor blockade
(c) Both
(d) Neither

39. Cardiotoxic side effects are particularly associated with:
(a) Tricyclic antidepressants
(b) Lithium salts
(c) Both
(d) Neither

40. Drugs reaching plasma via which route of administration may first undergo extensive hepatic degradation?
(a) Intravenous
(b) Intramuscular
(c) Sublingual
(d) Oral
(e) Subcutaneous

41. Which of the following is associated with supersensitivity of dopamine receptors in the basal ganglia?
(a) Tardive dyskinesia
(b) Parkinsonlike syndrome
(c) Both
(d) Neither

42. Weight loss is associated with which of the following drugs?
(a) Chlorpromazine
(b) Fluoxetine
(c) Diazepam
(d) Imipramine

43. Which of the following is useful in treating nausea of cancer chemotherapy?
(a) Dronabinol
(b) Nabilone
(c) Both
(d) Neither

44. Antipsychotics such as haloperidol are useful in treating toxic psychoses produced by:
(a) Amphetamine
(b) Cocaine
(c) Both
(d) Neither

45. Which drugs are effective in the absence of a functioning adrenal gland?
(a) Cortisone
(b) Dexamethasone
(c) Both
(d) Neither

46. Which of the following drugs acts through the release of formaldehyde in the urinary tract?
(a) Nitrofurantoin
(b) Ammonium chloride
(c) Methenamine
(d) Nalidixic acid
(e) None of the above

47. Which of the following is used to diminish heroin withdrawal symptoms?
(a) Clonidine
(b) Naloxone
(c) Both
(d) Neither

48. Which of the following causes decreased release of arachidonic acid from phospholipids?
(a) Glucocorticoids
(b) Aspirin
(c) Both
(d) Neither

49. Which of the following causes depressed formation of leukotrienes?
(a) Glucocorticoids
(b) Aspirin
(c) Both
(d) Neither

50. Which of the following causes depressed formation of prostaglandins?
(a) Glucocorticoids
(b) Aspirin
(c) Both
(d) Neither

51. Which of the following drugs is most likely to produce cardiac failure?
(a) Quinidine
(b) Diltiazen
(c) Procainamide
(d) Digoxin
(e) Phenytoin

52. Which of the following drugs may produce "paradoxical tachycardia"?
(a) Quinidine
(b) Diltiazem

(c) Procainamide
(d) Digoxin
(e) Phenytoin

53. Which of the following may result in a drug-induced lupus-erythematosus-like syndrome?
(a) Quinidine
(b) Diltiazem
(c) Procainamide
(d) Digoxin
(e) Phenytoin

54. Which of the following drugs exerts an inotropic effect via inhibition of phosphodiesterase?
(a) Aminophylline
(b) Amrinone
(c) Both
(d) Neither

55. Propranolol antagonizes the cardiac inotropic effect of which of the following drugs?
(a) Aminophylline
(b) Amrinone
(c) Both
(d) Neither

56. Which of the following may induce methemoglobinemia and hemolysis when administered to a subject with glucose-6-phosphate-dehydrogenase-deficient erythrocytes?
(a) Primaquine
(b) Sulfonamides
(c) Both
(d) Neither

57. Fat-soluble vitamins:
(a) Cause overdosage toxicity
(b) Are stored in liver
(c) Both
(d) Neither

58. Deficiency of which of the following substances causes the disease beriberi?
(a) Vitamin E
(b) Vitamin A
(c) Thiamine
(d) Nicotinic acid
(e) None of the above

59. Dose-limiting toxicity of anthracycline antitumor agents such as doxorubicin (Adriamycin) may be manifested as:
(a) Myelosuppression
(b) Congestive heart failure
(c) Nausea, vomiting
(d) Rashes
(e) Anaphylaxis

60. The increased usefulness of amoxicillin and clavulanic acid combinations is due to the fact that they:
(a) May be used safely in patients allergic to other penicillins
(b) Are better absorbed when taken orally
(c) Are effective against *Pseudomonas aeruginosa* infections
(d) Are effective against penicillinase-producing microorganisms
(e) None of the above

61. Prior to sensitivity studies, the most reasonable choice of an antibiotic to treat a *Staphylococcus aureus* infection acquired outside of the hospital would be:
(a) Oxacillin
(b) Penicillin G
(c) Ampicillin
(d) Carbenicillin
(e) Amoxicillin

62. The treatment of choice for a patient with Legionnaires' disease is:
(a) Penicillin G
(b) Cefotaxime
(c) Chloramphenicol
(d) Erythromycin
(e) Amikacin

63. Which of the following reduces blood pressure via suppression of angiotensin II formation?
(a) Captopril
(b) Propranolol
(c) Clonidine
(d) Guanethidine
(e) None of the above

64. Which of the following has antihypertensive effects associated with blockade of α-adrenoceptors?
(a) Captopril
(b) Propranolol
(c) Clonidine
(d) Guanethidine
(e) None of the above

65. Abrupt withdrawal of which of the following drugs may be accompanied by severe blood pressure elevation?
(a) Captopril
(b) Hydralazine
(c) Clonidine
(d) Hydrochlorothiazide
(e) None of the above

66. A patient receiving timolol and epinephrine instillation into the eye for glaucoma experienced dizziness associated with hypertension. The most likely explanation for this event is that timolol:
(a) Increased the release of norepinephrine
(b) Unmasked epinephrine's pressor response
(c) Prevented the urinary excretion of epinephrine

(d) Increased the activity of the enzymes monoamine oxidase and catechol-o-methyl transferase
(e) None of the above

67. Pseudomembranous colitis is believed to be due to a toxin produced by *Clostridium difficile*. Appropriate treatment of this condition would be:
(a) Intravenous vancomycin
(b) Intramuscular vancomycin
(c) Oral vancomycin
(d) Intravenous clindamycin
(e) Oral clindamycin

68. Which of the following statements about therapeutic doses of verapamil in *not* correct?
(a) Verapamil diminishes conduction velocity through the A-V node.
(b) Verapamil is used in the management of supraventricular tachycardia.
(c) Verapamil increases coronary blood flow by dilating coronary arteries.
(d) Verapamil has a positive inotropic effect.
(e) Verapamil has a negative chronotropic effect.

69. Neurotoxicity may be dose limiting for:
(a) 5-Fluorouracil
(b) Vincristine
(c) Doxorubicin (Adriamycin)
(d) Methotrexate
(e) Bleomycin

70. Which pharmacological action of hydralazine causes reduction of blood pressure in hypertensive patients?
(a) Increased renin release
(b) Enhanced inotropism
(c) Direct vasodilation
(d) Blockade of α-adrenoceptors
(e) Diminished sympathetic activity

71. Which of the following is one of the earliest dose-related signs or symptoms of aspirin toxicity in the adult?
(a) Respiratory depression
(b) Reye's syndrome
(c) Metabolic acidosis
(d) Tinnitus

72. Which of the following acts in the CNS?
(a) Clonidine
(b) Prazosin
(c) Both
(d) Neither

73. Which of the following promotes salt and water excretion?
(a) Clonidine
(b) Prazosin
(c) Both
(d) Neither

74. Which of the following inhibits norepinephrine release?
(a) Clonidine
(b) Prazosin
(c) Both
(d) Neither

75. Which of the following causes an initial syncopal reaction?
(a) Clonidine
(b) Prazosin
(c) Both
(d) Neither

76. Which of the following promotes uric acid excretion?
(a) Chlorothiazide
(b) Probenecid
(c) Allopurinol
(d) Furosemide
(e) None of the above

77. The drug of choice for type II hyperlipoproteinemia is:
(a) Nicotinic acid
(b) Gemfibrozil
(c) Cholestryramine
(d) D-Thyroxine

78. *N*-Acetylcysteine would be indicated for treatment of an overdose of which of the following?
(a) Aspirin
(b) Ibuprofen
(c) Acetaminophen
(d) Diflunisal
(e) Naproxen

79. A serious toxic effect associated with clozapine is:
(a) Nephrotoxicity
(b) Cardiotoxicity
(c) Agranulocytosis
(d) Hypertensive crisis

80. Nerve gases such as sarin and tabun are inhibitors of the enzyme:
(a) Acetylcholinesterase
(b) Monoamine oxidase
(c) Catechol-O-methyl transferase
(d) Choline acetyl transferase

81. Which of the following is used in the management of obsessive-compulsive disorder?
(a) Chlorpromazine
(b) Clozapine
(c) Clomipramine
(d) Cyclazocine

82. The combination of fluoxetine and a monoamine oxidase inhibitor:
(a) Increases antidepressant activity
(b) Decreases antidepressant activity

(c) Can be a potentially lethal interaction
(d) Causes no reported interaction

83. Selegiline is useful in Parkinson's disease because it inhibits:
(a) Dopamine metabolism
(b) Dopamine synthesis
(c) Acetylcholine metabolism
(d) Acetylcholine synthesis

84. Which nonsteroidal anti-inflammatory drug is available in IV formulation?
(a) Diclofenac
(b) Flurbiprofen
(c) Mefenamic acid
(d) Ketorolac

85. An H_1-receptor antihistamine reported not to cross the blood–brain barrier is:
(a) Astemizole
(b) Diphenhydramine
(c) Tripelennamine
(d) None of the above

86. Omeprazole is useful in the management of peptic ulcer disease because it:
(a) Blocks H_2 histamine receptors
(b) Inhibits the H^+/K^+ proton pump
(c) Neutralizes gastric acid
(d) Is anticholinergic

87. Hypercalcemia associated with neoplastic disease can be alleviated with:
(a) Gallium
(b) Ondansetron
(c) Idarubicin
(d) Carboplatin

88. The preferred drug for Lyme disease in children under age 8 years is:
(a) Tetracycline
(b) Erythromycin
(c) Amoxicillin
(d) Ceftriaxone

89. Foscarnet is effective against:
(a) Human immunodeficiency virus
(b) Herpes virus
(c) Hepatitis virus
(d) All of the above

90. Flumazenil reverses the sedation caused by:
(a) Lorazepam
(b) Meperidine
(c) Both
(d) Neither

91. Tacrine is indicated in the management of:
(a) Cholinergic crisis
(b) Alzheimer's disease
(c) Both
(d) Neither

92. The action of succinylcholine, compared with most nondepolarizing neuromuscular junction blockers, is best described as:
(a) Slower onset and longer duration
(b) Slower onset and shorter duration
(c) Faster onset and longer duration
(d) Faster onset and shorter duration

93. Multiple sclerosis symptoms may be alleviated by:
(a) Interferon-alfa
(b) Interferon beta-Ib
(c) Both
(d) Neither

94. Which of the following statements regarding risperidone is *not* true?
(a) May have slower onset of action than other neuroleptics
(b) May have decreased risk for tardive dyskinesia
(c) May cause sedation and orthostasis
(d) May be more effective in alleviating negative symptoms of schizophrenia.

95. Which of the following general anesthetics provides the most rapid induction?
(a) Desflurane
(b) Halothane
(c) Methoxyflurane
(d) All have equal rate of induction

96. The narcotic analgesic that is biotransformed to a long-acting metabolite with central nervous system toxicity is:
(a) Morphine
(b) Codeine
(c) Tramadol
(d) Meperidine

97. In persons who are physiologically dependent upon opiates, which narcotic antagonists will precipitate the abstinence syndrome?
(a) Pure antagonists
(b) Mixed antagonists
(c) Both
(d) Neither

98. Myopathy is a characteristic adverse effect of which hypolipemic drug?
(a) Lovastatin
(b) Cholestyramine
(c) Both
(d) Neither

99. Which of the following blocks angiotensin binding to receptors?
(a) Losartan
(b) Captopril
(c) Nifedipine
(d) Verapamil

100. The drug of choice for treating Lyme disease in adults is:
   (a) Chloramphenicol
   (b) Gentamicin
   (c) Doxycycline
   (d) Loracarbef
101. Which drug can increase the risk for vincristine neuropathy?
   (a) Methotrexate
   (b) Pegaspargase
   (c) Teniposide
   (d) Finasteride
102. Which is the shortest time interval that antitubercular drugs should be administered to persons infected with nonresistant mycobacteria?
   (a) Six days
   (b) Six weeks
   (c) Six months
   (d) Six years
103. Which antimicrobial increases the risk of ventricular dysrhythmias when given concurrently with astemizole or terfenidine?
   (a) Penicillin G
   (b) Ketoconazole
   (c) Isoniazid
   (d) Ciprofloxacin
104. Which antimicrobials cause erosion of cartilage in young animals?
   (a) Fluoroquinolones
   (b) Cephalosporins
   (c) Macrolides
   (d) Aminoglycosides
105. Which of the following statements regarding metformin is *not* correct?
   (a) Increases cellular uptake of glucose
   (b) Replaces insulin in the management of diabetes
   (c) Has lower risk for hypoglycemia than sulfonylureas
   (d) Can cause lactic acidosis
106. Which of the following statements regarding finasteride is *not* correct?
   (a) It can ameliorate prostatic hypertrophy.
   (b) Pregnant women should avoid all contact with this drug.
   (c) Increased libido can be a side effect.
   (d) It can interfere with screening for prostate cancer.
107. Which of the following may decrease myocardial damage of doxorubicin?
   (a) Leucovorin factor
   (b) Tacrolimus
   (c) Dexrazoxane
   (d) Vinorelbine

MULTIPLE TRUE-FALSE

From the list following the question, select all of the correct items and match them to the answer according to the following list:

A. If *only 1, 2, and 3* are correct
B. If *only 1 and 3* are correct
C. If *only 2 and 4* are correct
D. If *only 4* is correct
E. If *all* are correct

108. In which of the following conditions should narcotics be used with extreme caution or not at all?
   1. Head injury
   2. Pulmonary edema of left ventricular failure
   3. Emphysema
   4. Myocardial infarction
109. Sublingual administration of drugs:
   1. Results in the rapid achievement of therapeutic blood levels
   2. Is limited only to drugs that are not lipid soluble
   3. Is useful for drugs that are metabolized in the gastrointestinal tract
   4. Results primarily in effects to the brain
110. Benzodiazepines:
   1. Enhance the inhibitory actions of GABA, one of the brain's major inhibitory neurotransmitters
   2. Show cross-tolerance and cross-dependence with alcohol
   3. Are the most widely prescribed psychotherapeutic drugs
   4. Are effective in the treatment of most forms of depression.
111. Opiates produce their analgesic effects by:
   1. Inhibiting CNS pathways transmitting pain stimuli
   2. Inhibiting the sensitivity of peripheral pain receptors to chemical and physical stimuli
   3. Blunting the emotional reaction to pain stimuli
   4. Nonspecific inhibition of sensory pathways
112. These drugs may produce urinary retention.
   1. Belladonna alkaloids
   2. Tricyclic antidepressants
   3. Antihistamines
   4. Antipsychotic drugs
113. These drugs are useful in treating motion sickness.
   1. Belladonna alkaloids
   2. Tricyclic antidepressants
   3. Antihistamines
   4. Antipsychotic drugs
114. Carbamazepine is effective in the therapy of:
   1. Tonic–clonic convulsions
   2. Trigeminal neuralgia

3. Manic depressive disorder
4. Absence seizures

115. The adrenergic–neuronal blocking agent, guanethidine, should not be administered to patients receiving MAO inhibitors because:
    1. Central effects of guanethidine antagonize MAO action.
    2. Guanethidine will prevent the storage of MAO inhibitors.
    3. Guanethidine will prevent the metabolism of MAO inhibitors.
    4. Guanethidine may elicit a pressor response.
116. Patients with myasthenia gravis frequently exhibit:
    1. Improved muscle tone following the edrophonium test
    2. Decremental muscle response to repetitive nerve stimulation
    3. Antibodies to acetylcholine receptors
    4. High levels of plasma cholinesterase
117. Tardive dyskinesia is:
    1. Effectively controlled with benztropine
    2. A consequence of blocking the reuptake of dopamine by neurons in the basal ganglia
    3. Rapidly produced by all antipsychotic drugs
    4. Rarely reversible
118. Treatment for major depression includes:
    1. Electroconvulsive therapy (ECT)
    2. Methylphenidate
    3. Tranylcypromine
    4. Amphetamine
119. Lithium's side effects include:
    1. Constipation
    2. Tremor
    3. Weight loss
    4. Polyuria
120. Less muscle relaxant is required during anesthesia with:
    1. Nitrous oxide
    2. Enflurane
    3. Halothane
    4. Isoflurane
121. Drug combinations expected to have synergistic antibacterial actions include:
    1. Penicillin G and streptomycin
    2. Carbenecillin and gentamycin
    3. Trimethoprim and sulfamethoxazole
    4. Penicillin G and tetracycline
122. Overdose with which of the following analgesics is likely to produce coma, pinpoint pupils, and respiratory depression?
    1. Ibuprofen
    2. Meperidine
    3. Acetaminophen
    4. Morphine
123. Warfarinlike drugs:
    1. Are highly bound to plasma protein
    2. Reduce antithrombin III levels
    3. Interfere with the action of vitamin K
    4. Block the synthesis of thromboxane A_2
124. Which of the following is used in the treatment of supraventricular tachydysrhythmias?
    1. Digoxin
    2. Phenytoin
    3. Quinidine
    4. Lidocaine
125. Which of the following is used as a prophylactic against the occurrence of severe ventricular dysrhythmias following a myocardial infarction?
    1. Digoxin
    2. Phenytoin
    3. Quinidine
    4. Lidocaine
126. Which of the following drugs has (have) a high addiction liability?
    1. Barbiturates
    2. LSD (lysergic acid diethylamide)
    3. Meperidine
    4. PCP (phencyclidine)
127. Valproic acid:
    1. May produce hepatotoxicity
    2. Is used in the treatment of status epilepticus
    3. May raise plasma phenobarbital levels if chronically coadministered
    4. Is linked to a high incidence of gingival hyperplasia.
128. The signs and symptoms of withdrawal from physiological dependence on opiates include:
    1. Runny nose
    2. Hyperthermia
    3. Diarrhea
    4. Pupillary constriction
129. Chronic administration of which of the following may result in psychological dependence?
    1. Temazepam
    2. Lorazepam
    3. Oxazepam
    4. Chlordiazepoxide
130. Basic mechanisms of antimicrobial action include:
    1. Inhibition of bacterial cell wall synthesis
    2. Inhibition of bacterial protein synthesis
    3. Disruption of bacterial cell membranes
    4. Inhibition of nucleic acid synthesis
131. Which of the following is effective in reducing systemic heavy metal intoxication?
    1. Deferoxamine
    2. Calcium disodium edetate

3. Dimercaprol
4. Penicillamine

132. Which drug is useful in the treatment of Wilson's disease?
1. Deferoxamine
2. Calcium disodium edetate
3. Dimercaprol
4. Penicillamine

133. Which of the following could be expected in a case of severe aspirin overdose in a child?
1. Metabolic acidosis
2. Decreased respiration
3. Delirium, convulsions
4. Respiratory acidosis

134. Which of the following produces salt and water retention?
1. Clonidine
2. Hydralazine
3. Guanethidine
4. Minoxidil

135. Antihistamines associated with potentially lethal ventricular dysrhythmias are:
1. Cimetidine
2. Astemizole
3. Diphenhydramine
4. Terfenadine

136. Selective serotonin reuptake inhibitors include:
1. Fluoxetine
2. Sertraline
3. Paroxetine
4. Pargyline

137. The "serotonin syndrome" includes:
1. Delirium
2. Convulsions
3. Coma
4. Hypothermia

138. The "serotonin syndrome" is most likely to occur when selective serotonin reuptake inhibitors are given concurrently with:
1. Tricyclic antidepressants
2. Benzodiazepines
3. Phenothiazines
4. Monoamine oxidase inhibitors

139. Which of the following can induce folic acid deficiency?
1. Valproate
2. Lamotrigine
3. Carbamazepine
4. Phenytoin

140. Which of the following slow the rate of inactivation of lamotrigine?
1. Carbamazepine
2. Phenytoin
3. Phenobarbital
4. Valproate

141. Acetaminophen has similar efficacy to aspirin for which of the following effects?
1. Antipyretic
2. Anti-inflammatory
3. Analgesic
4. Antiplatelet

142. Drugs useful in the management of congestive heart failure include:
1. Angiotensin converting enzyme inhibitors
2. Beta-adrenergic blockers
3. Nitroprusside
4. Amrinone

143. Adverse effects of paclitaxel include:
1. Hypersensitivity
2. Granulocytopenia
3. Hair loss
4. Heart block

144. Which of the following can cause hyperkalemia?
1. Nifedipine
2. Triamterene
3. Cholestyramine
4. Quinapril

Identification Questions

Identify the item listed in questions 145–150 according to the following list:

A. If *only 1, 2, and 3* are correct

B. If *only 1 and 3* are correct

C. If *only 2 and 4* are correct

D. If *only 4* is correct

E. If *all* are correct

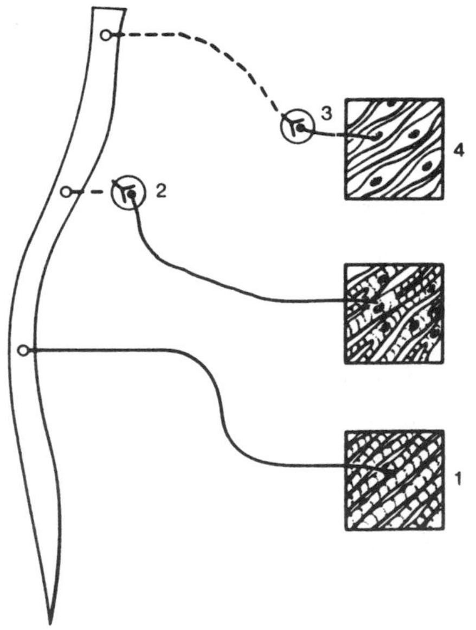

145. Acetylcholine release
146. Muscarinic receptors
147. Nicotinic receptors
148. Atropine inhibition

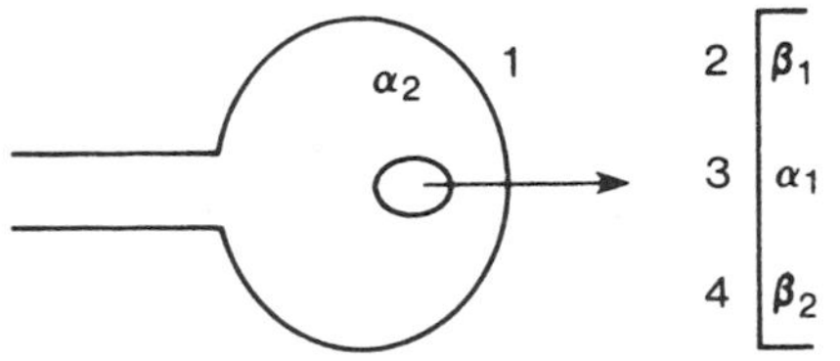

149. Epinephrine
150. Isoproterenol

Select the most appropriate choice for each question.

The following diagram presents the relationship between the recorded contraction of bronchial smooth muscle and the dose of injected acetylcholine (ACh). Identify drugs I and II from the list of choices.

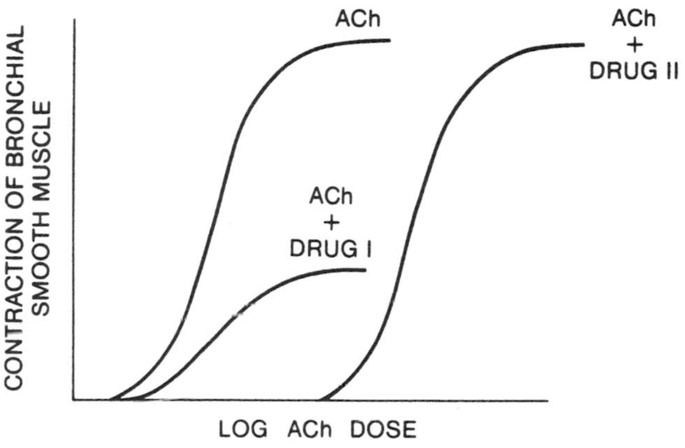

151. Drug I is:
   (a) Histamine
   (b) Atropine
   (c) Pilocarpine
   (d) Epinephrine
   (e) D-Tubocurarine
152. Drug II is:
   (a) Histamine
   (b) Atropine
   (c) Pilocarpine
   (d) Epinephrine
   (e) D-Tubocurarine

The following figure presents the relationship between heart rate and drug concentration in a vagotomized dog. Drug I is epinephrine. Identify drugs II, III, and IV from the list of choices.

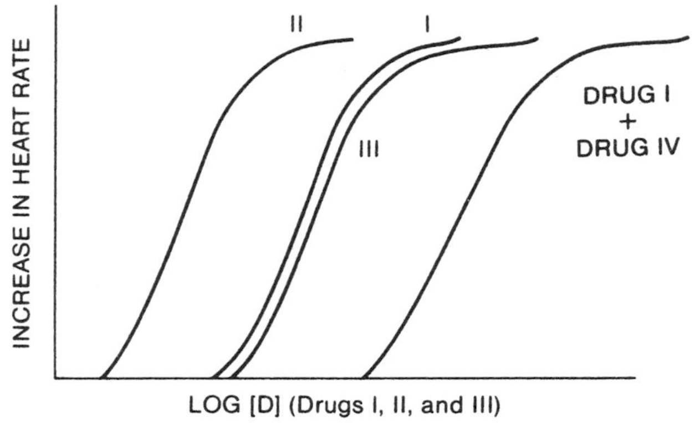

153. Drug II is:
   (a) Norepinephrine
   (b) Phenylephrine
   (c) Isoproterenol
   (d) Propranolol
   (e) None of the above
154. Drug III is:
   (a) Norepinephrine
   (b) Phenylephrine
   (c) Isoproterenol
   (d) Propranolol
   (e) None of the above
155. Drug IV is:
   (a) Norepinephrine
   (b) Phenylephrine
   (c) Isoproterenol
   (d) Propranolol
   (c) None of the above

ANSWERS TO PHARMACOLOGY QUESTIONS

1. b	**22.** a	**43.** c	**64.** e
2. a	**23.** d	**44.** c	**65.** c
3. a	**24.** b	**45.** c	**66.** b
4. c	**25.** b	**46.** c	**67.** c
5. d	**26.** b	**47.** a	**68.** d
6. b	**27.** c	**48.** a	**69.** b
7. c	**28.** d	**49.** a	**70.** c
8. c	**29.** b	**50.** c	**71.** d
9. c	**30.** c	**51.** b	**72.** a
10. c	**31.** c	**52.** a	**73.** d
11. c	**32.** d	**53.** c	**74.** a
12. d	**33.** a	**54.** c	**75.** b
13. c	**34.** b	**55.** d	**76.** b
14. c	**35.** c	**56.** c	**77.** c
15. a	**36.** c	**57.** c	**78.** c
16. b	**37.** a	**58.** c	**79.** c
17. c	**38.** d	**59.** b	**80.** a
18. c	**39.** c	**60.** d	**81.** c
19. d	**40.** d	**61.** a	**82.** c
20. a	**41.** a	**62.** d	**83.** a
21. e	**42.** b	**63.** a	**84.** d

85. a	**94.** a	**103.** b	**112.** E	**121.** A	**130.** E	**139.** D	**148.** D
86. b	**95.** a	**104.** a	**113.** B	**122.** C	**131.** E	**140.** D	**149.** E
87. a	**96.** d	**105.** b	**114.** A	**123.** B	**132.** D	**141.** B	**150.** C
88. c	**97.** c	**106.** c	**115.** D	**124.** B	**133.** B	**142.** E	**151.** d
89. b	**98.** a	**107.** c	**116.** A	**125.** D	**134.** E	**143.** E	**152.** b
90. a	**99.** a	**108.** B	**117.** D	**126.** B	**135.** C	**144.** C	**153.** c
91. b	**100.** c	**109.** B	**118.** B	**127.** B	**136.** A	**145.** E	**154.** a
92. d	**101.** c	**110.** A	**119.** C	**128.** A	**137.** A	**146.** D	**155.** d
93. b	**102.** c	**111.** B	**120.** C	**129.** E	**138.** D	**147.** A	

Rypins' Basic Sciences Review, 17th Edition,
edited by Edward D. Frohlich. Lippincott–Raven Publishers,
Philadelphia © 1997.

8

Behavioral Sciences

Ronald S. Krug, Ph.D.
David Ross Boyd Professor and
Interim Chairman
Department of Psychiatry and
Behavioral Sciences
University of Oklahoma Health Sciences Center
Oklahoma City, Oklahoma

INTRODUCTION

Behavioral Sciences Defined

Behavioral sciences is defined as the science of behavior. Because it is not the "art" of behavior, this topic belongs in the basic sciences section of medical education preparatory to the study of the clinical art of medicine.

It shares with other sciences use of the ***scientific method,*** or the generation of hypotheses about its content and the methodology for testing those hypotheses. The scientific method is a self-correcting style of thinking and inquiry. That is, from curiosity about and observation of the world, a general theory of how an event occurs is formulated. Hypotheses are then generated to test aspects of the theory, and, using appropriate controlled research design, the hypotheses are tested for their validity. Results are used to refine the theory, with the goal of replacing theoretical formulation with established fact.

The "behavioral" portion of behavioral sciences does *not* reflect the influence from the ***behaviorism*** school of psychology, which posited, "if you can't see it or measure it, it doesn't exist." The basic parameters of mental behavior, particularly as they contribute to the practice of medicine, are legitimate concerns for scientific study. These include thought processes, thought content, subjective emotional state, and perceptual phenomena. The static personality structure of individuals (their traits) as well as varying adaptations to fluctuating internal and external states (the ***dynamic*** aspects of human behavior) are also valid foci of scientific investigation. Also included are those phenomena that are expressions of the "collective man," such as society, culture, subculture, and mores.

Behavioral sciences in medical education is a body of knowledge that is continually argued and refined. A consensus of content is found in the publications of the Association of Behavioral Sciences in Medical Education (ABSAME) and in the constituency of the Behavioral Sciences committees of the National Board of Medical Examiners. Both have representation from throughout the United States and operate from the studied and organized conglomeration of data supplied by its changing membership. The academic discipline sources are varied. From the basic sciences of biochemistry, genetics, pharmacology, and physiology come data loosely termed behavioral biology, which is the relationship between molecular events and human behavior. From the social sciences of anthropology and sociology come cultural, group, and social system influences, and from psychology comes the information about abnormal behavior, assessment of behavior, developmental processes, personality, psycholinguistics, and psychophysiology.

Behavioral sciences has wide application to all of the subdivisions of medicine. Sabshin indicated, "Patients with psychiatric problems constitute a major portion of the work load for those ... in general medical practice.... More patients with mental illness are treated by health professionals than by mental health professionals...." The Institute of Medicine of the National Academy of Science reported that in a given year 60% of the mentally ill are seen by nonpsychiatric physicians, 20% are seen by mental health professionals, and 20% are seen by no one. Rakel reported psychofamilial patient problems as the third most common difficulty encountered in a family physician's office. Large-scale studies have validated the finding that 50% to 60% of adults randomly sampled report psychophysiologic symptomatology. Other large-scale studies have agreed that up to 80% of the American population is moderately to severely impaired by mental disorders (Midtown Manhattan Study) and a more recent NIMH survey (Kaplan and Sadock, 1991) documents a rate of 32.2% of diagnosable mental disorders in the general population. Obviously, it would be erroneous and perhaps dangerous to misconstrue behavioral sciences as simply, and only, an introduction to psychiatry.

Integration of Behavioral Sciences and Psychiatry

While we have noted that behavioral sciences is not an introduction to psychiatry, there are two practical ties between these fields. The first is academic history. For the most part, behavioral sciences was introduced through departments of psychiatry in medical schools. The second is an apparent similarity of content. Within behavioral sciences is a subsection of "abnormal behavior." Obviously, the diagnosis, intervention, and follow-up of many of these conditions are within the purview of psychiatry, not behavioral sciences. It should be remembered that the predisposers, precipitators, and maintainers of abnormal behavior may be orthogonal phenomena that call for different strategies. For example, a person may be genetically predisposed to alcoholism; however, that individual may begin to drink only because of the death of a child and continue to drink because of biochemical addiction to the drug. The genetic predisposition would have required genetic counseling, the precipitating stress would have required grief and bereavement work that provided more available and attractive alternatives than alcohol, and the biochemical addiction would demand medical detoxification from this class of depressant compounds. Some of these activities are the legitimate domain of behavioral scientists, and all are within the scope of the practicing physician regardless of medical specialty. It is only through applied research that the issues and answers surrounding predisposers, precipitators, and maintainers can be addressed.

RESEARCH METHODOLOGIES FOR THE STUDY OF HUMAN BEHAVIOR

Statistical Distributions

In research, a statement of significant difference is made based on statistical probabilities. The statement that the results are significant at the 0.05 level means that by chance alone the results are expected 5 times out of 100. The often-quoted statement should be remembered, "Statistics are like a light pole—they can be used for support as does the drunk or to illuminate a given area as does the sober person."

DISTRIBUTION STATISTICS

There are various statistics that describe the distribution of events (*i.e.*, scores). The major ones are measures of central tendency and measures of variation. The measures of central tendency are the ***mean*** ($\overline{X}$), the arithmetic average of all individual scores; the ***mode,*** the most frequent score; and the ***median,*** the point above and below which 50% of scores occur. For normal distributions, these are all the same point. One of the measures of variation is ***standard deviation*** (SD), the mathematical expression of the variability of all scores around the mean. Usually plus-and-minus-1 SD is considered to be "normal variation"; for example, if the mean IQ score is 100 and the SD is 10, then "normal" scores would be 90 through 110. ***Variance,*** the standard deviation squared, and ***range,*** the highest to the lowest scores of a distribution, are two other measures of variation.

NORMAL DISTRIBUTION

The ***normal distribution*** is the "bell-shaped" curve, which has been used to describe human traits. The curve is presented below. The percentage figures given in this diagram reflect the proportion of events that fall within a given standard deviation of the curve. Abnormality is defined as the amount of deviation from the mean or statistical average, not by social agreement.

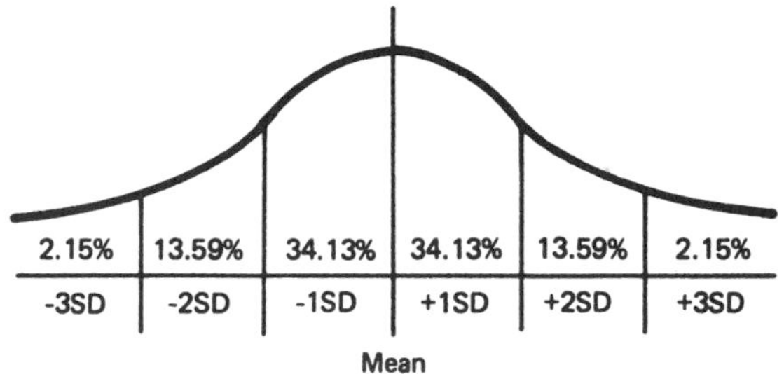

IRREGULAR DISTRIBUTIONS

Other distributions that do not have a "bell-shaped" or normal curve are:

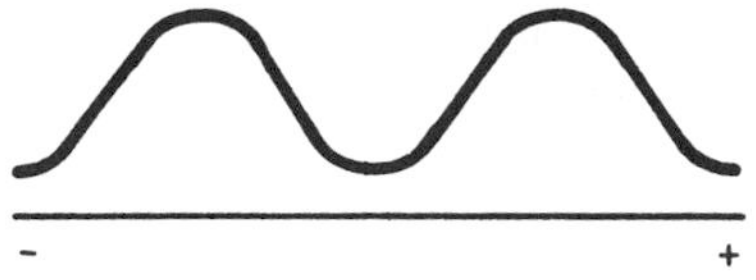

Bimodal

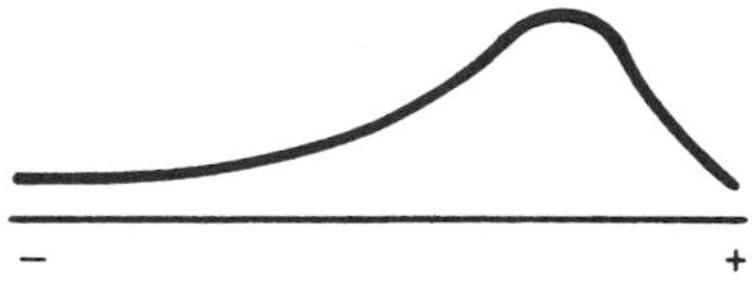

Skewed-negative

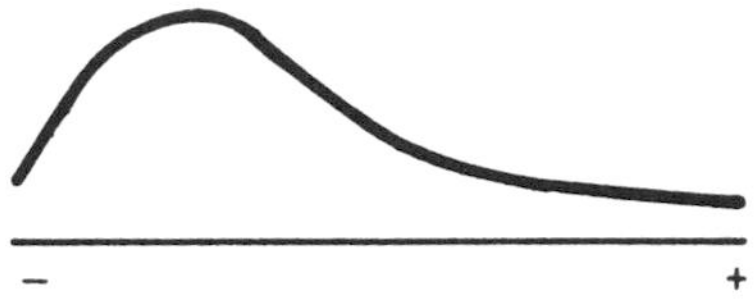

Skewed-positive

Skewed distributions are named in terms of their "tail."

Research Concepts

CONTROL GROUPS

Control groups are the core of experimental designs. These are groups that are as identical as possible to the experimental group upon which experimentation is done and only differ in the experimental treatment being applied. There are two major types of control groups.

No-treatment control groups are used, for example, with pathologic groups. In this design, the control group does not get an investigational treatment. After treatment is applied to the experimental group, the two groups are compared for improvement in the treated group. Use of such a design helps examine treatment efficacy relative to spontaneous remission rates.

Same-subject control groups are those in which measurement on the criterion of change is taken before a treatment is applied and again after the treatment. Scores are examined for significance of change. This design helps control extraneous factors, which might arise from using a matched control design of totally independent persons.

INDEPENDENT AND DEPENDENT VARIABLES

Independent variables are those that are manipulated (*e.g.*, a given medication). ***Dependent*** variables are those that reflect the effects of the independent variable (*e.g.*, decrease in a febrile condition after a certain medicine is administered).

VALIDITY

Validity refers to the true accuracy of the observed experimental effect. Using the above illustration, if the febrile condition decreased, was it the effect of the medication or the differential time of day the temperature reading was taken? Generally, cross validation of an experimenter's results by independent researchers is required before a given conclusion is accepted as valid.

RELIABILITY

Reliability means the regularity with which the phenomenon can be reproduced. Using the example from above, does the medication reduce the febrile condition 100% of the time it is administered or 50% of the time?

TRUE AND FALSE POSITIVES AND NEGATIVES

The concepts of true and false positives and negatives refer to the issue of accuracy of test results and are tied to the issues of sensitivity and specificity (below).

True positive: pathology present and results positive
True negative: pathology absent and results negative
False positive: pathology absent and results positive
False negative: pathology present and results negative

SENSITIVITY

Sensitivity is applied to a test of a given entity. A test is sensitive if it correctly picks up the *presence* of pathology in persons who have the pathology, a true positive. Sensitivity is expressed as a percentage. It is equal to the number of true positives divided by the number of true positives plus false negatives, multiplied by 100.

SPECIFICITY

Specificity is defined as the ability of a test to pick up the *absence* of pathology in a person who does not have the pathology, a true negative. Specificity is also expressed as a percentage. It is equal to the number of true negatives divided by the number of true negatives plus false positives, multiplied by 100.

EPIDEMIOLOGICAL CONCEPTS

Special statistics related to rates of occurrence of a phenomenon in a given population or sample from the entire population are important in behavioral sciences. There are four major epidemiologic statistics. ***Incidence*** is the rate of new cases of a phenomenon in a given group of persons. ***Prevalence*** is the rate of all cases of a phenomenon in a group. ***Morbidity*** is the ratio of the number of ill persons to the total population of a community. ***Mortality*** is the death rate in a given population.

Research Designs

The manner in which data are collected on a given research topic constitutes the research design.

LONGITUDINAL

Longitudinal studies track the same group of subjects over an extended time period. Periodic observations are made and changes in the group over time are tested for significance of change or are related through correlational statistics. This design can incorporate ''no-treatment'' or ''same-subject'' control groups and is employed when unpredictable extrapersonal events, like a world war, may confound results.

A special form of longitudinal study is the treatment follow-up design; for example, after patients have received a given treatment, does the treatment last or is it a temporary phenomenon? This is a particularly relevant research question when the treatment is expensive in physician's time, financial cost, or social–personal consequences.

CROSS-SECTIONAL

Cross-sectional designs examine different groups at various levels of a given variable all at the same time and compare the different groups for a given effect. For example, groups at ages 10, 20, 30, 40, 50, 60, and 70 years are administered IQ tests all on one day and results compared to evaluate the hypothesis that IQ decreases with age. This design does not control for the extrapersonal events (such as the fact that, as time goes by, the tendency is for more persons to get more education), which are controlled through the longitudinal design. This design is most applicable when one wishes to examine the effects of a given treatment on various levels of a variable, such as the response of different-aged carcinomas to a given chemotherapeutic regimen.

DOUBLE-BLIND

Double-blind designs are those in which neither the subject (S) nor the experimenter (E) knows if the treatment an S is receiving is true treatment or a ''placebo.'' This design is useful to control the subjective bias of both the S and E which frequently, without awareness, influences the outcome of research.

CROSS-OVER

Cross-over designs are a combination of no-treatment and same-subject control groups. In order to prove the efficiency of a given treatment, midway through the experiment, the experimental group is subjected to the events applied to the control group and vice versa. If the experimental treatment is effective, the respective positions of the two groups relative to the dependent variable will shift; or if treatment is permanent, the control group should approximate the experimental group. This is a powerful design that assures treatment effect and addresses the ethical issue of withholding a treatment from a group of persons (*e.g.*, patients with carcinoma not receiving a given type of chemotherapy that proves to be effective).

Research Statistics

Research statistics in behavioral sciences essentially test how similar or how different groups of subjects are.

MEASURES OF DIFFERENCE

Central to probability statistics based on the normal curve, is testing if an observation is significant or if it is a common, ''chance'' variation within the normal range. Distribution data characterized by a mean and standard deviation can be tested to see if two groups (*e.g.*, experimental and control) differ significantly on the dependent variable. This is done with the ***''t''*** test. This statistic compares the difference between the means of two samples using the standard deviations of each sample to ''pace off'' the distance between the two means. If the distributions don't overlap a great deal, it is concluded that the two groups are ''significantly different.'' The significance of the ''t'' value is determined by reference tables based on sample size and level of significance desired. The larger the sample and the lower the significance one is willing to accept, the smaller the ''t'' and vice versa.

The ***''F''*** statistic ***(Analysis of Variance*** or ***ANOVA)*** is similar to ''t'' except the ''F'' statistic can compare more than two means at a time (*e.g.*, different doses of a medication or the effects of different medications, time of day administered, and different doses of each on the dependent variable). The ''F'' statistic can reflect whether each of the independent variables is associated with the change in the dependent variable or whether it is an interaction among given variables that is significant.

MEASURES OF RELATIONSHIPS

In addition to statistics of central tendency and variation used to test differences between groups and to generally describe how a group of people present, there are also statistics of relationship between conditions.

The basic relationship statistic is the ***correlation coefficient*** (''r''). This statistic measures how two variables relate to or co-vary with each other. The ''r'' that is positive means, as one variable increases so does the other; the ''r'' that is negative means, as one variable increases the other decreases. The value of ''r'' can only range from 0.00 to 1.00; the higher the value, the stronger the relation. Therefore, ''r'' values can vary from -1.00 to $+1.00$. (An $r = -.85$ expresses a stronger relation than an $r = +.75$.) Correlational statistics can *never* be interpreted as cause–effect. There are three possible interpretations to all correlational data. If the ''r'' is between variables *a* and *b*, these are permissible interpretations: *a* leads to *b, b* leads to *a*, or *a* and *b* are related through a third variable, *c*. Correlations can be tested for significance of the size of the correlation (*i.e.*, significantly different from $r = 0$). One can also establish correlations among multiple variables. Multivariate analyses (*e.g.*, ***factor analysis***), multiple repression analysis, and so on are examples of this approach.

NONPARAMETRIC STATISTICS

The above measures of central tendency and relationships are parametric statistics. They are based on large samples and as such, have a great deal of power and generalizability to the overall population from which they were drawn. However, there are many studies in which the sample is small, and these require a special set of statistical analyses, referred to as nonparametric statistics. Results based on small samples and nonparametric statistics are not as powerful as those based on larger samples and parametric statistics. They are also not as amenable to generalization to the population as a whole.

PHENOMENOLOGY OF MENTAL PROCESS

Mental processes are those functions that constitute the concept of ''mind''; they are dimensions of behavior to which physicians attend as they evaluate the total person. These are the basic elements of mental functioning upon which the more complex and protean forms of human behavior are constructed. It is assumed that many are unique to man. Mental processes are not static events. They wax and wane, and they are in dynamic interchange with the person's internal and external environment.

Basic Concepts

MOTIVATION

Motivation is a concept that represents the energy that moves an individual to actively satisfy physical, psychological, and social needs. It is the ***drives*** or ***tension states*** created by ''survival'' needs as well as the ***impulses,*** or unexpected urges, over which the individual has little control. Other terms from various theories are ***libido*** and ***will. Primary needs*** are basically physiologic in origin, but through humans' symbolic and communication ability, psychological or social needs ***(secondary needs)*** also develop.

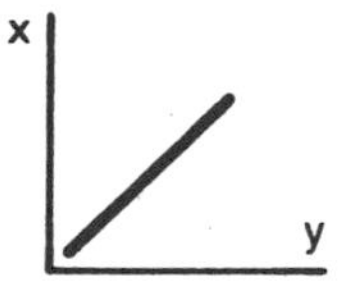

Fig. 8-1. Gradient. The graphic description of the relation between two variables.

GRADIENT

Gradient refers to the relationship between two elements as depicted by the slope of a line on a graph. For example, in Figure 8-1, as one progresses on the *x*-axis, the value of *y* increases. For example, if *x* represents a patient's distance from the hospital's surgical suite and *y* represents his anxiety levels then this gradient would state that the closer the patient is to the surgical suite, the more anxious he feels.

STRESS

Stress involves the disruption of a person's internal homeostatic state. If one's homeostatic balance is disrupted, the individual is understood to be stressed. ***Walter Cannon,*** writing in the 1940s, characterized the attempt to correct this lack of homeostasis as the ***fight or flight*** syndrome—demonstrated by increased blood sugar, dilated pupils, increased blood pressure, and increased muscle tone—to prepare the person for battle or rapid retreat. ***Hans Selye*** (1956) posited the ***general adaptation syndrome,*** which ultimately implicated activation of the entire endocrine system in response to somatic, psychological, or social stress. Arthur stated, ''Constant activation of the endocrine system can lead to adrenal exhaustion and deleterious bodily effects elsewhere from secondary processes such as elevated blood sugar.'' Selye's work is perhaps most applicable in those conditions where the stress emanates from an internal condition of the person from which it is not possible for the person to ''flee'' or that the individual cannot ''fight.'' Stress and immune function research has clearly shown that psychological stress can lead to increased susceptibility to disease by suppressing the immune response. However, mild stress can facilitate immune system activity; and, even **acute** moderate to severe stress does not always lead to increased susceptibility to illness. However, chronic stress, such as caring for a relative with Alzheimer's disease,

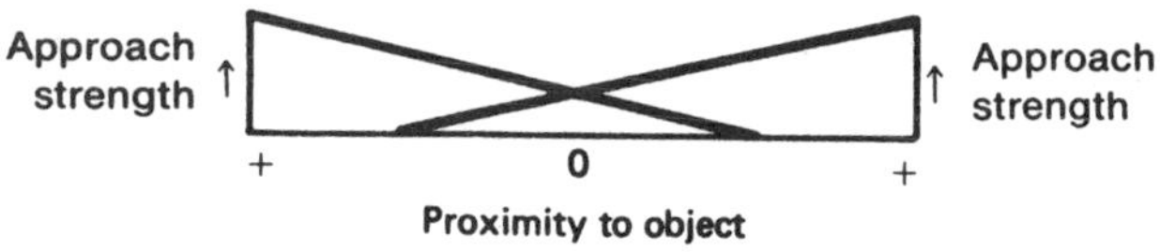

Fig. 8-2. Approach–approach conflict. Conflict generated by two equally positive objects.

can decrease immune cell function and increase incidence of illness in the caregivers. Social support tends to improve the overall health of persons who are vulnerable to stress. Three conditions seem to be most important in internal psychologically based stress: loss of significant objects (*e.g.,* a body part, loved one, occupation), injury or threat of injury (*e.g.,* surgery, illness, terminal disease, a robber with a gun), and frustration (*e.g.,* rejected lover, crowded living space, being kept sitting in a waiting room long after the appointment time). These three will be elucidated below.

CONFLICT

Conflict is present when two or more drives arise simultaneously (*e.g.,* to study for specialty board exams or to attend a desirable social event), or when two or more incompatible responses, including feelings, are aroused simultaneously (*e.g.,* love and hate toward one's parents). By definition, conflict is within the individual. Conflict can be classified into three types: ***approach–approach, avoidance–avoidance,*** and ***approach–avoidance.*** Figure 8-2 displays the schema for approach–approach conflicts. The conflict is maximal where the two gradients cross (*e.g.,* deciding whether to take a vacation in Tahiti or Hawaii). Once the individual has moved past the conflict point on either gradient (*e.g.,* once he has made a decision), no consequent difficulty arises because the level of the gradient of the nonchosen object decreases as the individual approaches the chosen object.

Figure 8-3 displays the schema for avoidance–avoidance conflict. Again, conflict is maximal where the gradients intersect. For example, the point where one decides to stop smoking in order to avoid lung cancer is the crisis point in the conflict of avoidance of health problems versus avoidance of stopping to smoke (avoidance of pleasure). However, in avoidance–avoidance conflict, once the individual makes a decision and moves towards an

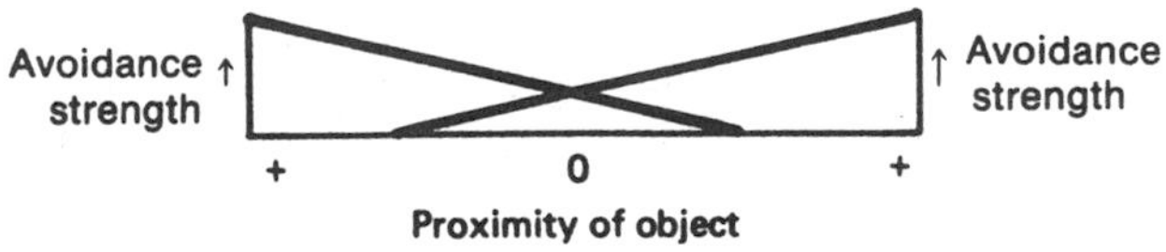

Fig. 8-3. Avoidance–avoidance conflict. Conflict generated by two equally negative objects.

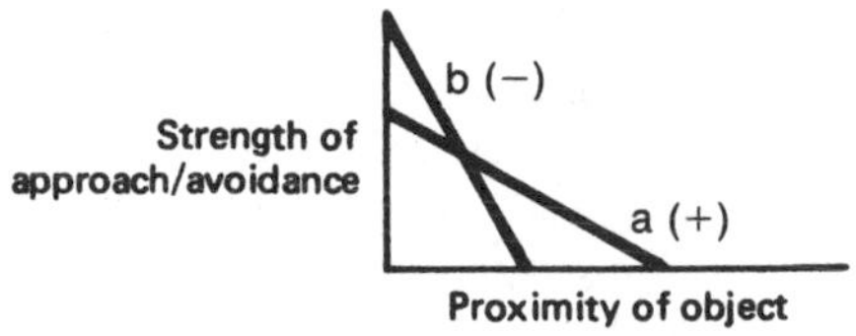

Fig. 8-4. Approach–avoidance conflict. Conflict generated by both positive and negative attributes residing within the same object.

object, the avoidance gradient increases and pushes the individual back into the conflict again.

Figure 8-4 demonstrates approach–avoidance conflicts. Here the same object, for example, marriage, has both approach (gradient *a*) and avoidance (gradient *b*) attributes. The person begins the approach gradient, making wedding plans, before encountering the avoidance gradient, awareness of losing freedom; again, the conflict is maximal where the two gradients cross. If the individual proceeds on the approach gradient, the avoidance increases; if the person retreats, the approach becomes more attractive once again. The resolution is either to increase the positive value or to decrease the negative value of the object so the gradients never cross.

ORGANIC–FUNCTIONAL

Organic–functional is a distinction that refers to the etiology of a given, usually "pathologic," human condition. ***Organic*** means the etiology is known, usually on the basis of one or more of the following conditions which affect the central nervous system (CNS) either directly or indirectly: metabolic, inflammatory, traumatic, toxic, infectious, neoplastic, congenital, degenerative, or vascular. (A handy memory aid, or mnemonic, is "MITTEN-CDV.") Behaviors that are organic in etiology can present to the physician as any of a number of psychiatric syndromes. However, organic brain dysfunction can usually be distinguished by a disordered sensorium or unique types of perceptual experiences discussed below. The term ***functional*** historically is derived from the fact that pathology could not be seen by using a light microscope. Today it implies that there is no known organic pathological condition that is responsible for the observed behavior pattern. Functional etiology can also imply a psychological or learned base to the behavior pattern observed by the physician. Functional pain, while sometimes inappropriately dismissed as "all in the head," does not make the experience of the pain any less for the patient who has it. This distinction is based in the historical concept of "separation of mind and body." That is, from a philosophical standpoint, the mind was regarded as the seat of the "soul"; and, since the soul could not be sick, the mind could not be ill like a body is sick. As research into the more molecular biological bases of all human behavior progresses, this distinction of functional versus organic etiology becomes less useful.

ACUTE–CHRONIC

The acute–chronic dimension used in behavioral sciences, specifically the pathologic conditions of behavior, is applied differently than in medicine as a whole. In psychiatry and behavioral sciences, ***acute*** implies that the condition is reversible and ***chronic*** means that it is not reversible. In certain situations, multiple acute episodes can produce a chronic–organic condition (*e.g.*, multiple acute alcohol intoxications can produce Korsakoff's psychosis).

"The Mind"

EMOTIONS

For this discussion, the words ***emotions*** and *affect* will be considered synonymous. Emotions accompany an alteration of the homeostatic state of the human organism. The alterations may be small and are often ignored by the person, or they may be large and overwhelming. The accompanying emotion can vary accordingly. Both large and small perturbations and their emotional concomitants are important because small, unnoticed changes can accumulate into a large, overwhelming situation. Emotions can be judged positive (*e.g.*, happy) or negative (*e.g.*, sad). However, because people usually do not seek assistance from the physician when they are happy, the following discussion will focus on the more disruptive emotions of anxiety–fear, anger–hostility, sadness, and disgust.

Anxiety–fear is the typical emotional response to some type of real or imagined injury or threat of injury. However, a distinction between fear and anxiety can be made. ***Fear*** as an emotion is related to a real thing that the frightened person recognizes and usually understands, and against which the person can make protective behavioral responses. ***Anxiety*** as an emotion is best understood as fear of something that the anxious person cannot identify. In anxiety, the symptoms of fear are experienced subjectively but are not linked to an object in the anxious person's awareness. The event responsible for the anxiety is said to be repressed. It is not that the anxious person will not tell the physician the source of experienced anxiety, but rather that he *cannot* because he or she has no awareness of the threatening object.

The subjective evidence of anxiety (*i.e.*, what the patient reports) includes statements like, "I'm nervous," "I'm scared," "I have butterflies in my stomach," or "My knees are shaky." The objective evidence (*i.e.*, what the physician sees) includes the following: excessive perspiration, fine motor tremor, speaking at the height of inspiration, head pulled back as if avoiding a blow to the face, eyes open wide so sclera is visible above and below the iris, eyebrows elevated leading to a wrinkled brow, frequent and rapid changes in body posture, fidgeting of the hands and feet, and, if the patient is sitting, the feet and lower legs positioned with one in front of the other as if to enable a "fast getaway."

The physiological correlates of anxiety include an epinephrinelike response peripherally. Overactivity of the sympathetic nervous system may result. Centrally, the locus ceruleus and the diencephalic limbic systems are implicated. These include excessive perspiration, skeletal muscle tension (*e.g.*, tension headaches, constriction of the back of the neck or chest, quivering voice, lower back pain), cardiovascular irritability (*e.g.*, transient dystolic hypertension, premature contractions, tachycardia, hypotension), genitourinary dysfunction (*e.g.*, urinary frequency, dysuria, erectile dysfunction in men, decreased vaginal lubrication in women), functional gastrointestinal disorders (*e.g.*, abdominal pain, anorexia, nausea, diarrhea, constipation), and respiratory difficulties. The extreme instance of the latter is known as the ***hyperventilation syndrome,*** which includes dyspnea; dizziness; paresthesias of the fingers, toes, and perioral area; and, in extreme cases, carpopedal spasm. Generally, hyperventilating patients subjectively report that they are oxygen deficient, but in fact their oxygen blood level is above normal. Appropriate intervention requires restoring a proper O_2–CO_2 balance.

Besides anxiety's role either as etiologic or, at least, an accompaniment of pathological behavior syndromes, there is a clear relationship between anxiety and performance, as expressed in Figure 8-5. To a certain degree, anxiety can enhance performance by making the person alert, active, and motivated. However, too much anxiety causes a decrease in performance.

The most common situations that provoke anxiety are as follows: ***anticipatory anxiety,*** where individuals frighten themselves with the unknown in advance of a given event (*e.g.*, stage fright), ***castration anxiety,*** which originated from psychoanalytic theory, meaning the anxiety/fear associated with the son's fear that the father will "cut off his penis" for "loving" the mother (today the concept is expanded to any situation where the person

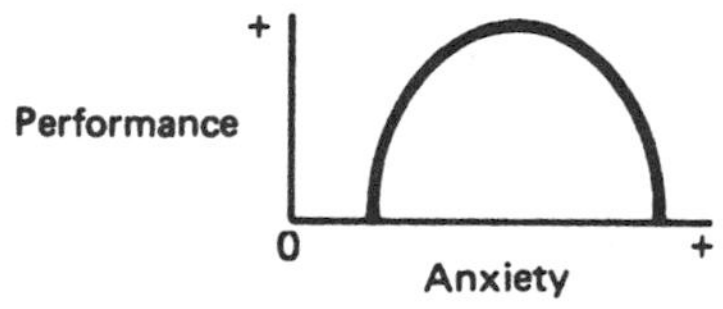

Fig. 8-5. Anxiety and performance. Mild to moderate anxiety enhances performance; however, higher levels of anxiety interfere with performance.

encounters threat from an authority figure such as a supervisor), ***separation anxiety,*** which is experienced when one is separated from another person who is needed (*e.g.*, the first day of school, frequently for both the child and the parents), ***stranger anxiety,*** which is a normal developmental event occurring in an infant between 6 and 12 months, when the infant is confronted with anyone who is "nonmother." This is frequently distressing (*i.e.*, anxiety provoking) for the nonmother figure, usually the father; however, stranger anxiety simply indicates that the child has begun to discriminate between objects. The child has developed object constancy.

These specific examples demonstrate the signal-alerting function of anxiety/fear. The anxiety/fear signals the individual that danger is present. It is frequently difficult for a person to "unlearn" anxiety/fear attached to a specific object that is no longer dangerous because the symptoms are so uncomfortable that the frightened/anxious person automatically avoids the source of the distress whenever the alerting signals are perceived. They never learn that the object is no longer a threat.

Anger as an emotional response usually has ***frustration*** as its stimulus. Frustration occurs when motivated (*i.e.*, goal-directed) behavior either is blocked or there is a challenge to obtaining the goal. The goal may be a real or symbolic object that will satisfy a given primary or secondary need (*e.g.*, pulling into a parking space and someone else blocks the entry). The aim of the resultant anger is to remove the blocking agent and allow the accomplishment of the drive. Anger is a drive discharge emotion in that the emotion, appropriately directed, allows for satisfaction of the frustrated drive/need state.

Anger is also related to ***hostility.*** The major distinction between anger and hostility is that anger is relatively short-lived if the frustrating stimulus is removed. Some authors suggest anger should not last longer than 20 minutes. Also, anger is not necessarily destructive, but is more aggressive. Hostility, however, is an emotional condition that pervades the person's entire behavioral repertoire, is present over extended periods of time (*e.g.*, years) and is physically or psychosocially destructive. Hostility may or may not be related to a specific frustrating stimulus or condition.

Subjective reports from the angry patient include statements like, "I'm mad," "I'm angry," or "I'm pissed off." Objective signs the physician can observe include narrowed eyelids, "knitted" eyebrows, flared nares, clenched teeth (*i.e.*, protruding masseter muscles), lips thin and tightly pursed, speaking in a loud, firm, clipped voice, head and neck jutted forward, protruding and throbbing temporal and neck blood vessels, rigid back, arms crossed tightly across the chest, and feet planted flatly and firmly on the floor.

The psychophysiologic concomitants of anger are peripherally epinephrine (and possibly norepinephrine) in nature. These include increased heart rate and blood pressure, dilated pupils, increased muscle tension, increased energy, constriction of peripheral vessels, and increased metabolic rate.

Primate studies have implicated the diencephalic–limbic system in anger. ***Rage*** reactions have been observed after intercollicular section and nociceptive stimulation in the posterior and lateral portions of the hypothalamus as well as other areas of the limbic system. Also, there appear to be modifying influences from the forebrain and rostral thalamic nuclei. Important considerations are the "forced activity" observed in ***temporal lobe epilepsy*** (also called partial complex seizures), and the absence of fear and aggression responses as well as the hypersexuality of the ***Kluver-Bucy syndrome*** associated with bilateral lesions of the amygdala and hippocampus. Testosterone is positively correlated with aggression; the neurotransmitters associated with aggressiveness include dopamine, norepinephrine, acetylcholine, serotonin, and β-endorphin.

Sadness as an emotional response usually has ***loss*** of a significant object as the etiologic event. The lost object may be a person, job, health, youth, or anything to which the individual is strongly attached. The subjective evidence for sadness is the patient's report that "I feel down," "I feel blue," or "I am sad." The objective evidence the physician can observe includes flaccid face, downcast gaze, sighing respiration, speaking at the end of expiration, head tilted down, shoulders slumped, decreased associative arm movement in walking, hands held loosely in the lap, legs crossed at the ankles, and general decreased amounts of body movements.

Sadness as an accompaniment of the ***mourning*** process is expected and must be distinguished from the ***depressive syndrome,*** which is characterized by dysphoria accompanied by dysfunctions in sleep, appetite, and weight; "libido"; concentration; and psychomotor activity, with feelings of guilt and worthlessness and suicidal ideation/impulses. Mourning should be completed in 6 to 12 months after major loss. If mourning extends into the second year, the physician should suspect that the patient is no longer mourning, but is depressed and should be treated accordingly. This holds true except in the loss of a child, in which case mourning goes on for years sometimes.

There are two important variations of sadness. The first is ***guilt,*** which can be conceptualized as a mixture of sadness plus anger turned back upon the self. The individual angrily blames the self for some event. For example, a mother whose child is born retarded may be sad over the "loss" of a "normal" child and may inappropriately assume the responsibility for the retardation with a statement such as, "If only I had (not) done. . . ." ***Shame,*** on the other hand, can be conceptualized as sadness in the face of external environment disapproval. For example, with the same mother noted above, the immediate family might say, "If only you had (not) done. . . ." Shame can also be viewed as the feeling one experiences in the presence of another's disgust.

There are five major descriptions that characterize emotions. First, they are ***bipolar:*** anxious–calm, angry/hostile–warm (similar to hate–love continuum), and sad–happy. Next, an emotion can be ***ambivalent*** in that an individual simultaneously experiences both ends of the bipolar continuum toward the same object. This is similar to the approach–avoidance conflict noted above (*e.g.,* loving and hating an individual at the same time). Third is the ability to express emotions either subjectively with words or objectively by facial expression, or both. Some persons have decreased or constricted expression, some have increased expression, and some demonstrate no emotional response. The absence of emotional expression is termed ***flat affect.*** Fourth is the ***appropriateness*** of an expressed emotion relative to the content to which it is attached. For example, it is generally appropriate to cry at the loss of a loved one, but not to laugh. Last, it is the rapidity of emotional change. All persons experience fluctuations in their emotional state; however, some individuals' emotions change markedly quite frequently (*e.g.,* every 30 seconds). This is termed ***liability*** of affect.

Disgust may also deserve attention. It is often a clue to the values held by a given individual. Disgust can be understood as the emotional accompaniment of a person encountering something distasteful. Its somatic expression may be significant in the evolution of certain symptoms (*i.e.,* nausea and vomiting). There is increasing evidence of its involvement in the development of compulsive behavior in some individuals. Disgust is recognized by the look of distaste on the face. The mouth is downturned at the corners, the nose wrinkled, and the tongue may protrude out and down as if the person has just tasted or smelled something offensive.

THOUGHT

Thinking is "mental" manipulation of symbolic processes usually for creative or problem-solving purposes. Since thoughts are intangible, thinking can only be judged objectively by verbal, written, or other products. For discussion purposes, thought will be divided into two separate portions: the process and the content.

Thought process, the first major division, describes *how* a person thinks. There is a given production rate, which may be inferred from the rapidity with which a person speaks, but geographic and cultural variations may be misleading. It is clearer to conceptualize production rate of thoughts as a person walking. ***Accelerated thought*** process is similar to a person descending a steep hill and about to lose balance. That person takes short rapid steps to prevent stumbling. The physician may try to intervene, but the person cannot help but continue rapidly downhill. ***Retarded thought process*** is similar to a person ascending a steep hill. The progress is slow and labored and, regardless of the physician's attempt to assist, the person maintains a slow pace. ***Blocking*** is exemplified by the person who, while walking, encounters sudden darkness in which the appropriate direction cannot be ascertained. This individual is confused, doesn't understand why the darkness occurred and can't extract himself from the darkness. Accelerated and retarded production rates generally accompany major affective disorders and certain organic conditions. Blocking is usually psychologically determined and precipitated by content issues that are in conflict; it is most common in major thought disorders.

When examining how a person thinks, besides rate there should be consideration of the ***continuity*** with which thoughts are connected. Most formal thought process is characterized by Aristotelian logic (*i.e.,* A → B → C → D . . . → Z). The term ***looseness of association*** refers to thought process that is non-Aristotelian, where associations between thoughts are formed on unique bases that have very loose connections. Sometimes this is called ***predicate logic*** (*e.g.,* von Damerus' Principle), where the association between thoughts is based on the objects of sentences (*i.e.,* "The Virgin Mary was a woman, I am a woman, I am the Virgin Mary"). In other forms, the associations between thoughts are on the basis of sounds and are called ***clang associations,*** like bang, rang, dang, sang, and clang. Another disorder of continuity is ***circumstantial*** thinking, in which the person produces every detail or circumstance surrounding a given event. For example, when asked, "What did you do this morning?" the person might respond, " I heard the alarm, opened my left eye, then my right eye, opened my mouth, yawned, stretched my right arm, then my left . . . . *(three hours later)* and then stood up at the side of the bed." These persons will eventually arrive at the end goal; however, the physician hardly has time to wait. ***Tangential*** thinking is that process characterized by the person slightly missing the goal. For instance, "Are you a good tennis player?" may elicit the answer, "I like to play tennis." While the questioner has some data relative to the inquiry, an "on-target" response was not made. The thought process known as ***perseveration*** is when persons repeat the same response regardless of the context of the question. (Q: "How old are you?" A: "30." Q: How many children do you have?" A: "30." Q: "How tall are you?" A: "30.")

Thought content, the second major division, is concerned with the message or meaning of the thoughts. The first consideration is the thought's ***relationship to reality,***

which is identified by three components: ***sense of reality*** (*e.g.*, knowing that the four-legged object on which one is sitting is a chair), ***testing reality*** (*e.g.*, validation with someone else or through functional experimentation that the object is, indeed, a chair), and ***adapting to reality*** (*e.g.*, using the chair to sit comfortably at a table to eat when the table is too high or low without it). The most significant aspect of relationship to reality is whether the individual is either realistic or ***autistic*** in thought content. Autistic means the individual has a private understanding of the world or external events which is not shared by others; for instance, Einstein's theory of relativity when initially proposed. If the autistic thinking becomes fixed in the face of contrary, overwhelming evidence and takes on a maladaptive or malevolent quality, the thought content is called delusional. ***Delusions*** are defined as false-fixed belief systems. Autistic thinking is characteristic of major thought disorders like schizophrenia.

The second aspect of thought content is the relative level of ***abstraction*** that an individual can attain. For example, upon request, can the individual abstract the common essence from examples of a general category (*e.g.*, an orange and banana are both fruit) and distill a general principle from a concrete example (*e.g.*, "A stitch in time saves nine" means prevention is cost effective)? If abstractability is impaired, the person can only identify superficial ***concrete*** qualities of diverse objects of a general class (*e.g.*, an orange and banana both have peelings) or can only repeat the example or give literal interpretation of the example (*e.g.*, "Sew a tear when it starts and it won't take as many stitches to fix"). While poor abstractability is found in functional and organic thought disorders, it is also characteristic of mental retardation and the thought processes of young children.

The next characteristic of thought content is whether the individual can develop ***insight.*** Can the person interdigitate relations between events in a cause–effect manner, or can the individual recognize stress events or internal conflicts and their subsequent emotional effects? Related to insight is ***judgment.*** Given insight, how does the person relate in social situations, generally exercise control over life, and judge the consequences of given situations and adjust to them?

Another significant element of thought content is the relative ***obsessional*** nature. That is, whether the same thought content characteristically intrudes uncontrollably into the person's awareness or whether characteristic thoughts are varied and rich in content.

It is useful to consider the major topics, themes, or issues that appear in a given patient. The physician stands back, so to speak, examines the patient's verbal landscape, and notes a title: "I constantly suffer at the hands of people who don't understand me," for example.

ORIENTATION

Orientation is knowing who and where one is at the present time. Some persons confuse orientation and memory. Orientation is the "who, what, when and where" of the *here and now.* Memory is the recall of the past. There are four dimensions of orientation that are considered: person, place, time, and situation.

Orientation to person means the individual knows who he is (*i.e.*, name, birthdate, can identify parts of the body or knows that the body belongs to himself). The phenomenon of ***depersonalization*** is a disorientation to person in which the body as a whole or parts of it seem dissociated from the "mind" (*e.g.*, the mind drifts from the body and observes events from the corner of the room). Two other disruptions in orientation to person are ***anosognosia,*** not knowing that one is ill, and ***autotopagnosia,*** not being able to correctly locate one's own body parts.

Orientation to place means the individual can locate himself geographically and spatially. If orientation to place is disrupted, the most common forms are ***derealization,*** a sensation of distortion of spatial relations and unreality, ***déjà vu,*** a feeling when in a strange environment that "I've been here before," and ***jamais vu,*** the reverse of déjà vu, where the individual is in a familiar environment and suddenly wonders, "Where am I?"

Orientation to time is the individual's ability to know present position in linear time; for example, day or night, morning or evening, day of the week, month, and year. The latter is emphasized because of the common assumption that if a person knows tha date and month, that person automatically knows the year. This is frequently untrue, particularly in the various forms of organic brain disorders and syndromes.

Orientation to situation is a synthesis of the above three. That is, to repeat the definition of orientation, does this person know who he or she is, where he is, when it is, and the present contextual situation that relates these three together?

CONSCIOUSNESS

Within behavioral sciences, the concept of conscious mental processes has three distinct definitions. First, consciousness is used to refer to the relative level of physiologic arousal. Second, it can mean that the person is physiologically alert, but there is a psychodynamic condition present that may grossly affect mental processes. Third, it is used to define whether a piece of data is in a person's awareness at the present time, with the assumption that the individual's physiological arousal level is normal and alert.

The first point (relative physiologic arousal) refers to the level of activation of the CNS and the associated non-fluctuating nature of consciousness. This aroused condition of the organism is intimately tied to the integrity and functioning of the ***reticular activating system (RAS).*** Apparently the RAS is also central to the behavioral ***alerting*** or ***orienting response,*** which is the primary determinant of ***attention.*** If the RAS is functioning in an activating manner, it is transmitting signals to other portions of the brain and the person is alert and attending or orienting to incoming stimuli. The RAS can also function in an inhibiting manner to suppress extraneous stimuli. This allows the person to attend more intensely to the object under consideration. However, if the RAS is compromised in function, the individual experiences conditions ranging from mental confusion, through clouding of consciousness, stupor (*i.e.,* the individual's senses are dulled and the person is capable of very little environmental interchange), to coma, where there is no awareness of the environment. If the inhibitory function of the RAS is impaired, the person may not be able to selectively attend to one stimulus at a time and may appear to be distractible. These alterations in physiologic alertness are common sequelae of CNS dysfunction and particularly ***traumatic head injury.*** In addition to the characteristic level of consciousness, fluctuating levels of consciousness (or attention) frequently accompany pathologic CNS conditions as well as psychologically based disorders. Organic conditions should be suspected if the person is well rested and is attempting to focus attention or concentrate, and cannot.

The second definition of consciousness implies that the person is physiologically alert; however, some psychologically based conflict has precipitated a condition in which the person seemingly functions in a "normal" manner but is unaware of massive amounts of personal experience. The most common of these conditions are ***fugue states,*** which are characterized by the assumption of a totally "new life" without being aware of a different earlier life (upon recovery of the earlier memory, the fugue life is forgotten) and ***dream*** or ***twilight states*** in which the physiologically alert person seems to focus all attention on an inner or far-off event. During the latter condition the person is relatively immobile and markedly unresponsive to environmental stimuli; amnesia for the event is expected. ***Somnambulism*** (*i.e.,* sleepwalking) is the third major type of psychologically based alteration in consciousness. It is similar to a short-lived fugue state, except that it begins while the person is asleep. Upon awakening, the individual has no recollection of the events that transpired during the sleepwalking episode.

The third definition of consciousness historically is derived from psychoanalytic theory, and recently from studies that focus on how the brain processes information, and it refers to whether given material is in the awareness of the person. Freud spoke of three levels; first, conscious material, which is in full awareness; second, preconscious material, which is not in awareness but can be readily recalled at will (*i.e.,* one's own telephone number); and third, unconscious material, which is not in awareness and cannot be brought into awareness without special techniques like hypnosis or free association.

SENSATION

Sensation is defined as the experience that results from stimulation of sensory nerve endings of any of the five senses: sight, sound, touch, smell/taste, and kinesthesia.

Primary sensation tends to provoke anxiety because of its "unknown" quality. This unknown disrupts the homeostatic condition of the person, which the person attempts to correct through understanding or perception as discussed below. Toxic conditions (*e.g.,* various drugs) and other neuropathologic conditions, such as irritating lesions of the visual cortex or migraine headache, can produce sensory phenomena. It is emphasized that primary sensations without environmental stimuli (*e.g.,* visual scotoma and "sparklers," tinnitus, foul odors) usually imply organic conditions. The primary sensory pathways, their projection sites in the brain, and behavioral correlates will be included in the discussion of the physiologic contributions to the determinants of behavior below.

Psychogenically based disorders of sensation are best represented by the phenomenon of chronic, psychogenic pain.

PERCEPTION

The understanding of sensory stimuli referred to above is the operational definition of perception. As stimuli enter the brain, in addition to the specific sensory nerve tracts that pass to the sensory cortical areas, there are collateral sensory inputs to the reticular formation which apparently activate the RAS. This activation results in ***attention*** to the stimulus and is called an ***orienting response.*** With attention and ***concentration*** on the nature of stimuli and past experience or frames of reference, the person "understands" or perceives the stimuli. For example, one is awakened in the night by a noise. Until the cause of the noise is perceived, arousal (*i.e.,* orienting response or attention) and anxiety remain at high levels. With perception, anxiety may change to fear or disappear depending upon the cause. The arousal may turn to concerted effort to deal with the perceived stimulus. Sometimes, for either organic or functional reasons, misperceptions of environmental stimuli occur. For example, a drape blown by a draft is perceived as someone entering a window, or the shadow of a leaf on a wall at night is perceived as a tarantula spider. These are ***illusions,*** defined as misinterpretations or misperceptions of real environmental events.

However, exteroceptive stimuli are not always necessary for perception to occur, as in imagination or dreaming. On occasion, internal stimuli like thoughts can become so intense that they are projected as perceptions onto the external world in the form of ***hallucinations.*** That is, the person perceives an imaginary or interoceptive event as an exteroceptive reality. Recent data from neuro-imaging techniques have demonstrated activity of specific functional brain regions when a person is hallucinating (*e.g.,* the occipital lobes are very active when visual hallucinations are occurring). While hallucinations are usually considered pathologic (auditory being more functionally based, and visual, tactile, olfactory/taste, and kinesthetic more organic) there are two forms of hallucinations that seem to be unrelated to significant pathologic conditions. In stages of sleep where control over "conscious" processes is marginal, hallucinations—particularly auditory types—are frequently reported. If a hallucination occurs as one enters sleep it is called a hypnagogic hallucination and if it occurs as one is gaining wakefulness it is called hypnopompic hallucination.

Advances in neuroscience confirm the statement that perception is a constructional process; it is not veridical. All of us literally see and hear the world differently. In that sense illusions are universal. We see what we believe.

MEMORY AND FORGETTING

Memory ***(mnesis)*** is the ability upon demand to bring into awareness past events and experiences. It is customary to divide the concept of memory into three arbitrary types based on how much time has elapsed since the original event occurred. ***Immediate memory*** or recall is the ability to reproduce data to which one has just been exposed; for example, finding a telephone number in a telephone book and having the number available for a few seconds, or the repetition of a serial set of numbers. This ability is apparently limited to seven "bits" or "chunks" of data. ***Recent*** or ***short-term memory*** is the ability to remember information after at least a ten-minute interval between exposure to and recollection of the data (*e.g.,* recollection of three independent items presented by an interviewer at the beginning of an interview, or notable news events that occurred within the last two weeks). ***Remote*** or ***long-term memory*** refers to the availability of information learned by the individual a considerable time before (*e.g.,* when was Pearl Harbor bombed, when was John F. Kennedy assassinated, who were the last 10 presidents of the United States?). REM sleep, discussed below, plays a central role in the memory process. During REM sleep, the day's events tend to be consolidated into the memory of the person.

Learning and memory for learned materials are clearly functional by the second month of an infant's life. Research also has demonstrated lasting memories as early as 2 years of age. Research also has established that both widespread neuroanatomical sites and numerous neurochemical processes are important in the mnestic process. Apparently the mesencephalic reticular system is important early in the memory process, and activation of the thalamic reticular system with attendant inhibition of the mesencephalic reticular system is crucial later in the memory process. The hippocampus appears to be particularly central to the transfer of information from short-term to long-term memory. Synthesis of ribonucleic acid (RNA) and protein is important, particularly in the formation and storage of long-term data. Recent work specifically involving research into ***Alzheimer's disease*** has documented the contribution of the CNS acetylcholine (ACh) neurotransmitter system in memory process. Studies have reported specific degeneration of the cholinergic neurons located in the nucleus basalis of Meynert. In the CNS, ACh is concentrated in the basal ganglia and the basal forebrain cholinergic complex. This concentration in these two areas is thought to play a pivotal part in memory processes.

Special states of memory include ***hypermnesia,*** which is unusual memory for detail of a specific or selected situation, ***iconic*** memory, which is the brief, detailed retention of visual stimuli, and ***eidetic*** ("photographic") memory, which is the unusual ability to glance at an object like a book page, look away, and recite it without error as if reading the page.

Forgetting ***(amnesia)*** is the inability to recall material to which one has been previously exposed. It is assumed that the forgetting of material has either a "dynamic" or functional base (*i.e.,* the information is "blocked" from awareness by psychological processes), or is organic. The most common types of amnesia are as follows. In ***patchy*** or ***lacunar*** amnesia, the person has intact memory around a given amnesic "hole," for example, the grandparents who can remember all grandchildren's names and birthdates except the one whose mother died at its birth. In ***anterograde*** amnesia, the person forgets all information following a given significant life event (*e.g.,* memory loss for 24 hours after being raped). ***Retrograde*** amnesia is the loss of memory for events preceding a significant life event (*e.g.,* 24 hours prior to being knocked unconscious from an automobile accident). ***Paramnesia*** (*e.g.,* retrospective falsification) is the distortion of remembered data. The person who experiences this is firmly convinced of the validity of the recollection. One specific instance of this phenomenon is called ***confabulation,*** characteristic of the organically based Korsakoff's psychosis, which is now called alcohol amnestic disorder. In confabulation, the individual weaves data from the here-and-now into

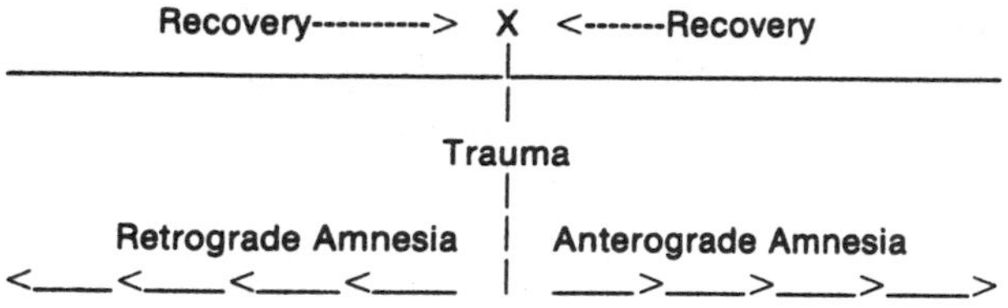

Fig. 8-6. Diagram of traumatic memory loss and its characteristic pattern of recovery.

the recalled experience. Sometimes the interwoven data is suggested by the physician as a way to test for confabulation.

In general, a memory defect is considered to be of psychogenic origin if the individual has no disturbed level of consciousness and there is no intellectual impairment. If recovery of lost memory is abrupt, a psychogenic etiology is implied. Organically based memory disorders have the following associations. Bilateral lesions of the hippocampus or mamillary bodies produce profound deficits, particularly in short-term memory. Long-term memory is usually unaffected by organic conditions unless accompanied by psychosis. If organic memory loss occurs, recovery is typically gradual and is regained from the extremes to the precipitating event (see Fig. 8-6).

INTELLIGENCE

The concept of intelligence is defined as the aggregate or global capacity of the individual to act purposely, to think rationally, and to deal effectively with his environment.

Intelligence is usually subdivided into two types: verbal and performance. These can be related to CNS lateralization of higher mental or cognitive processes in the brain with verbal abilities under greater executive control of the left hemisphere and nonverbal visual-spatial skills associated more predominantly with right-hemisphere functioning for most people, regardless of hand dominance.

A central issue in the discussion of intelligence involves the ***nature–nurture*** controversy: whether intelligence is determined by heredity or environment. Evidence in favor of the nature position includes twin studies, which have consistently shown a concordance rate between monozygotic twins that is higher than the rate for dizygotic twins, which, in turn, is higher than that of natural siblings. Also, an adopted child's IQ correlates higher with that of biological parents than with the IQ of adoptive parents.

For the nurture position, there is favorable evidence as well. Social, cultural, and interpersonal deprivation are correlated with low IQ scores. Rural, isolated, and mistreated children have lower IQ scores than matched urban, stimulated, and well-treated peers; minority children taught in inferior school systems who are moved to enriched schools have positive correlations between IQ scores and length of time in the enriched school system.

The ***intelligence quotient (IQ)*** is a mathematical expression of the relation between mental ability and age. IQ will be discussed in detail below under psychological assessment; however, dependent upon the particular IQ test administered, an average IQ is 100 with 10 to 15 points of variation on either side.

The distribution of intelligence is assumed to follow a normal, or ''bell-shaped,'' curve; however, because of early trauma, infections, or poor maternal prenatal health care, there is a higher than expected number of persons with lower intelligence in the population. Generally intelligence scores are grossly classified as below normal, normal, and above normal.

In the below-normal range are those persons diagnosed as having primary ***mental retardation.*** Primary mental retardation is a syndrome defined by low intelligence, poor social adaptation, and developmental problems. This definition excludes those persons whose intellectual ability is compromised by acquired brain dysfunction and related disorders. These are classified as having secondary mental retardation. The IQ distribution and functional classification according to the Diagnostic and Statistical Manual of Mental Disorders IV (DSM-IV) (American Psychiatric Association, 1994) is as follows:

IQ = below 20 or 25: ***profound*** mental retardation
IQ = 20–25 to 35–40: ***severe*** mental retardation
IQ = 35–40 to 50–55: ***moderate*** mental retardation
IQ = 50–55 to approximately 70: ***mild*** mental retardation
IQ = 70 to 89: ***borderline*** mental retardation

Another classification that is sometimes more useful is based on prognosis in self care (Pardes, 1985). This divides retarded individuals into the following classifications:

IQ = below 30: ***custodial*** (These persons cannot distinguish between safety and danger and therefore must live in a protected custodial environment.)
IQ = 30–50: ***trainable*** (Persons classified here can distinguish safety from danger; however, they cannot learn the essentials of symbolic communication, that is, reading, writing, and arithmetic.)
IQ = 50–70: ***educable*** (These individuals can learn the basics of symbolic communication but encounter difficulty in abstract thinking and complex judgment.)

The IQ range of 70 to 90 does not have a specific ''label''; however, these persons usually can be self-supporting financially and can care for their own personal needs. They can do minimal abstracting and can complete the basics of education.

Normal intelligence, then, is bordered by IQ scores of 90 and 109. The majority of persons fall within this range.

The person of above-average intelligence has an IQ score greater than 109. The classification according to Wechsler is as follows:

IQ = 110–119: ***bright*** normal
IQ = 120–129: ***superior***
IQ = 130 and above: ***very superior***

Recent research using brain-imaging techniques has demonstrated that persons with higher IQ use less mental energy (reflected by metabolism in the brain) to solve problems. The implication is that the brains of brighter persons work more efficiently than do those of persons who have lesser intelligence.

In addition to intelligence, there are persons with unique abilities. On the low-IQ end of this continuum, some persons have IQs in the range of "retarded" but show some dramatic, singular talent. These individuals are said to have the savant syndrome. Some have spectacular achievement in arithmetic calculation, artistic achievement, playing musical instruments, and calendar calculation for the remote past and distant future. Persons with Asperger's Syndrome also manifest this characteristic.

On the high end of the continuum are persons with IQs in the range of ***genius*** but who have some singular, outstanding deficit. For example, Albert Einstein, for all practical purposes, had an IQ that was so high as to be untestable. However, at age 15 his grades in history, geography, and language were poor and he left school with no diploma.

These aspects of the "mind" constitute what can be conceptualized as the phenomenology of mental process. The focus has been on delineating mental activity, which is the basis of an individual's interaction with the external environment. These parameters are conceptualized as biological "givens," which must function in a "normal" manner for the individual to be maximally adaptive in the world.

Frequently the physician must determine if a given individual's "mind" is functioning correctly. To do this in a valid manner, the physician must use a standard procedure that reflects the important dimensions of mental processes. This procedure is called the ***mental status examination*** and is discussed fully in the chapter on Psychiatry in *Rypins' Clinical Sciences Review*.

DETERMINANTS OF BEHAVIOR

The preceding section addressed the mental process of behavior. This section summarizes how behavior is influenced, beginning with genetic events and proceeding through biochemical influences, psychophysiologic parameters, learning, growth and development, sociocultural considerations, and psychosocial issues in current American society.

Genetic Influence on Human Behavior

Genetic factors are responsible for unique human conditions. Basic genetic concepts are as follows:

Alleles: alternative forms of a gene; each person has two alleles for a gene, one from each parent

Aneuploidy: a condition in which the number of chromosomes in a human differs from the normal 46, caused by the loss or addition of whole or parts of chromosomes.

Autosome: the 22 homologous pairs of nonsex chromosomes formed at the union of the sperm and the egg; because each complement of chromosomes from each parent is a chance assortment of half of each parent's chromosomes, every human is a unique genetic entity; also leads to an equal or random distribution of an autosomal trait between sexes

Centromere: the pale-staining primary constriction on each chromosome which divides the chromosome into two arm lengths

Chromosomes: the 23 pairs of "strands of genes" are present in virtually all cells of the body.

Corcordance rate: the rate at which each of pairs of persons has the same specific condition. The inheritability for a condition is inferred if the concordance rate for monozygotic twins is high compared to dizygotic twins, non-twin siblings, or adopted siblings

Dominant single-gene inheritance: when the genetic effect (*i.e.,* phenotypic expression) requires only one gene of a sperm–egg chromosome pair to carry a trait

Genes: the elemental unit of heredity composed of biochemical substance called deoxyribonucleic acid (DNA) provides hereditary information and controls.

Genotype: the genetic makeup of the person

Heterozygous: only one gene of sperm–egg chromosome pair carries a given trait

Homozygous: both corresponding genes of sperm–egg chromosome pair carry a given trait

Karyotype: the chromosome composition of the somatic or body cells

Linkage: genes whose loci are on the same chromosome; also refers to traits transmitted by different alleles found at the same chromosomal locus (*i.e.,* X-linked)

Mutations: alterations in the chemical composition of genes so new cells produce substances different from those produced by the cells that preceded the mutation; some are "spontaneous" (*i.e.,* unknown etiology), which are rare, and some are due to exposure to x rays, chemical actions, and so forth

Penetrance: the frequency at which a dominant or a homozygous recessive gene expresses itself phenotypically; lack of penetrance occurs when a dominant gene is not expressed phenotypically; incomplete penetrance occurs when a dominant gene is expressed in an attenuated manner

Phenotype: the expression of the genotype; unless special conditions are present, the genotype may not be observable or manifested as a phenotype.

Recessive: a trait or gene that is expressed only in those who are homozygous for that gene

Sex chromatin, or ***Barr body:*** a chromatin mass present in the somatic nuclei of normal females during interphase; normal males have no Barr bodies; thought to be inactivated by X chromosomes; number of Barr bodies is always fewer than the number of X chromosomes

Sex-linked: gene responsible for a trait is located on an X or Y sex chromosome; results in an unequal distribution of the given trait between the sexes

X chromosome: ''female'' chromosome (XX); can be provided by either the male or the female

Y chromosome: ''male'' chromosome (XY); can only be provided by the male

CHROMOSOMAL DISORDERS

Those behavioral disorders that have been established to be genetic in etiology can be divided into three major subgroups: sex chromosome disorders, inborn errors of metabolism, and translocation/nondisjunction errors.

Sex Chromosome Disorders. ***Turner's syndrome*** occurs in one per 3,000 to 5,000 girls and is characterized by underdeveloped external female genitalia, a small uterus, short stature, webbed neck, and usually a lack of ovaries. Often these girls show intellectual impairment but not usually severe mental retardation. The karyotype of these women shows 45 chromosomes with a sex chromosome constitution of XO, and there is no Barr body observed. Presumably this is due to nondisjunction of an X chromosome of one parent during gametogenesis.

Fragile X syndrome occurs when a mutation occurs on the X chromosome at the fragile site. It is the second most common cause of mental retardation (1 in 1,000 males and 1 in 2,000 females). The problems can range from very mild to severe.

Rett's disorder is a presumed X-linked dominant disorder leading to mental retardation in females. Beginning at about 1.5 years of age, neurologic deterioration progresses, with autistic-like movements, seizures, and spasticity ensuing.

Klinefelter's syndrome is an anomaly of males and is characterized by external male genitalia with small atrophic testes. These men are usually sterile, and they often have gynecomastia, sparse body hair, long legs, and an increased excretion of gonadotrophin. The syndrome occurs at a rate of one per 340 to 500 male births. Mental retardation is usually, but not invariably, present. The etiology is presumed to be nondisjunction of an X chromosome, leading to a karyotype of 47 chromosomes with an XXY sex chromosome constitution. There is a Barr body present, which is unusual for males.

XYY karyotype has led to a great deal of controversy because of a suggested link between this karyotype and criminality. These men—''supermales''—have been characterized as tall, displaying poor impulse control, and having disrupted interpersonal contacts and a greater than average sexual drive. If they have criminal histories, the criminality tends toward crimes of violence. The XYY karyotype has been demonstrated to have a higher prevalence rate in incarcerated men. Further research, however, has also demonstrated a high frequency of the karyotype among nonincarcerated males.

XXX karyotypes are women who are not exceptionally feminine, have no sexual abnormalities, and have many children. Most of these individuals are mentally retarded.

Inborn Errors of Metabolism. ***Phenylketonuria (PKU)*** results from insufficient amounts or absence of the enzyme phenylalanine hydroxylase, which oxidizes phenylalanine to tyrosine. As a consequence, phenylalanine is metabolized by alternate pathways, and either the excessive unmetabolized phenylalanine or the alternative metabolites alter brain metabolism. The disease can be diagnosed in the infant by detection of phenylpyruvic acid in the urine. Through dietary control (*i.e.*, low phenylalanine content), mental retardation can be prevented. Most states in the United States require urine testing of newborns for PKU. The incidence of the disease is about 1 per 16,000 births. If untreated, mental retardation appears at about six months. The ultimate result is severe retardation. This has an autosomal recessive transmission, and persons who are carriers have no clinical manifestations. However, carriers can be detected by their inability to rapidly metabolize test loads of phenylalanine.

Lesch-Nyhan disease is an autosomal recessive enzyme defect. It is accompanied by mental retardation and a tendency for the child to self-mutilate (*e.g.*, chew on lips, fingers, and toes).

Tay-Sachs disease is a disorder caused by a specific enzymatic deficiency. It has an autosomal recessive transmission, most prevalent in—but not confined to—Ashkenazi Jews. The disease is characterized by progressive mental deterioration, loss of visual function, cerebromacular degeneration, and accumulation of lipid substances throughout the CNS. The usual onset is from 4 to 8 months of age, with death by 3 years. The infants become hypotonic, display slow developmental progression, and are weak and apathetic. They become spastic with primitive postural reflexes, frequently have convulsions, and display progressive mental and physical deterioration. A cherry-red spot in the macula lutea of each retina can be discerned upon examination.

Translocation/Nondisjunction Errors. ***Down's syndrome*** (*i.e.*, "mongolism") is characterized by a prominence of the median folds of the eyelids, short stature, stubby hands and feet, and peculiarity of palm prints. Other congenital malformations, (*e.g.*, cardiovascular) may be present. Mental retardation is present. This condition represents the single most definable clinical entity causing severe mental retardation. There are two causes of Down's syndrome, which are phenotypically identical. The first type, trisomy 21, has chromosome 21 represented three times instead of two. This produces a karyotype with 47 chromosomes. Apparently this is due to nondisjunction of chromosome 21. The second type apparently is due to translocation of chromosomes 21 and 15. There are 46 chromosomes: the 21s are normal, one of the 15s is normal, and there is one large, unpaired chromosome that is interpreted as a fusion of 15 and 21. While it is not known *why* these alterations occur, it is known that they have a higher prevalence in offspring of older mothers and older fathers, and there is some relationship to exposure to x-ray radiation.

The Inheritability of Emotional Disorders. Genetic research in human behavior is conducted by three separate designs. ***Familial studies*** consider whether a given trait or traits "run in families." ***Twin studies*** look at the concordance rate of a given behavior or trait between monozygotic versus dizygotic twin groups. This method is most potent when the twins have been separated at birth and raised in different environments. ***Adoptive studies*** look at the concordance rates between the adopted child and the biologic versus adoptive parent for a given trait or behavior.

Schizophrenia, as with intelligence, has a concordance rate among family members that varies with the degree of genetic similarity. Franz Kallman's early work (1953) demonstrated that monozygotic twins raised together have a concordance rate of 86%, and monozygotics raised apart have a somewhat lower concordance rate; however, monozygotics reared apart have a higher rate than fraternals reared together, which is 15%. Other studies suggest concordance figures for monozygotics that range from 50% to 88%. Children of schizophrenic mothers who were raised away from the mother since day three were studied and found to experience significantly more difficulty on a number of relevant variables than did the controls (*e.g.*, total years incarcerated in mental institutions was 112 for children of schizophrenics versus 15 for children of nonschizophrenics). The degree of familial relationship to a schizophrenic yields a prevalence rate of schizophrenia as follows: monozygotic twin of one schizophrenic parent 47%, child of two schizophrenic parents 40%; dizygotic twin of a schizophrenic parent 12%; child of one schizophrenic parent 12%, nontwin sibling of a schizophrenic parent 8%, general population 1%.

Bipolar disorder (*i.e.*, manic-depressive illness) appears to be the major affective disorder that has a hereditary component. Concordance rates of 0.67 for monozygotic twins and 0.20 for dizygotic twins have been reported. Approximately 50% of all bipolar patients have at least one parent with a mood disorder. If one parent has a bipolar disorder, there is a 27% chance that the child will have a mood disorder. If both parents have bipolar disorder, there is between a 50% and 75% chance that an offspring will have a mood disorder. The recent data suggest that the genetic transmission may be on the X chromosome.

A number of other clinical behavioral syndromes appear to have genetic correlates. These include depressive disorder, dysthymic disorder, antisocial personality disorder, panic disorder, obsessive compulsive disorder, early-onset Alzheimer's disorder, Huntington's chorea, avoidant personality disorder, substance abuse disorders (alcoholism and dependence upon opiods, nicotine, marijuana, cocaine, anxiolytics, amphetamines, etc.; these appear to be mediated through a second version of the D2 receptor), enuresis, and attention deficit disorder, to name the most common. As research continues into the genetic bases of different behavioral complexes, recent research has documented genetic correlates in normal personality traits, shyness, and some types of homosexuality in both males and females.

In some of these, other factors appear to exert a stronger influence than the suggested genetic substrate.

Biochemical Determinants of Behavior (Neurotransmitters)

Neurotransmitters are biochemical substances that facilitate transmission of information from one neuron across the synapse to the next neuron, or from neuron to muscle fibers at the myoneural junction. Over 100 such substances have been identified to date. They are released from the presynaptic neuron into the synaptic cleft, where they attach to highly specific receptors at postsynaptic as well as presynaptic sites. They may be eliminated from the body through metabolism or reabsorbed by the presynaptic neuron. Their duration of action is very short. Different types of neurotransmitters are found in different areas of the nervous system. Some neurons may contain more than one transmitter substance. Research into the role of second-messenger systems in behavioral expression is beginning at this time.

Four general neurotransmitter systems appear to be the most important in understanding human behavior: ***monoamines,*** which are the catecholamines, dopamine (DA), norepinephrine (NE), and epinephrine (E), and the indolamine, serotonin (5-HT); ***acetylcholine*** (ACh); ***amino acids*** (*e.g.*, gamma-aminobutyric acid or GABA); and ***peptides*** (*i.e.*, endorphins, cholecystokinin, and neurotensin).

MONOAMINES

The ***catecholamines*** are formed by the breakdown of phenylalanine to tyrosine, tyrosine to 3,4-dihydroxyphenylalanine (DOPA), DOPA to dopamine, and dopamine to norepinephrine and then epinephrine.

In general, it appears that ***dopamine*** neurons selectively inhibit transmission of sensory information to enhance the signal-to-noise ratio. Dopamine also has a central role in reward mechanism. Its role in cocaine dependence is well established. Dopamine has been most associated clinically with the psychiatric disorder, schizophrenia.

There is strong evidence that the ***antipsychotic (neuroleptic) compounds*** have antidopaminergic effects, and that all antidopaminergic agents possess antipsychotic activity. This led to the ***dopamine hypothesis*** of the schizophrenias. It has been established that there are many different DA receptors. The role of D1 receptors in behavioral disorders is unclear. There has been demonstrated an increase in the number of D2 receptors in the caudate, putamen, and nucleus accumbens of schizophrenic patients. The clinical effects of antipsychotic drugs are related to their relative ability to block the D2 receptors. The D3 and D4 receptors are probably the site of action for the new atypical antipsychotic medications like clozapine. Other neurotransmitter systems are certainly involved in the schizophrenias since these disorders are extremely complex behavioral expressions.

The other most important behavioral correlate of the DA system is the appearance of ***Parkinsonism*** in persons who have deterioration in the nigrostriatal tract of the DA system. This may also be the system involved in ***tardive dyskinesia,*** a movement disorder secondary to relatively long-term maintenance on antipsychotic medications.

The ***norepinephrine*** (NE) cell bodies are found in the gigantocellular nucleus and, especially, in the ***locus ceruleus,*** but their highly branched axons project to all parts of the CNS. NE has been found to have inhibitory influences on some postsynaptic neurons and exciting effects on others. Therefore, it serves a modulating function within the CNS. Norepinephrine also plays a central role in the mobilization of the organism. There are some reports for increased levels of NE in the schizophrenias.

There is very strong evidence that this catecholamine plays an important role in the mood disorders such as the depressive syndrome. The mode of action of drugs that are most effective in the clinical management of depression all increase the available NE (and 5-HT; see below) at the receptor sites, probably by decreasing reabsorption. More recent evidence suggests that certain depressions may be associated with low NE synthesis and release, and others with low 5-HT. The ***catecholamine hypothesis*** of affective disorders suggests that depressions are associated with low levels of NE, and the manic syndrome is associated with excessive levels. More recent research suggests a more complicated interaction between NE and serotonin in mood disorders.

Other behavioral correlates of NE include anxiety, arousal, pain, and possibly components of the sleep cycle.

The role of ***epinephrine*** in stress is well recognized; however, little is known about epinephrine as a central neurotransmitter except in the locus ceruleus, where it inhibits firing of the neurons.

The neurotransmitter ***serotonin*** (5-HT), an ***indolamine,*** is synthesized from tryptophan. The majority of neurons that produce this substance are in the ***raphe nuclei.*** Its role in complex human behaviors is still poorly understood; however, 5-HT does play a role in pain, aggression, mood regulation, appetite, sleep, temperature control, cardiovascular components, and respiration.

The suspected role of 5-HT in affective disorders has been noted above, but the definition of that role is still unclear. Recent data implicate 5-HT in obsessive-compulsive behavior. 5-HT's role in the major thought disorders is unclear.

ACETYLCHOLINE

Today the most important role of ACh is in its link to Alzheimer's disease and, therefore, to memory and cognition. Present research into this disorder demonstrates reductions in choline acetyltransferase activity and the inability of brain tissue from Alzheimer's patients to synthesize acetylcholine.

The other behavioral role of ACh is in movement. When there is an imbalance between CNS levels of DA and ACh, Parkinsonlike movements appear.

AMINO ACIDS

GABA is probably the major inhibitory neurotransmitter in the CNS. Apparently, within the CNS its role is to modulate the activity of the other neurotransmitter systems.

A dysfunction in this modulation may be central to the

psychiatric syndrome called ***generalized anxiety disorder*** and, especially, in other syndromes involving panic.

PEPTIDES

The opioid peptide neurotransmitters emanate from one of three precursors: the β-endorphin/ACTH (adrenocorticotropic hormone) precursor, the enkephalin precursor, and the dynorphin/neo-endorphin precursor. The receptors of these neurotransmitter systems are distributed in the CNS close to the dopaminergic systems that have been implicated in the schizophrenias. All of these neurotransmitters seem to be important in the CNS systems that are responsive to stress.

Because of the location of peptide neurotransmitter systems in relation to dopaminergic systems, a great deal of research has been conducted relative to the role of peptides in the schizophrenias. Clinical studies provide no convincing support for an excess or deficiency of endorphin activity in schizophrenia. However, there may be an interactive effect between the peptide and dopamine systems. Because of the proximity of the two systems and the fact that neurotensin (NT) and cholecystokinin (CCK) coexist with dopamine in certain dopaminergic neurons, research in this important area is ongoing. Neuropeptides appear to coexist in all of the major neurotransmitter systems. In discussing peptides, increasingly a distinction is being made by investigators between neurotransmitters and neuromodulators.

Current speculation regarding ***narcotic addiction*** and the endorphin system involves the hypothesis that a constant external supply of morphine substances suppresses the natural production of endorphins. This constant external supply may also stimulate the CNS to produce additional receptors so that when that external supply is discontinued there is not enough endogenous substance to maintain a homeostatic state. Withdrawal, then, would be defined as an endorphin deficiency with an extended period of time to return to normal functioning level. This would, in part, account for the long-lasting depression and ***protracted abstinence syndrome*** common in narcotic withdrawal. A second hypothesis concerns congenital endorphin deficiency. Since congenital endorphin excess can be postulated from case studies of insensitivity to pain, such insensitivity being reversed by administration of a narcotic antagonist, it is logical the converse may occur. Such a finding would assist in understanding how some persons use narcotic substances without becoming addicted, and others report addictionlike ''craving'' behavior from first exposure.

Other important peptides and their behavioral correlates are cortisol, which is affected by mood states and stress; gonadotropin-releasing hormone (GRH), luteinizing hormone (LH), and follicle-stimulating hormone (FSH), all of which are important in sexual activity, sexual developmental stages, and sexual cycles; and melatonin, which is secreted by the pineal gland and is central to the wake-sleep cycle and strongly implicated in transient situations like ''jet-lag'' and more chronic clinical conditions like seasonal affective disorder.

Physiologic Determinants of Behavior

LIMBIC SYSTEM

The limbic system primarily is composed of the phylogenetically older cortex and associated structures: the ***hippocampus, fornix, mammillary bodies, anterior thalamic nuclei, cingulate gyrus, septal nuclei*** and ***amygdala.*** This system is arranged in circuits and influences behavioral expression regulated by the hypothalamus. Activities of the limbic system include modulation and coordination of the central processes of emotional elaboration, motivation, establishment of conditioned reflexes and memory storage. The major behavioral correlates of limbic system dysfunction are:

Bilateral lesions of the hippocampus produce profound deficits of short-term memory storage and retrieval.

Patients with irrepressible rage reactions demonstrate spiking on EEG tracings originating from the amygdala.

The Kluver-Bucy syndrome of submissive behavior, hypersexuality, visual agnosia, and oral exploration of objects—first noted in vicious monkeys after removal of the temporal lobes, uncus, amygdala, hippocampus and the tail of the caudate—has been demonstrated in humans with lesions to the amygdala. The amygdala also has links to brain areas involved in cognitive and sensory processing. Apparently it helps coordinate bodily reactions that serve as internal warnings.

Electrical stimulation of the septal region produces intense pleasure responses and pain/seizure blockade.

Electrical discharges from the uncus (*i.e.,* uncinate fits) are correlated with olfactory hallucinations of foul odors, such as feces or burning rubber, anxiety–fear (*e.g.,* ''empty feeling in the stomach''), jamais vu, or déjà vu.

The caudate nucleus helps regulate impulses involving sex, aggression, and various objects of disgust.

RETICULAR ACTIVATING SYSTEM

The RAS and its thalamic projections is one of the phylogenetically oldest parts of the brain involved with determining behavior. As noted in the section on consciousness, the RAS is intimately involved in ***arousal*** and ***attention.*** Most sensory and motor impulses pass through the RAS as they enter and exit the brain. Functionally, the RAS can, through diffuse activation, ''prime'' the entire brain to process stimuli; facilitate or inhibit sensory or motor stimuli; "filter" incoming information; and facilitate the active process of sleep through inhibition of the midbrain reticular system.

Based on evidence that all antipsychotic preparations have their effect in the RAS and limbic system, some theorists have postulated RAS dysfunction in the schizophrenias. In this framework, schizophrenia would be seen as the behavioral expression of improper filtration of environmental stimuli. The resultant stimulus influx overwhelms the schizophrenic's cortical function, reflected in the schizophrenic's inability to cope appropriately with the world.

CORTICAL SITES

Cortical sites are in executive control of much of human behavior. The left cerebral hemisphere is responsible for verbal abilities—with the exception of a very few right-hemisphere-dominant persons. Prerolandic areas are correlated with the motor act of speech. Dysfunction here results in ***motor*** or ***Broca's*** or ***expressive aphasia***—synonymous terms. Persons with such an aphasia usually are able to understand symbolic communication, but have difficulty expressing themselves freely in good grammatical form. Postrolandic areas (*i.e.,* temporal and parietal) appear to be in executive control of the comprehension of symbolic communication. Lesions here produce ***sensory*** or ***Wernicke's*** or ***receptive aphasia*** (also synonymous). ***Conduction aphasia*** results from lesions of the arcuate fasciculus. This results in a disconnection of the center of language production from the center of language comprehension. Neither production nor comprehension is severely impaired. These persons simply cannot repeat phrases. ***Global aphasia*** comes from impairment of the entire left hemisphere, usually from impairment of the blood supply of the left middle cerebral artery. Almost all language function is lost, with the person able to say only very routinized phrases like "hello" and "goodbye."

Damage to the right cerebral hemisphere in postrolandic areas is correlated with ***visual–spatial dysfunctions*** (*e.g.,* inability to follow a blueprint or road map) and ***construction dyspraxias,*** the inability to motorically reproduce a visual stimulus.

Sensorimotor abilities tend to be under control of the contralateral sensory/motor gyri of the cortex. ***Stereognosis*** is the ability to perceive spatial configuration of objects from tactile sense alone. This is characteristically under executive control of the contralateral postrolandic area. Dysfunction is called ***astereognosis.*** Audition is primarily contralateral in executive control, although there is an 80% to 20% split of fibers from the cochlea to the temporal lobes, with the 20% represented on the ipsilateral temporal cortex.

Vision is somewhat more complex. ***Visual fields*** are divided into quadrants. The right half of each retina and, therefore, the left visual field, is represented on the right occipital cortex. Conversely, the left half of each retina (the right visual field) is represented on the left occipital cortex. Fibers from the upper quadrants sweep through the temporal lobes, and fibers from the lower quadrants course through the parietal region. When corresponding fields in each eye are defective, it is called a ***homonymous hemianopsia*** if both upper and lower quadrants are defective. A homonymous hemianopsia implies either occipital lobe dysfunction or temporal and parietal dysfunction in the brain hemisphere contralateral to the field defect. Bilateral upper and lower outer field cuts imply dysfunction at the optic chiasm, usually tumors of the pituitary gland. Single-eye impairment suggests dysfunction anterior to the optic chiasm.

SENSORY DEPRIVATION

Sensory deprivation is a physiologic condition presumably tied to activity of the RAS. Sensory deprivation in the laboratory is attained through constant control of visual, auditory, olfactory, kinesthetic, thermal, tactile, and gustatory stimuli. When environmental sensory stimuli are decreased or removed, the RAS apparently can no longer maintain a homeostatic balance between internal and external reality. In perceptual terms, all external frames of reference to interpret cues are absent. The major correlates of sensory deprivation are profound anxiety; depression or hostility (*i.e.,* irritability); auditory, visual, and tactile hallucinations; depressed level of consciousness and alertness; and extreme stimulus hunger. The basic similarity between monotonous night driving, isolation for "brainwashing" or suggestability effects, and sensory deprivation is apparent.

SLEEP

Sleep behavior is an active physiologic process. Apparently, structures in the lower pons and medulla are responsible for initiating and/or maintaining sleep through synchronization of cerebral cortical rhythms. Serotonin production is correlated with sleep induction. Presumably these mechanisms act through inhibition of the midbrain reticular system. Sleep is divided into stages reflected by electroencephalogram (EEG) activity. Each progressive stage reflects deeper sleep (Hauri, 1977).

Stage 1: The EEG is characterized by low-voltage mixed frequency, but most predominant is theta activity (5 to 7 per second). This is the same wave form demonstrated by experienced mediators.

Stage 2: The EEG shows waxing and waning bursts of regular waves called sleep spindles. Sleep spindles are

12 to 14 per second and each spindle lasts 1 to 2 seconds. These are present against a background of low-voltage irregular rhythms.

Stage 3: High-voltage slow EEG activity is observed.

Stage 4: Continuous high-voltage slow EEG activity at about 1 per second is seen. ***Night terrors*** in children, ***enuresis*** and ***sleepwalking*** apparently all arise from stages 2, 3, and 4. These four stages are collectively referred to as non-REM sleep.

During ***rapid eye movement (REM),*** the background EEG is indistinguishable from stage 1, except that bursts of REM are recorded. Accompaniments of REM sleep include vivid visual dreams, penile tumescence in males from infancy through old age and vaginal lubrication in females, disappearance of torso EMG, and the greatest variability in activity of the autonomic nervous system (ANS). ***Nightmares*** arise here. ***Sedative–hypnotic medications*** reduce REM, and withdrawal of these medications results in ***REM rebound.*** REM deprivation is correlated with subsequent neural hyperexcitability and decreased electroconvulsive seizure threshold. Nonvisual dreams, similar to thoughts running through the mind, occur in other sleep stages.

Apparently, REM sleep interrupts non-REM sleep an average of every 90 minutes, with the amount of REM sleep increasing during the total sleep period. Over a lifetime, progressively less REM, and less sleep overall, is obtained, although in the adult and older person the amount of sleep spent in REM is about 20%. In the newborn and infant, the amount of REM is much higher. During a single, normal sleep period, individuals proceed regularly through consecutive stages of sleep, with few or no fully awake episodes during the period. Also with increased age, the trend is toward lighter sleep patterns and, therefore, more awakenings are to be expected. CNS–depressant drugs like alcohol produce similar effects at any age.

Sleep deprivation results in errors of omission (as opposed to errors of commission). When prolonged for more than 72 to 96 hours, the effects can be profound, resulting in a deliriumlike organic brain syndrome.

Disorders of sleep other than those noted above include ***narcolepsy,*** which is characterized by four symptoms: sudden onset of REM sleep resulting in excessive daytime sleepiness, ***cataplexy*** (a sudden loss of muscle control and tone) precipitated by strong emotion or excitement, sleep paralysis, and hypnagogic hallucinations. There is evidence for a recessive genetic component in narcolepsy as well as autoimmune factors. ***Sleep apnea*** syndromes, or sleep-induced respiratory impairment, are another group of disorders, characterized by three types: those associated with REM and non-REM (type A), those associated with non-REM only (type B), and those associated with REM and the transitions from wakefulness to stage 1, and transition to REM (type C). ***Drug dependency insomnia*** results from habitual use of hypnotics and tranquilizers. ***Nocturnal myoclonus*** is another sleep disorder that sometimes occurs with the "restless leg syndrome." ***Circadian rhythm disturbance,*** or "jet-lag," is a dissonance between the internal body clock and external time zone. In phase-lag syndrome, the individual has difficulty falling asleep; in phase-lead syndrome, the patient falls asleep and awakens too early. ***Pseudoinsomnia*** is a condition in which the patient sleeps 6 or more hours but believes (perhaps dreams) he is not sleeping. However, most insomnias relate to anxiety or depression.

CIRCADIAN RHYTHMS

Circadian rhythms are cyclic physiologic activities of the body which may have significant influence on behavior. The different rhythms have regulators of two origins. The first are ***endogenous regulators,*** which arise from within the person. With total isolation from atmospheric and/or other relevant influences, these will continue in a more or less regular fashion. The second are ***exogenous regulators,*** which originate outside the person. The major exogenous regulators that have been studied are the 24-hour light–dark cycle, the disruption of which is responsible for jet-lag; chemicals like alcohol, amphetamines and other drugs that can produce a new pattern in the circadian rhythms; and stress, emotional or physical, that can disrupt the normative rhythm.

The major circadian rhythms are the sleep–wakefulness period of the 24-hour day (the supra-chiasmatic nucleus plays a role in the day–night rhythms), menstrual cycle in women, adrenal steroid secretion, liver enzymes for metabolism, REM–non-REM variations in sleep, body temperature, heart rate, blood pressure, and cell reproduction and sensitivity. The latter rhythm has clinical significance for conventional radiation therapy, in that radiation of some tumors may kill more cancerous cells in the morning than at other times.

Acquisition of Behavior (Learning)

Genetic, biochemical, and physiologic determinants of behavior address "inborn" or "natural" events over which the individual has little control. The following discusses behaviors that either are acquired or strongly influenced by learning.

Learning is defined as the relatively permanent change in a behavioral tendency that occurs as a result of reinforced practice. This definition involves a number of assumptions. First, "change" implies that one can learn to do or learn not to do. Second, "behavioral tendency" implies that learning is inferred from behavior. Third, practice accompanied by reinforcement is the "cause" of acquisition and maintenance of a change in behavioral tendency. The neurophysiology of learning is a very exciting field of research by neurobiologists of various disciplines. For example, the formation of a memory trace involves a stimulus producing an electrical or chemical impulse, which passes through neurons and triggers formation of connections between synapses. When learning occurs in animals, synaptic connections have been shown to increase. Memory (previously learned material) has been demonstrated to be affected by the person's mood, emotional stress levels, fatigue, overload, and so forth.

REINFORCEMENT

Reinforcement has a central role in acquisition of most behavior. Two general types of reinforcement have been demonstrated. ***Primary reinforcements*** are those that address some type of primary need the organism has, such as food, sleep, or water. ***Secondary reinforcements*** are learned, such as money, a smile, verbal approval, or job promotion. Reinforcement is a "payoff" and is commonly conceptualized as ***positive*** when the person is *given* something that strengthens the response tendency, like food or money, or ***negative*** when something is *withdrawn,* which strengthens the response tendency (*e.g.,* pain, nagging, or other discomfort is removed). ***Punishment*** is classified as ***aversive*** stimulation and is usually only effective in suppressing behavior for a short while, or teaching the person who is punished to stay away from the punishing individual.

Also of considerable significance is the ***schedule of reinforcement.*** The person may be placed on an absolute reinforcement schedule, either reinforced every time the behavior occurs (which results in the reinforcement losing its effectiveness) or never reinforced for the behavior (which results in ***extinguishing*** a given behavior). Periodically the extinguished behavior will reoccur, "just to see if maybe it will work this time." This is called ***spontaneous recovery.*** Or the person may be placed on a ***partial reinforcement*** schedule. Partial reinforcement schedules produce the most stable behavior patterns and behavior resistant to extinction. The major schedules can be diagrammed as follows:

	Fixed	Variable
Interval		
Ratio		

Fixed-interval means reinforcement is available only after a given, consistent period of time has elapsed. This produces "bursts" of behavior immediately prior to the time reinforcement is available (*e.g.,* "cramming" for scheduled exams). This yields the fewest responses per unit of time and the least consistent rate of response (fourth place).

Variable-interval means reinforcement again is available after a period of time; however, the time period changes (*e.g.,* an instructor gives random "pop quizzes"). This improves response and consistency rates to third place.

Fixed-ratio improves response and consistency rates to second place. In this mode reward is available after a given constant amount of responding (*e.g.,* being reimbursed $5.00 per 100 stitches sewn).

Variable-ratio schedules produce the highest response and consistency rates. Again, reinforcement is available after the person produces a given number of responses; however, the response rate for "payoff" varies (*e.g.,* playing slot machines). This partial reinforcement schedule produces high rates of behavior because the person knows it's a variable-ratio reward system; therefore, the more responses, the sooner the reinforcement will appear—and maybe the ratio will be small "next time."

As a rule, the acquisition of behavior is maximal if practice is distributed over a series of trials rather than the same number of responses massed into fewer numbers of episodes.

TYPES OF LEARNING

Different types of learning are discussed below. These are ordered in terms of increasing complexity as well as chronological appearance:

Instincts. Instincts are defined as inborn predispositions to behave in a specific manner when appropriate stimulation is experienced. Today most writers refer to instincts as "primary drives" or "primary needs." While inborn and, therefore, not learned, their expression in humans is strongly modified by the milieu. Those instincts central to modern psychodynamic theories are sexuality, aggression, and dependence. Other writers include curiosity, mastery, nutrition, oxygen, and other vegetative functions. Whether called instincts, primary drives, or needs, they presumably originate from genetic, biochemical, or physiologic substrates; therefore, while they can be modified in expression (and actually, in some instances, suppressed for extended periods of time) they will recur given appropriate stimulation or through circadian fluctuation.

Imprinting. Imprinting was considered by ***Konrad Lorenz*** to be an innate mechanism that precipitated attachment to a significant parenting object, released by a set of stimuli at a critical time in neonates, and in which the role of reward was minimal. Lorenz adequately demonstrated the phenomenon in neonatal ducks and geese as they "imprinted" him as their "mother." Subsequent theoreticians have linked imprinting in lower animals to

bonding or ***attachment*** in human infants. While the analogy is obvious, whether the mechanisms are truly similar has not been established.

Classical Conditioning. Classical conditioning is the form of learning popularized by ***Pavlov,*** which is described as ***stimulus substitution.*** An event that does not produce a given effect is presented immediately prior to an event that will reliably produce a given effect. Overtime the first stimulus will become substituted for the second, and elicit the response. A clarifying example is a child who is only brought to the physician for immunizations. The child walks in the door, sees the doctor, is stuck with a needle, and begins to cry. With repetition, the child begins to cry when the doctor is first encountered. In classical conditioning terms, the needle stick is the ***unconditioned stimulus (UCS)*** that produces the cry, or ***unconditioned response (UCR).*** The physician is the ***conditioned stimulus (CS)*** and the cry on seeing the physician is the ***conditioned response (CR).*** The conditioning is the new link between the physician and the cry. Sometimes not only the physician, but also the waiting room, the nurse, the word ''doctor,'' the front door of the office, and all things associated with the needle stick begin to elicit the same conditioned response of crying. This is called ***stimulus generalization*** or ***stimulus gradient*** and is probably the factor responsible for the observation that hypertensive patients produce more hypertensive readings in the physician's office than in their home environment (so-called ''white coat'' hypertension).

Classical conditioning has been demonstrated in all animal life forms from unicellular animals through humans, both before and after birth. Classical conditioning is associated with sympathetic and parasympathetic responses of the ANS and, therefore, is not ordinarily under much cognitive control. There is an optimal time interval of 0.5 second separation between the CS and the UCS for the stimulus substitution to occur. Also, the UCS must occur regularly for the behavior to remain stable. If it does not, then extinction occurs (*i.e.,* weakening, and eventual disappearance of the CR). If the child does not experience the prick of the needle each time the physician is seen, soon the child will no longer cry when the physician enters the room. Heart rate, galvanic skin response, insulin shock, and immune reactions are a few of the responses that have been classically conditioned to neutral stimuli like a word or picture.

Classical conditioning may be the basic process by which certain early fears and emotional responses are acquired. Many authors feel the foundations of so-called ***psychosomatic illnesses*** are laid down in the infant through this process. There is some evidence that the ***placebo reaction*** alleviating pain may be a classically conditioned endorphin response.

Operant Conditioning. Operant, or instrumental, conditioning is frequently linked to the work of ***B. F. Skinner.*** It is the production of a given response through environmental reinforcement. For instance, the child stops crying and the physician gives the child a piece of candy, or the medical student diligently studies and receives an ''F.'' Later the same student doesn't study and receives an ''A.'' The student learns to ***discriminate*** which response the environment will differentially reinforce and thereafter does not study.

Operant conditioning is the general case of learning, and it affects all behavior, including activity of the ANS. ***Biofeedback*** is a direct outgrowth of operant conditioning. In biofeedback, a person receives positive secondary reinforcement (*e.g.,* a light or buzzer is activated for increasing periods of time, or a smile or approval from the experimenter) for controlling a body function, be the function under ANS control or not. The body function that is trained to appear is one that is incompatible with distress. For example, tension headache sufferers are trained to decrease frontalis muscle EMG. Biofeedback has been applied experimentally to a wide variety of medical problems including migraine and tension headaches, hypertension, and peripheral circulatory disorders. The technique, however, is still controversial as a therapeutic modality.

In direct opposition to classical conditioning, where the UCS (*i.e.,* the reinforcement) must always be present to ensure stable response patterns, in operant conditioning the reinforcement is present 100% of the time *only* during the response acquisition phase. After acquisition, a schedule of partial reinforcement (explained above) is instituted to maintain a stable response pattern. For example, parents who want to guarantee that children are disruptive should inconsistently provide either approval of the behavior or disapproval. Such partial reinforcement produces behaviors that are resistant to extinction.

A variant of operant conditioning is ***shaping.*** In this procedure, successive approximations of a complete behavior are developed through 100% reinforcement, and then a more complex form is developed and stabilized. For example, an elective mute child first would have *sounds* developed through 100% reinforcement and stabilized by partial reinforcement—then syllables, then words, then phrases, then sentences, and so forth. Shaping can also be used to decrease unwanted behaviors like toewalking: the child first is reinforced for partial toe-walking, then for partial sole walking, and then for flat foot walking.

Cognitive Learning. Cognitive learning, as opposed to conditioning, emphasizes the role of understanding. It assumes the individual is fully aware and attention is focused. (Data acquired by classical and operant conditioning may be employed to acquire material through this process.)

Piaget and associates have contributed significantly to our understanding of cognitive learning. Piaget emphasized that the cognitive apparatus to understand the world changes dramatically as a person matures. The child is not a miniature adult. Rather, the child at different ages and stages has different capacities to comprehend. The child is moved into more mature ways of understanding through the equilibration process, which has two components. First, ***assimilation*** means that the child, through active interchange with the environment, incorporates data from the external world. The child assimilates data until the extant mental structure can't manage the mass of assimilated data. At this point, ***accommodation*** takes place and the mental apparatus changes to the next more complex structure of cognitive processing and understanding. With this new structure the child assimilates more data until forced to accommodate the new mass of assimilated data to an even more complex cognitive structure.

In addition to the equilibration process, Piaget posited that physical maturation, active experience with environment, and social transmission of information were the essential elements for changing cognitive structure. Deprivation of any or all of these was believed to result in less than maximal cognitive functioning.

Piaget posited four stages of cognitive development:

Sensorimotor stage. During this stage, from birth to roughly 18 months, the infant employs senses and motor activity to interact with the environment. The focus is coordination of senses and movement. Pure sensations are relied upon; therefore, the infant operates on the principle, "out of sight out of mind," which explains why "peek-a-boo" can be a never-ending source of distraction and pleasure for the infant. During this stage, the infant moves beyond its body to interaction with the world. Continued practice produces more systematic and well-organized interaction. This sensorimotor period ends with the infant having an active interest in new behaviors and novel events. The infant has shifted from reflex activity to intentional means–ends action sequences, with independent motor systems purposely coordinated.

Preoperational stage. In this stage, roughly from 18 months to 7 years of age, the child relies specifically on perception and "intuition" in thought processes to comprehend the world. However, the conservation of identity of objects is not yet possible. For example, if one of two same-sized pieces of clay is elongated, it is reported to be "more" or "bigger" than the one that was not altered. The child at this stage can focus cognitive processes on only one dimension at a time.

Concrete operations stage. At this time, roughly from age 7 to 11–13 years, the child begins to abstract commonalities from tangible objects. When the child can see, touch, or gain images from objects, similarities between them can be extracted. This child can add and subtract elements to or from each other and yet conserve the essence of separate elements. Totally abstract discussions are not possible yet and "reversibility" in thought processes is difficult. The child is egocentric in both the preoperational and concrete operations stages; *i.e.,* everything happens "because of me." If untoward events occur during this time (*e.g.,* parent divorce or a parent dies) the child assumes the responsibility for the event.

Formal operations stage. This last stage, beginning at about 11 to 13 years of age, is characterized by the ability to indulge in abstract, conceptual thinking where tangible objects are not necessary for the conceptualization to occur. This individual can think in terms of relations and reversibility. Reflective conceptual cognitive reasoning and understanding is a reliable process at this stage. At this level of maturation, cognitive processes can be used to control emotions. Until this time the reverse has been the case.

Social Learning. Social learning theories focus on reciprocal ***interpersonal relations*** and those behaviors acquired as a result of ***modeling.*** The learner observes another person perform an act and models behavior after the observed person. The observer learns without the reinforcement necessary for conditioning-type learning. Indeed, vicarious reinforcement and vicarious extinction have been observed in children. If a child sees another rewarded for a behavior, the observing child will produce the same behavior—and vice versa with vicarious extinction. It is assumed that the integrated, conforming, social behavior which children acquire is based on observation either of peers being reinforced for producing a behavior or through imitation of parental behavior. Some of the most current controversial issues in social learning are those that involve the influence of media on children's behaviors (specifically sexuality, aggression, and violence observed on television) and peer influence in substance abuse.

While reinforcement—especially primary reinforcement—does not play a truly central role in social learning theories, it is important. Models may provide behavioral roles for others to follow; however, if primary or secondary reinforcement of the newly acquired behavior does not occur, it will soon extinguish.

Growth and Development

In addition to biochemical, physiologic, genetic, and learned influences on behavior, there is impact from the natural unfolding growth and development process. This process will be presented in two parts: the theories and the phenomenal observations.

THEORIES

Psychoanalytic. ***Psychoanalytic theory,*** associated most with Sigmund Freud and his cohorts, focuses on the ***intrapsychic*** aspects of the mind. Central to early psychoanalytic theory was the concept of ***libido,*** defined as "psychic" energy (*i.e.,* motivation) and presumed to emanate from tissue metabolism. During "psychosexual" development, this psychic energy, or libido, is invested (concentrated or "collected") in different somatic areas at different stages of maturation. There are five stages:

1. ***The oral sensory stage:*** Approximately from birth to 18 months, the child's major source of interest and gratification is the mouth, which serves as the major focus for exploration of the environment. "Oral receptivity" (*i.e.,* sucking) is characteristic of the early portion and "oral aggression" (*i.e.,* biting) is characteristic of the latter portion of this stage. The central psychological "personality" issues involve trusting others, the relative safety of the world, and dependency needs. "Separation anxiety" often has its roots in this period.
2. ***The anal musculoskeletal stage:*** Approximately from 18 months to 3 years of age, the anus and the musculoskeletal system are the major repository of libidinal energy and the primary source of gratification or pleasure. Personality issues of control (including excretory functions), mastery, attitudes about authority's rules, savings (holding on), and spending (letting go) are considered to emanate from this stage. The emotions of disgust and anger, from and toward others, have considerable influence in this period.
3. ***The phallic/urethral stage:*** From about 3 years to 6–7 years of age, libidinal energy is primarily invested in the sexual organs and sensual experience. Activity is concentrated in extension to others and awareness of sex differences. It is at this stage that the Oedipal/Electra complex develops and is, one hopes, resolved.

   Oedipal/Electra complex is a normal phase through which all persons pass. It encompasses the child's developing a "love" attachment to the parent of the opposite sex and a conflicting desire to "get rid of," as well as maintain a relationship with, the parent of the same sex so the son–mother or daughter–father love can be consummated. Characteristic of this phase is the child's saying to the loved parent, "I want to marry you when I grow up." Successful resolution of this conflict is through the child realizing the same-sexed parent is more powerful; therefore, attempts to "get rid of" that parent may precipitate dire consequences including removal or envy of the penis and loss of love, that is, ***castration anxiety.*** To resolve this, the child identifies with the same-sexed parent, gives up the opposite sexed parent as a primary love object, and says, "When I grow up I want to be like my (daddy/mommy) and marry a (woman/man) like you."

   Another way to understand this phase is that the child prematurely tries to take on adult responsibility. Normal resolution is achieved by the parents' reassurance that the child does not have to "grow up" yet. It is permissible for the child to remain a child for a while. Resolution that creates problems later includes issues of incest, loss of the child's same-sex parent so that "you're the man/woman of the house now," and so forth, in which cases the child prematurely assumes an adult role.
4. ***The latency stage:*** From approximately 7 to 12 years of age, libidinal energy is not concentrated in any specific body zone. It is characterized by same-sex peer relations and avoidance of opposite-sex interactions, although girls seem to be more interested in relations with boys than are boys to girls. Socialization, acquisition of social customs, and companionship are major issues.
5. ***The genital stage:*** From about 12 years of age to death, fully integrated, aware activities involve persons of the opposite sex and include romantic love. Fully established sexual identification, independence from parents, selecting a spouse, and vocational goals should be established during the early portions of this stage. The person who completes this stage well is referred to as a "Genital Character."

Throughout this maturational process, difficulty can be created through several mechanisms. First, ***fixation*** can occur at a particular stage of development, and little progress is made toward increasingly adaptive or mature levels of functioning. Second, normal progression through various stages occurs but during periods of stress, ***regression*** to an earlier stage of maturity can be observed. This is particularly true if a significant trauma occurred at an earlier stage producing a "weakness" or vulnerability. In this case, normal development may continue but later, under stress that is either literally or symbolically similar to the original trauma, the individual regresses to the stage at which the original trauma occurred. Because the content of the original trauma was ***repressed*** (*i.e.,* forgotten), the individual experiences the anxiety from the original threat without cognitive awareness of the frightening stimulus.

The concepts of conscious, preconscious, and unconscious as nonphysiologic referents stem from psychoanalytic theory. As noted above, ***conscious*** means material that is in present awareness of the person (*e.g.,* what is being read at this time), ***preconscious*** refers to material not presently in awareness (*e.g.,* one's phone number), and ***unconscious*** refers to material that is not in the person's awareness and cannot be brought into awareness without special techniques.

In addition to stages of development and levels of consciousness, Freud also posited the ***pleasure principle,*** meaning that people seek pleasure and avoid pain. The pleasure principle, modified by experience, is the ***reality principle,*** which allows for the delayed gratification of needs until an appropriate time.

Freud divided intrapsychic life—''mind''—or personality into three conceptual subdivisions: the ego, superego, and id. The ***ego*** is the portion that interfaces internal needs with the external reality. It has the most conscious awareness and operates predominantly by the reality principle. The functions that are characteristically assigned to the ego are as follows:

Reality is the relationship to, testing, and sense of whether one is operating in the real world or in delusion.

Object relations refers to whether one can establish and maintain long-term close, interpersonal relations with at least one other person.

Autonomous functioning is the ability to care for oneself and meet the ordinary demands of living. This includes ''conflict-free'' mental functions such as memory, mobility, and vocabulary.

Defense is protection of the ego from being overwhelmed by demands from the other sectors of the ''mind.'' (A partial list of ego defense mechanisms is presented below.)

Synthesis is the ability to integrate data about the self and portions of behavior into a meaningful integrated whole (*e.g.,* ''I am a physician'').

Identity usually refers to sexual identity (*i.e.,* maleness/femaleness) or, more broadly, to a sense of ''who am I?''

Thinking refers to those elements discussed above under the process of thought.

(A helpful mnemonic for ego functions is ''ROAD-SIT,'' comprised of the first letters of each word.)

The ***id*** is the repository of basically unconscious instinctual drives (*i.e.,* needs) and impulses. It operates on the pleasure principle and, therefore, constantly seeks immediate gratification of needs—which is unrealistic.

The ***superego*** is the ''conscience'' or value system that was acquired at a very young age from parents through introjection and identification. Because it is acquired at an early age, it is in pure form, usually irrational, punitive, and rigidly understood. Its function is control of instinctual needs (*i.e.,* id): ''Thou shalt not!''

The unconscious instincts of the id constantly seek gratification and are controlled by ego reality functioning and superego restrictiveness. In order for the ego to function in reality and not be overwhelmed by demands from the id, protective mental devices develop called ego defense mechanisms. These allow at least partial gratification of instinctual needs. All people have defense mechanisms, but some defense mechanisms are more healthy than others. The major ego defense mechanisms are as follows:

Repression is involuntary exclusion of material, particularly conflicted data, from conscious awareness. (Repression is considered to be the basic defense mechanism, operating in conjunction with one or more of the following.)

Suppression is the intentional exclusion of material from consciousness.

Introjection is the total assimilation of the values, attitudes, and prejudices from parents into one's own ego and, especially, the superego.

Identification, while similar to introjection, is less total or complete. It is modeling oneself after a significant other. It can also be the conforming to the values and attitudes of a group.

Displacement is employed when the object that will satisfy an instinctual need is changed. For example, a resident physician on the house staff may strike his spouse instead of the attending physician at whom the resident feels rage.

Projection is the attribution of one's own impulse and/or thoughts (particularly if they are unacceptable) to another person. This is the mechanism underlying scapegoating, the central core of prejudice.

Reaction formation is turning an impulse, feeling, or thought into its opposite (*e.g.,* persons who cannot accept their own sexual impulses may work as a censor of pornographic movies, thereby partially gratifying their sexual needs).

Sublimation is turning ''unacceptable'' impulses, thoughts, or feelings into socially acceptable ones (*e.g.,* an individual may have murderous rage as a characteristic feeling state, but become a butcher). Sublimation is one of the healthiest defense mechanisms because of constructive endproducts and elements of conscious decision making involved.

Compensation is employed when one encounters failure or frustration in one activity or arena, and overemphasizes another (*e.g.,* an uncoordinated child may overstress intellectual pursuits).

Denial is the failure to recognize or be aware of obvious and logical consequences of a thought, act, or situation (*e.g.,* the student who blatantly cheats on an exam while a proctor is observing the student). This is a rather primitive defense mechanism and is almost always pathologic in the adult.

Conversion is the somatic representation of conflicting impulses, feelings, or thoughts. The representation is in body functions under executive control of sensory nerves or the voluntary nervous system. The ***primary gain*** from a conversion reaction is neutralizing painful affect with the symptom being symbolic of the conflict; for instance, a student fearful of failing an exam may experience paralysis of the dominant hand. The student may gain a great deal of attention and sympathy from others—this is the ***secondary gain.*** This defense mechanism is always pathologic because it doesn't facilitate free function of the individual.

Somatization, in contrast to conversion, is the physical expression of conflicts through body parts under executive control of the ANS, both the sympathetic and parasympathetic branches (*e.g.,* peptic ulcer).

Regression is the return to an earlier level of maturation or personality development. As noted above, this usually occurs under periods of stress and can be expected to appear in certain specific situations. For example, at the birth of a sibling, an older sib may begin to behave below his or her achieved maturation level. Patients admitted to hospital characteristically become whining, demanding, and dependent. Elements of regression may be a normal, expected response to severe illness.

Dissociation is the responsible defense mechanism in ''multiple personalities.'' A group of thoughts, feelings, and actions is split off from the main portion of consciousness, that is, they are compartmentalized. One personality is ''good,'' the other is ''bad.'' More commonly, amnesia, fugue states, or feelings of unreality become manifest.

Rationalization is offering a socially acceptable and more-or-less logical reason for an act usually produced by unconscious or nonverbalized impulses (*e.g.,* ''I was drunk; therefore, I sexually approached my attending's spouse''). The person misleads the self as well as others.

Since psychoanalytic theory emanated from observations of and attempts to intervene in pathology, some concepts unique to management of patients are important. ***Transference*** refers to a situation in which the patient begins to inappropriately project thoughts, feelings, and impulses onto the health care provider which are derived from unconscious internal states of the patient, often those he holds toward other significant persons (*e.g.,* mother). Presumably these are from unmet needs that the patient is experiencing. Somewhat similar to transference is the behavior complex called ''acting out.'' Instead of dealing maturely with the transference the patient behaviorally expresses (*i.e.,* displaces) the impulses outside the treatment setting. In ***countertransference,*** the health care provider projects personal unmet needs, feelings, and impulses from unconscious processes onto the patient. ''Acting out'' by the professional may end in a malpractice suit or ''divorce.''

Psychosocial Model. The ***psychosocial model*** or theory also has psychoanalytic origins but emphasizes the person in interaction with the environment. ***Eric Erikson*** postulated eight stages in the psychosocial development of man. Each stage has a ''task'' for resolution before the next stage can be entered successfully. Defective resolution of a stage forms an inadequate foundation upon which subsequent stages are constructed. The stages and tasks follow. The ages at which these stages develop, particularly in adult years can be quite variable, depending on experience.

1. ***Trust versus mistrust*** (from birth to age 18 months): To know and feel that the world is intrinsically safe and trustworthy, the developing infant must have basic needs met appropriately (*e.g.,* the hungry infant must be able to trust that when it cries, it will be fed). There must be continuity between the infant's action and the world's reaction.
2. ***Autonomy versus shame and doubt*** (from age 18 months to 3 years): In this stage, the young child must attain confidence in his ability to operate in the world somewhat autonomously of parents or significant others. The child must not end this period doubting ''he (or she) can stand on his (or her) own two feet'' or ashamed of attempts to differentiate from significant others. Issues of self-control (including bodily functions) are primary at this stage, exemplified by toilet training and the automatic ''no'' of the ''terrible twos.'' Usually this is not obstructionism or rebellion, but rather the child's way of saying, ''I'm not you.''
3. ***Initiative versus guilt*** (from age 3 to about 6 years): At this stage, the child must achieve the ability to initiate independent activities in the world, and to effectively carry these activities to fruition without others overwhelming the plans through guilt induction. Disproportionate fear (*i.e.,* inadequate resolution of the Oedipal/Electra complex) and superego anger can combine to form guilt as an inadequate resolution of this stage.
4. ***Industry versus inferiority*** (from age 6 to about 11 years): Industry refers to the child's accomplishments of goals without parental support. The child

attends school with peers who are relative equals in ability to produce. If the child does not successfully compete in interaction with these peers without the support of the parents, then a sense of inferiority develops that can color the remaining stages of development. This frequently produces in children the overwhelming impression of having nothing to offer others.

5. ***Identity versus role confusion*** (from age 11 to about 18 years): During this phase, the young adult experiences extremely rapid physical/endocrine changes and simultaneously feels the impact of numerous new environmental influences. The major task is to develop fully a sense of personal identity, which includes the establishment of a solid sexual role. The adequate resolution must be, "I know myself, and I can make it as an adult." If, in the face of these extreme pressures, the young adult can't establish this sense, then adult role confusion develops.
6. ***Intimacy versus isolation*** (from age 18 to about 40 years): With foregoing stages mastered, the adult has the task of developing an intimate, trusting, and committed relationship with at least one other person. If, by the end of this stage, an individual has not established that intimate relationship, a pervasive state of singular isolation is experienced in which a person feels he (or she) can neither share his (or her) life with nor gain support from others.
7. ***Generativity versus stagnation*** (from age 40 to 65 years): Generativity refers both to establishment of offspring and the guidance of those children's development, and entrance into an occupational arena where accomplishment and continued growth are feasible. Without developing children as personal extensions of the self or developing opportunities for occupational advancement, individuals find little meaning in life and become stagnant. By the end of this stage, an individual must take active responsibility for himself or herself. That is, if at age 40 the person still attributes all responsibility for present conditions to parents and early childhood experiences, serious difficulty in adaptation usually occurs.
8. ***Integrity versus despair*** (age 65+): During this time, a person develops emotional integration, examines his (or her) life and begins to evaluate personal status. Hopefully the individual looks at the past, present, and future and perceives a continuity of which that person is proud. That is, the individual looks at his or her past life and says, "Given the various influences that were ongoing, I lived my life well and I'm happy with it." If this examination results in unrectifiable disapproval, despair is the consequence.

In summation, these theories—psychoanalytic and psychosocial—and the concepts that Piaget developed should not be regarded as adversarial. Instead they are different, but complementary, dimensions of human development. Freudian theory focuses on psychodynamic and psychosexual internal processes, Erikson examines interpersonal or psychosocial issues, and Piaget attends to development of cognition. There are other theories, but these are the most commonly encountered.

THE LIFE CYCLE OF GROWTH AND DEVELOPMENT

Pregnancy and Birth. From conception to birth, a number of variables have an impact on the fetus. High maternal emotional levels have been reported to result in high levels of ACTH, NE, and epinephrine substances in the fetal bloodstream, and concomitant irritability of the fetus has been observed. Maternal attitudes toward the pregnancy and the number of siblings predict postpartum childrearing practices (*e.g.,* Warm–Cold and Permissive–Restrictive).

An area of concern is maternal psychoactive drug use during pregnancy. During the embryonic stage (0 to 2 months) drugs can produce morphologic malformations. In the fetal stage (3 to 9 months) chemicals in the bloodstream apparently do not cause frank malformations; rather, the chemicals lead to brain damage or growth retardation since substances in the mother's blood readily cross via the placenta into the blood system of the fetus. A ***general withdrawal syndrome*** in neonates born to mothers who consistently use psychoactive drugs during pregnancy has been documented and a rating scale of severity established. This syndrome can be fatal to neonates if not appropriately managed, with fatality apparently due to pervasive CNS and behavioral hyperactivity resulting in dehydration and consequent febrile seizure activity. Long-term effects of neonatal addiction and the general withdrawal syndrome have not been fully established. Recent data regarding babies born to mothers who use "crack" cocaine during pregnancy document in these infants irritability, incessant crying, and a dislike of human contact. ***Fetal alcohol effects*** have resurfaced as a primary concern. These effects have been associated with maternal alcohol consumption during pregnancy. In severe cases, the ***fetal alcohol syndrome*** can include microcephaly, mental retardation, various system abnormalities, and stigmata suggestive of Down's syndrome. Low birth weights are common. In mild cases of maternal alcohol consumption, only behavioral hyperactivity may be seen in the offspring. No exclusive causal relationship between alcohol, or its metabolites alone, and the described syndromes have been definitely established in humans, suggesting interaction between alcohol and other idiosyncratic factors. There appears to be a dose-dependent relationship.

Fetuses have been observed to respond to loud noises with muscle contraction and increased heart rate. Also the following behaviors have been recorded: finger sucking at 28 weeks; flexing and changing of position; and different reflexes described below (grasp at 17 weeks and Moro at 25 weeks).

The utilization of CNS-depressant medications and anesthesias to assist the birth process is being scrutinized. The most common include inhalation anesthetics, barbituates, meperidine, ''major tranquilizers,'' and local anesthetics. Most of these drugs may affect maternal physiology and labor by changing the intrauterine environment; the newborn directly by altering activation of functions that have been dormant; or the neonate's behavior by altering EEG activity level and its behavioral correlates.

Due to these medication issues and suggested ''dehumanization'' of hospital births, natural or ***prepared childbirth*** is being reexamined. ***Lamaze*** and Dick-Reed have been major proponents of unmedicated labor and birth, with the father present and providing support for the delivering mother. Emotional support for the birthing mother during labor and delivery has been demonstrated to decrease problems during the delivery, and their newborns require fewer prolonged hospital stays.

At birth, neonatal function can be assessed by using the ***Apgar*** rating system. Assessment is done at 1 minute and 5 minutes using five indicators: heart rate, respiratory effort, muscle tone, reflex irritability, and color tone. Each indicator is rated on a three-point scale: 0 = no function; 1 = function present, but poor; 2 = function perfect. The 5-minute score, in combination with birth weight, has the best predictability. The following correlates have been suggested: 0 to 3 = likely death; 4 to 6 = serious subsequent problems; 7 to 9 = later attentional defects and possible learning disability; 10 = perfect functioning.

Infancy. The major abilities with which neonates can interact with the world are ***reflexes.*** The main primitive reflexes are as follows:

Babinski: When scratched on the lateral aspect of the sole of the foot, heel to toes, the infant responds with dorsiflexion of the big toe and fanning of the others. This response continues from birth to between 12 to 18 months of age, when it disappears in normal children.

Moro: Any sudden movement of the infant's head and neck stimulates a rapid abduction, extension and supination of the arms with opening of the hands. The fingers of the hands adopt a distinctive ''C'' formation of the thumb and index finger and other digits of the hand are extended. In normal infants, the reflex persists until 4 to 6 months of age. The reflex is absent in newborns with diffuse CNS depression and other brain stem disorders. Its persistence beyond 4 to 6 months of age has been associated with mental retardation and brain damage.

Eye blink: Tactile stimulation of eyelashes, tapping the bridge of the nose, a bright light, or a loud noise provokes the blink response.

Grasp: Palmar pressure causes a grasp response in infants from 1 month to 5 to 6 months of age. A similar response of plantar flexion can be elicited up to between 9 to 12 months of age by pressing an object on the sole of the foot behind the toes.

Crossed extensor: If the leg of a supine infant is extended by pressure exerted on the knee and the sole of the extended foot stimulated with a sharp object, the result is extension and slight abduction of the unstimulated limb. This reflex normally disappears by 2 months of age.

Deep tendon reflexes: The response of striated muscles to sudden stretching is termed a deep tendon reflex. Those characteristically tested in infants are: jaw jerk (C5), biceps (C5–C6), radical periosteal (C5–C6), triceps (C6–C8), knee (L2–L4), and ankle (S1–S2).

Suck: Stimulation of the perioral and oral area results in orientation to the stimulus and sucking behavior if the stimulus is encountered.

Normative motor control in the infant is always individually different and no developing infant is ''normal'' at all milestones of development. The following are presented as general guides (at ages in months):

1 month:	Can lift head briefly
2 months:	Can raise chest for brief periods
3 months:	Makes stepping motions, can lift the head and hold it above the body plane, and can retain a hold on objects
4 months:	Can sit on a lap, look around, and display some lumbar back curvature; the hands can be grasped together, played with, and unilateral open-handed approach to objects can be observed
5 months:	Can sit alone briefly and grasp objects in a one-hand directional motion
6 months:	Can do knee push or swimmer movements and can get up on hands
7 months:	Can roll over unassisted
8 months:	Can stand with help
9 months:	Can sit alone unassisted and make some progress on the stomach
10 months:	Can scoot backwards and is able to crawl
11 months:	Can stand holding on to furniture; can grasp an object in each hand and bring them together, and can use the thumb and

	opposing forefinger to pick up small objects
12 months:	At the end of the first year can pull to a stand, walk when led, take and release small objects, and place them in containers
15 months:	Can stand and walk alone
18 months:	Can walk forward and backward, throw a ball, feed self, and use a cup
24 months:	Can hold a pencil and draw with it

Social behavior development in the infant is characterized by appearance of selected behaviors. Appropriate ***social smiling*** appears at about two months. ***Stranger anxiety*** (*i.e.*, fear response to "nonmother" persons) normally appears between 6 to 12 months of age. (This indicates that the capability of Piagetian object constancy has developed.) During infancy, play activity is singular and concentrated in sensorimotor exercise. This moves the infant from reflexive–respondent behavior into controlled–purposive, externally directed activity. It has also been demonstrated that the mother's mood state significantly affects the infant's EEG activity and related behavior.

Verbalizations by the end of the first two years have reached an average frequency of 200 words. The acquisition of language is from early reflexive laughing and crying to self-motivated babbling, which appears at about 6 to 8 months of age. Words as meaningful symbols first appear at about the age of 12 months; however, a range of between 1 to 3 years is normal.

Toilet training is not feasible until sphincter control has developed at between 1.5 and 2.5 years of age. This is contrary to data that many American parents "toilet train" their children between 9 and 14 months. If a child is toilet trained prior to 18 months of age, it is the "mothering person" who has been trained to observe when elimination is imminent and, consequently, rushes the child to the "potty." In the latter stages of infancy, the ***terrible twos*** appear, in which the child responds with "No!" to any request. This behavior is the reflection of the infant's initial attempts to establish autonomy and reflects entrance into Erikson's second stage.

During the latter stages of infancy and extending into the first preschool year, the ***gender identity*** is established. Depending on how parents and significant others interact with the child and possibly differential brain functioning, he or she establishes the basic feeling of being male or female. This feeling is in part learned and set by the age of 3 years. It is the private experience of the child's sexuality.

Major problem areas for infants include maternal deprivation, which may precipitate the infant's withdrawal from all social interaction. If no mothering substitute is provided, the infant can enter an extremely withdrawn condition known as ***anaclitic depression,*** proceed to ***marasmus,*** and even die. Institutionally raised children display milder, but similar, withdrawn characteristics. Although they may not die, their ability to form close interpersonal relations in later life is seriously compromised. They are unresponsive and demonstrate retardation in cognitive, language, and motor development. In addition to maternal deprivation, highly nervous mothers have a higher prevalence of infants who demonstrate behavioral dysfunctions, such as sleep disorders, irritability, hyperactivity, and feeding disorders, and also prematurity.

Preschool. During the ***preschool age*** (2 to 5 years) psychomotor maturation involves development of gross and fine motor skills, and handedness is typically established.

Parental child-rearing attributes seem to be most influential here. The Warm–Cold and Restrictive–Permissive dimensions for exploratory behavior in parental child-rearing practices are correlated with characteristic behavior patterns in children. This relationship is characterized by Figure 8-7.

Play activities progress from individual play to ***parallel play,*** in which two children are in physical proximity; however, each is playing alone with his own toys and games. The only reliable interaction is one child taking a toy from the other, precipitating a relatively violent interchange.

During preschool years, the child is extremely ***egocentric;*** all understanding of events in the external world are referred to the self for causal relations (*e.g.*, "The sun came up because it's time for me to get up"). Serious problems often arise from this egocentricity. If parents argue or divorce during this stage, the child may assume personal responsibility for that event (*e.g.*, "My daddy left because I'm not lovable").

In these first 5 years, language has fully developed and that progression is presented here as a cohesive whole process. Language seems to have an underlying architecture regardless of the language spoken. Brain-imaging studies show the same areas are active regardless of the language a multilingual person speaks. The structure of language is roughly divided into ***phonemes, morphemes, syntax,*** and ***semantics.*** A phoneme is the smallest possible unit of language identifiable as a discrete sound. For example, in the word *pot*, the *p* (written) is a phoneme; the *k* sound of both words *cow* and *keep* is the same phoneme (K) even though the two words are spelled differently. A morpheme is comprised of several phonemes and is the smallest linguistic unit that can have independent meaning. The word *apples* has two morphemes: (1) *apple*, and (2) the *s* that makes it plural. Syntax is defined as the rules by which people speak and understand a lan-

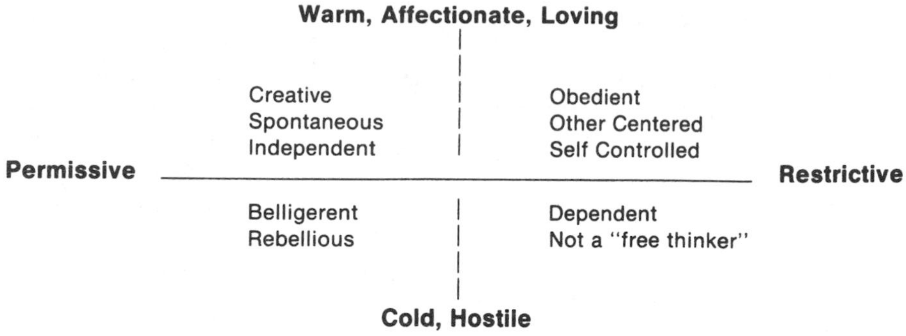

Fig. 8-7. Parental child-rearing dimensions and correlated child behavior.

guage. Syntax or grammar rules specify how morphemes are connected to produce meaningful units like phrases and sentences. Semantics is the inherent meaning, frequently involving emotional attachment, that is assigned to a particular piece of syntax. It is in this portion of language that major communication difficulty arises between persons, particularly if they are from different backgrounds. For example, the meaning of the word *white* is different depending on one's skin color (*e.g.,* black, red, white, or yellow), occupation (artist versus bleach manufacturer), and so forth.

Acquisition of language is interpersonal and represents an interplay between developmental process and the milieu within which a child is raised. Developmentally, prior to age 6 months, infants produce random sounds that are used in every known language. These sounds are identical, regardless of the infant's nationality, and are probably due to neuromuscular development of the throat and mouth. During the 6th to 12th month, when self-motivated babbling appears, apparently selective reinforcement by significant others shapes the infant's babbling into characteristic national language. The first words to appear are nouns, next are verbs, third are adjectives, and finally pronouns. Between 1 and 2 years of age, the phrases and sentences are simple and may be only one word (*e.g.,* "water"). Between 18 months and 2 years of age, the utterances become longer, with brief phrases and rudimentary sentences being assembled. By age 5, adult syntax (including past tenses, plurals and active as well as passive sentences) is established. Severely retarded persons are very slow to develop speech; however, for persons of normal and higher intellect, there is no correlation between the rapidity with which children talk and intelligence.

Issues in language development as influences on behavior include, especially, minority-majority issues. The majority of social institutions in America are white, Anglo-Saxon, and Protestant ("WASP"). Children who are not from a WASP background have been raised in a cultural milieu that has a different syntax than WASP, or that may assign a different semantic meaning to the WASP language. The result is that a minority child entering a majority school must become semantically bilingual and live in two different semantic worlds (the one of school and the one of home) in order to progress in WASP educational structure. Majority instructors frequently do not recognize this variance; therefore, when using a specific WASP word or phrase in the presence of a minority student, two things may occur: the student translates the word to and from minority semantics which gives the appearance of the student being slow, or the student may display a different emotional reaction to the word than the instructor expects, and, therefore, seems "strange" or "crazy."

Gender identification, the learned masculine or feminine public display of behaviors, develops during the preschool and school-age years.

School Age. By the time the child has reached ***school age*** (6 to 12 years of age), psychomotor development is complete and play activities have developed to a phase of ***cooperative*** interactional activity. In Erikson's framework, industry and adequacy in peer relations are of foremost importance. The beginning school years are when the child leaves the primary influence of parents and enters the control sphere of other adults—teachers—and peers. Typically, there is eager anticipation of school, which lasts for the first two years. The relationship children develop with teachers can be predicted by the child's relation to parents, that is, there is generalization between parents and teachers. Physical handicaps, eye–hand motor coordination difficulties, learning disabilities, perceptual problems, and hyperactivity can become barriers to adequate school performance which, in turn, will have an impact on the child's feeling of adequacy. Research suggests that males, children from lower classes, and children from minority groups—particularly if they also form a minority in the school—have a more difficult time adjusting to the WASP, sexist school situation characteristic of American public education.

During this stage, increased sexual exploration of self (*i.e.,* masturbatory activity) and others is normal. Because this age group is also characterized by same-sex interpersonal relations, same-sex sexual activity is also normally expected.

Sex role differences that began to appear in the previous stage are further defined and refined. Children learn at this time to regulate and sometimes to totally inhibit natural emotions. For instance, male children are taught not to cry (*i.e.,* not to demonstrate sad feelings: "big boys don't cry"); however, they are groomed to display aggressive, angry, hostile emotions. Conversely, female children learn that crying is perfectly permissible but that "nice girls never say *damn.*" As a consequence of this sex role training, males often display anger when they are sad, and females often cry when angry. Fortunately, several of the issues described above relating to language development, physical handicaps, physical orientation, and sex role differences are being perceived by educators and are being corrected.

Puberty and Adolescence. The onset of ***adolescence*** (from 12 to 17 years of age) is introduced by ***puberty:*** menstruation for females and seminal emissions for males. At puberty there is a physical growth spurt accompanied by radical endocrine shifts that control the onset of secondary sex characteristics (*i.e.,* distribution of body fat, pubic hair, voice changes, and facial hair in males). This endocrine shift also provides the overwhelming sexual drive observed in this phase. Females have an earlier onset of puberty than males, and there is evidence that onset of menses is occurring at younger ages, with the average age at 12.5 years and a normal range of 10.5 to 15 years of age. The onset of menses is apparently controlled in part by body size. Sperm production in males begins at about 14.5 years with a range of 12.5 to 16.5 years of age. Both masturbatory and interpersonal sexual activity heightens during this phase. Each year in America, there are approximately 30,000 pregnancies to females under the age of 15 years, and 1,000,000 to females between 15 and 19 years of age. About one third of these are aborted. About one half of unmarried mothers are teenagers. Teenage marriages frequently occur, 50% of which are because of pregnancy. While some of these are extremely stable and endure, one third end in divorce within four years.

During adolescence, a major achievement/milestone is for the young person to separate from the dependent role with parents. Cognitively, adolescents can meaningfully ask the question, "Why are things like they are?" but, because they have not fully developed delay of gratification, they want changes in perceived inequities now! In this constellation, the adolescent is faced with the necessity of separating from the parents, requiring affectional and emotional support needs, being associated with peers who share the perceived inequities and who can supply the support system. This configuration, in combination with the adolescent perception of personal invulnerability, contributes to high levels of illicit substance abuse, accidents (the leading cause of death among white teenagers), suicide (the second-leading cause of death), crimes of violence (peak at about 15 years of age), and homicide (the leading cause of death of black youth).

Throughout the above stages, ***moral development*** has also been maturing along with other psychosexual, psychosocial, and cognitive abilities. Depending on social model transmission, cognitive ability development, and other issues, the individual should have reached a high level of moral sophistication by the end of adolescence and entering into young adulthood. As with all developmental phases, persons may become fixated at one level or regress under special conditions of internal or external stress. ***Kohlberg*** (1973) provided the following framework for understanding moral development:

Stage 1: Punishment and obedience orientation. The physical consequences determine "goodness" or "badness" (*e.g.,* "It was bad because I got punished").
Stage 2: Instrumental relativist position. An action is right because it satisfied one's needs.
Stage 3: Interpersonal concordance. Good behavior is that which pleases or helps others and is approved by them.
Stage 4: Orientation to authority. Respect for law, authority, and order for their own sake.
Stage 5: Social contract orientation. Laws are agreements or contracts, and the contracts are what define right and wrong. Contracts are changeable.
Stage 6: Universal ethical principle orientation. Universal principles of justice prevail (*e.g.,* taking another's life is wrong).

Young Adulthood. In Erikson's framework, the major tasks during the young adult period (18 to 35 or 40 years of age) are developing an intimate relationship and establishing oneself in an occupational position. An intimate relationship in the United States usually implies love; according to Maslow, this is either ***B love*** or ***D love.*** "B" love is that which is based on each individual feeling personally secure—a full "genital" character in a psychodynamic framework. These persons like themselves, feel complete individually, and have an appreciation for "being." From this security and well-being, two persons choose each other to share their lives and create children from the union. Within this nuclear family, there is a maximum of respect for individuality with no ulterior motive to change the other person. Children in these families are guided, through warmth, permissiveness, and limit-setting, toward self-discovery and maximizing individual potential. "D" love is deficient love. In this framework, each person comes to the relationship out of perceived personal deficit and selects the other to fill the missing characteristic in the self. Such marriages frequently have an ulterior motive to alter the other person after the marriage has been established. Children in these nuclear families are acquired to fulfill needs the parents have (*e.g.,* to be an ''average'' family, to hold the marriage together, so the mother has ''something to do,'' and so forth). Such arrangements/dynamics predispose a nuclear family to later difficulties when the marriage partners can't or won't meet each other's needs, or the children leave the home.

The resolution to the second part of this Eriksonian phase, occupational choice—and particularly professional choice—is frequently based on irrational decisions. Early childhood or adolescent experiences often shape a premature decision, which is retained as an irrevocable law. Sometimes persons enter a particular field owing to familial or other social pressures (*e.g.,* ''All the women in this family have always been nurses.'') and maintain in their training ''until. . . .'' Unfortunately, ''until'' never comes and these persons frequently shift jobs at middle age. Terkel (1974) described four aspects of ***work:*** It influences the conception a person has about self and the surrounding world, it is used as a social locator, it can provide a source of power and autonomy, and it can be a source of major frustration and devaluation. In the United States, there is a work ethic that values and promotes productivity. While this orientation provides solid base to the economy, it creates considerable difficulty for youth who can't produce and the elderly who are forced into idleness at retirement age, particularly with regard to the first three of Terkel's items. Since ***socioeconomic status*** is based on income, education, and occupation, the young and old clearly wear a ''label'' of nonvalued lower socioeconomic status.

A major complicating factor, which develops for young adults, is forced incompatibility between marriage partners in Erikson's psychosocial context. Because extended-family structure in the United States is no longer the rule, each new nuclear family must quickly establish its own independent existence. This forces the husband to be preoccupied with work (*i.e.,* generativity), leaving the wife to raise the children and be the major source of warmth and intimacy. By the latter part of this stage, the husband frequently has established himself occupationally and wants to return to the family for the intimacy he has foregone while ''becoming a success.'' However, the wife has ''run out'' of intimacy and wants to begin her generativity. This decrease in extended-family dependence and psychosocial incompatibility certainly contributes to the observed increase in American divorce rates. About 1.5 million families in the United States have a separated or divorced person as head of the family, and those families involve more than 2.4 million children, 90% of whom live with their mothers. This condition, coupled with data presented earlier regarding sex role acquisition, egocentricity of youth, and so forth, provides a situation in which youth can become confused in identity, assume responsibility for the divorce of parents and, in frustration, act out maladaptively. Whether the increase in the number of wives entering the workforce over the past few decades will alter these astounding data remains to be seen.

Middle Age. As individuals enter the middle years (from 40 to 60 or 65 years of age), regardless of their previous occupational role—housewife or financial provider—they encounter the ***career clock*** phenomenon. They critically review accomplishments to date, reexamine the reasons for entering the role, and evaluate whether things should remain as they are. Frequently, the occupational, marital, social, and geographic status changes at this point because of no wish to carry through previous decisions that are inappropriate at this time. Others evaluate their present situations and find them unacceptable, yet do nothing to alter them, resulting in a subsequent life of desperation. Others evaluate, are happy with their present state, and continue with an integrity between previous, present, and anticipated future life-style. During this time, sex role stereotypes are better modulated, prejudices are relaxed, and overall tension levels are reduced. The issue of personal mortality is also confronted and, in the main, resolved. (This is often difficult for physicians.) Consistently, this age range is reported as the most gratifying for the majority of persons.

On the negative side, women who have overinvested in their children sometimes develop the ***empty nest syndrome*** and frequently experience a rather severe depressive episode when the last child is gone. Men at 45 to 54 years of age are at the peak of their earning power and careers; consequently, stress syndromes (*e.g.,* gastrointestinal distress, myocardial infarctions) may become manifest. Divorce also may occur due to waiting ''until the children are grown'' or to both persons being required to deal with each other rather than through the children.

Old Age. The technocracy in the United States has provided a socioeconomic climate which has drawn attention to the elderly of America. In this focus on the elderly, a number of myths have been generated. The most popular are as follows:

The elderly live alone in nursing homes. The reality is that 5% of elderly live in residential institutions, 60% own their own homes, and between 65% and 80% live with someone else. However, the percentage of elderly in nursing homes dramatically increases in the 75- to 85-year age group and increases more in the 85- to 95-year group.

The elderly are asexual. Realistically, 70% of elderly males and 20% of females report active sexuality. The disparity between males and females probably reflects the fact that males marry younger females and have a shorter life expectancy; therefore, more females are left without a sexual partner in later life.

The elderly are senile. While senility does have some correlation with plaque formation in the CNS, other determinants of senility are social isolation, forced inactivity, and lack of significant interpersonal involvement. One need only consider Albert Einstein to realize age per se has little to do with senility.

The realistic issues with which the elderly are confronted are multiple:

Mental processes: As persons age, two significant changes occur. First, reaction time slows. As a consequence, because quick sensorimotor reactions are the basis for performance items on most intelligence tests, there is an apparent but illusionary decrease in IQ as persons age. Second, immediate and recent memory are attenuated while remote memory is unimpaired. This results in older persons "boring" younger adults with repetition of remote data. However, young children are as fascinated with these recollections as they are with the retelling of fairy tales. While these acquisitional problems are relative and not absolute—older persons can and do learn—it does take longer for them to acquire new data.

Fixed income: 15% of American elderly are living on poverty level, fixed incomes that make them most vulnerable to fluctuations in national economics.

Chronic health conditions: About 85% of the elderly have at least one chronic health problem, twice as many are likely to be hospitalized, Medicare meets about 50% of total health care costs, 14% need assistance in their homes, 50% of the blind are 50 years of age or older, 25% of all prescribed drugs are consumed by the elderly, and 15% of the elderly make serious errors in the consumption of prescribed medication, mainly due to the recent memory problems (forgetting if and when they took medications).

Nutrition: Nutritional deficiencies affect about 10% of the elderly due to fixed income and rising food costs, loss of interest in preparing food and eating if they live alone, and compromised access to food based on transportation problems.

Transportation: The breakdown of extended families has led to the elderly being excluded from regular travel previously provided by their children. Health problems may limit the ability of the elderly to drive, and inadequate or expensive public transportation further limits mobility. In some studies, this is reported by the elderly as their major problem.

Inactivity: Enforced idleness is due to mandatory retirement with financial penalties for earning extra money, lack of mobility, and decreased social contacts as friends and relatives of the same age die.

The people who successfully age are those who actively planned for retirement, continue activities of the middle years, maintain an active social involvement, and provide themselves with continued growth experiences. The best predictors of successful aging are a good IQ, higher education, financial security, how active and integrated the individual was prior to onset of the rapid aging process, and the presence of an intimate relationship.

Interpersonal and Small-Group Determinants of Behavior

GROUP DYNAMICS

When an individual interacts with one or more persons, the needs of the single individual are placed in a context of the needs of the other. Usually, in such a setting, no single individual's needs are completely met. Group size dictates some basic influences on human behavior. Two interacting people—a ***dyad***—have an opportunity to develop intimacy and resolve differences when lack of consensus develops. Three people—a ***triad***—are involved in a more complex issue in that relations must be maintained at less than an intimate or dyadic level to avoid exclusion of one person. If dyadic intimacy does develop between persons in groups larger than two, priorities must be clearly established; for example, children in a family must understand they cannot destroy the marital bond and be the primary intimate object for one of the two parents. Likewise, parents must align solidly together for the child to mature appropriately. Triads always have the potential to move into the "drama triangle," where the roles of persecutor, victim, and rescuer are stable, but persons in the triangle assume different roles at different times. When more than three people interact, members tend to subdivide and form relationships with at least one other person in the group that are ***affiliative*** (*i.e.,* attraction) and ***differentiating*** (*i.e.,* repulsion). The affiliations and differentiations occur along multiple dimensions, such as sex, age, race, ethnicity, occupation, and socioeconomic status, as well as various combinations. These dimensions of affiliation and differentiation within a group frequently get superimposed upon the nature of the group.

The nature of the group is defined as whether the group has an end product, task, or goal—***task-oriented group***—or whether it assembles to support a given identity—***sentient group***—with no task or goal product expected.

Related to these affiliation–differentiation and task–sentient dimensions is the focus of the group; that is, does the group focus on the ***content–decision*** issue of a topic (more characteristic of task groups) or does the group focus on the ***process*** of how things are occurring? Typically, these content–process issues are always ongoing but difficult to attend to simultaneously. A neurosurgical team doing surgery is a task group focused on content–decision outcome issues. The outcome may be less acceptable if all team members are in the process of undercutting other members' effectiveness. That same team later in an informal setting discussing the outcome of the surgery, "rehashing" how well everyone performed and sharing personal feelings with each other, transforms to a sentient group, which is process oriented and no tangible product is expected.

LEADERSHIP

Leadership is tied to the nature, focus, and needs of the group. Leaders are typically polemically divided into authoritarian or democratic styles. ***Democratic leaders*** provide a setting in which group members are true contributors to decision making. Their groups perform consistently, display high morale, and produce when the leader is absent. They perceive themselves as an integral part of a whole. ***Authoritarian leaders*** have groups that have sporadic high performance when the leader is present, but noticeably diminished production when the leader is absent. Typically, in a group that is product-oriented but led by an authoritarian person who makes all meaningful decisions, the group concerns itself with irrelevant process issues or incidental content items. This group is not productive either in a task-oriented or a sentient sense.

Group needs and the consequent *expectation* by the group or the leader interact with the relative maturity of the group. Rioch has defined these issues as outlined in Table 8-1. Leaders who attempt to fulfill the fantasy demands of an immature group or who approach leadership from the fantasy/immature posture generally fail and the group either ostracizes the leader or deteriorates in functioning.

DESTRUCTIVE ISSUES

Other destructive variables to internal group structure are excessive competition and inappropriate aggression. Both of these variables not only interfere with group performance but, in some instances, also dissolve the extant group. The group, however, can extrude the offending member, close the group to the extruded person, and gain solidarity by closed-rank resistance to attempts from the extruded person either to rejoin or further destroy the group structure.

TABLE 8-1. Group Expectations

	GROUP EXPECTATIONS OF LEADER	
GROUP NEED	**Fantasy–Immature**	**Mature**
Dependency	Omnipotence	Dependable
Fight–Flight	Unbeatable	Courageous
Pairing/Affiliation	"Marvelous unborn"	Creative

GROUP AS A SYSTEM

A basic assumption underlying large and small groups is that a group is a relatively rigid, closed system that is tightly interdependent. Any alteration in the system, such as a person entering, exiting, or changing, requires compensatory alteration in other persons in the system to maintain stability.

Families can be viewed as such systems in which there are extremely stable roles that are resistant to change; however, the individual who fills a role can be variable (*e.g.,* the mothering role can be assumed by any family member). This role stability and resistance to change exists regardless of the relative functional adaptability or health of the family. Attempts to enter or alter the structure either are resisted or the system structure of the family group must change.

Family systems characterized by inclusion factors have changed considerably in the recent past. A ***nuclear family*** is a unit of procreation: mother, father, and children. ***Extended families*** are those in which there is inclusion of more than one unit of procreation, such as grandparents, parents, grandchildren, great grandchildren, aunts, and uncles. As a general rule, in America today most families are nuclear with only loose ties to other familial, procreative units. This weakening of bonds in extended family units has serious implications for a support system for orphaned, single, older, or new family members. Previously, new marriages in an extended family could rely on that system to provide support while the new family stabilized. Now new marriages must establish a stable nuclear family in an extremely short period of time.

ASSESSMENT OF BEHAVIOR

Observation of specific aspects of human behavior has been standardized by psychological tests. Because these are formal and consistent observations, normative data have been collected about performance of people. Consequently, any person's performance can be compared to the norms, and statements about that person's relative standing on a particular variable can be made. Normative data comprising the sample against which an individual's score is compared can be collected by selecting people ***randomly,*** where everyone in a given population has an equal opportunity to be selected for the sample on each draw from the population, or through ***stratification*** of the sample, where the sample is constituted to reflect relevant variables in the overall population at the rate the variables occur in the overall population (*e.g.*, including the percentage of Eskimos in the sample that reflects the incidence of Eskimos in the population).

The major types of psychological tests are described below. While some are administered in a group, individualized assessment is always more valid.

Developmental Scales

These are standard observations of the psychomotor/social development of infants and children. For example, the ***Denver Development Scale*** is applicable from birth to the age of six years, and provides data on gross developmental progress in personal–social, fine motor, language, and gross motor areas. The ***Vineland Social Maturity Scale*** is a standard interview, usually with the parent, about a child's socialization level that can be applied from birth to maturity.

Intelligence Tests

These are psychological tests that presumably reflect the concept of intelligence presented earlier. An IQ is derived by one of two methods. The first is the ***mental age concept,*** where a mental age (MA) score is derived from a standard test. That MA is divided by the person's chronological age (CA) and multiplied by 100 to yield the IQ. The formula is $MA/CA \times 100 = \text{IQ}$. The ***Stanford-Binet Intelligence Test*** is an example of this process.

The second method of IQ derivation, called the ***deviation IQ,*** is exemplified by the Wechsler scales: ***Wechsler Adult Intelligence Scale–Revised (WAIS-R)*** for those 16 years of age and older and the ***Wechsler Intelligence Scale for Children–Revised (WISC-R)*** for those under the age of 16. The IQ is derived from age subgroup norm tables; therefore, age-related factors that might contaminate scores are controlled. The Wechsler tests provide a ***verbal IQ (VIQ),*** a ***performance IQ (PIQ),*** and a ***full-scale IQ (FSIQ).*** The separate WAIS-R verbal scales that are combined to obtain the VIQ are ***Information,*** general fund of knowledge; ***Comprehension,*** social judgment; ***Arithmetic,*** mathematical ability; ***Similarities,*** ability to abstract commonalities from objects of a class; ***Digit Span,*** rote recall forward and backward; and ***Vocabulary,*** general vocabulary level. The timed WAIS-R performance scales that are combined to obtain the PIQ are ***Digit Symbol,*** a coding task; ***Picture Completion,*** visual recognition of incomplete pictures; ***Block Design,*** psychomotor reproduction of progressively more complex visual geometric designs; ***Picture Arrangement,*** visual appreciation of nonverbal social judgment situations; and ***Object Assembly,*** recognition of a gestalt from diverse parts of an object. The Verbal and Performance scales are combined through norm tables to provide the FSIQ. The IQ tests tend to be highly correlated with adequate education. The norms on IQ tests also tend to be nonhandicapped and "WASP"-biased; therefore, one must carefully interpret test results if the person examined is non-WASP, is poorly educated, or has a physical or mental handicap.

Achievement Tests

These are norm-based assessments that usually have been established on stratified representative national samples. They purport to reflect the amount an individual has "learned" or accomplished. The ***National Board of Medical Examiners*** tests are examples, as is the ***Wide Range Achievement Test (WRAT).*** The WRAT has subdivisions of reading, spelling, and arithmetic, with national norms applied from preschool through high school years.

Aptitude Scales

Ability or aptitude tests are those attempts to assess "native" endowment in areas like creativity, musical and artistic aptitude, and psychomotor coordination and speed.

Interest Tests

Scales like the ***Strong Vocational Interest Inventory*** were empirically derived by administering many diverse items to persons who were successful and satisfied in different occupations. Those items to which persons in a given vocation responded uniquely were combined into a scale. Persons who answer items in a similar manner are presumed to be good candidates for that vocation. In such empirical derivation, it is not necessary that item content have "face validity," *i.e.*, make sense.

Personality Scales

These tests presume to assess dimensions of stable intra- and interpersonal interaction patterns. They are typically subdivided into objective (*i.e.*, empirical) versus subjective (*i.e.*, projective) tests:

The Minnesota Multiphasic Personality Inventory (MMPI) is the best-known objective test. It is objective in that it was derived from empirical analysis and not theory. The MMPI has hundreds of true-false, mental disorder symptom-related questions, which are scored on ten clinical scales and three validity scales. It is not a true personality inventory because the clinical scales presumably reflect the relative absence or presence of psychopathology but not underlying personality dimensions. Use of the recently revised MMPI-2 is increasing because it offers numerous informative subscales in addition to the information mentioned above.

The Meyers-Briggs Inventory is an objective personality scale based on Jungian theory. The major dimensions reflected by this test are: Extroversion–Introversion, Sensing–Intuition, Feeling–Thinking, and Judgment–Perception.

These dimensions in combination, yield eight "types," which are personality descriptions, not degrees of psychopathology as with the MMPI. Norms are available for an individual's type as well as type compatibility in some special professions.

Other Objective Inventories include such tests as the California Personality Inventory (CPI), the Symptom Checklist-90 (SCL-90), the Brief Psychiatric Rating Scale (BPRS) (measures symptom complexes like grandiosity), and numerous special inventories to address a given behavioral trait, *e.g.*, the State-Trait Anxiety Scale and the Beck Depression Inventory (BDI).

The ***projective*** or ***subjective personality tests*** are those derived from personality theories and based on the ***projective hypothesis.*** The projective hypothesis states that given an ambiguous stimulus, people will structure the ambiguity according to their own needs and underlying dynamics. The clinician analyzes responses to the ambiguous stimuli and infers internal needs and underlying dynamics. The major projective tests are:

The Rorschach (known as the "ink blot test"), which is associated more with unconscious intrapersonal dynamics.

Thematic Apperception Test (TAT), which consists of ambiguous pictures of different persons and objects in vague settings about which the person creates a story. Again, the examiner infers from the stories the underlying personality needs and dimensions. The TAT reflects more interpersonal dynamics although some intrapersonal data can be obtained.

Children's Apperception Test (CAT), is similar to the TAT, which involves animals instead of humans in the vaguely structured pictures.

Other projective tests are the ***Draw-a-Person (DAP)*** and the ***Sentence Completion Test*** (*e.g.,* "Right now I feel. . . .").

Neuropsychological Tests

These are psychological instruments sensitive to cerebral (specifically, cortical) dysfunction. The ***Bender-Gestalt,*** a test of graphic reproduction of nine rather simple geometric designs, has been used for this purpose. The ***Halstead-Reitan battery,*** a combination of many different tests, has a long research and clinical history of proven utility in reflecting specific brain–behavior relationships. The ***Luria*** scales currently show promise in this regard. With biomedical advances (*e.g.,* CAT scans), the utility of these as primary differential diagnostic tools has decreased; however, they are helpful as noninvasive techniques for documenting relative progression of dysfunction or relative recovery of function after cerebral trauma. They are particularly meaningful in those situations where structural lesions are not present and other biomedical procedures cannot detect disease progression, for example, posttraumatic syndrome and its legal sequelae.

PSYCHOSOCIAL ISSUES IN HEALTH CARE DELIVERY

The following section addresses generic topics that have surfaced as major areas of concern in delivery of health care. They represent the interface between internal psychological/biological processes and social efforts to control them. For clarity, they have been divided into those issues associated with the patient versus those associated with the health care delivery system. However, in reality the issues are present for both the patient and the physician at all times in an interactive process.

Sociocultural Influences

The sociocultural milieu in which the patient is immersed defines for the patient what is "normal," allowed or sanctioned, how expression of allowed behavior is permitted, and how the patient can attend to illness. The cultural subgroup to which the patient belongs establishes the rewards and, through application of those rewards, controls behavior. While the term ***minority*** means a group that has less representation in the United States population, in the past it has been used to connote a value judgment of "weak" and "inferior" or "bad." It has been specifically applied to ethnic subgroups and has provided a basis for prejudice and negative discrimination. In health care this is exemplified by at least two classes of health care delivery: that applied to the majority (*i.e.,* private fee for service, private health insurance, Preferred Provider Options, Health Maintenance Organizations), and that delivered to the minority through a public health service model, which is government-subsidized and usually not considered to be as adequate or "caring" about the patient. In this instance, economic status plays a major role in defining "minority" or "majority."

Beliefs, attitudes, prejudice, and values are core psychosocial issues in health care delivery:

Beliefs are the cognitive information an individual accepts about an object. The belief may or may not be based in fact and varies in strength from an opinion, which is a lightly held belief, to a strong belief for which a person may die (*e.g.,* "women and children first").

Attitudes encompass the evaluative (*i.e.,* good–bad)

and affective aspects of responses toward a given object or situation. An attitude is defined as a predisposition to respond in a certain way. There are two basic components to an attitude: a belief portion and an affective part. For example, not only must a physician believe that the medical profession is worthwhile, but that physician also must derive a positive feeling from the practice of medicine. The belief and affect in turn determine behavior.

Stereotyping is having an attitude toward a group of persons that has little basis in fact or reality. ***Prejudice*** is an attitude that is harmful and based on the distortion of some small element of truth and frequently is directed toward a subgroup—usually a minority subgroup—of people. It is formed largely on an emotional basis without much thought. Within any group, prejudice toward those not in the group is common whether majority toward minority or vice versa. The distortion involves overgeneralization, oversimplification, and alteration of reality, and at times employs the phenomenon of ***scapegoating.*** In scapegoating (and prejudice), the defense mechanism of projection is used to project onto the victim qualities that the prejudiced persons are unconsciously ashamed or afraid of in themselves. The case against the scapegoat is justified by vices attributed (correctly or incorrectly) to the scapegoat. Usually the scapegoat is weak enough not to retaliate effectively but strong enough not to be easily victimized, easily accessible, and identifiable. It has been reported that persons who are subjected to scapegoating for protracted periods of time take on the attributes of the scapegoat role.

Typically, prejudice begins to appear at about the preschool age and is often conveyed by the parenting persons in the child's life. While influenced by cultural norms and the significant group to which the person belongs, prejudices also vary with socioeconomic status, education, and religious affiliation. Persons who are strongly prejudiced tend to have ***aggressive, authoritarian personalities*** that do not allow them to consider alternative views of the scapegoated object.

The alteration of prejudice, and other attitudes, is a complex process, which involves variations on the basic theme of extended exposure to the prejudiced object over time. Distorted facts are recognized and negative affects extinguished, and these are replaced with affiliative bonds. Other factors in attitude change include the creditability and prestige of the source, whether the source displays disinterest in changing the attitudes (*e.g.,* ''overheard'' conversations), whether the source argues a position against his own self-interest, the arousal of emotions other than fear or anger, and the intensity with which the prejudice is held.

Values are the personal guide an individual develops that give direction to life. They help the person relate to the world and take decisive personal action. Values are usually developed later in life as the result of considerations of various alternatives, and they usually have three aspects: choosing them consciously, prizing or feeling good about them, and acting on them.

The ***sick role*** significantly affects human behavior. People from different professional, socioeconomic, sexual, and ethnic backgrounds display illness differently. For example, health professionals frequently resist recognition of illness in themselves because of the ''omnipotent'' role forced on them by the culture and accepted by their own fear of disease. There is no more confining prison than being placed on or placing oneself on a pedestal. Women tend to seek more health care than men, even when the effects of pregnancy are controlled. Persons of lower socioeconomic levels do not seek as much preventive care as do those from the middle and upper classes. Consequently, hospital stays for poorer persons tend to be longer because illness progresses further in its course before care is sought. Basically, persons of lower socioeconomic status define illness when, in the course of dysfunction, there is impairment of earning power.

Ethnicity helps shape how individuals display their illness. Cultures that encourage open display of emotions (*e.g.,* Italians) will be volatile in expression, while less emotionally apparent cultures (*e.g.,* Chinese) will endure in quiet reservation. Ethnicity also determines what health care person is sought—medicine man, priest, chiropractor, physician, midwife, and so forth.

The psychosocial environment provides for additional considerations: ***Hollingshead and Redlick*** (1958) demonstrated that certain types of mental illness are more likely to receive medical treatment at earlier stages among the rich as compared to the poor and in cities compared with rural areas. There is a positive correlation between low socioeconomic status and severe symptom impairment, particularly schizophrenia. There does not seem to be a relationship between rural versus urban setting with regard to overall rates of mental disturbance. Rates for all functional psychosis tend to be higher in rural settings, and rates for neuroses and personality disorders appear higher for urban areas.

Holmes and Rahe (1967) established a strong relationship between ***life change events and illness.*** Their Social Readjustment Scale has proven effective in predicting relative mental and physical illness from cumulative life events such as divorce, Christmas holidays, and so forth.

Human Sexuality

Gender refers to sexual anatomy. The ***gender identity*** refers to the sexual role of the child in which it feels it belongs—either that of a man or woman. It is the private experience of sexuality. ***Gender identification*** means how the child, through modeling (*i.e.,* social learning),

TABLE 8-2. Sexual Stages

STAGE	FEMALE	MALE
Excitement	Vaginal ballooning Vaginal lubrication Nipple erection Clitoral erection	Penile erection Nipple erection
Plateau	Clitoral retraction Further vaginal ballooning HP, BP, Resp. increase	Testes increase in size Additional penile engorgement HR, BP, Resp. increase
Orgasm	Vagina and uterus contract at about $\frac{3}{4}$-sec. intervals for 3–15 contractions. HR, BP, Resp. may increase further	Ejaculation of seminal fluid: Marked penile and prostate contraction at .8 sec. for 3–4 major contractions. HR, BP, Resp. may increase further
Resolution	All changes return to unstimulated state within 30 min.	All changes return to unstimulated state within 30 min.

TABLE 8-3. Sex and the Elderly

STAGE	FEMALE	MALE
Excitement	Decreased vasocongestion Delayed vaginal lubrication	Decreased vasocongestion Increased time to erect
Plateau	Vaginal expansion is reduced	Increased duration of erection and activity without orgasm Full erection not until entering orgasmic phase
Orgasm	Contractile phase reduced in duration	Slower ejaculatory experience with decreased contractions Prostatic contractions are absent
Resolution	Very rapid return to unstimulated state	Very rapid detumescence of the penis

is taught to act, whether masculine or feminine. It is the public expression of the person's sexuality. These three can be independent of each other.

Sexual behavior that is accepted as normal in America includes sexual excitement from birth until death, masturbation from early adolescence until death, same-sex exploration in late childhood/early adolescence, and sexual behavior with opposite-sex persons from adolescence until death.

Masters and Johnson (1966) pioneered modern medicine's objective knowledge about adult human sexuality. Their work separates the human sexual response cycle into four phases. Table 8-2 summarizes the work of Sherfey (1972) and Sadock (1982).

In addition to these four phases, a ***refractory period*** after orgasm occurs for the male, during which time he cannot become erect or have additional orgasms. Females can be multiorgasmic. There are data in the literature that suggest some females may also have ejaculate at orgasm. These data are associated with the discussion of the ***"g" spot*** (for Graffenberg) in females.

The normal effects of ***aging*** on the human sexual response are shown in Table 8-3. In elderly males, if the erection is lost during the plateau phase, it may not be reachieved for up to an hour. In the man over 60 years of age, it has been observed that the refractory period is quite extended—to perhaps days—before the male can become erect again.

The human sexual response cycle is biologically stable and apparently correlated with normal biochemical/physiologic functioning. In the physiologically intact person, what is necessary is "friction and a frame of mind." Dysfunction can occur at any or all of the stages of the cycle for both males and females. These dysfunctions are noted in Table 8-4. Generally, if there is no underlying organic pathology, the etiology of these dysfunctions can be traced to inadequate education and social programming, getting out of the "here and now pleasure" and anxiously going into remembered past or projected future, or assuming a self-critical spectator role during sexual activity. It should also be noted that a number of primary

TABLE 8-4. Sexual Dysfunction

STAGE	FEMALE	MALE
Excitement	General sexual dysfunction ("frigidity") Vaginismus (strong vaginal contractions) Dyspareunia (painful intercourse)—usually organic base	Erectile dysfunction ("impotence") Dyspareunia (painful intercourse)—usually organic base
Orgasm	Inorgasmia (usually due to low trust level of partner)	Inorgasmia (performance anxiety) Premature ejaculation (inadequate learning or control)

physiologic illnesses (*e.g.,* diabetes melitis), aging, and drug use (prescription and otherwise) can produce identical sexual dysfunctions.

The utilization of behavioral modification techniques, resolution of physical abnormalities, and counseling toward improved communication between sexual partners (oriented to trust and taking personal responsibility for one's own pleasure), have resulted in high rates of resolution for many of these dysfunctions.

Besides the predominant heterosexual pattern, there are different sexual expressions, which form large subgroups within the population. ***Homosexuality*** is defined as emotional attachment to *and* physical/sexual preference for someone of the same sex. There is a growing body of data that suggests genetic and neuroanatomic substrates for some homosexual behavior. These data include higher concordance rates in monozygotic twins as opposed to the rate in dizygotic twins or adopted siblings (Bailey et al., 1991; 1993); correlations of the size of some brain structures with that of opposite-sexed persons (Levay, 1991); higher incidence of left-handedness; and so on. However, many writers view the different sexual preference as the result of early learning experiences based in either the gender identity formation prior to 3 years of age or role identification issues later in childhood. Some authors view the acquisition of sexual preference as similar to the acquisition of language. There is a biologic readiness upon which the preference (like the primary language) is acquired. Regardless of later preferences (or languages), there is the first acquisition, which is always present. As with language acquisition, the longer one stays with a sexual preference (or primary language), the more difficult it is to acquire a different one. Likewise, if one continues to practice the primary preference (language) while acquiring a different one, the new one is less well acquired.

Kinsey reported that 4% of adult, white males live an exclusive homosexual existence, and about 10% are "more or less" exclusively homosexual for at least three years between the ages of 16 and 65; 48% of male adolescents report same-sex genital play. According to Kinsey, there are a third to a quarter as many female ***(lesbians)*** as male homosexuals. Apparently, the discrepancy is correlated with relative definitions and differentially allowed or accepted behaviors between males and females in American society. Overall, the best estimate of adult homosexuality is that 10% of adults are homosexual. Of that 10%, 60% are males and 40% are females.

There are no valid data with regard to the number of practicing bisexual persons. However, the present AIDS epidemic strongly suggests this is a more prevalent behavior pattern than previously suspected.

The major medical concern regarding homosexuality is the prevalence of ***sexually transmitted diseases*** (STDs) among a subgroup of homosexual males who tend to be quite promiscuous and have a high STD rate. The advent of human immunodeficiency virus (HIV) and acquired immunodeficiency syndrome (AIDS) has led to concern regarding the sexual practices of some homosexual and bisexual males.

Transvestism is defined as intermittent, but regular, dressing in clothes of the opposite sex (*i.e.,* crossdressing), which is experienced as sexually pleasurable. In the United States, this syndrome is confined to males since females are allowed to crossdress with no social proscriptions.

In the above three conditions—heterosexuality, homosexuality, and transvestism—the gender identity is consistent with the gender (*i.e.,* biologic sex) and the major etiologic issue is gender identification.

Transsexuality apparently is due to gender ***identity inversion:*** the gender identity is opposite of the biologic sex. Since first memories, these persons feel as if they are the opposite-sexed person trapped in the body of the biologic sex of birth. They crossdress frequently from early childhood; it is not for sexual pleasure, but for role fulfillment. They usually are married with a family and, in middle years (30 to 50 years of age), seek cosmetic surgical intervention to align the external genitalia with internal feelings. These surgeries have been very successful from the patient's point of view.

Functionally based differences include ***pedophilia,*** which is defined as sexual interest in young children. This syndrome is predominantly heterosexual (95%) and is illegal in all states. There are high rates of having been sexually abused among pedophiliacs. ***Voyeurism*** is sexual gratification from watching sexual acts or looking at sexual organs. This is believed to be confined to males; however, differentially allowed (*i.e.,* prosecuted) behavior between males and females must be considered. ***Exhibitionism*** is the compulsive need to expose one's genitals, and it is usually only prosecuted in males. The act of exposure does not provide release of sexual tension, but the reaction from the female to the exposure does. Exacerbation of these syndromes apparently occurs when the male is faced with defeat, ego deflation, or other threat to adult functioning. Theoretically, these alternatives are taken because approaching a mature female in a situation where rejection is possible is too threatening.

While ***incest*** is verbalized as a universal taboo, high prevalence rates are reported. Incest is defined as sexual activity between close members of a family. Father (or stepfather) and daughter is most common by report, although mother–son and sibling (heterosexual and homosexual) are not infrequent patterns. Typically, it is reported that parent–child incest is correlated with a family constellation in which the same-sex parent as the child involved is an extremely poor and incompetent marriage partner who, at least passively, encourages and condones the relationship because it relieves that parent of unwanted and overwhelming responsibilities. Alcohol consumption is frequently involved in incest. While general statistics imply this is a phenomenon of persons of lower socioeconomic status, clinical experience suggests a differential legal prosecution and disposition rate among the social classes. Lower socioeconomic status persons go to jail while higher socioeconomic status persons are sent for mental health care from private professional persons.

Death and Dying

Death and the process of dying in the United States has become a hospital-focused issue because today few Americans die in their homes. ***Elizabeth Kübler-Ross*** pioneered the therapeutic work in death and dying. Since that time, the process stages identified by her (listed below) have been recognized to accompany any serious health loss of which the patient is informed. That is, if the patient is informed of a serious, though not fatal, illness, these stages can be observed, and until the patient works through the stages, compliance with proper medical regimens is not good.

THE ADULT

The stages of dealing with death in an adult are as follows:

Denial: The patient firmly insists there is a diagnostic error. Frequently, requests for independent validation are made or the patient disappears from the physician's practice. If the physician recognizes this stage and facilitates further evaluation, the patient usually will stay with the physician.

Anger: In this phase, the patient moves out of the denial stage and enters a phase of angrily asking the question, ''Why me?''

Bargaining: As the anger is dissipated, the patient attempts to strike compromises with the physician, self, or a diety. These frequently take the form of ''If I can live until (a given time or event), then I won't ask for more,'' or ''I'll do (usually a sacrifice).'' Temporary remissions during this phase frequently are interpreted by the patient as fulfillment of the bargain. These should be anticipated by medical personnel and carefully discussed with the patient to prevent overinterpretation.

Sadness or depression: During this stage, the patient becomes fully cognizant of the terminal nature of the condition and emotionally experiences the finality of the diagnosis. The anger and bargaining of previous stages is replaced with appropriate sadness, which accompanies any significant loss.

Acceptance: This is not a euphoric happiness, rather a condition in which the patient resolutely foregoes the sadness and depression, puts his or her life in order, and makes plans to live out the remainder of his or her life with the given situation. It is during this time that the dying person can truly say ''good-bye'' to surviving significant others.

Although these stages are listed as discrete entities, in reality they are fluid, and they overlap each other. The individual moves in and out of a given stage in a progression–regression pattern; however, there is usually predominance of one stage over the others. The issue for the physician is *how* to tell the patient of a serious condition, not *whether* to tell the patient. Collusion among health care personnel and relatives not to inform the patient of the true nature of the condition is ill-advised. It should be the patient's choice not to hear (*i.e.*, denial), not the physician's preference to withhold the information. Dying patients have also pointed up the serious error of the physician announcing to the patient what stage he is in as a way of circumventing dealing with the patient as a dying person; for example, ''Oh, you're in the stage of anger, you'll be out of it soon and start bargaining with me.''

THE CHILD

The dying child poses special issues. Because the child is in Piaget's preoperational or concrete-operations stage, the full, cognitive understanding of imminent death is not a true reality. The child comprehends it as going to sleep from which the child believes he or she will awaken. Dying children tend not to fear death, but rather they are most disturbed by separation from parents and mutilation that will make them different or that they may misperceive as punishment.

MANAGEMENT ISSUES

Commonly, physicians and other health care providers have avoided dealing with the dying patient by giving the patient no entree for discussion (busily making rounds and moving in and out of the patient's room quickly), geographically isolating the patient in a single room at the end of the hall or keeping the room door closed, making a contract with significant others not to inform the patient of the nature of the condition, extending unrealistic hope (*e.g.*, ''We're expecting a breakthrough any day,'' or automatically saying, ''You're going to be just fine.''), and maintaining a clouded sensorium in the patient through medication. Appropriate management of the dying patient tends to emphasize the opposite of these.

These realities, coupled with the American penchant

for keeping dying relatives isolated in social institutions, has led to the ***hospice*** movement, whereby persons with terminal illnesses are assisted in their dying process by involving the whole family as much as possible, allowing the patient to be afraid and discuss the fear, providing physical contact in a warm and supportive atmosphere, allowing the patient to talk and cry about the loss, managing temporary remissions without building unrealistic hope, providing as much dignity in the health care as is feasible, and using medications that provide pain relief without clouding the sensorium (*e.g.,* Brompton's mixture, a combination of narcotics and stimulants).

Grief and Bereavement

The persons remaining after the loss of a loved one through death or permanent separation (and, some authors report, after the loss of a body part like a limb, breast, or testicle) undergo predictable reactions. The grief and bereavement process reflects significant loss; therefore, it is related to the emotion of sadness. The expression of these reactions is culturally determined and varies by ethnic subgroup. It is expected that the normal process of mourning should be completed within 6 to 12 months after loss. Spouses and parents may not come to terms with their loss for up to 4 years. The bereavement of a child can normally take years, particularly if the loss was abrupt and unexpected. Grieving/mourning is a process—not a condition—and, as such, changes with time like a contusion that is in the process of resolution.

THE ADULT

The stages of the grief process for adults are as follows:

Acute disbelief or phase of protest: This may last for minutes, hours, or days, during which the individual is not fully aware the object is gone. It is a state of mental "shock" during which the person may intellectually know the loss has occurred but not affectively experience it. Anger is often projected toward the physician, relatives, and friends because these support people allowed the loved one to die or will not help the grieving person recover the loved one.

Grief work or phase of disorganization: In this second phase, the grieving person develops an emotional sense of loss. The world is experienced as empty, meaningless, and barren. The grieving person tends to withdraw from social contacts and isolates himself or herself. Initially, mental activity is almost exclusively involved with memories of the lost object. Frequently, the mourner will report feeling the "presence" of the individual in the room or close by. Waves of grief which seem to "come from nowhere" tend to overwhelm the grieving person. As this stage continues, the mental preoccupation with the lost one, the withdrawal/isolation, and the waves of grief diminish.

Resolution, or phase of reorganization: Through the first two phases, the mourner emerges with an acceptance that the loss is real. He or she has formed a new relationship with the lost object in terms of realistic memories, not vows to preserve the world as it was the day the loss occurred. This phase signals that the grieving individual is ready to return to the world and form relationships without experiencing guilt over fantasized unfaithfulness or what might have been.

AGE-RELATED GRIEVING

Humans react differently to the loss of another depending on their age and ability to comprehend the loss. The conditions listed below are common and normal accompaniments of mourning.

Infants may withdraw from social contact, refuse to eat, and die if a mother figure is lost and not replaced.

Children will frequently react with hyperactivity and assume a jocular attitude.

Adolescents and young adults will frequently react with hypersexuality, delinquent activity, and significant substance abuse.

Adults often develop psychosomatic illnesses or an exacerbation of a previous pathologic condition and are highly vulnerable to physical disease. Substance abuse is a potential problem.

Elderly adults, like infants, frequently withdraw from social contact and often die within the one year of mourning unless supportive steps are taken to involve them in the life process.

NORMAL VARIANTS

Anticipatory grief sometimes accompanies the death of someone who has had protracted illness. The grieving person has worked through the loss prior to the actual death and, frequently at the time of loss, is ready to begin establishing new, guilt-free relationships immediately. The major problems observed from this pattern are that the person may feel guilty because he or she is relieved at the death, and is not reacting as others expect. ***Delayed grief*** is the maintaining of the affectless shock from stage I until a protracted period of time after the death. Often delayed grief is triggered by accidentally finding a possession of the dead person. It is as if the possession or event has "slipped through" a defense mechanism and triggered the grief. Delayed grief reactions frequently appear in the person who was strong for the other grieving persons, made all funeral arrangements, and postponed mourning. Similarly, persons who have been separated from a parent at a young age and subsequently learn of that parent's death may experience a variant of a delayed grief reaction. They mourned the loss with the original separation and, with the final one, they experience the old grief—and also the anger that the parent died before a reuniting and resolution of desertion issues were managed. These delayed grief reactions can precipitate profound, acute clinical depression with impulsive suicidal acts. ***Anniversary reactions*** are exacerbations of the pain, sadness, and loss triggered by birthdays, or the wedding or death anniversary of the dead person. Usually these decrease in intensity with years; however, when they serve as a trigger for a delayed grief reaction, the initial grieving may be of equal or greater intensity than would have been expected with an immediate grief reaction.

ABNORMAL GRIEF PATTERNS

Abnormal variants of the grief process are usually of two types. First, the individual may become fixated in one of the age-related reaction patterns noted above and not move beyond it. For example, an adolescent may react to the loss of a sibling, friend, or parent with substance (*i.e.,* drug) abuse. The substance abuse becomes a defense against addressing the loss. Consequently, when the loss begins to surface (or the patient develops tolerance to the drug), drug use is increased to manage the uncomfortable feelings. Obviously, physicians who chronically medicate a grieving patient are preventing the patient from appropriately working through the grief and sometimes create iatrogenic addiction. Second, the adult patient may become fixated in the second stage of the grief process and not move into resolution. If grieving of a lost adult extends more than 12 months, the patient should be assumed to be clinically depressed and be treated appropriately.

Substance Abuse

Substance or drug abuse (also called chemical dependence) involves use of psychoactive chemicals taken for nonmedical reasons in a nonprescriptive pattern which is harmful to the person or society. Basically these are alcohol, narcotics, sedative–hypnotics, psychedelics, and stimulants. Definitions for substance abuse are not clear because substance abuse is socially defined and subject to social subgroup variation regarding "normal" or "deviant."

ALCOHOLISM

This is best defined as that pattern of alcohol consumption which results in dysfunction in one or more of five areas: marital, social, legal, occupational, or physical, *and* the person cannot stop drinking, that is, the individual has lost control of consumption. Problem drinking is defined as problems in any or all of the same five areas, but when the person is confronted with these as a result of alcohol consumption, the person can alter the drinking pattern so it no longer creates the problem.

ADDICTION

Addiction is defined as the nonprescriptive use of a drug harmful to society and/or self, that has the following properties: ***tolerance,*** increasing amounts of the drug are needed over time to achieve the same effect (a cellular, biochemical event), ***dependence,*** abrupt cessation of use of the drug precipitates a recognizable and characteristic withdrawal syndrome (a biochemical–physiologic condition), and ***habituation,*** the drug is taken for the psychological effect or it may be taken out of "habit."

PREVALENCE

Prevalence data for substances of abuse vary with time and the substance in question. However, the figures of 7% to 13% of adult Americans being alcoholics or having a drinking problem at some time in their lives appear to be stable consensual estimates. Data collected from graduating high school seniors reflect a consistent decrease each year since 1981 in the percentage of persons who are current users and occasional heavy drinkers. The percentage who have tried alcohol at some time by graduation from high school has remained stable at 92% (Alcohol and Health, 1990). What is true is that substance abuse is a significant health care problem and it extends to younger populations as well as to all socioeconomic and ethnic groups.

Persons with substance abuse problems have a high rate of comorbidity with other mental disorders. In persons diagnosed with alcoholism 37% have at least one additional psychiatric disorder; individuals who have been diagnosed with other substance abuse disorders have comorbidity rates as high as 53%.

ETIOLOGY

The etiologic theories of substance abuse (particularly alcoholism) fall into three major categories:

1. ***Physiologic*** and ***biologic*** models
   a. ***Genetotrophic*** issues include research on inherited metabolic defects that result in the need for greater than average consumption of certain foodstuffs such as alcohol. These studies also focus on genetically inherited metabolic differences in

tolerance to alcohol and its metabolites (*e.g.*, the flushing reaction to alcohol of many persons of Asian extraction).

b. ***Endocrine*** research data emphasize a defect that leads to episodic hypoglycemia. This produces emotional symptoms that stimulate drug taking to balance the system.

c. ***Normalizing effect*** of drugs. Multiple studies have demonstrated physiologic, biochemical, and neurophysiologic differences between substance abusers and nonabusers that disappear after acute drug ingestion. Unfortunately, no presubstance abuse measures have been available on these persons; therefore, it is not possible to know if observed differences are drug induced.

d. ***Genetic*** marker variables (*i.e.*, inherited color blindness, primary depression in female family members of male alcoholics, alcoholism and antisocial behavior patterns in male family members of female primary depressed persons), genetic mice strains that drink alcoholically, and concordance rates between adopted children and biologic, alcoholic parents all suggest a genetic component to substance abuse *for some persons.*

e. Recent research has documented ***evoked potential*** differences between 7-year-old male offspring of alcoholic men and matched controls.

f. Beta-***endorphin*** and salsolinol level differences between groups of alcoholic persons and matched controls suggest a self-medication of deficits in pain modulation systems of the body. All suggest a physiologic component to substance abuse for some persons.

2. ***Psychological models***

a. The ***psychodynamic model*** focuses on unconscious conflicts and low self-esteem as stress variables. The reinforcer of substance abuse is the stress reduction induced by the drug consumption.

b. ***Personality trait*** models have identified low stress tolerance, dependence, decreased self-image, insecurity, impulsiveness, and intolerance for delay of gratification, or deviant behaviors as traits associated with substance abuse.

Both the psychodynamic and personality trait models have only identified their core findings in persons who are substance dependent. They have neither examined the dependent persons prior to the substance dependence nor presented data on the number of persons who possess the traits and are not substance dependent.

It is important to know that there has *never* been a substance abuse personality identified, that is, a personality that, once identified, will predict substance abuse in all persons with the personality. Each time such a personality has been suggested, a significant number of persons who have the personality but no substance abuse are identified.

c. Behavioral ***learning models*** explain drug ingestion as a learned response that decreases felt stress. As a result of the chemical's properties and repeated use, the body becomes physiologically dependent, leading to continued drug use to avoid withdrawal.

d. ***Psychological dependence*** is a concept that has found popularity in the recent past and is defined as that individual who is self-medicating a psychological/psychosocial problem. Codependence refers to the relationship between a chemically dependent person and his or her significant other that allows and supports the dysfunctional substance use pattern.

3. ***Sociocultural models***

a. Cultural and ***socialization*** issues focus on cultural norms that promote substance abuse.

b. The ***cultural stress*** factors model relates substance abuse to the degree of stress and inner tension produced by the culture. It also explores the cultural drinking attitudes and the alternatives for stress management provided by the culture.

c. ***Familial*** pattern research is focused on role modeling, with social learning providing the basis for the substance abuse.

d. ***Environmental instabilities*** and crises produce change in individual life situations or social roles that precipitates instability, confusion, and stress. In this model drugs are taken as a mechanism to decrease these conditions.

DRUG EFFECTS AND TREATMENT

The effects of various psychoactive substances of abuse, their toxicology and some aspects of treatment are presented in Table 8-5. Different levels of drug toxicity involving different chemicals of abuse are frequently misdiagnosed as functional emotional disturbances. Most notably, psychedelics and stimulants have produced conditions similar to acute manic or paranoid schizophrenic reactions; and phencyclidine (PCP) can present as a dissociated, catatonic (*i.e.*, agitated or depressed) schizophrenic reaction. These toxic conditions can be complicated by unusually long abstinence syndromes from some drugs (sometimes weeks) presumably on a basis of the lipophilic binding properties or depletion of CNS neurotransmitter stores. Failure to obtain toxicologic studies on patients with distorted behavior patterns can result in improper medical regimens that exacerbate or prolong the episode rather than assist in its resolution. Sometimes

TABLE 8-5. Drug Effects

	ALCOHOL	NARCOTICS	SEDATIVE HYPNOTICS	PSYCHE-DELICS	PHEN-CYCLIDINE	STIMULANTS	MARI-JUANA
Physiologic Aspects							
Tolerance	X	X	X	X	X	X	X
Dependence	X	X	X			X	X
Habituation	X	X	X	X	X	X	X
Fatal in:							
a. Overdose	X	X	X	?	X	X	
b. Withdrawal from addiction	X		X				
Discomfort on withdrawal from addiction	X	X	X			X	?
Physiological Effects							
Pain blockade	X	X	X	X	X	X	?
Euphoria	X	X	X	X	X	X	X
Energy level							
Increase	?			?	X	X	
Decrease	X	X	X	?	X		X
Anxiety decrease	X	X	X		X		X
Perceptual changes (*e.g.*, hallucinations)	X			X	X	X	X
Psychomotor impairment	X	X	X		X		X
Time sense changes	X	X	X	?	?	X	X
Toxicologic test available	X	X	X		X	X	X
Treatment							
Titrated withdrawal recommended	X	X	X				
Chemical blockade of rewarding effects available	X	X					
Antagonist available		X					

Adapted from the National Institute on Drug Abuse Medical Monograph Series (1976).

inappropriate management due to inadequate diagnostic studies can be fatal.

Substance abuse treatment is both effective and cost-efficient. Treatment outcome studies have documented success rates as high as 92% in some populations, and have demonstrated that for every dollar spent, $12 is saved over the long term.

Violence

Violence may be a special case of uncontrolled aggression or a separate entity that has independent etiologies. While aggression can be directed toward a single person, groups of people, or an inanimate object, violence usually denotes interpersonal acts. For both aggression and violence, it is important to distinguish the ***intentionality*** of the act. That is, while war and crime are aggressive and violent acts, they are usually not premeditated to do harm to an individual person.

A form of violence that is increasing worldwide is terrorism. The perpetrators are usually a single or few individuals, acting on behalf of others, to make a statement of protest against a given organization or group of persons. Often these are claimed to be political acts; in reality, however, they are little more than mass murder. These are planned, premeditated acts that usually require a great deal of preparation and practice to execute. However, they also often are poorly thought out in the aftermath (*i.e.*, the perpetrators usually get caught). The underlying motive of terrorism is to tear apart the safety and security that people feel in their lives and create a sense of chaos and insecurity.

In the United States, reported juvenile crime has increased dramatically over the last few decades; one out of every nine youths below the age of 18 years will be arrested and will go through the court system. United States data reported regarding violence and school-age children suggest most school violence is predictable and occurs during school hours, at midweek, in February, between classes, and to a victim who is a seventh-grade, minority male in the school who has been victimized before. The offender is usually the same age and sex and is known to the victim.

Toch (1969) reported that the majority of adult acts of

violence fall into the following three categories: preservation of self-image (41%); pressure-removing (12%); as a manipulation tool (26%), *e.g.*, exploitation, bullying, self-defense, self-indulgence, norm-enforcing, cathartic, and so forth.

Specific data on the predictability of adult violence are not as clear as for youth. The major correlates are as follows. Most murders—about 25%—are a family affair in the heat of a quarrel. Repressive social conditions precipitate outbursts of violence. Violence is reported more in the lower SES groups and urban ghettos. Most violence is "race on race," not interracial; black on black is the highest, with white on white next. Also, more violence is reported among Catholics than Protestants. The most characteristic age of violence is 15 years old. Consistent delinquent and cruel behaviors have been demonstrated to have important genetic bases. Recent data show neurochemical correlates of violent behavior: low levels of 5-HIAA and high levels of MHPG; no changes in HVA have been associated with severe acting-out aggressive behavior.

Five special forms of violence are frequently seen by the physician: chemically induced, child abuse, domestic violence, elder abuse, and rape.

Chemically induced violence is most frequently associated with alcohol, stimulants—particularly amphetamines—or phencyclidine. There is a strong correlation between alcohol consumption and violence/aggression: 50% of all arrests, 24% of violent deaths, 50% to 64% of all homicides (killer or victim), 34% of all forcible rapes, and 41% of all assaults are alcohol-related.

Child abuse sometimes occurs during infancy, preschool, and subsequent school-age phases. Child abuse encompasses neglect, active physical trauma, and sexual abuse. Each state in the United States has laws against child abuse, which require physicians to report suspected child abuse and protect the physician from retaliatory acts. According to the National Center on Child Abuse and Neglect and researchers, parents reported for abuse of their children themselves were abused children, the parent seldom looks at or touches the child, the family is isolated (*e.g.*, unlisted phone number, no social club memberships, cannot be located, seems to trust no one, does not participate in school activities or events), the parents expect or demand behavior beyond the child's years or abilities, they don't care for the physical hygiene of the child, the parents over- or underreact to the child's condition, they appear to be misusing alcohol or other drugs, and they are overcritical of the child. These parents perceive the child's expression of needs as being purposeful acts of frustration and irritation to the parent (*e.g.*, a hungry child cries at night and the parents say, "That child won't let me sleep"). They are reluctant to give information about the child's injury or condition and are either unable to explain injuries or offer illogical or contradictory information. They appear to lack control or, at least, they fear losing control, and they generally know no other disciplinary techniques except physical punishment. Sometimes the parents are jealous of the child's interaction with the mothering figure, sometimes they self-righteously defend their right to use corporal punishment, and sometimes they are simply ineffective parents.

Characteristics of the ***abused*** or ***neglected*** child include obvious welts or skin injuries, inappropriate clothes for the weather, severely abnormal eating habits (*e.g.*, eating from garbage pails and drinking from toilet bowls) and begging or stealing food, and exhibiting extremes of behavior from aggression to extreme passivity/withdrawal. While these children appear overly mature, they also seem unduly afraid of parents and other adults. They generally cause trouble with peers, are wary of any physical contact, and are apprehensive around other children who are crying. They frequently engage in vandalism, sexual misconduct, and use alcohol and other drugs. Often these children need glasses or other medical attention, show severely retarded physical growth, and are often tired and without energy. Usually there is only one child in the family who is abused, and most research indicates that the abused child is either different in some way (*e.g.*, has a higher or lower IQ than others in the family or is physically handicapped) or is perceived by the family as "ugly."

Children who are the victims of violent child abuse tend to be more aggressive and violent with peers at school as early as kindergarten grades. There are developing data that soldiers who have developed Posttraumatic Stress Disorder (PTSD) after exposure to combat have higher rates of various types of child abuse in their backgrounds.

In general, child abuse occurs in a constellation of a ***culture/community*** that offers little support for the family unit and perceives children as having few rights; in a family with limited disciplinary knowledge except physical punishment; and with a child who is perceived as "different." Viewing child abuse simply as a function of parental pathology is naive.

Domestic violence by men has been reported at the rate of 4 million women per year. It apparently occurs in a three-stage cycle (Walker, 1984). In ***Phase I,*** which may last from a few days to years, the husband becomes increasingly critical, verbally abusive, and perhaps destructive to things (*e.g.*, throws a plate of food on the floor). This phase I build-up reaches a peak, at which time he enters phase II. ***Phase II*** is the violent beating of the wife. This phase is similar to a child's temper tantrum in that nothing the wife can say or do will intervene in the behavior, which may last from minutes to days. ***Phase III*** follows, during which the husband is extremely repentant and attentive and offers convincing statements that he will ''never do it again.'' This phase III behavior is the positive reinforcement that prevents the wife from pressing legal charges. Unless the wife does bring action at the first episode, the husband assumes her tacit agreement to participate in the activity. The great majority of wives do not obtain masochistic pleasure from the beating; rather, they usually stay in the relationship because of co-dependence issues (loneliness and financial considerations). The husbands are usually emotionally immature and insecure and the wives are the ''emotional glue that holds them together.'' The wives will usually tolerate the behavior until it begins to occur with the children.

Elder abuse is becoming a more recognized phenomenon. The estimated range is that 1 out of 8 to 1 out of 14 elderly are abused each year. The physical indicators include an injury that has not been cared for properly; cuts, lacerations, or puncture wounds; bruises, welts, discolorations bilaterally on upper arms, especially if old and new bruises coexist; poor hygiene, soiled clothes; poor health care (*e.g.*, gross decubiti); burns; and lack of necessary aids such as walking sticks, glasses, and so forth. Neglect is the most common form of elder abuse (58.5% in 1994).

The abuser is often the single female daughter caregiver who has been delivering the care for some time, has few resources to live elsewhere, and is not a voluntary caregiver. Characteristics include being reluctant to let the elderly person speak for himself or herself; having no assistance in the home; being indifferent to or angry at the victim; blaming the elderly person; having an aggressive behavioral stance; having been abused themselves; often having a substance abuse history; being socially isolated; withholding security and affection from the elderly person; and giving conflicting accounts to those presented by the elderly person.

The victim often protects the abuser and internalizes the blame for the abuse. Frequently this protection is done not only out of loyalty but also out of fear of abandonment or institutionalization.

In ***rape,*** the act is a violent—not a sexual—one. Characteristics of the noninstitutional (*i.e.*, nonprison) ***typical rapist*** include the following: 15 to 19 years of age, of a lower socioeconomic status, and sexually abused as a child (75%). Usually these men are sexually conservative and naive. The most frequent scenario is that the rape occurs in the victim's home (50%) by someone with whom the woman has at least a minimal acquaintance. Psychologically, the rape is best understood as a displacement onto the victim of anger or revenge toward a mother or other woman perceived as hostile/castrating/rejecting. Studies report that 25% of women will be raped at some time in their lives.

Recommendations for ***control of aggression*** (and perhaps violence) include the following: eliminate sources of frustration, don't reinforce aggressive behavior, reinforce nonaggressive behavior, eliminate associated objects (*e.g.*, toy guns), provide alternatives to violence, confront aggression/violence with an equal-strength, nonaggressive reaction, and decrease the use of physical punishment because it serves as a model of aggression.

Suicide

If aggression can't be directed appropriately, displaced, or scapegoated, it may be turned upon the self, and suicide occurs. Four different definitions or descriptions of suicide can be applied: (1) anyone who takes his own life, (2) taking one's own life when a given set of circumstances (*e.g.*, physical health, environmental conditions) are so hopeless that a person actively ''give up,'' (3) taking one's own life where unexpressed hostility toward others is involved, for example, ''I'll show you, you son-of-a-bitch, you'll miss me when I'm gone'' (Menninger wrote about this anger/self-destruction as simultaneously containing the wish to kill, the wish to be killed, and the wish to die), and (4) taking one's own life as an accompaniment of a serious depressive syndrome or other mental disorder.

The latter three definitions all incorporate the feeling of hopelessness for change: ''Things will never get any better and I don't want to continue like this.'' Feelings of hopelessness, helplessness, worthlessness, and loss of future orientation are the best predictors of active suicidal intent.

Statistically, approximately 26,000 to 30,000 persons in America are reported to commit suicide each year and about ten times that number attempt it. Children do commit suicide and in adolescents and college students (15 to 24 years of age) suicide is the *second* leading cause of death; accidents are first. It is likely that many accidents, particularly single-person vehicle deaths, are actually suicides. Suicide is also particularly problematic for older individuals. Elderly persons comprise 10% to 15% of the population and commit approximately 23% to 25% of the known suicides. Overall, suicide is one of the ten leading causes of death in America.

The demographics correlated with successful suicides are as follows. These are most significant: previous attempts; more males then females are successful (more females attempt it); single, widowed, or divorced; living alone; over 45 years of age; white; unemployed; a suicide note; poor health; early stages of recovery from depression (*i.e.*, energy and concentration levels have improved to where the individual can make plans and carry them through); and 25% to 36% are alcohol related. There are other correlates: eight out of ten have given a warning, hits all social classes (relative standing is difficult to ascertain because of differential recording), and it increases in incidence after a national crisis. It is commonly reported that physicians have a higher rate of suicide than the general population; however, if socioeconomic status is controlled, their rate is not significantly different. Recent research has documented that persons who are contemplating or have just attempted suicide have more of a particular serotonin receptor in their blood platelets than do controls.

Since suicide is a permanent solution to a temporary problem, appropriate management of the suicidal person should entail close supervision. Preferably, this is done by a close support system (*i.e.,* family or friends) on an ambulatory basis—admission to a mental hospital presupposes subsequent release, and the rate for suicidal persons discharged from mental hospitals is 34 times that of the general population. However, if no adequate ambulatory support system is available, hospitalization is indicated.

The Doctor–Patient Relationship

A major factor in the care of patients is the ***rapport*** that develops between the physician and the patient. Rapport is not simply, or necessarily, that "I like you"; rather, it is the understanding each has of the other and the cooperative effort to cure or control the patient's condition. That is, both the patient and the physician must be involved in the treatment process and the patient must actively attempt to "get well." This is best accomplished by the physician talking with the patient, not at him.

The verbal and nonverbal messages that physicians convey must be congruent and of a particular nature. The physician must be a warm, "nurturant parent." That does not necessarily mean totally permissive or all-giving. It does mean caring enough to sometimes set very specific boundaries (*e.g.,* "I won't let you kill yourself") and being honest (*e.g.,* "Your test results and examination suggest you have a malignancy"). The physician must maintain a mature adult reality with all patients. The physician must have an active, inventive mind to bring new solutions to patients' problems. It is quite clear from the literature that a major predictive factor in malpractice lawsuits is the quality of the doctor–patient relationship.

There are three major ***interviewing styles,*** which will predictably produce different outcomes with patients. There is no one correct style; however, each can be used differentially for specific purposes.

Laundry List: The physician asks a series of preprogrammed, structured questions, which effectively communicates to the patient, "I will tell you when to talk and what to talk about." This interview style is probably the least efficient in gathering data meaningful to the care of patients and certainly does the least to promote doctor–patient rapport. It is useful to structure persons with thought disorders or affective disorders, particularly mania, and to intervene in obsessive–compulsive verbal detail. That is, it can assist some patients by structuring their internal state and maintaining effective communication patterns.

Associative: In this style, the physician listens to and observes the patient. Any communication from the physician is associated to what the patient is presenting. The physician inserts minimal structure into the interview. This is considered the most efficient method of relevant data collection, first, because more pertinent information is elicited than by laundry list interviewing and, second, the best rapport is developed. Obviously, those conditions listed above for which a laundry list interview is indicated are those for which the associative interview is contraindicated.

Open-ended: This format is not truly appropriate for general medical interviewing because, it tends to focus on process rather than content issues. In true open-ended interviewing, whatever the patient wishes to verbalize is the topic at hand and no focus is necessary. This is useful in certain psychotherapeutic encounters, but not the majority of medical practice.

Some specific concepts for interviewing are as follows:

Support: any response, verbal or nonverbal, that demonstrates interest in, concern for, or understanding of the patient

Reassurance: a response that helps the patient feel good about himself, including feelings of merit and self-assurance

Empathy: a nonjudgmental response that shows the patient the doctor recognizes and accepts the patient's feelings, even though the doctor may personally disagree with them

Confrontation: a response that points out to the patient the patient's feelings or behavior; confrontation need not be a hostile or accusatory action

Reflection: a response that echos or mirrors a portion of what a patient has just said, which is generally intended to allow patients to become aware of what they have verbalized

Interpretation: a statement based on inference rather than on observation (*e.g.,* "Given those frustrating events, I assume you became angry").

Silence: Different types can be communicated—interested silence, disinterested silence, and withdrawn silence—however, silence can be a very effective communication device.

Summation: a response that reviews information given by the patient

Adherence Issues

Adherence to medical treatment is a significant issue in health care delivery, because research indicates that only 30% to 35% of patients totally follow their physician's recommendations, and 30% to 35% do not comply at all. Some studies have reported rates of adherence as low as 2% to 3%. The following variables have been documented as contributing to this issue and are probably rooted in the values of both the physician and patient.

Patients who have chronic illnesses (*e.g.*, cardiovascular disease, mental disorder, arthritis) tend to adhere less. Often they require long-term medication maintenance or use preventive medications which, when discontinued, do not produce immediate or noticeable effects. Adherence deteriorates with time. Young, elderly, and disadvantaged patients adhere less, as do persons who are described as hostile risk-takers and/or hypochondriacal. Patients who follow medical instructions perceive their physicians as caring, have a positive relationship with their doctor, are satisfied with their management, and believe they are ill. Patients selectively have better recall of information given at the beginning of an interaction than of information given at the end; unfortunately, most patients forget significant portions of what they are told shortly after leaving their physicians.

Medication variables that tend to decrease adherence include "lock top" dispensers. Adherence also decreases if more than three medications at a time are taken and if the medications are prescribed either more than four times per day or on an as needed basis. Adherence can be enhanced by correlating medication taking with daily activities such as meals, using cueing dispensers that have daily/hourly reminders, selecting medications with few side effects, and—most important—ensuring that the patient knows the name and action of the medication.

Treatment regimen variables that increase adherence include therapeutic recommendations that are easy to learn and carry out, take little time to complete, do not lead to social isolation, and do not increase fear. The more a patient is required to do, the more likely failure is to occur.

Physicians who obtain good compliance talk with their patients regarding the patient's feelings about the treatment (*e.g.*, prescribing multiple drugs may mean to patients that they are more ill). These physicians have a positive attitude toward both the drugs they prescribe and their patients, and they closely supervise the therapy prescribed. They give patients a specific appointment and keep the appointment on time, rather than having the patient "drop in" and keeping the patient waiting in the waiting room. Most important, the physician who has patients that adhere to therapy establishes a cooperative interpersonal working relationship whereby both the physician and the patient take responsibility for the patient's health care.

Assuring that a patient follows through with a referral is increased by a short referral time, referring the patient to a specific clinician, telephone reminders, and referring by letter, not telephone. Adherence in general can be improved by simplified treatment regimens, a tailored treatment plan, the use of reminders, clear and concise communications, educating the patient about the disease and mechanisms of action of medications, patient self-monitoring, and contracting with the patient regarding the patient's and physician's relative responsibilities and goals (Fuller and Gross, 1990).

Legal and Ethical Considerations

There are two basic philosophical positions from which medical ethics derive. The ***consequentialist*** position holds that an action is morally correct as a result of the function of its consequences. The most common consequentialist theory is *utilitarianism,* which holds that an action is morally correct if the consequences of the action produce the greatest amount of happiness for the greatest number of people. The ***deontologist*** position holds that an action is morally correct because of the rightness or wrongness of features or characteristics of the act itself, regardless of the consequences. From these two positions the major conflicts about medical ethics and ethical behavior develop. The major controversial ethical considerations today, as in the past, are those associated with life and death.

BIRTH CONTROL

A central issue of birth control is the physician's legal right to disseminate information or contraceptive devices to persons below the age of majority. While such information is available to adults in each state in the United States, some states maintain laws restricting the physician's dissemination of information to minors without parental consent.

ABORTION

The arguments about abortion are multifaceted but include these major points: public financing of abortion for indigent persons; the general ethics of performing elective abortions; whether a woman, without consent of the responsible man, should be able to receive an abortion; the physical or mental conditions under which abortions should be available.

THE PATIENT'S RIGHT TO DIE

These are central issues concerning a patient's right to die: First, if the patient is of sound mind, is in severe discomfort, or has a condition that, without medical support, will be fatal and the patient does not want the medical support, should it be withdrawn, particularly if the legal next-of-kin opposes the removal of life support system? Second, if the patient has only vital signs, which is clear indication that cortical death has occurred and that auxiliary life support systems are presumably maintaining basic physiologic functioning, by whose authority can the life support systems be withdrawn? A durable power of attorney for health may be appointed either by the patient prior to the loss of the patient's competence, or by the court should disagreement arise among family members. Physician-assisted suicide is currently a very significant controversy because it violates the basic medical ethic to always decide on the side of life, and, ''First, do no harm.'' However, it is ethically acceptable for a physician to gradually increase the appropriate medication for a patient, realizing that the medication may depress respiration and cause death (APA, 1995).

THE PATIENT'S RIGHT TO LIVE

While a patient's right to live is beginning to be a focal issue, as medical economics tighten it will become more critical. It encompasses the reality that as medical science advances, expensive technologies are developed. The available public health care dollar may not be able to subsidize these services for all persons who cannot personally afford them, and, if private, third-party health insurance carriers attempt to provide them, premium payments for all persons will increase dramatically. However, if a mechanism is not provided for the less affluent, then health care delivery for ''rich people'' and ''poor people'' will demonstrate more disparity than presently exists.

PARENTAL REFUSAL OF CHILD MEDICAL CARE

A life and death issue involves the emergent medical care of children whose parents reject medical intervention on religious or personal grounds. The basic legal maneuver to circumvent this difficulty has been to have the child declared a ward of the court and treatment effected. The aim is to provide care until the child is of legal and mental age to decide personally about medical intervention.

LEGAL ASPECTS

The legal issues that form a present, major focus are those that surround informed consent and the committed ''mentally ill'' person, although all patients are included.

Informed consent involves the patient knowing what a particular treatment regimen involves, including what specifically is being prescribed (*e.g.*, medicine, surgery), what options or alternative treatments are available, what the probable outcomes are, and what side effects are known to occur. The latter is particularly relevant both with antipsychotic medications and their association with tardive dyskinesia, as well as with the utilization of addictive drugs. If a patient is not physically or mentally able to comprehend the information, it is generally permissible to administer the least traumatic effective treatment if that treatment is responsible medical practice. As soon as the patient is able to comprehend the management, the patient must be fully informed. A better option, if available, is to discuss management with responsible family members and follow their wishes. In either case, documentation with time and date is essential. As far as the courts are concerned, if it is not documented in the patient's medical record, it did not happen.

Committed mentally ill adults legally are entitled to the following: they must have treatment available, they can refuse treatment, they can require a jury trial to determine sanity, and they retain their competence for conducting business transactions (*e.g.*, marriage, divorce, voting, driving). The words *sanity* and *competence* are legal, not psychiatric, terms. They refer to prediction of dangerousness to self and others, and most medical–psychological studies show that health care professionals cannot reliably and validly predict such dangerousness. The committed only lose the civil liberty to come and go. In most states, emergency detention can be effected by a physician or a law-enforcement person for 48 hours pending a hearing. A physician can detain only; a judge can commit.

With children, special rules exist: *physicians cannot detain*. Other than parents, only juvenile courts have authority over children. Children can be committed only if they are an imminent danger to self or others, they are unable to care for themselves in daily needs, or the parents have absolutely no control over the child and the child is a danger (*e.g.*, fire-setter).

Duty to warn derives from the Tarasoff Decision in 1976 and 1982, in which Tarasoff did not warn an eventual victim that Tarasoff's patient was threatening to kill the victim. Based on the decisions that came from this case, basically health professionals have the responsibility to warn a potential victim and the authorities that their patient is threatening violence. This breach of confidentiality is allowed. At this time the issue of duty to warn secondary to transmission of a potentially lethal disease like AIDS is not resolved.

Medical malpractice is usually established on the basis of the ***Four D's*** of malpractice: **D**ereliction (through negligence or omission) of a **D**uty that **D**irectly led to **D**amages. Usually malpractice can be averted by good documentation, informed consent, peer consultation, and practicing only within one's area of qualification.

REFERENCES

American Psychiatric Association: The Diagnostic and Statistical Manual of Mental Disorders, 4th ed. Washington, DC: Author, 1994

APA Ethics Newsletter. 9(2), 1995

Bailey JM, Pillard RC: A genetic study of male sexual orientation. Arch Gen Psychiatry 48:1089–1096, 1991

Bailey JM, Pillard RC, Neale MC, Agyei Y: Heritable factors influence sexual orientation in women. Arch Gen Psychiatry 50:217–223, 1993

Ezzel C: Brain feature linked to sexual orientation. Science News 140(9):134, 1991

Freidman RC, Downey J: Neurobiological and sexual orientation: current relationships. J Neuropsychiatry 5(2): 131–153, 144, 1993 References

Fuller M, Gross R: Adherence to medical regimens. In Wedding D (ed): Behavior and Medicine. St. Louis, MO: Mosby, 1990

Hauri P: The Sleep Disorders. Current Concepts: A Scope Publication. Kalamazoo, MI: Upjohn Pharmaceutical Company, 1977

Hollingshead AB, Redlich FC: Social Class and Mental Illness. New York: John Wiley & Sons, 1958

Holmes TH, Rahe RH: The social readjustment scale. J Psychosom Res 11:213, 1967

Kallman FJ: Heredity in Health and Mental Disorder. New York: Norton, 1953

Kaplan HI, Sadock BJ: Synopsis of Psychiatry: Behavioral Sciences and Clinical Psychiatry, 6th ed. Baltimore: Williams & Wilkins, 1991

Kohlberg L: The child as a moral philosopher. In Kirschenbaum H and Simon S (eds): Readings in Values Clarification. Minneapolis: Winston Press, 1973

LeVay S: A difference in hypothalamic structure between heterosexual and homosexual man. Science 253: 1034–1037, 1991

Masters WH, Johnson VE: Human Sexual Response. Boston: Little, Brown & Co, 1966

National Institute on Alcohol Abuse and Alcoholism: Alcohol and Health. Seventh Special Report to the U.S. Congress. Rockville, MD: Author, 1990

Pardes H: The syndrome of mental retardation. In Simons R (ed): Understanding Human Behavior in Health and Illness, 3rd ed. New York: Williams & Wilkins, 1985

Regier D: NIMH-Epidemiology Catchment Area Program. Arch Gen Psychiatry 45:981, 1988

Sadock VA: Sexual anatomy and physiology. In Grinspoon L (ed): Psychiatry 1982: Annual Review. Washington: American Psychiatric Press, 1982

Selye H: The Stress of Life. New York: McGraw-Hill, 1956

Sherfey MJ: The Nature and Evolution of Female Sexuality. New York: Random House, 1972

Srole L, Langner TS, Opler MK, Rennie TAC: Mental Health in the Metropolis: The Midtown Manhattan Study. New York: McGraw-Hill, 1962

Terkel S: Working: People Talk About What They Do All Day and How They Feel About What They Do. New York: Random House, 1974. Cited in Mumford E: The social significance of work and studies on the stress of life events. In Simons R (ed): Understanding Human Behavior in Health and Illness. New York: Williams & Wilkins, 1985

Toch HN: Violent Men. Chicago: Aldine Publishing Co., 1969

Walker L: Battered Women. New York: Springer Publishing, 1984

Wechsler D: Manual for the Wechsler Adult Intelligence Scale. New York: The Psychological Corporation, 1955

QUESTIONS IN THE BEHAVIORAL SCIENCES

Multiple-Choice Questions

1. The latency phase of psychoanalytic theory occurs at the same time as which of Erikson's stages?
   (a) Trust vs. mistrust
   (b) Identity vs. role confusion
   (c) Industry vs. inferiority
   (d) Autonomy vs. shame and doubt
   (e) Initiative vs. guilt
2. A 32-year-old housewife from an upper-middle-class background is married to an affluent junior executive who must travel a great deal. She does not work but pours herself into volunteer organizations, bridge club, working at the local orphanage, and visiting sick people in hospitals. In a social gathering she rather pointedly occupies the center of attention and generally gives the impression of "anything you can do, I can do better." She is also deathly afraid of riding on elevators. At which stage of Erikson's tasks of development is this woman fixated?
   (a) Initiative vs. guilt

(b) Industry vs. inferiority
(c) Identity vs. role confusion
(d) Intimacy vs. isolation
(e) Generativity vs. stagnation

3. Which of the following defense mechanisms would you naturally expect to occur as a psychological concomitant of physical illness, whereby the person is placed in a hospital?
(a) Symbolization
(b) Regression
(c) Isolation
(d) Compensation
(e) Introjection

4. According to the *Diagnostic and Statistical Manual of Mental Disorders,* Edition IV (DSM-IV), an IQ of 65 classifies a person as:
(a) Borderline mental retardation
(b) Mild mental retardation
(c) Moderate mental retardation
(d) Severe mental retardation
(e) Profound mental retardation

5. Which of the following is *not* expected after one hour of sensory deprivation?
(a) Anxiety
(b) Depression
(c) Hostility
(d) Fugue
(e) Hallucinations

6. A 14-year-old male is brought into your office by his mother. They have had an argument over the length of his hair. The boy reacts to you in a hostile, argumentative fashion even though you have reasonably long hair, a beard, and have not provoked the reaction from the young man. You would say that the phenomenon that is occurring is:
(a) Countertransference
(b) Transference
(c) Acting-out
(d) Regression
(e) Synthesis

7. With regard to children who have debilitating and terminal illness, their greatest fear is:
(a) Pain
(b) Death
(c) Separation from parents
(d) What will become of their pets
(e) Being anesthetized

8. In the prediction statistic, the correlation, the value that would have the most predictive power would be:
(a) +.95
(b) −.35
(c) 0
(d) −1.0
(e) +.65

9. Which of the following defense mechanisms is always pathologic?
(a) Rationalization
(b) Isolation
(c) Denial
(d) Disassociation
(e) Conversion

10. In a crisis management of persons who abuse drugs, there are certain drugs of abuse from which persons often die if they are abruptly withdrawn from the substance. Which of the following preparations constitutes a danger of death from abrupt withdrawal?
(a) Stimulants
(b) Sedative hypnotics
(c) Psychedelics
(d) Opiates
(e) Volatiles

11. In the grieving and mourning process we know that at different ages the mourning can take different forms. Which of the following is an *incorrect* statement?
(a) The infant might protest, deny, and detach himself.
(b) A child in the latency stage would probably be jocular and perhaps hypomanic.
(c) A child in the adolescent stage might turn to antisocial acting out.
(d) Middle-age persons quite frequently turn to hypochondriacal symptoms.
(e) Elderly persons typically are relieved and feel somewhat released.

12. The Thematic Apperception Test (TAT) is an example of what type of psychological test?
(a) Intelligence
(b) Achievement
(c) Ability
(d) Interest
(e) Personality

13. In speaking of orientation, four spheres are usually examined. All of the following are included *except:*
(a) Relationship of self to a place in time
(b) Awareness of self as a person
(c) Knowledge of geographic location
(d) Awareness of internal affective state
(e) Knowledge of present position in time

14. In terms of etiology, anxiety is usually viewed as repressed or forgotten:
(a) Fear
(b) Guilt
(c) Sorrow
(d) Grief
(e) Anger

15. All of the following are true statements about the memory process *except*:
    (a) Long-term memory is rarely defective in organicity unless accompanied by psychosis.
    (b) If memory loss occurs, recovery is typically from the extremes of loss to the precipitating event.
    (c) Memory is particularly disrupted with bilateral lesions of the hippocampus and/or mammillary bodies.
    (d) In general, memory defect is psychogenic if there is no disturbance of consciousness and no intellectual impairment.
    (e) If there is short-term memory loss and motivation and attention is good, it is suggestive of psychogenic involvement.
16. In Freudian theory, a child who has begun to be strongly attached to the parent of the opposite sex and display some ''fear'' of the parent of the same sex would be in which stage of psychosexual development?
    (a) Oral
    (b) Latent
    (c) Anal
    (d) Phallic/urethral
    (e) Genital
17. All of the following are considered to be functions of the ego *except:*
    (a) Personal values
    (b) Defense mechanisms
    (c) Object relations
    (d) Reality testing
    (e) Thought processes
18. In Erikson's theory of psychological tasks, which of the following is *not* a correct task?
    (a) Integrity vs. despair
    (b) Industry vs. inferiority
    (c) Intimacy vs. isolation
    (d) Generativity vs. stagnation
    (e) Identity vs. shame and doubt
19. The patient states: ''I feel uptight about my new job.'' This is an example of:
    (a) Objective evidence of anxiety
    (b) Subjective evidence of anxiety
    (c) Inappropriate effect
    (d) Repression of affect
    (e) A drive discharge emotion
20. All of the following are examples of psychophysiologic responses to anxiety *except*:
    (a) Excessive perspiration
    (b) Tension headaches, constriction in the chest, backache
    (c) Aphasia, apraxia, and a right homonymous hemianopsia
    (d) Dyspnea, dizziness, and paresthesias
    (e) Transient systolic hypertension, premature contractions, and tachycardia
21. A student did poorly on an examination. The student is afraid he will fail the course. On the next occasion he walks into the room in which the examination was given he experiences fear. This is an example of:
    (a) Classical conditioning learning
    (b) Social learning
    (c) Cognitive learning
    (d) Inhibition learning
    (e) Fixed-schedule learning
22. In learning theory, grades in an academic course would be an example of:
    (a) Acquisition
    (b) Generalization
    (c) Primary reinforcers
    (d) Secondary reinforcers
    (e) Ratio reinforcement
23. All of the statements below regarding adolescence (ages 13 to 18) are true *except:*
    (a) In Erikson's framework the basic task to be resolved is to develop affiliation with others.
    (b) Fifty percent of teenage marriages occur because of pregnancy.
    (c) One third of teenage marriages end in divorce within four years.
    (d) They are in Piaget's stage of formal operations.
    (e) Adolescents must maintain a sense of identity in the face of rapid changes.
24. Which of the following is most characteristic of the abuser of the elderly?
    (a) Encourages the elderly person to speak his or her mind.
    (b) Has cared for the elderly person for some time.
    (c) Lives separately from the abuse person.
    (d) Takes immaculate care of the house and the abused person.
    (e) Volunteered to take care of the abused person.
25. Which of the following is *not* associated with increased aggressive behavior?
    (a) Ablation of the amygdala
    (b) Destruction of the septum
    (c) Norepinephrine
    (d) Serotonin
    (e) Testosterone
26. All of the following behavioral conditions have demonstrated genetic correlates *except:*
    (a) Aggressive delinquent behavior
    (b) Bipolar disorder
    (c) Homosexuality
    (d) Pedophilia
    (e) Shyness

27. The consequentialist ethical stance is best represented by which of the following statements?
    (a) Abortion is always wrong.
    (b) Doctors infected with HIV should not be allowed to practice medicine.
    (c) I've decided to set the cutoff score on the examination so everyone passes the course.
    (d) Malpractice lawsuits should never be allowed to exceed $25,000.
    (e) Never let abused children return to the home of the parent who abused them.
28. Of the following, which is *not* one of the Four D's used to establish medical malpractice?
    (a) Damages resulted from the physician's behavior
    (b) Dereliction of action through neglect or omission
    (c) Direct linkage between cause and effect
    (d) Dispute of physician versus patient responsibility
    (e) Duty to act in a situation
29. Which of the following neurotransmitters is significantly involved with many different addictive disorders?
    (a) Dopamine
    (b) Endorphan
    (c) Epinephrine
    (d) GABA
    (e) Serotonin
30. Which of the following statements about violence is most correct?
    (a) Children who are physically abused are quiet and withdrawn at school.
    (b) Rage reactions are common with dysfunction of the hippocampus.
    (c) Suicide impulses and behaviors are correlated with serotonin levels.
    (d) The age at which most violence takes place is 23 years.
    (e) The object of terrorism is the overthrow of a governmental agency.

ANSWERS TO MULTIPLE-CHOICE QUESTIONS

1. c	**9.** e	**17.** a	**25.** a
2. a	**10.** b	**18.** e	**26.** d
3. b	**11.** e	**19.** b	**27.** c
4. b	**12.** e	**20.** c	**28.** d
5. d	**13.** d	**21.** a	**29.** a
6. b	**14.** a	**22.** d	**30.** c
7. c	**15.** e	**23.** a	
8. d	**16.** d	**24.** b	

Index

Note: Page numbers followed by *f* indicate figures; numbers followed by *t* indicate tabular material.